U0300903

坎贝尔骨科手术学
脊柱外科

Campbell's Operative Orthopaedics

第 14 版

（影印版）

Frederick M. Azar, MD

James H. Beaty, MD

人民卫生出版社

·北 京·

图书在版编目（CIP）数据

坎贝尔骨科手术学．脊柱外科：英文 /（美）弗雷德里克·M. 阿扎尔（Frederick M. Azar），（美）詹姆斯·H. 比蒂（James H. Beaty）主编．—影印本．—北京：人民卫生出版社，2021.12

ISBN 978-7-117-32523-3

Ⅰ. ①坎…　Ⅱ. ①弗…　②詹…　Ⅲ. ①骨科学－外科手术－英文②脊柱病－外科手术－英文　Ⅳ. ①R68 ②R681.5

中国版本图书馆 CIP 数据核字（2021）第 241763 号

人卫智网	**www.ipmph.com**	**医学教育、学术、考试、健康，购书智慧智能综合服务平台**
人卫官网	**www.pmph.com**	**人卫官方资讯发布平台**

图字：01-2021-6747 号

坎贝尔骨科手术学
脊 柱 外 科
Kanbeier Guke Shoushuxue
Jizhu Waike

主　　编：Frederick M. Azar　James H. Beaty
出版发行：人民卫生出版社（中继线 010-59780011）
地　　址：北京市朝阳区潘家园南里 19 号
邮　　编：100021
E - mail：pmph @ pmph.com
购书热线：010-59787592　010-59787584　010-65264830
印　　刷：三河市宏达印刷有限公司（胜利）
经　　销：新华书店
开　　本：889 × 1194　1/16　**印张：**35.5
字　　数：1690 千字
版　　次：2021 年 12 月第 1 版
印　　次：2022 年 1 月第 1 次印刷
标准书号：ISBN 978-7-117-32523-3
定　　价：499.00 元
打击盗版举报电话：010-59787491　E-mail：WQ @ pmph.com
质量问题联系电话：010-59787234　E-mail：zhiliang @ pmph.com

坎贝尔骨科手术学
脊柱外科

Campbell's Operative Orthopaedics

第 14 版

（影印版）

Frederick M. Azar, MD
Professor
Department of Orthopaedic Surgery and Biomedical Engineering University of Tennessee–Campbell Clinic
Chief of Staff, Campbell Clinic
Memphis, Tennessee

James H. Beaty, MD
Harold B. Boyd Professor and Chair
Department of Orthopaedic Surgery and Biomedical Engineering University of Tennessee–Campbell Clinic
Memphis, Tennessee

Editorial Assistance
Kay Daugherty ***and*** **Linda Jones**

人民卫生出版社
·北 京·

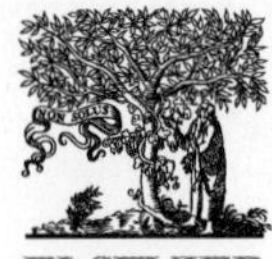

Elsevier (Singapore) Pte Ltd.
3 Killiney Road,
#08–01 Winsland House I,
Singapore 239519
Tel: (65) 6349–0200; Fax: (65) 6733–1817

Campbell's Operative Orthopaedics, 14E

ISBN: 978-0-323-67217-7

This English Reprint of Part Ⅻ from Campbell's Operative Orthopaedics, 14E by Frederick M. Azar and James H. Beaty was undertaken by People's Medical Publishing House and is published by arrangement with Elsevier (Singapore) Pte Ltd.
Part Ⅻ from Campbell's Operative Orthopaedics, 14E by Frederick M. Azar and James H. Beaty由人民卫生出版社进行影印，并根据人民卫生出版社与爱思唯尔（新加坡）私人有限公司的协议约定出版。

ISBN: 978-7-117-32523-3

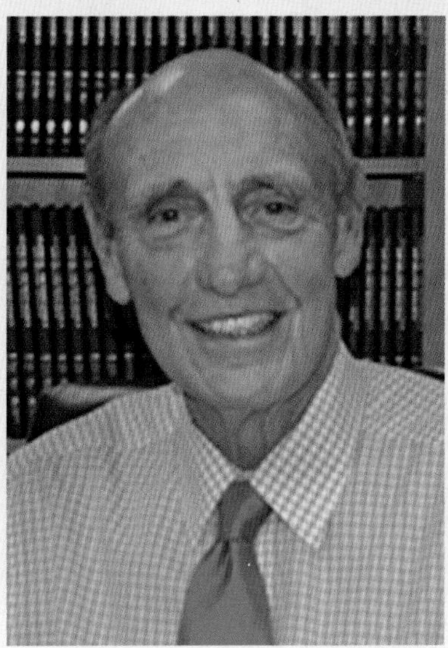

S. Terry Canale, MD

It is with humble appreciation and admiration that we dedicate this edition of *Campbell's Operative Orthopaedics* to Dr. S. Terry Canale, who served as editor or co-editor of five editions. He took great pride in this position and worked tirelessly to continue to improve "The Book." As noted by one of his co-editors, "Terry is probably the only person in the world who has read every word of multiple editions of *Campbell's Operative Orthopaedics*." He considered *Campbell's Operative Orthopaedics* an opportunity for worldwide orthopaedic education and made it a priority to ensure that each edition provided valuable and up-to-date information. His commitment to and enthusiasm for this work will continue to influence and inspire every future edition.

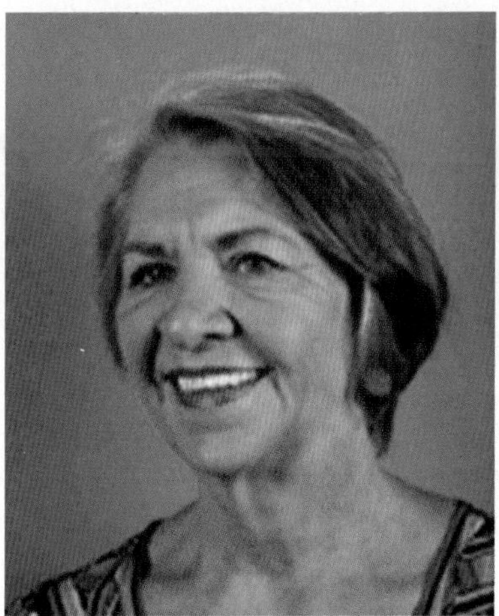

Kay C. Daugherty

It is with equal appreciation and regard that we dedicate this edition to Kay C. Daugherty, the managing editor of the last nine editions *Campbell's Operative Orthopaedics.* Over the last 40 years, she has faithfully and tirelessly edited, reshaped, and overseen all aspects of publication from manuscript preparation to proofing. She has a profound talent to put ideas and disjointed words into comprehensible text, ensuring that each revision maintains the gold standard in readability. Each edition is a testament to her dedication to excellence in writing and education. A favorite quote of Mrs. Daugherty to one of our late authors was, "I'll make a deal. I won't operate if you won't punctuate." We are grateful for her many years of continual service to the Campbell Foundation and for the publications yet to come.

CONTRIBUTORS

FREDERICK M. AZAR, MD
Professor
Director, Sports Medicine Fellowship
University of Tennessee–Campbell Clinic
Department of Orthopaedic Surgery and Biomedical Engineering
Chief-of-Staff, Campbell Clinic
Memphis, Tennessee

JAMES H. BEATY, MD
Harold B. Boyd Professor and Chair
University of Tennessee–Campbell Clinic
Department of Orthopaedic Surgery and Biomedical Engineering
Memphis, Tennessee

MICHAEL J. BEEBE, MD
Instructor
University of Tennessee–Campbell Clinic
Department of Orthopaedic Surgery and Biomedical Engineering
Memphis, Tennessee

CLAYTON C. BETTIN, MD
Assistant Professor
Director, Foot and Ankle Fellowship
Associate Residency Program Director
University of Tennessee–Campbell Clinic
Department of Orthopaedic Surgery and Biomedical Engineering
Memphis, Tennessee

TYLER J. BROLIN, MD
Assistant Professor
University of Tennessee–Campbell Clinic
Department of Orthopaedic Surgery and Biomedical Engineering
Memphis, Tennessee

JAMES H. CALANDRUCCIO, MD
Associate Professor
Director, Hand Fellowship
University of Tennessee–Campbell Clinic
Department of Orthopaedic Surgery and Biomedical Engineering
Memphis, Tennessee

DAVID L. CANNON, MD
Associate Professor
University of Tennessee–Campbell Clinic
Department of Orthopaedic Surgery and Biomedical Engineering
Memphis, Tennessee

KEVIN B. CLEVELAND, MD
Instructor
University of Tennessee–Campbell Clinic
Department of Orthopaedic Surgery and Biomedical Engineering
Memphis, Tennessee

ANDREW H. CRENSHAW JR., MD
Professor Emeritus
University of Tennessee–Campbell Clinic
Department of Orthopaedic Surgery and Biomedical Engineering
Memphis, Tennessee

JOHN R. CROCKARELL, MD
Professor
University of Tennessee–Campbell Clinic
Department of Orthopaedic Surgery and Biomedical Engineering
Memphis, Tennessee

GREGORY D. DABOV, MD
Assistant Professor
University of Tennessee–Campbell Clinic
Department of Orthopaedic Surgery and Biomedical Engineering
Memphis, Tennessee

MARCUS C. FORD, MD
Instructor
University of Tennessee–Campbell Clinic
Department of Orthopaedic Surgery and Biomedical Engineering
Memphis, Tennessee

RAYMOND J. GARDOCKI, MD
Assistant Professor
University of Tennessee–Campbell Clinic
Department of Orthopaedic Surgery and Biomedical Engineering
Memphis, Tennessee

BENJAMIN J. GREAR, MD
Instructor
University of Tennessee–Campbell Clinic
Department of Orthopaedic Surgery and Biomedical Engineering
Memphis, Tennessee

JAMES L. GUYTON, MD
Associate Professor
University of Tennessee–Campbell Clinic
Department of Orthopaedic Surgery and Biomedical Engineering
Memphis, Tennessee

JAMES W. HARKESS, MD
Associate Professor
University of Tennessee–Campbell Clinic
Department of Orthopaedic Surgery and Biomedical Engineering
Memphis, Tennessee

ROBERT K. HECK JR., MD
Associate Professor
University of Tennessee–Campbell Clinic
Department of Orthopaedic Surgery and Biomedical Engineering
Memphis, Tennessee

MARK T. JOBE, MD
Associate Professor
University of Tennessee–Campbell Clinic
Department of Orthopaedic Surgery and Biomedical Engineering
Memphis, Tennessee

DEREK M. KELLY, MD
Professor
Director, Pediatric Orthopaedic Fellowship
Director, Resident Education
University of Tennessee–Campbell Clinic
Department of Orthopaedic Surgery and Biomedical Engineering
Memphis, Tennessee

SANTOS F. MARTINEZ, MD
Assistant Professor
University of Tennessee–Campbell Clinic
Department of Orthopaedic Surgery and Biomedical Engineering
Memphis, Tennessee

ANTHONY A. MASCIOLI, MD
Assistant Professor
University of Tennessee–Campbell Clinic
Department of Orthopaedic Surgery and Biomedical Engineering
Memphis, Tennessee

BENJAMIN M. MAUCK, MD
Assistant Professor
Director, Hand Fellowship
University of Tennessee–Campbell Clinic
Department of Orthopaedic Surgery and Biomedical Engineering
Memphis, Tennessee

MARC J. MIHALKO, MD
Assistant Professor
University of Tennessee–Campbell Clinic
Department of Orthopaedic Surgery and Biomedical Engineering
Memphis, Tennessee

WILLIAM M. MIHALKO, MD PhD
Professor, H.R. Hyde Chair of Excellence in Rehabilitation Engineering
Director, Biomedical Engineering
University of Tennessee–Campbell Clinic
Department of Orthopaedic Surgery and Biomedical Engineering
Memphis, Tennessee

ROBERT H. MILLER III, MD
Associate Professor
University of Tennessee–Campbell Clinic
Department of Orthopaedic Surgery and Biomedical Engineering
Memphis, Tennessee

G. ANDREW MURPHY, MD
Associate Professor
University of Tennessee–Campbell Clinic
Department of Orthopaedic Surgery and Biomedical Engineering
Memphis, Tennessee

ASHLEY L. PARK, MD
Clinical Assistant Professor
University of Tennessee–Campbell Clinic
Department of Orthopaedic Surgery and Biomedical Engineering
Memphis, Tennessee

EDWARD A. PEREZ, MD
Associate Professor
University of Tennessee–Campbell Clinic
Department of Orthopaedic Surgery and Biomedical Engineering
Memphis, Tennessee

BARRY B. PHILLIPS, MD
Professor
University of Tennessee–Campbell Clinic
Department of Orthopaedic Surgery and Biomedical Engineering
Memphis, Tennessee

DAVID R. RICHARDSON, MD
Associate Professor
University of Tennessee–Campbell Clinic
Department of Orthopaedic Surgery and Biomedical Engineering
Memphis, Tennessee

MATTHEW I. RUDLOFF, MD
Assistant Professor
Co-Director, Trauma Fellowship
University of Tennessee–Campbell Clinic
Department of Orthopaedic Surgery and Biomedical Engineering
Memphis, Tennessee

JEFFREY R. SAWYER, MD
Professor
Co-Director, Pediatric Orthopaedic Fellowship
University of Tennessee–Campbell Clinic
Department of Orthopaedic Surgery and Biomedical Engineering
Memphis, Tennessee

BENJAMIN W. SHEFFER, MD
Assistant Professor
University of Tennessee–Campbell Clinic
Department of Orthopaedic Surgery and Biomedical Engineering
Memphis, Tennessee

DAVID D. SPENCE, MD
Assistant Professor
University of Tennessee–Campbell Clinic
Department of Orthopaedic Surgery and Biomedical Engineering
Memphis, Tennessee

NORFLEET B. THOMPSON, MD
Instructor
University of Tennessee–Campbell Clinic
Department of Orthopaedic Surgery and Biomedical Engineering
Memphis, Tennessee

THOMAS W. THROCKMORTON, MD
Professor
Co-Director, Sports Medicine Fellowship
University of Tennessee–Campbell Clinic
Department of Orthopaedic Surgery and Biomedical Engineering
Memphis, Tennessee

PATRICK C. TOY, MD
Associate Professor
University of Tennessee–Campbell Clinic
Department of Orthopaedic Surgery and Biomedical Engineering
Memphis, Tennessee

WILLIAM C. WARNER JR., MD
Professor
University of Tennessee–Campbell Clinic
Department of Orthopaedic Surgery and Biomedical Engineering
Memphis, Tennessee

JOHN C. WEINLEIN, MD
Assistant Professor
Director, Trauma Fellowship
University of Tennessee–Campbell Clinic
Department of Orthopaedic Surgery and Biomedical Engineering
Memphis, Tennessee

WILLIAM J. WELLER, MD
Instructor
University of Tennessee–Campbell Clinic
Department of Orthopaedic Surgery and Biomedical Engineering
Memphis, Tennessee

A. PAIGE WHITTLE, MD
Associate Professor
University of Tennessee–Campbell Clinic
Department of Orthopaedic Surgery and Biomedical Engineering
Memphis, Tennessee

KEITH D. WILLIAMS, MD
Associate Professor
University of Tennessee–Campbell Clinic
Department of Orthopaedic Surgery and Biomedical Engineering
Memphis, Tennessee

DEXTER H. WITTE III, MD
Clinical Assistant Professor in Radiology
University of Tennessee–Campbell Clinic
Department of Orthopaedic Surgery and Biomedical Engineering
Memphis, Tennessee

PREFACE

When Dr. Willis Campbell published the first edition of *Campbell's Operative Orthopaedics* in 1939, he could not have envisioned that over 80 years later it would have evolved into a four-volume text and earned the accolade of the "bible of orthopaedics" as a mainstay in orthopaedic practices and educational institutions all over the world. This expansion from some 400 pages in the first edition to over 4,500 pages in this 14th edition has not changed Dr. Campbell's original intent: "to present to the student, the general practitioner, and the surgeon the subject of orthopaedic surgery in a simple and comprehensive manner." In each edition since the first, authors and editors have worked diligently to fulfill these objectives. This would have not been possible without the hard work of our contributors who always strive to present the most up-to-date information while retaining "tried and true" techniques and tips. The scope of this text continues to expand in the hope that the information will be relevant to physicians no matter their location or resources.

As always, this edition also is the result of the collaboration of a group of "behind the scenes" individuals who are involved in the actual production process. The Campbell Foundation staff—Kay Daugherty, Linda Jones, and Tonya Priggel—contributed their considerable talents to editing often confusing and complex author contributions, searching the literature for obscure references, and, in general, "herding the cats." Special thanks to Kay and Linda who have worked on multiple editions of *Campbell's Operative Orthopaedics* (nine editions for Kay and six for Linda). They probably know more about orthopaedics than most of us, and they certainly know how to make it more understandable. Thanks, too, to the Elsevier personnel who provided guidance and assistance throughout the publication process: John Casey, Senior Project Manager; Jennifer Ehlers, Senior Content Development Specialist; and Belinda Kuhn, Senior Content Strategist.

We are especially appreciative of our spouses, Julie Azar and Terry Beaty, and our families for their patience and support as we worked through this project.

The preparation and publication of this 14th edition was fraught with difficulties because of the worldwide pandemic and social unrest, but our contributors and other personnel worked tirelessly, often in creative and innovative ways, to bring it to fruition. It is our hope that these efforts have provided a text that is informative and valuable to all orthopaedists as they continue to refine and improve methods that will ensure the best outcomes for their patients.

Frederick M. Azar, MD
James H. Beaty, MD

CONTENTS

CHAPTER 1

ANATOMIC APPROACHES TO THE SPINE

Raymond J. Gardocki

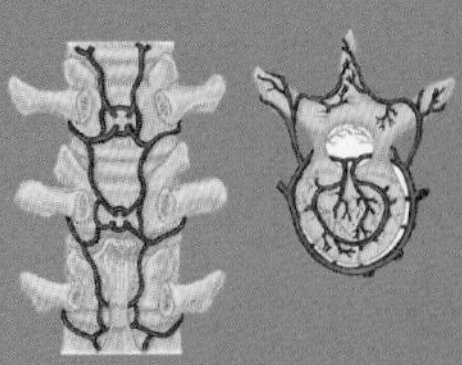

ANATOMY OF VERTEBRAL COLUMN

The vertebral column comprises 33 vertebrae divided into five sections (7 cervical, 12 thoracic, 5 lumbar, 5 sacral, and 4 coccygeal) (Fig. 1.1). The sacral and coccygeal vertebrae are fused, which typically allows for 24 mobile segments. Congenital anomalies and variations in segmentation are common. The cervical and lumbar segments develop lordosis as an erect posture is acquired. The thoracic and sacral segments maintain kyphotic postures, which are found in utero, and serve as attachment points for the rib cage and pelvic girdle. In general, each mobile vertebral body increases in size when moving from cranial to caudal. A typical vertebra comprises an anterior body and a posterior arch that enclose the vertebral canal. The neural arch is composed of two pedicles laterally and two laminae posteriorly that are united to form the spinous process. To either side of the arch of the vertebral body is a transverse process and superior and inferior articular processes. The articular processes articulate with adjacent vertebrae to form synovial joints. The relative orientation of the articular processes accounts for the degree of flexion, extension, or rotation possible in each segment of the vertebral column. The spinous and transverse processes serve as levers for the numerous muscles attached to them. The length of the vertebral column averages 72 cm in men and 7 to 10 cm less in women. The vertebral canal extends throughout the length of the column and provides protection for the spinal cord, conus medullaris, and cauda equina.

ANATOMY OF SPINAL JOINTS

The individual vertebrae are connected by joints between the neural arches and between the bodies. The joints between the neural arches are the zygapophyseal joints or facet joints. They exist between the inferior articular process of one vertebra and the superior articular process of the vertebra immediately caudal. These are synovial joints with surfaces covered by articular cartilage, a synovial membrane bridging the margins of the articular cartilage, and a joint capsule enclosing them. The branches of the posterior primary rami innervate these joints.

The interbody joints contain specialized structures called *intervertebral discs*. These discs are found throughout the vertebral column except between the first and second cervical vertebrae. The discs are designed to accommodate movement, weight bearing, and shock by being strong but deformable. Each disc contains a pair of vertebral endplates with a central nucleus pulposus and a peripheral ring of annulus fibrosus sandwiched between them. They form a secondary cartilaginous joint or symphysis at each vertebral level.

The vertebral endplates are 1-mm thick sheets of cartilage-fibrocartilage and hyaline cartilage with an increased ratio of fibrocartilage with increasing age. The nucleus pulposus is a semifluid mass of mucoid material, 70% to 90% water, with proteoglycan constituting 65% and collagen constituting 15% to 20% of the dry weight. The annulus fibrosus consists of 12 concentric lamellae, with alternating orientation of collagen fibers in successive lamellae to withstand multidirectional strain. The annulus is 60% to 70% water, with collagen constituting 50% to 60% and proteoglycan about 20% of the dry weight. With age, the proportions of proteoglycan and water decrease. The annulus and nucleus merge in a junctional zone without a strict demarcation. The discs are the largest avascular structures in the body and depend on diffusion from a specialized network of endplate blood vessels for nutrition.

ANATOMY OF SPINAL CORD AND NERVES

The spinal cord is shorter than the vertebral column and terminates as the conus medullaris at the second lumbar vertebra in adults and the third lumbar vertebra in neonates. From the conus, a fibrous cord called the *filum terminale* extends to the dorsum of the first coccygeal segment. The spinal cord is enclosed in three protective membranes—the pia, arachnoid, and dura mater. The pia and arachnoid membranes are separated by the subarachnoid space, which contains the cerebrospinal fluid. The spinal cord has enlargements in the cervical and lumbar regions that correlate with the brachial plexus and lumbar plexus. Within the spinal

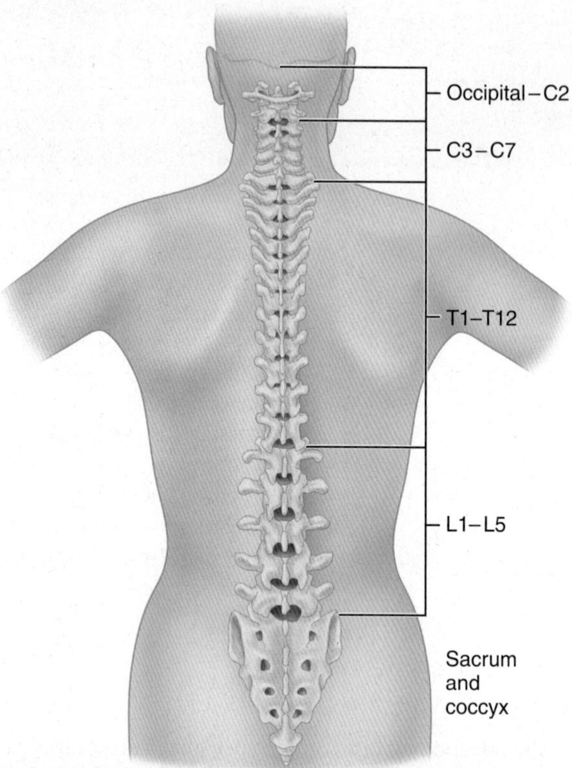

FIGURE 1.1 Vertebral column: upper cervical vertebrae (occiput to C2), lower cervical vertebrae (C3-7), thoracic vertebrae (T1-12), lumbar vertebrae (L1-5), sacrum, and coccyx.

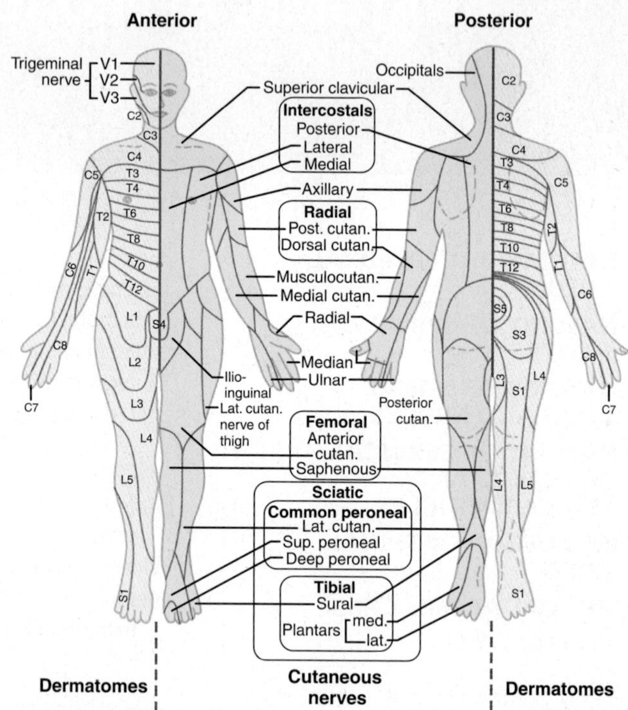

FIGURE 1.2 Dermatomal and sensory distribution. (Redrawn from Patton HD, Sundsten JW, Crill WE, et al, editors: *Introduction to basic neurology*, Philadelphia, 1976, WB Saunders.)

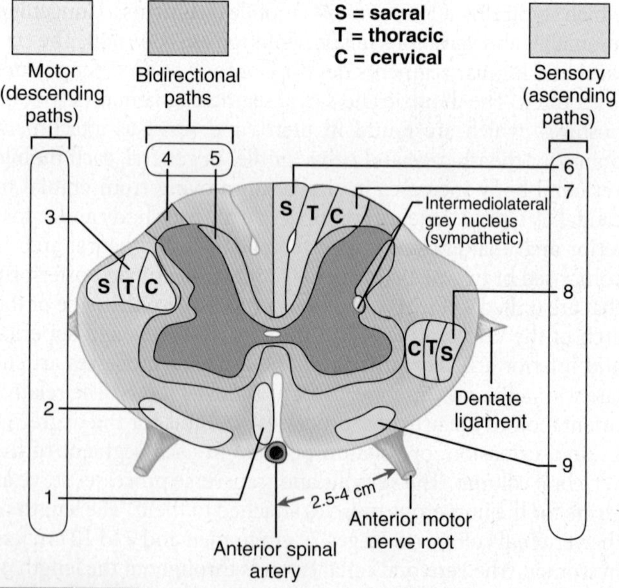

FIGURE 1.3 Schematic cross section of cervical spinal cord. (Redrawn from Patton HD, Sundsten JW, Crill WE, et al, editors: *Introduction to basic neurology*, Philadelphia, 1976, WB Saunders.)

cord are tracts of ascending (sensory) and descending (motor) nerve fibers. These pathways typically are arranged with cervical tracts located centrally and thoracic, lumbar, and sacral tracts located progressively peripheral. This accounts for the clinical findings of central cord syndrome and syrinx. Understanding the location of these tracts aids in understanding different spinal cord syndromes (Figs. 1.2 and 1.3; Table 1.1).

Spinal nerves exit the canal at each level. Spinal nerves C2-7 exit above the pedicle for which they are named (the C6 nerve root exits the foramen between the C5 and C6 pedicles). The C8 nerve root exits the foramen between the C7 and T1 pedicles. All spinal nerves caudal to C8 exit the foramen below the pedicle for which they are named (the L4 nerve root exits the foramen between the L4 and L5 pedicles). The final dermatomal and sensory nerve distributions are shown in Figure 1.2. Because the spinal cord is shorter than the vertebral column, the spinal nerves course more vertically as one moves caudally. Each level gives off a dorsal (sensory) root and a ventral (mostly motor) root, which combine to form the mixed spinal nerve. The dorsal root of each spinal nerve has a ganglion located near the exit zone of each foramen. This dorsal root ganglion is the synapse point for the ascending sensory cell bodies. This structure is sensitive to pressure and heat and can cause a dysesthetic pain response if manipulated.

ANATOMY OF CERVICAL, THORACIC, AND LUMBAR PEDICLES

Numerous studies have documented the anatomic morphology of the cervical, thoracic, and lumbar vertebrae. Advanced internal fixation techniques, including pedicle screws, have been developed and used extensively in spine surgery, not only for traumatic injuries but also for degenerative conditions. As the role for anterior and posterior spinal instrumentation continues to evolve, understanding the morphologic characteristics of the human vertebrae is crucial in avoiding complications during fixation.

Placement of screws in the cervical pedicles is controversial and carries more risk than anterior plate or lateral mass fixation. Although cervical pedicles can be suitable for screw fixation, uniformly sized cervical pedicle screws cannot be used at

TABLE 1.1

Ascending and Descending (Motor) Tracts

NUMBER (FIG. 1.3)	PATH	FUNCTION	SIDE OF BODY
1	Anterior corticospinal tract	Skilled movement	Opposite
2	Vestibulospinal tract	Facilitates extensor muscle tone	Same
3	Lateral corticospinal (pyramidal tract)	Skilled movement	Same
4	Dorsolateral fasciculus	Pain and temperature	Bidirectional
5	Fasciculus proprius	Short spinal connections	Bidirectional
6	Fasciculus gracilis	Position/fine touch	Same
7	Fasciculus cuneatus	Position/fine touch	Same
8	Lateral spinothalamic tract	Pain and temperature	Opposite
9	Anterior spinothalamic tract	Light touch	Opposite

Modified from Patton HD, Sundsten JW, Crill WE, Swanson PD, editors: *Introduction to basic neurology*, Philadelphia, 1976, WB Saunders.

every level. Screw placement in the pedicles at C3, C4, and C5 requires smaller screws (<4.5 mm) and more care in placement than those of the other cervical vertebrae. CT measurements of cervical pedicle morphology found that C2 and C7 pedicles had larger mean interdiameters than all other cervical vertebrae, and that C3 had the smallest mean interdiameter. The outer pedicle width-to-height ratio increased from C2 to C7, indicating that pedicles in the upper cervical spine (C2-4) are elongated, whereas pedicles in the lower cervical spine (C6-7) are rounded. It also is crucial to know that cervical pedicles angle medially at all levels, with the most medial angulation at C5 and the least at C2 and C7. The pedicles slope upward at C2 and C3, are parallel at C4 and C5, and are angled downward at C6 and C7.

The vertebral artery from C3 to C6 is at significant risk for iatrogenic injury during pedicle screw placement. The pedicle cortex is not uniformly thick. The thinnest portion of the cortex (the lateral cortex) protects the vertebral artery, and the medial cortex toward the spinal cord is almost twice as thick as the lateral cortex. Variations in the course of the vertebral artery also place it at risk during placement of pedicle screws. At the C2 and C7-T1 levels, the vertebral artery is less at risk during pedicle screw fixation. The vertebral artery follows a more posterior and lateral course at C2, whereas at C7-T1 it is outside the transverse foramen.

Pedicle dimensions and angles change progressively from the upper thoracic spine distally. A thorough knowledge of these relationships is important when considering the use of the pedicle as a screw purchase site. A study of 2905 pedicle measurements made from T1 to L5 found that pedicles were widest at L5 and narrowest at T5 in the horizontal plane (Fig. 1.4). The widest pedicles in the sagittal plane were at T11, and the narrowest were at T1. Because of the oval shape of the pedicle, the sagittal plane width was generally larger than the horizontal plane width. The largest pedicle angle in the horizontal plane was at L5. In the sagittal plane, the pedicles angle caudal at L5 and cephalad at L3-T1. The depth to the anterior cortex was significantly longer along the pedicle axis than along a line parallel to the midline of the vertebral body at all levels except T12 and L1.

The thoracic pedicle is a convoluted, three-dimensional structure that is filled mostly with cancellous bone (62% to 79%). Panjabi et al. showed that the cortical shell is of variable density throughout its perimeter and that the lateral wall is significantly thinner than the medial wall. This seemed to be true for all levels of thoracic vertebrae.

The locations for screw insertion have been identified and described in several studies. The respective facet joint space and the middle of the transverse process are the most important reference points. An opening is made in the pedicle with a drill or handheld curet, after which a self-tapping screw is passed through the pedicle into the vertebral body. The pedicles of the thoracic and lumbar vertebrae are tube-like bony structures that connect the anterior and posterior columns of the spine. Medial to the medial wall of the pedicle lies the dural sac. Inferior to the medial wall of the pedicle is the nerve root in the neural foramen. The lumbar roots usually are situated in the upper third of the foramen; it is more dangerous to penetrate the pedicle medially or inferiorly as opposed to laterally or superiorly.

We use three techniques for open localization of the pedicle: (1) the intersection technique, (2) the pars interarticularis technique, and (3) the mammillary process technique. It is important in preoperative planning to assess individual spinal anatomy with the use of high-quality anteroposterior and lateral radiographs of the lumbar and thoracic spine and axial CT or MRI at the level of the pedicle. In the lumbar spine, coaxial fluoroscopy images are a reliable guide to the true bony cortex of the pedicle. The intersection technique is perhaps the most commonly used method of localizing the pedicle. It involves dropping a line from the lateral aspect of the facet joint, which intersects a line that bisects the transverse process at a spot overlying the pedicle (Fig. 1.5). The pars interarticularis is the area of bone where the pedicle connects to the lamina. Because the laminae and the pars interarticularis can be identified easily at surgery, they provide landmarks by which a pedicular drill starting point can be made. The mammillary process technique is based on a small prominence of bone at the base of the transverse process. This mammillary process can be used as a starting point for transpedicular drilling. Usually, the mammillary process is more lateral than the intersection technique starting point, which also is more lateral than the pars interarticularis starting point. Thus, different angles must be used when drilling from these sites. With the help of preoperative CT scanning or MRI at the level of the pedicle and intraoperative fluoroscopy, the angle of the pedicle to the sagittal and horizontal planes can be determined.

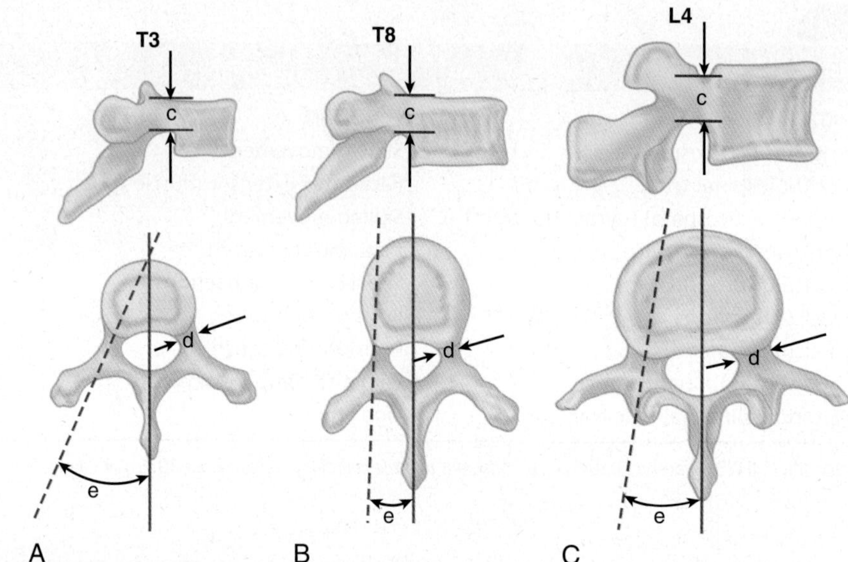

FIGURE 1.4 Pedicle dimensions of T3 **(A)**, T8 **(B)**, and L4 **(C)** vertebrae. Vertical diameter *(c)* increases from 0.7 to 1.5 cm, horizontal diameter *(d)* increases from 0.7 to 1.6 cm with minimum of 0.5 cm in T5. Direction is almost sagittal from T4 to L4. Angle *(e)* seldom extends beyond 10 degrees. More proximally, direction is more oblique: T1 = 36 degrees, T2 = 34 degrees, T3 = 23 degrees. L5 is oblique (30 degrees) but is large and easy to drill. (Redrawn from Roy-Camille R, Saillant G, Mazel CH: Plating of thoracic, thoracolumbar, and lumbar injuries with pedicle screw plates, *Orthop Clin North Am* 17:147, 1986.)

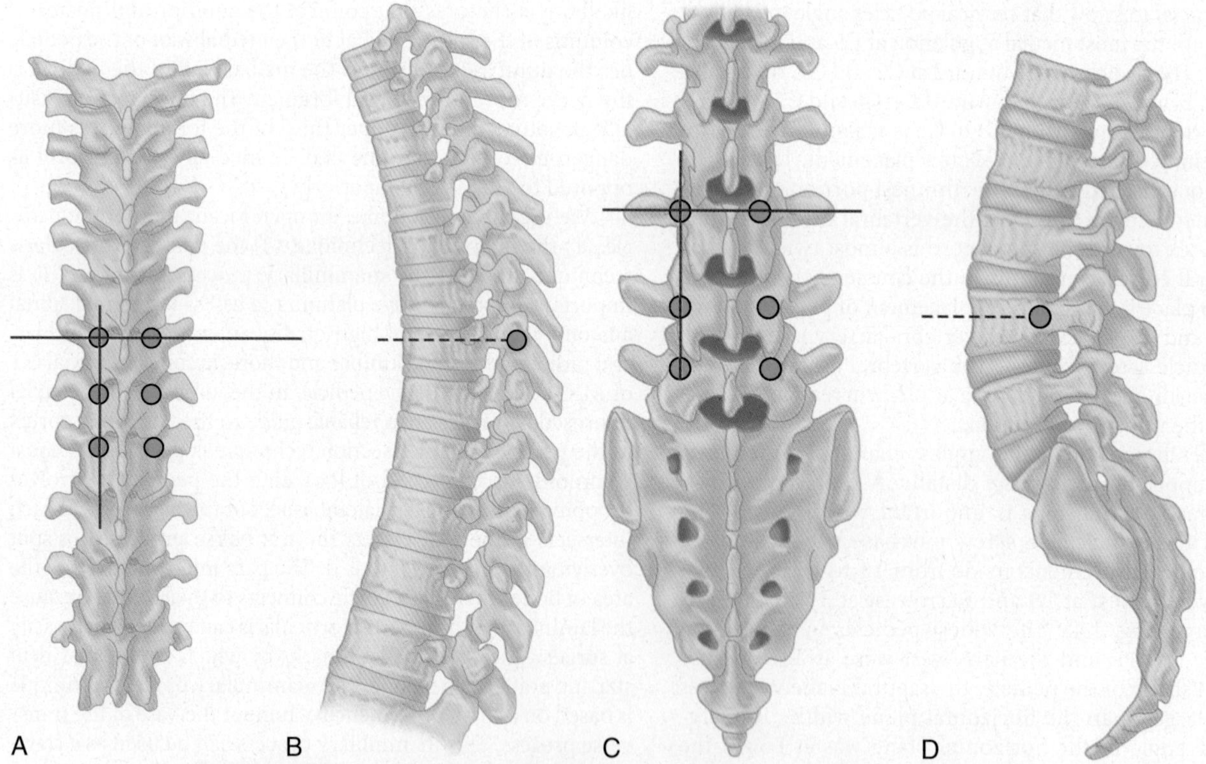

FIGURE 1.5 A and B, Anteroposterior and lateral views of pedicle entrance point in thoracic spine at intersection of lines drawn through middle of inferior articular facets and middle of insertion of transverse processes (1 mm below facet joint). C and D, Anteroposterior and lateral views of pedicle entrance point in lumbar spine at intersection of two lines. On typical bony crest, it is 1 mm below articular joint. (Redrawn from Roy-Camille R, Saillant G, Mazel CH: Plating of thoracic, thoracolumbar, and lumbar injuries with pedicle screw plates, *Orthop Clin North Am* 17:147, 1986).

For percutaneous pedicle screw placement, we use fluoroscopy that is orthogonal to the target vertebral body in the anteroposterior and lateral planes and allows clear visualization of the medial wall of the pedicle and pedicle/vertebral body junction. A Jamshidi needle typically is docked on the pedicle of interest at the lamina/pedicle junction on the anteroposterior view (9 o'clock position for left pedicles and 3 o'clock position for right pedicles). For the most cephalad screw of a construct in the lumbar spine, we prefer to place the starting point slightly below midline on the anteroposterior view (8 o'clock for left pedicles and 4 o'clock for right pedicles) to limit encroachment of the next cephalad facet joint. Under anteroposterior imaging, the needle is then advanced down the pedicle 20 to 25 mm at a trajectory that will allow the tip of the needle to be placed at the pedicle/vertebral body junction without violating the medial wall of the pedicle. When seated, the needle should pass obliquely across the pedicle with the tip just lateral to the medial wall on the anteroposterior view and just deep to the base of the pedicle on the lateral view. This will allow passage of a guidewire into the vertebral body and placement of a cannulated percutaneous pedicle screw using a Seldinger technique. The technique of connecting rod passage depends on the implant manufacturer.

Midline cortical screw placement is another technique that can be used as a slightly less invasive means of fixation in conjunction with a spinous process splitting or limited midline approach and with a posterior lumbar interbody fusion when a posterolateral fusion is not performed. The initial screw starting point is at the medial caudal border of the target pedicle on true anteroposterior view of the target vertebrae (Fig. 1.6). A burr is used to dimple the cortical bone at the entry site. A pedicle awl is then used to traverse the pedicle in a medial-to-lateral and caudal-to-cranial trajectory, taking care not to violate the cortical wall of the pedicle as seen on anteroposterior and lateral fluoroscopy. Once the track is formed, it should be tapped to the size of the screw that will be inserted to prevent fracture of the thick cortical bone of the pars. A sound is used to confirm bony continuity along the screw path, and markers can be inserted to confirm position with imaging. The desired decompression and interbody fusion is then performed and cortical bone screws placed at the end of the case.

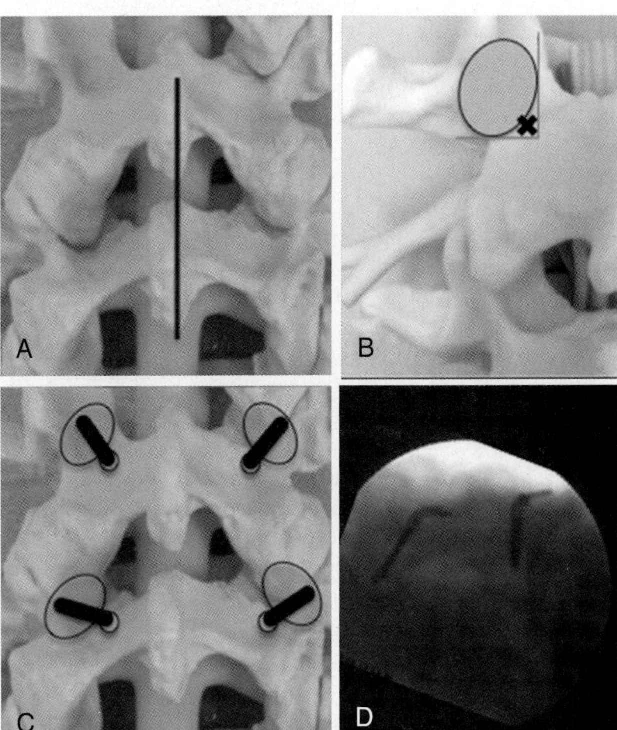

FIGURE 1.6 Midline cortical screw placement. A, Incision. B, Starting point at intersection of medial and caudal aspect of pedicle. C, Cortical bone trajectory. D, Proper positioning of marker pins. (From Mizuno M, Kuraishi K, Umeda Y, et al: Midline lumbar fusion with cortical bone trajectory screw, Neurol Med Chir [Tokyo] 54:716, 2014.)

CIRCULATION OF SPINAL CORD

The arterial supply to the spinal cord has been determined from gross anatomic dissection, latex arterial injections, and intercostal arteriography. Dommisse contributed significantly to knowledge of the blood supply, stating that the principles that govern the blood supply of the cord are constant, whereas the patterns vary with the individual. He emphasized the following factors:

1. *Dependence on three vessels.* These are the anterior median longitudinal arterial trunk and a pair of posterolateral trunks near the posterior nerve rootlets.
2. *Relative demands of gray matter and white matter.* The longitudinal arterial trunks are largest in the cervical and lumbar regions near the ganglionic enlargements and are much smaller in the thoracic region. This is because the metabolic demands of the gray matter are greater than those of the white matter, which contains fewer capillary networks.
3. *Medullary feeder (radicular) arteries of the cord.* These arteries reinforce the longitudinal arterial channels. There are 2 to 17 anteriorly and 6 to 25 posteriorly. The vertebral arteries supply 80% of the radicular arteries in the neck; arteries in the thoracic and lumbar areas arise from the aorta. The lateral sacral, the fifth lumbar, the iliolumbar, and the middle sacral arteries are important in the sacral region.
4. *Supplementary source of blood supply to the spinal cord.* The vertebral and posterior inferior cerebellar arteries are important sources of arterial supply. Sacral medullary feeders arise from the lateral sacral arteries and accompany the distal roots of the cauda equina. The flow in these vessels seems reversible and the volume adjustable in response to the metabolic demands.
5. *Segmental arteries of the spine.* At every vertebral level, a pair of segmental arteries supplies the extraspinal and intraspinal structures. The thoracic and lumbar segmental arteries arise from the aorta; the cervical segmental arteries arise from the vertebral arteries and the costocervical and thyrocervical trunks. In 60% of individuals, an additional source arises from the ascending pharyngeal branch of the external carotid artery. The lateral sacral arteries and, to a lesser extent, the fifth lumbar, iliolumbar, and middle sacral arteries supply segmental vessels in the sacral region.
6. *"Distribution point" of the segmental arteries.* The segmental arteries divide into numerous branches at the intervertebral foramen, which has been termed the *distribution point* (Fig. 1.7). A second anastomotic network lies within the spinal canal in the loose connective tissue of the extradural space. This occurs at all levels, with the greatest concentration in the cervical and lumbar regions. The presence of the rich anastomotic channels offers alternative pathways for arterial flow, preserving spinal cord circulation after the ligation of segmental arteries.
7. *Artery of Adamkiewicz.* The artery of Adamkiewicz is the largest of the feeders of the lumbar cord; it is located on

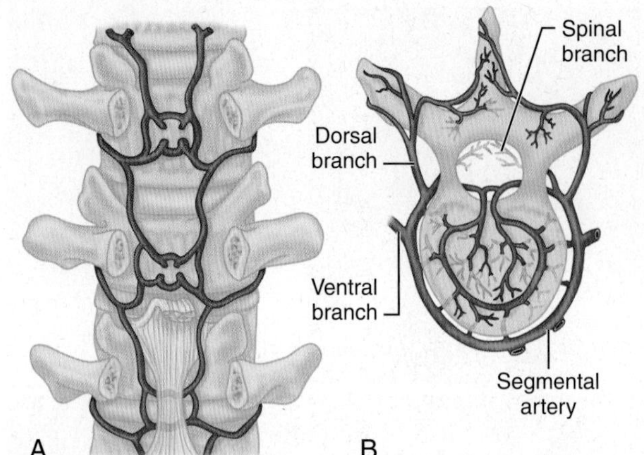

FIGURE 1.7 **Vertebral blood supply. A, Posterior view; laminae removed to show anastomosing spinal branches of segmental arteries. B, Cross-sectional view; anastomosing arterial supply of vertebral body, spinal canal, and posterior elements.** (Redrawn from Bullough PG, Oheneba BA: *Atlas of spinal diseases*, Philadelphia, 1988, JB Lippincott.)

the left side, usually at the level of T9-11 (in 80% of individuals). The anterior longitudinal arterial channel of the cord rather than any single medullary feeder is crucial. The preservation of this large feeder does not ensure continued satisfactory circulation for the spinal cord. In principle, it would seem of practical value to protect and preserve each contributing artery as far as is surgically possible.

8. *Variability of patterns of supply of the spinal cord.* The variability of blood supply is a striking feature, yet there is absolute conformity with a principle of a rich supply for the cervical and lumbar cord enlargements. The supply for the thoracic cord from approximately T4 to T9 is much poorer.
9. *Direction of flow in the blood vessels of the spinal cord.* The three longitudinal arterial channels of the spinal cord can be compared with the circle of Willis at the base of the brain, but it is more extensive and more complicated, although it functions with identical principles. These channels permit reversal of flow and alterations in the volume of blood flow in response to metabolic demands. This internal arterial circle of the cord is surrounded by at least two outer arterial circles, the first of which is situated in the extradural space and the second in the extravertebral tissue planes. By virtue of the latter, the spinal cord enjoys reserve sources of blood supply through a degree of anastomosis lacking in the inner circle. The "outlet points" are limited, however, to the perforating sulcal arteries and the pial arteries of the cord.

The blood supply to the spinal cord is rich, but the spinal canal is narrowest and the blood supply is poorest at T4-9. T4-9 should be considered the critical vascular zone of the spinal cord, a zone in which interference with the circulation is most likely to result in paraplegia.

The dominance of the anterior spinal artery system has been challenged by the fact that many anterior spinal surgeries have been performed in recent years with no increase in the incidence of paralysis. This would seem to indicate that a rich anastomotic supply does exist and that it protects the spinal cord. The evidence suggests that the posterior spinal arteries may be as important as the anterior system but are as yet poorly understood. Venous drainage of the spinal cord is more difficult

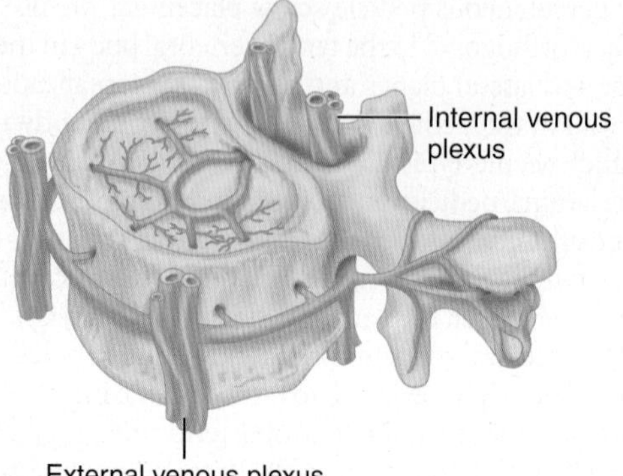

FIGURE 1.8 **Venous drainage of vertebral bodies and formation of internal and external vertebral venous plexuses.** (Redrawn from Bullough PG, Oheneba BA: *Atlas of spinal diseases*, Philadelphia, 1988, JB Lippincott.)

to define clearly than is the arterial supply (Fig. 1.8). It is well known that the venous system is highly variable. Dommisse pointed out that there are two sets of veins: veins of the spinal cord and veins that fall within the plexiform network of Batson. The veins of the spinal cord are a small component of the entire system and drain into the plexus of Batson. The Batson plexus is a large and complex venous channel extending from the base of the skull to the coccyx. It communicates directly with the superior and inferior vena cava system and the azygos system. The longitudinal venous trunks of the spinal cord are the anterior and posterior venous channels, which are the counterparts of the arterial trunks. The three components of the Batson plexus are the extradural vertebral venous plexus; the extravertebral venous plexus, which includes the segmental veins of the neck, the intercostal veins, the azygos communications in the thorax and pelvis, the lumbar veins, and the communications with the inferior vena caval system; and the veins of the bony structures of the spinal column. The venous system plays no specific role in the metabolism of the spinal cord; it communicates directly with the venous system draining the head, chest, and abdomen. This interconnection allows metastatic spread of neoplastic or infectious disease from the pelvis to the vertebral column.

During anterior spinal surgery, we empirically follow these principles: (1) ligate segmental spinal arteries only as necessary to gain exposure; (2) ligate segmental spinal arteries near the aorta rather than near the vertebral foramina; (3) ligate segmental spinal arteries on one side only when possible, leaving the circulation intact on the opposite side; and (4) limit dissection in the vertebral foramina to a single level when possible so that collateral circulation is disturbed as little as possible.

SURGICAL APPROACHES

ANTERIOR APPROACHES

With the posterior approach for correction of spinal deformities well established, more attention has been placed on the anterior approach to the spinal column. Many pioneers in the field of anterior spinal surgery recognized that anterior spinal cord decompression was necessary in spinal tuberculosis and that laminectomy not only failed to relieve anterior pressure but also removed important posterior stability and produced worsening of kyphosis. Advances in major surgical procedures, including anesthesia and intensive care, have made it possible to perform anterior spinal surgery with acceptable safety.

In general, anterior approaches to the spine are indicated for decompression of the neural elements (spinal cord, conus medullaris, cauda equina, or nerve roots) when anterior neural compression has been documented by myelography, postmyelogram CT, or MRI. Many pathologic entities can cause significant compression of the neural elements, including traumatic, neoplastic, inflammatory, degenerative, and congenital lesions. In the lumbar spine, this indication has been expanded to include anterior interbody fusions for discogenic pain and instability.

In many centers, a team approach is preferred to employ the skills of an orthopaedic surgeon, neurosurgeon, thoracic surgeon, or head and neck surgeon. The orthopaedic surgeon still must have a working knowledge of the underlying viscera, fluid balance, physiology, and other elements of intensive care. These approaches should be used with care and only in appropriate circumstances. Potential dangers include iatrogenic injury to vascular, visceral, or neurologic structures. Complications of anterior spine surgery are rare; however, there is a high risk of significant morbidity, and these approaches should be used with care and only in appropriate circumstances.

The choice of approach depends on the preference and experience of the surgeon, the patient's age and medical condition, the segment of the spine involved, the underlying pathologic process, and the presence or absence of signs of neural compression. Commonly accepted indications for anterior approaches are listed in Box 1.1.

BOX 1.1

Relative Indications for Anterior Spinal Approaches

1. Traumatic
   a. Fractures with documented neurocompression secondary to bone or disc fragments anterior to dura
   b. Incomplete spinal cord injury (for cord recovery) with anterior extradural compression
   c. Complete spinal cord injury (for root recovery) with anterior extradural compression
   d. Late pain or paralysis after remote injuries with anterior extradural compression
   e. Herniated intervertebral disc
2. Infectious
   a. Open biopsy for diagnosis
   b. Debridement and anterior strut grafting
3. Degenerative
   a. Cervical spondylitic radiculopathy
   b. Cervical spondylitic myelopathy
   c. Thoracic disc herniation
   d. Cervical, thoracic, and lumbar interbody fusions
4. Neoplastic
   a. Extradural metastatic disease
   b. Primary vertebral body tumor
5. Deformity
   a. Kyphosis—congenital or acquired
   b. Scoliosis—congenital, acquired, or idiopathic

ANTERIOR APPROACH, OCCIPUT TO C3

The anterior approach to the upper cervical spine (occiput to C3) can be transoral or retropharyngeal, depending on the pathologic process present and the experience of the surgeon.

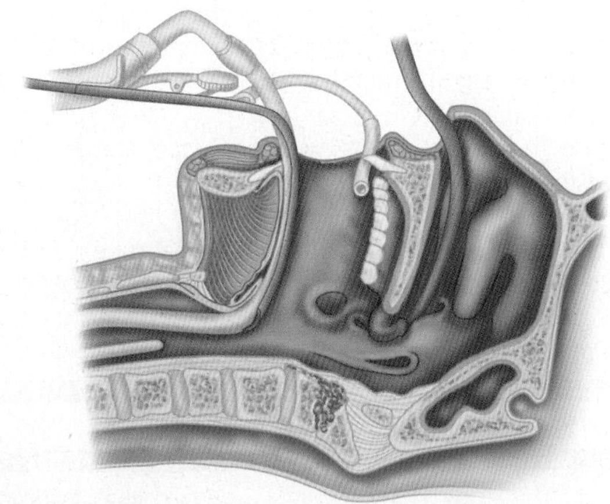

FIGURE 1.9 **Anterior transoral approach (see text).** (Redrawn from Spetzler RF: Transoral approach to the upper cervical spine. In Evarts CM, editor: *Surgery of the musculoskeletal system,* New York, 1983, Churchill Livingstone.) **SEE TECHNIQUE 1.1.**

ANTERIOR TRANSORAL APPROACH

TECHNIQUE 1.1 ***Figure 1.9***

(SPETZLER)

- Position the patient supine using a Mayfield head-holding device or with skeletal traction through Gardner-Wells tongs. Monitoring of the spinal cord through somatosensory evoked potentials is recommended. The surgeon may sit directly over the patient's head.
- Pass a red rubber catheter down each nostril and suture it to the uvula. Apply traction to the catheters to pull the uvula and soft palate out of the operative field, taking care not to cause necrosis of the septal cartilage by excessive pressure.
- Insert a McGarver retractor into the open mouth and use it to retract and hold the endotracheal tube out of the way. The operating microscope is useful to improve the limited exposure.
- Prepare the oropharynx with hexachlorophene (pHiso-Hex) and povidone-iodine (Betadine).
- Palpate the anterior ring of C1 beneath the posterior pharynx and make an incision in the wall of the posterior pharynx from the superior aspect of C1 to the top of C3.
- Obtain hemostasis with bipolar electrocautery, taking care not to overcauterize, producing thermal necrosis of tissue and increased risk of infection.
- With a periosteal elevator, subperiosteally dissect the edges of the pharyngeal incision from the anterior ring of C1 and the anterior aspect of C2. Use traction stitches to maintain the flaps out of the way.
- Under direct vision, with the operating microscope or with magnification loupes and headlights, perform a meticulous debridement of C1 and C2 with a high-speed air drill, rongeur, or curet. When approaching the posterior longitudinal ligament, a diamond burr is safer to use in removing the last remnant of bone.
- When adequate debridement of infected bone and necrotic tissue has been accomplished, decompress the upper cervical spinal cord.

- If the cervical spine is to be fused anteriorly, harvest a corticocancellous graft from the patient's iliac crest, fashion it to fit, and insert it.
- Irrigate the operative site with antibiotic solution and close the posterior pharynx in layers.

POSTOPERATIVE CARE An endotracheal tube is left in place overnight to maintain an adequate airway. A halo vest can be applied, or skeletal traction may be maintained before mobilization.

ANTERIOR RETROPHARYNGEAL APPROACH

The anterior retropharyngeal approach to the upper cervical spine, as described by McAfee et al., is excellent for anterior debridement of the upper cervical spine and allows placement of bone grafts for stabilization if necessary. In contrast to the transoral approach, it is entirely extramucosal and is reported to have fewer complications of wound infection and neurologic deficit.

TECHNIQUE 1.2

(MCAFEE ET AL.)

- Position the patient supine, preferably on a turning frame with skeletal traction through tongs or a halo ring. Somatosensory evoked potential monitoring of cord function is suggested during the procedure.
- Perform fiberoptic nasotracheal intubation to prevent excessive motion of the neck and to keep the oropharynx free of tubes that could depress the mandible and interfere with subsequent exposure.
- Make a right-sided transverse skin incision in the submandibular region with a vertical extension as long as required to provide adequate exposure (Fig. 1.10A). If the approach does not have to be extended below the level of the fifth cervical vertebra, there is no increased risk of damage to the recurrent laryngeal nerve.
- Carry the dissection through the platysma muscle with the enveloping superficial fascia of the neck and mobilize flaps from this area.
- Identify the marginal mandibular branch of the seventh nerve with the help of a nerve stimulator and ligate the retromandibular veins superiorly.
- Keep the dissection deep to the retromandibular vein to prevent injury to the superficial branches of the facial nerve.
- Ligate the retromandibular vein as it joins the internal jugular vein.
- Mobilize the anterior border of the sternocleidomastoid muscle by longitudinally dividing the superficial layer of the deep cervical fascia. Feel for the pulsations of the carotid artery and protect the contents of the carotid sheath.
- Resect the submandibular gland (Fig. 1.10B) and ligate the duct to prevent formation of a salivary fistula.
- Identify the digastric and stylohyoid muscles and tag and divide the tendon of the former. The facial nerve can be injured by superior retraction on the stylohyoid muscle; however, by dividing the digastric and stylohyoid muscles, the hyoid bone and hypopharynx can be mobilized medially, preventing exposure of the esophagus, hypopharynx, and nasopharynx.
- Identify the hypoglossal nerve and retract it superiorly.
- Continue dissection to the retropharyngeal space between the carotid sheath laterally and the larynx and pharynx medially. Increase exposure by ligating branches of the carotid artery and internal jugular vein, which prevent retraction of the carotid sheath laterally (Fig. 1.10C and D).
- Identify and mobilize the superior laryngeal nerve.
- Following adequate retraction of the carotid sheath laterally, divide the alar and prevertebral fascial layers longitudinally to expose the longus colli muscles. Take care to maintain the head in a neutral position and identify the midline accurately.
- Remove the longus colli muscles subperiosteally from the anterior aspect of the arch of C1 and the body of C2, avoiding injury to the vertebral arteries.
- Meticulously debride the involved osseous structures (Fig. 1.10E); if needed, perform bone grafting with autogenous iliac or fibular bone.
- Close the wound over suction drains and repair the digastric tendon. Close the platysma and skin flaps in layers.

POSTOPERATIVE CARE The patient is maintained in skeletal traction with the head of the bed elevated to reduce swelling. Intubation is continued until pharyngeal edema has resolved, usually by 48 hours. The patient can be extubated and mobilized in a halo vest, or, if indicated, a posterior stabilization procedure can be done before mobilization.

EXTENDED MAXILLOTOMY AND SUBTOTAL MAXILLECTOMY

Cocke et al. described an extended maxillotomy and subtotal maxillectomy as an alternative to the transoral approach for exposure and removal of tumor or bone anteriorly at the base of the skull and cervical spine to C5. This procedure is technically demanding and requires a thorough knowledge of head and neck anatomy. It should be performed by a team of surgeons, including an otolaryngologist, a neurosurgeon, and an orthopaedist.

Before surgery, the size, position, and extent of the tumor or bone to be removed should be determined using the appropriate imaging techniques. Three to 5 days before the surgery, nasal, oral, and pharyngeal secretions are cultured to determine the proper antibiotics needed. Cephalosporin and aminoglycoside antibiotics are given before and after surgery if the floral cultures are normal and are adjusted if the flora is abnormal or resistant to these drugs.

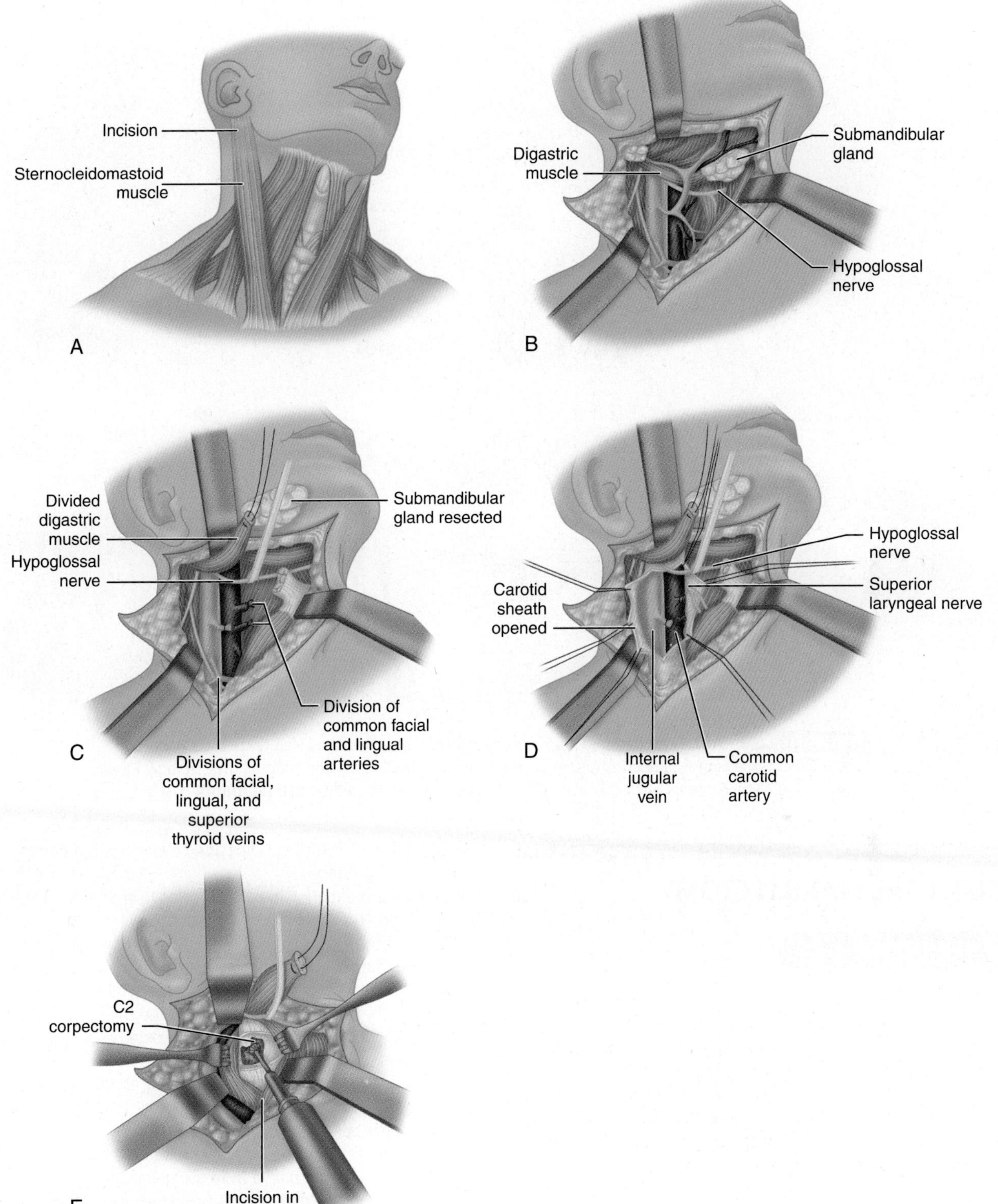

FIGURE 1.10 **A-E, Anterior retropharyngeal approach (see text).** (Redrawn from McAfee PC, Bohlman HH, Riley LH Jr, et al: The anterior retropharyngeal approach to the upper part of the cervical spine, *J Bone Joint Surg* 69A:1371, 1987.) **SEE TECHNIQUE 1.2.**

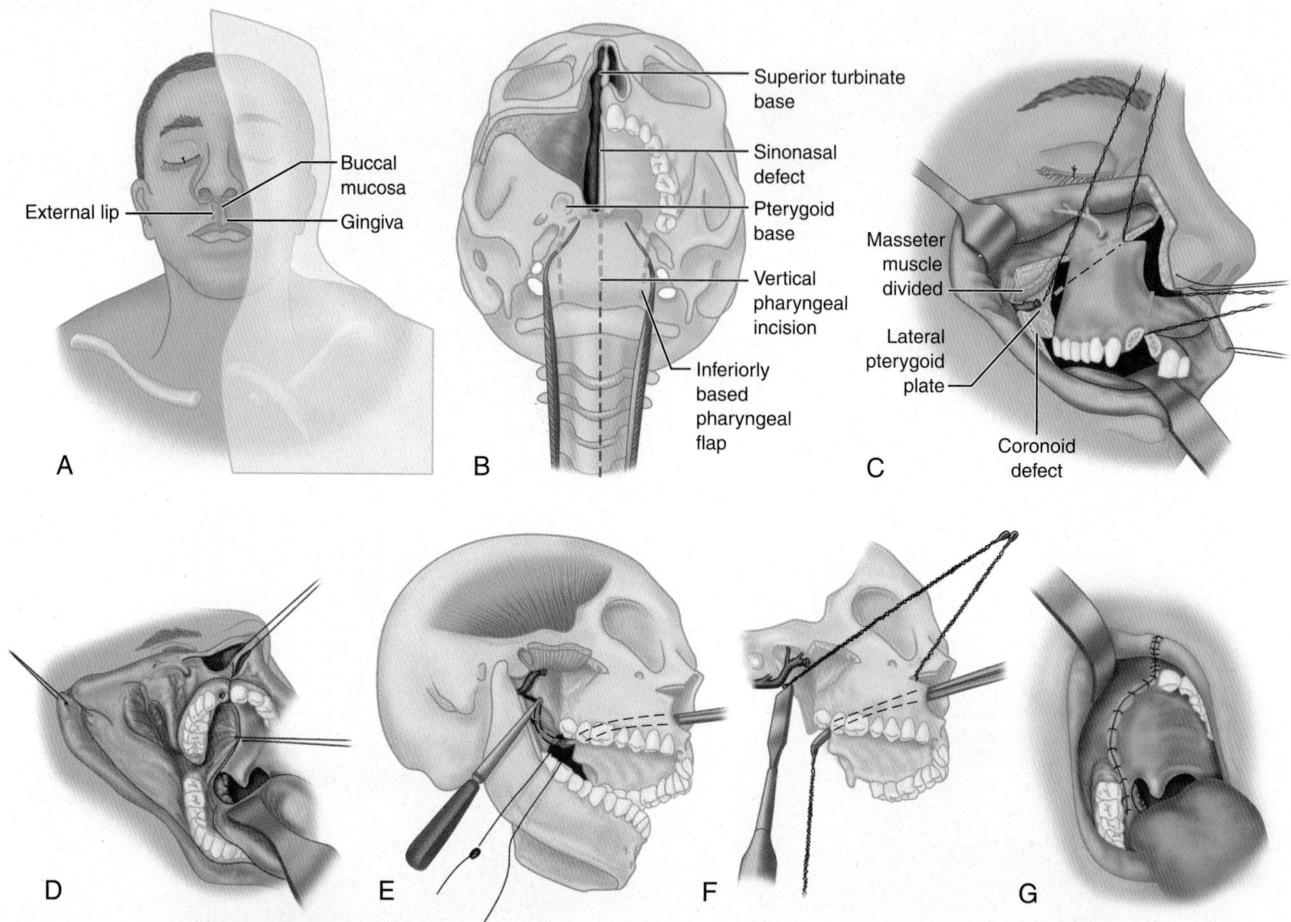

FIGURE 1.11 **A-G, Extended maxillotomy and subtotal maxillectomy (see text).** (Redrawn from Cocke EW Jr, Robertson JH, Robertson JR, et al: The extended maxillotomy and subtotal maxillectomy for excision of skull base tumors, *Arch Otolaryngol Head Neck Surg* 116:92, 1990.) **SEE TECHNIQUE 1.3.**

SUBTOTAL MAXILLECTOMY

TECHNIQUE 1.3

(COCKE ET AL.)

- Position the patient on the operating table with the head elevated 25 degrees. Intubate the patient orally and move the tube to the contralateral side of the mouth.
- Perform a percutaneous endoscopic gastrostomy if the wound is to be left open or if problems are anticipated.
- Perform a tracheostomy if the exposure may be limited or if there are severe pulmonary problems. This step usually is unnecessary.
- Insert a Foley catheter and suture the eyelids closed with 6-0 nylon.
- Infiltrate the soft tissues of the upper lip, cheek, gingiva, palate, pterygoid fossa, nasopharynx, nasal septum, nasal floor, and lateral nasal wall with 1% lidocaine and 1:100,000 epinephrine.
- Pack each nasal cavity with cottonoid strips saturated with 4% cocaine and 1% phenylephrine.
- Prepare the skin with povidone-iodine and then alcohol. Drape the operative site with cloth drapes held in place with sutures or surgical clips and covered with a transparent surgical drape.
- Expose the superior maxilla through a modified Weber-Ferguson skin incision (Fig. 1.11A). Make a vertical incision through the upper lip in the philtrum from the nasolabial groove to the vermilion border. Extend the lower end to the midline and vertically in the midline through the buccal mucosa to the gingivobuccal gutter. Divide the upper lip and ligate the labial arteries. Extend the external skin incision transversely from the upper end of the lip incision in the nasolabial groove to beyond the nasal ala and superiorly along the nasofacial groove to the lower eyelid.
- Extract the central incisor tooth.
- Make a vertical midline incision through the mucoperiosteum of the anterior maxilla from the gingivobuccal gutter to the central incisor defect and transversely through the buccal gingiva adjacent to the teeth to the retromolar region.
- Elevate the skin, subcutaneous tissues, periosteum, and mucoperiosteum of the maxilla to expose the anterior and lateral walls of the maxilla, nasal bone, piriform aperture of the nose, inferior orbital nerve, malar bone, and masseter muscle (Fig. 1.11D).
- Divide the anterior margin of the masseter muscle at its malar attachment and remove a wedge of malar bone. Use this wedge to accommodate the Gigli saw as it divides the maxilla (Fig. 1.11E and F).

- Make an incision in the lingual, hard palate mucoperiosteum adjacent to the teeth from the central incisor defect to join the retromolar incision.
- Extend the retromolar incision medial to the mandible lateral to the tonsil and to the retropharyngeal space to the level of the hyoid bone or lower pharynx, if necessary.
- Elevate the mucoperiosteum of the hard palate from the central incisor defect and alveolar ridge to and beyond the midline of the hard palate.
- Detach the soft palate with its nasal lining from the posterior margin of the hard palate.
- Divide and electrocoagulate the greater palatine vessels and nerves. Pack the palatine foramen with bone wax.
- Retract the mucoperiosteum of the hard palate, soft palate, anterior tonsillar pillar, tonsil, and pharynx medially from the prevertebral fascia. It is usually unnecessary to detach and retract the soft palate from the posterior or lateral pharyngeal walls.
- Expose the nasal cavity by detaching the nasal soft tissues from the lateral margin and base of the nasal piriform aperture (Fig. 1.11B).
- Remove a bony wedge of the ascending process of the maxilla to accommodate the upper Gigli saw (Fig. 1.11E).
- Remove the coronoid process of the mandible above the level of entrance of the inferior alveolar vessels and nerves, after dividing its temporalis muscle attachment, to expose the lateral pterygoid plate and the internal maxillary artery.
- Divide the pterygoid muscles with a Shaw knife or the cutting current of the Bovie cautery until the sharp, posterior bone edge of the lateral pterygoid plate is seen or palpated.
- Mobilize, clip, ligate, and divide the internal maxillary artery near the pterygoid plate.
- Direct the suture behind the lateral pterygoid plate into the nasopharynx and behind the posterior margin of the hard palate into the oropharynx (Fig. 1.11F).
- Pass a Kelly forceps through the nose to behind the hard palate to retrieve the medial end of the silk suture in the ligature carrier.
- Attach a Gigli saw to the lateral end of the suture and thread the saw into position to divide the upper maxilla.
- Position the upper Gigli saw (Fig. 1.11E and F) using a sharp-pointed, medium-size, curved, right-angle ligature carrier threaded with No. 2 black silk suture.
- Engage the medial arm of the saw into the ascending process wedge and its lateral arm into the malar wedge. Take care to position the saw as high as possible behind the pterygoid plate. Use a broad periosteal elevator beneath the saw on the pterygoid plate to maintain the elevated position (Fig. 1.11F).
- Position the lower Gigli saw by passing a Kelly forceps (Fig. 1.11E) through the nose into the nasopharynx behind the posterior nares of the hard palate. Engage the saw between the blades of the clamp and thread it through the nose into position for division of the hard palate (Fig. 1.11C).
- Divide the bony walls of the maxilla (Fig. 1.11C). First divide the hard palate and then the upper maxilla. Avoid entangling the saws and protect the soft tissues from injury.
- Remove the maxilla after division of its muscle attachments.
- Ligate the distal end of the internal maxillary artery.
- Place traction sutures in the soft tissues of the lip on either side of the initial lip incision and in the mucoperiosteum of the hard and soft palates. The posterior pharynx is now fully exposed.
- Infiltrate the mucous membrane covering the posterior wall of the nasopharynx, oropharynx, and the tonsillar area to the level of the hyoid bone with 1% lidocaine and epinephrine 1:100,000.
- Make a vertical midline incision through the soft tissues of the posterior wall of the nasopharynx extending from the sphenoidal sinus to the foramen magnum. Another option is to make a transverse incision from the sphenoidal sinus to the lateral nasopharyngeal wall posterior to the eustachian tube along the lateral pharyngeal wall inferiorly, posterior to the posterior tonsillar pillar behind the soft palate (Fig. 1.11B).
- Duplicate this incision on the opposite side, producing an inferiorly based pharyngeal flap (Fig. 1.11B).
- Make a more extensive exposure by extending the lateral pharyngeal wall incision through the anterior tonsillar pillar to join the retromolar incision. Extend this incision into the retropharyngeal space and retract the anterior tonsillar pillar, tonsil, and soft palate toward the midline with a traction suture. It is unnecessary to separate the soft palate completely from the pharyngeal wall.
- Extend the pharyngeal wall incision inferiorly to the level of the hyoid bone or beyond.
- Elevate, divide, and separate the superior constrictor muscle, prevertebral fascia, longus capitis muscle, and anterior longitudinal ligaments from the bony skull base and upper cervical spine ventrally.
- Expose the amount of bone to be operated on from the foramen magnum to C5. Use an operating microscope or loupe magnification for improved vision.
- Remove the offending bone with a high-speed burr, avoiding penetration of the dura.
- Close the nasopharyngeal mucous membrane and the subcutaneous tissue in one layer with interrupted sutures.
- Use a split-thickness skin or dermal graft from the thigh to resurface the buccal mucosa and any defects in the nasal surface of the hard palate.
- Use a quilting stitch to hold the graft in place without packing.
- Replace the zygoma and stabilize it with wire if it was mobilized.
- Return the maxilla to its original position and hold it in place with wire or compression plates.
- Place a nylon sack impregnated with antibiotic into the nasal cavity.
- Close the oral cavity incision with vertical interrupted mattress 3-0 polyglycolic acid sutures (Fig. 1.11G).
- Close the facial wound with 5-0 chromic and 6-0 nylon sutures.

EXTENDED MAXILLOTOMY

TECHNIQUE 1.4

- Expose the base of the skull and upper cervical spine as by the maxillectomy technique but omit the extraction of the central incisor and the gingivolingual incision.
- Use a degloving procedure for elevation of the facial skin over the maxilla and nose to avoid facial scars.

- Divide the fibromuscular attachment of the soft palate to the pterygoid plate and hard palate, exposing the nasopharynx.
- Place the upper Gigli saw with the aid of a ligature carrier for division of the maxilla beneath the infraorbital nerve.
- Elevate the mucoperiosteum of the adjacent floor of the nose from the piriform aperture to the soft palate. Extend this elevation medially to the nasal septum and laterally to the inferior turbinate.
- Divide the bone of the nasal floor with a Stryker saw without lacerating the underlying hard palate periosteum.
- Hinge the maxilla on the hard palate, nasal mucoperiosteum, and soft palate, and rotate it medially.

POSTOPERATIVE CARE Continuous spinal fluid drainage is maintained, and the head is elevated 45 degrees if the dura was repaired or replaced. These procedures are omitted if there was no dural tear or defect. An ice cap is used on the cheek and temple to reduce edema. Antibiotic therapy is continued until the risk of infection is minimized. Half-strength hydrogen peroxide is used for mouth irrigation to help keep the oral cavity clean. The endotracheal tube is removed when the risk of occlusion by swelling is minimized. The nasopharyngeal cavity is cleaned with saline twice daily for 2 months after pack removal. Facial sutures are removed at 4 to 6 days, and oral sutures are removed at 2 weeks.

ANTERIOR APPROACH, C3 TO C7

Exposure of the middle and lower cervical region of the spine is most commonly done through an anterior approach medial to the carotid sheath. A thorough knowledge of anatomic fascial planes allows a safe, direct approach to this area. The most frequent complication of the anterior approach is vocal cord paralysis caused by injury to the recurrent laryngeal nerve. Injury to the recurrent laryngeal nerve may be less common on the left side because the nerve has a more vertical course and lies in a protected position within the esophagotracheal groove. On the right, the nerve leaves the main trunk of the vagus nerve and passes anterior to and under the subclavian artery, whereas on the left it passes under and posterior to the aorta at the site of origin of the ligamentum arteriosum. The nerve runs upward, having a variable relationship with the inferior thyroid artery, making the recurrent laryngeal nerve on the right side highly vulnerable to injury if the inferior thyroid vessels are not ligated as laterally as possible or if the midline structures along with the recurrent laryngeal nerve are not retracted intermittently.

The shorter, more lateral position of the right recurrent laryngeal nerve places it at risk for injury from direct trauma or from the retraction that is necessary to expose the anterior cervical vertebrae. A left-sided exposure medial to the carotid artery and internal jugular vein can be used to minimize the risk of injury. Although many spine surgeons use the right-sided approach with a low incidence of symptomatic paralysis of the recurrent laryngeal nerve, the incidence of temporary, partial, or asymptomatic paralysis may be underestimated. We believe that using the left-sided approach may reduce the risk of such injuries.

ANTERIOR APPROACH, C3 TO C7

TECHNIQUE 1.5

(SOUTHWICK AND ROBINSON)

As with other approaches to the cervical spine, skeletal traction is suggested, and spinal cord monitoring can be used at the surgeon's discretion. Exposure can be carried out through either a transverse or a longitudinal incision, depending on the surgeon's preference (Fig. 1.12A). We generally use a transverse incision for one- and two-level approaches and a longitudinal incision for approaches involving three levels or more. A left-sided skin incision is preferred because of the more constant anatomy of the recurrent laryngeal nerve and the lower risk of inadvertent injury to the nerve. In general, an incision three to four fingerbreadths above the clavicle is needed to expose C3-5; an incision two to three fingerbreadths above the clavicle allows exposure of C5-7. On rare occasions, this approach

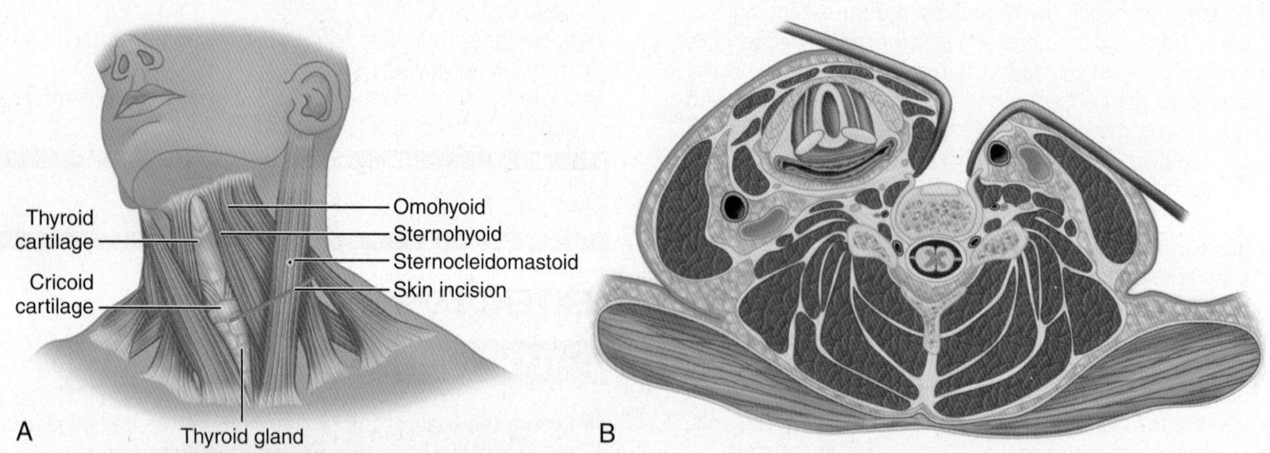

FIGURE 1.12 Anterior approach to C3-7 (see text). **A,** Incision. **B,** Thyroid gland, trachea, and esophagus have been retracted medially, and carotid sheath and its contents have been retracted laterally in opposite direction. **SEE TECHNIQUE 1.5.**

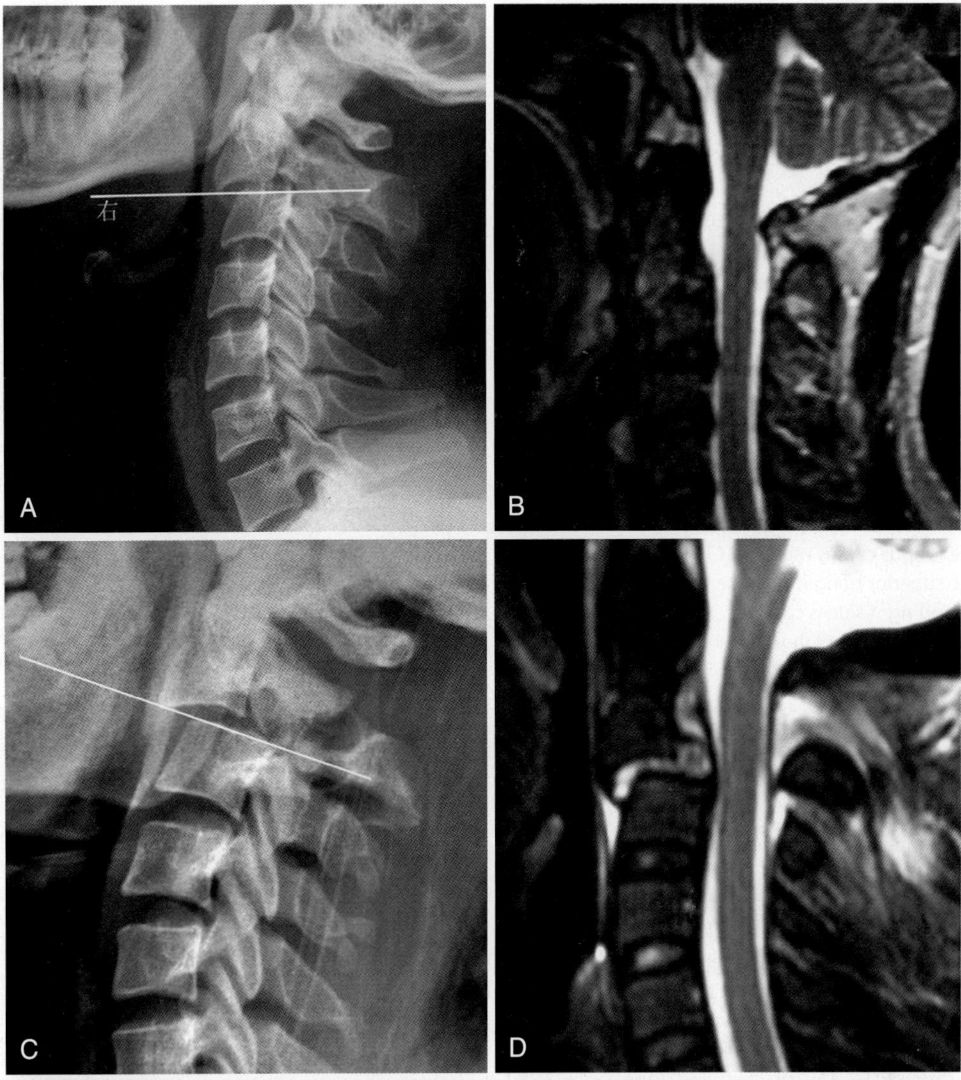

FIGURE 1.13 Lateral extension radiograph **(A)** and T2-weighted magnetic resonance image **(B)**. A line based on the C3 upper endplate is drawn on a lateral extension radiograph of the cervical spine. Candidates for the subaxial anterior approach should have a mandibular angle higher than the line. Lateral extension radiograph **(C)** and T2-weighted magnetic resonance image **(D)**. A large chin with a mandibular angle that extends over the line may make it difficult to reach C2 with the subaxial anterior approach. (From Zhang Y, Zhang J, Wang X, et al: Application of the cervical subaxial anterior approach at C2 in select patients, *Orthopedics* 36:e554, 2013.)

can be used to access C2-3 in individuals with long, thin necks when a line drawn through the C2-3 disc space passes below the mandibular angle on lateral preoperative radiographs (Fig. 1.13).

- Center a transverse incision over the medial border of the sternocleidomastoid muscle. Infiltration of the skin and subcutaneous tissue with a 1:500,000 epinephrine solution assists with hemostasis.
- Incise the platysma muscle in line with the skin incision or open it vertically for more exposure.
- Identify the anterior border of the sternocleidomastoid muscle and longitudinally incise the superficial layer of the deep cervical fascia; localize the carotid pulse by palpation.
- Carefully divide the middle layer of deep cervical fascia that encloses the omohyoid medial to the carotid sheath.
- As the sternomastoid and carotid sheath are retracted laterally, the anterior aspect of the cervical spine can be palpated. Identify the esophagus lying posterior to the trachea and retract the trachea, esophagus, and thyroid medially (Fig. 1.12B).
- Bluntly divide the deep layers of the deep cervical fascia, consisting of the pretracheal and prevertebral fascia overlying the longus colli muscles.
- Subperiosteally reflect the longus colli from the anterior aspect of the spine out laterally to the level of the uncovertebral joints. The resulting exposure is sufficient for wide debridement and bone grafting.
- Close the wound over a drain to prevent hematoma formation and possible airway obstruction.
- Approximate the platysma and skin edges in routine fashion.

ANTEROLATERAL APPROACH, C2 TO C7

Chibbaro et al. and Bruneau et al. described an anterolateral approach to the cervical spine that allows decompression of the body and roots that are affected with unilateral myelopathy and/

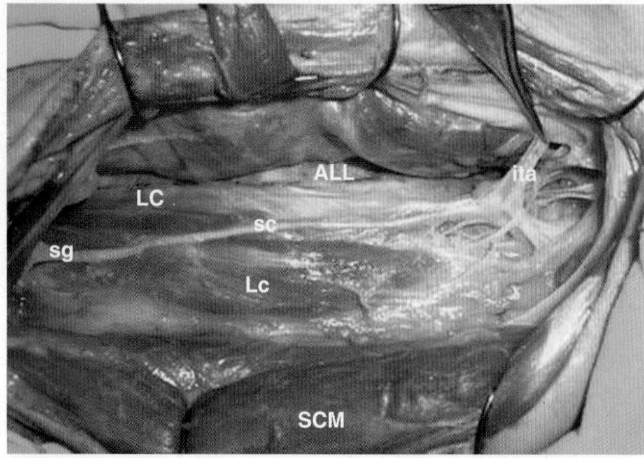

FIGURE 1.14 Anatomic dissection showing the relation of the cervical sympathetic chain *(sc)* to the longus coli muscle *(Lc)*. Also shown are the sternocleidomastoid muscle (SCM), the anterior longitudinal ligament *(ALL)*, the longus capitis muscle *(LC)*, the inferior thyroidal artery *(ita)*, and the superior ganglion of the sympathetic trunk *(sg)*. (Left side is cranial and right side is caudal.) (From Civelek E, Karasu A, Cansever T, et al: Surgical anatomy of the cervical sympathetic trunk during anterolateral approach to the cervical spine, *Eur Spine J* 17:991, 2008.)

or radiculopathy. This technique allows the removal of a wedge of cervical vertebra without the need for grafting or instrumentation. This technique also allows the direct exposure of the vertebral artery and veins by direct exposure of the vertebral foramen. It is recommended for elderly patients and smokers with unilateral anterior or lateral bony compression without instability. Cited advantages of this technique include wide decompression at a single level or multiple levels while providing direct vision of the vertebral artery and nerve roots. A disadvantage is the difficulty of the dissection with the potential injury to the vertebral artery, veins, XI cranial nerve, and the sympathetic chain, which can result in Horner syndrome (ptosis, ipsilateral miosis, and anhidrosis). In 459 procedures done since 1992, Chibbaro et al. noted no vertebral artery injury, cerebrospinal fluid leaks, dysphagia, or nerve root palsy; however, 14 patients (3%) developed Horner syndrome, which became permanent in four, and three had infections. The frequency of Horner syndrome reported in the literature is as high as 4%. The authors stressed that there is a steep learning curve with this procedure. From anatomic studies, Civelek et al. determined that the cervical sympathetic chain was on average 11.6 mm from the medial border of the longus coli muscle (Fig. 1.14). The superior ganglion was always at the level of C4, whereas the intermediate ganglion varied at its level of the cervical spine. The greatest risk to the sympathetic chain is during sectioning of the longus coli muscle transversely and dissection of the prevertebral fascia.

We have no experience with this procedure.

ANTEROLATERAL APPROACH, C2 TO C7

TECHNIQUE 1.6

(BRUNEAU ET AL., CHIBBARO ET AL.)

- Place the patient supine with the head rotated to the side opposite the incision and the neck in extension. Prepare and drape the neck as for any usual anterior cervical disc surgery.
- Identify the involved level radiographically.
- Make a longitudinal incision along the medial border of the sternocleidomastoid muscle. (At the C2-3 level, the incision extends to the tip of the mastoid process superiorly and to the sternal notch for exposure of C7-T1 inferiorly.)
- Incise the platysma muscle along the plane of the skin incision.
- Open the space between the sternocleidomastoid muscle and the internal jugular vein with sharp dissection. Retract the sternocleidomastoid muscle laterally and the undissected great vessels, trachea, and esophagus medially (Fig. 1.15A).
- Identify the fatty sheath surrounding cranial nerve XI and expose the nerve from C2 to C4.
- Identify the transverse processes with a finger.
- Divide the aponeurosis of the longus coli longitudinally to identify the sympathetic chain, which lies on top of the longus coli.
- Retract the aponeurosis and the sympathetic chain laterally.
- Divide the longus coli longitudinally at the interval of the junction of the vertebral body and the transverse processes.
- Take care to be sure the vertebral artery is not entering at an abnormally high level such as C3, C4, or C5.
- Clear the transverse processes and the lateral aspect of the vertebral body. Confirm the level of dissection radiographically.
- Subperiosteally dissect the lateral aspect of the uncovertebral joint and medial border of the vertebral artery.
- Open the vertebral foramen laterally by removing the anterior portion of the transverse foramen with a Kerrison rongeur. This frees the cervical root from the dural root to the vertebral artery margin.
- Confirm the level of decompression again radiographically.
- Make an oblique corpectomy in the vertebra using a burr for longitudinal removal of bone from upper to lower disc spaces (Fig. 1.15B to D).
- Start with a longitudinal trench just medial to the vertebral artery and continue the bone removal medially. Preserve the posterior cortex until the wedge is completed.
- Resect the posterior cortex and the posterior longitudinal ligament to decompress the cord.
- Recheck the decompression radiographically.
- Obtain good hemostasis, irrigate the wound, and remove the retractors. The tissues will fall into place.
- Close the subcutaneous tissue and skin as desired.
- A drain can be used if necessary.
- Immobilization with a collar may be desired for soft-tissue healing.

ANTERIOR APPROACH TO CERVICOTHORACIC JUNCTION, C7 TO T1

There is no ready anterior access to the cervicothoracic junction. The rapid transition from cervical lordosis to thoracic kyphosis results in an abrupt change in the depth of the wound. Also, this is a confluent area of vital structures that are not readily retracted. The three approaches to this area are (1) the low anterior cervical approach, (2) the high transthoracic approach, and (3) the transsternal approach.

The low anterior cervical approach provides access to T1 at the inferior extent and the lower cervical spine at the

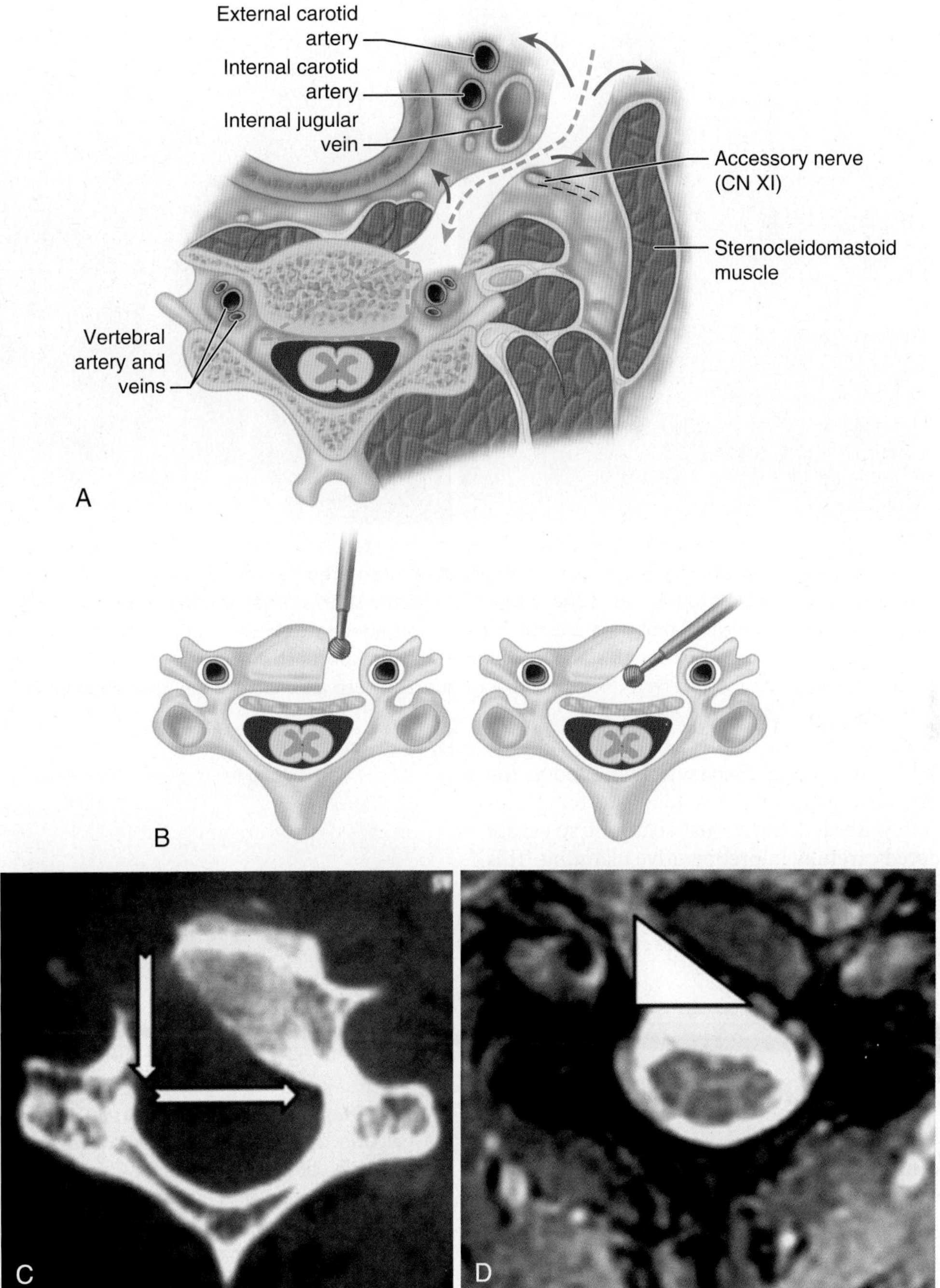

FIGURE 1.15 **A,** Anterolateral approach to the cervical spine through the interval between the sternocleidomastoid laterally and along the internal jugular vein medially with the other vascular structures including the internal carotid and external carotid. The XI cranial nerve is identified at C2 to 4 *(CN XI)*. The longus coli aponeurosis is longitudinally opened and the sympathetic chain is identified and carefully protected while exposing the uncovertebral joints and the anterior surface of the transverse process. The foramen is opened over the vertebral artery. **B,** Bony exposure through wedge-shaped lateral decompression. **C,** CT after wedge decompression. **D,** Postoperative MRI showing decompression. (From Chibbaro S, Mirone G, Bresson D, George B: Cervical spine lateral approach for myeloradiculopathy: technique and pitfalls, *Surg Neurol* 72:318, 2009.) **SEE TECHNIQUE 1.6.**

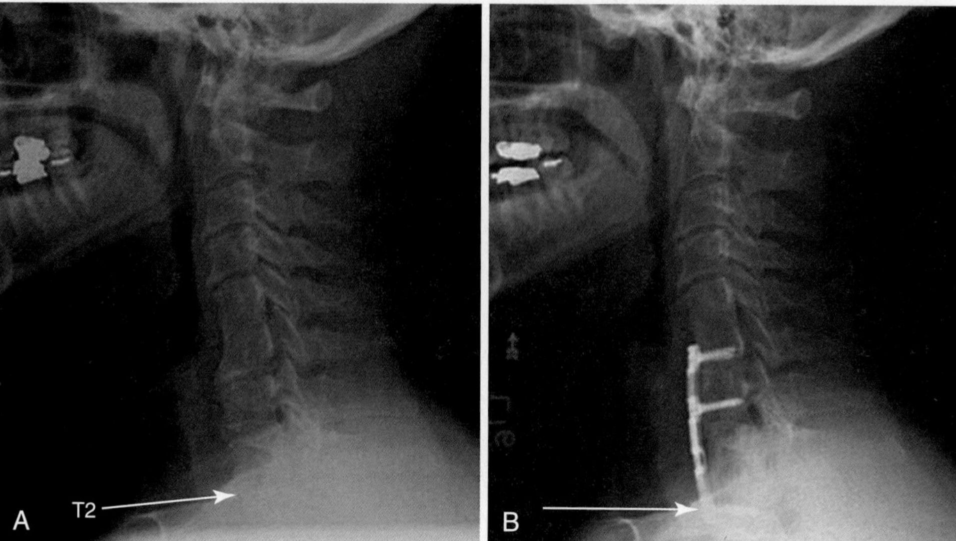

FIGURE 1.16 Criterion of Cho et al. for use of the standard Smith-Robinson approach for upper thoracic anterior fusion. **A,** On a preoperative lateral radiograph, a line drawn from the intended skin incision to the top of the manubrium (at the suprasternal notch) to the level of the disc space (T1-2) indicated that this trajectory would allow adequate exposure of the cervicothoracic junction. **B,** Fusion done through standard Smith-Robinson approach. (From Cho W, Buchowski JM, Park Y, et al: Surgical approach to the cervicothoracic junction. Can a standard Smith-Robinson approach be utilized? *J Spinal Disord Tech* 25:264, 2012.)

superior extent of the dissection. Exposure is limited at the upper thoracic region but generally is adequate for placement of a strut graft if needed. Individual anatomic structure should be considered carefully in preoperative planning. This approach can be used if the lowest instrumented vertebra can be seen on a lateral radiograph and a line passing from the planned skin incision site to this level on the spine lies cephalad to the manubrium (Fig. 1.16).

LOW ANTERIOR CERVICAL APPROACH

TECHNIQUE 1.7

- Enter on the left side by a transverse incision placed one fingerbreadth above the clavicle.
- Extend it well across the midline, taking particular care when dissecting around the carotid sheath in the area of entry of the thoracic duct. The latter approaches the jugular vein from its lateral side, but variations are common.
- Further steps in exposure follow those of the conventional anterior cervical approach.

HIGH TRANSTHORACIC APPROACH

TECHNIQUE 1.8

- A kyphotic deformity of the thoracic spine tends to force the cervical spine into the chest, in which instance a high transthoracic approach is a logical choice.

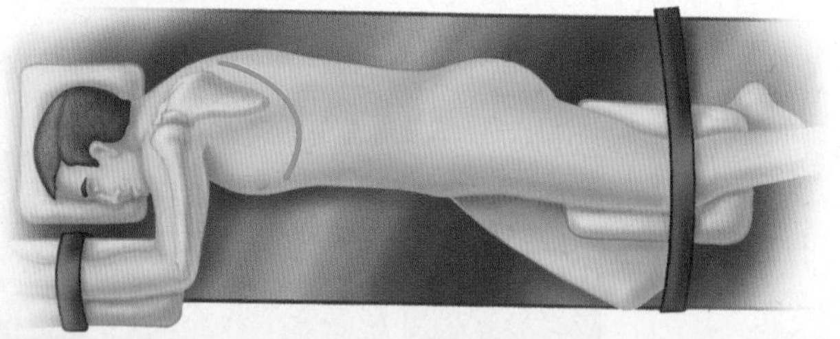

FIGURE 1.17 Patient positioning and periscapular incision for high transthoracic approach. **SEE TECHNIQUE 1.8.**

- Make a periscapular incision (Fig. 1.17) and remove the second or third rib; removing the latter is necessary to provide sufficient working space in a child or if a kyphotic deformity is present. This exposes the interval between C6 and T4. Excision of the first or second rib is adequate in adults or in the absence of an exaggerated kyphosis.

For equal exposure of the thoracic and cervical spine from C4 to T4, the sternal splitting approach is recommended; it is commonly used in cardiac surgery.

TRANSSTERNAL APPROACH

TECHNIQUE 1.9

- Make a Y-shaped or straight incision with the vertical segment passing along the midsternal area from the suprasternal notch to just below the xiphoid process (Fig. 1.18A).

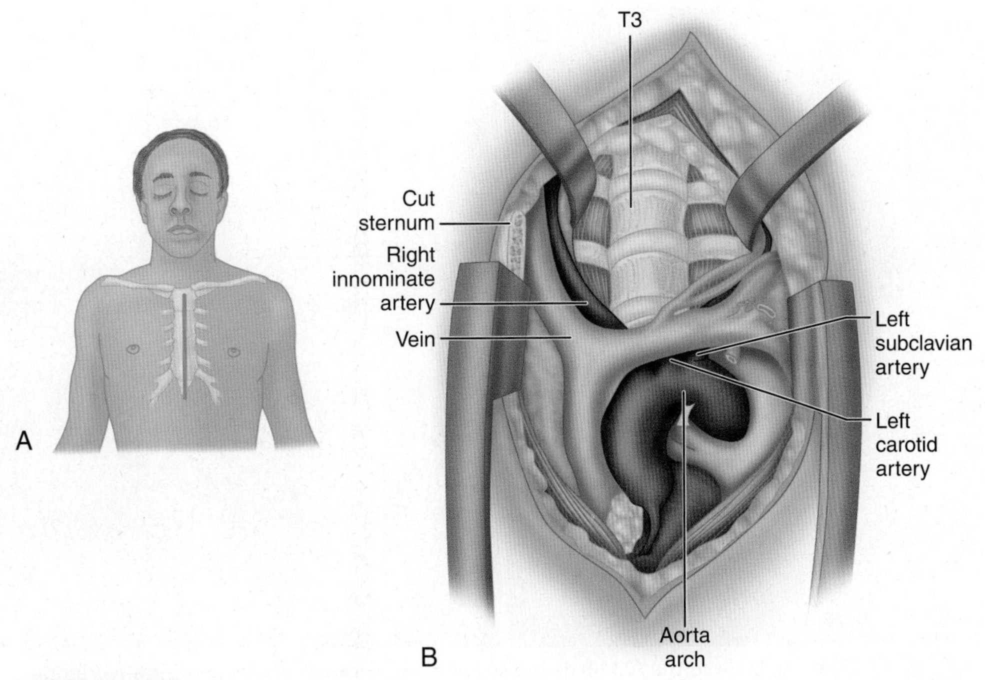

FIGURE 1.18 **Transsternal approach to cervicothoracic spine (see text). A, Incision. B, Approach completed.** (Redrawn from Pierce DS, Nickel VH, editors: *The total care of spinal cord injuries,* Boston, 1977, Little, Brown.) **SEE TECHNIQUE 1.9.**

- Extend the proximal end diagonally to the right and left along the base of the neck for a short distance. To avoid entering the abdominal cavity, take care to keep the dissection beneath the periosteum while exposing the distal end of the sternum. At the proximal end of the sternal notch, avoid the inferior thyroid vein.
- By blunt dissection, reflect the parietal pleura from the posterior surfaces of the sternum and costal cartilages and develop a space. Pass one finger or an instrument above and below the suprasternal space, insert a Gigli saw, and split the sternum. Spread the split sternum and gain access to the center of the chest (Fig. 1.18B). In children, the upper portion of the exposure is posterior to the thymus and bounded by the innominate and carotid arteries and their venous counterparts.
- Develop the left side of this area bluntly.
- In patients with kyphotic deformity, the innominate vein now may be divided as it crosses the field; it may be very tense and subject to rupture. Fang et al. recommended this division. A disadvantage of ligation is that it leaves a slight postoperative enlargement of the left upper extremity that is not apparent unless carefully assessed.
- This approach provides limited access, and its success depends on accuracy in preoperative interpretation of the deformity and a high degree of surgical precision.

MODIFIED ANTERIOR APPROACH TO CERVICOTHORACIC JUNCTION

Several authors have described an anterior approach to the cervical thoracic junction using a combined full median sternotomy and a cervical incision. Others have combined this approach with osteotomy of the clavicle or resection of the left sternoclavicular joint. The approach described by Darling et al. provides excellent exposure from C3 to T4 without the associated morbidity related to the division of the manubrium or the innominate vein. This procedure is technically simple and avoids the risk of injury to the subclavian vessels that can occur with resection of the clavicle or sternoclavicular junction. Mai et al. developed an MRI-based algorithm to evaluate the accessibility of a vertebral disc space with this approach and identified patient factors that may affect accessibility. Caudal disc space accessibility was first evaluated on radiographs: a straight line was drawn through and parallel to the disc space that passes just above the suprasternal notch. The mid-sagittal T2 MRI image was used to identify the most caudal accessible disc space (Fig. 1.19A). If the suprasternal notch could not be adequately identified, the MR scout midline image was used (Fig. 1.19B). In 93% of 180 patients, the algorithm successfully identified the most caudal accessible disc. Age and body mass index were major determinants of accessibility.

TECHNIQUE 1.10

(DARLING ET AL.)

- Place the patient supine. If the neck is stable, place a sandbag transversely behind the shoulders to extend the neck and position the head in a head ring turned to the right. The left side is used to protect the left recurrent laryngeal nerve.
- Make an incision along the anterior border of the left sternocleidomastoid muscle to the sternal notch and continue in the midline to the level of the third costal cartilage.

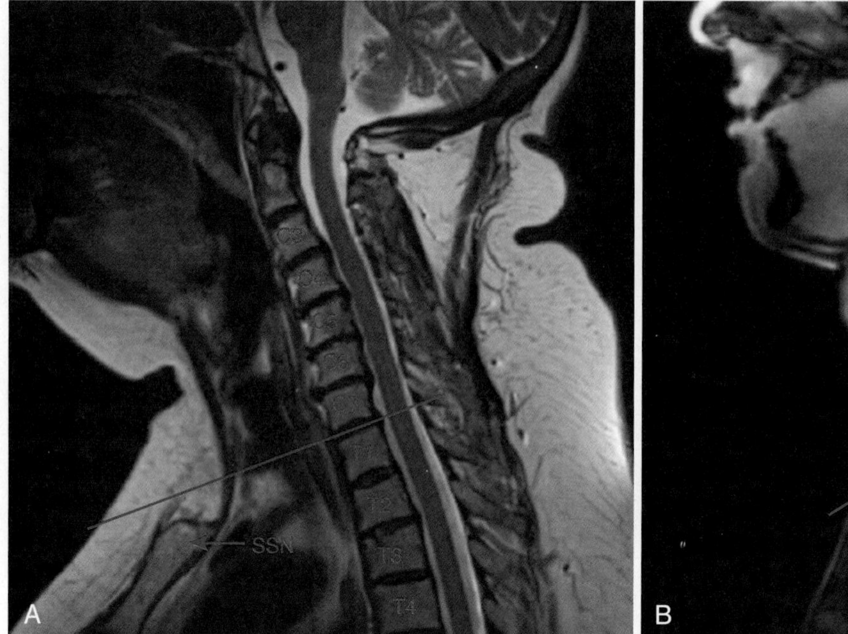

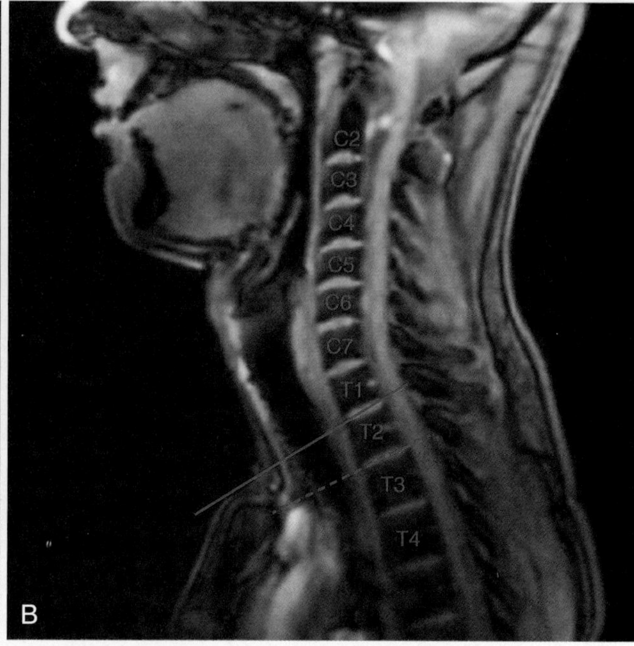

FIGURE 1.19 **A, Mid-sagittal T2 MRI demonstrating a line drawn parallel to the intervertebral space parallel above the most caudal accessible spinal level (C7-T1) as determined by the suprasternal notch (SSN). B, Mid-sagittal SCOUT MRI demonstrating the T1-T2 space as the most caudal accessible level.** (From Mai HT, Mitchell SM, Jenkins TJ, et al: Accessibility of the cervicothoracic junction through an anterior approach. An MRI-based algorithm, *Spine* 41:69, 2016.)

- Divide the platysma in the line of the incision, retract the sternocleidomastoid laterally, and divide the omohyoid muscle.
- Retract the carotid sheath laterally, enter the prevertebral space, and develop a plane of dissection.
- Gently retract the esophagus, trachea, and adjacent recurrent laryngeal nerve to the right and elevate them away from the vertebral column.
- Incise the sternal fascia and divide the sternum in the midline from the sternal notch to the level of the second intercostal space.
- Retract the sternum laterally to the left through the synostosis between the manubrium and body of the sternum.
- Divide the strap muscles near their origin from the sternum to permit reconstruction, connecting the two portions of the incision. Do not divide the sternocleidomastoid muscle.
- Place a small chest retractor and open the partial sternotomy.
- Ligate and divide the inferior thyroid artery and middle and inferior thyroid veins. Take care not to injure the recurrent laryngeal nerve or the superior laryngeal nerve through pressure or traction.
- Dissect the thymus and mediastinal fat away from the left innominate vein.
- If exposure to T3-4 is required, divide the thymic and left innominate veins, if necessary, to expose the level of the aortic arch anteriorly and T4-5 posteriorly (Fig. 1.20). In completing the dissection, avoid injuring the thoracic duct as it ascends to the left of the esophagus from the level of T4 to its junction with the left internal jugular and subclavian veins.
- After spinal decompression and stabilization are completed, close the wound by approximating the manubrium with two or three heavy-gauge stainless steel wires using standard techniques.
- Reattach the strap muscles to the sternum and close the presternal fascia.
- Drain the prevertebral space with a soft Silastic drain through a separate stab wound and attach the drain to closed suction.
- Close the platysma and skin.

ANTERIOR APPROACH TO THE CERVICOTHORACIC JUNCTION WITHOUT STERNOTOMY

Pointillart et al. reported that exposure of the cervicothoracic junction can be achieved with the usual anterior approach without a sternotomy. They noted that exposure of T3 and T4 may require a median manubrial resection.

TECHNIQUE 1.11

(POINTILLART ET AL.)

- Incise the skin along the medial border of the sternocleidomastoid muscle and extend it distally over the manubrium (Fig. 1.21A).
- Begin the dissection as in a standard anterior cervical approach, then extend it caudally by following the vessel-free area anterior to the vertebrae along the deep cervical fascia.

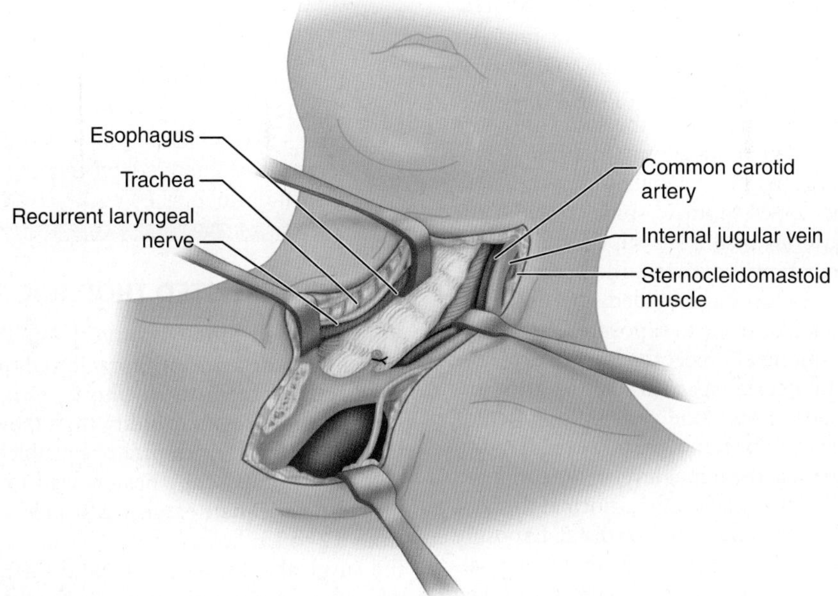

FIGURE 1.20 **Modified anterior approach to cervicothoracic junction.** (Redrawn from Darling GE, McBroom R, Perrin R: Modified anterior approach to the cervicothoracic junction, *Spine* 20:1519, 1995.) **SEE TECHNIQUE 1.10.**

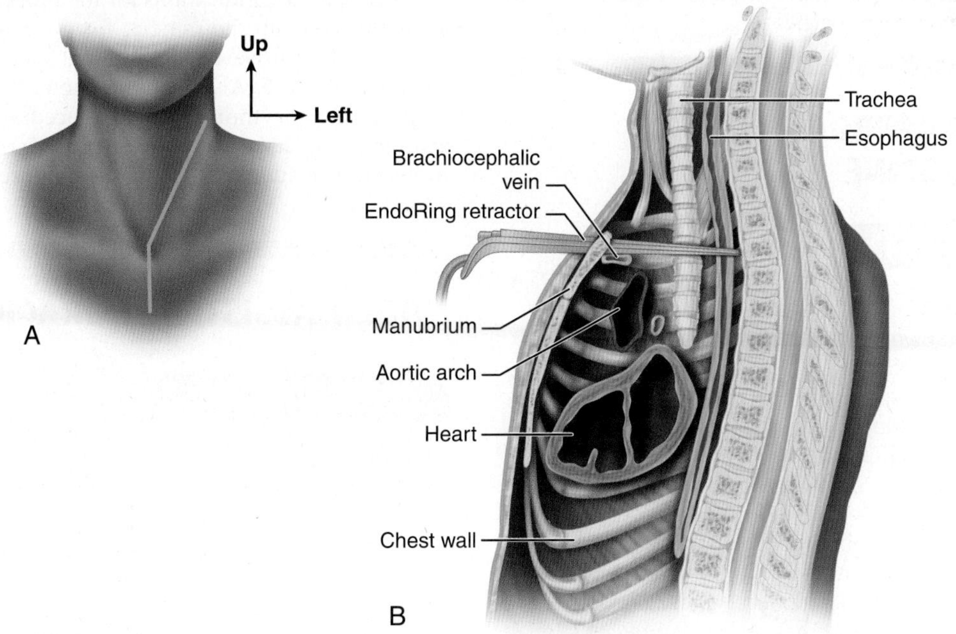

FIGURE 1.21 **Anterior approach to cervicothoracic junction without sternotomy. A, Incision for exposure at cervicothoracic junction. B, Sagittal section of the chest reflecting the thoracic spine exposure possible with upper manubrium resection and retraction.** (Redrawn from Pointillart V, Aurouer N, Gangnet N, Vital JM: Anterior approach to the cervicothoracic junction without sternotomy: a report of 37 cases, *Spine* 32:2875, 2009.) **SEE TECHNIQUE 1.11.**

- Identify and cut the sternal ends of the sternocleidomastoid muscle and infrahyoid muscles 2 cm from their sternal insertions.
- Expose the manubrium to the medial portion of the sternoclavicular joint.
- Use finger dissection to free the posterior aspect of the manubrium for resection.
- With a high-speed drill, resect the manubrium down to the posterior cortex to allow the exposure desired (Fig. 1.21B). Excise the remaining bone with a Kerrison rongeur to complete the exposure.
- Cut the sternoclavicular ligament with scissors.
- Retract the retrosternal fat and large vessels caudally and anteriorly to expose the upper thoracic vertebrae.

ANTERIOR APPROACH TO THE THORACIC SPINE

The transthoracic approach to the thoracic spine provides direct access to the vertebral bodies T2-12. The midthoracic vertebral bodies are best exposed by this approach, whereas views of the upper and lower extremes of the spine are more limited. In general, a left-sided thoracotomy incision is preferred, although some surgeons favor a right-sided thoracotomy for approaching the upper thoracic spine to avoid the subclavian and carotid arteries in the left superior mediastinum. In a left-sided thoracotomy approach, the heart may be retracted anteriorly, whereas in a right-sided approach, the liver may present a significant obstacle to exposure. The level of the incision should be positioned to meet the level of exposure required. Ordinarily, an intercostal space is selected at or just above the involved segment. If only one vertebral segment is involved, the rib at that level can be removed; however, if multiple levels are involved, the rib at the upper level of the proposed dissection should be removed. Because of the normal thoracic kyphosis, dissection is easier from proximal to distal. Exposure is improved by resection of a rib, and the rib provides a satisfactory bone graft, but resection is unnecessary if a limited exposure is adequate for biopsy, decompression, or fusion. The transthoracic approach adds a significant operative risk and is more hazardous than the more commonly used posterior or posterolateral approaches. The increased risk of thoracotomy must be weighed against the more limited exposure provided by alternative posterior approaches.

ANTERIOR APPROACH TO THE THORACIC SPINE

TECHNIQUE 1.12

- Place the patient in the lateral decubitus position with the right side down; an inflatable beanbag is helpful in maintaining the patient's position, and the table can be flexed to increase exposure (Fig. 1.22A).
- Make an incision over the rib corresponding to the involved vertebra and expose it subperiosteally. Use electrocautery to maintain hemostasis during the exposure.
- Disarticulate the rib from the transverse process and the hemifacets of the vertebral body. Identify and preserve the intercostal nerve lying along the inferior aspect of the rib as it localizes the neural foramen leading into the spinal canal. Incise the parietal pleura and reflect it off of the spine, usually one vertebra above and one below the involved segment, to allow adequate exposure for debridement and grafting (Fig. 1.22B).
- Identify the segmental vessels that cross the midportion of each vertebral body and ligate and divide these (Fig. 1.22C).
- Carefully reflect the periosteum overlying the spine with elevators to expose the involved vertebrae.
- Use a small elevator to delineate the pedicle of the vertebra and a Kerrison rongeur to remove the pedicle, exposing the dural sac.
- Identify the disc spaces above and below the vertebrae and incise the annulus. Remove disc material using rongeurs and curets.
- An entire cross-section of the vertebral body is developed, and the anterior margin of the neural canal is identified with the posterior longitudinal ligament lying in the slight concavity on the back of the vertebral body.
- Expose sufficient segmental vessels and disc spaces to accomplish the intended procedure—usually corpectomy and strut grafting.

VIDEO-ASSISTED THORACIC SURGERY

Video-assisted thoracic surgery (VATS) has been used successfully in the anterior thoracic and thoracolumbar spine for treatment of scoliosis, kyphosis, tumors, and fractures and seems to have less morbidity than the standard thoracotomy, which can result in respiratory problems or pain after thoracotomy. Thoracoscopy has evolved rapidly and is capable of providing adequate exposure to all levels of the thoracic spine from T2 to L1; however, the learning curve is significant, and the surgical team always should include a thoracic surgeon who is competent in thoracoscopy and a spine surgeon who is well trained in endoscopic techniques.

Reported complications include intercostal neuralgia, atelectasis, excessive epidural blood loss (2500 mL), and temporary paraparesis related to operative positioning.

Although the indications for the thoracoscopic approach apparently remain the same as for open thoracotomy, some procedures require extensive internal fixation and may not be suitable for VATS. Also, patients should be informed before surgery that the thoracoscopic procedure may have to be abandoned in favor of an open procedure. Relative contraindications include preexisting pleural disease from previous surgeries.

VIDEO-ASSISTED THORACIC SURGERY

TECHNIQUE 1.13

(MACK ET AL.)

- Routine intraoperative monitoring for thoracic procedures is used, including an arterial pressure line, pulse oximeter, and end-tidal carbon dioxide measurement. Somatosensory evoked potentials should be monitored routinely for patients undergoing spinal deformity correction or corpectomy.
- Place the initial trocar in the seventh intercostal space in the posterior axillary line. Place a 10-mm, 30-degree angled rigid telescope through the 10-mm trocar. Use a 0-degree end-viewing scope and a 30-degree scope for direct vision of the intervertebral disc space to avoid impeding surgical instrumentation or obscuring the operative field. Mack et al. recommended placing the viewing port in the posterior axillary line directly over the spine and two or three access sites for working ports in the anterior axillary line to allow better access to the spine. This "reverse L" arrangement can be moved cephalad or caudad, depending on the level of the thoracic spine to be approached.
- Use the portals for placement of surgical instruments (Fig. 1.23).

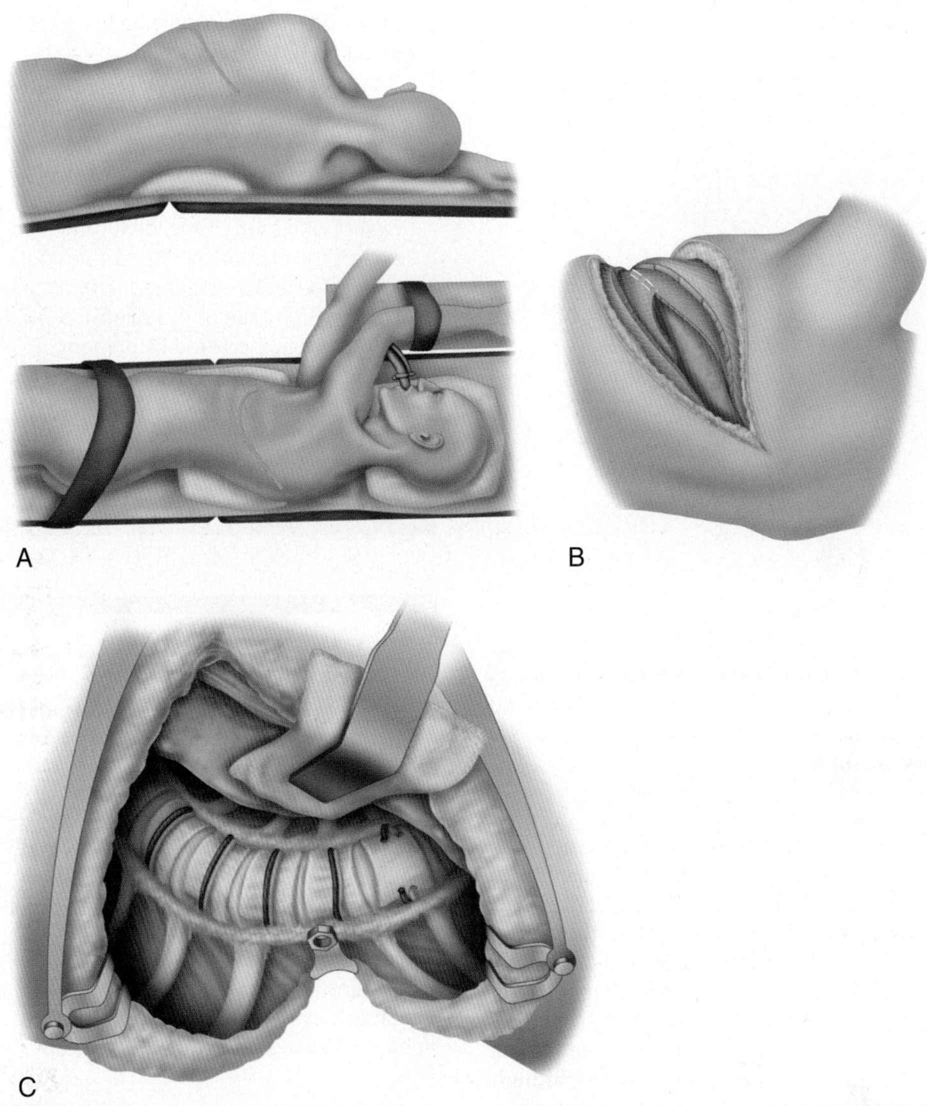

FIGURE 1.22 Transthoracic approach (see text). **A,** Positioning of patient and incision. **B,** Rib removal and division of pleura, exposing lung. **C,** Exposure of spine and division of segmental vessels over one vertebral body **SEE TECHNIQUE 1.12.**

- Rotate the patient anteriorly and place the patient in a Trendelenburg position for the lower thoracic spine or reverse Trendelenburg for the upper thoracic spine.
- The lung usually falls away from the operative field when completely collapsed, obviating the need for retraction instruments.
- A departure from the standard VATS approach is the positioning of the operative team. Operative procedures routinely are performed by a spine surgeon and thoracic surgeon. In contrast to other VATS procedures in which the surgeon and assistant are positioned on opposite sides of the operating table, both surgeons are positioned on the anterior side of the patient viewing a monitor on the opposite side. In addition, the camera and the viewing field are rotated 90 degrees from the standard VATS approach so that the spine is viewed horizontally.
- Perform an initial exploratory thoracoscopy to determine the correct spinal level for operative intervention.
- Count the ribs by "palpation" with a blunt grasping instrument.
- When the target level has been defined, place a 20-gauge long needle percutaneously into the disc space from the lateral aspect and confirm radiographically.
- When the correct level is ascertained, perform the specific spinal procedure.

ANTERIOR APPROACH TO THE THORACOLUMBAR JUNCTION

Occasionally, it may be necessary to expose simultaneously the lower thoracic and upper lumbar vertebral bodies. Technically, this is a more difficult exposure because of the diaphragm and the increased risk involved in simultaneous exposure of the thoracic cavity and the retroperitoneal space. In most instances, thoracic lesions should be exposed through the chest, whereas lesions predominantly involving the upper lumbar spine can

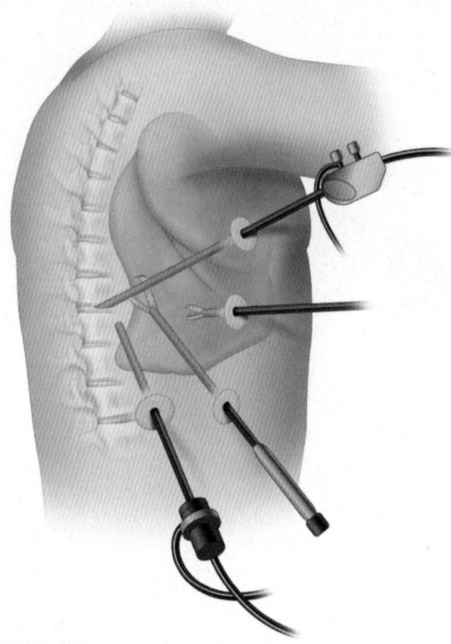

FIGURE 1.23 Thoracoscopic instrument placement for thoracic spine procedures. (Redrawn from Regan JJ, McAfee PC, Mack MJ, editors: *Atlas of endoscopic spine surgery*, St. Louis, 1995, Quality Medical Publishing.) **SEE TECHNIQUE 1.13.**

be exposed through an anterior retroperitoneal incision. The diaphragm is a dome-shaped organ that is muscular in the periphery and tendinous in the center. Posteriorly, it originates from the upper lumbar vertebrae through crura, the arcuate ligaments, and the 12th ribs. Anteriorly and laterally, it attaches to the cartilaginous ends of the lower six ribs and xiphoid. The diaphragm is innervated by the phrenic nerve, which descends through the thoracic cavity on the pericardium. The phrenic nerve joins the diaphragm adjacent to the fibrous pericardium, dividing into three major branches that extend peripherally in anterolateral and posterior directions. Division of these major branches may interfere with diaphragmatic function. It is best to make an incision around the periphery of the diaphragm to minimize interference with function when making a thoracoabdominal approach to the spine. We recommend a left-sided approach at the thoracolumbar junction because the vena cava on the right is less tolerant of dissection and may result in troublesome hemorrhage, and the liver may be hard to retract.

ANTERIOR APPROACH TO THE THORACOLUMBAR JUNCTION

TECHNIQUE 1.14

- Place the patient in the right lateral decubitus position and place supports beneath the buttock and shoulder.
- Make the incision curvilinear with ability to extend the cephalad or the caudal end (Fig. 1.24A).
- To gain the best access to the interval of T12-L1, resect the 10th rib, which allows exposure between T10 and L2. The only difficulty is in identifying the diaphragm as a separate structure; it tends to approximate closely the wall of the thoracic cage, allowing the edge of the lung to penetrate into the space beneath the knife as the pleura is divided (Fig. 1.24B).
- Take care in entering the abdominal cavity. Because the transversalis fascia and the peritoneum do not diverge, dissect with caution and identify the two cavities on either side of the diaphragm. To achieve confluence of the two cavities, reflect the diaphragm from the lower ribs and the crus from the side of the spine (Fig. 1.24C).
- Alternatively, incise the diaphragm 2.5 cm away from its insertion and tag it with sutures for later accurate closure.
- Incise the prevertebral fascia.
- Identify the segmental arteries and veins over the midportion of each vertebral body. Isolate these, ligate them in the midline, and expose the bone as previously described.

MINIMALLY INVASIVE APPROACH TO THE THORACOLUMBAR JUNCTION

Although a variant of the lateral retropleural thoracotomy, the minimally invasive lateral extracelomic (retroperitoneal/retropleural) approach can provide adequate exposure of the thoracolumbar junction to allow vertebrectomy and canal decompression from T10 to L2 without the need to enter the pleural or peritoneal cavities and avoid the morbidities associated with retropleural thoracotomy. It combines the positive attributes of both the anterolateral transthoracic approach and the lateral extra-cavitary approach and is particularly useful for centrally located pathologies such as central thoracic disc herniation.

TECHNIQUE 1.15

- With the patient in a lateral decubitus position and under fluoroscopic guidance, make a 6-cm oblique incision (following the trajectory of the rib at the index level) at the midaxillary line.
- The side of the approach is chosen according to the vertebral level and the location of the abnormality, but the left-sided approach is preferred to avoid retraction of the liver and vena cava on the right.
- Dissect subperiosteally approximately 5 cm of the rib immediately overlying the target level from the underlying pleura and neurovascular bundle and remove it. Set aside the portion of resected rib for use as autograft.
- Once the parietal pleura is exposed, develop the plane between the endothoracic fascia and the pleura, taking care not to enter the pleural or peritoneal cavities (Fig. 1.25A).
- Use a sponge stick or finger dissection to bluntly mobilize the pleura anteriorly along with the diaphragm until the lateral side of the vertebral body and adjacent discs are exposed.
- If the target levels include L1, divide the medial and lateral arcuate ligaments off the costal and lumbar attachments

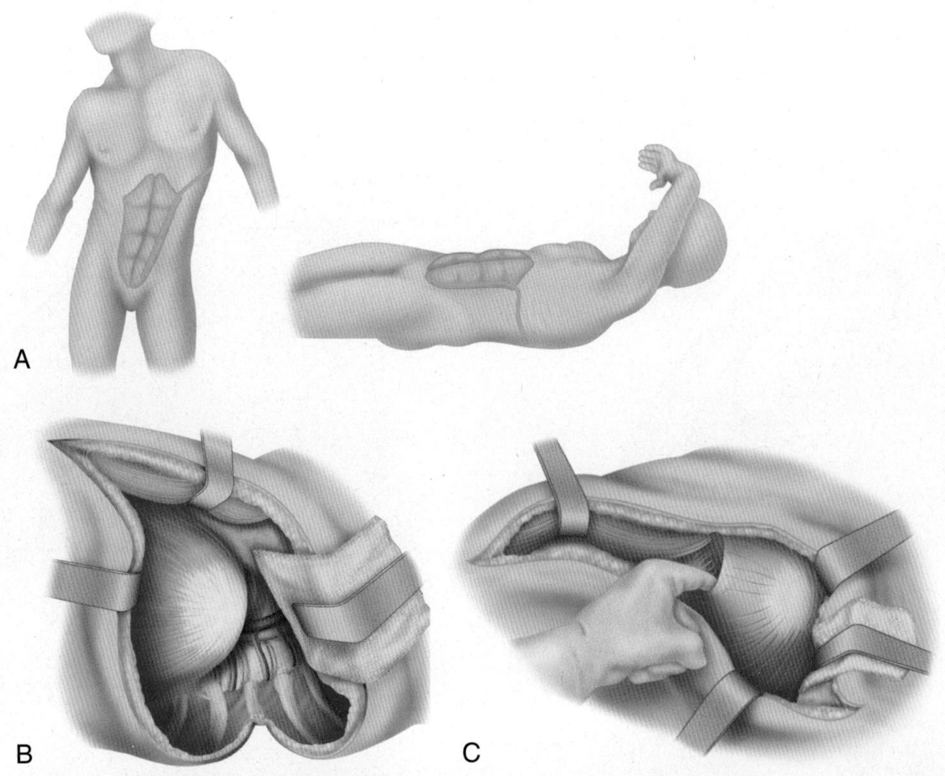

FIGURE 1.24 Thoracolumbar approach (see text). **A,** Skin incision. **B,** Transthoracic detachment of diaphragm. **C,** Retroperitoneal detachment of diaphragm. **SEE TECHNIQUE 1.14.**

to adequately mobilize the diaphragm. If more anterior access or exposure of L2 is needed, fully transect the crus of the diaphragm connecting the retropleural and retroperitoneal spaces.

- Retract the aorta and hemiazygos vein anteriorly. Insert sequential tubular dilators and place a tube retractor system over the largest dilator and secure it with a flexible table-mounted arm assembly (Fig. 1.25B).
- Under magnification, remove the rib head and the costovertebral ligaments at the corresponding level and complete the desired procedure with direct observation of the dura laterally and ventrally.
- If the pleural cavity is not violated, there is no need for a chest tube, and postoperative mobilization can begin immediately.

ANTERIOR RETROPERITONEAL APPROACH, L1 TO L5

The anterior retroperitoneal approach to the lumbar vertebral bodies is a modification of the anterolateral approach commonly used by general surgeons for sympathectomy. It is an excellent approach that should be considered for extensive resection, debridement, or grafting at multiple levels in the lumbar spine. Depending on which portion of the lumbar spine is to be approached, the incision may be varied in placement between the 12th rib and the superior aspect of the iliac crest. The major dissection in this approach is behind the kidney in the potential space between the renal fascia and the quadratus lumborum and psoas muscles.

ANTERIOR RETROPERITONEAL APPROACH, L1 TO L5

TECHNIQUE 1.16

- Position the patient in the lateral decubitus position, generally with the right side down. The approach is made most often from the left side to avoid the liver and the inferior vena cava, which is more difficult to repair than the aorta if vascular injury occurs during the approach to the spine.
- Flex the table to increase exposure between the 12th rib and the iliac crest. Flex the hips slightly to release tension on the psoas muscle.
- Make an oblique incision over the 12th rib from the lateral border of the quadratus lumborum to the lateral border of the rectus abdominis muscle to allow exposure of the first and second lumbar vertebrae (Fig. 1.26A).
- Alternatively, place the incision several fingerbreadths below and parallel to the costal margin when exposure of the lower lumbar vertebrae (L3-5) is necessary.
- Use electrocautery to divide the subcutaneous tissue, fascia, and muscle of the external oblique, internal oblique, transversus abdominis, and transversalis fascia in line with the skin incision (Fig. 1.26B and C).
- Carefully protect the peritoneum and reflect it anteriorly by blunt dissection. If the peritoneum is entered during the approach, it must be repaired.

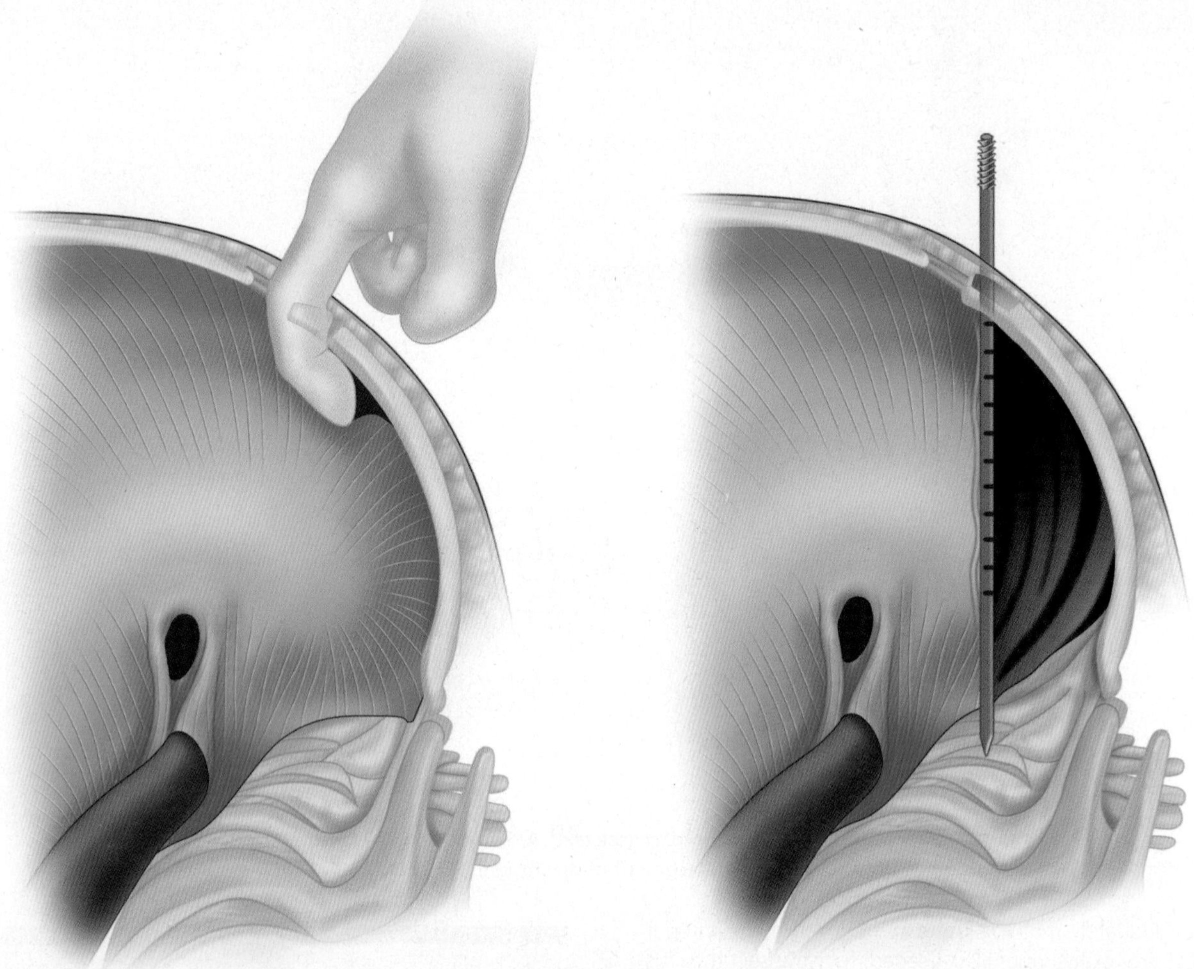

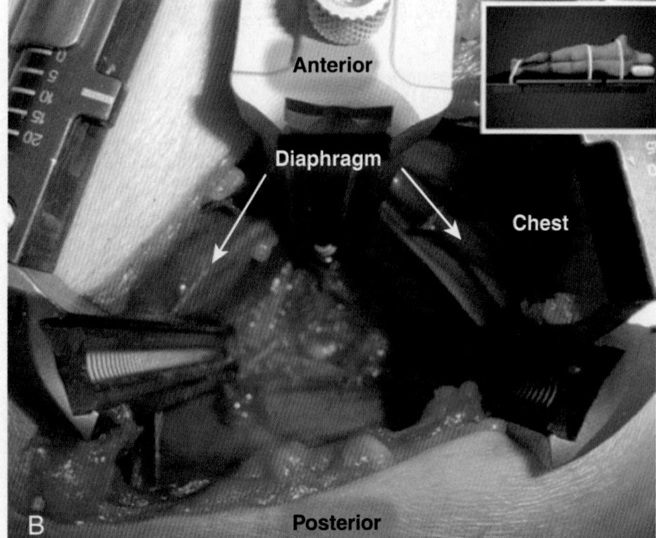

FIGURE 1.25 Minimally invasive lateral extracelomic approach. **A,** Diaphragm looking from caudal to cranial demonstrating blunt dissection with the aid of a finger to develop the extracelomic space *(left)*. The diaphragm is retracted anteriorly once the costal and lumbar attachments have been mobilized *(right)*. **B,** Cadaver specimen in the right lateral decubitus position *(inset)* demonstrating the view through the tubular retractor when placed in the extracelomic space. (A from NuVasive, Inc. B from Dakwar E, Ahmadian A, Uribe JS: The anatomical relationship of the diaphragm to the thoracolumbar junction during minimally invasive lateral extracelomic (retropleural/retroperitoneal) approach. Laboratory investigation, *J Neurosurg Spine* 16:359, 2012.) **SEE TECHNIQUE 1.15.**

- Identify the psoas muscle in the retroperitoneal space and allow the ureter to fall anteriorly with the retroperitoneal fat.
- The sympathetic chain is found between the vertebral bodies and the psoas muscle laterally, whereas the genitofemoral nerve lies on the anterior aspect of the psoas muscle.
- Place a Finochietto rib retractor between the costal margin and the iliac crest to aid exposure.
- Palpate the vertebral bodies from T12 to L5 and identify and protect with a Deaver retractor the great vessels lying anterior to the spine. The lumbar segmental vessels lie in the midportion of the vertebral bodies, and the relatively avascular discs are prominent on each adjacent side of the vessels (Fig. 1.26D).
- When the appropriate involved vertebra is identified, elevate the psoas muscle bluntly off the lumbar vertebrae and retract it laterally to the level of the transverse process with a Richardson retractor. Sometimes, removal of the transverse process with a rongeur is helpful in allowing adequate retraction of the psoas muscle.
- Ligate and divide the lumbar segmental vessel overlying the involved vertebra.
- Delineate the pedicle of the involved vertebra with a small elevator and locate the neural foramen with the exiting nerve root. Bipolar coagulation of vessels around the neural foramen is recommended.
- Remove the pedicle with an angled Kerrison rongeur and expose the dura.
- After completion of the spinal procedure, obtain meticulous hemostasis and close the wound in layers over a drain in the retroperitoneal space.

PERCUTANEOUS LATERAL APPROACH TO LUMBAR SPINE, L1 TO L4-5 (DLIF OR XLIF)

Ozgur et al. first described the technique of extreme lateral interbody fusion (XLIF) as a refinement of the laparoscopic lateral approach. The primary use for this approach has been the placement of an anterior lumbar interbody graft for degenerative disc disease without central canal stenosis, scoliosis, or spondylolisthesis. Park et al. analyzed the distance from a

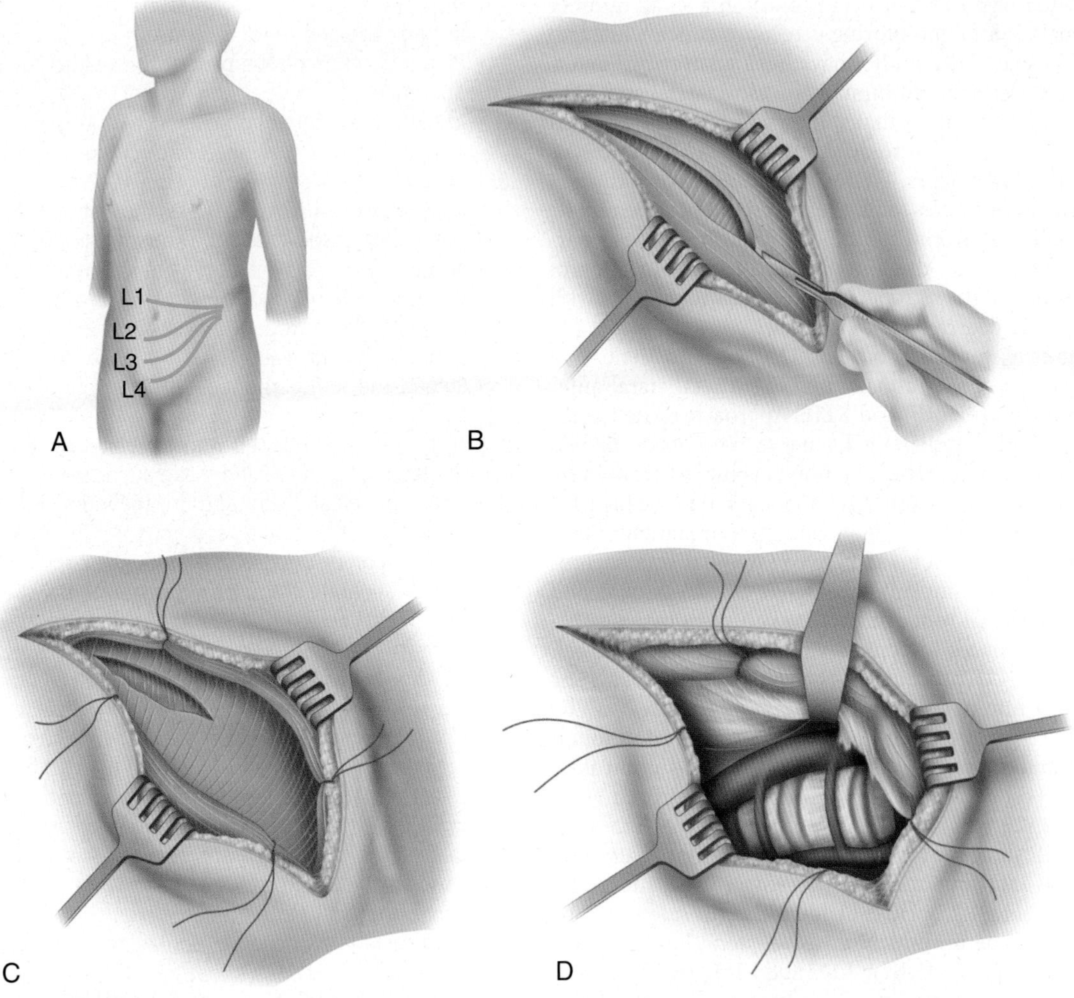

FIGURE 1.26 Anterior retroperitoneal approach (see text). **A,** Skin incisions for lumbar vertebrae. **B,** Incision of fibers of external oblique muscle. **C,** Incision into fibers of internal oblique muscle. **D,** Exposure of spine before ligation of segmental vessels **SEE TECHNIQUE 1.16.**

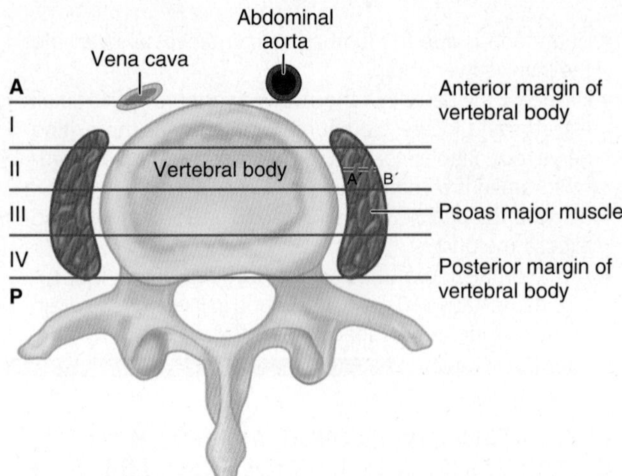

FIGURE 1.27 **Zones of the lumbar vertebral body.** (Redrawn from Hu WK, He SS, Zhang SC, et al: An MRI study of psoas major and abdominal large vessels with respect to the X/DLIF approach, *Eur Spine J* 20:557–562, 2011.)

guidewire placed in 10 human cadavers using the usual lateral approach and concluded that the intrapsoas nerves are a safe distance from the radiographic center of the disc in most cases. Because of the risk of nerve injury in a small number of individuals, neural monitoring is recommended while traversing the psoas. MRI studies have been analyzed to determine the safe zones for a minimally invasive lateral approach in both normal and abnormal spines. Most levels evaluated (247) were normal, 18 were degenerative, and 19 were scoliotic. On the MR images, the overlap between the adjacent neurovascular structures and the vertebral body endplate gradually increased from L1-2 to L4-5, resulting in a very narrow safe zone at L4-5. Alteration in the anatomic location of the nerve root and the retroperitoneal vessels in patients with scoliosis further decreases this safe zone.

Knight et al. reported that 13 (22%) of 58 patients had complications after a minimally invasive direct lateral anterior lumbar fusion (DLIF) and XLIF. Approach-related complications included ipsilateral L4 nerve root injury in two patients, irritation of the lateral femoral cutaneous nerve in six patients, significant psoas spasm that lengthened the hospital stay in one patient, and less significant psoas irritation in five. Major complications occurred in five (8.6%) patients, including reoperation for implant subsidence in one patient and persistence of the L4 root injury at 1 year in two patients. No significant differences in complications were noted between the XLIF and DLIF procedures. Nayar et al. compared 1292 patients with minimally invasive lateral approaches to 768 patients with standard open posterior approaches and found that the lateral approach was associated with a significantly lower rate of reoperation than the posterior approach at 30 days and at 2 years.

Using MR images of the lumbar spine with the vertebral body divided into four zones, each being 25% of the vertebral diameter (Fig. 1.27), Hu et al. identified the safe zones for approach using the minimally invasive lateral lumbar interbody fusion to be zones II-III at L1-2 and L2-3, zone II at L3-4, and zones I-II on the left at L4-5, and zone II on the right at L4-5 (Fig. 1.28A and B). Benglis et al. evaluated the position of the lumbar plexus in the psoas muscle of three fresh frozen human cadavers and noted that the lumbar plexus rests on the dorsal surface of the psoas muscle in a cleft created by the transverse process/vertebral body junction. The plexus progressed in a dorsal fashion from near the posterior aspect of the vertebral body at L1-2 to 0.28 of the vertebral diameter at L4-5 (Fig. 1.29). The plexus was at the greatest risk of injury at the L4-5 level.

PERCUTANEOUS LATERAL APPROACH, L1 TO L4-5

TECHNIQUE 1.17

(OZGUR ET AL.)

- After the induction of a general endotracheal anesthesia, place the patient in a right lateral decubitus position on a radiolucent operating table.
- Adjust the patient so a true 90-degree lateral image can be obtained with image intensification.
- Secure the patient in this position with taping and a bean bag or similar device.
- Adjust the table to allow maximal distance between the left rib cage and the iliac crest.
- Prepare and drape the patient for a direct lateral lumbar approach.
- Identify the midlateral position of the disc space to be entered using a Kirschner wire marker and fluoroscopic imaging (Fig. 1.30). Mark this point on the skin.
- Make a second mark posterior to the first mark at the border of the erector spinae and the abdominal oblique muscles.
- Make a 2-cm skin incision at this second mark and use blunt dissection with the index finger through the muscle layers to the retroperitoneal space; avoid entering the peritoneum (Fig. 1.31A).
- Sweep the retroperitoneal space anteriorly and palpate the psoas muscle (Fig. 1.31B).
- Turn the index finger up in a direct lateral position toward the lateral skin mark and make an incision at this mark.
- Insert the initial dilator and use the index finger to safely direct the dilator to the psoas muscle (Fig. 1.31C); confirm the position of the dilator with fluoroscopy.
- Gently separate the psoas with the initial dilator, using blunt dissection at the level determined to be in the safe zone for the level to be accessed.
- Monitor the progress of the dilator in the psoas muscle using electromyography. The stimulus necessary to elicit an electromyography response will vary with the distance from the nerve. Threshold values of more than 10 mA indicate a distance that is safe for the nerves and adequate for working.
- Take care to minimize trauma to the psoas muscle.
- Observe the progress of the dilator directly to check for nerves that may lie in the safe zone.
- Continue the dissection by spreading the midpsoas fibers laterally (Fig. 1.31D).
- Avoid the genitofemoral nerve by observing it directly until the disc is reached.
- Reconfirm placement of the initial dilator with fluoroscopy.

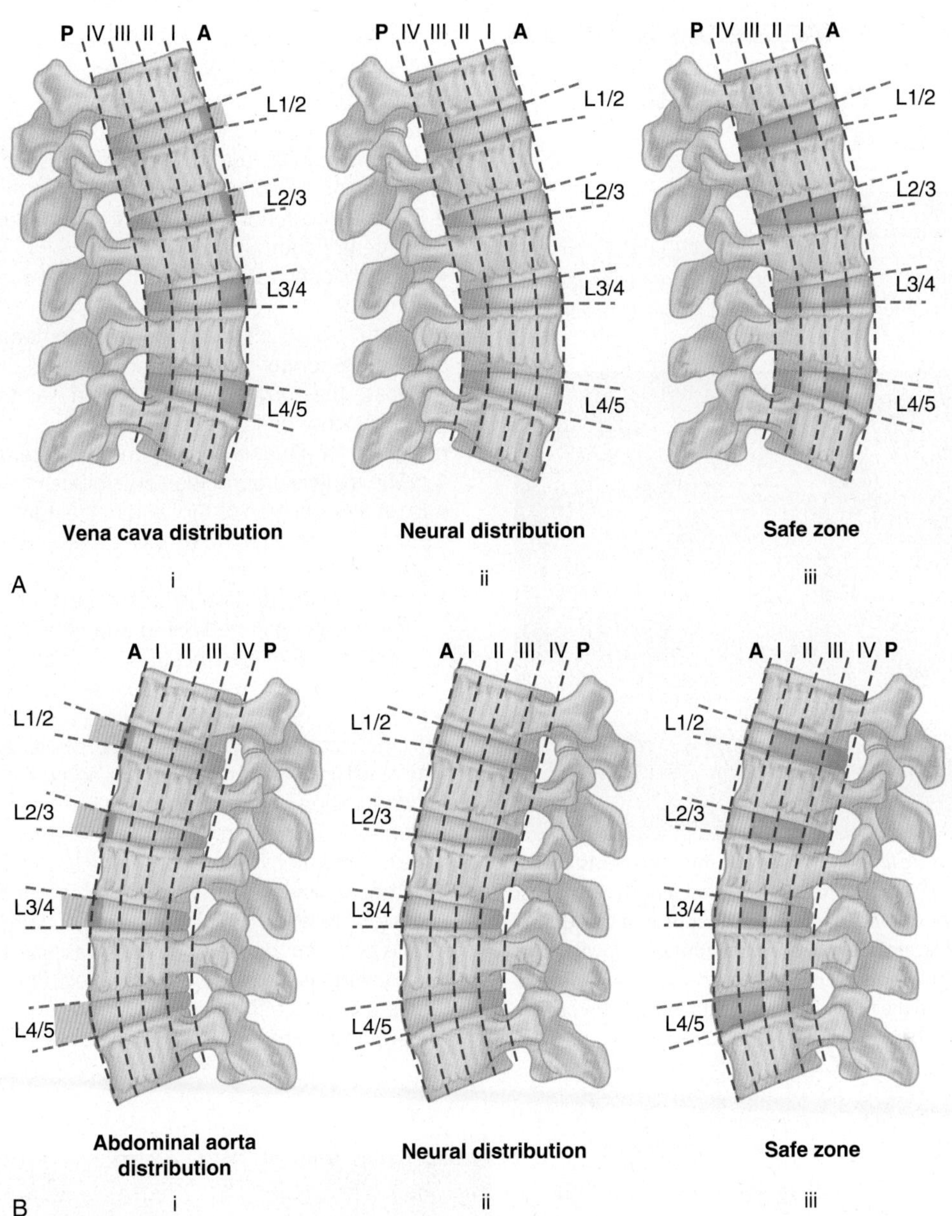

FIGURE 1.28 **A,** Right-sided XLIF approach as related to anatomic structure: *i,* vena cava distribution; *ii,* neural distribution; *iii,* safe zone. **B,** Left-sided extreme lateral interbody fusion (XLIF) approach associated with anatomic structures: *i,* distribution of abdominal aorta; *ii,* neural distribution; *iii,* safe zone. (From Hu WK, He SS, Zhang SC, et al: An MRI study of psoas major and abdominal large vessels with respect to the X/DLIF approach, *Eur Spine J* 20:557–562, 2011.)

- Introduce subsequent dilators until the retractor can be inserted (Fig. 1.32). (This instrument varies with the system used.) Expand the retractor blades to minimize nerve pressure and maximize disc exposure.
- Confirm the final position with anteroposterior and lateral fluoroscopy before excising the disc.

ANTERIOR TRANSPERITONEAL APPROACH TO THE LUMBOSACRAL JUNCTION, L5 TO S1

Transperitoneal exposure of the lumbar spine is an alternative to the retroperitoneal approach. The advantage of the transperitoneal route is a more extensive exposure, especially at the L5-S1 level. A disadvantage is that the great vessels and hypogastric nerve plexus must be mobilized before the spine is exposed. The superior hypogastric plexus contains the sympathetic function for the urogenital systems, and damage of this structure in men can cause complications such as retrograde ejaculation; however, damage to the superior hypogastric plexus should not produce impotence or failure of erection. Injury to the hypogastric plexus can be avoided by careful opening of the posterior peritoneum and blunt dissection of the prevertebral tissue from left to right and by opening the posterior peritoneum higher over the bifurcation of the aorta and extending the opening down over the sacral promontory. In addition, electrocautery should be kept to a minimum when dissecting within the aortic bifurcation, and until the annulus of the L5-S1 disc is clearly exposed, no transverse scalpel cuts on the front of the disc should be made.

ANTERIOR TRANSPERITONEAL APPROACH, L5 TO S1

TECHNIQUE 1.18

- Position the patient supine on the operating table and make a vertical midline or a transverse incision (Fig. 1.33A).

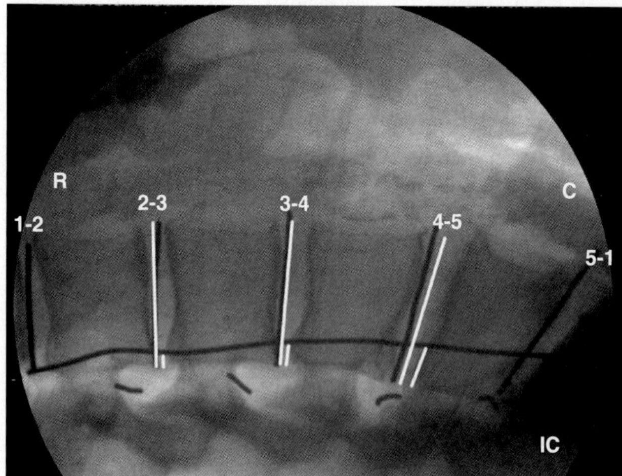

FIGURE 1.29 *White lines* show the ratio measurements: plexus to posterior endplate *(short white line)* to total length of the disc *(long white line)*. *Longitudinal dark line* is the course of the lumbar plexus as seen in the lateral view of a frozen human cadaver spine. (From Benglis DM Jr, Vanni S, Levi AD: An anatomical study of the lumbosacral plexus as related to the minimally invasive transpsoas approach to the lumbar spine, *J Neurosurg Spine* 10:139, 2009.)

The transverse incision is cosmetically superior and gives excellent exposure; it requires transection of the rectus abdominis sheath.

- Identify and open the sheath and transect the rectus abdominis muscle. The posterior rectus sheath, abdominal fascia, and peritoneum are conjoined in this area.
- Open the posterior rectus sheath and abdominal fascia to the peritoneum.
- Carefully open the peritoneum to avoid damage to bowel content.
- Carefully pack off the abdominal contents and identify the posterior peritoneum over the sacral promontory.
- Palpate the aorta and the common iliac vessels through the posterior peritoneum.
- Make a longitudinal incision in the posterior peritoneum in the midline around the aortic bifurcation.
- Extend the incision distally and to the right along the right common iliac artery to its bifurcation at the external and internal iliac arteries.
- Identify the right ureter, crossing the right iliac artery, and curve the incision medially to avoid this structure.
- Avoid the use of electrocautery anterior to the L5-S1 disc space to prevent damage to the superior hypogastric plexus.
- The left common iliac vein often lies as a flat structure across the L5-S1 disc within the aortic bifurcation. After identification of the left common iliac artery and vein, use blunt dissection to the right of the artery and hypogastric plexus and mobilize the soft tissue from left to right.
- Carefully dissect the middle sacral artery and vein from left to right (Fig. 1.33B). Longitudinal blunt dissection allows better mobilization of these vascular structures.
- If bleeding is encountered, use direct finger and sponge pressure rather than electrocautery. If electrocautery is used in this area, we recommend the bipolar rather than

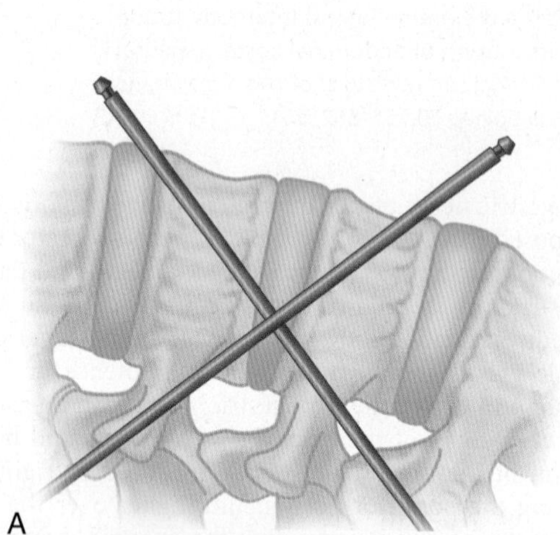

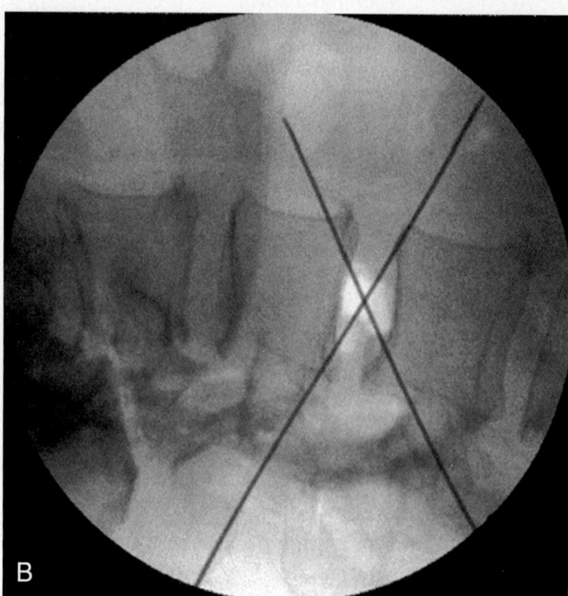

FIGURE 1.30 Percutaneous lateral approach to L1 to L4-5. **A,** Patient positioning and placement of Kirschner wires. **B,** Fluoroscopic image showing wire placement. (Redrawn from Ozgur BM, Aryan JE, Pimenta L, Taylor WR: Extreme lateral interbody fusion (XLIF): a novel surgical technique for anterior lumbar interbody fusion, *Spine J* 6:435, 2006.) **SEE TECHNIQUE 1.17.**

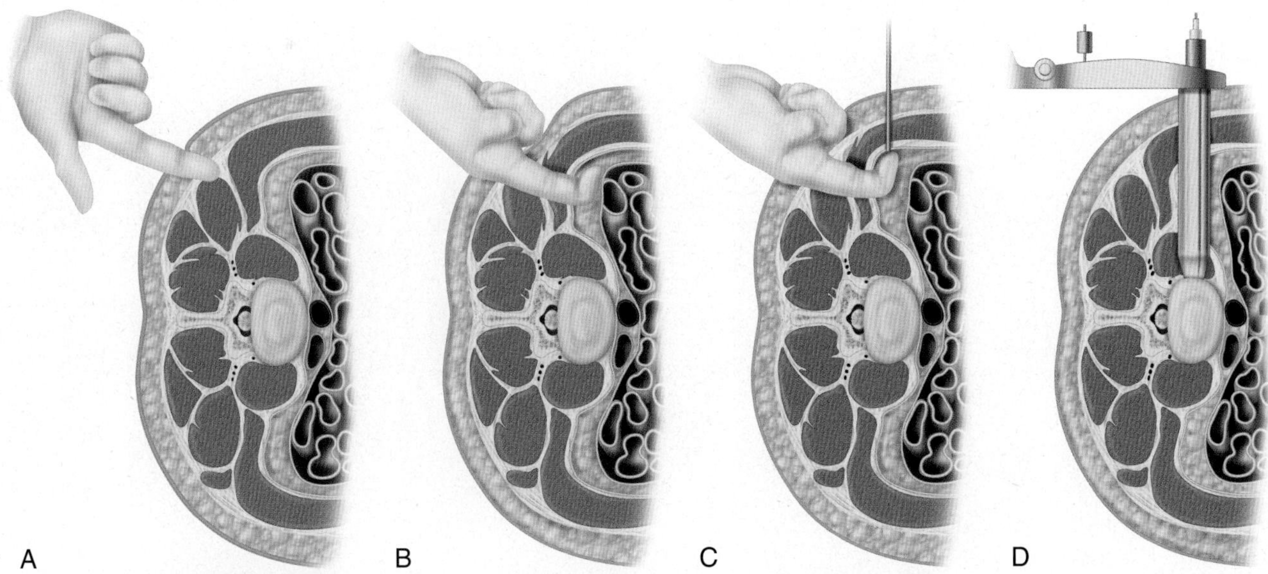

FIGURE 1.31 Percutaneous lateral approach to L1 to L4-5. **A,** Surgeon's index finger inserted into paraspinal incision site. **B,** Identification of retroperitoneal space. **C,** Guidance of the initial dilator into position. **D,** Retractor inserted into retroperitoneal space, penetrating the psoas major, positioned directly on the lateral intervertebral disc space. (Redrawn from Ozgur BM, Aryan JE, Pimenta L, Taylor WR: Extreme lateral interbody fusion (XLIF): a novel surgical technique for anterior lumbar interbody fusion, *Spine J* 6:435, 2006.) **SEE TECHNIQUE 1.17.**

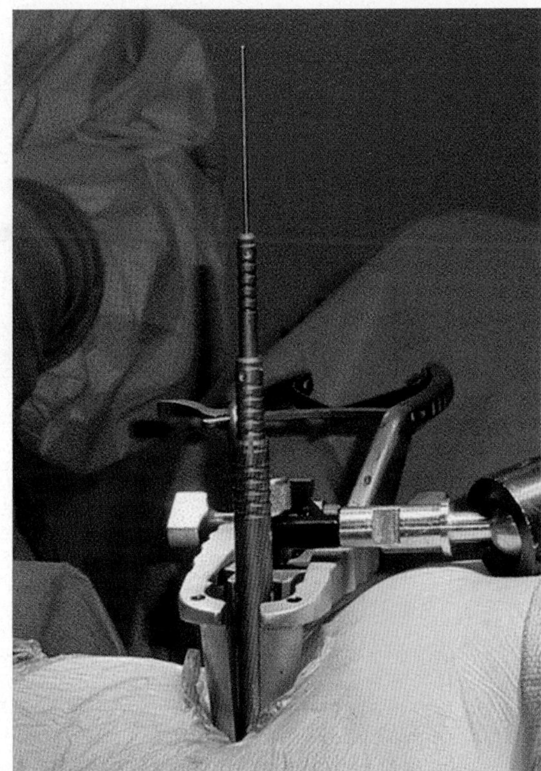

FIGURE 1.32 Operative photograph of laterally inserted dilators. With patient in lateral decubitus position, sequentially larger dilators are shown inserted, penetrating the psoas major, and resting on the desired disc space. (From Ozgur BM, Aryan JE, Pimenta L, Taylor WR: Extreme lateral interbody fusion (XLIF): a novel surgical technique for anterior lumbar interbody fusion, *Spine J* 6:435, 2006.) **SEE TECHNIQUE 1.17.**

the unipolar machine because there is less likelihood of injuring the hypogastric plexus with a thermal burn.

- After adequate exposure of the L5-S1 disc, obtain a radiograph after inserting a 22-gauge spinal needle into the disc space. Because the L5-S1 disc and the sacrum often are angled horizontally, the body of L5 may be mistaken for the sacrum.
- Further development of the exposure proceeds as in other anterior approaches to the lumbar vertebrae.

OBLIQUE APPROACH FOR LUMBAR INTERBODY FUSION, L1-L5 AND L5-S1

The approach for oblique lumbar interbody fusion (OLIF) accesses the spine between the anterior vessels and the psoas muscles, avoiding both sets of structures to allow efficient clearance of disc space and application of a large interbody device to provide distraction for foraminal decompression and endplate preparation (Fig. 1.34). Advocates of the OLIF approach cite two shortcomings of anterior lumbar interbody fusion (ALIF) and posterior lumbar interbody fusion (XLIF) that are avoided by OLIF: iliac vessel and peritoneal injury with ALIF and psoas muscle splitting and limited lower lumbar spine access with XLIF. A study of 812 patients with this approach reported a 4% intraoperative/in-hospital complication rate, no abdominal or urologic injuries, and three each vascular and neurologic injuries. Woods et al. reported an overall complication rate of 12% in 11 patients who had OLIF at L1-L5, L5-S1, or both. The most common

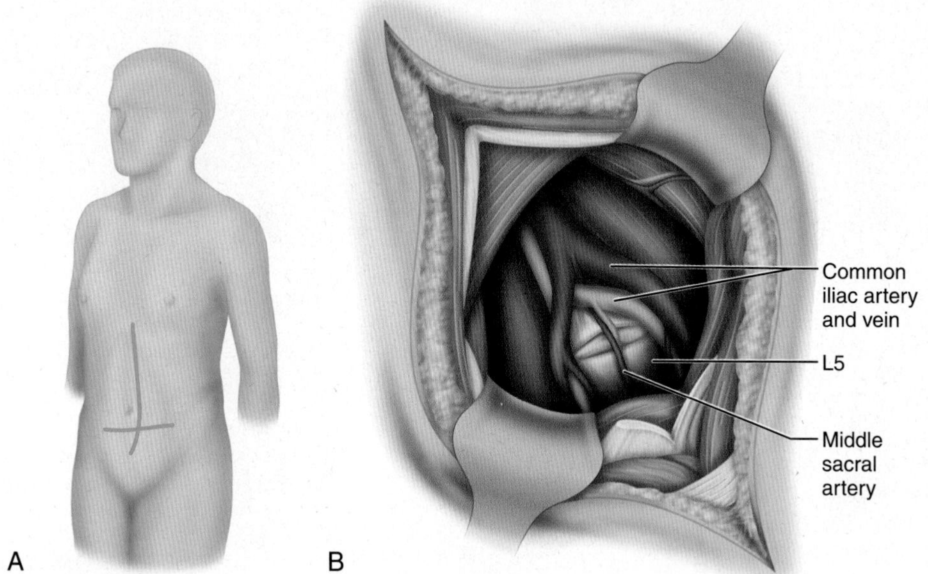

FIGURE 1.33 Transperitoneal approach to lumbar and lumbosacral spine (see text). **A,** Median longitudinal or transverse Pfannenstiel incision. **B,** Dissection of middle sacral artery and vein **SEE TECHNIQUE 1.18**.

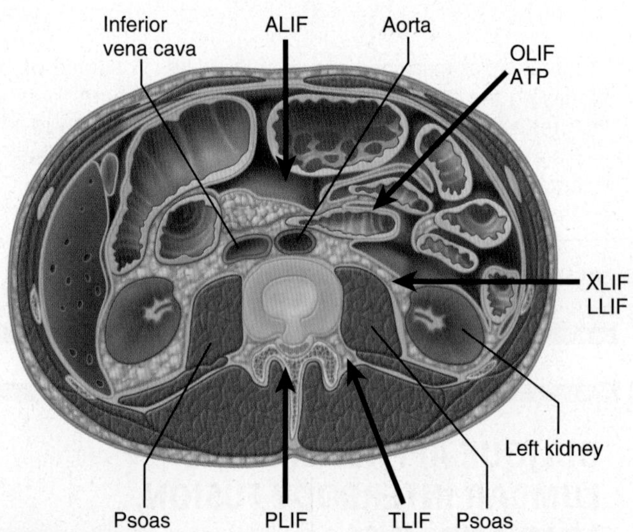

FIGURE 1.34 **Zones of approach for lumbar interbody fusion.** ***ALIF,*** **Anterior lumbar interbody fusion;** ***ATP,*** **anterior to psoas;** ***LLIF,*** **lateral lumbar interbody fusion;** ***OLIF,*** **oblique lumbar interbody fusion;** ***PLIF,*** **posterior lumbar interbody fusion;** ***XLIF,*** **extreme lateral interbody fusion.** (From Phan K, Maharaj M Assem Y, et al: Review of early clinical results and complications associated with oblique lumbar interbody fusion (OLIF), *J Clin Neurosci* 31:23, 2016.)

complications were subsidence (4.4%), postoperative ileus (2.9%), and vascular injury (2.9%). Fusion was successful in 98% of patients. Another cited advantage of this approach is that it can be done without costly neuromonitoring or an additional surgeon.

TECHNIQUE 1.19

(MEHREN ET AL.)

- Place the patient in a right-sided lateral decubitus position that is tilted slightly backward, depending on the target level, to get access to the physiologic corridor between the psoas muscle and vena cava anteriorly (Fig. 1.35).
- Under fluoroscopy, mark the center of the disc on the skin.
- Make a 4-cm skin incision centered in the projection of the target segment, parallel to the external oblique muscle fibers.
- Dissect the external and internal oblique muscles and the transverse abdominal muscle along the direction of the fibers with a blunt, muscle-splitting technique.
- Access the retroperitoneal space by blunt dissection along the retroperitoneal fat tissue.
- Mobilize the peritoneal sac anteriorly.
- With the anterior longitudinal ligament as a medial landmark, identify the border of the psoas muscle as a lateral landmark; retract the psoas muscle at the disc space level (Fig. 1.36).
- Take care to protect the genitofemoral nerve, which courses on top of the psoas muscle, and the sympathetic chain in the anterior third of the vertebral body. If necessary, mobilize the sympathetic chain anteriorly.
- For multilevel fusions, enlarge the incision up to 6 cm or use the same 4-cm incision in a "sliding window" technique that takes advantage of the mobility of the abdominal wall.
- Use Langenbeck hooks or self-retaining retractors for further exposure and preparation of the target area.
- Confirm the correct level with fluoroscopy.

L5-S1 EXPOSURE—KIM ET AL.

- If L5-S1 interbody fusion is planned, tilt the operating table to place the patient supine.
- Check to be sure that a line drawn parallel to the L5-S1 disc passes above the pubic symphysis on a lateral pelvic radiograph to ensure adequate access to the back of the disc space.
- When the left common iliac vessel is exposed in the medial side of the psoas muscle in the retroperitoneal space, check the location of the left iliac artery with the fingers; check the sacral promontory with the index finger and apply dissection with a sponge stick.
- When the L5-S1 disc is exposed, check the level with a guide pin and the C-arm.
- If the level is correct, discectomy, endplate preparation, and interbody fusion are done as usual.

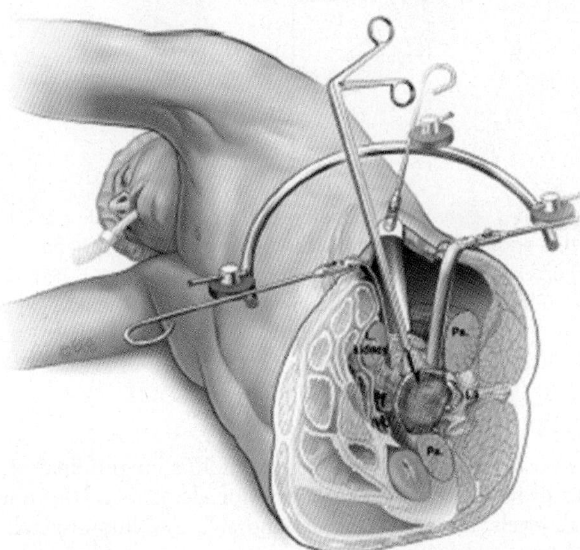

FIGURE 1.35 Patient positioning and exposure for the oblique lateral lumbar fusion. (From Phan K, Maharaj M Assem Y, et al: Review of early clinical results and complications associated with oblique lumbar interbody fusion (OLIF), *J Clin Neurosci* 31:23, 2016.)

VIDEO-ASSISTED LUMBAR SURGERY

Standard anterior approaches to the lower lumbar and lumbosacral spine include the anterior transperitoneal, anterolateral extraperitoneal, and anterior retroperitoneal approaches. As with thoracoscopy, the endoscopic technique is evolving rapidly in terms of its role in procedures involving the anterior aspect of the lumbar spine. Transperitoneal laparoscopic approaches, which have been used for discectomy or fusion, are true endoscopic procedures that are performed with carbon dioxide insufflation and may be impeded by abdominal wall adhesions. Complications include vascular and peritoneal injuries. McAfee et al. described a minimally invasive anterior retroperitoneal approach to the lumbar spine using an endoscopic technique, and Onimus et al. described a less invasive, standard midline, extraperitoneal approach that fully preserves the abdominal innervation and is optimized with video assistance. This procedure avoids peritoneal complications, and it is anterior and midline oriented, giving direct access to the anterior aspect of the

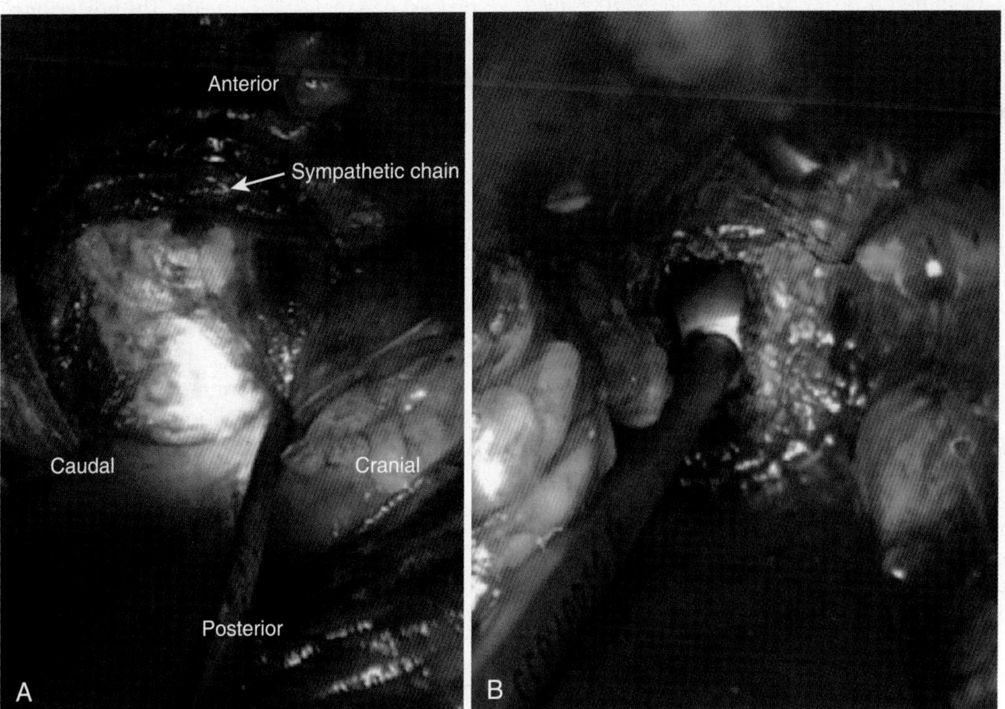

FIGURE 1.36 Oblique anterolateral approach to the lumbar spine. Psoas muscle is retracted by a Langenbeck hook to expose the anterolateral aspect of the disc space. (From Mehren C, Mayer HM, Zandanell C, et al: The oblique anterolateral approach to the lumbar spine provides access to the lumbar spine with few early complications, *Clin Orthop Relat Res* 474:2020, 2016.)

disc. Video assistance allows for a smaller incision, improved lighting, and easier presacral dissection. In addition, good exposure of the vertebral endplates is achieved, allowing a better resection and perhaps, although not reported, an improved fusion rate. In addition, surgical assistants can observe the operation despite the small incision and, if necessary, the incision can be extended cephalad or caudad if conversion to a laparotomy is necessary.

VIDEO-ASSISTED LUMBAR SURGERY

TECHNIQUE 1.20

(ONIMUS ET AL.)

- Place the patient supine and angulate the operative table to place the lumbar spine in slight extension.
- Make a 4-cm vertical incision on the midline at the umbilicus for the L4-5 approach and halfway between the umbilicus and the pubic symphysis for the L5-S1 approach. In women, a more cosmetic horizontal suprapubic incision is available for the L5-S1 approach.
- After division of the linea alba, dissect on the left side between the posterior sheath of the rectus abdominis and posterior aspect of this muscle.
- Divide the posterior sheath at the lateral edge of the rectus returning to the subperitoneal fascia. The division begins at the linea arcuata. Use blunt dissection with a finger and dissecting swabs.
- The next landmark is the prominence of the psoas muscle and the iliac vessels. Reflect the ureter and peritoneum together. The lateral cleavage of the peritoneum can be increased by use of an inflatable balloon.
- Introduce a 10-mm endoscope through a lateral portal between the umbilicus and anterior superior iliac spine for exposure of L5-S1 and at the level of the umbilicus for exposure of L4-5. Introduction of the endoscope gives good exposure of the prevertebral area and allows the operation to be continued under endoscopic and direct vision.
- Expose the anterior aspect of the intervertebral disc by blunt dissection through the midline incision.
- For exposure of L5-S1, hemoclip the middle sacral vessels and divide them. Retract the common iliac vessels cranially with a specially designed retractor that is introduced through the midline incision and held in position by two Steinmann pins inserted in L5 and S1.
- For exposure of L4-5, retract the iliac vessels caudally. Divide the iliolumbar vein to allow caudal retraction of the left iliac vein.
- More acute endoscopic exposure of the vertebral plates is possible by using a 30-degree angulated arthroscope.
- Intervertebral distraction allows iliac autogenous graft insertion. The procedure can be completed with disc and vertebral plate resection.
- Close the wound on a retroperitoneal suction tube inserted through the endoscope's lateral port.

POSTOPERATIVE CARE Standing and ambulation are allowed 2 to 3 days after surgery. A body jacket orthosis is worn for 3 months.

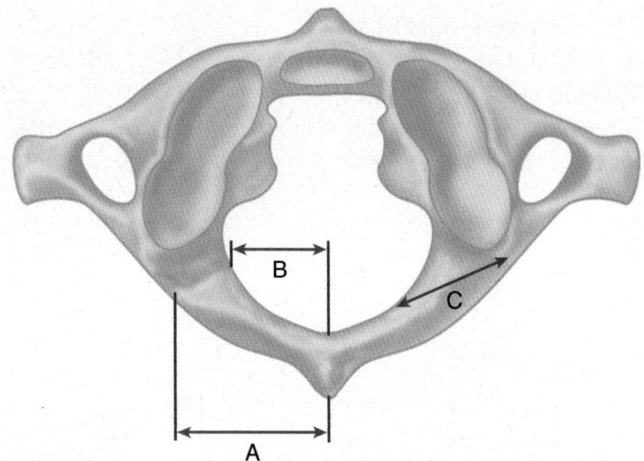

FIGURE 1.37 **Distance between the posterior midline and the medial end of the vertebral artery groove at outer *(A)* and inner *(B)* cortex and the length of vertebral artery groove *(C)*.** (Redrawn from Gupta T: Quantitative anatomy of vertebral artery groove on the posterior arch of atlas in relation to spinal surgical procedures, *Surg Radiol Anat* 30:239, 2008.)

POSTERIOR APPROACHES

The posterior approach through a midline longitudinal incision provides access to the posterior elements of the spine at all levels, including cervical, thoracic, and lumbosacral. It is the most direct access to the spinous processes, laminae, and facets. In addition, the spinal canal can be explored and decompressed over a large area after laminectomy. Under most circumstances, the choice of approach to the spine should be dictated by the site of the primary pathologic condition. Posterior approaches to the spine rarely are indicated when the anterior spinal column is the site of an infectious process or a metastatic disease. The posterior elements usually are not involved in the pathologic process and provide stabilization for the uninvolved structures of the spinal column. Removal of the uninvolved posterior elements, as in laminectomy, may result in subluxation, dislocation, or severe angulation of the spine, causing increased compression of the neural elements and worsening of any neurologic deficit. Posterior approaches to the spine commonly are used for degenerative or traumatic spinal disorders and allow excellent exposure to perform a wide variety of fusion techniques, with or without internal stabilization. Gupta measured the distance from the midline of C1 to the vertebral artery groove in 55 adult vertebrae and found that at least 1.5 cm of the posterior arch could be safely exposed without mobilization of the vertebral artery (Fig. 1.37). With mobilization of the vertebral artery, another 10 mm of arch could be exposed in either direction.

POSTERIOR APPROACH TO THE CERVICAL SPINE, OCCIPUT TO C2

TECHNIQUE 1.21

- Position the patient prone on a turning frame with skeletal traction through tongs, avoiding excessive pressure on the eyes. Alternatively, a three-point head rest can be

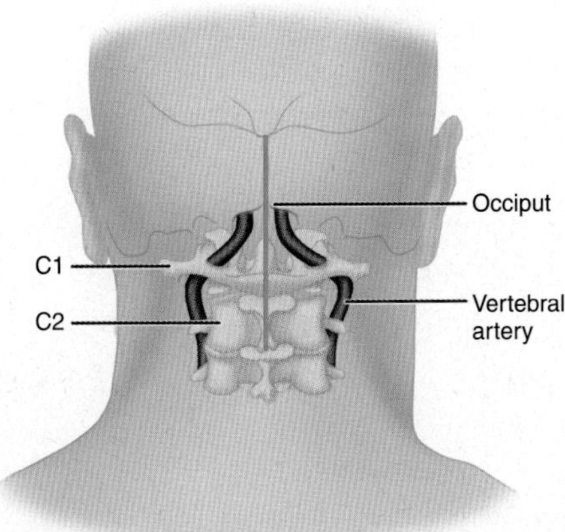

FIGURE 1.38 Posterior approach to upper cervical spine (see text). **SEE TECHNIQUE 1.21.**

used to provide rigid immobilization of the cervical spine during surgery.

- After routine skin preparation, attach the drapes to the neck with stay sutures or staples.
- Make a midline longitudinal skin incision from the occiput to C2 (Fig. 1.38). Infiltration of the skin and subcutaneous tissue with a dilute 1:500,000 epinephrine solution helps to provide hemostasis.
- Using electrocautery and elevators, expose the posterior elements subperiosteally and insert self-retaining retractors.
- It is important to deepen the incision in the midline through the thin white median raphe and avoid cutting muscle tissue. The median raphe of the cervical spine is a wandering avascular ligament and does not follow a straight midline incision. In children, do not expose any spinal levels unnecessarily to avoid spontaneous fusion at adjacent levels, including the occiput.
- When exposing the upper cervical spine, do not carry the dissection farther than 1.5 cm laterally on either side to avoid the vertebral arteries.
- When necessary, expose the occiput with elevators and insert the self-retaining retractors to expose the base of the skull and the dorsal spine of C2. The area in between contains the ring of C1; this is often deep compared with the spinous process of C2.
- While maintaining lateral retraction of the soft tissues, identify the posterior tubercle of C1 longitudinally in the midline and begin subperiosteal dissection to the bone. Often the ring of C1 is thin, and direct pressure can fracture it or cause the instrument to slip off the ring and penetrate the atlantooccipital membrane. The dura may be vulnerable on the superior and the inferior edges of the ring of C1.
- The second cervical ganglion is an important landmark on the ring of C1 laterally. It lies approximately 1.5 cm laterally on the lamina of C1 in the groove for the vertebral artery. There is little, if any, indication for dissection lateral to this groove.
- The vertebral artery may be damaged by penetration of the atlantooccipital membrane off the superior border of the ring of C1 more lateral than the usually safe 1.5 cm from the midline.

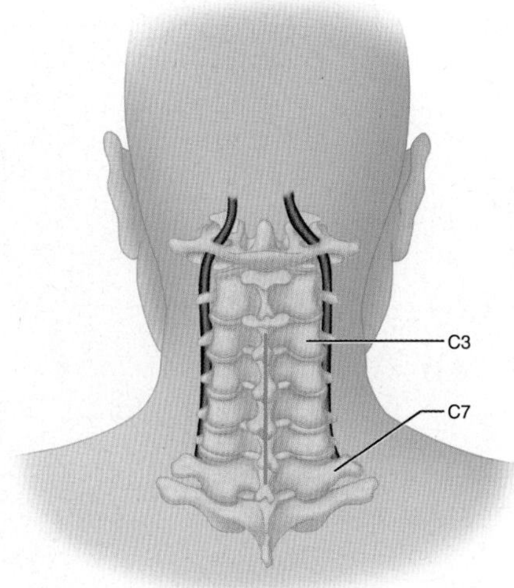

FIGURE 1.39 Posterior approach to lower cervical spine (see text). **SEE TECHNIQUE 1.22.**

- Below C2, the lateral margins of the facet joints are the safe lateral extent of dissection.
- After exposure of the posterior occiput, the ring of C1, and the posterior elements of C2, the intended surgical procedure may be performed.
- After this, the wound is closed in layers over a drain.

POSTERIOR APPROACH TO THE CERVICAL SPINE, C3 TO C7

TECHNIQUE 1.22

- Position the patient prone on a turning frame with skeletal traction through tongs or with the head positioned in the three-point head fixation device that is attached to the table.
- The large spinous processes of C2 and C7 are prominent and can be identified by palpation. It is important to note on preoperative radiographs any posterior element deficiencies, such as an occult spina bifida, before exposure of the posterior elements.
- Make a midline skin incision over the appropriate vertebrae (Fig. 1.39) and inject the skin and subcutaneous tissues with a 1:500,000 epinephrine solution to aid in hemostasis.
- Deepen the dissection in the midline using the electrocautery knife and staying within the thin white median raphe to avoid cutting the vascular muscle tissue (Fig. 1.40). It is helpful to maintain tension on the soft tissue by inserting self-retaining retractors.
- Using electrocautery and elevators, detach the ligamentous attachments to the spinous processes and expose the posterior elements subperiosteally to the lateral edge of

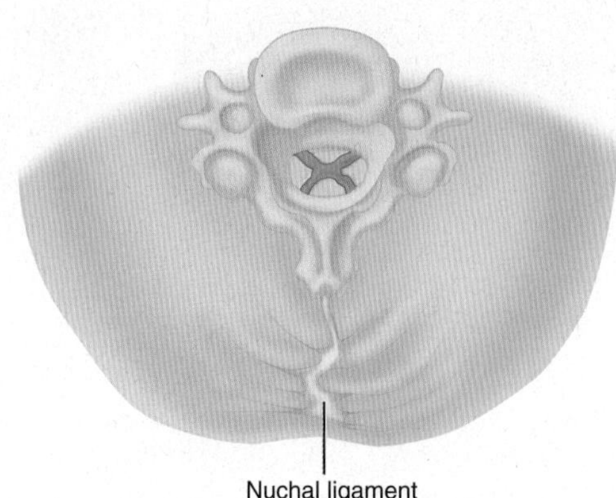

FIGURE 1.40 Posterior approach to lower cervical spine. Nuchal ligament is irregular. To maintain dry field, surgeon must stay within ligament. **SEE TECHNIQUE 1.22.**

the facet joints, which is the extent of dissection on either side of the midline.

- After identifying the lateral edge of the facet joint, pack each level with a taped sponge to keep blood loss to a minimum.
- It is helpful to expose the spinous processes distal to proximal because the muscles can be stripped from the spinous processes in the acute angle between their insertions and the bone. If exposure in the opposite direction is attempted, the knife blade or periosteal elevator would tend to follow the direction of the fibers into the muscle and divide the vessels, increasing hemorrhage.

POSTERIOR APPROACH TO THE THORACIC SPINE, T1 TO T12

The posterior approach to the thoracic spine can be made through a standard midline longitudinal exposure with reflection of the erector spinae muscle laterally to the tips of the transverse processes. Alternatively, the thoracic vertebrae can be approached through a costotransversectomy when direct access to the transverse processes and pedicles of the thoracic spine and limited access to the vertebral bodies are indicated. Costotransversectomy should be considered for simple biopsy or local debridement. This approach does not provide the working operative area or length of exposure to the thoracic vertebral bodies that is afforded by a transthoracic approach or the mid-longitudinal posterior approach.

TECHNIQUE 1.23

- Position the patient prone on a padded spinal operating frame.
- Make a long midline incision over the area to be exposed (Fig. 1.41). Infiltration of the skin, subcutaneous tissue, and erector spinae to the level of the laminae with 1:500,000 epinephrine solution helps provide hemostasis.

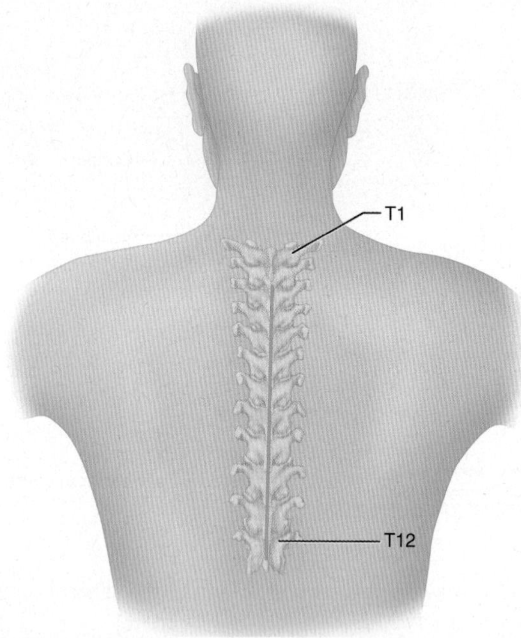

FIGURE 1.41 Posterior approach to thoracic spine (see text). **SEE TECHNIQUE 1.23.**

- Deepen the dissection in the midline using a scalpel or the electrocautery knife through the superficial and lumbodorsal fasciae to the tips of the spinous processes.
- Expose subperiosteally the posterior elements by reflecting the erector spinae muscle laterally to the tips of the transverse processes distal to proximal, using periosteal elevators.
- Repeat the procedure until the desired number of vertebrae is exposed; where both sides of the spine require exposure, use the same technique on each side.
- Pack each segment with a taped sponge immediately after exposure to lessen bleeding.
- After satisfactory exposure of the posterior elements, obtain a radiograph to confirm proper localization of the intended level.
- After completion of the spinal procedure, close the wound in layers over a suction drain.

MINIMALLY INVASIVE APPROACHES TO THE POSTERIOR SPINE

All the posterior approaches to the spine can be made in a minimally invasive fashion when only a limited area of dissection is needed within the lateral recess, canal, or lumbar intervertebral foramen. The adaptation typically involves dilating through the posterior overlying fascia (thoracolumbar) and musculature, followed by inserting down to the spine a fixed or adjustable tubular retractor that is attached to a table-mounted retractor arm. The location of the incision is critical in a minimally invasive approach and depends on the exact procedure since the smaller field of view and working portal limit the surgical corridor. A 2-cm error in placement of the incision when using a 20-mm retractor is a 100% error. Planning the location of the incision based on preoperative imaging (MRI and/or CT) and fluoroscopic localization of the incision is mandatory for minimally invasive posterior approaches.

COSTOTRANSVERSECTOMY

TECHNIQUE 1.24

- Place the patient prone on a padded spinal operating frame.
- Make a straight longitudinal incision about 2.5 inches (6.3 cm) lateral to the spinous processes centered over the level of the desired vertebral dissection (Fig. 1.42A). (Alternatively, make a curved incision with its apex lateral to the midline.)
- Palpate the slight depression between the dorsal paraspinal muscle mass and the prominent posterior angle of the rib and center the incision over this groove lateral to the spinous processes.
- Deepen the dissection through the subcutaneous tissues and the trapezius and latissimus dorsi muscles and the lumbodorsal fasciae, which are divided longitudinally.
- Dissect the paraspinal muscles sharply from their insertions on the ribs and transverse processes and retract them medially.
- Expose the transverse process and posterior aspects of the associated rib subperiosteally and remove a section of rib 5 to 7.5 cm long at the level of involvement. The rib generally is transected with rib cutters about 3.5 inches (~9 cm) lateral to the vertebra at its prominent posterior angle. The costotransverse ligament and joint capsule are strong and increase the inherent stability of the thoracic spine.
- Remain subperiosteal and extrapleural during this part of the exposure and protect the intercostal neurovascular bundle. Anterior to the transverse process is the vertebral pedicle, and above and below the pedicle lie the neural foramina. The nerve roots emerge from the superior portion of the foramina, giving off a dorsal and ventral ramus. The ventral ramus becomes the intercostal nerve and is joined by the intercostal vessels.
- When the pedicles, neural foramina, and neurovascular structures have been identified, proceed with dissection directly anteriorly on the pedicle to the vertebral body along a path that is relatively free of major vessels or nerves (Fig. 1.42B).
- Carefully dissect the parietal pleura with elevators anteriorly to expose the anterolateral aspect of the vertebral body, raising the sympathetic trunk and parietal pleura.
- Exposure can be increased by removal of the transverse process, pedicle, and facet joints as necessary.
- After completion of the spinal procedure, fill the wound with saline and inflate the lungs to check for air leaks.
- Close the wound in layers over a drain to prevent hematoma collection.
- Obtain a chest radiograph to document the absence of air in the pleural space, which may occur if the pleura is inadvertently entered during the exposure.

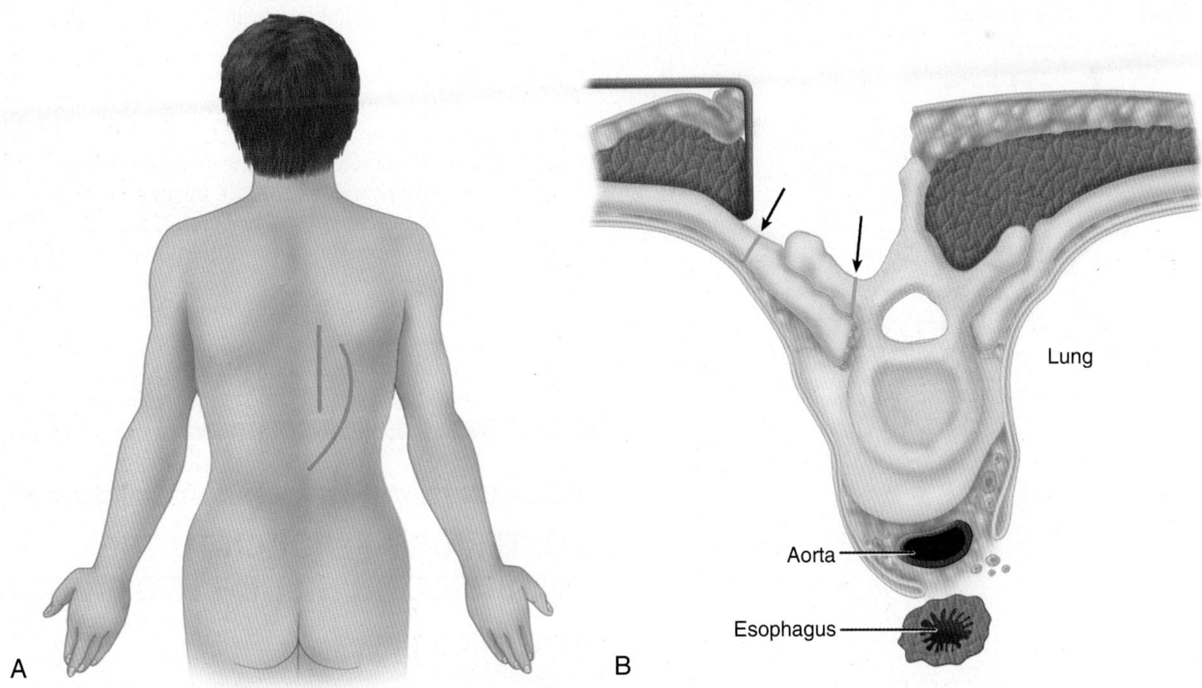

FIGURE 1.42 Costotransversectomy. **A,** Straight longitudinal incision about 2.5 inches (6.3 cm) lateral to spinous processes, centered over level of vertebral dissection. Alternative curved incision also shown. **B,** Resection of costotransverse articulation. **SEE TECHNIQUE 1.24.**

POSTERIOR APPROACH TO THE LUMBAR SPINE, L1 TO L5

The posterior approach to the lumbar spine provides access directly to the spinous processes, laminae, and facet joints at all levels. In addition, the transverse processes and pedicles can be reached through this approach. Wiltse and Spencer refined the paraspinal approach to the lumbar spine, which involves a longitudinal separation of the sacrospinalis muscle group to expose the posterolateral aspect of the lumbar spine. This approach is especially useful in removing far-lateral disc herniation, decompressing a "far out" syndrome, and inserting pedicle screws.

TECHNIQUE 1.25

- Position the patient prone or in the kneeling position on a padded spinal frame. By allowing the abdomen to hang free, intravenous pressure is decreased and blood loss is decreased as a result of collapse of the epidural venous plexus.
- Make a midline skin incision centered over the involved lumbar segment (Fig. 1.43). Infiltrating the skin and subcutaneous tissue with 1:500,000 epinephrine aids hemostasis.
- Carry the dissection down in the midline through the skin, subcutaneous tissue, and lumbodorsal fascia to the tips of the spinous processes. Use self-retaining retractors to maintain tension on soft tissues during exposure.
- Subperiosteally expose the posterior elements from distal to proximal using electrocautery and periosteal elevators to detach the muscles from the posterior elements.
- Pack each segment with a taped sponge immediately after exposure to lessen bleeding.

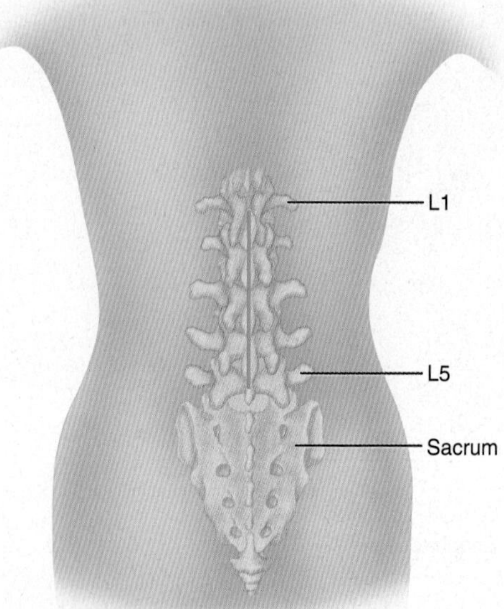

FIGURE 1.43 Posterior approach to lumbar spine (see text). **SEE TECHNIQUE 1.25.**

- If the procedure requires exposure of both sides of the spine, use the same technique on each side.
- We recommend accurate localization of the involved segment with a permanent radiograph in the operating room.
- After completion of the spinal procedure, close the wound in layers over a drain.

PARASPINAL APPROACH TO LUMBAR SPINE

TECHNIQUE 1.26

(WILTSE AND SPENCER)

- Position the patient prone or in the kneeling position on a spinal frame. By allowing the abdomen to hang free, intravenous pressure is decreased and blood loss is decreased as a result of collapse of the epidural venous plexus.
- Make a midline skin incision centered over the involved lower lumbar segment (Fig. 1.44A). Infiltration with 1:500,000 epinephrine helps to provide hemostasis.
- Carry dissection down to the lumbodorsal fascia and retract the skin and subcutaneous tissue laterally on either side.
- Make a fascial incision approximately 2 cm lateral to the midline (Fig. 1.44B and C).
- After the fascial layers have been divided, a natural cleavage plane is entered lying between the multifidus and longissimus muscles. Using blunt finger dissection between the muscle groups (Fig. 1.44D and E), palpate the facet joints at L4-5. Place self-retaining Gelpi retractors between the two muscle groups.
- Using electrocautery or an elevator, separate the transverse fibers of the multifidus from their heavy fascial attachments.
- Expose the lumbar transverse processes, facet joints, and laminae subperiosteally and denude them of soft tissue. Avoid carrying the dissection anterior to the transverse processes because the exiting spinal nerves lie just in front of the transverse processes and can be injured.
- Use bipolar cautery to control bleeding from the lumbar arteries and veins coursing above the base of the transverse processes.
- Perform unilateral or bilateral decompression and fusion of the lumbosacral spine.
- Close the wound over a suction drain and suture the skin flaps down to the fascia to remove dead space.

POSTERIOR APPROACH TO THE LUMBOSACRAL SPINE, L1 TO SACRUM

TECHNIQUE 1.27

(WAGONER)

- Make a longitudinal incision over the spinous processes of the appropriate vertebrae and incise the superficial fascia,

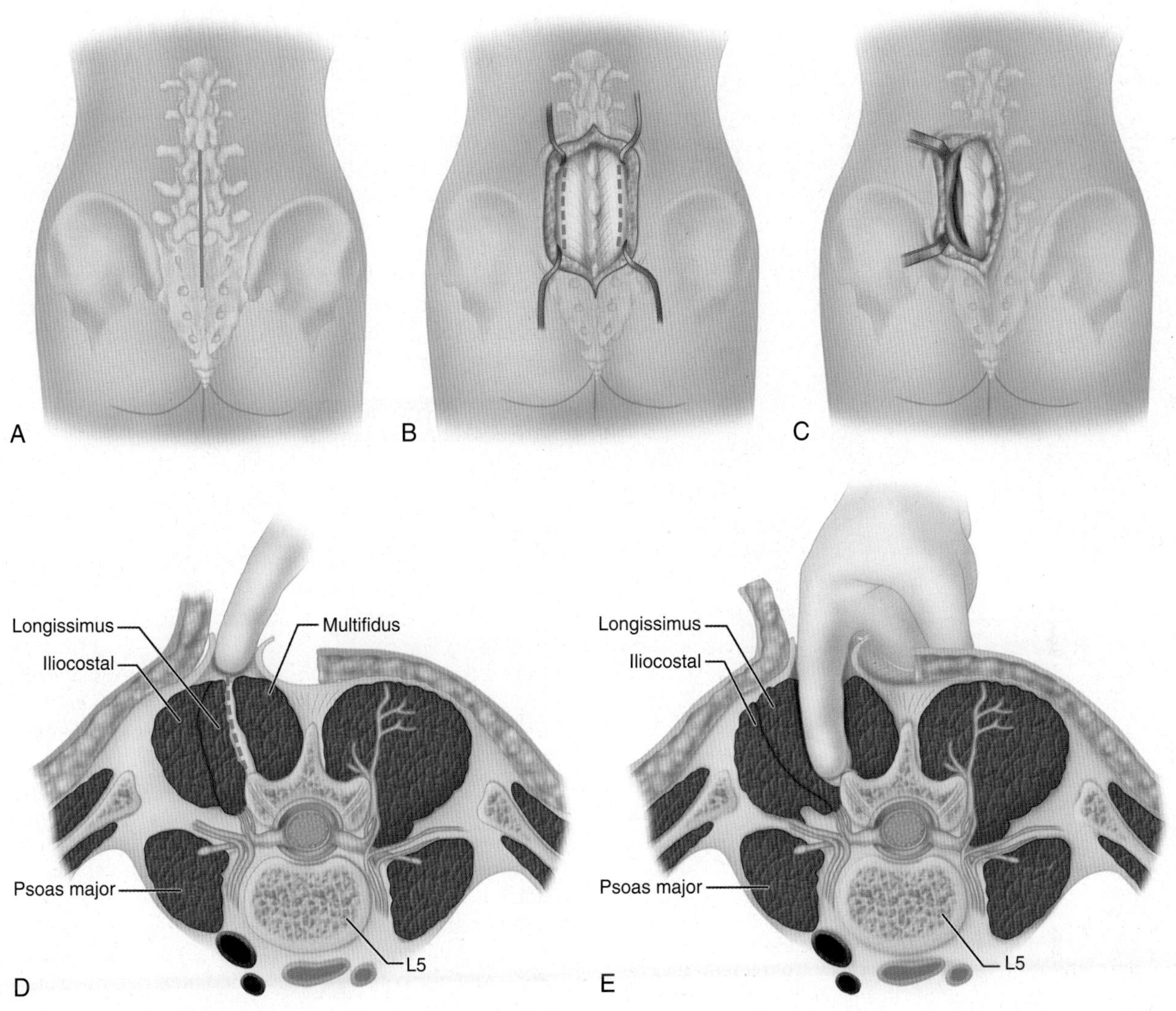

FIGURE 1.44 Paraspinal approach to lumbar spine (see text). **A,** Midline skin incision. **B** and **C,** Fascial incisions. **D** and **E,** Blunt finger dissection between muscle groups to palpate facet joints. (Redrawn from Wiltse LL, Spencer CW: New uses and refinements of the paraspinal approach of the lumbar spine, *Spine* 13:696, 1988.) **SEE TECHNIQUE 1.26.**

the lumbodorsal fascia, and the supraspinous ligament longitudinally, precisely over the tips of the processes.

- With a scalpel, divide longitudinally the ligament between the two spinous processes in the most distal part of the wound.
- Insert a small, blunt periosteal elevator through this opening so that its end rests on the junction of the spinous process with the lamina of the more proximal vertebra (Fig. 1.45A). Move the handle of the elevator proximally and laterally to place under tension the muscles attached to this spinous process.
- With a scalpel moving from distal to proximal, strip the muscles subperiosteally from the lateral surface of the process.
- Place the end of the elevator in the wound so that its end rests on the junction of the spinous process with the lamina of the next most proximal vertebra and repeat the procedure as described.
- Repeat the procedure until the desired number of vertebrae have been exposed (Fig. 1.45B).
- For operations requiring exposure of both sides of the spine, use the same technique on each side.
- This approach exposes the spinous processes and medial part of the laminae.
- Increase the exposure, if desired, by further subperiosteal reflection along the laminae; expose the posterior surface of the laminae and the articular facets.
- Pack each segment with a tape sponge immediately after exposure to lessen bleeding.
- Divide the supraspinous ligament precisely over the tip of the spinous processes and denude subperiosteally the sides of the processes because this route leads through a

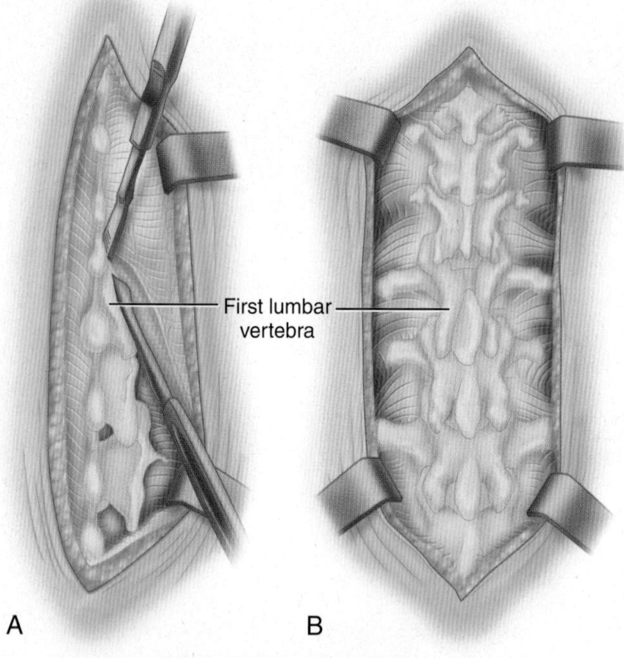

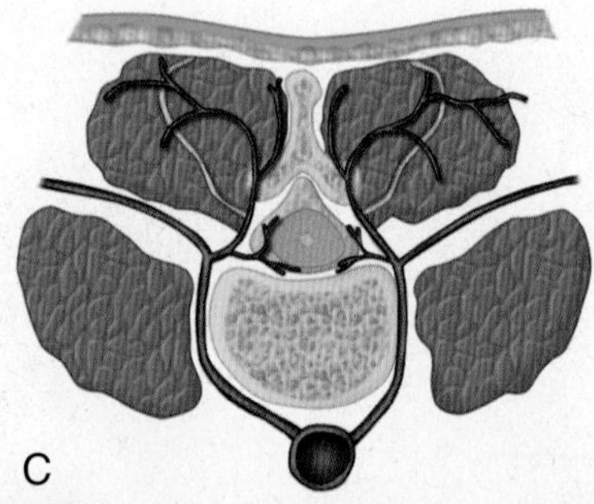

FIGURE 1.45 Approach to posterior aspect of spine. **A,** Muscle insertions are freed subperiosteally from lateral side of spinous processes and interspinous ligaments; dissection proceeds proximally, with periosteal elevator being held against bases of spinous processes. **B,** Spinous processes, laminae, and articular facets exposed. **C,** Courses of arteries supplying posterior spinal muscles, showing proximity of internal muscular branches to spinous processes. (Modified from Wagoner G: A technique for lessening hemorrhage in operations on the spine, *J Bone Joint Surg* 19:469, 1937.) **SEE TECHNIQUE 1.27.**

relatively avascular field; otherwise, the arterial supply to the muscles is encountered (Fig. 1.45C).

- Blood loss can be decreased further by using electrocautery and a suction apparatus. Replace blood as it is lost.
- Expose the spinous processes from distal to proximal as just described because the muscles can then be stripped from the spinous processes in the acute angle between their insertions and the bone.
- If exposure in the opposite direction is attempted, the knife blade or periosteal elevator tends to follow the direction of the fibers into the muscle and divides the vessels, increasing hemorrhage.

POSTERIOR APPROACH TO THE SACRUM AND SACROILIAC JOINT

The posterior sacrum and sacroiliac joint are approached most commonly through a standard posterior exposure; however, the access to the sacroiliac joint is limited. Ebraheim et al. described a transosseous approach to the sacroiliac joint that they suggested improves access for debridement and arthrodesis with only minimal soft-tissue dissection and iliac bone resection. Indications include trauma, infection, degenerative disease, and inflammatory processes. This approach allows direct exposure of the corresponding sacral articular surfaces.

TECHNIQUE 1.28

(EBRAHEIM ET AL.)

- Place the patient prone on padded bolsters or a spinal frame.
- Make an incision beginning at the level of the posterior superior iliac spine and extending distal to the midpoint between the posterior superior iliac spine and the posterior inferior iliac spine.
- Extend the incision laterally and distally approximately 5 cm (Fig. 1.46A).
- Divide the superficial fascia and incise the gluteus medius muscle along the line of the skin incision.
- Sharply dissect the origin of the gluteus maximus from the posterior ilium.
- Subperiosteally elevate the gluteal musculature laterally and identify the superior border of the greater sciatic notch.
- Insert one or two Steinmann pins into the ilium to assist in retracting the gluteus maximus laterally and distally. It is important not to injure the superior gluteal neurovascular bundle.
- Expose the posterior external surface of the ilium between the posterior superior iliac spine above and the superior border of the greater sciatic notch below.
- Elevate a right-angle triangular bone window from the posterior ilium using an osteotome or power saw and remove the articular cartilage from the sacrum and ilium (Fig. 1.46B). Debride the joint with curets.
- After removal of the articular cartilage, place the previously elevated bone window into its original position and carefully tamp it back into place.
- Accurate localization of the bone window in the iliac crest is important to avoid laceration to the superior gluteal artery, which may retract into the pelvis, making hemostasis difficult. Injury to the superior gluteal nerve may denervate the gluteus medius, leading to dysfunction in hip abduction. The dimensions of the right-angle triangle in the outer table of the posterior ilium are illustrated in Fig. 1.46B.

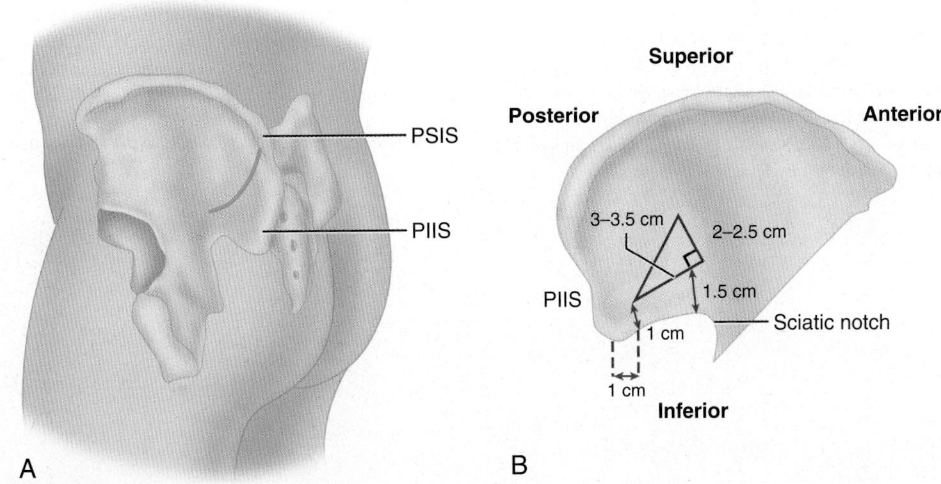

FIGURE 1.46 Posterior approach to sacroiliac joint. **A,** Skin incision. **B,** Right triangle on outer table of posterior ilium. *PIIS,* Posterior inferior iliac spine; *PSIS,* posterior superior iliac spine. (Redrawn from Ebraheim NA, Lu J, Biyani A, et al: Anatomic considerations for posterior approach to the sacroiliac joint, *Spine* 21:2709, 1996.) **SEE TECHNIQUE 1.28.**

REFERENCES

Abe K, Orita S, Mannoji C, et al.: Perioperative complications in 155 patients who underwent oblique lateral interbody fusion surgery: perspectives and indications from a retrospective, multicenter survey, *Spine (Phila Pa 1976)* 42:55, 2017.

Adkins DE, Sandhu FA, Voyadzis JM: Minimally invasive lateral approach to the thoracolumbar junction for corpectomy, *J Clin Neurosci* 20:1289, 2013.

Baaj AA, Papadimitriou K, Amin AG, et al.: Surgical anatomy of the diaphragm in the anterolateral approach to the spine: a cadaveric study, *J Spinal Disord Tech* 27:220, 2014.

Cheung KMC, Mak KC, Luk KDK: Anterior approach to cervical spine, *Spine* 37:E297, 2012.

Cho W, Buchowski JM, Park Y, et al.: Surgical approach to the cervicothoracic junction. can a standard smith-robinson approach be utilized? *J Spinal Disord Tech* 25:264, 2012.

Dakwar E, Ahmadian A, Uribe JS: The anatomical relationship of the diaphragm to the thoracolumbar junction during the minimally invasive lateral extracoelomic (retropleural/retroperitoneal) approach. laboratory investigation, *J Neurosurg Spine* 16:359, 2012.

Elsamadicy AA, Adogwa O, Behrens S, et al.: Impact of surgical approach on complication rates after elective spinal fusion (≥3 levels) for adult spine deformity, *J Spine Surg* 3:31, 2017.

Fuentes S, Malikov S, Blondel B, et al.: Cervicosternotomy as an anterior approach to the upper thoracic and cervicothoracic spinal junction, *J Neurosurg Spine* 12:160, 2010.

Gavriliu TS, Japie EM, Ghita RA, et al.: Burnei's anterior transthoracic retropleural approach of the thoracic spine: a new operative technique in the treatment of spinal disorders, *J Med Life* 8:160, 2015.

Harel R, Stylianou P, Knoller N: Cervical spine surgery: approach-related complications, *World Neurosurg* 94:1, 2016.

Hu WK, He SS, Zhang SC, et al.: An MRI study of psoas major and abdominal large vessels with respect to the X/DLIF approach, *Eur Spine J* 20:557–562, 2011.

Kapetanakis S, Gkasdaris G, Angoules AG, et al.: Transforaminal percutaneous endoscopic discectomy using transforaminal endoscopic spine system: technique pitfalls that a beginner should avoid, *World J Orthop* 8:874, 2017.

Katz AD, Mancini N, Karukonda T, et al.: Approach-based comparative and predictor analysis of 30-day readmission, reoperation, and morbidity in patients undergoing lumbar interbody fusion using the ACS-NSQIP dataset, *Spine (Phila Pa 1976)*, 2018. Epub ahead of print.

Kaye ID, Passias P: Minimally invasive surgery (MIS) approaches to thoracolumbar trauma, *Bull Hosp Jt Dis* 76(2013):71, 2018.

Kim KT, Jo DJ, Lee SH, et al.: Oblique retroperitoneal approach for lumbar interbody fusion from L1 to S1 in adult spine deformity, *Neurosurg Rev* 41:355, 2018.

Le Huec JC, Tournier C, Aunoble S, et al.: Video-assisted treatment of thoracolumbar junction fractures using a specific distractor for reduction: prospective study of 50 cases, *Eur J Spine* 19(Suppl 2):S27, 2010.

Li JX, Phan K, Mobbs R: Oblique lumbar interbody fusion: technical aspects, operative outcomes, and complications, *World Neurosurg* 98:113, 2017.

Litré CF, Duntze J, Benhima Y, et al.: Anterior minimally invasive extrapleural retroperitoneal approach to the thoraco-lumbar junction of the spine, *Orthop Traumatol Surg Res* 99:94, 2013.

Liu C, Wang J: Learning curve of minimally invasive surgery oblique lumbar interboy fusion for degenerative lumbar diseases, *World Neurosurg*, 2018. Epub ahead of print.

Mai HT, Mitchell SM, Jenkins TJ, et al.: Accessibility of the cervicothoracic junction through an anterior approach. an MRI-based algorithm, *Spine* 41:69, 2016.

Mehren C, Mayer HM, Zandanell C, et al.: The oblique anterolateral approach to the lumbar spine provides access to the lumbar spine with few early complications, *Clin Orthop Relat Res* 474:2020, 2016.

Nayar G, Wang T, Stanley EW, et al.: Minimally invasive lateral access surgery and reoperation rates: a multi-institution retrospective review of 2060 patients, *World Neurosurg* 116:e744, 2018.

Park DK, Lee MJ, Lin EL, et al.: The relationship of intrapsoas nerves during a transpsoas approach to the lumbar spine: anatomic study, *J Spinal Disord Tech* 23:223, 2010.

Phan K, Maharaj M, Assem Y, et al.: Review of early clinical results and complications associated with oblique lumbar interbody fusion (OLIF), *J Clin Neurosci* 31:23, 2016.

Salzmann SN, Derman PB, Lampe LP, et al.: Cervical spinal fusion: 16-year trends in epidemiology, indications, and in-hospital outcomes by surgical approach, *World Neurosurg* 113:e280, 2018.

Sen RD, White-Dzuro G, Ruzevick J, et al.: Intra- and peri-operative complications associated with endoscopic spine surgery: a multi-institutional study, *World Neurosurg*, 2018. Epub ahead of print.

Silvestre C, Mac-Thiong JM, Hilmi R, et al.: Complications and morbidities of mini-open anterior retroperitoneal lumbar interbody fusion: oblique lumbar interbody fusion in 179 patients, *Asian Spine J* 6:89, 2012.

Song Y, Tharin S, Divi V, et al.: Anterolateral approach to the upper cervical spine: case report and operative technique, *Head Neck* 37:E115, 2015.

Woods KRM, Billys JB, Hynes RA: Technical description of oblique lateral interbody fusion at L1-L5 (OLIF25) and at L5-S1 (OLIF51) and evaluation of complication and fusion rates, *Spine J* 17:545, 2017.

Yue JK, Upadhyayula PS, Deng H, et al.: Risk factors for 30-day outcomes in elective anterior versus posterior cervical fusion: a matched cohort analysis, *J Craniovertebr Junction Spine* 8:222, 2017.

Zhang Y, Zhang J, Wang X, et al.: Application of the cervical subaxial anterior approach at C2 in select patients, *Orthopedics* 36:e554, 2013.

The complete list of references is available online at Expert Consult.com.

CHAPTER 2

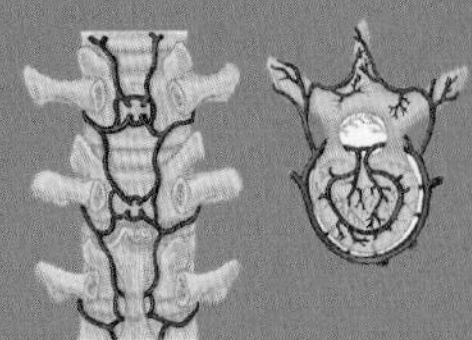

DEGENERATIVE DISORDERS OF THE CERVICAL SPINE

Raymond J. Gardocki, Ashley L. Park

OVERVIEW OF DISC DEGENERATION AND HERNIATION IN THE CERVICAL SPINE

Cervical degenerative disc disease (DDD) is not a specific diagnosis but a pathophysiologic process that incorporates a spectrum of disease states. Manifestations of cervical DDD can range from neck pain and headache to cervical radiculopathy and/or myelopathy. Fortunately, most of these pathologies can be managed nonoperatively; they may require surgical intervention if the symptoms and signs are found to be persistent or progressive. The clinician's job is to determine the most specific diagnosis that explains the symptoms so that the optimal treatment can be applied.

Axial spine pain, which should be distinguished from disc degeneration, is the most frequent musculoskeletal complaint. Axial spine pain—whether cervical, thoracic, or lumbar—often is attributed to disc degeneration. Disc degeneration does not always cause pain, but it can lead to internal disc derangement or disc herniation. Each of these diagnoses has unique clinical findings and treatments.

The genetic influence on disc degeneration may be attributed to a small effect from each of multiple genes or possibly a relatively large effect of a smaller number of genes. To date, several specific gene loci have been identified that are associated with disc degeneration. This association of a specific gene with degenerative disc changes has been confirmed. Other variations in the aggrecan gene, metalloproteinase-3 gene, collagen type IX, and alpha 2 and 3 gene forms also have been associated with disc pathology and symptoms.

Nonspecific axial pain is an international health issue of major significance and should be discriminated from pain associated with a disc herniation. Approximately 80% of individuals are affected by this symptom at some time in their lives. Impairments of the back and spine are ranked as the most frequent cause of limitation of activity in individuals younger than 45 years old by the National Center for Health Statistics (www.cdc.gov/nchs). Axial pain typically described as discogenic pain may not even arise from the disc itself.

Nonanatomic factors, specifically work perception and psychosocial factors, are intimately intertwined with physical complaints. Compounding the diagnostic and treatment difficulties is the high incidence of significant abnormalities shown by imaging studies, which in asymptomatic matched controls is 76%. Optimal outcome primarily depends on "proper patient selection"; such patients can be difficult to identify. Until the pathologic process is better described and reliable criteria for the diagnosis are determined, improvement in treatment outcomes will change slowly.

DISC AND SPINE ANATOMY

The intervertebral disc has a complex structure; the nucleus pulposus has an organized matrix, which is laid down by relatively few cells. The central gelatinous nucleus is contained around the periphery by the collagenous anulus, the cartilaginous anulus, and the cartilage endplates cephalad and caudad. Collagen fibers continue from the anulus to the surrounding tissues, tying into the vertebral body along its rim and into the anterior and posterior longitudinal ligaments and the hyaline cartilage endplates superiorly and inferiorly. The cartilage endplates are secured to the osseous endplate by the calcified cartilage. Few, if any, collagen fibers cross this boundary. The anulus has a lamellar structure with interconnections between adjacent layers of collagen fibrils (Fig. 2.1).

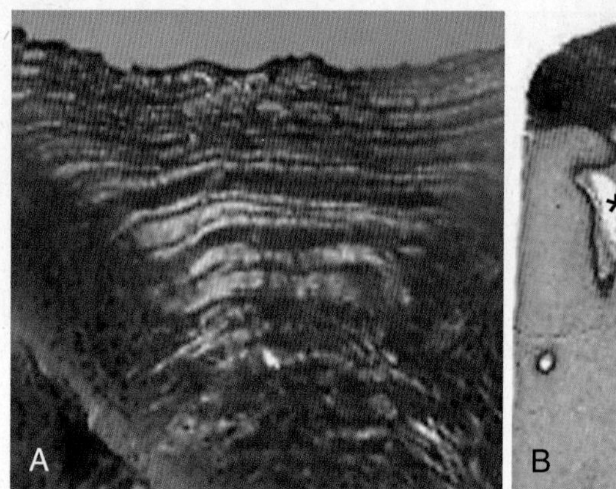

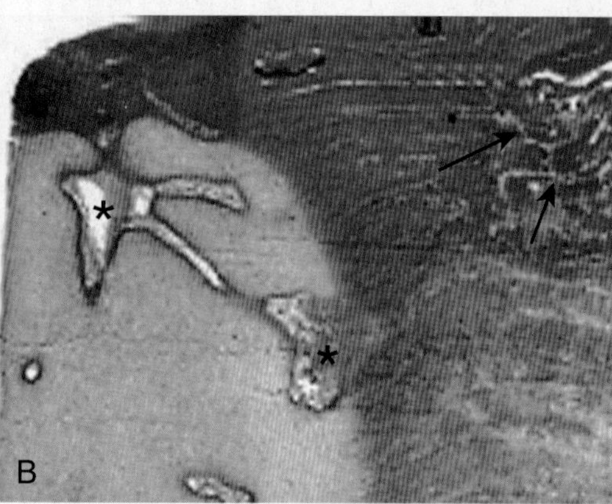

FIGURE 2.1 Histologic findings of human intervertebral discs. **A,** Specimen from 30-month-old child shows how regular concentric lamellae can be seen when specimen is viewed with polarized light. **B,** Specimen from neonate shows how outer aspect of anulus fibrosus and cartilage endplate are vascularized with blood vessels *(arrows)* and vascular channels *(asterisks).* (**A** and **B** stained with hematoxylin and eosin; original magnification, ×10 **[A]** and ×30 **[B]**. From Roberts S, Evans H, Trivedi J, et al: Histology and pathology of the human intervertebral disc, *J Bone Joint Surg* 88A[Suppl 2]:10, 2006.)

At birth, the disc has some direct blood supply contained within the cartilaginous endplates and the anulus. These vessels recede in the first years of life, and by adulthood there is no appreciable blood supply to the disc. Over time, for reasons not well understood, the water content of the gelatinous nucleus matrix decreases, with a decreased and altered proteoglycan composition. These changes lead to a more fibrous consistency of the nucleus, which ultimately fissures. Blood vessels grow into the disc through these outer fissures, with an increase in cellular proliferation and formation of cell clusters. Also, there is an increase in cell death, the mechanism of which is unknown. The cartilage endplates become thinned, with fissuring occurring with subsequent sclerosis of the subchondral endplates. The above-enumerated changes are quite similar if not identical to the changes of disc degeneration. Herniated discs have a greater number of senescent cells than nonherniated discs and have higher concentrations of matrix metalloproteinases.

The normal adult disc has a large amount of extracellular matrix and a few cells that account for about 1% by volume. These cells are of two phenotypes: anulus cells and nucleus cells. The anulus cells are more elongated and appear more like fibroblasts, whereas nucleus cells are oval and resemble chondrocytes. These two cell types behave differently and may be able to sense mechanical stresses. In culture, they respond differently to loads and produce different matrix proteins. The anulus cells produce predominantly type I collagen, whereas nucleus cells synthesize type II collagen. The characteristics of these cell types under normal and abnormal circumstances are beginning to be determined, and much is known, but this is beyond the scope of this chapter; however, this information is necessary to understand and subsequently treat disc disorders.

The cells within the disc are sustained by diffusion of nutrients into the disc through the porous central concavity of the vertebral endplate. Histologic studies have shown regions where the marrow spaces are in direct contact with the cartilage and that the central portion of the endplate is permeable to dye. Motion and weight bearing are believed to be helpful in maintaining this diffusion. The metabolic turnover of the disc is relatively high when its avascularity is considered but slow compared with other tissues. The glycosaminoglycan turnover in the disc is quite slow, requiring 500 days.

NEURAL ELEMENTS

The organization of the neural elements is strictly maintained throughout the entire neural system, even within the conus medullaris and cauda equina distally. The orientation of the nerve roots in the dural sac and at the conus medullaris follows a highly organized pattern, with the most cephalad roots lying lateral and the most caudad lying centrally. The motor roots are ventral to the sensory roots at all levels. The arachnoid mater holds the roots in these positions.

The pedicle is the key to understanding surgical spinal anatomy. The relation of the pedicle to the neural elements varies by region within the spinal column. In the cervical region, there are seven vertebrae but eight cervical roots. Accepted nomenclature allows each cervical root to exit cephalad to the pedicle of the vertebra for which it is named (e.g., the C6 nerve root exits above, or cephalad to, the C6 pedicle). This relationship changes in the thoracic spine because the C8 root exits between the C7 and T1 pedicles, requiring the T1 root to exit caudal (or below) the pedicle for which it is named. This relationship is maintained throughout the remaining more caudal segments. The naming of the disc levels is different, in that all levels where discs are present are named for the vertebral level immediately cephalad (i.e., the C6 disc is immediately caudal to the C6 vertebra, and disc pathology at that level typically would involve the C7 nerve root).

NATURAL HISTORY OF DISC DISEASE

One theory of spinal degeneration assumes that all spines degenerate and that current methods of treatment are for symptomatic relief, not for a cure. The degenerative process has been divided into three separate stages with relatively distinct findings. The first stage is dysfunction, which is seen in individuals 15 to 45 years old. It is characterized by circumferential and radial tears in the disc anulus and localized synovitis of the facet joints. The next stage is instability. This

TABLE 2.1

Spectrum of Pathologic Changes in Facet Joints and Discs and Interaction of These Changes

PHASES OF SPINAL DEGENERATION	FACET JOINTS		PATHOLOGIC RESULT		INTERVERTEBRAL DISC
Dysfunction	Synovitis	→	Dysfunction	←	Circumferential tears
	Hypermobility		↓	↖	
	Continuing degeneration	↗	Herniation	←	Radial tears
Instability	Capsular laxity	→	Instability	←	Internal disruption
	Subluxation	→	Lateral nerve entrapment	←	Disc resorption
Stabilization	Enlargement of articular processes	→	One-level stenosis	←	Osteophytes
		↳	Multilevel spondylosis and stenosis	↙	

Modified from Kirkaldy-Willis WH, editor: *Managing low back pain*, New York, 1983, Churchill Livingstone.

stage, found in 35- to 70-year-old patients, is characterized by internal disruption of the disc, progressive disc resorption, degeneration of the facet joints with capsular laxity, subluxation, and joint erosion. The final stage, present in patients older than 60 years, is stabilization. In this stage, the progressive development of hypertrophic bone around the disc and facet joints leads to segmental stiffening or frank ankylosis (Table 2.1).

Each spinal segment degenerates at a different rate. As one level is in the dysfunction stage, another may be entering the stabilization stage. Disc herniation in this scheme is considered a complication of disc degeneration in the dysfunction and instability stages. Spinal stenosis from degenerative arthritis in this scheme is a complication of bony overgrowth compromising neural tissue in the late instability and early stabilization stages.

In general, the literature supports an active care approach, minimizing centrally acting medications. The judicious use of epidural steroids also is supported for short-term relief but does not have effect on long-term outcomes. Nonprogressive neurologic deficits can be treated nonoperatively with expected improvement clinically. If surgery is necessary, it usually can be delayed 6 to 12 weeks to allow adequate opportunity for improvement. The important exceptions are patients with cervical myelopathy or progressive neurologic deficits, who are best treated surgically.

The natural history of DDD is one of recurrent episodes of pain followed by periods of significant or complete relief. The frequency and intensity of symptoms helps determine the aggressiveness of intervention.

Before a discussion of diagnostic studies, axial spine pain with radiation of radicular pain to one or more extremities must be considered. Understanding certain symptoms must be juxtaposed to a rudimentary understanding of certain pathophysiologic entities. It is doubtful if there is any other area of orthopaedics in which accurate diagnosis is as difficult or the proper treatment as challenging as in patients with persistent neck and arm or low back and leg pain. Although many patients have a clear diagnosis properly arrived at by careful history and physical examination with confirmatory imaging studies, more patients with pain have absent neurologic findings other than sensory changes and have normal imaging studies or studies that do not support the clinical complaints and findings. Inability to easily determine an appropriate diagnosis in a patient does not relieve the physician of the obligation to recommend treatment or to direct the patient to a setting where such treatment is available. Careful assessment of these patients to determine if they have problems that can be successfully treated (operatively or nonoperatively) is imperative to avoid overtreatment and undertreatment.

Operative treatment can benefit a patient if it corrects a deformity, corrects instability, relieves neural compression, or treats a combination of these problems. Obtaining a history and completing a physical examination to determine a diagnosis that should be supported by other diagnostic studies is a useful approach; conversely, matching the diagnosis and treatment to the results of diagnostic studies, as can often be done in other subspecialties of orthopaedics (e.g., treating extremity pain based on a radiograph that shows a fracture), is risky because numerous studies have documented abnormal imaging in asymptomatic populations.

DIAGNOSTIC STUDIES

RADIOGRAPHY

The simplest and most readily available diagnostic tests for cervical pain are anteroposterior and lateral radiographs of the involved spinal region. On lateral radiographs bony abnormalities, such as subluxation, congenital narrowing, or fracture, can be identified. Soft-tissue swelling may be visible. Anteroposterior radiographs can reveal uncovertebral arthritis; potential abnormalities can be identified by looking at the relationships between pedicles and the spinous processes. Obtaining other views, such as flexion and extension radiographs, can reveal if instability is present. Oblique views show the foramen. These simple radiographs show a relatively high incidence of abnormal findings.

MYELOGRAPHY

The value of myelography is the ability to check all spinal regions for abnormality and to define intraspinal lesions; it may be unnecessary if clinical and CT or MRI findings are in complete agreement. The primary indications for myelography are inability to get an MRI, suspicion of an intraspinal lesion, patients with spinal instrumentation causing artifact, or questionable diagnosis resulting from conflicting clinical

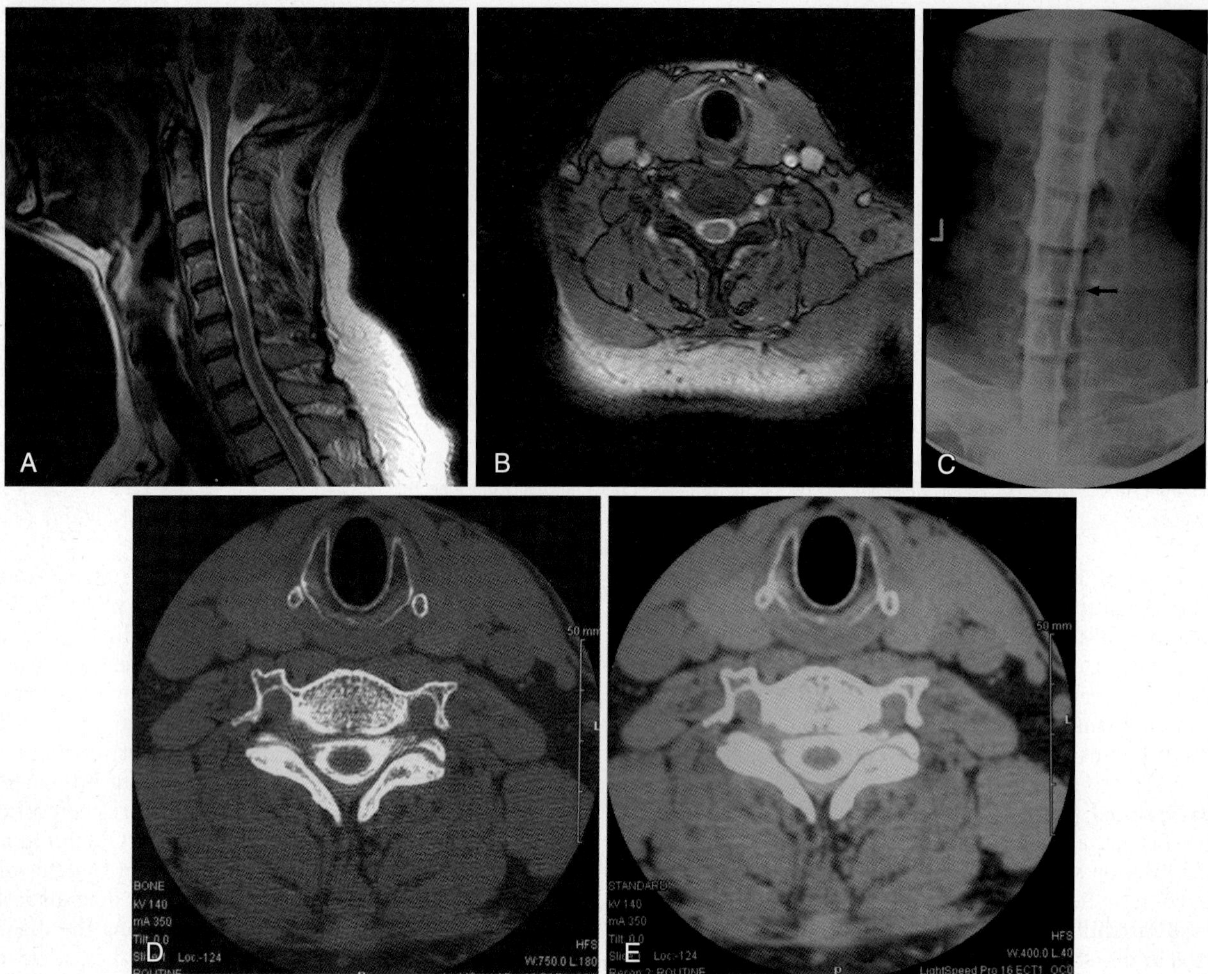

FIGURE 2.2 Forty-five-year-old patient with right C7 radiculopathy clinically. **A and B,** MRI was inconclusive for disc herniation. **C-E,** Postmyelogram CT clearly reveals right intraforaminal disc herniation.

findings and other studies (Fig. 2.2). In addition, myelography is valuable in a previously operated spine and in patients with marked bony degenerative change that may be underestimated on MRI. Myelography is improved by the use of postmyelography CT, in this setting and in evaluating spinal stenosis.

Several contrast agents have been used for myelography: air, oil contrast, and water-soluble (absorbable) contrast agents, including metrizamide (Amipaque), iohexol (Omnipaque), and iopamidol (Isovue-M). Because these nonionic agents are absorbable, the discomforts of removing them and the severity of the postmyelography headache have decreased.

COMPUTED TOMOGRAPHY

Most clinicians now agree that CT is an extremely useful diagnostic tool in the evaluation of spinal disease. The current technology and computer software have made possible the ability to reformat the standard axial cuts in almost any direction and magnify the images so that exact measurements of various structures can be made. Software is available to evaluate the density of a selected vertebra and compare it with vertebrae of the normal population to give a numerically reproducible estimate of vertebral density to quantitate osteopenia.

Numerous types of CT studies for the spine are available. One must be careful in ordering the study to ensure that the areas of clinical concern are included. Sagittal, axial, and coronal cuts allow a three-dimensional view of the cervical spine. Location markers allow finer scrutiny of the area of pathology.

MAGNETIC RESONANCE IMAGING

MRI is currently the standard for advanced imaging of the spine and is superior to CT in most circumstances, in particular, identification of infections, tumors, and degenerative changes within the discs. More importantly, MRI is superior for imaging the disc and directly imaging neural structures. Also, MRI typically shows the entire region of study (i.e., cervical, thoracic, or lumbar). Of particular value is the ability to image the nerve root in the foramen (especially with foramen specific oblique cuts), which is difficult even with postmyelography CT because the subarachnoid space and the contrast agent do not extend fully through the foramen. Despite this superiority, there are circumstances in which MRI and CT, with or without myelography, can be used in a complementary fashion.

One of the difficulties with MRI is showing anatomy that is abnormal but which may be asymptomatic. MRI evidence of disc degeneration has been reported in the cervical spine in 25% of patients younger than 40 years and in 60% of patients 60 years and older. The demonstrated findings must be carefully correlated with the clinical impression. The importance of this concept cannot be overstated. The best way to obtain meaningful clinical information from MRI of the spine is to have a specific question before the study. This question is derived from a patient's history and a careful physical examination, and is posed using the parameters of (1) neural compression, (2) instability, and (3) deformity. In each case, the specific location of the abnormality should be suspected before MRI and confirmed with the study. Ideally an advanced imaging study should be used for confirmation, not reevaluation. Only abnormalities in one or a combination of these categories are important, because operative techniques can treat only these problems. Failure to interpret an imaging study in this way, especially MRI, which is sensitive to anatomic abnormalities, would inevitably lead to poor clinical choices and outcomes.

A newer MRI imaging technique—diffusion tensor imaging—is based on the diffusion rate of water in tissue and has been reported to demonstrate spinal cord impairment in patients with early stage cervical spondylosis before it is visible on plain MRI scans (see discussion of cervical spondylotic myelopathy). The information it provides can be helpful in early identification of patients in whom operative treatment is indicated.

OTHER DIAGNOSTIC TESTS

Numerous diagnostic tests, in addition to radiography, myelography, CT, and MRI, have been used in the diagnosis of intervertebral disc disease. The primary advantage of these tests is to rule out diseases other than primary disc herniation, spinal stenosis, and spinal arthritis.

Electromyography and nerve conduction velocity can be helpful if a patient has a history and physical examination suggestive of radiculopathy at either the cervical or the lumbar level with inconclusive imaging studies. One advantage of electromyography is in the identification of peripheral nerve dysfunction and diffuse neurologic involvement indicating higher or lower lesions. Paraspinal muscles in a patient with a previous posterior open surgical approach usually are abnormal and are not a reliable diagnostic finding.

Bone scans are another procedure in which positive findings usually are not indicative of intervertebral disc disease—but they can confirm neoplastic, traumatic, and arthritic problems in the spine. Various laboratory tests, such as a complete blood cell count, differential white blood cell count, C-reactive protein, biochemical profile, urinalysis, serum protein electrophoresis, and erythrocyte sedimentation rate, are extremely good screening procedures for other causes of pain in the spine. Rheumatoid screening studies, such as rheumatoid arthritis, antinuclear antibody, lupus erythematosus cell preparation, and HLA-B27, also are useful when indicated by the clinical picture.

INJECTION STUDIES

Whenever a diagnosis is in doubt, and the complaints seem real or the pathologic condition is diffuse, identification of the source of pain is problematic. The use of local anesthetics or contrast media in various specific anatomic areas can be helpful. These agents are relatively simple, safe, and minimally painful. Contrast media such as diatrizoate meglumine (Hypaque), iothalamate meglumine (Conray), iohexol (Omnipaque), iopamidol, and metrizamide (Amipaque) have been used for discography and blocks with no reported ill effects. Reports of neurologic complications with contrast media used for discography and subsequent chymopapain injection are well documented. The best choice of a contrast medium for documenting structures outside the subarachnoid space is an absorbable medium with low reactivity because it might be injected inadvertently into the subarachnoid space. Iohexol and metrizamide are the least reactive, most widely accepted, and best tolerated of the currently available contrast media. Local anesthetics, such as lidocaine (Xylocaine), tetracaine (Pontocaine), and bupivacaine (Marcaine), are used frequently epidurally and intradurally. The use of bupivacaine should be limited to low concentrations and low volumes because of reports of death after epidural anesthesia using concentrations of 0.75% or higher.

Spinal arachnoiditis was associated in past years with the use of epidural methylprednisolone acetate (Depo-Medrol). This complication was thought to be caused by the use of the suspending agent, polyethylene glycol, which has since been eliminated from the Depo-Medrol preparation. For epidural injections, we prefer the use of Celestone Soluspan, which is a mixture of betamethasone sodium phosphate and betamethasone acetate. Celestone Soluspan provides immediate and long-term duration of action, is highly soluble, and contains no harmful preservatives. Celestone should not be mixed with local anesthetics containing preservatives such as parabens or phenol because flocculation and clogging of the suspension can occur. If Celestone is not available, other commonly used preparations for spinal injections include methylprednisolone (Depo-Medrol) and triamcinolone acetonide (Kenalog), all of which are particulate corticosteroids (Table 2.2). Isotonic saline is the only other injectable medium used frequently around the spine with no reported adverse reactions.

When discrete, well-controlled injection techniques directed at specific targets in and around the spine are used, grading the degree of pain before and after a spinal injection is helpful in determining the location of the pain generator. The patient is asked to grade the degree of pain on a 0-to-10 scale before and at various intervals after the spinal injection (Box 2.1). If a spinal injection done under fluoroscopic control results in an 80% or more decrease in the level of pain, which corresponds to the duration of action of the anesthetic agent used, we presume the target area injected to be the pain generator. Less pain reduction, 50% to 65%, does not constitute a positive response.

EPIDURAL STEROID INJECTIONS

Epidural injections in the spine were developed to diagnose and treat spinal pain. Information obtained from epidural injections can be helpful in confirming pain generators that are responsible for a patient's discomfort. Structural abnormalities do not always cause pain, and diagnostic injections can help to correlate abnormalities seen on imaging studies with associated pain complaints. In addition, epidural injections can provide pain relief during the recovery of disc or nerve root injuries and allow patients to increase their level of physical activity. Epidural steroid injections in the treatment of disc herniation and radiculitis are performed based on the pathophysiologic mechanism of reducing inflammation; however, the evidence suggests that local anesthetics with or without steroids are equally as effective as steroids alone in many settings. Because severe pain from an acute disc injury with or without radiculopathy often is time limited, therapeutic injections help to manage pain and may alleviate or decrease the need for oral analgesics.

TABLE 2.2

Common Corticosteroids Used in Spinal Interventions Compared With Hydrocortisone

	HYDROCORTISONE	METHYLPREDNISOLONE (DEPO-MEDROL)	TRIAMCINOLONE ACETONIDE (KENALOG)	BETAMETHASONE SODIUM PHOSPHATE AND ACETATE (CELESTONE SOLUSPAN)
Relative antiinflammatory potency	1	5	5	25
pH	5.0-7.0	7.0-8.0	4.5-6.5	6.8-7.2
Onset	Fast	Slow	Moderate	Fast
Duration of action	Short	Intermediate	Intermediate	Long
Concentration (mg/mL)	50	40-80	20	6
Relative mineralocorticoid activity	2+	0	0	0

From el Abd O: Steroids in spine interventions. In Slipman CW, Derby D, Simeone FA, Mayer TG, editors: *Interventional spine: an algorithmic approach*, Philadelphia, 2008, Elsevier.

BOX 2.1

Pain Scale and Diary

0 No pain
1 Mild pain that you are aware of but not bothered by
2 Moderate pain that you can tolerate without medication
3 Moderate pain that is discomforting and requires medication
4-5 More severe pain and you begin to feel antisocial
6 Severe pain
7-9 Intensely severe pain
10 Most severe pain (you might contemplate suicide because of it)

Activity	Comments	Location of Pain	Time	Severity of Pain (0-10)

Steroids prepared for intramuscular injection also have been used frequently in the epidural space with few and usually transient complications. There are conflicting reports on the short- and long-term quality-of-life outcomes and the cost-effectiveness of cervical epidural steroid injections. A cost-effectiveness analysis of steroid injection compared to conservative management for patients with radiculopathy or neck pain found that at short-term follow-up (3 months) steroid injections produced greater improvement in quality-of-life scores at a lower cost. Epstein, however, warned against cervical epidural steroid injections, citing several serious complications, including epidural hematomas, infection, inadvertent intramedullary cord injections, and cord, brainstem, and cerebellar strokes. Other cited adverse reactions include procedural-related pain, steroid side effects, and vasovagal reactions, which are relatively minor and self-limited. We have found these complications and reactions to be rare.

The most adverse immediate reaction during an epidural injection is a vasovagal reaction. Dural puncture has been estimated to occur in 0.5% to 5% of patients having cervical or lumbar epidural steroid injections. The anesthesiology literature reported a 7.5% to 75% incidence of postdural puncture (positional) headaches, with the highest estimates associated with the use of 16- and 18-gauge needles. Headache without dural puncture has been estimated to occur in 2% of patients and is attributed to air injected into the epidural space, increased intrathecal pressure from fluid around the dural sac, and possibly an undetected dural puncture. Some minor common complaints caused by corticosteroids injected into the epidural space include nonpositional headaches, facial flushing, insomnia, low-grade fever, and transient increased back or lower extremity pain. Epidural corticosteroid injections are contraindicated in the presence of infection at the injection site, systemic infection, bleeding diathesis, uncontrolled diabetes mellitus, and congestive heart failure.

We perform epidural corticosteroid injections in a fluoroscopy suite equipped with resuscitative and monitoring equipment. Intravenous access is established in all patients with a minimum of a 20-gauge angiocatheter placed in the upper extremity. Mild sedation is achieved through intravenous access with the patient remaining alert and responsive. We recommend the use of fluoroscopy for diagnostic and therapeutic epidural injections for several reasons. Epidural injections performed without fluoroscopic guidance are not always made into the epidural space or the intended interspace. Even in experienced hands, needle misplacement occurs in 40% of epidural injections when done without fluoroscopic guidance. Accidental intravascular injections also can occur, and the absence of blood return with needle aspiration before injection is an unreliable indicator of this complication. In the presence of anatomic anomalies, such as a midline epidural septum or multiple separate epidural compartments, the desired flow of epidural injectants to the presumed pain generator is restricted and remains undetected without fluoroscopy. In addition, if an injection fails to relieve pain, it would be impossible without fluoroscopy to determine whether the failure was caused by a genuine poor response or by improper needle placement.

CERVICAL EPIDURAL INJECTION

Cervical epidural steroid injections have been used with some success to treat cervical spondylosis associated with acute disc disruption and radiculopathies, cervical strain syndromes with associated myofascial pain, postlaminectomy cervical pain, reflex sympathetic dystrophy, postherpetic neuralgia, acute viral brachial plexitis, and muscle contraction headaches. The best results with cervical epidural steroid injections have been in patients with acute disc herniations or well-defined radicular symptoms and in patients with limited myofascial pain. In a group of 70 patients with herniated cervical discs without myelopathy for which conservative management failed to relieve symptoms, cervical epidural steroid injections provided significant pain relief and avoided surgery in 63%. Better outcomes were noted in patients older than 50 years and those who received the injections earlier (<100 days from diagnosis). Preoperative opioid use has been suggested to be associated with worse patient-reported outcomes. Wei et al. found that pre-injection opioid use was associated with slightly higher odds of worse disability and leg/arm pain; however, increased pre-injection opioid use did not affect long-term outcomes.

At this time, extreme caution is needed when performing cervical transforaminal injections because of the increasing number of reports of catastrophic neurologic complications involving injury to the spinal cord and brainstem after such injections. These injuries are the result of intraarterial injection into either a reinforcing radicular artery or the vertebral artery, as well as intra-arterial corticosteroid injection with distal embolization. Injection into a radicular artery is an unavoidable complication but one that can be recognized by using real-time monitoring of a test dose of contrast medium. In the case of intraarterial injection, the procedure should be aborted to avoid injury to the spinal cord.

More recent research demonstrated an alternative mechanism of injury. In a mouse model, several particulate steroids had an immediate and massive effect on microvascular perfusion because of the formation of red blood cell aggregates associated with the transformation of red blood cells into spiculated red blood cells.

INTERLAMINAR CERVICAL EPIDURAL INJECTION

TECHNIQUE 2.1

- Place the patient prone on a pain management table. We use a low-attenuated carbon fiber tabletop that allows better imaging and permits unobstructed C-arm viewing. For optimal placement and comfort, place the patient's face in a cervical prone cutout cushion.
- Cervical epidural injections using a paramedian approach should be done routinely at the C7-T1 interspace unless previous surgery of the posterior cervical spine has been done at that level, in which case the C6-7 or T1-2 level is injected. Aseptically prepare the skin area with isopropyl alcohol and povidone-iodine several segments above and below the laminar interspace to be injected. If the patient is allergic to povidone-iodine, use chlorhexidine gluconate (Hibiclens).
- Drape the area in sterile fashion.
- Using anteroposterior fluoroscopic imaging, identify the target laminar interspace. With the use of a 27-gauge, ¼-inch needle, anesthetize the skin so that a skin wheal is raised over the target interspace on the side of the patient's pain with 1 to 2 mL of 1% preservative-free lidocaine without epinephrine. To diminish the burning discomfort of the anesthetic, mix 3 mL of 8.4% sodium bicarbonate in a 30-mL bottle of 1% preservative-free lidocaine without epinephrine. Nick the skin with an 18-gauge hypodermic needle. Under fluoroscopic control, insert and advance a 22-gauge, 3½-inch spinal needle in a vertical fashion until contact is made with the upper edge of the T1 lamina 1 to 2 mm lateral to the midline.
- Anesthetize the lamina with 1 to 2 mL of 1% preservative-free lidocaine without epinephrine. Anesthetize the soft tissues with 2 mL of 1% preservative-free lidocaine without epinephrine as the spinal needle is withdrawn.
- Insert an 18-gauge, 3½-inch Tuohy epidural needle and advance it vertically within the anesthetized soft-tissue track until contact is made with the T1 lamina under fluoroscopy.
- "Walk off" the lamina with the Tuohy needle onto the ligamentum flavum. Remove the stylet from the Tuohy needle, and attach a 10-mL syringe filled halfway with air and sterile saline. Advance the Tuohy needle into the epidural space using the loss-of-resistance technique. When loss of resistance has been achieved, aspirate to check for blood or cerebrospinal fluid (CSF). If neither blood nor CSF is evident, remove the syringe from the Tuohy needle and attach a 5-mL syringe containing 1.5 mL of nonionic contrast dye.
- Confirm epidural placement by producing an epidurogram with the nonionic contrast agent (Fig. 2.3). To confirm proper placement further, adjust the C-arm to view the area from a lateral perspective. A spot radiograph can be obtained to document placement.
- Inject a test dose of 1 to 2 mL of 1% preservative-free lidocaine without epinephrine and wait 3 minutes. If the patient does not complain of warmth, burning, or significant paresthesias or show signs of apnea, place a 10-mL syringe on the Tuohy needle and slowly inject 2 mL of 1% preservative-free lidocaine without epinephrine and 2 mL of 6 mg/mL Celestone Soluspan slowly into the epidural space. If Celestone Soluspan cannot be obtained, 40 mg/mL of triamcinolone is a good substitute.

ZYGAPOPHYSEAL (FACET) JOINT INJECTIONS

The facet joint can be a source of back or neck pain; the exact cause of the pain is unknown. Theories include meniscoid entrapment and extrapment, synovial impingement, chondromalacia facetae, capsular and synovial inflammation, and mechanical injury to the joint capsule. Osteoarthritis is another cause of facet joint pain; however, the incidence of facet joint arthropathy is equal in symptomatic and asymptomatic patients. As with other osteoarthritic joints, radiographic changes correlate poorly with pain.

Although the history and physical examination may suggest that the facet joint is the cause of spine pain, no noninvasive pathognomonic findings distinguish facet joint–mediated pain from other sources of spine pain. Fluoroscopically guided facet joint injections are commonly considered the "gold standard" for isolating or excluding the facet joint as a source of spine or extremity pain.

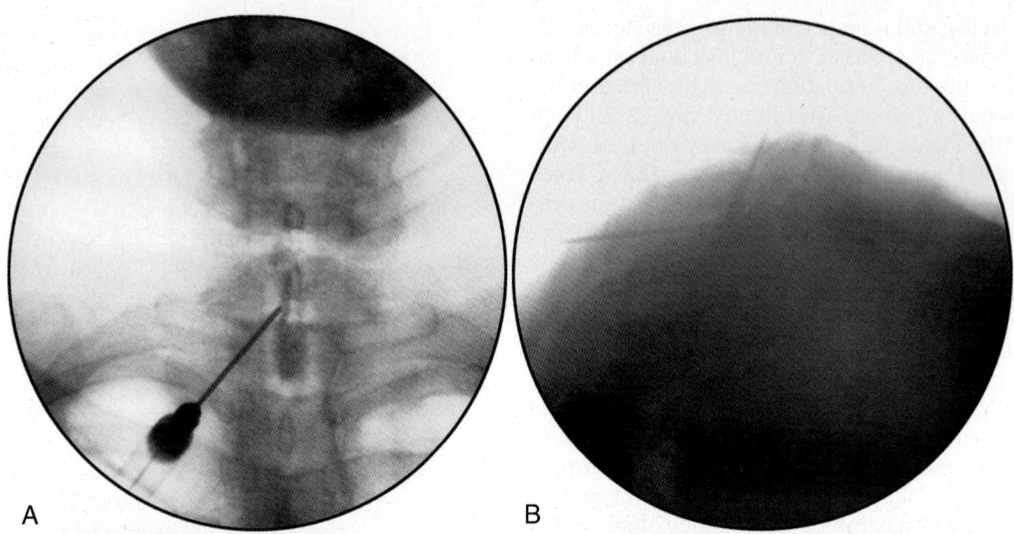

FIGURE 2.3 **A,** Posteroanterior view of cervical interlaminar epidurogram showing characteristic C7-T1 epidural contrast flow pattern. **B,** Lateral radiograph of cervical epidurogram. **SEE TECHNIQUE 2.1.**

Clinical suspicion of facet joint pain by a spine specialist remains the major indicator for diagnostic injection, which should be done only in patients who have had pain for more than 4 weeks and only after appropriate conservative measures have failed to provide relief. Facet joint injection procedures may help to focus treatment on a specific spinal segment and provide adequate pain relief to allow progression in therapy. Either intraarticular or medial branch blocks can be used for diagnostic purposes. Although injection of cortisone into the facet joint was a popular procedure through most of the 1970s and 1980s, many investigators have found no evidence that this effectively treats low back pain caused by a facet joint. The only controlled study on the use of intraarticular corticosteroids in the cervical spine found no added benefit from intraarticular betamethasone over bupivacaine.

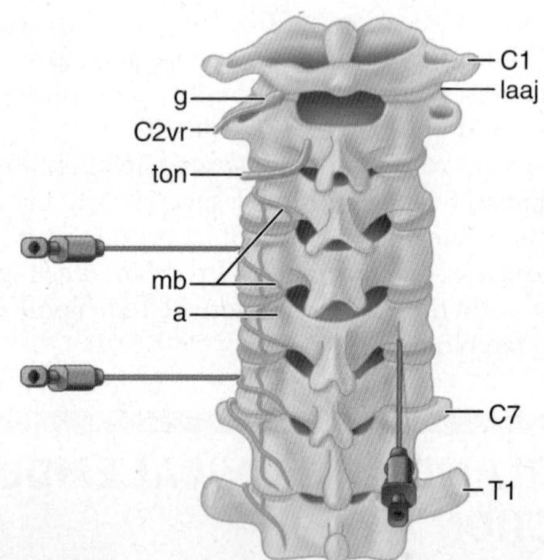

FIGURE 2.4 Proper needle placement for posterior approach to C4 and C6 medial branch blocks. Second cervical ganglion *(g)*, third occipital nerve *(ton)*, C2 ventral ramus *(C2vr)*, and lateral atlantoaxial joint *(laaj)* are noted. *a*, Articular facet; *mb*, medial branch. **SEE TECHNIQUE 2.2.**

CERVICAL MEDIAL BRANCH BLOCK INJECTION

TECHNIQUE 2.2

- Place the patient prone on the pain management table. Rotate the patient's neck so that the symptomatic side is down. This allows the vertebral artery to be positioned further beneath the articular pillar, creates greater accentuation of the cervical waists, and prevents the jaw from being superimposed. Aseptically prepare and drape the side to be injected.
- Identify the target location using anteroposteriorly directed fluoroscopy. Each cervical facet joint from C3-4 to C7-T1 is supplied from the medial nerve branch above and below the joint that curves consistently around the "waist" of the articular pillar of the same numbered vertebrae (Fig. 2.4). To block the C6 facet joint nerve supply, anesthetize the C6 and C7 medial branches.
- Insert a 22- or 25-gauge, 3½-inch spinal needle perpendicular to the pain management table and advance it under fluoroscopic control ventrally and medially until contact is made with periosteum. Direct the spinal needle laterally until the needle tip reaches the lateral margin of the waist of the articular pillar and then direct the needle until it rests at the deepest point of the articular pillar's concavity under fluoroscopy.
- Remove the stylet. If there is a negative aspirate, inject 0.5 mL of 0.75% preservative-free bupivacaine.

CERVICAL DISCOGRAPHY

The approach to the cervical spine differs from the approaches used for discography of the lumbar and thoracic spine. The cervical spine is approached anteriorly rather than posteriorly.

Complications associated with cervical discography because of the surrounding anatomy include injury to the trachea, esophagus, carotid artery, and jugular veins and spinal cord injury and pneumothorax. Discitis is a concern in the cervical spine; disc infection often originates from the gram-negative and anaerobic flora of the esophagus.

Traditionally, the approach to the cervical intervertebral discs has been via a paralaryngeal route that requires displacement of the trachea and esophagus away from the site of entry. A more lateral approach that is gaining popularity bypasses these structures and does not require such displacement.

CERVICAL DISCOGRAPHY

TECHNIQUE 2.3

(FALCO)

- Place the patient supine on the procedure table.
- Insert an angiocatheter into the upper extremity and begin intravenous antibiotic infusion. Alternatively, intradiscal antibiotics can be given during surgery.
- Sedate the patient, and prepare and drape the skin sterilely, including the anterolateral aspect of the neck.
- Under fluoroscopic imaging, identify the intervertebral discs with aligned endplates and sharp margins of the intervertebral discs. Approach the paralaryngeal area from the right, using a finger to displace the esophagus and trachea to the left and the carotid artery to the right. With the other hand, insert a 2- or 3½-inch spinal needle over the finger through the skin and into the outer anulus of the disc. Advance the needle into the center of the disc, using anteroposterior and lateral fluoroscopic guidance.
- An alternative method is a more lateral approach to the cervical spine using a single needle. This approach may reduce the incidence of infection by passing the needle posterior to the trachea and esophagus en route to the disc space. Position the patient or the C-arm to place the cervical spine in an oblique position for optimal foraminal exposure and continue adjusting until the endplates, disc space, and uncovertebral process are in sharp focus (Fig. 2.5).
- Insert a 2- or 3½-inch needle into the skin and advance it until the tip makes contact with the subjacent uncovertebral process. "Walk off" the needle just anterior to the uncovertebral process. Advance the needle into the center of the disc, using anteroposterior and lateral fluoroscopic guidance.
- After needle placement with either technique, the rest of the procedure is essentially the same as that described for thoracic or lumbar discography (Chapter 3).
- Inject either saline or a nonionic contrast dye into each disc.
- Record any pain response as none, dissimilar, similar, or exact in relationship to the patient's typical pain. Record intradiscal pressures to assist in determining if the disc is the cause of the pain.
- Perform radiography and CT of the cervical spine on completion of the study.

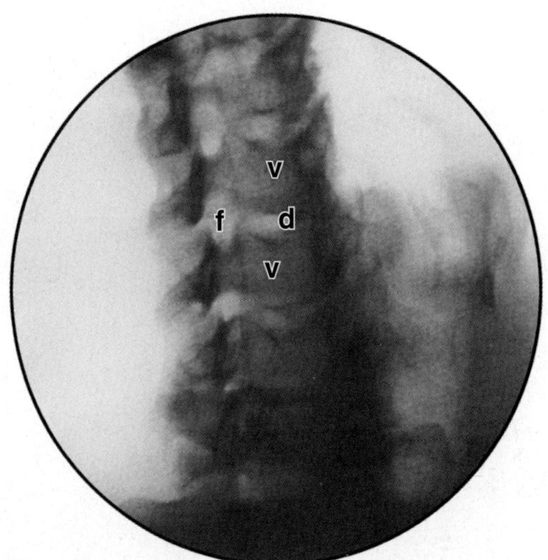

FIGURE 2.5 Foraminal position for performing cervical discography with anterolateral approach. *d*, Intervertebral disc; *f*, foramen; *v*, vertebral body. (Courtesy of Frank J. E. Falco, MD.) **SEE TECHNIQUE 2.3.**

CERVICAL DISC DISEASE

Herniation of the cervical intervertebral disc with spinal cord compression has been identified since Key detailed the pathologic findings of two cases of cord compression by "intervertebral substance" in 1838. Cervical disc disease is slightly more common in men. Factors associated with the injury are frequent heavy lifting on the job, cigarette smoking, and frequent diving from a board. Patients with cervical disc disease also are likely to have lumbar disc disease. MRI has shown increasing cervical disc degeneration with age.

The pathophysiology of cervical disc disease is the same as DDD in other areas of the spine as described by Kirkaldy-Willis. Physiologic changes in the nucleus are followed by progressive annular degeneration. Frank extrusion of nuclear material can occur as a complication of this normal degenerative process. As the disc degeneration proceeds, hypermobility of the segment can result in instability or degenerative arthritic changes or both. In contrast to those in the lumbar spine, these hypertrophic changes are predominantly at the uncovertebral joint (uncinate process) (Fig. 2.6). Hypertrophic changes eventually develop around the facet joints and vertebral bodies. Progressive stiffening of the cervical spine and loss of motion are the usual result in the end stages. Hypertrophic spurring anteriorly occasionally results in dysphagia. Increased amounts of matrix metalloproteinases, nitric oxide, prostaglandin E_2, and interleukin-6 have been identified in disc material removed from cervical disc hernias, suggesting that these products are involved in the biochemistry of disc degeneration. These substances also are implicated in pain production.

The classic approach to discs in this region has been posteriorly with laminectomy. Anterior cervical discectomy with fusion is still the most commonly performed procedure when the disc is removed anteriorly to avoid disc space collapse, but the reported results of disc arthroplasty have it challenging the gold standard of ACDF. Foraminotomy is the classic procedure of choice when the disc fragment is lateral and can be removed posteriorly but fully endoscopic foraminotomy is

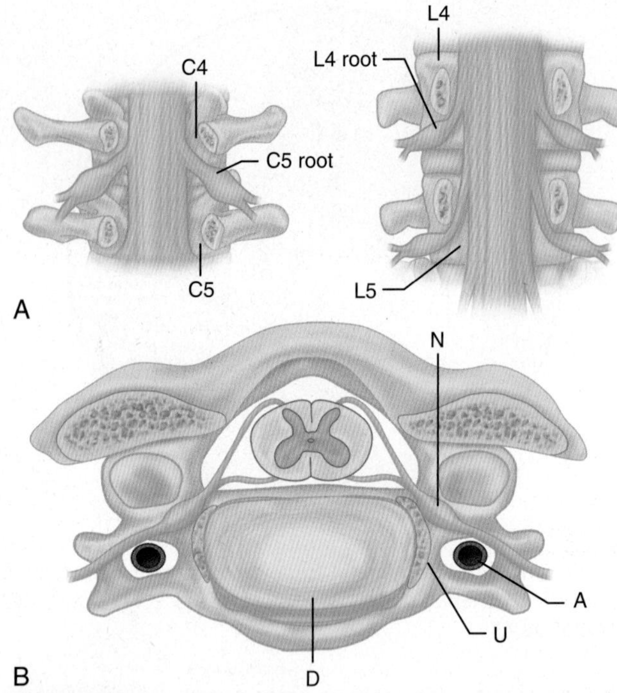

FIGURE 2.6 **A,** Comparison of points at which nerve roots emerge from cervical and lumbar spine. **B,** Cross-sectional view of cervical spine at level of disc *(D)*. Uncinate process *(U)* forms ventral wall of foramen. Root *(N)* exits dorsal to vertebral artery *(A)*.

showing promise to be the procedure that provides the least immediate morbidity and quickest recovery.

SIGNS AND SYMPTOMS

The signs and symptoms of cervical intervertebral disc disease are best separated into symptoms related to the spine itself, symptoms related to nerve root compression, and symptoms of myelopathy. Several authors reported that when the disc is punctured anteriorly for the purpose of discography, pain is noted in the neck and shoulder. Complaints of neck pain, medial scapular pain, and shoulder pain are probably related to primary pain around the disc and spine. Anatomic studies have indicated cervical disc and ligamentous innervations. This has been inferred to be similar in the cervical spine to that of the lumbar spine, with its sinuvertebral nerve.

Symptoms of root compression usually are associated with pain radiating into the arm or chest with numbness in the fingers and motor weakness. Cervical disc disease also can mimic cardiac disease with chest and arm pain. Usually the radicular symptoms are intermittent and combined with more frequent neck and shoulder pain.

The signs of midline cervical spinal cord compression (myelopathy) are unique and varied. The pain is poorly localized and aching and may be only a minor complaint. Occasional sharp pain or generalized tingling may be described with neck extension. This is similar to the Lhermitte sign in multiple sclerosis. The pain can be in the shoulder and pelvic girdles; it is occasionally associated with a generalized feeling of weakness in the lower extremities and a feeling of instability. Global numbness in the upper extremities and difficulty with fine motor coordination are common findings. Gait disturbances and difficulty with tandem gait may be the first symptoms.

BOX 2.2

C5 Nerve Root Compression

Sensory Deficit
Upper lateral arm and elbow

Motor Weakness
Deltoid
Biceps (variable)

Reflex Change
Biceps (variable)

Indicative of C4-5 disc rupture or other pathologic condition at that level.

BOX 2.3

C6 Nerve Root Compression

Sensory Deficit
Lateral forearm, thumb, and index finger

Motor Weakness
Biceps
Extensor carpi radialis longus and brevis

Reflex Change
Biceps
Brachioradialis

Indicative of C5-6 disc herniation or other local pathologic condition at that level.

BOX 2.4

C7 Nerve Root Compression

Sensory Deficit
Middle finger (variable because of overlap)

Motor Weakness
Triceps
Wrist flexors (flexor carpi radialis)
Finger extensors (variable)

Reflex Change
Triceps

Indicative of C6-7 disc rupture or other pathologic condition at that level.

In patients with predominant cervical spondylosis, symptoms of vertebral artery compression also may be found, including dizziness, tinnitus, intermittent blurring of vision, and occasional episodes of retroocular pain. The signs of lateral root pressure from a disc or osteophytes are predominantly neurologic (Boxes 2.2 to 2.6). By evaluating multiple motor groups, multiple levels of deep tendon reflexes, and sensory abnormalities, the level of the lesion can be localized as accurately as any other lesion in the nervous system. The multiple innervation of muscles sometimes can lead to confusion in determining the exact root involved. For this reason, MRI or other studies done for imaging confirmation of the clinical impression usually are helpful.

Rupture of the C4-5 disc with compression of the C5 nerve root should result in weakness in the deltoid and biceps

BOX 2.5

C8 Nerve Root Compression

Sensory Deficit
Ring finger, little finger, and ulnar border of palm

Motor Weakness
Interossei
Finger flexors (variable)
Flexor carpi ulnaris (variable)

Reflex Change
None

Indicative of C7-T1 disc rupture or other pathologic condition at that level.

BOX 2.6

T1 Nerve Root Compression

Sensory Deficit
Medial aspect of elbow

Motor Weakness
Interossei

Reflex Change
None

Indicative of T1-2 disc rupture or other pathologic condition at that level.

muscles. The deltoid is almost entirely innervated by C5, but the biceps has dual innervation. The biceps reflex may be diminished with injury to this nerve root, although it also has a C6 component, and this must be considered. Sensory testing should show a patch on the lateral aspect of the proximal arm to be diminished (Fig. 2.7).

Rupture of the C5-6 disc with compression of the C6 root can be confused with other root levels because of dual innervation of structures. Weakness may be noted in the biceps and extensor carpi radialis longus and brevis. As mentioned earlier, the biceps is dually innervated by C5 and C6, whereas the long extensors are dually innervated by C6 and C7. The brachioradialis and biceps reflexes also may be diminished at this level. Sensory testing usually indicates a decreased sensibility over the lateral proximal forearm, thumb, and index finger.

Rupture of the C6-7 disc with compression of the C7 root frequently results in weakness of the triceps. Weakness of the wrist flexors, especially the flexor carpi radialis, also is more indicative of C7 root problems. Extensor digitorum communis weakness also can indicate C7 root involvement and may be more readily apparent because of the normal relative weakness of this muscle compared with the triceps. Weakness of the flexor carpi ulnaris usually is caused more by C8 lesions. As mentioned earlier, finger extensors also may be weakened in that they have C7 and C8 innervation. The triceps reflex may be diminished. Sensation is diminished in the middle finger. C7 sensibility varies because it is so narrow, and overlap is prominent. Definite sensibility change can be difficult to document.

Rupture between C7 and T1 with compression of the C8 nerve root results in no reflex changes. Weakness may be noted in the finger flexors and in the interossei of the hand. Sensibility is lost on the ulnar border of the palm, including the ring and little fingers. Compression of the T1 nerve root produces weakness of the interosseous muscles, decreased sensibility around the medial aspect of the elbow, and no reflex changes.

Care should be taken in the examination of the extremity when radicular problems are encountered, to rule out more distal compression syndromes in the upper extremities, such as thoracic outlet syndrome, carpal tunnel syndrome, and cubital tunnel syndrome. The lower extremities should be examined with special attention to long tract signs indicating myelopathy.

Although no tests for movement of the upper extremity correspond with straight-leg raising tests in the lower extremity, the Spurling test is a maneuver that is 95% sensitive and 94% specific for diagnosing cervical nerve root pathology. A positive Spurling sign occurs when pain radiates in a dermatomal distribution ipsilaterally when the examiner turns the patient's head to the affected side while extending the neck and applying downward pressure on the head.

The shoulder abduction relief sign is another clinical sign that can be helpful in diagnosing cervical root compression syndromes. The test consists of shoulder abduction and elbow flexion with placement of the hand on the top of the head. This maneuver should relieve the arm pain caused by radicular compression. If this position is allowed to persist for 1 or 2 minutes and pain is increased, more distal compressive neuropathies, such as a tardy ulnar nerve syndrome (cubital tunnel syndrome) or primary shoulder pathologic conditions, often are the cause. This is a very good test for distinguishing cervical pathology from shoulder pathology.

Cervical paraspinal spasm and limitation of neck motion are frequent findings of cervical spine disease but do not indicate a specific pathologic process. Special maneuvers involving neck motion can be helpful in the selection of conservative treatment and identification of pathologic processes. The distraction test, which involves the examiner placing the hands on the occiput and jaw and distracting the cervical spine in the neutral position, can relieve root compression pain, but also can increase pain caused by ligamentous injury. Neck extension and flexion with or without traction can be helpful in selecting conservative therapies.

Patients relieved of pain with the neck extended, with or without traction, usually have hyperextension syndromes with ligamentous injury posteriorly, whereas patients relieved of pain with distraction and neck flexion are more likely to have nerve root compression caused by a soft ruptured disc or (more likely) hypertrophic spurs in the neural foramina. Pain usually is increased in any condition with compression. One must be careful before applying compression or distraction to ensure no cervical instability or fracture is present. One also must be careful in interpreting the distraction test to ensure the temporomandibular joint is not diseased or injured, because distraction also would increase the pain in this area.

The signs of midline disc herniation are those of spinal cord compression. If the lesion is high in the cervical region, paresthesias, weakness, atrophy, and occasionally fasciculations may occur in the hands. A Hoffman sign (upper cervical spinal cord) or the inverted radial reflex also may be present when the pathology is at or above the C5/6 level. Most commonly, however, the first and most prominent symptoms

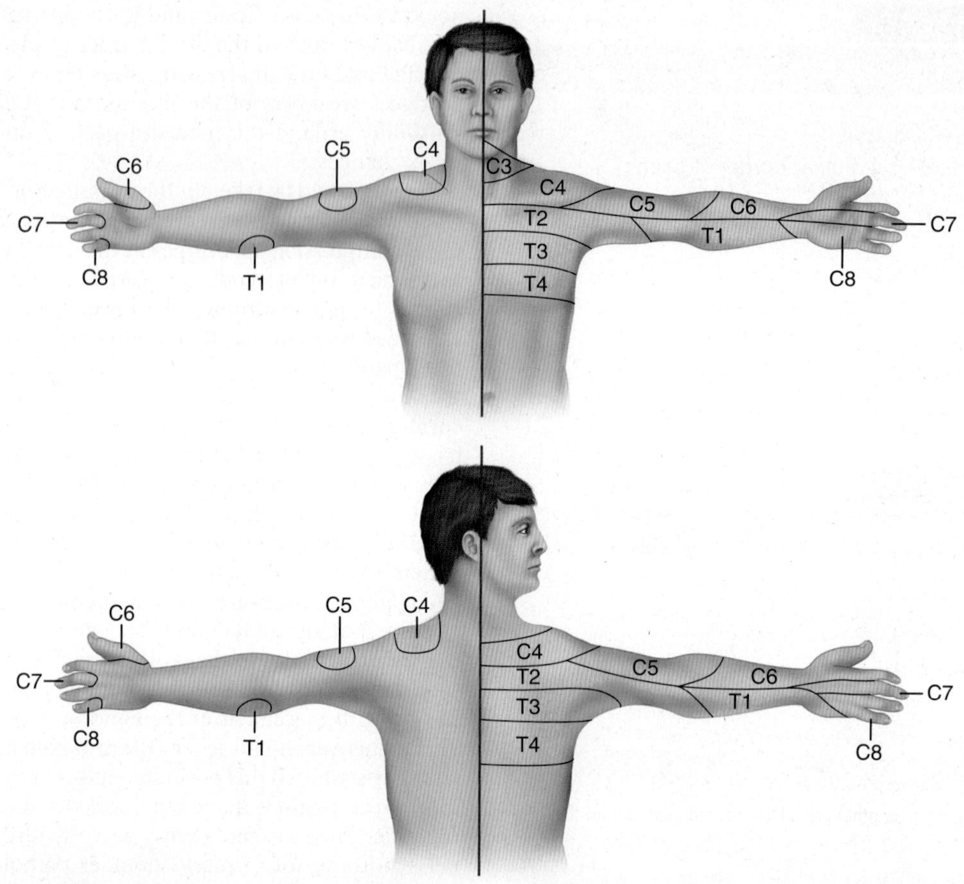

FIGURE 2.7 Anterior and posterior cervical dermatomes.

are those of involvement of the corticospinal tract; less commonly, the posterior columns are affected. The primary signs are sustained clonus, hyperactive reflexes, and the Babinski reflex. Less significant findings are varying degrees of spasticity, weakness in the legs, and impairment of proprioception. Equilibrium may be grossly disturbed, but sense of pain and temperature sense rarely are lost and usually are of little localizing value.

DIFFERENTIAL DIAGNOSIS

The differential diagnosis of cervical disc disease is best separated into extrinsic and intrinsic factors. Extrinsic factors generally include disease processes extrinsic to the neck resulting in symptoms similar to primary neck problems. Included in this group are tumors of the chest; nerve compression syndromes distal to the spine; degenerative processes, such as shoulder and upper extremity arthritis; temporomandibular joint syndrome; and lesions around the shoulder, such as acute and chronic rotator cuff tears and impingement syndromes. Intrinsic problems primarily consist of lesions directly associated with the cervical spine, the most common being cervical disc degeneration with concomitant disc herniation or later development of hypertrophic arthritis. Congenital factors, such as spinal stenosis in the cervical region, also may produce symptoms. Primary and secondary tumors of the cervical spine and fractures of the cervical vertebrae also should be considered as intrinsic lesions.

Odom et al. categorized cervical disc disease into four groups: (1) unilateral soft disc protrusion with nerve root compression; (2) foraminal spur, or hard disc, with nerve root compression; (3) medial soft disc protrusion with spinal cord compression; and (4) transverse ridge or cervical spondylosis with spinal cord compression. Soft disc herniations usually affect one level, whereas hard disc herniations can affect multiple levels. Central lesions usually result in cord compression symptoms, and lateral lesions usually result in radicular symptoms.

Most of the soft disc herniations in the series of Odom et al. occurred at the C6 interspace (70%) and C5 interspace (24%). Only six occurred at the C7 interspace. Foraminal spurs also were found predominantly at the C6 interspace (48%). The C5 interspace (39%) and C7 interspace (13%) accounted for the remaining levels where foraminal spurs were found. These investigators also noted the incidence of medial soft disc protrusion with myelopathy to be rare (14 of 246 patients).

CONFIRMATORY IMAGING

Radiographic evaluation of the cervical spine frequently shows loss of normal cervical lordosis. Disc space narrowing and hypertrophic changes frequently increase with age but are not indicative of cervical disc rupture. Usually radiographs are most helpful to rule out other problems. Oblique radiographs of the cervical spine may reveal foraminal encroachment.

MRI of the cervical spine has rapidly become the major diagnostic procedure for neck, arm, and shoulder symptoms. MRI should confirm the objective clinical findings.

Asymptomatic findings should be expected to increase with the age of the patient. Cervical myelography usually is indicated only after noninvasive evaluation by MRI fails to reveal the cause or level of the lesion or the patient is unable to obtain an MRI. If MRI is inconclusive, electromyography or nerve conduction velocity may be indicated to show active radiculopathy before proceeding with myelography, especially if the history and physical examination are not strongly supportive of the presence of radiculopathy.

Cervical discography is a controversial technique with limited benefits. It is not indicated in frank disc rupture, spondylosis, or spinal stenosis. The primary use is in patients with persistent neck pain without localized neurologic findings in whom standard MRI, myelography, and CT scan are inconclusive. Some investigators maintain that isolated painful discs can be identified in some patients by discography. A degenerative disc without pain on injection is not likely to be the source of the patient's complaint. Cervical discography requires considerable care and caution. It should be considered a preoperative test in patients in whom an anterior disc excision and interbody fusion are considered for primary neck and shoulder pain. Assessing the psychosocial well-being of a patient is recommended before proceeding with operative treatment. Great care is required in the technique and in the interpretation if reproducible results are desired. Cervical root blocks also have been suggested for the localization and confirmation of symptomatic root compression when used in conjunction with cervical discography. Facet joint injections also should be considered before fusion as a therapeutic and diagnostic procedure. These procedures were described earlier in this chapter.

When a component of dynamic cord compression is present, myelography remains a valuable tool, although dynamic MRI has reduced the role of myelography. Myelography is performed for ruptured cervical discs. Considerable attention must be paid to the flow of the column of contrast medium with the neck in hyperextended, neutral, and flexed positions. One cannot conclude that spinal cord compression is not present until one is certain that the cephalad flow of the medium is not obstructed with the neck acutely hyperextended. The neck should be hyperextended carefully because of the danger of further damage to the spinal cord. Cervical dynamic instability can be shown because the cephalad flow of contrast material is blocked between the lamina of the cephalad level and the disc or body of the caudal level.

NONOPERATIVE TREATMENT

As discussed earlier, most patients with symptomatic cervical disc herniations respond well to nonoperative treatment, including some patients with nonprogressive radicular weakness (between 70% and 80%). Reasonably good evidence shows that acute disc herniations decrease in size over time in the cervical region. Many conservative treatment methods for neck pain are used for multiple diagnoses. The primary purpose of the cervical spine and associated musculature is to support and mobilize the head while providing a conduit for the nervous system. The forces on the cervical spine are much smaller than on the lower spinal levels. The cervical spine is vulnerable to muscular tension forces, postural fatigue, and excessive motion. Most nonoperative treatments focus on one or more of these factors. The best primary treatment is short periods of rest, massage, ice, and antiinflammatory agents (glucocorticoids or nonsteroidal antiinflammatory) with active mobilization as soon as possible. The position of the neck for comfort is essential for relief of pain. The position of greatest relief may suggest the offending pathologic process or mechanism of injury. Patients with hyperflexion injuries usually are more comfortable with the neck in extension over a small roll under the neck. No specific position indicates lateral disc herniation, although most patients tolerate the neutral position best. Patients with spondylosis (hard disc) are most comfortable with the neck in flexion.

Cervical traction can be helpful in selected patients. Care must be exercised in instructing the patient in the proper use of traction. It should be applied to the head in the position of maximal pain relief. Traction never should be continued if it increases pain. The weights should rarely exceed 10 lb (weight of the head). The proper head halter and duration of traction sessions should be chosen to prevent irritation of the temporomandibular joint. Traction applied by a patient-controlled pneumatic force, which is more mobile than halter-type units, avoids irritation of the temporomandibular joint. Traction also should allow general relaxation of the patient. "Poor man's" traction is a simple method of evaluating the efficacy of cervical traction. It uses the weight of the unsupported head for the traction weight (about 10 lb). For extension traction, the patient is supine and the head is allowed to extend gently off the examining table or bed. For flexion, the same procedure is repeated in the prone position. The patient continues the exercise in the position that is most comfortable for 5 to 10 minutes several times daily.

The postural aspects of neck pain can be treated with more frequent changes in position and ergonomic changes in the work area to prevent fatigue and encourage good posture. Techniques to minimize or relieve tension also are helpful.

Cervical braces usually limit excessive motion. Similar to traction, they should be tailored to the most comfortable neck position. Except in cases of trauma, use of an orthosis should be limited to prevent atrophy of the musculature. They may be most helpful for patients who are very active.

Neck and shoulder exercises are most beneficial as the acute pain subsides. Isometric exercises are helpful in the acute phase. Occasionally, shoulder problems, such as adhesive capsulitis, may be found concomitantly with cervical spondylosis; complete immobilization of the painful extremity should be avoided. Physical therapy should be initiated.

OPERATIVE TREATMENT

The primary indications for operative treatment of cervical disc disease are (1) failure of nonoperative pain management; (2) increasing and significant neurologic deficit; and (3) cervical myelopathy, which predictably progresses, based on natural history studies. In most patients, the persistence of pain is the primary indication. The intensity of the persistent pain should be severe enough to interfere consistently with the patient's desired activity and greater than would reasonably be expected after operative treatment. The approach chosen should be determined by the location and type of lesion. Soft lateral discs are easily removed with the posterior approach, whereas soft central or hard discs (central or lateral) probably are best treated with an anterior approach. Any controversy that existed relative to the need for fusion with anterior discectomy essentially has been

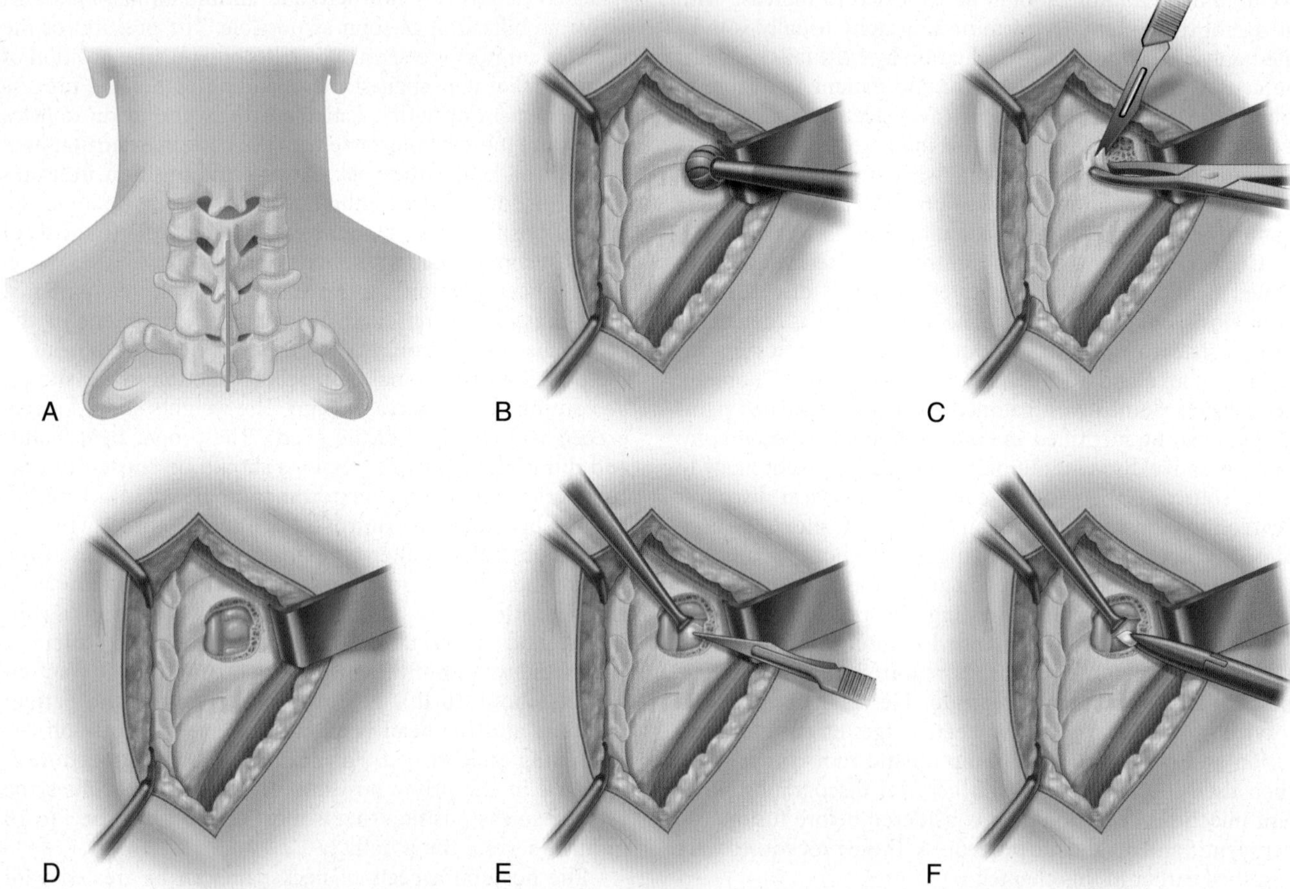

FIGURE 2.8 Technique of removal of disc between fifth and sixth cervical vertebrae. **A,** Midline incision extending from spinous process of C5 to that of C6. **B,** Paraspinal muscles have been dissected from laminae and retracted laterally. Hole is to be drilled with high-speed burr (see text). **C,** Ligamentum flavum is being dissected. **D,** Defect measuring about 1.3 cm has been made (see text) to expose nerve root and lateral aspect of dura. **E,** Nerve root has been separated from nucleus and retracted superiorly to expose herniated disc. **F,** Longitudinal ligament has been incised, and loose fragment of nucleus is being removed. **SEE TECHNIQUE 2.4.**

resolved with long-term follow-up studies of patients without fusion, such as that by Yamamoto et al. Osteophytes that were not removed at surgery frequently have been shown to be reabsorbed at the level of fusion. The use of a graft also prevents the collapse of the disc space and maintains adequate foraminal size.

REMOVAL OF POSTEROLATERAL HERNIATIONS BY POSTERIOR APPROACH (POSTERIOR CERVICAL FORAMINOTOMY)

TECHNIQUE 2.4

- With the patient under general endotracheal anesthesia in the prone position and the head in a Mayfield positioner, flex the neck to decrease the cervical lordosis as much as possible. The upright position for surgery decreases venous bleeding, but we are reluctant to recommend its use because of concern regarding the possibility of air embolism and cerebral hypoxia in the event of a significant decline in blood pressure. Usually a slight reverse Trendelenburg position works well in posterior cervical surgery, coupled with careful dissection to minimize bleeding. The shoulders are retracted inferiorly with tape if imaging of the lower cervical levels is contemplated. This imaging is needed if a microsurgical technique using tubular retractors is chosen (see Technique 2.5).
- Appropriately prepare and drape the operative field.
- Make a midline incision centered on the spinous process tip of the cephalad level involved (Fig. 2.8A) and 2 cm in length. Retract the edges of this incision and the skin withdraws in a cephalad direction so that the wound becomes properly placed.
- Divide the ligamentum nuchae longitudinally to expose the tips of the spinous processes above and below the designated area. The correct position is reasonably well ensured by palpation of the last bifid spinous process, which usually is C6. It must be verified intraoperatively, however, by a marker attached to the spinous process and documented on the lateral cervical spine radiograph.

- Dissect subperiosteally the paravertebral muscles from the laminae on the side of the lesion and retract them with a self-retaining retractor or with the help of an assistant using a hand-held retractor (Fig. 2.8B).
- With a small high-speed burr, drill away the caudal edge of the lateral portion of the lamina cephalad to the interspace (see Fig. 2.8B). Usually minimal bone removal from the cephalad edge of the lateral portion of the caudal lamina is needed. Only a small amount of the medial portion of the facet needs to be removed in most patients. A small Kerrison rongeur (1 to 2 mm) can be used to enlarge this keyhole as needed.
- Sharply excise the ligamentum flavum with a small Kerrison rongeur and identify the nerve root, which is commonly displaced posteriorly and flattened by pressure from the underlying disc fragments (Fig. 2.8C). Removal of additional bone along the dorsal aspect of the foramen and immediately above and below the nerve root often is beneficial at this point (Fig. 2.8D).
- When the bony removal has been completed, we prefer to use the operative microscope for the remainder of the procedure. This allows more delicate work around the neural elements, while minimizing additional bone removal, and allows better hemostasis.
- The herniated nucleus pulposus most often lies slightly caudal to the center of the nerve root but occasionally is cephalad. Gently retract the nerve root superiorly to expose the extruded nuclear fragments or a distended posterior longitudinal ligament (Fig. 2.8E). The nerve root should not be retracted in a caudal direction. If additional exposure is needed, remove more bone rather than risk nerve root or spinal cord injury from traction on the root. To control troublesome venous oozing at this point, use bipolar cautery if possible. Otherwise, place tiny pledgets of cotton and thrombin-soaked absorbable gelatin sponge (Gelfoam) above and below the nerve root. Do not pack the pledgets tightly around the nerve. The nerve root can be retracted slightly in a cephalad direction to allow incision of the posterior longitudinal ligament over the herniated nucleus pulposus in a cruciate manner to permit the removal of the disc fragments (Fig. 2.8F).
- After removal of all visible loose fragments, it is imperative to search thoroughly for additional fragments laterally and medially. Ensure that the nerve root is thoroughly decompressed by inserting a probe in the intervertebral foramen. If the nerve root still seems to be tight, remove more bone from the articular facets until the nerve root is completely free. Because recurrence is so rare, do not curet the intervertebral space.
- Remove any cotton pledgets and Gelfoam after meticulous hemostasis has been achieved. Hemostasis must be complete because postoperative hemorrhage can produce cord compression and quadriplegia.
- Close the wound by suturing the fascia to the supraspinous ligament with interrupted sutures and then suturing the subcutaneous layers and skin.

POSTOPERATIVE CARE Neurologic function is closely monitored after surgery. Discharge is permitted when the patient is ambulatory, which usually is the same day as surgery. Pain should be controlled with oral medication. Radicular pain relief usually is dramatic and prompt, although hypesthesia can persist for weeks or months. The patient is allowed to return to clerical work when comfortable and to manual labor after 6 weeks. As a rule, neither support nor physical therapy is necessary, and the patient's future activity is not restricted. Isometric neck exercises, upper extremity range-of-motion exercises, and posterior shoulder girdle exercises can be useful for patients in whom atrophy or inactivity has been considerable. A soft cervical collar can help relieve immediate postoperative pain.

MINIMALLY INVASIVE POSTERIOR APPROACHES TO THE CERVICAL SPINE

Because of the extensive subperiosteal stripping of the paraspinal musculature required for open posterior approaches, which can result in significant postoperative pain, muscle spasm, and dysfunction, less invasive procedures have been developed. Cited advantages of these "minimally invasive" techniques include shorter operative time, fewer operative risks, less blood loss, less postoperative pain, and earlier return to activity. The advent of muscle-splitting tubular retractor systems and improvements in endoscopic technology have led to the development of microendoscopic and full-endoscopic techniques for posterior cervical foraminotomy and fusion. Indications for minimally invasive posterior cervical procedures include radiculopathy caused by lateral disc herniation or foraminal stenosis, persistent or recurrent nerve root symptoms after anterior cervical discectomy, and cervical disc disease in patients for whom anterior approaches are contraindicated (e.g., those with anterior neck infection, tracheostomy, prior irradiation, previous radical neck surgery or neoplasm). Contraindications are much the same as those for open treatment and include pure axial neck pain without neurologic symptoms, gross cervical instability, symptomatic central disc herniation, and kyphotic deformity that would make posterior decompression ineffective.

A number of studies have reported the efficacy and safety of minimally invasive cervical procedures. In a systematic review and meta-analysis including 14 studies and 1216 patients, Sahai et al. found that minimally invasive posterior cervical foraminotomy resulted in significantly greater improvement in visual analog scale (VAS) scores compared to anterior cervical discectomy and fusion (ACDF), while rates of complications and reoperations were similar. In a comparison of microendoscopic laminotomy with conventional laminoplasty for cervical spondylotic myelopathy, neurologic outcomes were similar at 5-year follow-up, but patients with microendoscopic laminotomy had significantly less postoperative axial pain and improved subaxial cervical lordosis. In a comparison of microendoscopic selective laminectomy (46 patients) to conventional laminoplasty (41 patients) in patients with degenerative cervical myelopathy, Oshima et al. reported that microendoscopic laminectomy resulted in better outcomes in terms of postoperative range of motion, axial pain, and quality of life, although both procedures showed good neurologic improvement.

One cited disadvantage of minimally invasive techniques is the learning curve required to become proficient. Reported numbers of cases required range from 0 to 50. In a study at our institution, the mean operative time steadily decreased over the first 50 procedures to approximately 60% of the initial times, where it plateaued for both the transforaminal and interlaminar approaches (mean time 65 minutes), but there was no difference in the frequency of reoperation over the length of the learning curve.

MINIMALLY INVASIVE POSTERIOR CERVICAL FORAMINOTOMY WITH TUBULAR DISTRACTORS

TECHNIQUE 2.5

(GALA, O'TOOLE, VOYADZIS, AND FESSLER)

- After induction of general anesthesia, place the patient in Mayfield three-point head fixation. Progressively flex the operating table to bring the patient into a semi-sitting position so that the head is flexed but not rotated and the long axis of the cervical spine is perpendicular to the floor. The seated position allows decreased blood accumulation in the operative field, reduces blood loss and operative times, and improves lateral fluoroscopic images because of the gravity-dependent positioning of the shoulders.
- Secure the Mayfield frame to a table-mounted crossbar and fold the patient's arms across the lap or chest, depending on body habitus. Pad the legs, hands, and arms to prevent positional neural injury.
- Confirm the operative level on lateral fluoroscopy while holding a long Kirschner wire or Steinmann pin over the lateral side of the patient's neck.
- Mark an 18-mm longitudinal incision approximately 1.5 cm off the midline on the operative side and inject it with local anesthesia.
- Through a stab incision, advance a Kirschner wire slowly through the musculature under fluoroscopic guidance and dock it at the inferomedial edge of the rostral lateral mass of the level of interest (Fig. 2.9A). Be sure to identify and palpate bone and do not penetrate the interlaminar space where the laterally thinned ligamentum flavum may not protect against iatrogenic dural or spinal cord injury.
- Complete the incision approximately 1 cm rostral and caudal to the wire entry point and remove the wire.
- Incise the cervical fascia equal to the length of the incision with monopolar cautery or scissors so that muscle dilation can be done in a safe and controlled fashion.
- Reinsert the Kirschner wire under fluoroscopy and serially place the muscle dilators or, as an alternative, place the first dilator instead of the wire (Fig. 2.9B).
- After dilation is complete, place a 16- or 18-mm tubular retractor over the dilators and fix it over the laminofacet junction with a table-mounted flexible retractor arm (Fig. 2.9C); remove the dilators.
- Attach a 25-degree angled glass-rod endoscope to the camera, insert it, and attach it to the tube with a cylindrical plastic friction couple.
- Use monopolar cautery and pituitary rongeurs to clear the remaining soft tissue off the lateral mass and lamina, taking care to start the dissection over solid bone laterally.
- Use a small up-angled curet to gently detach the ligamentum flavum from the undersurface of the inferior edge of the lamina and use a Kerrison punch with a small footplate to begin the laminotomy (Fig. 2.9D,E).
- Subsequent steps differ little from the open procedure. Depending on the degree of facet hypertrophy, use the Kerrison punch to complete most of the laminotomy and early foraminotomy or use a drill if required. Using a fine-cutting bit and adjustable guard sleeve makes drilling around critical neural structures easier.
- After the laminotomy, remove the ligamentum flavum medially to identify the lateral edge of the dura and proximal portion of the nerve root. Bony resection should follow the nerve root into the foramen through a partial medial facetectomy. To maintain biomechanical integrity, preserve at least 50% of the facet.
- Carefully coagulate and incise the venous plexus overlying the nerve root.
- Use a fine-angled dissector to palpate the space ventral to the nerve root for osteophytes or disc fragments. If an osteophyte is present, use a down-angled curet to tamp the material farther ventrally into the disc space or fragment it for subsequent removal. For a soft disc herniation, use a nerve hook passed ventrally and inferiorly to the root to gently tease the fragment away from the nerve; remove it with a pituitary rongeur (Fig. 2.9F,G).
- Inspect the foramen a final time for any further signs of compression and irrigate the field with antibiotic-impregnated solution. Obtain hemostasis with bipolar cautery, bone wax, or commercial hemostatic agent.
- Remove the tube and inject local anesthetic into the fascia and muscles surrounding the incision.
- Close the wound with one or two absorbable stitches for the fascia, two or three inverted stitches for the subcutaneous layer, and a running subcuticular stitch and skin adhesive for the final skin closure.
- Place the patient supine and remove the Mayfield frame.

POSTOPERATIVE CARE The patient is mobilized as soon as possible. No cervical collar of any type is necessary. If medically stable, patients are typically discharged after 2 to 3 hours.

Ruetten et al. described an all-endoscopic technique for posterior cervical foraminotomy using a 25-degree angled 5.9-mm arthroscope, with a working canal of 3.1-mm diameter. They reported no serious complications in 91 patients, of whom only three had recurrence of symptoms. Postoperative pain was significantly reduced compared with a similar group of patients with open foraminotomy, and return to work was significantly quicker (19 days compared with 34 days).

FULL-ENDOSCOPIC POSTERIOR CERVICAL FORAMINOTOMY

TECHNIQUE 2.6

(RUETTEN ET AL.)

- With the patient prone and after induction of general anesthesia, mark the line of spinal joints under radiographic control, as for a conventional open foraminotomy.
- Determine the location of the correct segment, make the skin incision, and insert a dilator onto the facet joint.

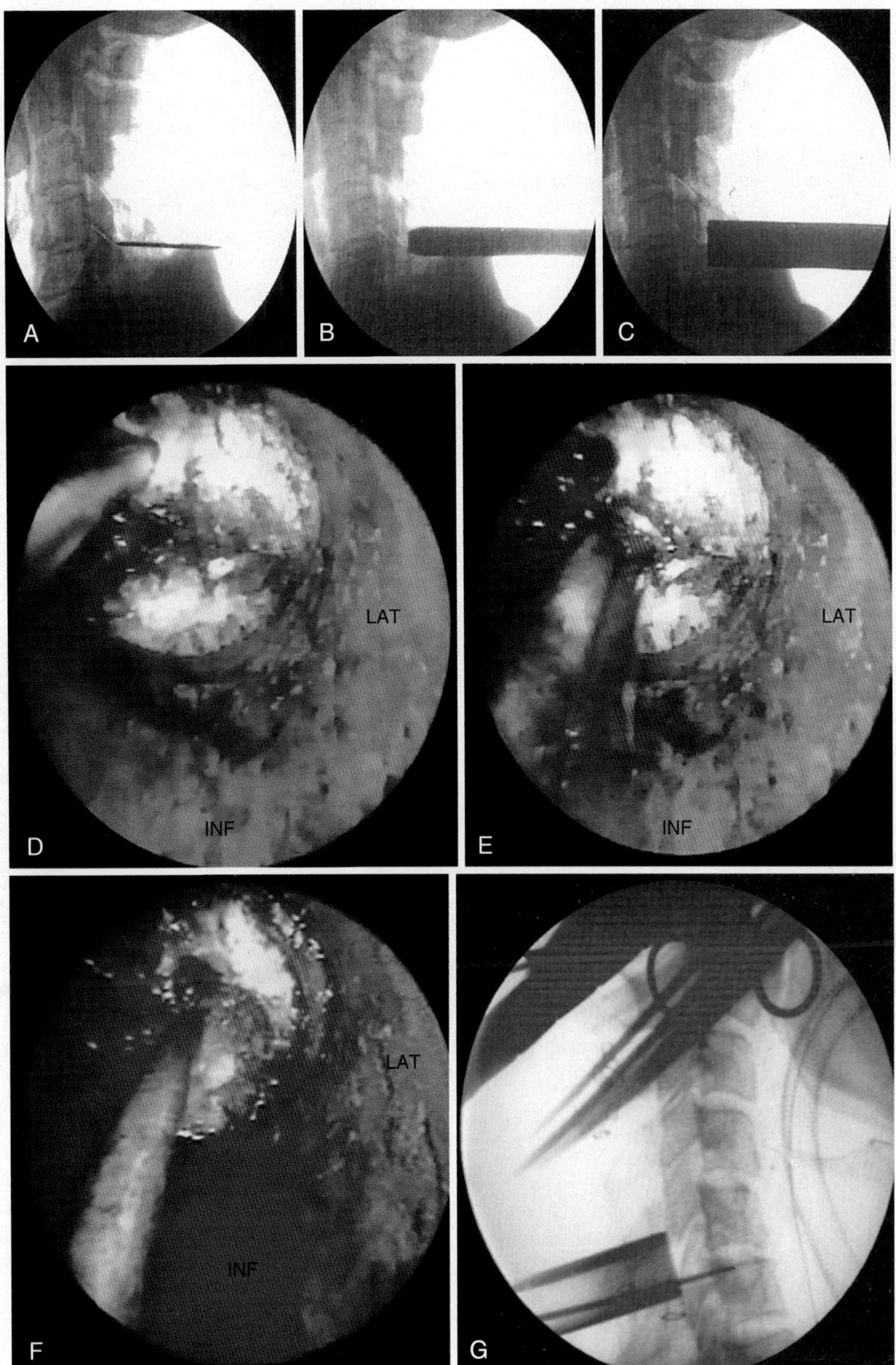

FIGURE 2.9 Minimally invasive posterior cervical foraminotomy with tubular distractors. **A,** Kirschner wire identification of area of interest. **B,** Placement of serial dilators. **C,** Placement of tubular retractor. **D** and **E,** Laminotomy and foraminotomy. **F** and **G,** Disc removal and nerve root decompression. (From Fessler RG, Khoo LT: Minimally invasive cervical microendoscopic foraminotomy: an initial clinical experience, *Neurosurgery* 51[Suppl 2]:37, 2002.) **SEE TECHNIQUE 2.5.**

- Insert the operating sheath over the dilator and remove the dilator.
- Prepare the joint segment and ligamentum flavum with bipolar electrocautery and pituitary rongeurs. Begin the foraminotomy by bone resection at the medial joint segments, resection of the lateral ligamentum flavum, and identification of the lateral edge of the dura and branching of the spinal nerve. It is helpful to start just medial to the facet joint and identify the insertion of the ligamentum flavum to delineate the cephalad and caudal extent of drill work and then work laterally.

- Use 3-mm drills and bone punches inserted through the endoscopic working canal for bone resection.
- Use bipolar radiofrequency to coagulate the venous plexus.
- Depending on the particular pathology, extend the foraminotomy laterally or craniocaudally as needed. Take care to prevent excessive resection of the articular process.
- After completion of the foraminotomy, remove all instruments and close the skin. No drainage is required.

POSTOPERATIVE CARE A soft brace is worn for 5 days.

TISSUE-SPARING POSTERIOR CERVICAL FUSION

McCormack and Dhawan described a technique for tissue-sparing posterior cervical fusion, for which they developed a simple, disposable instrument set. The instruments and technique minimize soft-tissue disruption and facilitate access for cervical facet joint cartilage decortication. A small incision is used to insert an elongated access chisel into the appropriate facet, which, confined by facet anatomy, serves as a post extending out through a minimal skin incision. The surgeon uses the post to apply rotatory decorticators to the medial lamina and rostral and caudal lateral mass. A guide tube inserted after the chisel facilitates rasping of the facet cartilaginous endplates, a task which is difficult with open posterior fusion techniques. Most soft-tissue dissection of the lamina and spinous process required with lateral mass fixation or interspinous wiring is avoided. This technique is proposed for select patients who do not require laminectomy. The facet access and decortication instruments also can be used with other posterior spine approaches to improve facet cartilage decortication.

TECHNIQUE 2.7

(MCCORMACK AND DHAWAN)

- Make an incision just off midline and typically two to three levels below the target level, depending on facet anatomy (Fig. 2.10A). An externally placed Steinmann pin aligned with the intended facet under fluoroscopy can guide the rostral to caudal placement of the skin incision.
- Carry the incision through the subcutaneous tissue and ligamentum nuchae.
- Insert the access chisel through the incision into the facet at the target level and advance it until it abuts the pedicle of the rostral vertebra (Fig. 2.10B,C).
- Advance the decortication trephine over the access chisel to dissect fascia and muscle attachments off of the lateral lamina and lateral mass under visual guidance (Fig. 2.10D).
- Decorticate the lateral mass and lamina above and below the facet.
- Place the guide tube over the access chisel and advance it into the facet joint (see Fig. 2.10A). The guide tube maintains facet distraction, provides visualization, and serves as a working channel.
- Remove the access chisel and decorticate the facet articular surfaces with the rasps and burrs. Insert bone graft material through the guide tube and place it into the decorticated bed.
- Withdraw all instruments.
- Multiple levels can be treated using one small incision, depending on facet joint trajectory (Figs. 2.10A,E).
- Repeat the procedure on the contralateral side.

RESULTS

In few, if any, operations in orthopaedic surgery are the results better than after the removal of a lateral herniated cervical disc. With either open or minimally invasive techniques, approximately 90% of patients have good results with relatively few complications.

ANTERIOR CERVICAL ARTHRODESIS

Anterior cervical discectomy with interbody fusion has gained wide acceptance by both orthopaedic surgeons and neurosurgeons in the management of refractory symptoms of cervical disc disease. The literature attests to a low incidence of major complications and postoperative morbidity and a high degree of success in relieving these symptoms. The fundamental difference in the many techniques is whether surgery is limited to simple discectomy and interbody fusion or whether an attempt is made to enter the spinal canal to remove osteophytes or otherwise decompress the spinal cord and nerve roots.

Extreme care must be exercised in anterior fusion of the cervical spine because of significant potential complications, including injury to the cervical viscera and neurologic and vascular injury. Dysphagia is one of the most common postoperative complications of anterior fusion, with nearly 90% occurrence in one retrospective study; however, rates of dysphagia lasting longer than 3 months appear to be low. Yee et al., in a systematic review of the literature, found a pooled incidence of less than 1%. Reported causes of complications related to fusion by the drill and dowel method include operation of a drill without the protection of the drill guard, which allowed the drill to enter the spinal canal; displacement of a dowel bone graft into the spinal canal, either during surgery or postoperatively, which damaged the cervical cord; and the use of electrocoagulation on the posterior longitudinal ligament. The use of a tricortical iliac graft is recommended for interbody fusions.

Anterior discectomy and interbody fusion has a wide application, producing excellent results in virtually all forms of cervical disc disease and spondylosis, regardless of the objective neurologic signs. Despite subtle differences in surgical technique, the intent of the procedure is discectomy and interbody fusion with no attempt to remove osteophytes. The extent to which the posterior and posterolateral osteophytes with spondylosis contribute to the symptoms of cervical disc disease and the indications for removing them have not been completely defined. Often the discrepancy between the degree of bony spurring or other radiographic changes and the symptoms present is striking. Also, the level of neurologic involvement does

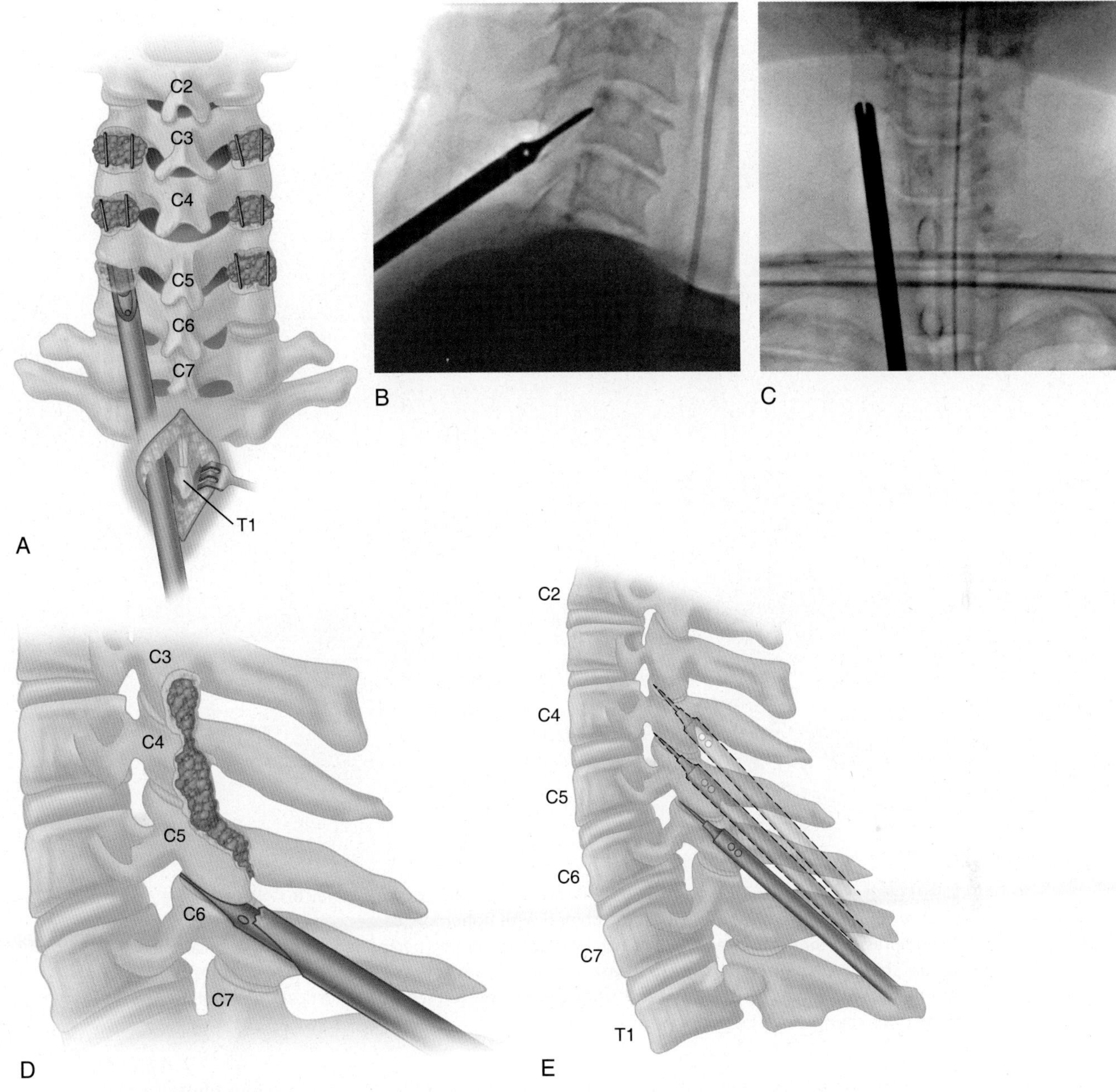

FIGURE 2.10 Tissue-sparing posterior cervical fusion. **A,** Midline minimally invasive incision at C7-T1 with superior two-level access. Posteroanterior view shows guide tube over decortication rasp. Facets are decorticated with medial-to-lateral angulation, avoiding medial nerve. Intraoperative anteroposterior (**B**) and lateral (**C**) fluoroscopy images showing facet chisel properly positioned in C5-6 facet. On lateral view, radiolucent hole is at posterior facet border. **D,** Lateral cervical view with decortication trephine over access chisel to decorticate superior and inferior lateral masses at C5-6. **E,** Lateral cervical view of guide tube at lower level C5-6 with access to several superior levels through one minimally invasive incision. (From McCormack BM, Dhawan R: Novel instrumentation and technique for tissue sparing posterior cervical fusion, *J Clin Neurosci* 34:299, 2016.) **SEE TECHNIQUE 2.7.**

not always coincide with the site of the greatest radiographic findings. Because plain radiographs cannot provide the necessary information for identifying the level or levels of neural compression, either MRI or CT myelography when indicated is strongly recommended in operative planning; both provide the detailed diagnostic information necessary. In descending order of frequency, the disc levels involved with degenerative changes are C5, C6, and C4. Correlation of the patient's symptoms with diagnostic studies is crucial because 14% of asymptomatic patients younger than 40 years of age and 28% of those older than 40 years have significant abnormalities, as shown on MRI studies. The symptoms of the degenerative processes are related to the interplay of multiple aspects of the disease process and not solely to the amount of bony spurs present. Observation of patients who have had fusions shows that

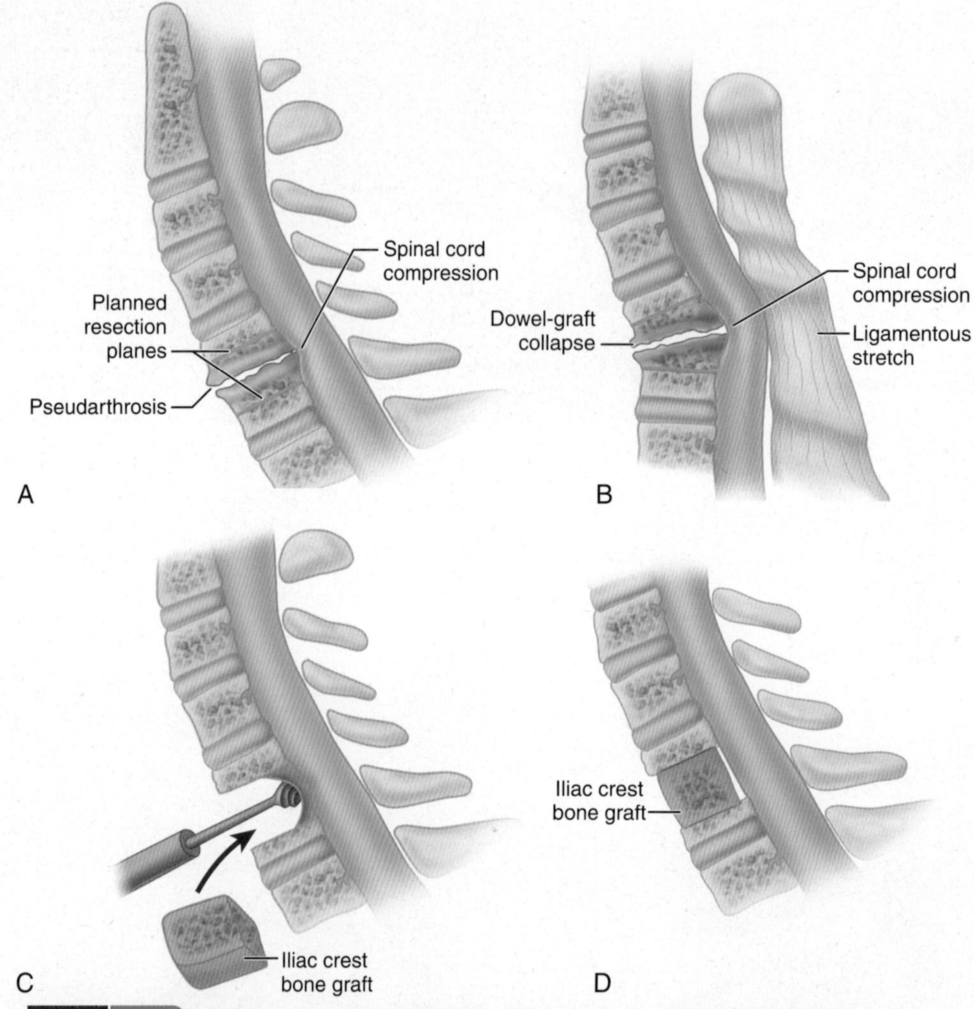

FIGURE 2.11 **A,** Typical nonunion with fibrocartilage compromising canal. **B,** Collapse of graft leads to sharp angular kyphosis, which, combined with nonunion, causes compression of cord. **C,** Decompression through anterior approach. Hemicorporectomy performed cephalad and caudad to disc space with high-speed burr to create parallel surfaces of cancellous bone. Decompression completed with angled curets. **D,** Anterior bone grafting performed with tricortical Smith-Robinson bone graft countersunk into position.

a significant percentage of osteophytes but not all will be spontaneously resorbed postoperatively in the presence of a stable interbody fusion.

In our experience, simple discectomy and interbody fusion without removal of the posterior longitudinal ligament or osteophytes has been adequate in the treatment of neural compression caused by soft disc material. If the compression of neural tissue, especially the spinal cord, is caused by large osteophytes or an ossified posterior longitudinal ligament, direct decompression by removal of the compressing structures has given superior results and is recommended (Fig. 2.11). This is especially true if the T2 sequences on MRI demonstrate cord signal abnormality. In the hands of skilled surgeons, with the use of an operating microscope, a high-speed burr, small angled curets, and small Kerrison rongeurs, safe anterior excision of osteophytes and other offending structures from the spinal canal can be completed before grafting and stabilization. In selected instances, monitoring of somatosensory and motor evoked potentials is useful, primarily in patients with myelopathy or spinal cord signal abnormality, to minimize the risk of spinal cord injury from positioning or hypotension while the exposure and initial phase of decompression is being completed.

GENERAL COMPLICATIONS

For every anatomic structure present in the neck there is a possibility of a surgical error; however, poor results also occur because of poor indications and surgical technique.

The *wrong patient* may be operated on because the neck is a common target for psychogenic pain. Careful preoperative evaluation is essential to rule out a hysterical personality or a chronic anxiety state. In the absence of significant neurologic findings to localize the level of pathologic condition, great care in evaluating the patient's pain is essential. The relatively high incidence of imaging abnormalities in asymptomatic volunteers should be kept in mind. Adjunctive studies, including discography, may be of benefit. Disc degeneration may be a multifocal disease in the cervical spine; therefore, even if an examination seems to point to a single level, it is possible that within a short time other segments will become symptomatic and surgery will be of no long-term benefit. With multiple-level disc degeneration, results have not been gratifying. The best results are obtained with a single segment discectomy and fusion for definite nerve root impairment, spinal cord compression, or, less commonly, localized disc disease without root compression. Fusions of more than two segments performed for pain relief alone produce fair or poor results; improvement, not cure, is the best possible result.

The operation can be done at the *wrong level* if an incorrect vertebral count is made at surgery. Use of a localization film with a metal marker is mandatory, and the first or second cervical vertebra should always be shown on this check film. The marker needle should be directed cranially so that the tip butts the vertebra above and avoids the theca. Additionally, by placing two right-angle bends, beginning 1 cm proximal to the tip of the spinal needle, penetration of the needle beyond a depth of 1 cm is prevented.

The operation may be done in the *wrong way*; for example, the recurrent laryngeal nerve, esophagus, or pharynx can be injured by retractors. Sympathetic nervous system injuries are avoided by dissecting in the correct planes. Keeping the dissection medial to the carotid avoids the sympathetic nervous system. An approach from the left was thought to be less likely to damage the recurrent laryngeal nerve. However, this has not been proved in more recent studies. A cadaver study showed that a right-sided approach involves retraction and manipulation of the nerve for optimal exposure, while on the left the nerve is already in the tracheoesophageal groove and out of the surgical field, which requires minimal direct mobilization of the nerve. One large series suggested that compression of the recurrent laryngeal nerve may well be caused by endotracheal tube position combined with tracheal retraction and may be decreased by deflating and reinflating the endotracheal tube cuff after retractor placement to allow the tube to reposition itself within the trachea. Instruments can tear the dura or compress neural tissue and must be used with extreme caution in removing the posterior disc fragments and osteophytes. Small, angled curets and Kerrison rongeurs should be sharp to prevent the need for excessive force and loss of control of the instruments. Grafts must be accurately measured and tightly fitted under compression.

The operation may be done at the *wrong time*. Timing of an operation is important; surgery should not be delayed if root conduction is significantly impaired. In patients in whom the clinical findings are purely subjective, consideration usually is given to delaying surgery until any possible litigation is settled. However, this can lead to chronic pain patterns that are difficult to eradicate. We rarely treat surgically patients who do not have objectively demonstrated neural compression or neurologic deficits. Otherwise results seem, at best, unpredictable.

POSTOPERATIVE COMPLICATIONS

All anterior surgical wounds are best drained to decrease the risks of a retropharyngeal hematoma, which can produce obstruction of the airway with its subsequent complications. A soft, closed-suction drainage system usually is inserted deep into the wound. Airway obstruction, although rare, typically occurs 12 to 36 hours postoperatively. Maximal swelling occurs 24 to 48 hours after the procedure.

Extrusion of a graft is most commonly seen in the treatment of fracture-dislocations of the neck with posterior instability. This is not common in fusions for disc degeneration when posterior stability of the ligamentous structures is not impaired. At this clinic, anterior plate stabilization and cervical orthosis for 6 to 8 weeks or posterior internal fixation is a routine adjunct when posterior ligamentous stability is lost for any reason and the anterior approach for arthrodesis is necessary. At times anterior stabilization combined with external fixation with a halo vest is used. Use of the halo vest may preclude the need for posterior internal fixation.

A rectangular graft provides the best stability when compared with other graft types. Unless the graft extrudes more than 50% of its depth, or unless it causes dysphagia, revision surgery usually is not indicated. The extruded portion will be resorbed, and the graft will ossify as the arthrodesis heals. If healing time is protracted, external immobilization time should be adjusted accordingly.

Complications related to anterior instrumentation have been reported. Locking-type plate devices minimize the risk of screws backing out and esophageal or tracheal perforation. This type of device also precludes the need for bicortical drilling and thereby decreases the risk for spinal cord injury during drilling or screw placement.

Nonunion of an anterior cervical fusion is unusual. With multiple-level interbody fusions, however, the pseudarthrosis rate increases in a nonlinear fashion. For single-level fusions the literature reports a 3% to 7% nonunion rate even with autograft bone. Similar pseudarthrosis rates are noted with single-level fusions using allograft. With autogenous iliac tricortical grafts, the nonunion rate in two-level interbody fusions without anterior instrumentation ranges from 12% to 18%. However, the addition of stable internal fixation reduces this significantly. This also is true for three or more level fusions. Allograft bone should not be used for multiple-level interbody fusions without anterior plating because of a high nonunion rate. Multiple-level anterior fusions using adjunctive anterior plate fixation with allograft bone can provide satisfactory fusion rates, although the results are not as good as with autograft. When nonunions occur, typically they occur at the caudalmost segment.

If a cervical pseudarthrosis is determined to be symptomatic, usually it is best managed by posterior cervical fusion. If a significant anterior pathologic condition persists, satisfactory revision anterior surgery can be performed (see Fig. 2.11).

When anterior cervical arthrodesis is being done for traumatic disorders with resultant instability from ligamentous tears or posterior element fractures, postoperative treatment must be planned to accommodate this added factor. The postoperative care described here usually applies to arthrodesis for "stable" degenerative or other nontraumatic conditions. If cervical instability is present, or if two or more disc levels are fused, such as with corpectomy, anterior internal fixation and immobilization are routinely used.

Three basic techniques have been used for anterior cervical disc excision and fusion. The Cloward technique involves making a round hole centered at the disc space. A slightly larger, round iliac crest plug is inserted into the disc space hole. The Smith-Robinson technique involves inserting a tricortical strut of iliac crest into the disc space after removing the disc and cartilaginous endplate. The graft is inserted with the cancellous side facing the cord (posterior). This technique has been modified by fashioning the tricortical graft to be thicker in its midportion and inserting the graft with the cancellous portion facing anteriorly. The Bailey-Badgley technique involves the creation of a slot in the superior and inferior vertebral bodies. This technique is most applicable to reconstruction when one or more vertebral bodies are excised for tumor, stenosis, or other extensive pathologic conditions. This technique has been modified by using a keystone graft that increases the surface area of the graft by 30% and allows more complete locking of the graft. Biomechanically, the Smith-Robinson technique provides the greatest stability and least risk of extrusion compared with the Cloward and Bailey-Badgley types of fusions.

A left-sided approach was recommended for years to avoid recurrent laryngeal nerve injury. More recent studies, however, have shown no difference in injury rate to this nerve when comparing approaches. Approach side should be chosen based on the surgeon's comfort. Patients who have dysphagia, dysphonia, or a history of prior neck surgery on preoperative examination should undergo an evaluation of vocal cords and swallowing. If a paralyzed vocal cord is identified, the approach should be on the ipsilateral side of vocal cord paralysis.

SMITH-ROBINSON ANTERIOR CERVICAL FUSION

TECHNIQUE 2.8

(SMITH-ROBINSON ET AL.)

- Place the patient supine on the operating table with a small roll in the interscapular area.
- Apply a head halter if anterior plate fixation is to be used. Apply 5 to 10 pounds of traction to the head halter if so desired. Otherwise, the halter is not necessary because the distraction pins and the retraction set can be used to open the disc space and allow exposure.
- Rotate the patient's head slightly to the side opposite the planned approach.
- Mark the anterior cervical skin, preferably using an existing curved skin crease, before placing the adhesive surgical field drape. The hyoid (C3), thyroid cartilage (C4-5), and cricoid cartilage (C6) are useful landmarks. The transverse-type skin incision can be used, even for three-level corpectomies if it is well placed; otherwise, an incision along the sternocleidomastoid border is useful. Throughout the exposure, meticulous hemostasis should be maintained to allow better identification of dissection planes and important anatomic structures.
- After sharply dividing the skin, sharply dissect the subcutaneous layer off the anterior fascia of the platysma to allow mobility of the wound to the desired level.
- Divide the platysma vertically near the midline by lifting it between two pairs of forceps and dividing it sharply in the cephalad and caudal directions. This allows exposure of the sternocleidomastoid border.
- Develop the interval just medial to the sternocleidomastoid to allow palpation and exposure of the carotid sheath and the overlying omohyoid muscle.
- Mobilize the omohyoid and retract caudally for access cephalad to C5 or mobilize cranially for access to C5 or caudal levels.
- Sharply divide the pretracheal fascia medial to the carotid sheath. Take care to avoid any dissection lateral to the carotid sheath that would place the sympathetic chain at risk.
- Once the pretracheal fascia has been incised, adequately develop the prevertebral space using blunt finger dissection directed medially and posteriorly.
- Place blunt hand-held retractors medially to view the paired longus colli muscles. To avoid injury to the midline structures, use bipolar cautery and small key-type elevators to subperiosteally elevate the longus colli so that self-retaining retractors can be placed deep to the medial borders of these muscles.
- Obtain a localization radiograph using a prebent spinal needle to mark the disc space before proceeding with disc excision or corpectomy.
- If the superior or inferior thyroid vessels limit exposure, ligate and divide the vessels.
- When elevating the longus colli muscles, do not extend laterally to the transverse processes to avoid the sympathetic chain and the vertebral artery. This dissection, however, must extend laterally enough to expose the anterior aspect of the uncovertebral joints bilaterally.
- Place self-retaining retractor blades deep to the longus colli bilaterally and attach to the self-retaining retractor.
- For single-level discectomy, distraction pins can be inserted. For multiple-level procedures or if screw fixation is planned, the distraction pins are best avoided because of potential microfracture at the pin sites that will compromise screw purchase.
- Once all levels are adequately exposed, use a No. 11 blade scalpel to remove the anterior anulus at each level, cutting toward the midline from each uncovertebral joint.
- Remove the anulus with pituitary rongeurs and curets to allow exposure of each uncinate process, which appears as a slight upward curve of the endplate of the caudal segment. This marks the safe extent of lateral dissection to avoid the vertebral artery. Remove the anterior one half to two thirds of the disc at each level in this way.
- Use an operating microscope for safe removal of the posterior disc, osteophytes, or posterior longitudinal ligament as needed.
- With a high-speed burr, remove the anterior lip of the cephalad vertebra to a level matching the subchondral bone at midbody level (Fig. 2.12). This forms a completely flat surface and enhances visibility for removing the remaining disc material and the cartilaginous endplates to the level of the posterior longitudinal ligament.
- If preoperative imaging demonstrates a soft disc fragment and this is found without violation of the posterior longitudinal ligament, further exploration of the canal is not warranted.
- If necessary, perform foraminotomy to remove uncovertebral tissue with small Kerrison rongeurs. If a defect through the posterior longitudinal ligament is found, enlarge it and explore the canal for additional fragments.
- If the surgical plan calls for complete removal of the posterior longitudinal ligament, complete all corpectomies first.

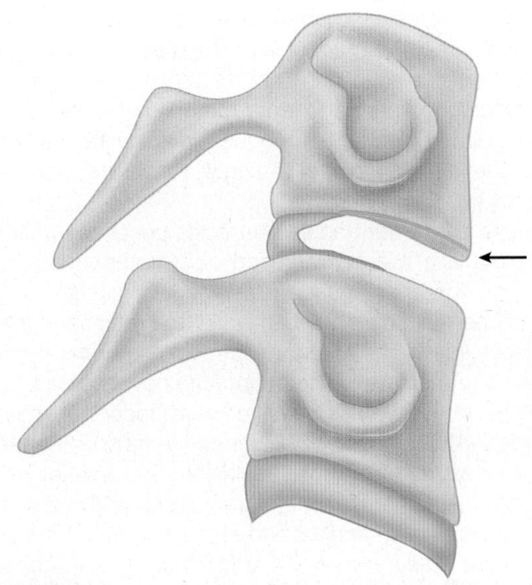

FIGURE 2.12 Diagram of bone removal with high-speed burr of anterior lip of cephalad vertebra to level matching subchondral bone at midbody level. **SEE TECHNIQUE 2.8.**

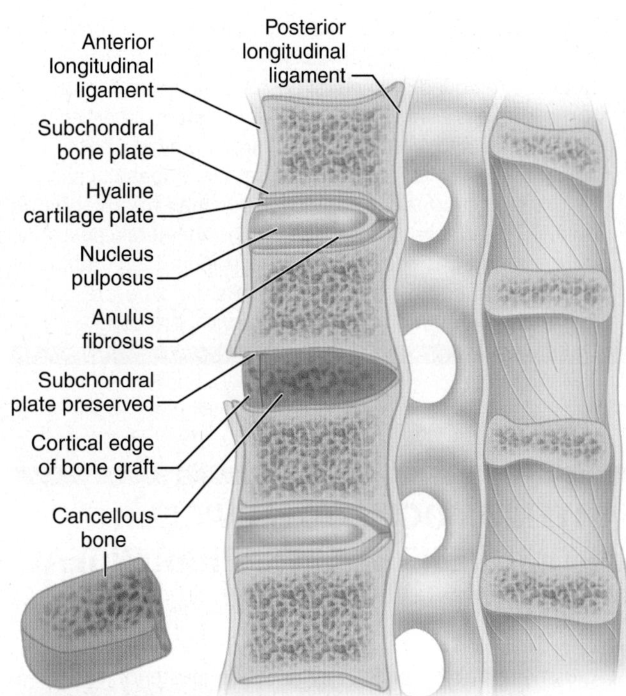

FIGURE 2.13 Technique of Robinson et al. for anterior fusion of cervical spine. **SEE TECHNIQUE 2.8.**

- To perform the corpectomies, use a high-speed burr to create a lateral gutter at the level of the uncinate process bilaterally that extends from one disc space to the next.
- Remove the midline bone to the same depth as the gutters and continue posteriorly until the brisk bleeding of cancellous bone gives way to cortical bone. Usually there will be significant bleeding from the posterior midpoint of the body that can be easily controlled with bipolar cautery once the cortical bone has been drilled away. Do not use unipolar cautery in close proximity to neural tissue.
- Thin the cortical bone with the high-speed burr and remove with angled curets, or remove carefully with the burr. If necessary, remove the posterior longitudinal ligament by lifting it anteriorly with a small blunt hook and opening the epidural space with a 1-mm Kerrison rongeur. This must be done with excellent visualization and care to avoid dural injury.
- After the epidural space is entered, remove the posterior longitudinal ligament entirely if needed. If the canal is significantly compromised, carefully free it from the underlying dura with blunt dissection.
- Perform foraminotomies at this time and remove osteophytes if necessary. A small blunt probe should pass easily anterolaterally after foraminotomy. When possible, preserve the posterior longitudinal ligament to enhance construct stability.
- Carefully prepare the adjacent endplates so that all cartilage is removed, subchondral bone is preserved, the entire decompression is the width of the endplate between the uncinate processes, and the endplates are parallel to one another.
- Carefully measure the anterior to posterior dimension at each endplate. The graft depth should be 3 to 4 mm less than the shorter of the two to allow the graft to be recessed 2 mm anteriorly and not compromise the spinal canal posteriorly. Also, carefully measure the length of graft needed in the cephalad to caudal dimension. Remember to measure with and without traction being applied through the head halter so that the graft will be under proper compression. Also, make sure at this point that endplates are parallel to one another.
- Remove the disc laterally to allow visualization of the uncinate process bilaterally, which will appear as a slight upturning of the endplate and marks the safe extent of lateral decompression.
- Obtain a tricortical iliac graft using a small oscillating saw (Fig. 2.13).
- During preparation of the endplate, take care to preserve the anterior cortex of the cephalad and caudal vertebrae.
- Fashion the bone graft to the appropriate depth. Position the graft with the cancellous surface directed posteriorly and bevel the cephalad and caudal posterior margins slightly to facilitate impaction. With traction applied, impact the graft into place so that the cortical portion is recessed 1 to 2 mm posterior to the anterior cortex of the vertebral bodies. There should be 2 mm of free space between the posterior margin of the graft and the spinal canal. The graft should fit snugly even when traction is being applied.
- Release traction and check the fit of the graft using a Kocher clamp to grasp it. Repeat this procedure for each additional disc space.
- Apply anterior cervical plate instrumentation if necessary with all traction released. Various systems are available and should be placed according to the manufacturer's recommendations.
- Obtain intraoperative radiographs to verify graft and hardware position.
- Close the platysmal layer over a soft, closed-suction drain and close the skin and subcutaneous layers. Apply a thin dressing. Place the patient in a cervical orthosis before extubation.

POSTOPERATIVE CARE The patient is allowed to be out of bed later on the day of surgery. If a drain is used, it should be removed on the first postoperative day. The cervical orthosis is continued 4 to 6 weeks after discectomy patients and 8 to 12 weeks after corpectomy, depending on patient compliance and radiographic appearance of the graft. Occasionally a soft collar is helpful for an additional 1 or 2 weeks. Flexion and extension lateral cervical spine radiographs should reveal no evidence of motion at the fusion site, and trabeculation should be present before discontinuation of the rigid cervical orthosis.

ANTERIOR OCCIPITOCERVICAL ARTHRODESIS BY EXTRAPHARYNGEAL EXPOSURE

Rarely, an anterior occipitocervical fusion is required for a grossly unstable cervical spine when posterior fusion is not feasible, such as in patients who have had extensive laminectomies and for rheumatoid arthritis, traumatic quadriparesis, neoplastic metastasis to the spine, and congenital abnormalities. This operation is a cranial extension of the approach described by Robinson and Smith and by Bailey and Badgley; it permits access to the base of the occiput and the anterior aspect of all the cervical vertebrae. We have no experience with this procedure.

TECHNIQUE 2.9

(DE ANDRADE AND MACNAB)

- Maintain initial spinal stability by applying a cranial halo device with the patient on a turning frame. Keep the patient on the frame and maintain the traction throughout the operation.
- Make the exposure from the right side with an incision coursing along the anterior border of the sternocleidomastoid muscle from above the angle of the mandible to below the cricoid cartilage (Fig. 2.14A).
- Divide the platysma and deep cervical fascia in line with the incision and expose the anterior border of the sternocleidomastoid. Take care not to injure the spinal accessory nerve as it enters the anterior aspect of the sternocleidomastoid at the level of the transverse process of the atlas (Fig. 2.14B).
- Retract the sternocleidomastoid laterally and the pretracheal strap muscles anteriorly and palpate the carotid artery in its sheath. Expose the latter.
- Divide the omohyoid muscle as it crosses at the level of the cricoid cartilage (see Fig. 2.14B).
- Identify the digastric muscle and hypoglossal nerve at the cranial end of the wound (see Fig. 2.14B). Bluntly dissect the retropharyngeal space and enter it at the level of the thyroid cartilage.
- Divide the superior thyroid, lingual, and facial arteries and veins to gain access to the retropharyngeal space in the upper part of the wound.
- Continue blunt dissection in the retropharyngeal space and palpate the anterior arch of the atlas and the anterior tubercle in the midline. Continue above this area with the exploring finger and enter the hollow at the base of the occiput. Dissection cannot be carried farther cephalad because of the pharyngeal tubercle, to which the pharynx is attached (Fig. 2.14C).
- Insert a broad right-angled retractor under the pharynx and displace it anterosuperiorly. Use intermittent traction on the pharyngeal and laryngeal branches of the vagus nerve during this maneuver to minimize the risk of hoarseness. The anterior aspect of the upper cervical spine and the base of the occiput are now exposed.
- Coagulate the profuse plexus of veins under the anterior border of the longus colli. Separate the muscles from the anterior aspect of the spine by incising the anterior longitudinal ligament vertically and transversely and expose the anterior arch of C1 and the bodies of C2 and C3. The working space is approximately 4 cm because the hypoglossal nerve exits from the skull through the anterior condyloid foramen about 2 cm lateral to the midline (Fig. 2.14D).
- Roughen the anterior surface of the base of the occiput and upper cervical vertebrae with a curet.
- Obtain from the iliac crest slivers of fresh autogenous cancellous bone and place them on the anterior surface of the vertebrae to be fused. Make the slivers no thicker than 4.2 mm to prevent excessive bulging into the pharynx.
- Close the wound by suturing the platysma and skin only with a suction drain left in the retropharyngeal space for 48 hours.

POSTOPERATIVE CARE The patient is kept on a turning frame, and traction is maintained for 6 weeks. A tracheostomy set must be kept by the bedside in case upper airway obstruction occurs. For earlier ambulation a halo vest can be applied; the halo vest is removed 16 weeks after the operation. Consolidation of the graft should occur by this time.

FIBULAR STRUT GRAFT IN CERVICAL SPINE ARTHRODESIS WITH CORPECTOMY

When performing a corpectomy, it is important to evaluate the vertebral arteries on axial images of the MRI or CT. An anomalous vertebral artery can course medially into the body, putting it at risk during removal of the vertebral body.

TECHNIQUE 2.10

(WHITECLOUD AND LAROCCA)

- Use the surgical approach of Robinson et al. (see Technique 2.8). As described in that technique, self-retaining retractors are helpful. These can be placed for cephalad and caudal retraction, as well as midline retraction achieved by placing the blades deep to the longus colli muscles that have been elevated.

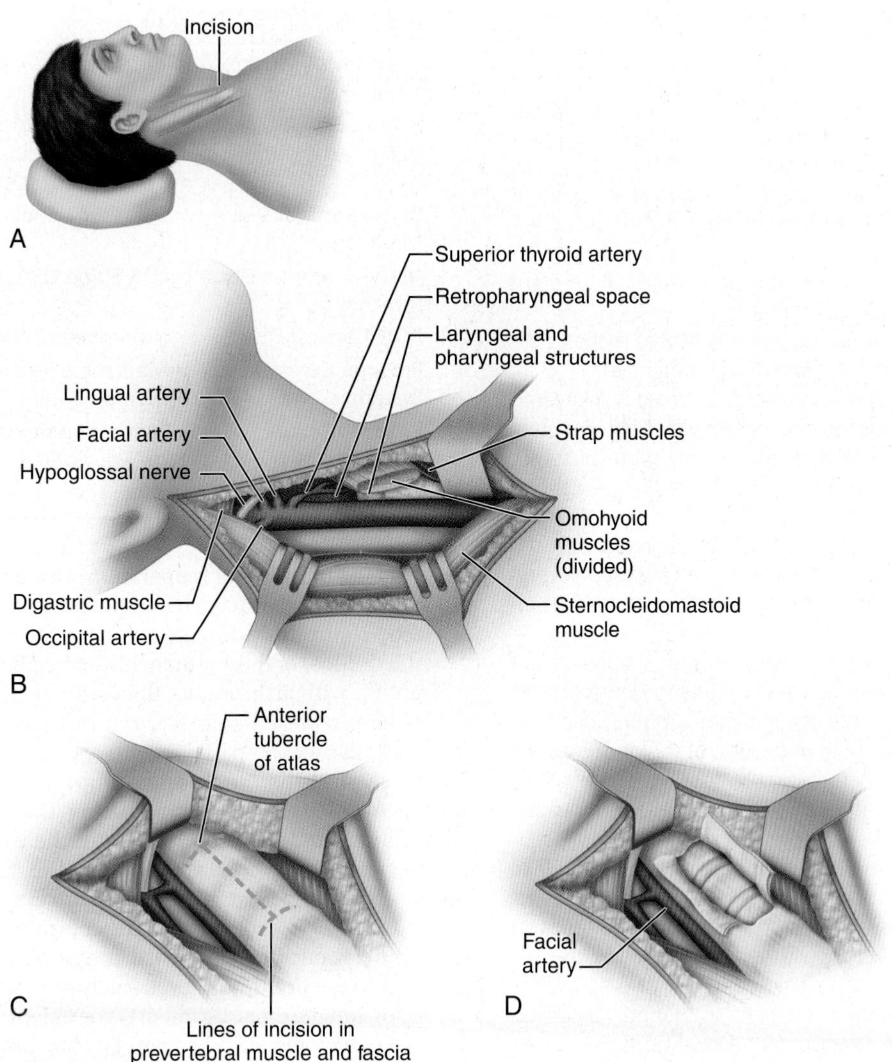

FIGURE 2.14 Technique of de Andrade and Macnab for anterior occipitocervical arthrodesis. **SEE TECHNIQUE 2.9.**

- Remove a rectangular segment of the anterior longitudinal ligament and remove the anterior anulus at each disc level that is to be excised.
- Remove the anterior half to two thirds of the disc with a curet and pituitary rongeurs and identify the uncovertebral joints at each level laterally.
- With the uncovertebral joints clearly identified with the operating microscope, use a high-speed burr, small curets, and small Kerrison rongeurs to remove the remaining disc material back to the posterior longitudinal ligament at each disc level and remove the intervening vertebral bodies as described in Technique 2.8.
- The width of the trough should be maintained at the width between the uncinate processes. The medial portion of the uncinate process can be removed, but removal should not be carried lateral to the uncinate process because this endangers the vertebral artery.
- Carry the dissection through the vertebral body until the posterior cortex is encountered. The bleeding pattern of the bone will change from a cancellous pattern to a cortical pattern at this point.
- Perform the vertebrectomy and the posterior discectomy at each level with the aid of the operating microscope or loupe magnification with the use of a headlight.
- Maintain meticulous hemostasis and use bipolar cautery on the posterior soft-tissue structures, such as the posterior longitudinal ligament.
- Apply bone wax to the cancellous surfaces laterally on the edges of the trough.
- Maintain the sides of the trough in a parasagittal plane.
- When the posterior cortex has been reached and thinned to paper thickness, use a small curet to pull the bone anteriorly, detaching it from the posterior longitudinal ligament. In this fashion, the posterior longitudinal ligament can be thinned and pathologic processes, such as ossification of the posterior longitudinal ligament where spinal cord compression occurs, can be treated.

- Remove the posterior longitudinal ligament by thinning it and developing a plane just ventral to the dura. The dura can be quite attenuated in some circumstances and is easily torn. Exercise great caution during this portion of the procedure. Small curets, small Kerrison rongeurs, and micro blunt hook and micro blunt dissector are quite useful in removing the posterior longitudinal ligament and osteophytes at the posterior aspect of the uncovertebral joints.
- On completion of the decompression, use a full segment of fibula for strut graft placement.
- Place the fibular graft into prepared notches in the vertebra at both ends of the segment to be spanned.
- Notch the fibular graft at each end so that it will key into the prepared notch in each endplate. Place the endplate recess at the cephalad endplate slightly more posterior than the recess through the endplate at the caudal end to make graft insertion easier.
- Prepare the superior and inferior endplates to accept the graft by removing the cartilaginous endplate and preparing the notches. Preserve the anterior portion of the vertebral cortex to prevent graft dislodgment anteriorly.
- After the fibular graft has been cut and shaped to appropriate dimensions, increase the traction on the head and insert the graft into the superior vertebra, using an impactor to sink the inferior portion of the graft into the endplate recess, and pull distally, locking it into place. Two thirds of the graft then comes to lie posterior to the anterior aspect of the vertebral column.
- Anterior cervical plate fixation is added for stability. Take care in selecting proper plate length so that the screws will not be too close to the graft-recipient site interface.
- Check the graft position with radiographs and close the wound over soft, closed-suction drains in layers.
- Plating provides adequate stability so that only a cervical orthosis is needed after surgery. However, if screw purchase is not acceptable, halo vest immobilization should be used with the uninstrumented fibular technique or a posterior stabilizing procedure with mass screws should be considered.

POSTOPERATIVE CARE Depending on the type of internal fixation, initial immobilization is continued with an orthosis for 6 to 8 weeks, depending on healing demonstrated on radiograph. The time required for fusion will understandably be longer with cortical bone than with a corticocancellous bone graft. Prolonged immobilization may be necessary.

POSTERIOR CERVICAL ARTHRODESIS

The techniques of posterior arthrodesis of the cervical spine are discussed in the section on fractures, dislocations, and fracture-dislocations of the cervical spine (see chapter 5).

CERVICAL DISC ARTHROPLASTY

Several cervical arthroplasty devices have been approved by the US Food and Drug Administration (FDA) and more are in the approval process (Table 2.3; Fig. 2.15). The primary argument favoring these devices is that, by avoiding anterior fusion, adjacent segment degeneration can be minimized, reducing the need for reoperation. This benefit of cervical disc arthroplasty appears to be supported by a number of randomized, controlled comparisons of arthroplasty and standard ACDF. Most of these studies also noted better maintenance of motion with arthroplasty than with arthrodesis. Other studies have reported a quicker return to work (approximately 2 weeks earlier) by patients with arthroplasty. The indications for cervical disc arthroplasty appear to be similar to those for ACDF (see chapter 5). Using the published contraindications and indications listed in the trials of four different cervical disc arthroplasty devices (Box 2.7), a review of 167 consecutive patients who had cervical spine surgery identified 95 (57%) who had absolute contraindications to this procedure. Kani and Chew listed anterior compressive pathology at the vertebral body level (such as ossification of the posterior longitudinal ligament), coexistent posterior compressive pathology (such as from facet arthrosis), and segmental instability (43.5 mm sagittal plane translation on dynamic cervical spine radiographs) as contraindications to cervical disc arthroplasty. Osteopenia and concurrent lumbar degenerative disease have been reported to increase the risk of development of adjacent segment disease after cervical disc arthroplasty. Reported complications include implant migration, heterotopic ossification, and recurrent radiculopathy. Metal-on-metal disc replacements also have been found to result in a lymphocytic reaction, similar to that with metal-on-metal hip prostheses, in a few patients.

TABLE 2.3

United States Food and Drug Administration–Approved Cervical Disc Replacement Devices

Device	Manufacturer
ActivL Artificial Disc	B. Braun Aesculap Implant Systems, LLC, Center Valley, PA
Bryan Cervical Disc Medtronic	Sofamor Danek, Memphis, TN
Mobi-C Cervical Disc Prosthesis	LDR Spine USA, Inc, Austin, TX
PCM Cervical Disc	NuVasive, Inc San, Diego, CA
Prestige Cervical Disc System	Medtronic Sofamor Danek, Memphis, TN
Prodisc-C	Synthes Spine, Westchester, PA
Secure-C Artificial Cervical Disc	Globus Medical, Inc, Audubon, PA

There are several additional considerations if cervical arthroplasty is to be recommended. The patient should be informed of the current expected or possible benefits and the current uncertainties involved with the procedure. Also, from an anatomic standpoint, the condition of the facets should be essentially normal because arthroplasty treats only one of the three joints at each motion segment. If there is significant disc space narrowing with facet overload and facet degeneration noted on CT, then cervical arthroplasty at this time cannot be recommended. Also, as with virtually any spine implant, the quality of the patient's bone may preclude disc replacement if osteoporosis is present.

Proper implant position and size are crucial to the function and potential failure of each device. As described by Kani and Chew, an ideal cervical disc (Fig. 2.16A,B) should have a height similar to adjacent normal discs, provide as much

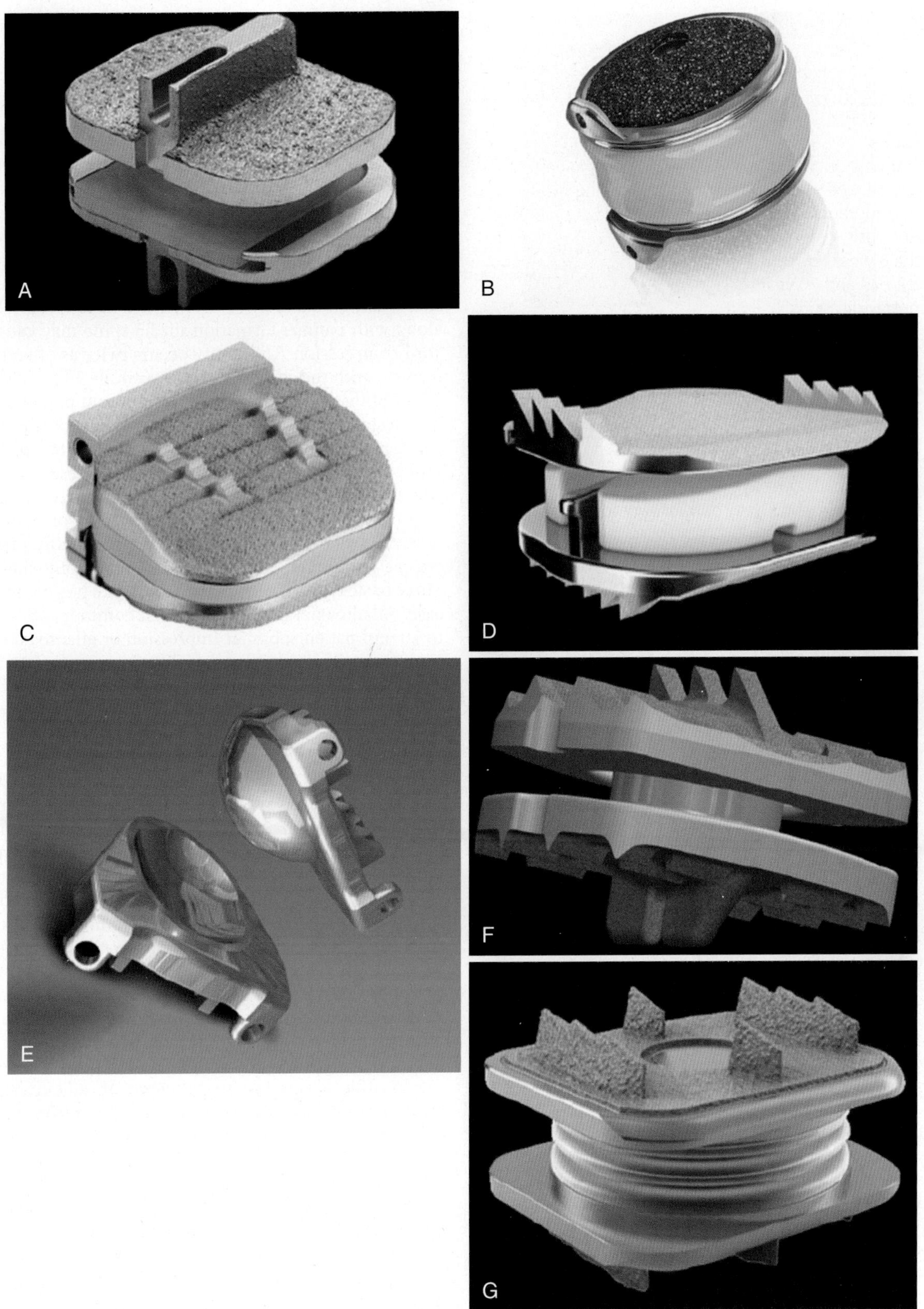

FIGURE 2.15 Cervical total disc replacements. **A,** Prodisc-C (Johnson and Johnson). **B,** Bryan Cervical Disc (Medtronic). **C,** PCM Cervical Disc (Medtronic). **D,** Mobi-C Cervical Disc (Zimmer Biomet). **E,** Prestige LP (Medtronic). **F,** SimplifyDisc (Simplify Medical). **G,** M6-C Artifical Cervical Disc (Spinal Kinetics.). (From Nunley PD, Coric D, Frank KA, et al: Cervical disc arthroplasty: current evidence and real-world application, *Neurosurgery* 83:1087, 2018.)

BOX 2.7

Indications and Contraindications for Cervical Disc Replacement

Indications

- Symptomatic cervical disc disease at one or two vertebral levels between C3-T1 confirmed by imaging (MRI, CT, or myelography) showing herniated nucleus pulposus, spondylosis, or loss of disc height
- Failed ≥ 6 weeks of conservative therapy
- Between 20 and 70 years of age
- No contraindications

Contraindications

- ≥3 vertebral levels requiring treatment
- Cervical instability (translation >3 mm and/or >11-degree rotational difference to that or either adjacent level)
- Known allergy to implant materials (titanium, polyethylene, cobalt, chromium, and molybdenum)
- Cervical fusion adjacent to the level to be treated
- Posttraumatic vertebral body deficiency/deformity
- Facet joint degeneration
- Neck or arm pain of unknown etiology
- Axial neck pain as the solitary presenting symptom
- Severe spondylosis (bridging osteophytes, disc height loss >50%, and absence of motion <2 degrees)
- Osteoporosis/osteopenia
- Prior surgery at the level to be treated
- Active malignancy; history of invasive malignancy, unless treated and asymptomatic for at least 5 years
- Systemic disease (acquired immune deficiency syndrome, human immunodeficiency virus, hepatitis B or C, and insulin-dependent diabetes)
- Other metabolic bone disease (i.e., Paget disease and osteomalacia)
- Morbid obesity (body mass index [BMI] >40 or weight >100 lb over ideal body weight)
- Pregnant or trying to become pregnant in next 3 years
- Active local/systemic infection
- Presently on medications that can interfere with bone/soft-tissue healing (i.e., corticosteroids)
- Autoimmune spondyloarthropathies (rheumatoid arthritis)

From Auerbach JD, Jones KJ, Fras CI, et al: The prevalence of indications and contraindications to cervical total disc replacement, *Spine J* 8:711, 2008.

surface coverage of the opposing endplates as possible, and be centrally positioned in both the sagittal and coronal planes. Prostheses that are undersized (Fig. 2.16C,D) increase stress concentrations per unit area and may increase the risk of subsidence. Inadequate coverage of the endplates by an undersized prosthesis may predispose to heterotopic ossification and posterior osteophyte formation, which ultimately restrict cervical segmental motion. Prostheses that are not centrally positioned on anteroposterior and lateral radiographs can lead to adjacent segment degeneration and scoliosis. Malpositioning of the implant in the coronal plane (see Fig. 2.16C) may cause unilateral neural foraminal narrowing with resultant radiculopathy. Overstuffing the disc space with an oversized implant (Fig. 2.16E) results in distraction of the facet joints, which can cause axial neck pain and referred scapular pain and decrease cervical spine segmental motion. The reader is referred to the specific technique guides for these parameters. Our experience with these devices is limited at this time, and their ultimate value for patient care has not been determined.

RHEUMATOID ARTHRITIS OF THE SPINE

Rheumatoid arthritis is a systemic inflammatory disorder caused by lymphoproliferative disease within synovium, which results in cartilaginous destruction, periarticular erosions, and attenuation of ligaments and tendons. The latter along with pannus formation in the spine may cause spinal cord compression. This entity occurs twice as often in young women, with the age at diagnosis typically 30 to 50 years old. Cervical instability is the most serious and potentially lethal manifestation of rheumatoid arthritis, with radiographic changes or instability present in 19% to 88% of patients. Lumbar or thoracic pathology rarely is present in patients with rheumatoid arthritis. Risk factors for developing cervical involvement are an older age at onset, more active synovitis, higher levels of C-reactive protein, rapidly progressive erosive peripheral joint disease, and early joint subluxation. Three basic types of cervical instability are present in this disease. Atlantoaxial instability is most common, affecting 19% to 70% of patients; basilar impression or atlantoaxial impaction occurs in 38%; and subaxial subluxation occurs in 7% to 29%. These pathologies are less frequent today with the use of modern rheumatologic medical treatments.

CLINICAL EVALUATION

Pain, neurologic sequelae, and instability often are the presenting symptoms. Approximately 61% of patients undergoing total joint replacement were reported to have instability in the cervical spine; 50% of these patients had no symptoms attributable to the neck preoperatively. Neck pain is reported by 40% to 88% of patients with rheumatoid arthritis of the spine, and 7% to 58% have neurologic findings. Axial neck pain usually is occipital and may be associated with headaches. Myelopathic symptoms include early weakness and gait disturbance, with frequent tripping or clumsiness. Hand function may be impaired, with coordination disturbances that cause difficulty differentiating coins or buttoning clothing. Sensory changes and bowel and bladder incontinence are late myelopathic symptoms. In patients with atlantoaxial instability, vertebrobasilar insufficiency resulting from kinking of the vertebral arteries can cause vertigo, tinnitus, or visual disturbances that lead to loss of equilibrium. Neurologic evaluation in patients with rheumatoid arthritis can be difficult. Tendon ruptures, severe joint disturbances, and previous surgery can make it difficult to distinguish radicular and myelopathic symptoms from peripheral disease involvement. Any findings consistent with myelopathy should stimulate further investigation.

DIAGNOSTIC IMAGING

RADIOGRAPHY

Radiographs should include anteroposterior, lateral, odontoid, and lateral flexion and extension views. Instability and potential for neurologic sequelae are correlated best with the posterior atlantodens interval, which is determined by

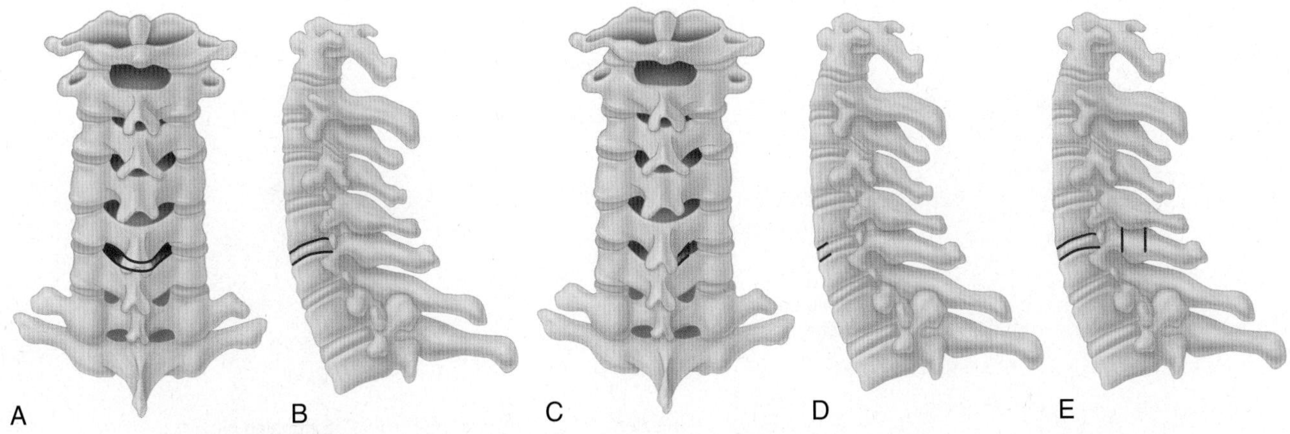

FIGURE 2.16 **A** and **B**, Ideal size and positioning of cervical disc prosthesis. **C** and **D**, Undersized and eccentrically positioned prosthesis. **E**, Oversized implant. (From Kani KK, Chew FS: Cervical disc arthroplasty: review and update for radiologists, *Semin Roentgenol* 54:113, 2019.)

measuring the distance between the ventral surface of the lamina of C1 and the dorsal aspect of the odontoid; the interval should be more than 14 mm. This measurement is 97% sensitive for the presence of paralysis. In patients with preoperative paralysis caused by atlantoaxial subluxation, recovery is not expected if the spinal canal diameter is less than 10 mm. If basilar impression is coexistent, significant recovery occurs only if the space available for the cord is at least 13 mm. Therefore when patients have a posterior atlantodens interval of 14 mm or less, decompression must be considered because of the risk of paralysis from their atlantoaxial instability. Remember that the posterior atlantodens interval measured on a radiograph does not represent the actual space available for the cord because the soft tissues are not included in the measurement.

The atlantodens interval is determined by measuring the distance between the posterior edge of the anterior ring of C1 and the anterior edge of the odontoid. Normally this distance should be 3.5 mm or less in an adult. An atlantodens interval of more than 10 mm is clinically significant and suggests transverse ligament disruption; however, this measurement is not useful in predicting neurologic sequelae caused by instability, possibly because of the natural history of atlantoaxial instability. As atlantoaxial instability progresses, subsequent vertical instability develops. As this superior migration occurs, the atlantodens interval decreases. Despite significant progression of instability and potential neurologic deficit, the atlantodens interval does not increase further. Posterior subluxation is best determined by acute angulation of the cord and upper cervical spine as identified by sagittal reformatted CT, lateral air contrast tomography, or preferably MRI. Lateral subluxation implies some rotation of the atlas and is present when the lateral masses of C1 are 2 mm or more laterally than those of C2.

Atlantoaxial impaction is measured using the McGregor line (Fig. 2.17). This line is constructed from the base of the hard palate to the outer cortical table of the occiput. The tip of the odontoid is measured perpendicular to this line. Superior migration is considered present in men if the tip of the odontoid is 4.5 mm above this line. Ranawat et al. described a method of determining the degree of settling on the lateral radiograph using the minimal distance between a line drawn from the center of the anterior arch to the center of the posterior arch of the atlas and a vertical line drawn along the posterior aspect of the odontoid from the center of the pedicles of C2. They reported that the normal value was 15 mm for women and 17 mm for men, with less than 13 mm considered abnormal (Fig. 2.18). To determine vertebral settling, Redlund-Johnell and Pettersson used the minimal distance between the McGregor line and the midpoint of the inferior margin of the body of the axis on the lateral radiograph in the neutral position (Fig. 2.19). They noted the normal value to be 34 mm or more for men and 29 mm or more for women (100 patients each). In a comparative study of these two screening methods, the Redlund-Johnell method was found to be better for diagnosing basilar impression.

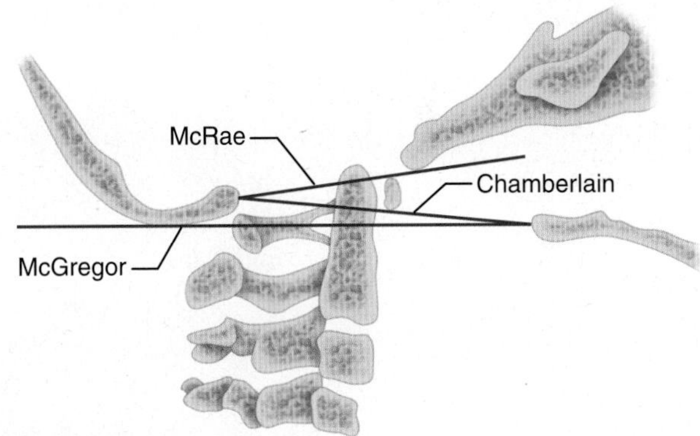

FIGURE 2.17 Drawing of base of skull and upper spine showing McGregor, McRae, and Chamberlain lines.

Subaxial subluxations produce a cascading, or “staircase,” appearance of the spine. Any slippage of 4 mm or more, or 20% of the adjacent vertebral body, is considered significant. Measurement of sagittal spinal canal diameter is most useful and should be more than 13 mm. The risk of spinal cord compression and injury is higher in patients with smaller canal diameters.

COMPUTED TOMOGRAPHIC MYELOGRAPHY AND MAGNETIC RESONANCE IMAGING

Three-dimensional imaging is useful in patients who have a neurologic deficit or radiographic evidence of instability. MRI

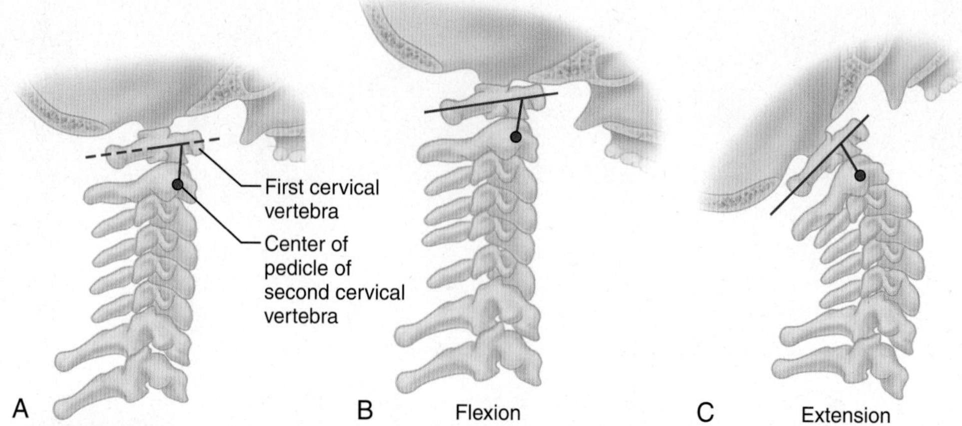

FIGURE 2.18 Ranawat et al. measurement of superior migration in rheumatoid arthritis. **A,** Diameter of ring of first cervical vertebra and distance from center of pedicle of second cervical vertebra to this diameter are measured. **B** and **C,** Measurement of superior migration is unchanged in flexion or extension of spine.

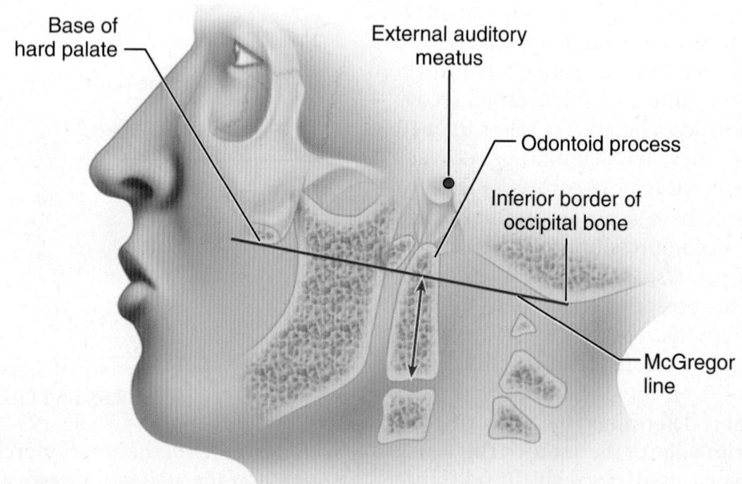

FIGURE 2.19 Redlund-Johnell determination of vertebral settling in rheumatoid arthritis. Distance is measured between McGregor line and midpoint of base of C2.

or CT myelography helps delineate the true space available for the cord. MRI is excellent for viewing soft tissues and the neural elements, but myelography followed by CT gives similar information. In addition to bony compression, pannus further decreases the space available for the cord by 3 mm or more in approximately 66% of patients. Determining the cervicomedullary angle is helpful in identifying vertical instability. A line drawn along the dorsal surface of the odontoid intersects a line drawn ventral and parallel to the medulla. This angle normally should be 135 to 175 degrees, with angles less than 135 degrees suggesting atlantoaxial impaction and correlating with the presence of myelopathy. MRI has been shown to be 100% accurate in identifying vertical settling, and it is currently the most definitive, least invasive test for cord compression. Flexion and extension MRI also has been used to determine dynamic compression of the spinal cord. Data from anatomic studies indicate that the space available for the cord should be 14 mm at the foramen magnum, 13 mm at the atlantoaxial articulation, and 12 mm in the subaxial cervical spine.

CERVICAL INSTABILITY

Cervical disease has an early onset and is correlated with appendicular disease activity. Other factors that predict more severe spinal involvement include longer duration of disease, positive rheumatoid factor, use of steroids, and male sex. Patients with rheumatoid arthritis have a shorter life expectancy than the normal population. When cervical myelopathy is established, mortality is common if this condition remains untreated. Of 21 patients refusing surgery for cervical instability, all 21 died within 7 years of the onset of myelopathy. The incidence of sudden death from the combination of basilar impression and atlantoaxial instability is about 10%.

Atlantoaxial subluxation is the most common instability, with a reported incidence of 11% to 46% of cases at necropsy. Atlantoaxial subluxation can be anterior, posterior, or lateral, with anterior instability predominating. Posterior instability may occur in 20% and lateral instability in 7% of patients. This instability results from erosive synovitis of the atlantoaxial, atlanto-odontoid, and atlantooccipital joints. Basilar impression, vertical settling, or atlantoaxial impaction is the settling of the skull onto the atlas and the atlas onto the axis as a result of erosive arthritis and bone loss. This settling can result in vertebral arterial thrombosis. According to Ranawat et al., atlantoaxial instability is present in 38% of patients with rheumatoid arthritis; however, its frequency increases with disease severity (0% in mild disease, 52% in moderate disease, and 88% in severe disease in a report by Oda et al.). Subaxial subluxations are more subtle and frequently multiple, affecting 10% to 20% of patients with rheumatoid arthritis. They are believed to result from synovitis of the facet joints and uncovertebral joints, accompanied by erosion of the ventral endplates. They may result in root compression from foraminal narrowing. Myelography, postmyelography reformatted CT, and MRI all show root cutoff and partial or complete block. Postmyelography reformatted CT and MRI are clearly superior in identifying soft-tissue obstructions and cord compression. Absolute subluxation distances of clinical significance are unknown for this problem.

The signs and symptoms of these instability patterns include pain, stiffness, pyramidal tract involvement, vertebrobasilar insufficiency, root findings, and symptoms similar to the Lhermitte sign in multiple sclerosis. Early clinical manifestations include Hoffmann and Babinski signs and hyperreflexia.

NONOPERATIVE TREATMENT

Disease-modifying antirheumatic medications are changing the course of this disease. Early use of nonbiologic or biologic antirheumatic drugs can be beneficial in avoiding irreversible injury. The use of a combination of these medications has been shown to prevent or retard the development of anterior atlantoaxial subluxation and other cervical spine lesions in patients with an early diagnosis of rheumatoid arthritis. Patients should be under the care of a rheumatologist once the diagnosis is made.

Goals of nonoperative treatment include preventing neurologic injury, avoiding sudden death, minimizing pain, and maximizing function. Many patients, despite radiographic abnormalities, remain asymptomatic, and supportive treatment and close observation are necessary. Medical management during disease flares is important for patient comfort and should be coordinated with a rheumatologist. A cervical orthosis is helpful in some patients if pain persists. Isometric exercises help stabilize the neck without excessive motion and may help alleviate mechanical symptoms. Yearly follow-up with five-view radiographs is indicated to detect instability so that stabilization can be done before neurologic deficits develop.

OPERATIVE TREATMENT

The indications for operative treatment are neurologic impairment, instability, and pain. Fusion is recommended for patients, with or without neurologic deficits, who have atlantoaxial subluxation and a posterior atlantoodontoid interval of 14 mm or less, atlantoaxial subluxation with at least 5 mm of basilar invagination, or subaxial subluxation with a sagittal spinal canal diameter of 14 mm or less. Axial imaging that shows compression of the spinal cord to a diameter of less than 6 mm also is an indication for surgery.

Atlantoaxial subluxation is best treated by posterior C1 and C2 fusion. When the subluxation is reducible, fusion may be accomplished by a posterior wiring technique (Gallie or Brooks wiring, see Technique 5.12), Magerl transarticular screws (see Technique 5.11), or Harms C1-2 lateral mass fixation (see Technique 5.9). When the atlantoaxial subluxation is not reducible, posterior wiring techniques are contraindicated and screw fixation as described by Magerl or Harms should be used in combination with a C1 laminectomy if decompression is needed. Occipitocervical fusion also may be considered when adequate fixation cannot be achieved in C1. The need for a halo vest postoperatively should be based on the stability of the surgical fixation, bone quality, and compliance of the patient.

Preoperative planning for transarticular screws or C1 lateral mass fixation must include CT with sagittal and axial reconstructions to determine if ample lateral masses are present for fixation and to see if there are anomalies of the vertebral arteries. Stabilization alone should result in some decrease of pannus, and odontoid excision is unnecessary, unless anterior compression persists after fusion or if compression is purely bony.

In patients with basilar impression, a trial of halo or tong traction for reduction is an option, if tolerated. If reduction is accomplished, a posterior occipitocervical fusion is done. If reduction is impossible, posterior fusion is done after anterior transoral decompression or posterior decompression that includes decompression of the foramen magnum. Posterior stabilization can be obtained with wiring and cancellous struts, Luque rods, lateral mass plates, Y-plates, and newer rod-screw or rod-hook systems. The prognosis is guarded in patients with preoperative neurologic deficits, and basilar impression is associated with poorer recovery of function. As a result, aggressive treatment is indicated to prevent neurologic deficits when progressive atlantoaxial impaction is identified.

Symptomatic subaxial subluxation is best treated by surgical stabilization anteriorly or posteriorly. Anteriorly, stabilization can be achieved by discectomy or corpectomy and fusion using a cage and autograft or allograft, structural allograft, or tricortical autogenous bone graft, depending on the pathology. In their comparative analysis of anterior fusion with allograft or intervertebral cage involving 6130 patients, Pirkle et al. found that the nonunion rate with cages (5%) was higher than that with allografts (2%) and concluded that the increased rate of nonunion with intervertebral cages suggests the superiority of allograft over cages in ACDF. Posteriorly, fusion is done using wires, plates, or mass screws and rods and autogenous bone grafting. Halo traction can be used to reduce subluxations preoperatively, especially in patients with myelopathy or paraplegia. Anterior decompression and fusion are preferred for irreducible subluxations and in patients who require a decompression. Supplementation with posterior instrumentation should be considered for patients who require multilevel anterior procedures and in patients with poor bone quality.

The mortality associated with surgery for rheumatoid arthritis patients is between 5% and 10% and is higher in patients with cardiovascular disease or atlantoaxial impaction. The complication rate also is high; 25% of patients will have wound complications.

Boden and Clark developed a treatment algorithm for atlantoaxial subluxation (Fig. 2.20). The techniques for occipitocervical, atlantoaxial, and subaxial posterior cervical fusion are described in chapter 5.

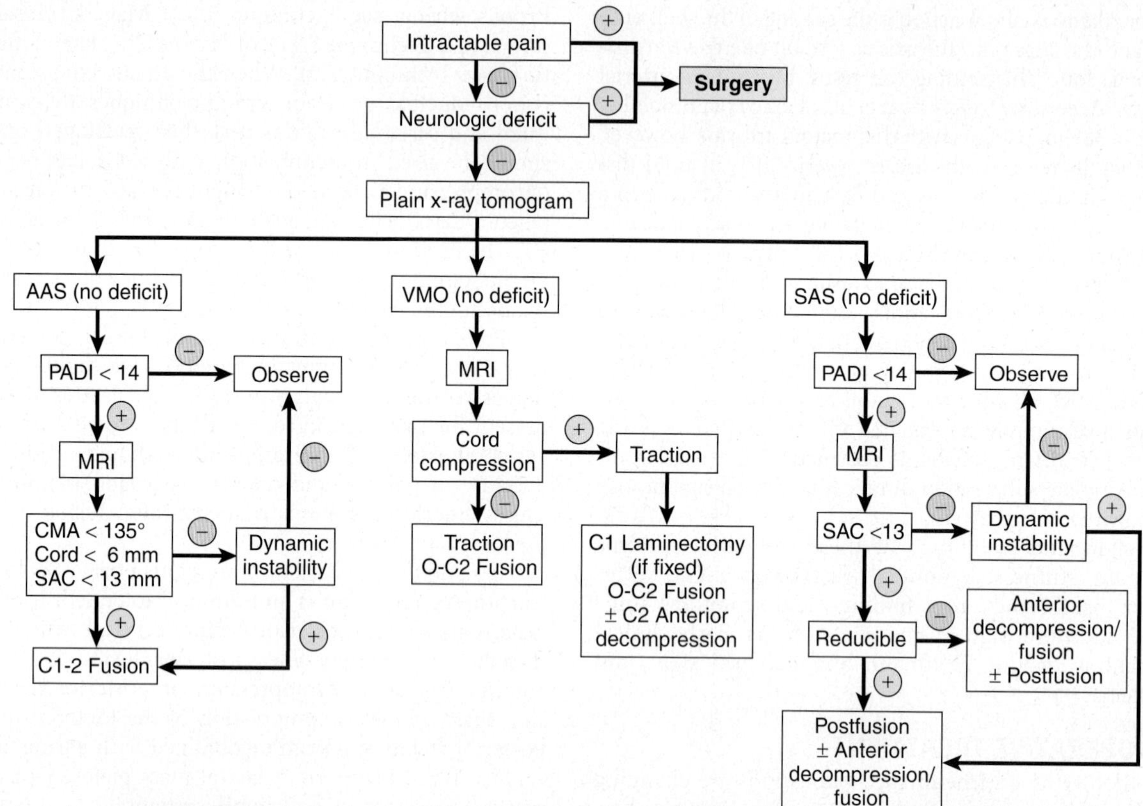

FIGURE 2.20 Algorithm for evaluation and management of rheumatoid arthritis of cervical spine. *AAS*, Atlantoaxial subluxation; *CMA*, cervicomedullary angle; *PADI*, posterior atlantodental interval; *SAC*, space available for cord; *SAS*, subaxial subluxation; *VMO*, vertical migration of odontoid. (From Boden SD, Clark CR: Rheumatoid arthritis of the cervical spine. In *The Cervical Spine Research Society, Editorial Committee: The cervical spine*, ed 3, Philadelphia, 1998, Lippincott-Raven.)

Pain is decreased after surgery in 90% to 97% of patients. Peppelman et al. reported that neurologic function improved in 95% of patients with atlantoaxial subluxations, in 76% of patients with combined atlantoaxial subluxation and atlantoaxial impaction, and in 94% of patients with subaxial subluxations. Atlantoaxial subluxations have a poor prognosis for neurologic recovery, with several studies reporting improvement of function of one Ranawat class in only 40% to 50% of patients. The severity of the preoperative neurologic deficit also influenced results.

ANKYLOSING SPONDYLITIS OF THE CERVICAL SPINE

Ankylosing spondylitis is a chronic inflammatory disease of unknown etiology. It is a seronegative spondyloarthropathy that primarily affects the axial skeleton, sacroiliac joints, and pelvis. Less commonly, involvement of peripheral joints, eyes (iritis or uveitis), heart, and lungs can occur. Inflammation of the spinal joints and enthesopathies cause chronic pain and stiffness and can lead to progressive ankylosis of the spine in patients with long-standing disease. Ankylosing spondylitis typically affects young adults between the ages 20 and 40 years, with a male to female ratio of 1:3. The average onset of symptoms occurs at 23 years of age; there can be an 8.5- to 11.4-year delay from initial symptoms to diagnosis. There is a known association with the HLA-B27 antigen. Of patients who have ankylosing spondylitis, 88% to 96% are HLA-B27 positive, but only 5% of the HLA-B27 population develops ankylosing spondylitis.

In the cervical spine, ankylosing spondylitis can lead to progressive deformity, causing disabling functional deficits. In addition, fused sections of the spine make it more susceptible to fracture, pseudarthrosis, or spondylodiscitis. Long stiff segments of autofused spine can also provoke accelerated degeneration in adjacent mobile segments.

To aid in surgical planning for the sites and levels of osteotomies in the treatment of ankylosing spondylitis, Wang et al. proposed a classification system based on radiographic findings. They described four types according to the location of the apex: type I (lumbar), type II (thoracolumbar), type III (thoracic), and type IV (cervical or cervicothoracic junction). This classification has not been validated at this time.

DIAGNOSIS

In the vertebral bodies, inflammatory resorption of bone at the enthesis causes periarticular osteopenia. This resorption initially is seen as a "squaring off" of the corners of the vertebral bodies. Subsequent ossification occurs in the anulus fibrosis, sparing the anterior longitudinal ligament and disc and giving the "bamboo spine" appearance on radiographs. The posterior elements are similarly affected, with ossification of the facet joints, interspinous and supraspinous ligaments, and ligamentum flavum. Atlantoaxial instability must be identified, especially in any patient having surgery for conditions associated with ankylosing spondylitis. Because of the stiff subaxial spine, instability occurs in 25% to 90% of patients with ankylosing spondylitis.

Distorted anatomy from disc ossification, ectopic bone, and sclerosis can make the spinal fractures difficult to see on plain radiographs, and these injuries often are missed. A widened anterior disc space, which creates an unstable configuration that is prone to translation, late neurologic loss, and slow healing, may be the only obvious radiographic finding. Imaging with MRI, CT, or bone scan may be helpful in making the diagnosis. Ankylosing spondylitis patients diagnosed with spine fractures should have the entire spine imaged to rule out associated fractures at other levels.

Characteristic MRI findings suggestive of cervical spondylotic myelopathy, such as increased signal intensity of the spinal cord on T2-weighted imaging, typically occur late in the course of the disease and are predictive of poor neurologic outcome even with decompression surgery. Clinical studies have shown that conventional MRI for the evaluation of cervical spine myelopathy has a poor correlation with the symptoms and prognosis, with a diagnostic sensitivity between 15% and 65% in patients with major signs and symptoms. A newer imaging technique—diffusion tensor imaging—had been reported to demonstrate spinal cord impairment in patients with early stage cervical spondylosis before it is visible on plain MRI scans. Diffusion tensor imaging is based on the diffusion rate of water in tissue, making it sensitive to disease processes altering the water movement in the cervical spinal cord at a microscopic level beyond conventional MRI. The information it provides can be helpful in early identification of patients in whom operative treatment is indicated.

TREATMENT

Treatment is directed at maintaining flexibility and maintaining spinal alignment with exercises and posture. Sleeping supine on a firm mattress with one pillow may help maintain sagittal alignment. Medications used in the treatment of ankylosing spondylitis fall into three categories. The first includes nonsteroidal antiinflammatory drugs that relieve pain by decreasing joint inflammation. The second group comprises disease-modifying antirheumatic drugs such as minocycline, sulfasalazine, and methotrexate. This is an unrelated group of drugs found to slow the disease process, but they do not provide a cure. Finally, tumor necrosis factor-α blockers have been shown to be effective.

Operative management in patients with ankylosing spondylitis is indicated to decrease pain and improve function. Total hip arthroplasties are the most common surgical interventions performed in this population, followed by spinal osteotomies to correct sagittal imbalances.

Spinal fractures in patients with ankylosing spondylitis are always serious and frequently are life-threatening injuries. In patients with ankylosing spondylitis, cervical spine fracture is a leading cause of in-hospital mortality. Spine osteopenia that is common in this population combined with fused segments make patients more vulnerable to fractures, especially from minor trauma. It should be up to the treating physician to prove that the patient with ankylosis does not have a fracture after trauma. Spinal precautions and immobilization in a position accommodating the patient's posture is very important. Fractures usually occur in the lower cervical spine, frequently are unstable, and usually are discovered late. Persistent pain may be the only finding until late neurologic loss occurs. In patients with established kyphosis, the deformity may suddenly improve. The patient's previous deformity may be unknown to individuals providing emergency care. Any perceived change in spinal alignment, even if the result of trivial trauma, should be considered a fracture in a patient with ankylosing spondylitis. The standard procedure is to immobilize the patient in the position in which he or she is found because extension may result in sudden neurologic loss.

Surgical stabilization of fractures in patients with ankylosing spondylitis is associated with a high complication rate but has been shown to improve survival in this population. For stabilization of cervical fractures, combined anterior and posterior or long posterior constructs are recommended because of the poor bone quality. Yan et al. reported successful fusion of lower cervical spine fractures in 35 patients after pedicle screw fixation and autologous bone grafting through a single posterior approach. Anterior-only stabilization procedures are prone to failure; we recommend that they be avoided. The morbidity and mortality associated with these procedures in patients with ankylosing spondylitis are very high because of the comorbidities many of these patients have. Guo et al., however, reported successful fusion in nine of 10 patients treated with a single anterior approach followed by postoperative immobilization with a cervical collar and suggested that this technique can yield acceptable results in properly selected patients.

OSTEOTOMY OF THE CERVICAL SPINE

In patients with chin-on-chest deformity, often the mandible is so near the sternum that opening the mouth and chewing properly are difficult. Cervicodorsal kyphosis usually can be treated satisfactorily by lumbar osteotomy, which provides a compensatory lumbar lordosis and results in an erect posture. Cervical osteotomy may be indicated, however, (1) to elevate the chin from the sternum, improving the appearance, the ability to eat, and the ability to see ahead; (2) to prevent atlantoaxial and cervical subluxations and dislocations, which result from the weight of the head being carried forward by gravity; (3) to relieve tracheal and esophageal distortion, which causes dyspnea and dysphagia; and (4) to prevent irritation of the spinal cord tracts or excessive traction on the nerve roots, which causes neurologic disturbances.

The appropriate level for osteotomy is determined by the deformity and the degree of ossification of the anterior longitudinal ligament. Law successfully performed osteotomies at the levels of C3-4, C5-6, and C6-7, fixing the spine internally with the plates devised by Wilson and Straub for use in lumbosacral arthrodesis. Wiring of the spinal processes (see chapter 5), or use of a halo alone, also should be effective. In the osteotomy technique described by Simmons (Fig. 2.21), decompression is done first and is extended into the neural foramina. After decompression and resection of the inferior aspect of the pedicles, extension manipulation is done. The operation is done with the patient sitting on a stool or in a dental chair and inclined forward with the arms resting on an operating table (Fig. 2.22). Overcorrection of the deformity

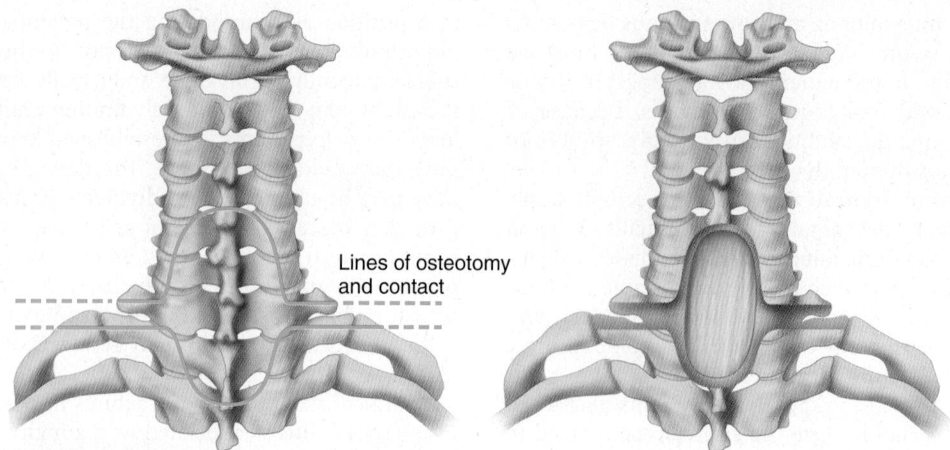

FIGURE 2.21 Extent of resection of cervical laminae for safe osteotomy. Lateral resections are beveled toward each other so that opposing surfaces are parallel and in apposition after extension osteotomy.

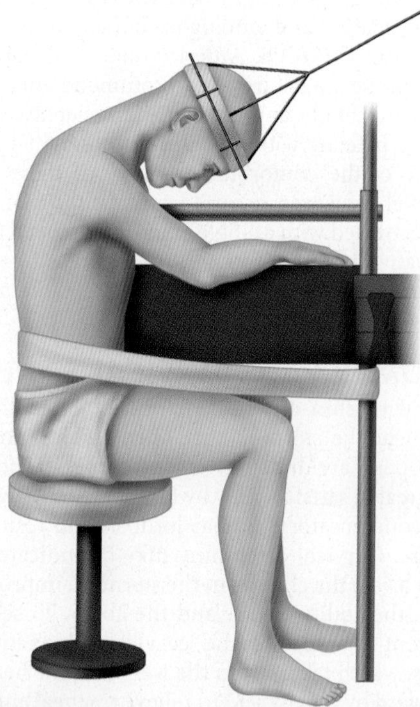

FIGURE 2.22 Position of patient for cervical osteotomy: sitting on stool with head suspended by halo and traction allows abdomen to be completely free of external pressure.

must be avoided because otherwise the trachea and esophagus could be overstretched and become obstructed. If halo stabilization alone is used, postoperative neurologic symptoms are treated by lessening correction; if internal fixation is used for more postoperative stability, reoperation is required for adjustment of correction. The halo is worn for 3 months, and a Philadelphia collar or similar orthosis is worn an additional 6 to 8 weeks.

REFERENCES

OVERVIEW OF DISC DEGENERATION AND HERNIATION

Badhiwala JH, Ahuja CS, Akbar MA, et al.: Degenerative cervical myelopathy — update and future directions, *Nat Rev Neurol* 16:108, 2020.

DISC AND SPINE ANATOMY

Dunbar L, Vidakovic H, Löffler S, et al.: Anterior cervical spine blood supply: a cadaveric study, *Surg Radiol Anat* 41:607, 2019.

Lee HJ, Kim JH, Kim IS, et al.: Anatomical evaluation of the vertebral artery (V2) and its influence in cervical spine surgery, *Clin Neurol Neurosurg* 174:80, 2018.

Rajabian A, Walsh M, Quraishi NA: Right- versus left-sided exposures of the recurrent laryngeal nerve and considerations of cervical spinal surgical corridor: a fresh-cadaveric surgical anatomy of RLN pertinent to spine, *Spine* 45:10, 2020.

NATURAL HISTORY OF DISC DISEASE

Hu P, He Z, Cui J, et al.: Pathological changes of cervical spinal canal in cervical spondylotic myelopathy: a retrospective study on 39 cases, *Clin Neurol Neurosurg* 181:133, 2019.

Hutton MJ, Bayer JH, Powell J, Sharp DJ: Modic vertebral body changes: the natural history as assessed by consecutive magnetic resonance imaging, *Spine* 36:2304, 2011.

Nouri A, Martin AR, Mikulis D, et al.: Magnetic resonance imaging assessment of degenerative cervical myelopathy: a review of structural changes and measurement techniques, *Neurosurg Focus* 40(6):E5, 2016.

Pesce A, Wierzbicki V, Piccione E, et al.: Adjacent segment pathology: natural history or effect of anterior cervical discectomy and fusion? A 10-year follow-up radiological multicenter study using an evaluation scale of the ageing spine, *Eur J Orthop Surg Traumatol* 27:503, 2017.

IMAGING STUDIES

Nukala M, Abraham J, Khandige G, et al.: Efficacy of diffusion tensor imaging in identification of degenerative cervical spondylotic myelopathy, *Eur J Radiol Open* 6:16, 2019.

Schöller K, Siller S, Brem C, et al.: Diffusion tensor imaging for surgical planning in patients with cervical spondylotic myelopathy, *J Neurol Surg Cent Eur Neurosurg* 81:001, 2020.

Toktas Z, Tanrikulu B, Koban O, et al.: Diffusion tensor imaging of cervical spinal cord: a quantitative diagnostic tool in cervical spondylotic myelopathy, *J Craniovertebr Junction Spine* 7:26, 2016.

INJECTION STUDIES

Alvin MD, Mehta V, Halabi HA, et al.: Cost-effectiveness of cervical epidural steroid injections: a 3-month pilot study, *Global Spine J* 9:143, 2019.

Bogduk N: *International Spine Intervention Society practice guidelines for spinal diagnostic and treatment procedures*, San Francisco, 2004, International Spine Intervention Society.

Chen B, Rispoli L, Stitik TP, et al.: Optimal needle entry angle for cervical transforaminal epidural injections, *Pain Physician* 17:139, 2014.

Cohen-Adad J, Buchbinder B, Oaklander AL: Cervical spinal cord injection of epidural corticosteroids: comprehensive longitudinal study including multiparametric magnetic resonance imaging, *Pain* 153:2292, 2012.

Epstein NE: Major risks and complications of cervical epidural steroid injections: an updated review, *Surg Neurol Int* 9:86, 2018.

Falco FJ, Manchikanti L, Datta S, et al.: Systematic review of the therapeutic effectiveness of cervical facet joint interventions: an update, *Pain Physician* 15:E839, 2012.

Gerling MC, Radcliff K, Isaacs R, et al.: Trends in nonoperative treatment modalities prior to cervical surgery and impact on patient-derived outcomes: two-year analysis of 1522 patients from the prospective spine treatment outcome study, *Int J Spine Surg* 12:250, 2018.

Gill JS, Aner M, Jyotsna N, et al.: Contralateral oblique view is superior to lateral view for interlaminar cervical and cervicothoracic epidural access, *Pain Med* 16:68, 2015.

Hoang JK, Massoglia DP, Apostol MA, et al.: CT-guided cervical transforaminal steroid injections: where should the needle tip be located? *AJNR Am J Neuroradiol* 34:688, 2013.

Laemmel E, Segal N, Mirshahi M, Azzaene D, et al.: Deleterious effects of intra-arterial administration of particulate steroids on microvascular perfusion in a mouse model, *Radiology* 279:731, 2016.

Manchikanti L, Abdi S, Atluri S, et al.: An update of comprehensive evidence-based guidelines for interventional techniques in chronic spinal pain. Part II: guidance and recommendations, *Pain Physician* 16(Suppl 2):S49, 2013.

Manchikanti L, Cash KA, Pampati V, et al.: The effectiveness of fluoroscopic cervical interlaminar epidural injections in managing chronic cervical disc herniation and radiculitis: preliminary results of a randomized, double-blind, controlled trial, *Pain Physician* 13:223, 2010.

Manchikanti L, Cash KA, Pampati V, et al.: A randomized, double-blind, active control trial of fluoroscopic cervical interlaminar epidural injections in chronic pain of cervical disc herniation: results of a 2-year follow-up, *Pain Physician* 16:465, 2013.

Manchikanti L, Malla Y, Cash KA, Pampati V: Do the gaps in the ligamentum flavum in the cervical spine translate into dural punctures? An analysis of 4,396 fluoroscopic interlaminar epidural injections, *Pain Physician* 18:259, 2015.

Manchikanti L, Singh V, Pampati V, et al.: Comparison of the efficacy of caudal, interlaminar, and transforaminal epidural injections in managing disc herniation: is one method superior to the other? *Korean J Pain* 28:11, 2015.

Mehta P, Syrop I, Singh JR, Kirschner J: Systematic review of the efficacy of particulate versus nonparticulate corticosteroids in epidural injections, *PMR* 9:502, 2017.

Nishio I: Cervical transforaminal epidural steroid injections: a proposal for opitimizing the preprocedural evaluation with available imaging, *Reg Anesth Pain Med* 39:546, 2014.

Obernauer J, Galiano K, Gruber H, et al.: Ultrasound-guided versus computed tomography-controlled facet joint injections in the middle and lower cervical spine: a prospective randomized clinical trial, *Med Ultrason* 15:10, 2013.

Pampati V, et al.: Cervical epidural injections in chronic discogenic neck pain without disc herniation or radiculitis: preliminary results of a randomized, double-blind, controlled trial, *Pain Physician* 13:E265, 2010.

Park CH, Lee SH: Contrast dispersion pattern and efficacy of computed tomography-guided cervical transforaminal epidural steroid injection, *Pain Physician* 17:487, 2014.

Schneider BJ, Maybin S, Sturos E: Safety and complications of cervical epidural steroid injections, *Phys Med Rehabil Clin N Am* 29:155, 2018.

Shipley K, Riew KD, Gilula LA: Fluoroscopically guided extraforaminal cervical nerve root blocks: analysis of epidural flow of the injectate with respect to needle tip position, *Global Spine J* 4:7, 2014.

Vasudeva V, Chi J: Defining the role of epidural steroid injections in the treatment of radicular pain from degenerative cervical disk disease, *Neurosurgery* 76:N16, 2015.

Wald JT, Maus TP, Diehn FE, et al.: CT-guided cervical transforaminal epidural steroid injections: technical insights, *J Neuroradiol* 41:211, 2014.

Wald JT, Maus TP, Geske JR, et al.: Immediate pain response does not predict long-term outcome of CT-guided cervical transforaminal epidural steroid injections, *AJNR Am J Neuroradiol* 34:1665, 2013.

SURGERY—TECHNIQUES, OUTCOMES, COMPLICATIONS

Alvin MD, Qureshi S, Klineberg E, et al.: Cervical degenerative disease: systematic review of economic analyses, *Spine* 39(22 Suppl 1):S53, 2014.

Buerba RA, Giles E, Webb ML, et al.: Increased risk of complications after anterior cervical discectomy and fusion in the elderly: an analysis of 6253 patients in the American College of Surgeons National Surgical Quality Improvement Program database, *Spine* 39:2062, 2014.

Bydon M, Mathios D, Macki M, et al.: Long-term patient outcomes after posterior cervical foraminotomy: an analysis of 151 cases, *J Neurosurg Spine* 21:727, 2014.

Cardoso MJ, Mendelsohn A, Rosner MK: Cervical hybrid arthroplasty with 2 unique fusion techniques, *J Neurosurg Spine* 15:48, 2011.

Caridi JM, Pumberger M, Hughes AP: Cervical radiculopathy: a review, *HSS J* 7:265, 2011.

Chen Q, Brahimaj BC, Khanna R, et al.: Posterior atlantoaxial fusion: a comprehensive review of surgical techniques and relevant vascular anomalies, *J Spine Surg* 6:164, 2020.

Cho W, Buchowski JM, Park Y, et al.: Surgical approach to the cervicothoracic junction: can a standard Smith-Robinson approach be utilized? *J Spinal Disord Tech* 25:264, 2012.

Cho SK, Riew KD: Adjacent segment disease following cervical spine surgery, *J Am Acad Orthop Surg* 21:3, 2013.

Cole T, Veeravagu A, Zhang M, et al.: Anterior versus posterior approach for multilevel degenerative cervical disease: a retrospective propensity score-matched study of the MarketScan database, *Spine* 40:1033, 2015.

Dohrmann G, Hsieh JC: Long-term results of anterior versus posterior operations for herniated cervical discs: analysis of 6000 patients, *Med Princ Pract* 23:70, 2014.

Fineberg SJ, Ahmadinia K, Oglesby M, et al.: Hospital outcomes and complications of anterior and posterior cervical fusion with bone morphogenetic protein, *Spine* 38:1304, 2013.

Graham RS, Samsell BJ, Proffer A, et al.: Evaluation of glycerol-reserved bone allografts in cervical spine fusion: a prospective, randomized controlled trial, *J Neurosurg Spine* 22:1, 2015.

Gutman G, Rosenzweig DH, Golan JD: Surgical treatment of cervical radioculopathy: meta-analysis of randomized controlled trials, *Spine* 43:E365, 2018.

Guyer RD, Ohnmeiss DD, Blumenthal SL, et al.: In which cases do surgeons specializing in total disc replacement perform fusion in patients with cervical spine symptoms? *Eur Spine J*, 2020 Jan 2, [Epub ahead of print].

Hirai T, Yoshii T, Sakai K, et al.: Long-term results of a prospective study of anterior decompression with fusion and posterior decompression with laminoplasty for treatment of cervical spondylotic myelopathy, *J Orthop Sci* 23:32, 2018.

Hsu WK: Outcomes following nonoperative and operative treatment for cervical disc herniations in National Football League athletes, *Spine* 36:800, 2010.

Ishak B, Younsi A, Wieckhusen C, et al.: Accuracy and revision rate of intraoperative computed tomography point-to-point navigation for lateral mass and pedicle screw placement: 11-year single-center experience in 1054 patients, *Neurosurg Rev* 42:895, 2019.

Johnson MD, Matur AV, Asghar F, et al.: Right versus left approach to anterior cervical discectomy and fusion: an anatomic versus historic debate, *World Neurosurg* 135:135, 2020.

Lawrence BD, Jacobs WB, Norvell DC, et al.: Anterior versus posterior approach for treatment of cervical spondylotic myelopathy: a systematic review, *Spine* 38(22 Suppl 1):S173, 2013.

Lovecchio F, Hsu WK, Smith TR, et al.: Predictors of thirty-day readmission after anterior cervical fusion, *Spine* 39:127, 2014.

Lubelski D, Healy AT, Silverstein MP, et al.: Reoperation rates after anterior cervical discectomy and fusion versus posterior cervical foraminotomy: a propensity-matched analysis, *Spine J* 15:1277, 2015.

McCormack BM, Dhawan R: Novel instrumentation and technique for tissue sparing posterior cervical fusion, *J Clin Neurosci* 34:299, 2016.

Maulucci CM, Ghobrial GM, Sharan AD, et al.: Correlation of posterior occipitocervical angle and surgical outcomes for occipitocervical fusion, *Evid Based Spine Care J* 592:163, 2014.

McAnany S, Noureldin MN, Elboghdady IM, et al.: Mesenchymal stem cell allograft as a fusion adjunct in one and two level anterior cervical discectomy and fusion: a matched cohort analysis, *Spine J* 16:163, 2016.

Miller LE, Block JE: Safety and effectiveness of bone allografts in anterior cervical discectomy and fusion surgery, *Spine* 36:2045, 2011.

Nanda A, Sharma M, Sonig A, et al.: Surgical complications of anterior cervical diskectomy and fusion for cervical degenerative disk disease: a single surgeon's experience of 1,576 patients, *World Neurosurg* 82:1380, 2014.

Narain AS, Hijji FY, Haws BE, et al.: Impact of body mass index on surgical outcomes, narcotics consumption, and hospital costs following anterior cervical discectomy and fusion, *J Neurosurg Spine* 28:160, 2018.

Onyewu O, Manchikanti L, Falco FJ, et al.: An update of the appraisal of the accuracy and utility of cervical discography in chronic neck pain, *Pain Physician* 15:E777, 2012.

Pahys JM, Pahys JR, Cho SK, et al.: Methods to decrease postoperative infections following posterior cervical spine surgery, *J Bone Joint Surg* 95A:549, 2013.

Pirkle S, Kaskovich S, Cook DJ, et al.: Cages in ACDF are associated with a higher nonunion rate than allograft: a stratified comparative analysis of 6130 patients, *Spine* 44:384, 2019.

Raizman NM, Yu WD, Jenkins MV, et al.: Traumatic C4-C5 unilateral facet dislocation with posterior disc herniation above a prior anterior fusion, *Am J Orthop* 41:E85, 2012.

Shau DN, Bible JE, Samade R, et al.: Utility of postoperative radiographs for cervical spine fusion: a comprehensive evaluation of operative technique, surgical indication, and duration since surgery, *Spine* 37:1994, 2012.

Singh K, Marquez-Lara A, Nandyala SV, et al.: Incidence and risk factors for dysphagia after anterior cervical fusion, *Spine* 38:1820, 2013.

Skovrlj B, Gologorsky Y, Haque R, et al.: Complications, outcomes, and need for fusion after minimally invasive posterior cervical foraminotomy and microdiscectomy, *Spine J* 14:2405, 2014.

Srinivasan D, La Marca F, Than KD, et al.: Perioperative characteristics and complications in obese patients undergoing anterior cervical fusion surgery, *J Clin Neurosci* 21:1159, 2014.

Tannoury CA, An HS: Complications with the use of bone morphogenetic protein 2 (BMP-2) in spine surgery, *Spine J* 14:552, 2014.

Tschugg A, Neururer S, Scheufler KM, et al.: Comparison of posterior foraminotomy and anterior foraminotomy with fusion for treating spondylotic foraminal stenosis of the cervical spine: study protocol for a randomized controlled trial (ForaC), *Trials* 15:437, 2014.

Wang TY, Lubelski D, Abdullah KG, et al.: Rates of anterior cervical discectomy and fusion after initial posterior cervical foraminotomy, *Spine J* 15:971, 2015.

Williams BJ, Smith JS, Fu KM, et al.: Does BMP increase the incidence of perioperative complications in spinal fusion? A comparison of 55,862 cases of spinal fusion with and without BMP, *Spine* 36:1685, 2011.

Wang Y, Zheng GQ, Zhang YG, et al.: Proposal of a new treatment-oriented classification system for spinal deformity in ankylosing spondylitis, *Spine Deform* 6:366, 2018.

Wysham KD, Murray SG, Hills N, et al.: Cervical spinal fracture and other diagnoses associated with mortality in hospitalized ankylosing spondylitis patients, *Arthritis Care Res* 69:271, 2017.

Yee TJ, Swong K, Park P: Complications of anterior cervical spine surgery: a systematic review of the literature, *J Spine Surg* 6:302, 2020.

Yan L, Luo Z, He B, et al.: Posterior pedicle screw fixation to treat lower cervical fractures associated with ankylosing spondylitis: a retrospective study of 35 cases, *BMC Musculoskelet Disord* 18:81, 2017.

You J, Tang X, Gao W, et al.: Factors predicting adjacent segment disease after anterior cervical discectomy and fusion treating cervical spondylotic myelopathy: a retrospective study with 5-year follow-up, *Medicine (Baltim)* 97:e12893, 2018.

Yuan X, Wei C, Xu W, et al.: Comparison of laminectomy and fusion vs laminoplasty in the treatment of multilevel cervical spondylotic myelopathy: a meta-analysis, *Medicine (Baltim)* 98:e14971, 2019.

MINIMALLY INVASIVE SURGERY

Ahn Y: Endoscopic spine discectomy: indications and outcomes, *Int Orthop* 43:909, 2019.

Branch BC, Hilton Jr DL, Watts C: Minimally invasive tubular access for posterior cervical foraminotomy, *Surg Neurol Int* 6:81, 2015.

Burkhardt BW, Oertel JM: Endoscopic spinal surgery using a new tubular retractor with 15 mm outer diameter, *Br J Neurosurg* 33:514, 2019.

Clark JG, Abdullah KG, Steinmetz MP, et al.: Minimally invasive versus open cervical foraminotomy: a systematic review, *Global Spine J* 1:9, 2011.

Epstein NE: Learning curves for minimally invasive spine surgeries: are they worth it? *Surg Neurol Int* 8:61, 2017.

Gutman G, Rosenzweig DH, Golan JD: Surgical treatment of cervical radiculopathy: meta-analysis of randomized controlled trials, *Spine* 43:E65, 2018.

Hussain I, Schmidt FA, Kirnaz S, et al.: MIS approaches in the cervical spine, *J Spine Surg* 5(Suppl 1):S74, 2019.

Jeon JK, Oh CH, Chung D, et al.: Prevertebral vascular esophageal consideration during percutaneous cervical disc procedures, *Spine* 39:275, 2014.

Lee S, Park JH: Minimally invasive cervical pedicle screw placement with a freehand technique through the posterolateral approach using a tubular retractor: a technical note, *Oper Neurosurg (Hagerstown)* 17:E166, 2019.

Mansfield HE, Canar WJ, Gerard CS, O'Toole JE: Single-level anterior cervical discectomy and fusion versus minimally invasive posterior cervical foraminotomy for patients with cervical radiculopathy: a cost analysis, *Neurosurg Focus* 37:E9, 2014.

McAnany SJ, Kim JS, Overley SC, et al.: A meta-analysis of cervical foraminotomy: open versus minimally invasive techniques, *Spine J* 15:849, 2015.

Minamide A, Yoshida M, Simpson AK, et al.: Microendoscopic laminotomy versus conventional laminoplasty for cervical spondylotic myelopathy: 5-year follow-up study, *J Neurosurg Spine* 27:403, 2017.

Ross MN, Ross DA: Minimally invasive cervical laminectomy for cervical spondylotic myelopathy, *Clin Spine Surg* 31:331, 2018.

Sahai N, Changoor S, Dunn CJ, et al.: Minimally invasive posterior cervical foraminotomy as an alternative to anterior cervical discectomy and fusion for unilateral cervical radiculopathy: a systematic review and meta-analysis, *Spine* 44:1731, 2019.

Song Z, Zhang Z, Hao J, et al.: Microsurgery or open cervical foraminotomy for cervical radiculopathy? A systematic review, *Int Orthop* 40:1335, 2016.

Wu PF, Li YW, Wang B, et al.: Complications of full-endoscopic versus microendoscopic foraminotomy for cervical radiculopathy: a systematic review and meta-analysis, *World Neurosurg* 114:217, 2018.

Wu PF, Li YW, Wang B, et al.: Posterior cervical foraminotomy via full-endoscopic versus microendoscopic approach for radiculopathy: a systematic review and meta-analysis, *Pain Physician* 22(1):41, 2019.

CERVICAL DISC ARTHROPLASTY

Bevevino A, Lehman Jr RA, Kang DG, et al.: The effect of cervical posterior foraminotomy on segmental range of motion in the setting of total disc arthroplasty, *Spine* 39:1572, 2014.

Brody MJ, Patel AA, Ghanayem AJ, et al.: The effect of posterior decompressive procedures on segmental range of motion after cervical total disc arthroplasty, *Spine* 39:1558, 2014.

Cheng L, Nie L, Li M, et al.: Superiority of the BRYAN disc prosthesis for cervical myelopathy: a randomized study with 3-year followup, *Clin Orthop Relat Res* 469:3408, 2011.

Coric D, Nunley PD, Guyer RD, et al.: Prospective, randomized multicenter study of cervical arthroplasty: 269 patients from the Kineflex-C artificial disc investigational device exemption study with a minimum 2-year follow-up, *J Neurosurg Spine* 15:348, 2011.

Garrido BJ, Wilhite J, Nakano M, et al.: Adjacent-level cervical ossification after Bryan cervical disc arthroplasty compared with anterior cervical discectomy and fusion, *J Bone Joint Surg* 93:1185, 2011.

Ghobrial GM, Lavelle WF, Florman JE, et al.: Symptomatic adjacent level disease requiring surgery: analysis of 10-year results from a prospective, randomized, clinical trial comparing cervical disc arthroplasty to anterior cervical fusion, *Neurosurgery* 84:347, 2019.

Guyer RD, Shellock J, MacLennan B, et al.: Early failure of metal-on-metal artifical disc prostheses associated with lymphocytic reaction: diagnosis and treatment experience in four cases, *Spine* 36:E492, 2011.

Hu Y, Lv G, Ren S, et al.: Mid- to long-term outcomes of cervical disc arthroplasty versus anterior cervical discectomy and fusion for treatment of symptomatic cervical disc disease: a systematic review and meta-analysis of eight prospective randomized controlled trials, *PloS One* 11: e0149312, 2016.

Jawahar A, Cavanaugh DA, Kerr 3rd EJ, et al.: Total disc arthroplasty does not affect the incidence of adjacent segment degeneration in cervical spine: results of 93 patients in three prospective randomized clinical trials, *Spine J* 10:1043, 2010.

Jiang H, Zhu Z, Qiu Y, et al.: Cervical disc arthroplasty versus fusion for single-level symptomatic cervical disc disease: a meta-analysis of randomized controlled trials, *Arch Orthop Trauma Surg* 132:141, 2012.

Joaquim AF, Makhni MC, Riew D: Evidence-based use of arthroplasty in cervical degenerative disc disease, *Int Orthop* 43:767, 2019.

Kani KK, Chew FS: Cervical disc arthroplasty: review and update for radiologists, *Semin Roentgenol* 54:113, 2019.

Kelly MP, Mok JM, Frisch RF, et al.: Adjacent segment motion after anterior cervical discectomy and fusion versus Prodisc-c cervical total disk arthroplasty: analysis from a randomized, controlled trial, *Spine* 36:1171, 2011.

Kim SW, Paik SH, Castro PA, et al.: Analysis of factors that may influence range of motion after cervical disc arthroplasty, *Spine J* 10:683, 2010.

Koreckij TD, Sapan D, Gandhi SD, Park DK: Cervical disk arthroplasty, *J Am Acad Orthop Surg* 27:e96, 2019.

Luo J, Hongbo Wang H, Peng J, et al.: Rate of adjacent segment degeneration of cervical disc arthroplasty versus fusion: meta-analysis of randomized controlled trials, 113:225, 2018.

MacDowall A, Moreira CN, Marques C, et al.: Artificial disc replacement versus fusion in patients with cervical degenerative disc disease and radiculopathy: a randomized controlled trial with 5-year outcomes, *J Neuro Spine* 30:323, 2019.

Nabhan A, Ishak B, Steudel WI, et al.: Assessment of adjacent-segment mobility after cervical disc replacement versus fusion: RCT with 1 year's results, *Eur Spine J* 20:934, 2011.

Nunley PD, Coric D, Frank KA, et al.: Cervical disc arthroplasty: current evidence and real-world application, *Neurosurgery* 83:1087, 2018.

Nunley PD, Hawahar A, Kerr 3rd EJ, et al.: Factors affecting the incidence of symptomatic adjacent level disease in cervical spine after total disc arthroplasty: 2-4 years follow-up of 3 prospective randomized trials, *Spine* 37:445, 2012.

Sasso RC, Anderson PA, Riew KD, Heller JG: Results of cervical arthroplasty compared with anterior discectomy and fusion: four-year clinical outcomes in a prospective, randomized controlled trial, *J Bone Joint Surg* 93A:1684, 2011.

Stadler 3rd JA, Wong AP, Graham RB, Liu JC: Complications associated with posterior approaches in minimally invasive spine decompression, *Neurosurg Clin N Am* 25:233, 2014.

Sundseth J, Fredriks OA, Kolstad F, et al.: The Norwegian Cervical Arthroplasty Trial (NORCAT): 2-year clinical outcome after single-level cervical arthroplasty versus fusion—a prospective, single-blinded, randomized, controlled multicenter study, *Eur Spine J* 26:1255, 2017.

Upadhyayula PS, Yue JK, Curtis EI, et al.: A matched cohort comparison of cervical disc arthroplasty versus anterior cervical discectomy and fusion: evaluating perioperative outcomes, *J Clin Neurosci* 43:235, 2017.

White NA, Moreno DP, Brown PJ, et al.: Effects of cervical arthrodesis and arthroplasty on neck response during a simulated frontal automobile collision, *Spine J* 14:2195, 2014.

Zhang X, Zhang X, Chen C, et al.: Randomized, controlled, multicenter, clinical trial comparing BRYAN cervical disc arthroplasty with anterior cervical decompression and fusion in China, *Spine* 37:433, 2012.

Zindrick M, Harris MB, Humphreys SC, et al.: Cervical disc arthroplasty, *J Am Acad Orthop Surg* 18:631, 2010.

RHEUMATOID ARTHRITIS OF THE SPINE

Ferrante A, Ciccia F, Giammalva GR, et al.: The craniovertebral junction in rheumatoid arthritis: state of the art, *Acta Neurochir Suppl* 125:79, 2019.

Han MH, Ryu JI, Kim CH, et al.: Factors that predict risk of cervical instability in rheumatoid arthritis patients, *Spine* 42:966, 2017.

Horowitz JA, Puvanesarajah V, Jain A, et al.: Rheumatoid arthritis is associated with an increased risk of postoperative infection and revision surgery in elderly patients undergoing anterior cervical fusion, *Spine* 43(17):E1040, 2018.

Joaquim AF, Ghizoni E, Tedeschi H, et al.: Radiological evaluation of cervical spine involvement in rheumatoid arthritis, *Neurosurg Focus* 38:E4, 2015.

Kim HJ, Nemani VM, Riew KD, Brasington R: Cervical spine disease in rheumatoid arthritis: incidence, manifestations, and therapy, *Curr Rheumatol Rep* 17:9, 2015.

Li J, Goldstein PA: Images in aesthesiology: cranial settling: a cervical spine complication of rheumatoid arthritis, *Anesthesiology* 123:668, 2015.

Narváez J, Narváez JA, Serrallonga M, et al.: Subaxial cervical spine involvement in symptomatic rheumatoid arthritis patients: comparison with cervical spondylosis, *Semin Arthritis Rheum* 45:9, 2015.

Söderman T, Olerud C, Shalabi A, et al.: Static and dynamic CT imaging of the cervical spine in patients with rheumatoid arthritis, *Skeletal Radiol* 44:241, 2015.

Stein BE, Hassanzadeh H, Jain A, et al.: Changing trends in cervical spine fusions in patients with rheumatoid arthritis, *Spine* 39:1178, 2014.

Terashima Y, Yurube T, Hirata H, et al.: Predictive risk factors of cervical spine instabilities in rheumatoid arthritis: a prospective multicenter over 10-year cohort study, *Spine* 42:556, 2017.

Wasserman BR, Moskovich R, Razi AE: Rheumatoid arthritis of the cervical spine—clinical considerations, *Bull NYU Hosp Jt Dis* 69:136, 2011.

Yurube T, Sumi M, Nishida K, et al.: Incidence and aggravation of cervical spine instabilities in rheumatoid arthritis: a prospective minimum 5-year follow-up study of patients initially without cervical involvement, *Spine* 37:2136, 2012.

Yurube T, Sumi M, Nishida K, et al.: Accelerated development of cervical spine instabilities in rheumatoid arthritis: a prospective minimum 5-year cohort study, *PloS One* 9:e88970, 2014.

Zhang T, Pope J: Cervical spine involvement in rheumatoid arthritis over time: results from a meta-analysis, *Arthritis Res Ther* 17:148, 2015.

Zhu S, Xu W, Luo Y, et al.: Cervical spine involvement risk factors in rheumatoid arthritis: a meta-analysis, *Int J Rheum Dis* 20:541, 2017.

ANKYLOSING SPONDYLITIS OF THE CERVICAL SPINE

Baraliakos X, Listing J, von der Recke A, Braun J: The natural course of radiographic progression in ankylosing spondylitis: differences between genders and appearance of characteristic radiographic features, *Curr Rheumatol Rep* 13:383, 2011.

Guo Q, Cui Y, Wang L, et al.: Single anterior approach for cervical spine fractures at C5-T1 complicating ankylosing spondylitis, *Clin Neurol Neurosurg* 147:1, 2016.

Koller H, Koller J, Mayer M, et al.: Osteotomies in ankylosing spondylitis: where, how many, and how much? *Eur Spine J* 27(Suppl 1):70, 2018.

Lin B, Zhang B, Li ZM, Li QS: Corrective surgery for deformity of the upper cervical spine due to ankylosing spondylitis, *Indian J Orthop* 48:211, 2014.

Mehdian SM, Boreham B, Hammett T: Cervical osteotomy in ankylosing spondylitis, *Eur Spine J* 21:2713, 2012.

Wang Y, Zheng GQ, Zhang YG, et al.: Proposal of a new treatment-oriented classification system for spinal deformity in ankylosing spondylitis, *Spine Deform* 6:366, 2018.

Wysham KD, Murray SG, Hills N, et al.: Cervical spinal fracture and other diagnoses associated with mortality in hospitalized ankylosing spondylitis patients, *Arthritis Care Res* 69:271, 2017.

Yan L, Luo Z, He B, et al.: Posterior pedicle screw fixation to treat lower cervical fractures associated with ankylosing spondylitis: a retrospective study of 35 cases, *BMC Musculoskelet Disord* 18:81, 2017.

Yang J, Huang Z, Grevitt M, et al.: Precise bending rod technique a novel method for precise correction of ankylosing spondylitis kyphosis, *J Spinal Disord Tech* 29:E452, 2016.

The complete list of references is available online at ExpertConsult.com.

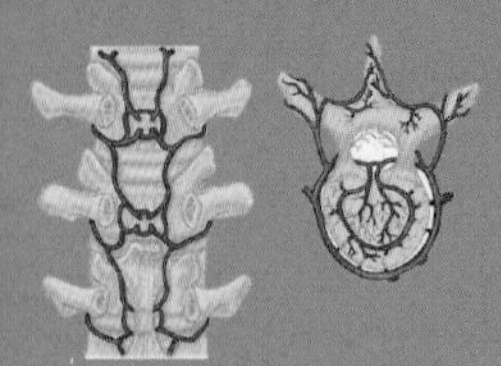

CHAPTER 3

DEGENERATIVE DISORDERS OF THE THORACIC AND LUMBAR SPINE

Raymond J. Gardocki, Ashley L. Park

OVERVIEW OF LUMBAR AND THORACIC DISC DEGENERATION AND HERNIATION

Despite an improving understanding of degenerative disc disease on the basis of its natural history and basic science, treatment results of this entity vary greatly. There is no lack of treatment options for degenerative discs; what we tend to lack is understanding of the specific cause(s) of the patient's chief complaint. Despite the fact that William Kirkaldy-Willis has described the spectrum of disc degeneration and its pathologic progression, the clinical correlation of history, physical examination, and imaging that yields a specific diagnosis remains the greatest challenge. Over the past several decades, studies of patients with back and/or leg pain have led to improved treatment of the patients in whom a specific diagnosis was possible. This group remains the minority of patients who are evaluated for low back or leg pain. Complex psychosocial issues, depression, and secondary gain are a few of the non-anatomic problems that must be considered when evaluating these patients. In addition, the number of anatomic causes for these symptoms, whether real or perceived, has increased as understanding and diagnostic capabilities have increased.

Axial spine pain, which should be distinguished from disc degeneration, is the most frequent musculoskeletal complaint. Axial spine pain—whether cervical, thoracic, or lumbar—often is attributed to disc degeneration. This degenerative process does not always cause pain, but it can lead to internal disc derangement, disc herniation, facet arthrosis, degenerative spondylolisthesis, and stenosis that can be seen on imaging. Each of these pathologic processes has unique clinical findings and treatments. Outcomes of treatment for each of these specific pathologic entities also vary greatly despite their being from the same etiologic spectrum. The understanding of disc degeneration and the associated pathologies has changed markedly over the past several years.

The genetic influence on disc degeneration may be caused by a small effect from each of multiple genes or possibly a relatively large effect from a smaller number of genes. To date, several specific gene loci have been identified that are associated with disc degeneration. This association of a specific gene with degenerative disc changes has been confirmed. Other variations in the aggrecan gene, metalloproteinase-3 gene, collagen type IX, and alpha 2 and 3 gene forms also have been associated with disc pathology and symptoms. The understanding of symptoms and treatment success for disc herniations has surpassed those related to disc degeneration alone.

Nonspecific axial pain is an international health issue of major significance and should be discriminated from pain associated with a disc herniation. Approximately 80% of individuals are affected by this symptom at some time in their lives. Impairments of the back and spine are ranked as the most frequent cause of limitation of activity in individuals younger than 45 years old by the National Center for Health Statistics (www.cdc.gov/nchs). Physicians who treat patients with spinal disorders and spine-related complaints must distinguish the complaint of back pain, which several epidemiologic studies reveal to be relatively constant, from disability attributed to back pain. Although back pain as a presenting complaint may account for only 2% of the patients seen by a general practitioner, the cost to society and the patient in terms of lost work time, compensation, and treatment is staggering.

The total cost of low back pain in the United States is greater than $100 billion per year; one third are direct costs for care, with the remaining costs resulting from decreased productivity, lost wages, and absenteeism. Also, only about 5% of patients accounted for 75% of the costs. Typically, about 90% of patients return to work by 3 months, with most returning to work by 1 month. Patients off work for 6 months have only a 50/50 probability of ever returning to work, whereas at 1 year this probability decreases to 25%.

Nonanatomic factors, specifically work perception and psychosocial factors, are intimately intertwined with physical complaints. Compounding the diagnostic and treatment difficulties is the high incidence of significant abnormalities shown by imaging studies, which in asymptomatic matched controls is 76%. Identified risk factors for radiographically apparent disc disorders of the lumbar spine include genetic factors, age, gender, smoking, increased intra-abdominal fat, metabolic syndrome, and, to a minimal degree, occupational exposure, but not socioeconomic factors. In contrast is the importance of socioeconomic factors for the development of low back pain and disability. Job dissatisfaction, physically strenuous work, psychologically stressful work, low educational attainment, and workers' compensation insurance all are associated with low back pain or disability. These data suggest that aggressive treatment between 4 weeks and 6 months is necessary for patients with low back pain. Consideration of socioeconomic factors is an important component of appropriate patient evaluation because there is an inextricable link between an individual's socioeconomic status and his or her health.

Optimal outcome primarily depends on "proper patient selection," which so far has defied satisfactory definition. Until the pathologic process is better described and reliable criteria for the diagnosis are determined, improvement in treatment outcomes will change slowly.

DISC AND SPINE ANATOMY

The anatomy of the spine and discs is discussed in detail in chapter 1.

NEURAL ELEMENTS

The organization of the neural elements is strictly maintained throughout the entire neural system, even within the conus medullaris and cauda equina distally. The orientation of the nerve roots in the dural sac and at the conus medullaris follows a highly organized pattern, with the most cephalad roots lying lateral and the most caudad lying centrally. The motor roots are ventral to the sensory roots at all levels. The arachnoid mater holds the roots in these positions.

The pedicle is the key to understanding surgical spinal anatomy. The relation of the pedicle to the neural elements varies by region within the spinal column. In the thoracic and lumbar spine, the named root exits below the named pedicle. Discs are formally named for the vertebral bodies between which they lie (e.g., the L4-5 disc is between the L4 and L5 vertebral bodies). This allows slightly more specificity in describing the discs if there is an anatomic variant (e.g., L4-S1) and less confusion than having the vertebral body, nerve root, and disc sharing the same name. Despite being less specific, the disc often is informally named for the vertebral level immediately cephalad (e.g., the L4 disc is immediately caudal to the L4 vertebra). In the lumbar spine, lateral recess

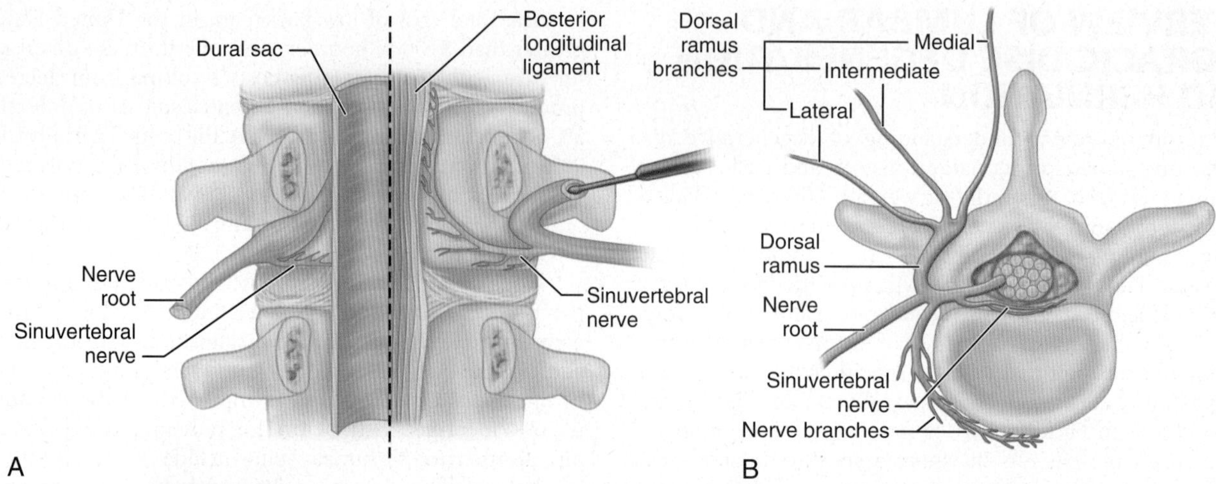

FIGURE 3.1 **A,** Dorsal view of lumbar spinal segment with lamina and facets removed. On left side, dura and root exiting at that level remain. On right side, dura has been resected and root is elevated. Sinuvertebral nerve with its course and innervation of posterior longitudinal ligament is usually obscured by nerve root and dura. **B,** Cross-sectional view of spine at level of endplate and disc. Note that sinuvertebral nerve innervates dorsal surface of disc and posterior longitudinal ligament. Additional nerve branches from ventral ramus innervate more ventral surface of disc and anterior longitudinal ligament. Dorsal ramus arises from root immediately on leaving foramen. This ramus divides into lateral, intermediate, and medial branches. Medial branch supplies primary innervation to facet joints dorsally.

pathology, such as lateral recess stenosis or posterolateral disc herniation, typically involves the next nerve root exiting caudal to that disc; for example, an L4-5 posterolateral disc herniation would be expected to cause L5 nerve root symptoms.

At the level of the intervertebral foramen is the dorsal root ganglion (DRG). The DRG lies within the outer confines of the foramen. Distal to the ganglion, three distinct branches arise; the most prominent and important is the ventral ramus, which supplies all structures ventral to the neural canal. The second branch, the sinuvertebral nerve, is a small filamentous nerve that originates from the ventral ramus and progresses medially over the posterior aspect of the disc and vertebral bodies, innervating these structures and the posterior longitudinal ligament. The third branch is the dorsal ramus. This branch courses dorsally, piercing the intertransverse ligament near the pars interarticularis. Three branches from the dorsal ramus innervate the structures dorsal to the neural canal. The lateral and intermediate branches provide innervation to the posterior musculature and skin. The medial branch separates into three branches to innervate the facet joint at that level and the adjacent levels above and below (Fig. 3.1).

Disc innervation is through afferent axons with cell bodies within the DRG. Nociceptive signals are transmitted to the spinal cord by neurons from the DRG. Animal studies have revealed two paths between the annulus and the DRG: one from the sinuvertebral nerve and another along the paravertebral sympathetic trunk. The sinuvertebral nerve is a recurrent branch of the ventral ramus that connects back to the posterior disc at each level. The paired ganglia chains of the sympathetic trunks have axons that course through the gray rami communicantes to the spinal nerve. The disc is innervated by fibers from multiple levels. In animal models, the lateral annulus was found to be innervated by fibers coursing from the index level and two additional superior levels through the sinuvertebral nerves. Also, there was innervation through the sympathetic trunk by the DRG from the three levels even more superior than the sinuvertebral innervations. Contralateral DRG involvement also occurs through both pathways. Similar nonsegmental, multilevel innervation patterns also have been reported for the ventral disc surface. These complex multilevel innervations would help explain the pain patterns encountered clinically if similar patterns are present in humans. Also, innervations of the disc from the vertebral endplate have been shown. Intraosseous nerves follow the osseous vasculature. This endplate innervation is through a branch of the sinuvertebral nerve, the basivertebral nerve. This nerve enters the foramen, and the nerve fibers enter the vertebral margin with the vessels. The density of innervation is similar to that seen in the outer annulus, which suggests that the endplates are as important to pain generation as is the annulus.

NATURAL HISTORY OF DISC DISEASE

One theory of spinal degeneration assumes that all spines degenerate and that current methods of treatment are for symptomatic relief, not for cure. The degenerative process has been divided into three separate stages with relatively distinct findings. The first stage is dysfunction, which is seen in individuals 15 to 45 years old. It is characterized by circumferential and radial tears in the disc annulus and localized synovitis of the facet joints. The next stage is instability. This stage, found in 35- to 70-year-old individuals, is characterized by internal disruption of the disc, progressive disc resorption, and degeneration of the facet joints with capsular laxity, subluxation, and joint erosion. The final stage, present in individuals older than 60 years, is stabilization. In this stage, the progressive development of hypertrophic bone around the disc and facet joints leads to segmental stiffening or frank ankylosis.

Each spinal segment degenerates at a different rate. As one level is in the dysfunction stage, another may be entering the stabilization stage. Disc herniation in this scheme is considered a complication of disc degeneration in the dysfunction and instability stages. Spinal stenosis from degenerative arthritis in this scheme is a complication of bony overgrowth compromising neural tissue in the late instability and early stabilization stages.

Long-term follow-up studies of lumbar disc herniations have documented several principles, the foremost being that generally symptomatic lumbar disc herniation (which is only one of the consequences of disc degeneration) has a favorable outcome in most patients. The primary benefit of surgery has been noted to occur early on in the first year after surgery, but with time the statistical significance of the improvement appears to be lost. In general, the literature supports an active care approach, minimizing centrally acting medications. The judicious use of epidural steroids also is supported, but long-term results and repeated use is questionable. Nonprogressive neurologic deficits originating from the lumbar spine (except cauda equina syndrome) can be treated nonoperatively with expected clinical improvement. If surgery is necessary, it usually can be delayed 6 to 12 weeks to allow adequate opportunity for improvement. Some patients are best treated surgically, and this is discussed in the section dealing specifically with operative treatment of lumbar disc herniation.

The natural history of degenerative disc disease is one of recurrent episodes of pain followed by periods of significant or complete relief.

Before a discussion of diagnostic studies, axial spine pain with radiation to one or more extremities must be considered. Also, understanding certain pathophysiologic entities must be juxtaposed to other entities of which only a rudimentary understanding exists. It is doubtful there is any other area of orthopaedics in which accurate diagnosis is as difficult or the proper treatment as challenging as in patients with persistent neck and arm or low back and leg pain. Although many patients have clear diagnoses properly arrived at by careful history and physical examination with confirmatory imaging studies, many patients with pain have absent neurologic findings other than sensory changes and have normal imaging studies or studies that do not support the clinical complaints and findings. Inability to easily determine an appropriate diagnosis does not relieve the physician of the obligation to recommend treatment or to direct the patient to a setting where such treatment is available. Careful assessment of these patients to determine if they have problems that can be orthopaedically treated (operatively or nonoperatively) is imperative to avoid both overtreatment and undertreatment.

Operative treatment can benefit a patient if it corrects a deformity, corrects instability, relieves neural compression, or treats a combination of these problems directly attributable to the patient's complaint. Obtaining a history and completing a physical examination to determine a diagnosis that should be supported by other diagnostic studies is fundamental; conversely, matching the diagnosis and treatment to the results of diagnostic studies, as often can be done in other subspecialties of orthopaedics (e.g., treating extremity pain based on a radiograph that shows a fracture), is more complex and difficult. The history, physical examination, and imaging studies must all confirm the same pathologic process as the source of symptoms if surgical intervention is to be reproducibly successful.

AXIAL LUMBAR PAIN

Axial lumbar pain occurs at some point in the lives of most people. Appropriate treatment for what can be at times excruciating pain generally should begin with evaluation for a significant spinal pathologic process. This pathologic process being absent, a brief (1 to 3 days) period of bed rest with institution of an antiinflammatory regimen and rapid progression to an active exercise regimen with an anticipated return to full activity should be expected and encouraged. Generally, patients treated in this manner improve significantly in 4 to 8 weeks. Diagnostic studies, including radiographs, often are not helpful because they add little information. More sophisticated imaging with CT and MRI or other studies have even less utility initially. An overdependence on the diagnosis of disc herniation can occur with early use of these diagnostic studies, which show disc herniations in 20% to 36% of normal volunteers. General imaging guidelines have been developed to help identify patients for whom radiography is indicated (Box 3.1).

Patients should understand that persistence of some pain does not indicate treatment failure, necessitating further measures; however, it is important for treating physicians to recognize that the longer a patient is limited by pain, the less likely he or she is to return to full activity.

For patients who do not respond to treatment regimens, early recognition that other issues may be involved is essential. Careful reassessment of complaints and reexamination for new information or findings and inconsistencies are necessary. Many studies of occupational back pain have revealed that depression, occupational mental stress, job satisfaction, intensity of concentration, anxiety, and marital status can be

BOX 3.1

Selective Indications for Radiography in Acute Low Back Pain

- Age >50 years
- Significant trauma
- Neuromuscular deficits
- Unexplained weight loss (10 lb in 6 months)
- Suspicion of ankylosing spondylitis
- Drug or alcohol abuse
- History of cancer
- Use of corticosteroids
- Temperature ≥37.8°C (≥100°F)
- Recent visit (≤1 month) for same problem and no improvement
- Patient seeking compensation for back pain

TABLE 3.1

Classification for Spinal Nerve and Thecal Sac Deformation on Magnetic Resonance Imaging

SPINAL NERVE DEFORMATION IN LATERAL RECESS OR INTERVERTEBRAL FORAMEN	
0—absent	No visible disc material contacting or deforming nerve
I—minimal	Contact with disc material deforming nerve but displacement <2 mm
II—moderate	Contact with disc material displacing ≥2 mm; nerve is still visible and not obscured by disc material
III—severe	Contact with disc material completely obscuring nerve
THECAL SAC DEFORMATION IN VERTEBRAL CANAL	
0—absent	No visible disc material contacting or deforming thecal sac
I—minimal	Disc material in contact with thecal sac
II—moderate	Disc material deforming thecal sac; anteroposterior distance of thecal sac ≥7 mm
III—severe	Disc material deforming thecal sac; anteroposterior distance of thecal sac <7 mm

From Beattie PF, Myers SP, Stratford P, et al: Associations between patient report of symptoms and anatomical impairment visible on lumbar magnetic resonance imaging, *Spine* 25:819–828, 2000.

related to complaints of pain and disability. The role of these factors as causal or consequential of the symptoms remains an area of continued study; however, there is some evidence that the psychologic stresses occur before complaints of pain in some patients. Another finding that is evident from the literature is the inability of physicians to detect psychosocial factors adequately without using specific instruments designed for this purpose in patients with back pain. In one study, experienced spinal surgeons were able to identify distressed patients only 26% of the time based on patient interviews. Given the difficulty of identifying patients with psychosocial distress, being aware of the high incidence of incidental abnormal findings on imaging studies underscores the need for critical individual review of these studies by treating physicians. Severe nerve compression shown by MRI or CT correlates with symptoms of distal leg pain; however, mild-to-moderate nerve compression (Table 3.1), disc degeneration or bulging, and central stenosis do not correlate significantly with specific pain patterns.

DIAGNOSTIC STUDIES

RADIOGRAPHY

The simplest and most readily available diagnostic tests for lumbar pain are anteroposterior and lateral radiographs of the involved spinal region. These simple radiographs show a relatively high incidence of abnormal findings; however, spinal radiographs on the initial visit for acute low back pain may not contribute to patient care and are not always cost effective. Plain radiographs may be considered only after the initial therapy fails, especially in patients younger than 45 years old.

There is insignificant correlation between back pain and the radiographic findings of lumbar lordosis, transitional vertebra, disc space narrowing, disc vacuum sign, and claw spurs. In addition, the entity of disc space narrowing is extremely difficult to quantify in all but operated backs or in obviously abnormal circumstances. A study of 321 patients found that only when traction spurs or obvious disc space narrowing or both were present did the incidence of severe back and leg pain, leg weakness, and numbness increase. These positive findings had no relationship to heavy lifting, vehicular exposure, or exposure to vibrating equipment. Other studies have shown some relationship between back pain and the findings of spondylolysis, spondylolisthesis, and adult scoliosis, but these findings also can be observed in spine radiographs of asymptomatic patients.

Special radiographic views can be helpful in further defining the initial clinical radiographic impression. Oblique views are useful in defining further spondylolisthesis and spondylolysis but are of limited use in facet syndrome and hypertrophic arthritis of the lumbar spine. Lateral flexion and extension radiographs may reveal segmental instability. The interpretation of these views depends on patient cooperation, patient positioning, and reproducible technique. Lateral lumbar flexion views are valid only if done in the seated position, which maximizes lumbar kyphosis. The Ferguson view (20-degree caudocephalic anteroposterior radiograph) has been shown to be of value in the diagnosis of the "far out syndrome," that is, fifth root compression produced by a large transverse process of the fifth lumbar vertebra against the ala of the sacrum. Angled caudal views localized to areas of concern may show evidence of facet or laminar pathologic conditions.

MYELOGRAPHY

The value of myelography is the ability to check all spinal regions for abnormality and to define intraspinal lesions; it may be unnecessary if clinical and CT or MRI findings are in complete agreement. The primary indications for myelography are suspicion of an intraspinal lesion, patients with spinal instrumentation, or questionable diagnosis resulting from conflicting clinical findings and other studies. In addition, myelography is valuable in a previously operated spine and in patients with marked bony degenerative change that may be underestimated on MRI. Myelography is improved by the use of postmyelography CT in this setting and in evaluating spinal stenosis.

Several contrast agents have been used for myelography: air, oil contrast, and water-soluble (absorbable) contrast agents, including metrizamide (Amipaque), iohexol (Omnipaque), and iopamidol (Isovue-M). Because these nonionic agents are absorbable, the discomfort of removing them and the severity of the postmyelography headache have decreased.

Arachnoiditis is a severe complication that has been attributed occasionally to the combination of iophendylate and blood in the cerebrospinal fluid (CSF). This diagnosis usually is confirmed only by repeat myelography. Attempts at surgical neurolysis have resulted in only short-term relief and a return of symptoms within 6 to 12 months after the procedure. Time may decrease the effects of this serious problem in some patients, but progressive paralysis has been reported in rare instances. Arachnoiditis also can be caused by tuberculosis and other types of meningitis. Arachnoiditis has not been noted to be related to the use of a water-soluble contrast agent, with or without injection, in the presence of a bloody tap.

Water-soluble contrast media are now the standard agents for myelography. Their advantages include absorption by the body, enhanced definition of structures, tolerance, and the ability to vary the dosage for different contrasts. Similar to iophendylate, they are meningeal irritants, but they have not been associated with arachnoiditis. The complications of these agents include nausea, vomiting, confusion, and seizures. Rare complications include stroke, paralysis, and death. Iohexol and iopamidol have significantly lower complication rates than metrizamide. The more common complications seem to be related to patient hydration, phenothiazines, tricyclic antidepressants, and migration of contrast material into the cranial vault. Many reported complications can be prevented or minimized by using the lowest possible dose to achieve the desired degree of contrast. Adequate hydration and discontinuation of phenothiazines and tricyclic antidepressants before, during, and after the procedure also should minimize the incidence of the more common reactions. Likewise, maintenance of at least a 30-degree elevation of the patient's head until the contrast material is absorbed should help prevent reactions. Complete information about these agents and the dosages required is found in their package inserts.

Iohexol is a nonionic contrast medium approved for thoracic and lumbar myelography. The incidence of reactions to this medium is low. The most common reactions are headache (<20%), pain (8%), nausea (6%), and vomiting (3%). Serious reactions are rare and include mental disturbances and aseptic meningitis (0.01%). Good hydration is essential to minimize the common reactions. The use of phenothiazine antinauseants is contraindicated when this medium is employed. Management before and after the procedure is the same as for metrizamide.

Air contrast is used rarely and probably should be used only in situations in which myelography is mandatory and the patient is extremely allergic to iodized materials. The resolution from such a procedure is poor. Air epidurography in conjunction with CT has been suggested in patients in whom further definition between postoperative scar and recurrent disc material is required.

Myelographic technique begins with a careful explanation of the procedure to the patient before its initiation. Hydration of the patient before the procedure may minimize postmyelographic complaints. Heavy sedation rarely is needed. Proper equipment, including a fluoroscopic unit with a spot film device, image intensification, tilt table, and television monitoring, is useful. The type of needle selected also influences the risk of postdural puncture headaches, which can be severe. Smaller gauge needles (22- or 25-gauge) have been found to result in a lower incidence of postdural puncture headaches. Also, use of a Whitacre-type needle with a blunter tip and side port opening results in fewer postdural puncture headache complaints.

The most common technical complications of myelography are significant retention of contrast medium (oil contrast only), persistent headache from a dural leak, and epidural injection. These problems usually are minor. Persistent dural leaks usually are responsive to a blood patch. With the use of a water-soluble contrast medium, the persistent abnormalities caused by retained medium and epidural injection are eliminated.

MYELOGRAPHY

TECHNIQUE 3.1

- Place the patient prone on the fluoroscopic table. Use of an abdominal pillow is optional. Prepare the back in the usual surgical fashion.
- Determine needle placement by the suspected pathologic level. Placement of the needle cephalad to L2-3 is more dangerous because of the risk of damaging the conus medullaris.
- Infiltrate the selected area of injection with a local anesthetic. Use the smallest gauge needle that can be well placed. If a Whitacre-type needle is used, a 19-gauge needle may be placed through the skin, subcutaneous tissue, and fascia to form a track because this relatively blunt needle cannot penetrate these structures well. Midline needle placement usually minimizes lateral nerve root irritation and epidural injection. Advance the needle with the bevel parallel to the long axis of the body. Subarachnoid placement can be enhanced by tilting the patient up to increase intraspinal pressure and minimize the epidural space.
- When the dura and arachnoid have been punctured, turn the bevel of the needle cephalad. A clear continuous flow of CSF should continue with the patient prone. Manometric studies can be done at this time if desired or indicated. Remove a volume of CSF equal to the planned injection volume for laboratory evaluation as indicated by the clinical suspicions. In most patients, a cell count, differential white blood cell count, and protein analysis are performed.
- Inject a test dose of the contrast material under fluoroscopic control to confirm a subarachnoid injection. If a mixed subdural-subarachnoid injection is suspected, change the needle depth; occasionally, a lateral radiograph may be required to confirm the proper depth. If flow is good, inject the contrast material slowly.
- Ensure continued subarachnoid injection by occasionally aspirating as the injection continues. The usual dose of iohexol for lumbar myelography in an adult is 10 to 15 mL with a concentration of 170 to 190 mg/mL. Higher concentrations of water-soluble contrast are required if higher areas of the spine are to be demonstrated. Consult the package insert of the contrast agent used. The needle can be removed if a water-soluble contrast agent (iohexol) is used.
- Allow the contrast material to flow caudally for the best views of the lumbar roots and distal sac. Make spot films in the anteroposterior, lateral, and oblique projections. A full lumbar examination should include thoracic evaluation to about the level of T7 because lesions at the thoracic level may mimic lumbar disc disease. Take additional spot films as the contrast proceeds cranially.
- If a total or cervical myelogram is desired, allow the contrast to proceed cranially. Extend the neck and head maximally to prevent or minimize intracranial migration of the contrast medium.
- If blood is present in the initial tap, aborting the procedure if the CSF does not clear rapidly is best. It can be attempted again in several days if the patient has no

symptoms related to the first tap and is well hydrated. If the proper needle position is confirmed in the anteroposterior and lateral views, and CSF flow is minimal or absent, suspect a neoplastic process. Place the needle at a higher or lower level as indicated by the circumstances. If attempts to obtain CSF continue to fail, abandon the procedure and reevaluate the clinical situation.

COMPUTED TOMOGRAPHY

CT can be a useful diagnostic tool in the evaluation of spinal disease (Fig. 3.2). The current technology and computer software have made possible the ability to reformat the standard axial cuts in almost any direction and magnify the images so that exact measurements of various structures can be made. Software is available to evaluate the density of a selected vertebra and compare it with vertebrae of the normal population to give a numerically reproducible estimate of vertebral density to quantitate osteopenia.

Numerous types of CT studies for the spine are available. One must be careful when ordering the study to ensure that the areas of clinical concern are included. The most common routine for lumbar disc herniations consists of making serial cuts through the last three lumbar intervertebral discs. If the equipment has a tilting gantry, an attempt is made to keep the axis of the cuts parallel with the discs. Frequently, the gantry cannot tilt enough, however, to allow a parallel beam through the lowest disc space. This technique does not allow demonstration of the canal at the pedicles. Another method involves making cuts through the discs without tilting the gantry. The entire canal is not shown, and the lower cuts frequently have the lower and upper endplates of adjacent vertebrae superimposed in the same view.

The most complex method consists of making multiple parallel cuts at equal intervals. This allows computer reconstruction of the images in different planes, usually sagittal and coronal. These reformatted views allow an almost three-dimensional view of the spine and most of its structures. The greatest benefit of this technique is the ability to see beyond the limits of the dural sac and root sleeves. The diagnosis of foraminal encroachment by bone or disc material can be made in the face of a normal myelogram. The proper procedure can be chosen that fits all of the pathologic conditions involved.

Optimal reformatted CT should include enlarged axial and sagittal views with clear notation as to laterality and sequence of cuts. Several sections of the axial cuts should include the local soft tissue and contiguous abdominal contents. Finally, a set of images adjusted for improved bony detail should be included for evaluation of the facet joints and the lateral recesses. This

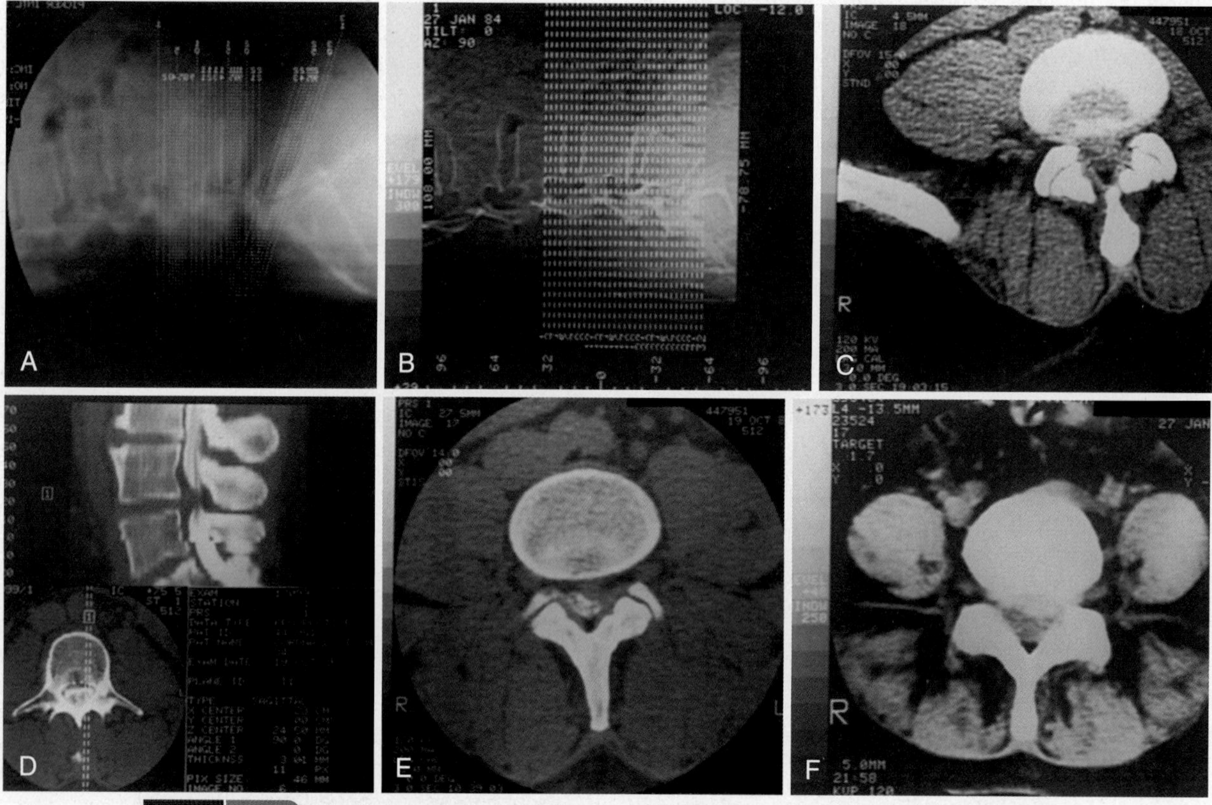

FIGURE 3.2 **A,** CT scan scout view of lumbar disc herniation at lumbar disc level showing angled gantry technique. **B,** CT scan scout view of straight gantry technique. **C,** CT scan of lumbar disc herniation at L4-5 disc level showing cross-sectional anatomy with gantry straight. **D,** CT scan of L4-5 disc herniation at lumbar disc level showing cross-sectional, sagittal, and coronal anatomy using computerized reformatted technique. **E,** CT scan of L4-5 disc herniation at lumbar disc level showing cross-sectional anatomy 2 hours after metrizamide myelography. **F,** CT scan of lumbar disc herniation at L4-5 disc level showing cross-sectional anatomy after intravenous injection for greater soft-tissue contrast.

study should be centered on the level of greatest clinical concern. The study can be enhanced further if done after water contrast myelography or with intravenous injection of a contrast medium. Enhancement techniques are especially useful if the spine being evaluated has been operated on previously.

This noninvasive, painless outpatient procedure can supply more information about spinal disease than was previously available with a battery of invasive and noninvasive tests usually requiring hospitalization. CT does not show intraspinal tumors or arachnoiditis and is unable to differentiate scar from recurrent disc herniation. The use of intravenous contrast medium (Fig. 3.2F) followed by CT can improve the definition between scar and disc herniation. Myelography is still required to show intraspinal tumors and to "run" the spine to detect occult or unsuspected lesions. The development of low-dose metrizamide or iohexol myelography with reformatted CT done as an outpatient procedure allows maximal information to be obtained with minimal time, risk, discomfort, and cost.

MAGNETIC RESONANCE IMAGING

MRI is currently the standard for advanced imaging of the spine and is superior to CT in most circumstances, in particular identification of infections, tumors, and degenerative changes within the discs (Fig. 3.3). More important, MRI is superior for imaging the disc and directly images neural structures. Also, MRI typically shows the entire region of study (cervical, thoracic, or lumbar). Of particular value is the ability to image the nerve root in the foramen, which is difficult even with postmyelography CT because the subarachnoid space and the contrast agent do not extend fully through the foramen. Despite this superiority, there are circumstances in which MRI and CT, with or without myelography, can be used in a complementary fashion.

One of the difficulties with MRI is showing anatomy that is abnormal but may be asymptomatic. MRI evidence of disc degeneration has been reported in the cervical spine in 25% of patients younger than 40 years and in 60% of patients 60 years and older, and lumbar disc degeneration was found in 35% of patients 20 to 39 years old and in 100% of patients older than 50. The demonstrated findings must be carefully correlated with the clinical impression. The importance of this concept cannot be overstated. The best way to obtain meaningful clinical information from MRI of the spine is to have a specific question before the study. This question is derived from the patient's history and careful physical examination and is posed using the parameters of (1) neural compression, (2) instability, and (3) deformity. In each case the specific location of the abnormality should be suspected before MRI and confirmed with the study. Only abnormalities in one or a combination of these categories are important, and operative techniques can treat only these problems. Failure to interpret an imaging study in this way, especially MRI, which is sensitive to anatomic abnormalities, would inevitably lead to poor clinical choices and outcomes.

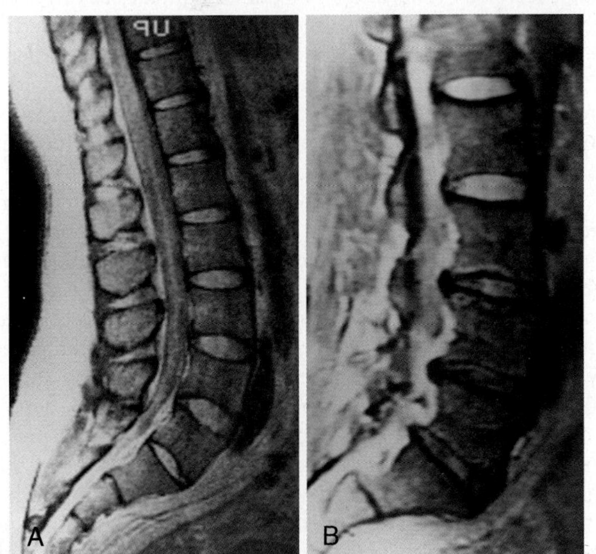

FIGURE 3.3 MRI of lumbar spine. **A,** Normal T2-weighted image. **B,** T2-weighted image showing degenerative bulging or herniated discs, or both, at L3-4, L4-5, and L5-S1.

OTHER DIAGNOSTIC TESTS

Numerous diagnostic tests have been used in the diagnosis of intervertebral disc disease in addition to radiography, myelography, CT, and MRI. The primary advantage of these tests is to rule out diseases other than primary disc herniation, spinal stenosis, and spinal arthritis.

Electromyography is the most notable of these tests. One advantage of electromyography is in the identification of peripheral neuropathy and diffuse neurologic involvement indicating higher or lower lesions. Electromyography and nerve conduction velocity can be helpful if a patient has a history and physical examination suggestive of radiculopathy at either the cervical or lumbar level with inconclusive imaging studies. Paraspinal muscles in a patient with a previous posterior operation usually are abnormal and are not a reliable diagnostic finding.

Bone scans are another procedure in which positive findings usually are not indicative of intervertebral disc disease, but they can confirm neoplastic, traumatic, and arthritic problems in the spine. Various laboratory tests, such as a complete blood cell count, differential white blood cell count, C-reactive protein, biochemical profile, urinalysis, serum protein electrophoresis, and erythrocyte sedimentation rate, are extremely good screening procedures for other causes of pain in the spine. Rheumatoid screening studies, such as those for rheumatoid arthritis, antinuclear antibody, lupus erythematosus cell preparation, and HLA-B27, also are useful when indicated by the clinical picture.

Some tests that were developed to enhance the diagnosis of intervertebral disc disease have been surpassed by more advanced technology. Lumbar venography and ultrasonographic measurement of the intervertebral canal are two examples.

INJECTION STUDIES

Whenever a diagnosis is in doubt and the complaints seem real or the pathologic condition is diffuse, identification of the source of pain is problematic. The use of local anesthetics or contrast media in various specific anatomic areas can be helpful. These agents are relatively simple, safe, and minimally painful. Contrast media such as diatrizoate meglumine (Hypaque), iothalamate meglumine (Conray), iohexol (Omnipaque), iopamidol, and metrizamide (Amipaque) have been used for discography and blocks with no reported ill effects. Reports of neurologic complications with contrast media used for discography and subsequent chymopapain injection are well documented. The best choice of a contrast medium for documenting structures outside the subarachnoid space is an absorbable medium with low reactivity, because it might be injected inadvertently into the subarachnoid space. Iohexol and metrizamide are the least reactive, most widely accepted, and best tolerated of the currently available contrast media. Local anesthetics, such as lidocaine (Xylocaine), tetracaine (Pontocaine), and bupivacaine (Marcaine), are used frequently epidurally and intradurally. The use of bupivacaine should be limited to low concentrations and low volumes because of reports of death after epidural anesthesia using concentrations of 0.75% or higher.

Steroids prepared for intramuscular injection also have been used frequently in the epidural space with few and usually transient complications. Spinal arachnoiditis in past years was associated with the use of epidural methylprednisolone acetate (Depo-Medrol). This complication was thought to be caused by the use of the suspending agent, polyethylene glycol, which has since been eliminated from the Depo-Medrol preparation. For epidural injections, we prefer the use of Celestone Soluspan, which is a mixture of betamethasone sodium phosphate and betamethasone acetate. Celestone Soluspan provides immediate and long-term duration of action, is highly soluble, and contains no harmful preservatives. Celestone should not be mixed with local anesthetics containing preservatives such as parabens or phenol because flocculation and clogging of the suspension can occur. If Celestone is not available, other commonly used preparations for spinal injections include methylprednisolone (Depo-Medrol) and triamcinolone acetonide (Kenalog). Isotonic saline is the only other injectable medium used frequently around the spine with no reported adverse reactions. All substrates injected into the epidural space should be preservative free.

Steroids and local anesthesia are generally used in combination for antiinflammatory and analgesic effects. It is theorized that the lipophilic characteristic of the steroid permits sustained release from the abundant epidural fat, which is where the steroid is injected. Cells exposed to the steroid synthesize a phospholipase A2-inhibitory glycoprotein (termed lipomodulin) and inhibit the inflammatory pathway. Phospholipase A2, which is an inflammatory enzyme, converts membrane phospholipids into arachidonic acid and subsequently controls lipoxygenase, leading to the formation of leukotrienes. The steroid also reduces nerve swelling and upregulates the transcription of antiinflammatory genes, in contrast to local analgesics, which are responsible for immediate pain relief.

When discrete, well-controlled injection techniques directed at specific targets in and around the spine are used, grading the degree of pain before and after a spinal injection is helpful in determining the location of the pain generator. The patient is asked to grade the degree of pain on a 0-to-10 scale before and at various intervals after the spinal injection (see Box 2.1). If a spinal injection done under fluoroscopic control results in an 80% or more decrease in the level of pain, which corresponds to the duration of action of the anesthetic agent used, we presume the target area injected to be the pain generator. Less pain reduction, 50% to 65%, does not constitute a positive response.

EPIDURAL CORTISONE INJECTIONS

Epidural injections in the cervical, thoracic, and lumbosacral spine were developed to diagnose and treat spinal pain. Information obtained from epidural injections can be helpful in confirming pain generators that are responsible for a patient's discomfort. Structural abnormalities do not always cause pain, and diagnostic injections can help to correlate abnormalities seen on imaging studies with associated pain complaints. In addition, epidural injections can provide pain relief during the recovery of disc or nerve root injuries and allow patients to increase their level of physical activity. Because severe pain from an acute disc injury, with or without radiculopathy, often is time limited, therapeutic injections can help to manage pain and may alleviate or decrease the need for oral analgesics.

A retrospective study comparing interlaminar to transforaminal epidural injections for symptomatic lumbar intervertebral disc herniations found that transforaminal injections resulted in better short-term pain improvement and fewer long-term operative interventions.

A number of randomized, double-blind, controlled studies have been done to evaluate the effectiveness of lumbar interlaminar injections, as well as caudal epidural injections, in the treatment of chronic discogenic pain with and without radiculitis. Overall these studies indicate that a high percentage of patients receiving the injections have significant pain relief and functional improvement. The question still remains whether there is any significant long-term benefit to these injections.

Few serious complications occur in patients receiving epidural corticosteroid injections; however, epidural abscess, epidural hematoma, durocutaneous fistula, and Cushing syndrome have been reported as individual case reports. The most adverse immediate reaction during an epidural injection is a vasovagal reaction, although this is much more common with cervical injections. Dural puncture has been estimated to occur in 0.5% to 5% of patients having cervical or lumbar epidural steroid injections. Some minor, common complaints caused by corticosteroid injected into the epidural space include nonpositional headaches, facial flushing, insomnia, low-grade fever, and transient increased back or lower extremity pain. Major adverse events can occur with epidural injections, but these are rare, their true incidence is unknown, and they have been described only in case reports. Several large series involving nearly 5000 patients with over 8000 transforaminal lumbar epidural injections reported no major adverse events and a less than 1% incidence of postinjection headache; the most frequent sequela was increased leg or back pain, which also occurred in less than 1% of patients.

Epidural corticosteroid injections are contraindicated in the presence of infection at the injection site, systemic infection, bleeding diathesis, uncontrolled diabetes mellitus, and congestive heart failure.

When considering epidural steroid injections, several preexisting conditions should be checked to avoid complications. These conditions include coagulopathy or concurrent anticoagulation therapy, systemic infection, local skin infection at the puncture site, hypersensitivity to administered agents, and pregnancy. According to a consensus statement by the Society of Interventional Radiology, epidural steroid injection is classified as a category 2 procedure, that is, a moderate risk for bleeding (between a low-bleeding-risk procedure, in which bleeding is easily detected and controllable, and a significant-bleeding-risk procedure, in which bleeding is difficult to detect or control). For category 2 procedures, the international normalized ratio (INR) and platelet count should be adjusted to less than 1.5 and more than 50,000/μL, respectively. If a patient is taking anticoagulants, the medication should be withheld in consultation with the prescribing physician. Warfarin should be withheld 5 days before epidural steroid injection, and the patient's INR should be rechecked before the procedure. Low-molecular-weight heparin therapy should be stopped 24 hours before epidural steroid injection, whereas heparin does not need to be withheld because it is a short-acting agent (the half-life of heparin is 23 minutes to 2.48 hours). Fondaparinux (Arixtra, Glaxo Smith Kline, London) should be withheld for 2 to 5 days before the procedure, clopidogrel (Plavix, Handok, Seoul) for 5 days, and ticlopidine (Ticlid, Roche, Basel, Switzerland) for 5 days. Nonsteroidal antiinflammatory drugs, including aspirin, do not have to be stopped before epidural steroid injections.

We perform epidural corticosteroid injections in a fluoroscopy suite equipped with resuscitative and monitoring equipment. Intravenous access is established in all patients with a 20-gauge angiocatheter placed in the upper extremity. Mild sedation is achieved through intravenous access. We recommend the use of fluoroscopy for diagnostic and therapeutic epidural injections for several reasons. Epidural injections performed without fluoroscopic guidance are not always made into the epidural space or the intended interspace. Even in experienced hands, needle misplacement occurs in 40% of caudal and 30% of lumbar epidural injections when done without fluoroscopic guidance. Accidental intravascular injections also can occur, and the absence of blood return with needle aspiration before injection is an unreliable indicator of this complication. In the presence of anatomic anomalies, such as a midline epidural septum or multiple separate epidural compartments, the desired flow of epidural injectants to the presumed pain generator is restricted and remains undetected without fluoroscopy. In addition, if an injection fails to relieve pain, it would be impossible without fluoroscopy to determine whether the failure was caused by a genuine poor response or by improper needle placement.

THORACIC EPIDURAL INJECTION

Epidural steroid injections in the thoracic spine have been shown to provide relief from thoracic radicular pain secondary to disc herniations, trauma, diabetic neuropathy, herpes zoster, and idiopathic thoracic neuralgia, although reports in the literature are few.

INTERLAMINAR THORACIC EPIDURAL INJECTION

TECHNIQUE 3.2

- A paramedian rather than a midline approach is used because of the angulation of the spinous processes.
- Place the patient prone on a pain management table. The preparation of the patient and equipment are identical to that used for interlaminar cervical epidural injections (see Technique 2.1). Aseptically prepare the skin area several segments above and below the interspace to be injected. Drape the area in sterile fashion.
- Identify the target laminar interspace using anteroposterior fluoroscopic guidance.
- Anesthetize the skin over the target interspace on the side of the patient's pain. Under fluoroscopic control, insert and advance a 22-gauge, 3½-inch spinal needle to the superior edge of the target lamina. Anesthetize the lamina and the soft tissues as the spinal needle is withdrawn.
- Mark the skin with an 18-gauge hypodermic needle and insert an 18-gauge, 3½-inch Tuohy epidural needle, and advance it at a 50- to 60-degree angle to the axis of the spine and a 15- to 30-degree angle toward the midline until contact with the lamina is made. To view the thoracic interspace better, position the C-arm so that the fluoroscopy beam is in the same plane as the Tuohy epidural needle.
- "Walk off" the lamina with the Tuohy needle into the ligamentum flavum. Remove the stylet from the Tuohy needle and, using the loss-of-resistance technique, advance it into the epidural space. When loss of resistance has been achieved, aspirate to check for blood or CSF. If neither blood nor CSF is evident, inject 1.5 mL of nonionic contrast dye to confirm epidural placement.
- To confirm proper placement further, adjust the C-arm to view the area from a lateral projection (Fig. 3.4). A spot radiograph or epidurogram can be obtained. Inject

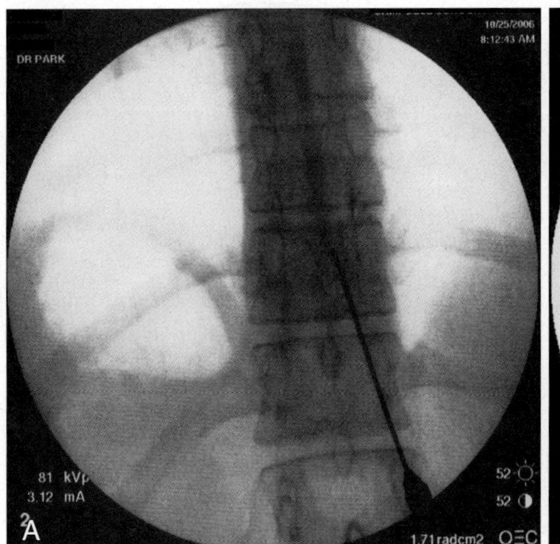

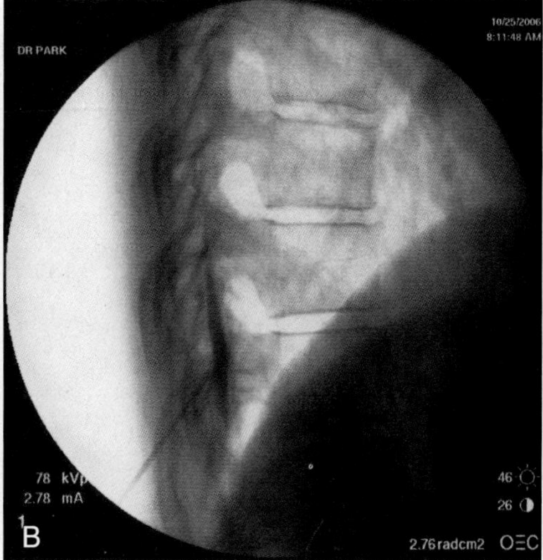

FIGURE 3.4 A, Posteroanterior view of thoracic interlaminar epidurogram showing characteristic contrast flow pattern. B, Lateral radiograph of thoracic epidurogram. **SEE TECHNIQUE 3.2.**

2 mL of 1% preservative-free lidocaine without epinephrine and 2 mL of 6 mg/mL Celestone Soluspan slowly into the epidural space.

LUMBAR EPIDURAL INJECTION

Certain clinical trends are apparent with lumbar epidural steroid injections. When nerve root injury is associated with a disc herniation or lateral bony stenosis, most patients who received substantial relief of leg pain from a well-placed transforaminal injection, even if temporary, benefit from surgery for the radicular pain. Patients who do not respond and who have had radicular pain for at least 12 months are unlikely to benefit from surgery. Patients with back and leg pain of an acute nature (<3 months) respond better to epidural corticosteroids. Unless a significant reinjury results in an acute disc or nerve root injury, postsurgical patients tend to respond poorly to epidural corticosteroids.

INTERLAMINAR LUMBAR EPIDURAL INJECTION

TECHNIQUE 3.3

- Place the patient prone on a pain management table. Aseptically prepare the skin area with isopropyl alcohol and povidone-iodine several segments above and below the laminar interspace to be injected. Drape the area in a sterile fashion.
- Under anteroposterior fluoroscopy guidance, identify the target laminar interspace. Using a 27-gauge, ¼-inch needle, anesthetize the skin over the target interspace on the side of the patient's pain with 1 to 2 mL of 1% preservative-free lidocaine without epinephrine.
- Insert a 22-gauge, 3½-inch spinal needle vertically until contact is made with the upper edge of the inferior lamina at the target interspace, 1 to 2 cm lateral to the caudal tip of the inferior spinous process under fluoroscopy. Anesthetize the lamina with 2 mL of 1% preservative-free lidocaine without epinephrine. Anesthetize the soft tissue with 2 mL of 1% lidocaine as the spinal needle is withdrawn.
- Nick the skin with an 18-gauge hypodermic needle and insert a 17-gauge, 3½-inch Tuohy epidural needle and advance it vertically within the anesthetized soft-tissue track until contact with the lamina has been made under fluoroscopy.
- "Walk off" the lamina with the Tuohy needle onto the ligamentum flavum. Remove the stylet from the Tuohy needle and attach a 10-mL syringe filled halfway with air and sterile saline to the Tuohy needle. Advance the Tuohy needle into the epidural space using the loss-of-resistance technique. Avoid lateral needle placement to decrease the likelihood of encountering an epidural vein or adjacent nerve root. Remove the stylet when loss of resistance has been achieved. Aspirate to check for blood or CSF. If neither blood nor CSF is present, remove the syringe from the Tuohy needle and attach a 5-mL syringe containing 2 mL of nonionic contrast dye.
- Confirm epidural placement by producing an epidurogram with the nonionic contrast agent (Fig. 3.5). A spot radiograph can be taken to document placement.
- Remove the 5-mL syringe and place on the Tuohy needle a 10-mL syringe containing 2 mL of 1% preservative-free lidocaine and 2 mL of 6 mg/mL Celestone Soluspan. Inject the corticosteroid preparation slowly into the epidural space.

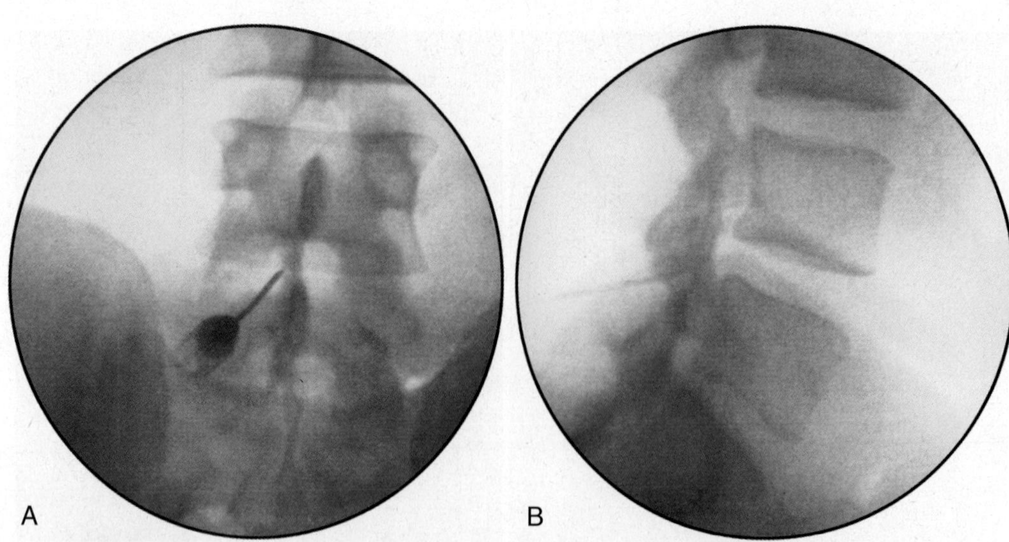

FIGURE 3.5 **A,** Posteroanterior view of lumbar interlaminar epidurogram showing characteristic contrast flow pattern. **B,** Lateral radiograph of lumbar epidurogram. **SEE TECHNIQUE 3.3.**

TRANSFORAMINAL LUMBAR AND SACRAL EPIDURAL INJECTION

TECHNIQUE 3.4

- Place the patient prone on a pain management table. Aseptically prepare the skin area with isopropyl alcohol and povidone-iodine several segments above and below the interspace to be injected. Drape the area in sterile fashion.
- Under anteroposterior fluoroscopic guidance, identify the target interspace. Anesthetize the soft tissues over the lateral border and midway between the two adjacent transverse processes at the target interspace.
- Insert a 22-gauge, 4¾ inch spinal needle and advance it within the anesthetized soft-tissue track under fluoroscopy until contact is made with the lower edge of the superior transverse process near its junction with the superior articular process.
- Retract the spinal needle 2 to 3 mm, redirect it toward the base of the appropriate pedicle, and advance it slowly to the 6-o'clock position of the pedicle under fluoroscopy. Adjust the C-arm to a lateral projection to confirm the position and then return the C-arm to the anteroposterior view.
- Remove the stylet. Inject 1 mL of nonionic contrast agent slowly to produce a perineurosheathogram (Fig. 3.6). After an adequate dye pattern is observed, inject slowly a 2-mL volume containing 1 mL of 0.75% preservative-free bupivacaine and 1 mL of 6 mg/mL Celestone Soluspan.
- The S1 nerve root also can be injected using the transforaminal approach.
- With the patient prone on the pain management table and after appropriate aseptic preparation, direct the C-arm so that the fluoroscopy beam is in a cephalocaudad and lateral-to-medial direction so that the anterior and posterior S1 foramina are aligned.
- Anesthetize the soft tissues and the dorsal aspect of the sacrum with 2 to 3 mL of 1% preservative-free lidocaine without epinephrine. Insert a 22-gauge, 3½-inch spinal needle, and advance it within the anesthetized soft-tissue track under fluoroscopy until contact is made with posterior sacral bone slightly lateral and inferior to the S1 pedicle. "Walk" the spinal needle off the sacrum into the posterior S1 foramen to the medial edge of the pedicle.
- Adjust the C-arm to a lateral projection to confirm the position and return it to the anteroposterior view.
- Remove the stylet. Inject 1 mL of nonionic contrast slowly to produce a perineurosheathogram (Fig. 3.7). After an adequate dye pattern of the S1 nerve root is obtained, insert a 2-mL volume containing 1 mL of 0.75% preservative-free bupivacaine and 1 mL of 6 mg/mL Celestone Soluspan.

CAUDAL SACRAL EPIDURAL INJECTION

TECHNIQUE 3.5

- Place the patient prone on a pain management table. Aseptically prepare the skin area from the lumbosacral junction to the coccyx with isopropyl alcohol and povidone-iodine. Drape the area in sterile fashion.
- Try to identify by palpation the sacral hiatus, which is located between the two horns of the sacral cornua. The sacral hiatus can be best observed by directing the fluoroscopic beam laterally.
- Anesthetize the soft tissues and the dorsal aspect of the sacrum with 2 to 3 mL of 1% preservative-free lidocaine without epinephrine. Keep the C-arm positioned so that the fluoroscopic beam remains lateral.
- Insert a 22-gauge, 3½-inch spinal needle between the sacral cornua at about 45 degrees, with the bevel of

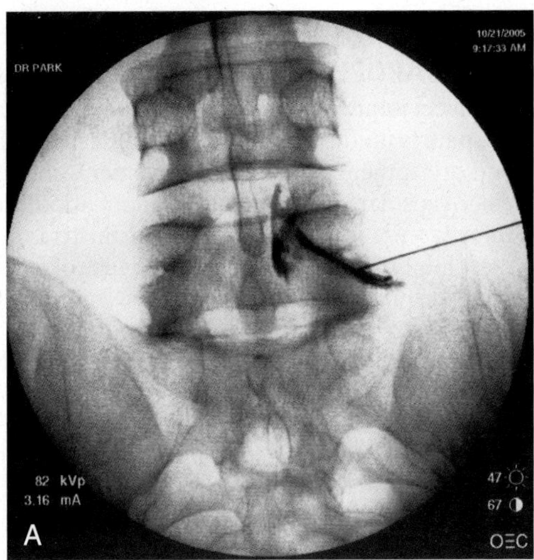

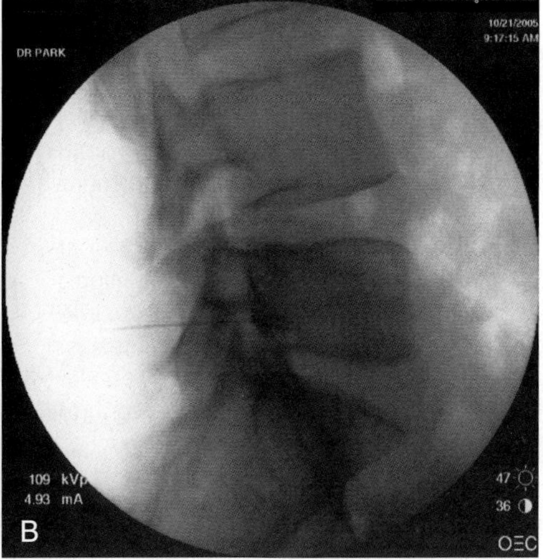

FIGURE 3.6 **A,** Right L5 selective nerve root injection contrast pattern. **B,** Lateral radiograph of L5 selective nerve block contrast flow pattern in anterior epidural space. **SEE TECHNIQUE 3.4.**

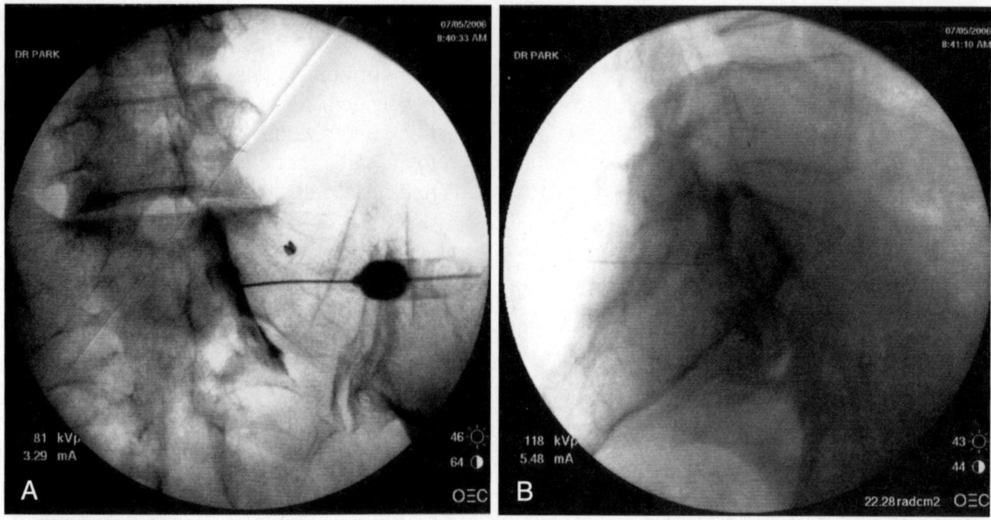

FIGURE 3.7 **A,** Right S1 selective nerve root injection contrast pattern with perineurosheathogram. **B,** Lateral radiograph of S1 contrast flow in sacral epidural space. **SEE TECHNIQUE 3.4.**

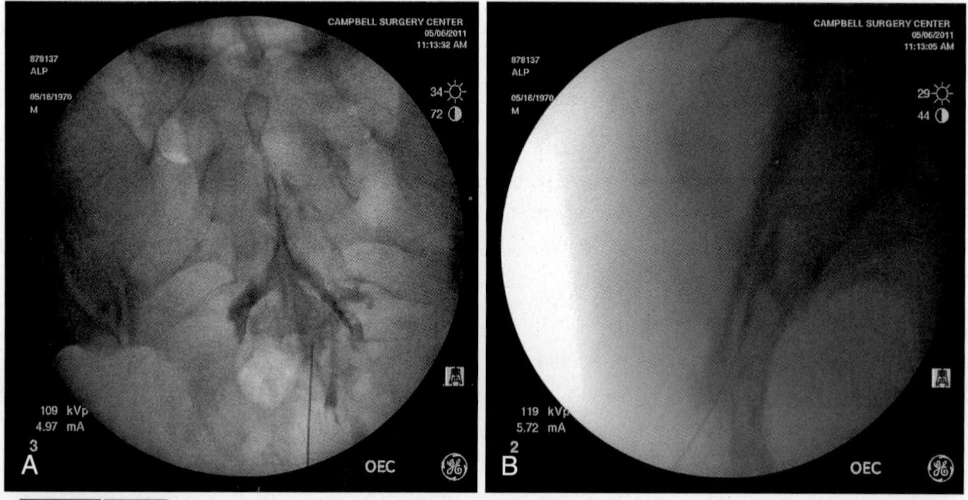

FIGURE 3.8 Fluoroscopic view (caudal approach) of lumbar epidural injection. **SEE TECHNIQUE 3.5.**

the spinal needle facing ventrally until contact with the sacrum is made. Using fluoroscopic guidance, redirect the spinal needle more cephalad, horizontal, and parallel to the table, advancing it into the sacral canal through the sacrococcygeal ligament and into the epidural space (Fig. 3.8).

- Remove the stylet. Aspirate to check for blood or CSF. If neither blood nor CSF is evident, inject 2 mL of nonionic contrast dye to confirm placement. Move the C-arm into the anteroposterior position and look for the characteristic "Christmas tree" pattern of epidural flow. If a vascular pattern is seen, reposition the spinal needle and confirm epidural placement with nonionic contrast dye.
- When the correct contrast pattern is obtained, slowly inject a 10-mL volume containing 3 mL of 1% preservative-free lidocaine without epinephrine, 3 mL of 6 mg/mL Celestone Soluspan, and 4 mL of sterile normal saline.

ZYGAPOPHYSEAL (FACET) JOINT INJECTIONS

The facet joint can be a source of back pain; the exact cause of the pain is unknown. Theories include meniscoid entrapment and extrapment, synovial impingement, chondromalacia facetae, capsular and synovial inflammation, and mechanical injury to the joint capsule. Osteoarthritis is another cause of facet joint pain; however, the incidence of facet joint arthropathy is equal in symptomatic and asymptomatic patients. As with other osteoarthritic joints, radiographic changes correlate poorly with pain. Although the history and physical examination may suggest that the facet joint is the cause of spine pain, no noninvasive pathognomonic findings distinguish facet joint–mediated pain from other sources of spine pain. Fluoroscopically guided facet joint injections are commonly considered the "gold standard" for isolating or excluding the facet joint as a source of spine or extremity pain.

Clinical suspicion of facet joint pain by a spine specialist remains the major indicator for diagnostic injection, which should be done only in patients who have had pain for more than 4 weeks and only after appropriate conservative measures have failed to provide relief. Facet joint injection procedures may help to focus treatment on a specific spinal segment and provide adequate pain relief to allow progression in therapy. Either intraarticular or medial branch blocks can be used for diagnostic purposes. Although injection of cortisone into the facet joint was a popular procedure through most of the 1970s and 1980s, many investigators have found no evidence that this effectively treats low back pain caused by a facet joint. The only controlled study on the use of intraarticular corticosteroids in the cervical spine found no added benefit from intraarticular betamethasone over bupivacaine.

LUMBAR FACET JOINT

LUMBAR INTRAARTICULAR INJECTION

TECHNIQUE 3.6

- Place the patient prone on a pain management table. Aseptically prepare and drape the patient.
- Under fluoroscopic guidance, identify the target segment to be injected. Upper lumbar facet joints are oriented in the sagittal (vertical) plane and often can be seen on direct anteroposterior views, whereas the lower lumbar facet joints, especially at L5-S1, are obliquely oriented and require an ipsilateral oblique rotation of the C-arm to be seen.
- Position the C-arm under fluoroscopy until the joint silhouette first appears. Insert and advance a 22- or 25-gauge, 3½-inch spinal needle toward the target joint along the axis of the fluoroscopy beam until contact is made with the articular processes of the joint. Enter the joint cavity through the softer capsule and advance the needle only a few millimeters. Capsular penetration is perceived as a subtle change of resistance. If midpoint needle entry is difficult, redirect the spinal needle to the superior or inferior joint recesses.
- Confirm placement with less than 0.1 mL of nonionic contrast dye with a 3-mL syringe to minimize injection pressure under fluoroscopic guidance. When intraarticular placement has been verified, inject a total volume of 1 mL of injectant (local anesthetic with or without corticosteroids) into the joint.

LUMBAR MEDIAL BRANCH BLOCK INJECTION

TECHNIQUE 3.7

- Place the patient prone on a pain management table. Aseptically prepare and drape the area to be injected.

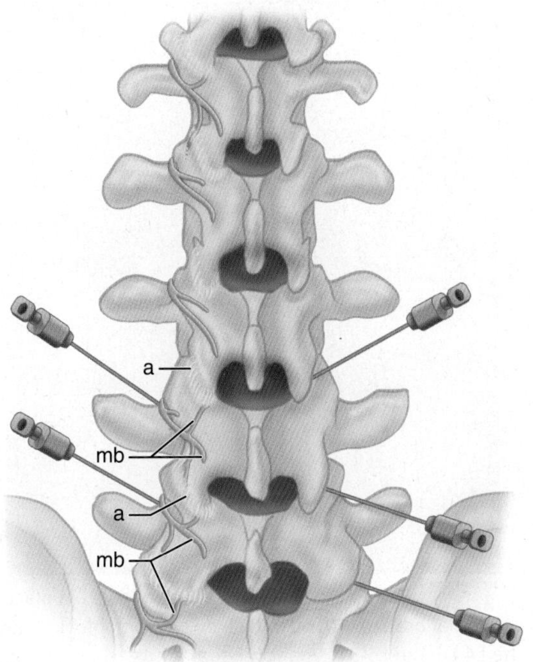

FIGURE 3.9 Posterior view of lumbar spine showing location of medial branches *(mb)* of dorsal rami, which innervate lumbar facet joints *(a)*. Needle position for L3 and L4 medial branch. Blocks shown on left half of diagram would be used to anesthetize L4-5 facet joint. Right half of diagram shows L3-4, L4-5, and L5-S1 intraarticular facet joint injection positions. **SEE TECHNIQUE 3.7.**

- Because there is dual innervation of each lumbar facet joint, two medial branch blocks are required. The medial branches cross the transverse processes below their origin (Fig. 3.9). The L4-5 facet joint is anesthetized by blocking the L3 medial branch at the transverse process of L4 and the L4 medial branch at the transverse process of L5. In the case of the L5-S1 facet joint, anesthetize the L4 medial branch as it passes over the L5 transverse process and the L5 medial branch as it passes across the sacral ala.
- Using anteroposterior fluoroscopic imaging, identify the target transverse process. For L1 through L4 medial branch blocks, penetrate the skin using a 22- or 25-gauge, 3½-inch spinal needle lateral and superior to the target location.
- Under fluoroscopic guidance, advance the spinal needle until contact is made with the dorsal superior and medial aspects of the base of the transverse process so that the needle rests against the periosteum. To ensure optimal spinal needle placement, reposition the C-arm so that the fluoroscopy beam is ipsilateral oblique and the "Scotty dog" is seen. Position the spinal needle in the middle of the "eye" of the Scotty dog. Slowly inject (over 30 seconds) 0.5 mL of 0.75% bupivacaine.
- To inject the L5 medial branch (more correctly, the L5 dorsal ramus), position the patient prone on the pain management table with the fluoroscopic beam in the anteroposterior projection (Fig. 3.10).

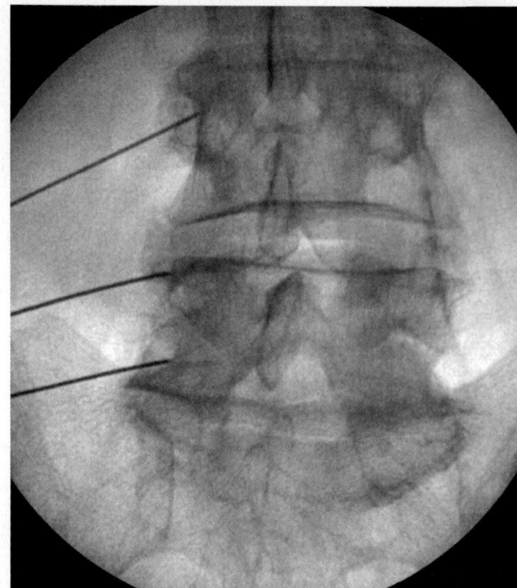

FIGURE 3.10 Posteroanterior view of needles in place for L3 and L4 medial branch blocks, and L5 dorsal rami block to anesthetize the L4-L5 and L5-S1 zygapophyseal joints.

- Identify the sacral ala. Rotate the C-arm 15 to 20 degrees ipsilateral obliquely to maximize exposure between the junction of the sacral ala and the superior process of S1. Insert a 22- or 25-gauge, 3½-inch spinal needle directly into the osseous landmarks approximately 5 mm below the superior junction of the sacral ala with the superior articular process of the sacrum under fluoroscopy. Rest the spinal needle on the periosteum and position the bevel of the spinal needle medial and away from the foramen to minimize flow through the L5 or S1 foramen. Slowly inject 0.5 mL of 0.75% bupivacaine.

SACROILIAC JOINT

The sacroiliac joint remains a controversial source of primary low back pain despite validated scientific studies. It often is overlooked as a source of low back pain because its anatomic location makes it difficult to examine in isolation and many provocative tests place mechanical stresses on contiguous structures. In addition, several other structures may refer pain to the sacroiliac joint.

Similar to other synovial joints, the sacroiliac joint moves; however, sacroiliac joint movement is involuntary and is caused by shear, compression, and other indirect forces. Muscles involved with secondary sacroiliac joint motion include the erectae spinae, quadratus lumborum, psoas major and minor, piriformis, latissimus dorsi, obliquus abdominis, and gluteal. Imbalances in any of these muscles as a result of central facilitation may cause them to function in a shortened state that tends to inhibit their antagonists reflexively. Theoretically, dysfunctional movement patterns may result. Postural changes and body weight also can create motion through the sacroiliac joint.

Because of the wide range of segmental innervation (L2-S2) of the sacroiliac joint, there are myriad referral zone patterns. In studies of asymptomatic subjects, the most constant referral zone was localized to a 3- × 10-cm area just inferior to the ipsilateral posterior superior iliac spine (PSIS) (Fig. 3.11); however, pain may be referred to the buttocks, groin, posterior thigh, calf, and foot.

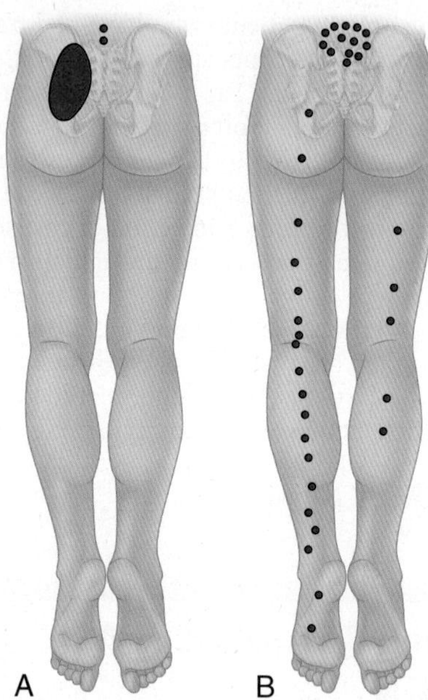

FIGURE 3.11 Pain diagram. **A,** Patient-reported pain diagram consistent with sacroiliac joint dysfunction. **B,** Patient-reported diagram inconsistent with sacroiliac joint dysfunction. (From Fortin JD, Dwyer AP, West S, et al: Sacroiliac joint: pain referral maps upon applying a new injection/arthrography technique, part I: asymptomatic volunteers, *Spine* 19:1475–1482, 1994.)

Sacroiliac dysfunction, also called sacroiliac joint mechanical pain or sacroiliac joint syndrome, is the most common painful condition of this joint. The true prevalence of mediated pain from sacroiliac joint dysfunction is unknown; however, several studies indicated that it is more common than expected. Because no specific or pathognomonic historical facts or physical examination tests accurately identify the sacroiliac joint as a source of pain, diagnosis is one of exclusion. Sacroiliac joint dysfunction should be considered, however, if an injury was caused by a direct fall on the buttocks, a rear-end motor vehicle accident with the ipsilateral foot on the brake at the moment of impact, a broadside motor vehicle accident with a blow to the lateral aspect of the pelvic ring, or a fall in a hole with one leg in the hole and the other extended outside. Lumbar rotation and axial loading that can occur during ballet or ice skating is another common mechanism of injury. Although controversial, the risk of sacroiliac joint dysfunction may be increased in individuals with lumbar fusion or hip pathology. Other causes include insufficiency stress fractures; fatigue stress fractures; metabolic processes, such as deposition diseases; degenerative joint disease; infection; and inflammatory conditions, such as ankylosing spondylitis, psoriatic arthritis, and Reiter disease. The diagnosis of sacroiliac joint pain can be confirmed if symptoms are reproduced on distention of the joint capsule by provocative injection and subsequently abated with an analgesic block.

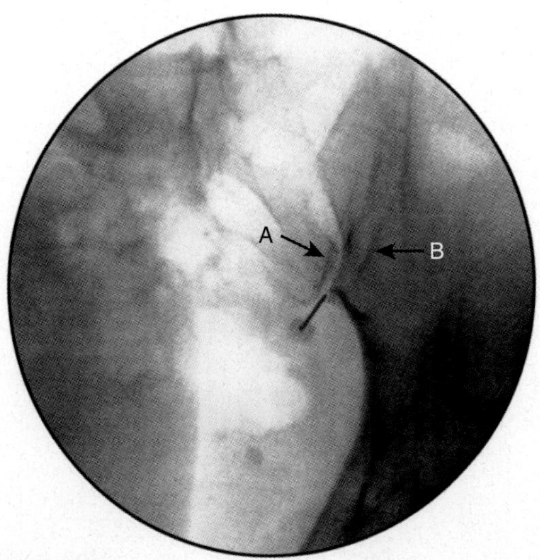

FIGURE 3.12 Sacroiliac joint injection showing medial *(A)* and lateral *(B)* joint planes (silhouettes). Entry into joint is achieved above most posteroinferior aspect of joint. **SEE TECHNIQUE 3.8.**

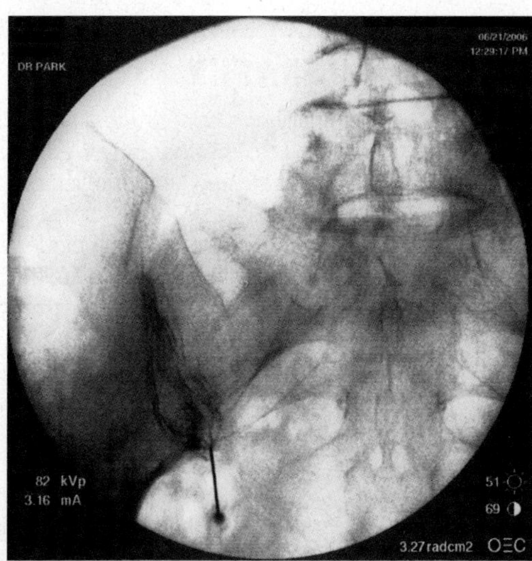

FIGURE 3.13 Left sacroiliac joint contrast pattern. **SEE TECHNIQUE 3.8.**

SACROILIAC JOINT INJECTION

TECHNIQUE 3.8

- Place the patient prone on a pain management table. Aseptically prepare and drape the side to be injected. Rotate the C-arm until the medial (posterior) joint line is seen.
- Use a 27-gauge, ¼-inch needle to anesthetize the skin of the buttock 1 to 3 cm inferior to the lowest aspect of the joint. Using fluoroscopy, insert a 22-gauge, 3½-inch spinal needle until the needle rests 1 cm above the most posteroinferior aspect of the joint (Fig. 3.12). Rarely, a larger spinal needle is required in obese patients. Advance the spinal needle into the sacroiliac joint until capsular penetration occurs.
- Confirm intraarticular placement under fluoroscopy with 0.5 mL of nonionic contrast dye (Fig. 3.13). A spot radiograph can be taken to document placement. Inject a 2-mL volume containing 1 mL of 0.75% preservative-free bupivacaine and 1 mL of 6 mg/mL Celestone Soluspan into the joint.

DISCOGRAPHY

Discography has been used since the late 1940s for the experimental and clinical evaluation of disc disease in the cervical and lumbar regions of the spine. Since that time, discography has had a limited but important role in the evaluation of suspected disc pathology.

The clinical usefulness of the data obtained from discography is controversial. Although early studies concluded that lumbar discography was an unreliable diagnostic tool, with a 37% false-positive rate, later studies found a 0% false-positive rate for discography and concluded that, with current technique and a standardized protocol, discography was a highly reliable test.

The most important aspect of discography is provocative testing for concordant pain (i.e., pain that corresponds to a patient's usual pain) to provide information regarding the clinical significance of the disc abnormality. Although difficult to standardize, this testing distinguishes discography from other anatomic imaging techniques. If the patient is unable to distinguish customary pain from any other pain, the procedure is of no value. In patients who have a concordant response without evidence of a radial annular fissure on discography, CT should be considered because some discs that appear normal on discography show disruption on a CT scan.

Indications for lumbar discography include operative planning of spinal fusion, testing of the structural integrity of an adjacent disc to a known abnormality such as spondylolisthesis or fusion, identifying a painful disc among multiple degenerative discs, ruling out secondary internal disc disruption or suspected lateral or recurrent disc herniation, and determining the primary symptom-producing level when chemonucleolysis is being considered. Lumbar discography is most useful as a test to exclude levels from operative intervention rather than as a primary indication for operative fusion in patients with axial back pain. Thoracic discography can be a useful tool in the investigation of thoracic, chest, and upper abdominal pain. Degenerative thoracic disc disease, with or without herniation, has a highly variable clinical presentation, frequently mimicking visceral conditions and causing back or musculoskeletal pain. Discography also may be justified in medicolegal situations to establish a more definitive diagnosis even though treatment may not be planned on that disc.

Compression of the spinal cord, stenosis of the roots, bleeding disorders, allergy to the injectable material, and active infection are contraindications to diagnostic discography procedures. Although the risk of complications from discography is low, potential problems include discitis, nerve root injury, subarachnoid puncture, chemical meningitis, bleeding, and allergic reactions. In addition, in the cervical region, retropharyngeal and epidural abscess can occur. Pneumothorax is a risk in the cervical and thoracic regions.

LUMBAR DISCOGRAPHY

Lumbar discography originally was done using a transdural technique in a manner similar to myelography with a lumbar puncture. The difference between lumbar myelography and discography was that the needle used for the latter was advanced through the thecal sac. The technique later was modified, consisting of an extradural, extralaminar approach that avoided the thecal sac, and it was refined further to enable entry into the L5-S1 disc using a two-needle technique to maneuver around the iliac crest.

A patient's response during the procedure is the most important aspect of the study. Pain alone does not determine if a disc is the cause of the back pain. The concordance of the pain in regard to the quality and location are paramount in determining whether the disc is a true pain generator. A control disc is necessary to validate a positive finding on discography.

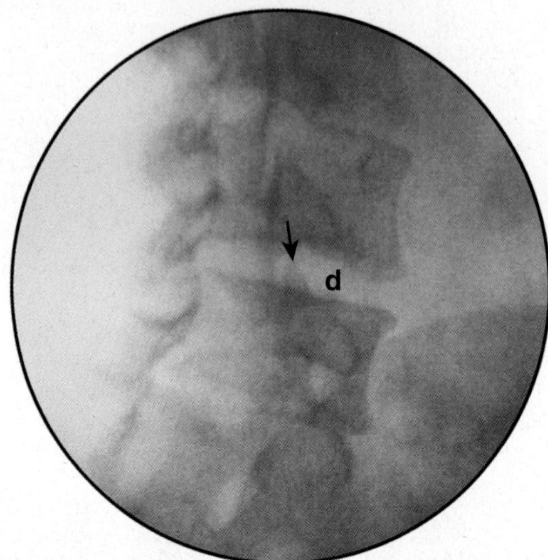

FIGURE 3.14 **Lumbar spine in oblique position with superior articular process *(arrow)* dividing disc space *(d)* in half.** (Courtesy Frank J. E. Falco, MD.) **SEE TECHNIQUE 3.9.**

TECHNIQUE 3.9

(FALCO)

- Place the patient on a procedure or fluoroscopic table.
- Insert an angiocatheter into the upper extremity and infuse intravenous antibiotics to prevent discitis. Some physicians prefer to give antibiotics intradiscally during the procedure.
- Place the patient in a modified lateral decubitus position with the symptomatic side down to avoid having the patient confuse the pain caused by the needle with the actual pain on that same side. This position also allows for easier fluoroscopic imaging of the intervertebral discs and mobilizes the bowel away from the needle path.
- Sedate the patient with a short-acting agent. It is best to avoid analgesic agents that may alter the pain response.
- Prepare and drape the skin sterilely, including the lumbosacral region.
- Under fluoroscopic control, identify the intervertebral discs. Adjust the patient's position or the C-arm so that the lumbar spine is in an oblique position with the superior articular process dividing the intervertebral space in half (Fig. 3.14).
- Anesthetize the skin overlying the superior articular process with 1 to 2 mL of 1% lidocaine if necessary.
- Advance a single 6-inch spinal needle (or longer, depending on the patient's size) through the skin and deeper soft tissues to the outer annulus of the disc. The disc entry point is just anterior to the base of the superior articular process and just above the superior endplate of the vertebral body, which allows the needle to pass safely by the exiting nerve root (Fig. 3.15). Advance the needle into the central third of the disc, using anteroposterior and lateral fluoroscopic imaging.
- Confirm the position of the needle tip within the central third of the disc with anteroposterior and lateral fluoroscopic imaging. Inject either saline or nonionic contrast dye into each disc.
- Record any pain that the patient experiences during the injection as none, dissimilar, similar, or exact in relationship to the patient's typical low back pain. Record intradiscal pressures to assist in determining if the disc is the cause of the pain.

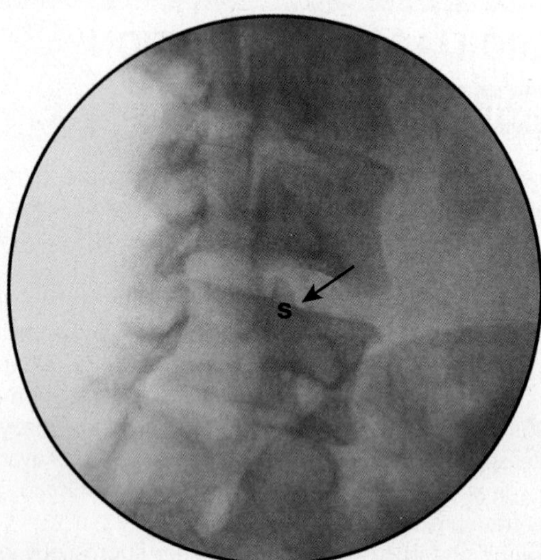

FIGURE 3.15 **Disc entry point is just anterior *(arrow)* to base of superior articular process *(s)* and just above superior endplate of vertebral body.** (Courtesy Frank J. E. Falco, MD.) **SEE TECHNIQUE 3.9.**

- Obtain radiographs of the lumbar spine on completion of the study, paying particular attention to the contrast-enhanced disc. Obtain a CT scan if necessary to assess disc anatomy further.
- An alternative method is a two-needle technique in which a 6- or 8-inch spinal needle is passed through a shorter introducer needle (typically 3½ inches) into the disc in the same manner as a single needle. This approach may reduce the incidence of infection by allowing the procedure needle to pass into the disc space without ever penetrating the skin. The introducer needle also may assist in more accurate needle placement, reducing the risk of injuring the exiting nerve root. The two-needle approach may require more time than the single-needle technique, and the larger introducer needle could cause more pain to the patient.

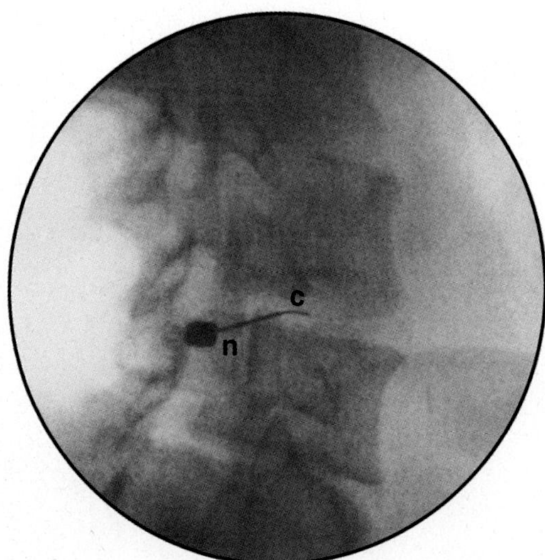

FIGURE 3.16 Curved procedure needle *(c)* passing through straight introducer needle *(n)*. (Courtesy Frank J. E. Falco, MD.) **SEE TECHNIQUE 3.9.**

- The two-needle technique often is used to enter the L5-S1 disc space with one modification. The procedure needle typically is curved (Fig. 3.16). To bypass the iliac crest, the introducer needle is advanced at an angle that places the needle tip in a position that does not line up with the L5-S1 disc space, which makes it difficult, if not impossible, for a straight procedure needle to advance into the L5-S1 disc. A curved procedure needle allows the needle tip to align with the L5-S1 disc as it is advanced toward and into the disc adjusting for malalignment.

THORACIC DISCOGRAPHY

Thoracic discography has been refined to provide a technique that is reproducible and safe. A posterolateral extralaminar approach similar to lumbar discography is used with a single-needle technique. The significant difference between thoracic and lumbar discography is the potential for complications because of the surrounding anatomy of the thoracic spine. In contrast to lumbar discography, which typically is performed in the mid to lower lumbar spine below the spinal cord and lungs, thoracic discography has the inherent risk of pneumothorax and direct spinal cord trauma; other complications include discitis and bleeding. Essentially the same protocol is used for thoracic discography as for lumbar discography.

TECHNIQUE 3.10

(FALCO)

- Place the patient in a modified lateral decubitus position on the procedure table with the symptomatic side down.
- Begin antibiotics through the intravenous catheter. Alternatively, intradiscal antibiotics may be given during the procedure.

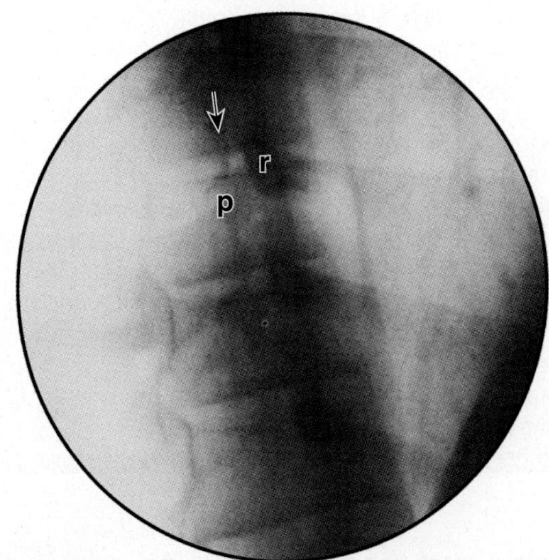

FIGURE 3.17 Oblique position with superior articular process *(arrow)* dividing thoracic intervertebral space in half. *p*, Pedicle; *r*, rib head. (Courtesy Frank J. E. Falco, MD.) **SEE TECHNIQUE 3.10.**

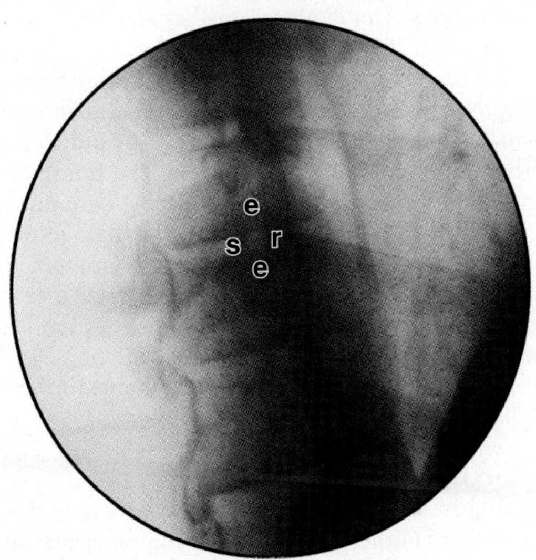

FIGURE 3.18 Thoracic endplates *(e)*, superior articular process *(s)*, and rib head *(r)* form box. (Courtesy Frank J. E. Falco, MD.)

- Sedate the patient and prepare and drape the skin in a sterile manner.

  Using fluoroscopic imaging, identify the intervertebral thoracic discs. Move the patient or adjust the C-arm obliquely to position the superior articular process so that it divides the intervertebral space in half (Fig. 3.17). At this point, the intervertebral discs and endplates, subjacent superior articular process, and adjacent rib head should be in clear view. The endplates, the superior articular process, and the rib head form a "box" (Fig. 3.18) that delineates a safe pathway into the disc, avoiding the spinal cord and lung. Keep the needle tip within the confines of this "box" while advancing it into the annulus.
- After proper positioning and exposure, anesthetize the skin overlying the superior articular process with 1 to 2 mL of 1% lidocaine if necessary.

- Advance a single 6-inch spinal needle (a shorter or longer needle can be used, depending on the patient's size) through the skin and the deeper soft tissues into the outer annulus within the "box" just anterior to the base of the superior articular process and just above the superior endplate. Continue into the central third of the disc, using anteroposterior and lateral fluoroscopic guidance.
- Inject either saline or a nonionic contrast dye into each disc in the same manner as for lumbar discography.
- Record any pain response and analyze for reproduction of concordant pain using the same protocol as for lumbar discography.
- Obtain radiographs and CT scan of the thoracic spine on completion of the study.

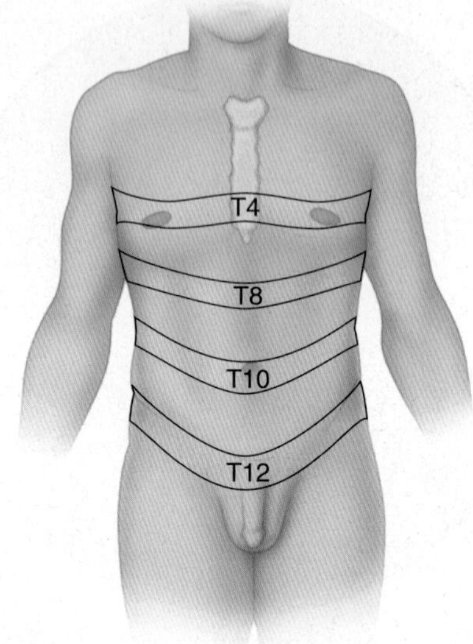

FIGURE 3.19 Sensory dermatomes of trunk region.

THORACIC DISC DISEASE

The thoracic spine is the least common location for disc pathology. Since the 1960s, many approaches have been described and validated through clinical experience. It is apparent that posterior laminectomy has no role in the operative treatment of this problem. Other posterior approaches, such as costotransversectomy, have good indications.

Symptomatic thoracic disc herniations remain rare, with an estimated incidence of one in 1 million individuals per year. They represent 0.25% to 0.75% of the total incidence of symptomatic disc herniations. The most common age at onset is between the fourth and sixth decades. As with the other areas of the spine, the incidence of asymptomatic disc herniations is high; an estimated 37% of thoracic disc herniations are asymptomatic. Operative treatment of thoracic disc herniations is indicated in rare patients with acute disc herniation with myelopathic findings attributable to the lesion, especially progressive neurologic symptoms.

SIGNS AND SYMPTOMS

The natural history of symptomatic thoracic disc disease is similar to that in other areas, in that symptoms and function typically improve with conservative treatment and time. The clinical course can vary, however, and a high index of suspicion must be maintained to make the correct diagnosis. The differential diagnosis for the symptoms of thoracic disc herniations is fairly extensive and includes nonspinal causes occurring with the cardiopulmonary, gastrointestinal, and musculoskeletal systems. Spinal causes of similar symptoms can occur with infectious, neoplastic, degenerative, and metabolic problems within the spinal column and the spinal cord.

Two general patient populations have been documented in the literature. The smaller group of patients is younger and has a relatively short history of symptoms, often with a history of trauma. Typically, an acute soft disc herniation with either acute spinal cord compression or radiculopathy is present. Outcome generally is favorable with operative or nonoperative treatment. The larger group of patients has a longer history, often more than 6 to 12 months of symptoms, which result from chronic spinal cord or root compression. Disc degeneration, often with calcification of the disc, is the underlying process.

Pain is the most common presenting feature of thoracic disc herniations. Two patterns of pain are apparent: one is axial, and the other is bandlike radicular pain along the course of the intercostal nerve. The T10 dermatomal level is the most commonly reported distribution, regardless of the level of involvement. This is a band extending around the lower lateral thorax and caudad to the level of the umbilicus. This radicular pattern is more common with upper thoracic and lateral disc herniations. Some axial pain often occurs with this pattern as well. Associated sensory changes of paresthesias and dysesthesia in a dermatomal distribution also occur (Fig. 3.19). High thoracic discs (T2 to T5) can manifest similarly to cervical disc disease with upper arm pain, paresthesias, radiculopathy, and Horner syndrome. Myelopathy also may occur. Complaints of weakness, which may be generalized by the patient, typically involving both lower extremities occur in the form of mild paraparesis. Sustained clonus, a positive Babinski sign, and wide-based and spastic gait all are signs of myelopathy. Bowel and bladder dysfunction occur in only 15% to 20% of these patients. The neurologic evaluation of patients with thoracic disc herniations must be meticulous because there are few localizing findings. Abdominal reflexes, cremasteric reflex, dermatomal sensory evaluation, rectus abdominis contraction symmetry, lower extremity reflexes and strength and sensory examinations, and determination of long tract findings all are important.

CONFIRMATORY IMAGING

Plain radiographs are helpful to evaluate traumatic injuries and to determine potential osseous morphologic variations that may help to localize findings, especially on intraoperative films, if these become necessary. MRI is the most important and useful imaging method to show thoracic disc herniations. In addition to the disc herniation, neoplastic or infectious pathology can be seen. The presence of intradural pathology, including disc fragments, also usually is shown on MRI. The spinal cord signal may indicate the presence of inflammation or myelomalacia as well. Despite all of these advantages, MRI may underestimate the thoracic disc herniation, which often is calcified and has low signal intensity on T1- and T2-weighted sequences.

Myelography followed by CT also can be useful in evaluating the bony anatomy and more accurately assessing the calcified portion of the herniated thoracic disc. Regardless of the imaging methods used, the appearance and presence of a thoracic disc herniation must be carefully considered and correlated with the patient's complaints and detailed examination findings. Relief of pain with thoracic transforaminal epidural can confirm the source of pain and is a good predictor of improvement with surgical intervention.

TREATMENT RESULTS

As mentioned previously, nonoperative treatment usually is effective. A specific regimen cannot be recommended for all patients; however, the principles of short-term rest, pain relief, antiinflammatory agents, and progressive directed activity restoration seem most appropriate. These measures generally should be continued at least 6 to 12 weeks if feasible. If neurologic deficits progress or manifest as myelopathy, or if pain remains at an intolerable level, surgery should be recommended. The initial procedure recommended for this lesion was posterior thoracic laminectomy and disc excision. At least half of the lesions have been identified as being central, making the excision from this approach extremely difficult, and the results were disheartening. Most series reported fewer than half of the patients improving, with some becoming worse after posterior laminectomy and discectomy. Recent studies suggest that lateral rachiotomy (modified costotransversectomy) or an anterior transthoracic approach for discectomy produces considerably better results with no evidence of worsening after the procedure.

Video-assisted thoracic surgery (VATS) has been used in several series to remove central thoracic disc herniations successfully without the need for a thoracotomy or fusion.

The most promising and least invasive technique for surgical treatment of thoracic disc herniation is awake transforaminal endoscopic discectomy. It can be used to treat thoracic herniations of the midline without the morbidity of chest surgery, fusion, or even general anesthesia.

OPERATIVE TREATMENT

The best operative approach for these lesions depends on the specific characteristics of the disc herniation and on the particular experience of the surgeon. Simple laminectomy has no role in the treatment of thoracic disc herniations. Posterior approaches, including costotransversectomy, transpedicular, transfacet pedicle-sparing, transdural, and lateral extracavitary approaches, all have been used successfully. Anterior approaches via thoracotomy, a transsternal approach, retropleural approach, or VATS also have been used successfully (Fig. 3.20). More recently, a number of minimally invasive posterior and anterior techniques have been developed, most using a series of muscle dilators, tubular retractors, and microscope visualization. The surgical intervention with the least morbidity is awake transforaminal endoscopic discectomy when used for herniations accessible by that approach.

COSTOTRANSVERSECTOMY

Costotransversectomy is probably best suited for thoracic disc herniations that are predominantly lateral or herniations that are suspected to be extruded or sequestered. Central disc herniations are probably best approached transthoracically. Some surgeons have recommended subsequent fusion after disc removal anteriorly or laterally.

THORACIC COSTOTRANSVERSECTOMY

TECHNIQUE 3.11

- The operation usually is done with the patient under general anesthesia with a double-lumen endotracheal tube or a Carlen tube to allow lung deflation on the side of approach.
- Place the patient prone and make a long midline incision or a curved incision convex to the midline centered over the side of involvement.
- Expose the spine in the usual manner out to the ribs.
- Remove a section of rib 5.0 to 7.5 cm long at the level of involvement, avoiding damage to the intercostal nerve and artery.
- Carry the resection into the lateral side of the disc, exposing it for removal. Additional exposure can be made by laminectomy and excision of the pedicle and facet joint. Fusion is unnecessary unless more than one facet joint is removed.
- Close the wound in layers.

POSTOPERATIVE CARE Postoperative care is similar to that for lumbar disc excision without fusion (see Technique 3.16).

THORACIC DISC EXCISION

Because of the relative age of patients with thoracic disc ruptures, special care must be taken to identify patients with pulmonary problems. In these patients, the anterior approach can be detrimental medically, making a posterolateral approach safer. Patients with midline protrusions probably are best treated with the transthoracic approach to ensure complete disc removal.

THORACIC DISCECTOMY—ANTERIOR APPROACH

TECHNIQUE 3.12

- The operation is done with the patient under general anesthesia, using a double-lumen endotracheal tube for lung deflation on the side of the approach.
- Place the patient in a lateral decubitus position. A left-sided anterior approach usually is preferred, making the operative procedure easier, if the herniation is central.
- Make a skin incision along the line of the rib that corresponds to the second thoracic vertebra above the involved intervertebral disc except for approaches to the upper five thoracic segments, where the approach is through the third rib. The skin incision is best determined by correlating preoperative imaging with intraoperative fluoroscopy.
- Cut the rib subperiosteally at its posterior and anterior ends and insert a rib retractor. Save the rib for grafting later in the procedure. One can decide on an extrapleural or transpleural approach depending on familiarity and

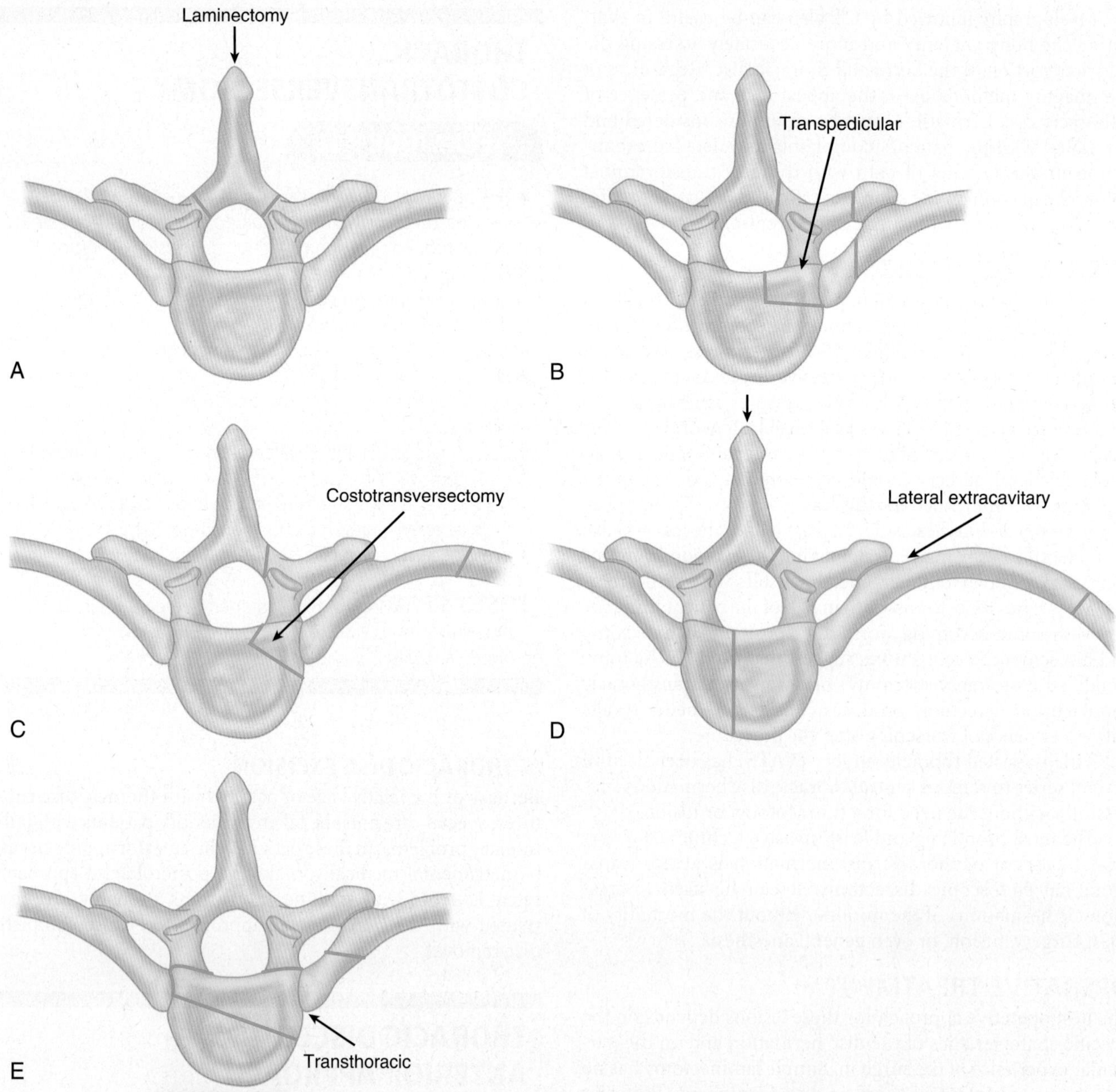

FIGURE 3.20 **A to E,** Exposure of thoracic disc provided by standard laminectomy **(A)**, transpedicular approach **(B)**, costotransversectomy approach **(C)**, lateral extracavitary approach **(D)**, and transthoracic approach **(E)**.

ease. Exposure of the thoracic vertebrae should give adequate access to the front and opposite side.

- Dissect the great vessels free of the spine.
- Ligate the intersegmental vessels near the great vessels and not near the foramen. One should be able to insert the tip of a finger against the opposite side of the disc when the vascular mobilization is complete. Exposure of the intervertebral disc without disturbing more than three segmental vessels is preferable to avoid ischemic problems in the spinal cord.
- In the thoracolumbar region, strip the diaphragm from the 11th and 12th ribs. The anterior longitudinal ligament usually is sectioned to allow spreading of the intervertebral disc space. Remove the disc as completely as possible if fusion is planned. The use of an operating microscope or loupe magnification eases the removal of the disc near the posterior longitudinal ligament. Use curets and Kerrison rongeurs to remove the disc back to the posterior longitudinal ligament. When using this technique with fusion, removal of most of the disc is straightforward. As the posterior portion of the disc, including the herniation, is removed, however, the technique becomes more difficult. As mentioned previously, the herniation and surrounding disc usually are calcified and must be removed either piecemeal or with a high-speed drill. Careful dissection to develop a plane between tissue to be removed and the ventral dura is required. This

is best done with blunt Penfield-type dissectors and small curets of various designs and orientations. Even if a drill is used, the removal of the posteriormost tissue should be done with hand instruments, not powered instruments. Expect significant bleeding from the epidural veins, which usually are congested at the level of herniation.

- After removal of the disc, strip the endplates of their cartilage.
- Make a slot on the margin of the superior endplate to accept the graft material. Preserve the subchondral bone on both sides of the disc space. Insert iliac, tibial, or rib grafts into the disc space. If multiple short rib grafts are used, they can be tied together with heavy suture material when the maximal number of grafts has been inserted. This helps maintain vertical alignment for all such grafts.
- Close the wound in the usual manner and use standard chest drainage.
- Alternatively, if fusion is not desired, a more limited resection using an operating microscope can be done.
- Also, the minimally invasive lateral retroperitoneal/retropleural approach as described in chapter 1 can be used for herniations from T10-11 to L1-2.
- After the vascular mobilization, resect the rib head to allow observation of the pedicle and foramen caudal to the disc space. The cephalad portion of the pedicle can be removed with a high-speed burr and Kerrison rongeurs, exposing the posterolateral aspect of the disc. This allows for careful, blunt development of the plane ventral to the dura with removal of the disc herniation and preservation of the anterior majority of the disc and limits the need for fusion. A similar technique using VATS is described in Technique 3.13.
- The transthoracic approach removing a rib two levels above the level of the lesion can be used up to T5. The transthoracic approach from T2 to T5 is best made by excision of the third or fourth rib and elevation of the scapula by sectioning of attachments of the serratus anterior and trapezius from the scapula. The approach to the T1-2 disc is best made from the neck with a sternum-splitting incision.

POSTOPERATIVE CARE Postoperative care is the same as for a thoracotomy. The patient is allowed to walk after the chest tubes are removed. Extension in any position is prohibited. A brace or body cast that limits extension should be used if the stability of the graft is questionable. The graft usually is stable without support if only one disc space is removed. Postoperative care is the same as for anterior corpectomy and fusion if more than one disc level is removed. If no fusion is done, the patient is mobilized as pain permits without a brace.

THORACOSCOPIC DISC EXCISION

In the fields of general surgery and thoracic surgery, the development of laparoscopic surgical techniques and VATS has allowed significant improvements to be made with respect to decreasing pain, duration of hospitalization, and recovery times for a variety of procedures (Fig. 3.21). Microsurgical and endoscopic operative techniques are highly technical, and they should be performed by a surgeon who is proficient in this technique and in the use of thoracoscopic equipment and with the assistance of an experienced thoracic surgeon. Ideally, the procedure should first be done on cadavers or live animals.

THORACOSCOPIC THORACIC DISCECTOMY

TECHNIQUE 3.13

(ROSENTHAL ET AL.)

- Place the patient in the left lateral decubitus position to allow a right-sided approach and displacement of the aorta and heart to the left.
- Insert four trocars in a triangular fashion along the middle axillary line converging on the disc space. Introduce a rigid endoscope with a 30-degree optic angle attached to a video camera into one of the trocars, leaving the other three as working channels.
- Deflate the lung using a Carlen tube or similar method.
- Split the parietal pleura starting at the medial part of the intervertebral space and extending up to the costovertebral process.
- Preserve and mobilize the segmental arteries and sympathetic nerve out of the operating field.
- Drill away the rib head and lateral portion of the pedicle. Remove the remaining pedicle with Kerrison rongeurs to improve exposure to the spinal canal. Removing the superior posterior portion of the vertebra caudal to the disc space allows safer removal of the disc material, which can be pulled anteriorly and inferiorly away from the spinal canal to be removed. Use endoscopic instruments for surgery in the portals.
- Remove the disc posteriorly and the posterior longitudinal ligament, restricting bone and disc removal to the posterior third of the intervertebral space and costovertebral area to maintain stability.
- Insert chest tubes in the standard fashion and set them to water suction; close the portals.

POSTOPERATIVE CARE The patient is rapidly mobilized as tolerated by the chest tubes. Discharge is possible after the chest tubes have been removed and the patient is ambulating well.

MINIMALLY INVASIVE THORACIC DISCECTOMY

TECHNIQUE 3.14

- Place the patient in the lateral decubitus position with the affected side up.
- Localize an incision over the disc space of interest. A 5-cm portion of rib can be resected if it is overlying the disc, or the approach can sometimes be performed without rib resection. Using blunt finger dissection, make a retropleural approach down to the spine and dock a minimally invasive retractor system on the disc space and rib head of interest. Sometimes the pleura must be opened, but this does not change the exposure significantly because the retractor can safely retract the lung while being insufflated.

- Complete the procedure as in an open discectomy through a thoracotomy using the self-retaining retractor (many different styles are available).
- Once the procedure is finished there is no need for a chest tube if the pleura is not violated.
- Close the rib base and subcutaneous tissues in layers.

This approach can be extended down to L1-2 by mobilizing the diaphragm off the rib and transverse process attachments.

POSTOPERATIVE CARE The patient is mobilized the day of surgery and is discharged when ambulating well.

THORACIC ENDOSCOPIC DISC EXCISION

TRANSFORAMINAL ENDOSCOPIC THORACIC DISCECTOMY

The awake transforaminal endoscopic approach using the outside-in technique to the thoracic spine allows resection of disc material that can begin midline and be extended laterally to either side. This approach typically can reach herniations from T4 to L4 in most people, does not require violation of the chest cavity, usually does not require fusion, and does not even require general anesthesia, making it the least invasive approach for removal of a thoracic disc herniation.

A diagnostic transforaminal epidural injection at the site of the herniation can confirm the diagnosis and ensure enough space between the rib, transverse process, and facet joint for the endoscopic approach. If the patient gets profound relief from the transforaminal epidural, it is a good predictor of surgical outcome, and endoscopic surgery can be planned if the pain from the thoracic disc herniation returns.

TECHNIQUE 3.15

- Plan the approach to the appropriate thoracic foramen on preoperative axial imaging.
- Place the patient prone on a radiolucent table.
- Advance an 18- to 20-gauge needle into the foramen at the level of the herniation based on the preoperative imaging plan.
- Place a guide wire through the needle and remove the needle.
- Anesthetize the skin and subcutaneous tissue with 8 mL 1% lidocaine with epinephrine and use a no. 11 blade to make a 1-cm incision.
- Place dilators over the guidewire and advance them into the foramen under fluoroscopic guidance.
- Some systems allow reaming of the foramen with percutaneous reamers under fluoroscopic guidance. Alternatively, advance the operative cannula into the foramen and open the foramen with a diamond burr under direct light-based endoscopic visualization. This technique is best for surgeons who are more comfortable with bony resection under direct visualization, and it is our preferred technique.
- Remove bone vigorously to allow space to work and avoid tension on the dura. Remove a significant amount of superior articular process, pedicle, and posterior end plates as needed.
- Adjust fluid flow through the endoscope to control epidural bleeding.
- After the bony anatomy of the arch formed by the inferior pedicle and superior articular process is visualized, identify the herniation.
- Use instruments to remove disc material from the subanular space and push disc material away from the dura into the cavity created by the drilling.
- Decompression is complete when the undersurface of the thoracic dura is seen pulsating to heartbeat and the patient notes resolution of his or her typical thoracic radicular pain.
- Suction excess fluid from the wound and infiltrate the epidural space with 1 mL of steroid and 2 mL of 0.25% Marcaine.
- Remove the operative cannula, close the skin with a single subcuticular stitch, and close the wound with a dab of skin glue. Ask the patient to transfer himself or herself to the gurney.

POSTOPERATIVE CARE The patient is limited in bending, lifting, and twisting, but may shower the day of the procedure. Patients are typically discharged from the surgery center as soon as they can ambulate independently and void. Driving is delayed until postoperative day 2 or until narcotics are discontinued, but this procedure is commonly done with only nonsteroidal antiinflammatory medications for postoperative pain control. Patients are allowed to begin a trunk stabilization therapy program at 2 weeks after surgery and advance as tolerated.

LUMBAR DISC DISEASE

SIGNS AND SYMPTOMS

Although back pain is common from the second decade of life on, intervertebral disc disease and disc herniation are most prominent in otherwise healthy people in the third and fourth decades of life. Most people relate their back and leg pain to a traumatic incident, but close questioning frequently reveals that the patient has had intermittent episodes of back pain for many months or even years before the onset of severe leg pain. In many instances, the back pain is relatively fleeting and is relieved by rest. Heavy exertion, repetitive bending, twisting, or heavy lifting often brings on axial back pain. In other instances, an inciting event cannot be elicited. The pain usually begins in the lower back, radiating to the sacroiliac region and buttocks. The pain can radiate down the posterior thigh. Back and posterior thigh pain of this type can be elicited from many areas of the spine, including the facet joints, longitudinal ligaments, and periosteum of the vertebra. Radicular pain usually extends below the knee and follows the dermatome of the involved nerve root (Fig. 3.22).

The usual history of lumbar disc herniation is of repetitive lower back and buttock pain, relieved by a short period of rest. This pain is suddenly exacerbated, often by a flexion

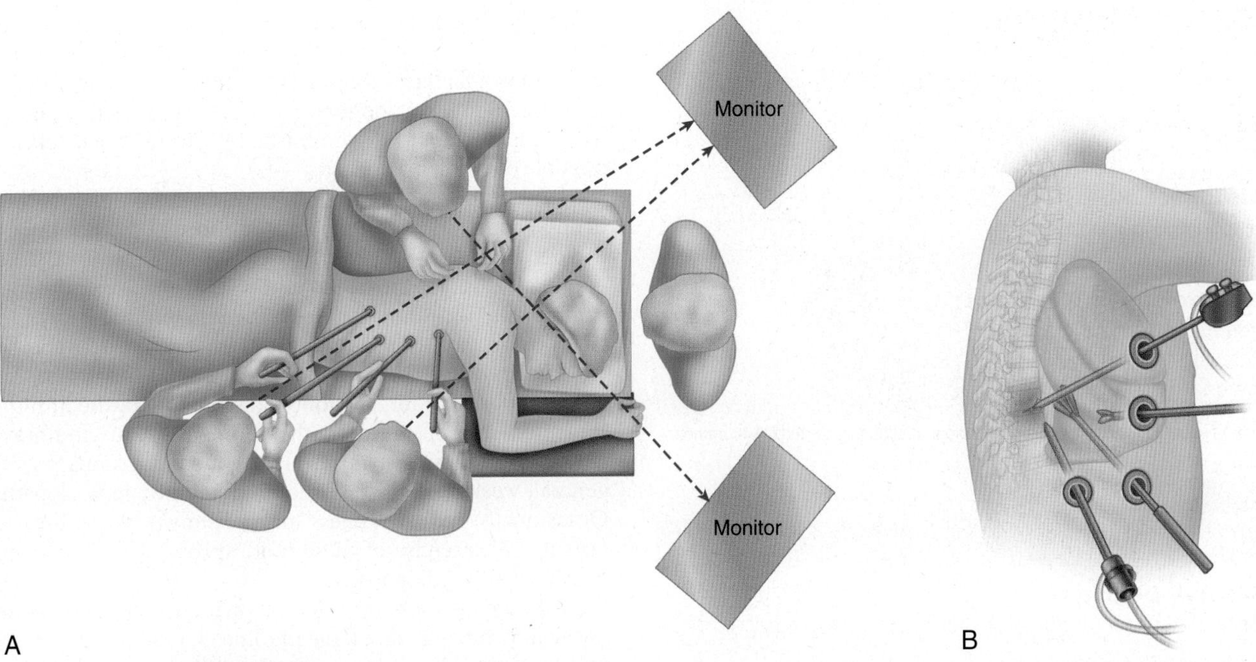

FIGURE 3.21 Video-assisted thoracic surgery. **A,** Patient positioned in left lateral decubitus position and portal positions marked. **B,** Portals.

episode, with the appearance of leg pain. Most radicular pain from nerve root compression caused by a herniated nucleus pulposus is evidenced by leg pain equal to, or in many cases greater than, the degree of back pain. Whenever leg pain is minimal and back pain is predominant, great care should be taken before making the diagnosis of a symptomatic herniated intervertebral disc. The pain from disc herniation usually varies, increasing with activity, especially sitting and driving.

The pain can be decreased by rest, especially in the semi-Fowler position, and can be exacerbated by straining, sneezing, or coughing. Whenever the pattern of pain is bizarre or the pain is uniform in intensity, a diagnosis of symptomatic herniated disc should be viewed with some skepticism.

Other symptoms of disc herniation include weakness and paresthesias. In most patients, the weakness is intermittent, varies with activity, and is localized to the neurologic level of involvement. Paresthesias also vary and are limited to the dermatome of the involved nerve root. Whenever these complaints are generalized, the diagnosis of a simple unilateral disc herniation should be questioned.

Numbness and weakness in the involved leg and occasionally pain in the groin or testis can be associated with a high or midline lumbar disc herniation. If a fragment is large or the herniation is high, symptoms of pressure on the entire cauda equina can occur with development of cauda equina syndrome. These symptoms include numbness and weakness in both legs, rectal pain, numbness in the perineum, and paralysis of the sphincters. This diagnosis should be the primary consideration in patients who complain of sudden loss of bowel or bladder control. Whenever the diagnosis of cauda equina syndrome is caused by an acute midline herniation, evaluation and treatment should be aggressive.

The physical findings with disc disease vary because of the time intervals involved. Usually patients with acute pain show evidence of marked paraspinal spasm that is sustained during walking or motion. A scoliosis or a list in the lumbar spine may be present, and in many patients the normal lumbar lordosis is lost. As the acute episode subsides, the degree of spasm diminishes remarkably, and the loss of normal lumbar lordosis may be the only telltale sign. Point tenderness may be present over the spinous process at the level of the disc involved, and pain may extend laterally in some patients.

If there is nerve root irritation, it centers over the length of the sciatic nerve, in the sciatic notch, and more distally in the popliteal space. In addition, stretch of the sciatic nerve at the knee should reproduce buttock, thigh, and leg pain (i.e., pain distal to the knee). A Lasègue sign usually is positive on the involved side. A positive Lasègue sign or straight-leg raising should elicit buttock and leg pain distal to the knee. Occasionally, if leg pain is significant, the patient leans back from an upright sitting position and assumes the tripod position to relieve the pain. This is referred to as the "flip sign." Contralateral leg pain produced by straight-leg raising should be regarded as pathognomonic of a herniated intervertebral disc. The absence of a positive Lasègue sign should make one skeptical of the diagnosis, although older individuals may not have a positive Lasègue sign and tend toward more claudicatory symptoms. Likewise, inappropriate findings and inconsistencies in the examination usually are nonorganic in origin (see discussion of nonspecific axial pain). If the leg pain has persisted for any length of time, atrophy of the involved limb may be present, as shown by asymmetric girth of the thigh or calf. The neurologic examination varies as determined by the level of root involvement (Boxes 3.2 to 3.4).

Unilateral disc herniation at L3-4 usually compresses the L4 root as it crosses the disc before exiting at the L4-5 intervertebral foramen below the L4 pedicle. Pain may be localized around the medial side of the leg. Numbness may be present over the anteromedial aspect of the leg. The anterior tibial muscle may be weak, as evidenced by inability

BOX 3.2

L4 Root Compression*

Sensory Deficit
Posterolateral thigh, anterior knee, and medial leg

Motor Weakness
Quadriceps (variable)
Hip adductors (variable)

Anterior Tibial Weakness
Reflex change
Patellar tendon
Anterior tibial tendon (variable)

* Indicative of L3-4 disc herniation or pathologic condition localized to L4 foramen.

BOX 3.3

L5 Root Compression*

Sensory Deficit
Anterolateral leg, dorsum of the foot, and great toe

Motor Weakness
Extensor hallucis longus
Gluteus medius
Extensor digitorum longus and brevis

Reflex Change
Usually none
Posterior tibial (difficult to elicit)

* Indicative of L4-5 disc herniation or pathologic condition localized to L5 foramen.

BOX 3.4

S1 Root Compression*

Sensory Deficit
Lateral malleolus, lateral foot, heel, and web of fourth and fifth toes

Motor Weakness
Peroneus longus and brevis
Gastrocnemius-soleus complex
Gluteus maximus

Reflex Change
Achilles tendon (gastrocnemius-soleus complex)

* Indicative of L5-S1 disc herniation or pathologic condition localized to S1 foramen.

to heel walk. The quadriceps and hip adductor group, both innervated from L2, L3, and L4, also may be weak and, in extended ruptures, atrophic. Reflex testing may reveal a diminished or absent patellar tendon reflex (L2, L3, and L4) or anterior tibial tendon reflex (L4). Sensory testing may show diminished sensibility over the L4 dermatome, the isolated portion of which is the medial leg (see Fig. 3.22) and the autonomous zone of which is at the level of the medial malleolus.

Unilateral disc herniation at L4-5 results in compression of the L5 root. L5 root radiculopathy should produce pain in the dermatomal pattern. Numbness, when present, follows the L5 dermatome along the anterolateral aspect of the leg and the dorsum of the foot, including the great toe. The autonomous zone for this nerve is the dorsal first web of the foot and the dorsum of the third toe. Weakness may involve the extensor hallucis longus (L5), gluteus medius (L5), or extensor digitorum longus and brevis (L5). Reflex change usually is not found. A diminished posterior tibial reflex is possible but difficult to elicit.

With unilateral rupture of the disc at L5-S1, the findings of an S1 radiculopathy are noted. Pain and numbness involve the dermatome of S1. The S1 dermatome includes the lateral malleolus and the lateral and plantar surface of the foot, occasionally including the heel. There is numbness over the lateral aspect of the leg and, more important, over the lateral aspect of the foot, including the lateral three toes. The autonomous zone for this root is the dorsum of the fifth toe. Weakness may be shown in the peroneus longus and brevis (S1), gastrocnemius-soleus (S1), or gluteus maximus (S1). In general, weakness is not a usual finding in S1 radiculopathy. Occasionally, mild weakness may be shown by asymmetric fatigue with exercise of these motor groups. The ankle jerk usually is reduced or absent.

Massive extrusion of a disc involving the entire diameter of the lumbar canal or a large midline extrusion can produce pain in the back, legs, and occasionally perineum. Both legs may be paralyzed, the sphincters may be incontinent, and the ankle jerks may be absent.

More than 95% of the ruptures of the lumbar intervertebral discs occur at L4-5 or L5-S1. Ruptures at higher levels in many patients are not associated with a positive straight-leg raising test. In these instances, a positive femoral stretch test can be helpful. This test is done by placing the patient prone and acutely flexing the knee while placing the hand in the popliteal fossa. When this procedure results in anterior thigh pain, the result is positive and a high lesion should be suspected. In addition, these lesions may occur with a more diffuse neurologic complaint without significant localizing neurologic signs.

Often the neurologic signs associated with disc disease vary over time. If the patient has been up and walking for a period of time, the neurologic findings may be much more pronounced than if he or she has been at bed rest for several days, decreasing the pressure on the nerve root and allowing the nerve to resume its normal function. In addition, various conservative treatments can change the physical signs of disc disease.

Comparative bilateral examination of a patient with back and leg pain is essential in finding a clear-cut pattern of signs and symptoms. The evaluation commonly may change. Adverse changes in the examination may warrant more aggressive therapy, whereas improvement of the symptoms or signs should signal a resolution of the problem. Early symptoms or signs suggesting cauda equina syndrome or severe or progressive neurologic deficit should be treated aggressively from the onset.

DIFFERENTIAL DIAGNOSIS

The differential diagnosis of back and leg pain is extremely lengthy and complex. It includes diseases intrinsic to the spine and diseases involving adjacent organs but causing pain referred to the back or leg. For simplicity, lesions can be categorized as being extrinsic or intrinsic to the spine. Extrinsic lesions include diseases of the urogenital system, gastrointestinal system, vascular system, endocrine system, nervous system not localized to the spine, and extrinsic musculoskeletal

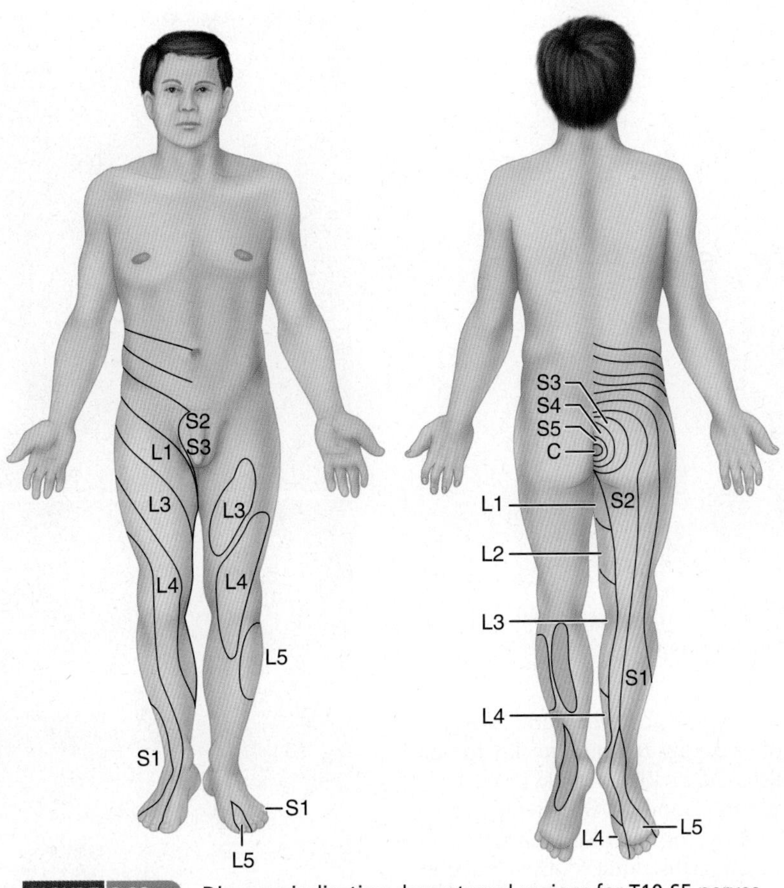

FIGURE 3.22 Diagram indicating dermatomal regions for T10-S5 nerves.

system. These lesions include infections, tumors, metabolic disturbances, congenital abnormalities, and associated diseases of aging. Intrinsic lesions involve diseases that arise primarily in the spine. They include diseases of the spinal musculoskeletal system, the local hematopoietic system, and the local neurologic system. These conditions include trauma, tumors, infections, diseases of aging, and immune diseases affecting the spine or spinal nerves.

Although the predominant cause of back and leg pain in healthy individuals usually is lumbar disc disease, one must be extremely cautious to avoid a misdiagnosis, particularly given the high incidence of disc herniations present in asymptomatic patients as discussed previously. A full physical examination must be completed before making a presumptive diagnosis of herniated disc disease. Common diseases that can mimic disc disease include ankylosing spondylitis, multiple myeloma, vascular insufficiency, arthritis of the hip, osteoporosis with stress fractures, extradural tumors, peripheral neuropathy, and herpes zoster. Infrequent but reported causes of sciatica not related to disc herniation include synovial cysts, rupture of the medial head of the gastrocnemius, sacroiliac joint dysfunction, lesions in the sacrum and pelvis, and fracture of the ischial tuberosity.

CONFIRMATORY IMAGING

Although the diagnosis of a herniated lumbar disc should be suspected from the history and physical examination, imaging studies are necessary to rule out other causes, such as a tumor or infection. Plain radiographs are of limited use in the diagnosis because they do not show disc herniations or other intraspinal lesions, but they can show infection, tumors, or other anomalies and should be obtained, especially if surgery is planned. Currently, the most useful test for diagnosing a herniated lumbar disc is MRI (Figs. 3.23 and 3.24). Since the advent of MRI, myelography is used much less frequently, although in some situations it may help to show subtle lesions. When myelography is used, it should be followed by CT.

NONOPERATIVE TREATMENT

The number and variety of nonoperative therapies for back and leg pain are diverse and overwhelming. Treatments range from simple rest to expensive traction apparatus. All of these therapies are reported with glowing accounts of miraculous "cures"; few have been evaluated scientifically. In addition, the natural history of lumbar disc herniation is characterized by exacerbations and remissions with eventual improvement of extremity complaints in most cases, which can make any intervention appear successful to the patient. Finally, several distinct symptom complexes seem to be associated with disc disease. Few, if any, studies have isolated the response to specific and anatomically distinct diagnoses.

The simplest treatment for acute back pain is rest; generally 2 days of bed rest are better than a longer period. Biomechanical studies indicate that lying in a semi-Fowler position (i.e., on the side with the hips and knees flexed) with a pillow between the legs should relieve most pressure on the disc and nerve roots. Muscle spasm can be controlled by the application of ice, preferably with a massage over the muscles in spasm. Pain relief

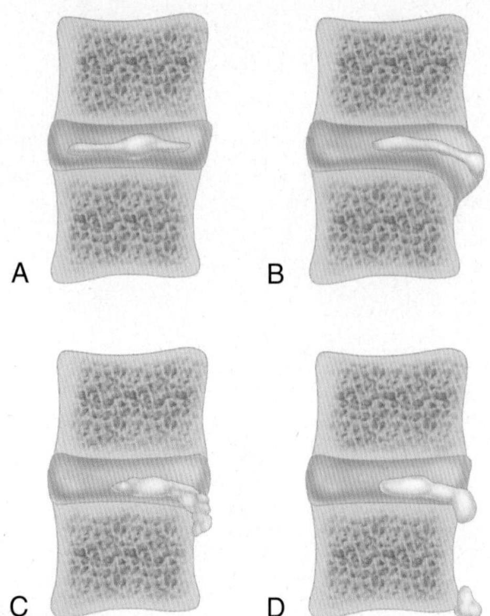

FIGURE 3.23 Types of disc herniation. **A,** Normal bulge. **B,** Protrusion. **C,** Extrusion. **D,** Sequestration.

and antiinflammatory effect can be achieved with NSAIDs. Most acute exacerbations of back pain respond quickly to this therapy. As the pain diminishes, the patient should be encouraged to begin isometric abdominal and lower extremity exercises. Walking within the limits of comfort also is encouraged. Sitting, especially riding in a car, is discouraged. Continuation of ordinary activities within the limits permitted by pain has been shown to lead to a quicker recovery.

Education in proper posture and body mechanics is helpful in returning the patient to the usual level of activity after the acute exacerbation has improved. This education can take many forms, from individual instruction to group instruction. Back education of this type is now usually referred to as "back school." Although the concept is excellent, the quality and quantity of information provided may vary widely. The work of Bergquist-Ullman and Larsson and others indicates that patient education of this type is extremely beneficial in decreasing the amount of time lost from work initially but does little to decrease the incidence of recurrence of symptoms or length of time lost from work during recurrences. The combination of back education and combined physical therapy is superior to placebo treatment. Physical therapy can help improve activity level and physical function but should be discontinued if it aggravates the radiculopathy.

Numerous medications have been used with various results in subacute and chronic back and leg pain syndromes. The current trend seems to be moving away from the use of strong narcotics and muscle relaxants in the outpatient treatment of these syndromes. This is especially true in the instances of chronic back and leg pain where drug habituation and increased depression are frequent. Oral steroids used briefly can be beneficial as potent antiinflammatory agents. The many types of NSAIDs also are helpful when aspirin is not tolerated or is of little help. Numerous NSAIDs are available for the treatment of low back pain. When depression is prominent, mood elevators such as nortriptyline can be beneficial in reducing sleep disturbance and anxiety without increasing depression. Nortriptyline also decreases the need for narcotic medication.

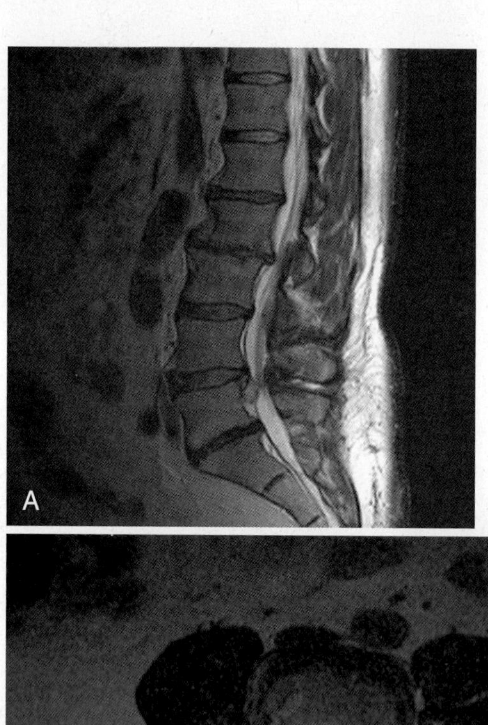

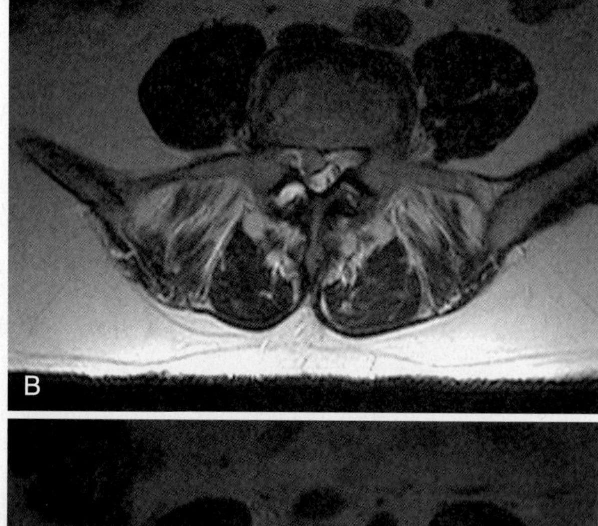

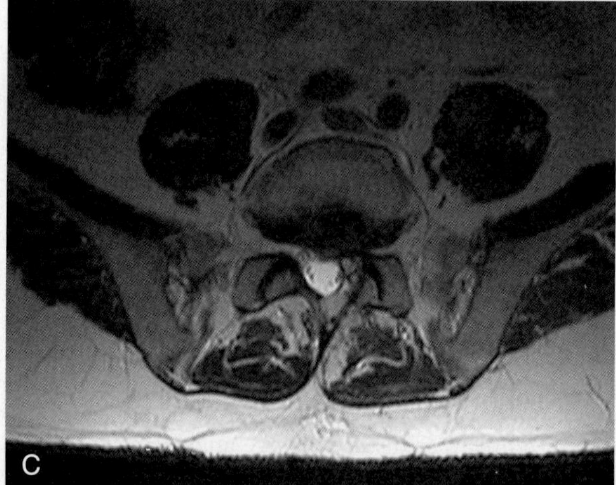

FIGURE 3.24 Sixty-one-year-old patient with right L5 radiculopathy. **A,** T2 sagittal MR image reveals sequestered L4 herniated disc fragment. **B,** T2 axial MR image shows the fragment between L5 pedicles. **C,** This patient also had asymptomatic left L5 disc extrusion.

Physical therapy should be used judiciously. The exercises should be fitted to the symptoms and not forced as an absolute group of activities. Patients with acute back and thigh pain eased by passive extension of the spine in the prone position can benefit from extension exercises rather than flexion exercises. Improvement in symptoms with extension indicates a good prognosis with conservative care. Patients whose pain is increased by passive extension may be improved by flexion exercises. These exercises should not be forced in the face of increased pain. This may avoid further disc extrusion. Any exercise that increases pain should be discontinued. Lower extremity exercises can increase strength and relieve stress on the back, but they also can exacerbate lower extremity arthritis. The true benefit of such treatments may be in the promotion of good posture and body mechanics rather than of strength. Numerous treatment methods have been advanced for the treatment of back pain. Some patients respond to the use of transcutaneous electrical nerve stimulation. Others do well with traction varying from skin traction in bed with 5 to 8 lb to body inversion with forces of more than 100 lb. Back braces or corsets may be helpful to other patients. Ultrasound and diathermy are other treatments used in acute back pain. The scientific efficacy of many of these treatments has not been proved.

As discussed earlier, the natural history of lumbar disc disease generally is favorable. Although low-back pain can result in significant disability, approximately 95% of patients return to their previous employment within 3 months of symptom onset. Failure to return to work within 3 months has been identified as a poor prognostic sign. Longer periods of disability equate to lower probability of returning to work: in patients with total disability lasting a year, the likelihood of returning to work is 21%, and in those with disability lasting 2 years the likelihood is less than 2%. Obesity and smoking have been shown to correlate unfavorably with low back pain and may adversely affect the progression of symptoms.

OPERATIVE TREATMENT

If nonoperative treatment for lumbar disc disease fails, the next consideration is operative treatment. Before this step is taken, the surgeon must be sure of the diagnosis. The patient must be certain that the degree of pain and impairment warrants such a step. The surgeon and the patient must realize that disc surgery is not a cure but may provide symptomatic relief. It neither stops the pathologic processes that allowed the herniation to occur nor restores the disc to a normal state. The patient still must practice good posture and body mechanics after surgery. Activities involving repetitive bending, twisting, and lifting with the spine in flexion may have to be curtailed or eliminated. If prolonged relief is to be expected, some permanent modification in the patient's lifestyle may be necessary, although often no specific limitations are applied.

The key to good results in disc surgery is appropriate patient selection. The optimal patient is one with predominant (if not only) unilateral leg pain extending below the knee that has been present for at least 6 weeks. The pain should have been decreased by rest, antiinflammatory medication, or even epidural steroids but should have returned to the initial levels after a minimum of 6 to 8 weeks of conservative care. Physical examination should reveal signs of sciatic irritation and possibly objective evidence of localizing neurologic impairment. CT, lumbar MRI, or myelography should confirm the level of involvement consistent with the patient's examination.

Operative disc removal is mandatory and urgent only in patients with cauda equina syndrome; other disc excisions should be considered elective. The elective status of surgery should allow a thorough evaluation to confirm the diagnosis, level of involvement, and physical and psychologic status of the patient. Frequently, if there is a rush to the operating room to relieve pain without proper investigation, the patient and the physician later regret the decision.

Regardless of the method chosen to treat a disc rupture surgically, the patient should be aware that the procedure is predominantly for the symptomatic relief of leg pain. Patients with predominantly back pain may not experience relief.

■ MICRODISCECTOMY

Most disc surgery is performed with the patient under general endotracheal anesthesia, although local anesthesia has been used with minimal complications. Patient positioning varies with the operative technique and surgeon. To position the patient in a modified kneeling position, a specialized frame or custom frame is popular. Positioning the patient in this manner allows the abdomen to hang free, minimizing epidural venous dilation and bleeding (Fig. 3.25). A headlamp allows the surgeon to direct light into the lateral recesses where a large proportion of the surgery may be required. The addition of loupe magnification also greatly improves the identification and exposure of various structures. Most surgeons also use an operative microscope to improve visibility further. The primary benefit of an operating microscope compared with loupes is the narrowed interocular distance while maintaining binocular vision and the view afforded the assistant. Radiographic confirmation of the proper level is necessary. Care should be taken to protect neural structures. Epidural bleeding should be controlled with bipolar electrocautery. Any sponge, pack, or cottonoid patty placed in the wound should extend to the outside. Pituitary rongeurs should be marked at a point equal to the maximal allowable disc depth to prevent injury of viscera or great vessels.

MICROSCOPIC LUMBAR DISC EXCISION

Microscopic lumbar disc excision has replaced the standard open laminectomy as the procedure of choice for herniated lumbar disc. This procedure can be done on an outpatient basis and allows better lighting, magnification, and angle of view with a much smaller exposure. Because of the limited dissection required, there is less postoperative pain and a shorter postoperative stay.

Microscopic lumbar discectomy requires an operating microscope with a 400-mm lens, a variety of small-angled Kerrison rongeurs of appropriate length, microinstruments, and preferably a combination suction/nerve root retractor. The procedure is performed with the patient prone. A specialized frame (see Fig. 3.25) previously described can be used, or the patient can be positioned on chest rolls. There are several advantages to using a specialized table, such as an Andrews table: (1) it allows the belly to hang free where venous blood will pool, which results in decreased venous epidural bleeding intraoperatively; (2) the knee-chest position maximizes the lumbar kyphosis, placing the ligamentum flavum on slight tension that allows for easier removal but also opens the interlaminar space, which may provide greater canal access with less bone removal; and (3) the small footprint of the bed enables the operating microscope to be placed at the foot, which not only makes access to the ocular lens easier for both the surgeon and assistant standing on opposite sides of the table but also allows the fluoroscope to be moved into the surgical field for imaging without having to move the microscope base itself.

The microscope can be used from skin incision to closure. The initial dissection can be done under direct vision,

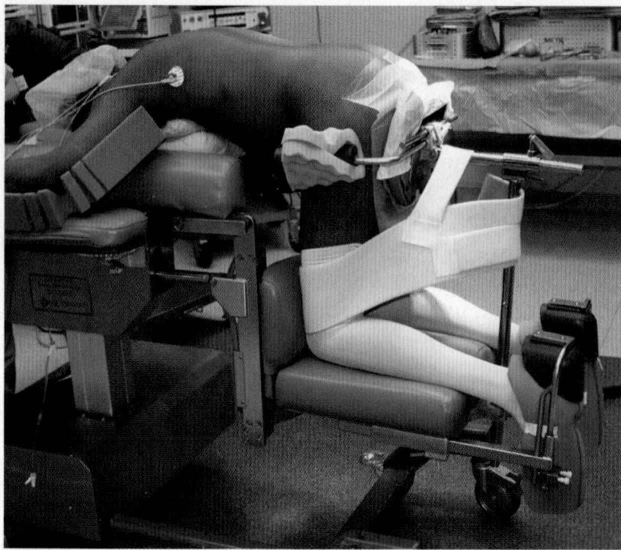

FIGURE 3.25 Knee-chest position for lumbar disc excision allows abdomen to be completely free of external pressure.

however. A lateral radiograph is taken to confirm the level, but fluoroscopy is much quicker when used for localization. Fluoroscopy is essential for localization when using tubular retractors because the field of view is smaller, making the available margin for error in placing the skin incision less.

TUBULAR TECHNIQUES

Tubular techniques have been developed with the purported advantage of shortened hospital stay, faster return to activity, and fewer wound issues. These techniques generally are variations of the microdiscectomy technique using a tubular retractor rather than the McCulloch and different types of bayoneted instruments. This remains another alternative technique. The basic principles remain the same as with microdiscectomy. The less-invasive tubular retractors have been used in a transmuscular fashion, allowing disc excision with less soft-tissue damage because of the more precise exposure; however, better objective clinical results have not been shown with this technique.

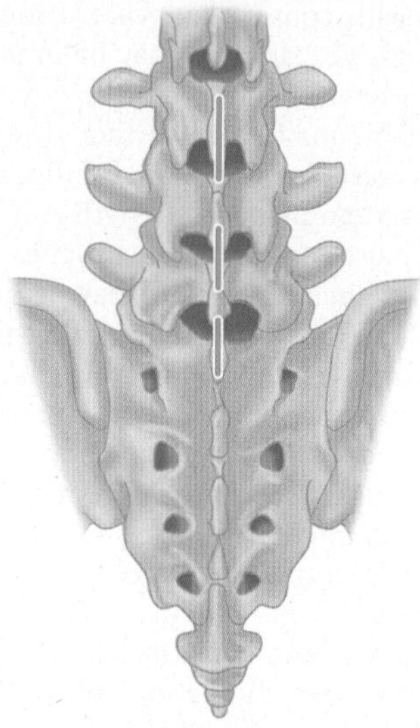

FIGURE 3.26 Incision for microscopic lumbar disc excision. (From Gardocki RG: Microscopic lumbar discectomy. In Canale ST, Beaty JH, Azar FM, editors: *Campbell's core procedures*, Philadelphia, Elsevier, 2016.) **SEE TECHNIQUE 3.16.**

MICROSCOPIC LUMBAR DISCECTOMY

TECHNIQUE 3.16

APPROACH FOR USE OF MCCULLOCH RETRACTOR

- Infiltrate the operative field (paraspinous muscle, subcutaneous tissue, and skin) with 10 mL of 0.25% bupivacaine with epinephrine for preemptive analgesia and hemostasis.
- Make the incision from the midspinous process of the upper vertebra to the superior margin of the spinous process of the lower vertebra at the involved level. This usually results in a 1-inch (25- to 30-mm) skin incision. This incision may need to be moved slightly higher for higher lumbar levels (Fig. 3.26).
- Maintain meticulous hemostasis with electrocautery as the dissection is carried to the fascia.
- Incise the fascia at the midline using electrocautery. Insert a periosteal elevator in the midline incision. Using gentle lateral movements, elevate the deep fascia and muscle subperiosteally from the spinous processes and lamina on the involved side only.
- Obtain a lateral radiograph with a metal clamp attached to the spinous process to verify the level.
- With a Cobb elevator, gently sweep the remaining muscular attachments off in a lateral direction to expose the interlaminar space and the edge of each lamina. A sharp elevator makes this task easier. Meticulously cauterize all bleeding points.
- Insert the appropriate length McCulloch-type retractor into the wound with the shorter spike medial and the flat blade lateral and adjust the microscope. Shaving down the flat blades of the retractor to produce a narrower retractor can help minimize the incision size and collateral soft-tissue damage but increase pressure on soft tissues at the edge of the blades.

APPROACH FOR USE OF TUBULAR RETRACTOR

- Alternatively, the approach can be made using a tubular retractor, which further minimizes damage to the paraspinal muscles and prevents detachment of the lumbodorsal fascia from the supraspinous ligament. A curved drill is required for visualization when drilling bone through the tubular retractor because of the narrower operating corridor.
- With fluoroscopic guidance, place an 18-gauge needle through the skin and into the paraspinous muscles with a trajectory toward the target disc space, approximately the radius of the final retractor diameter away from the edge of the spinous process (e.g., 8 mm off the edge of the spinous process if the ultimate tubular retractor diameter will be 16 mm) to prevent conflict between the spinous process and tubular retractor. It is essential that the needle be orthogonal with the target disc because it

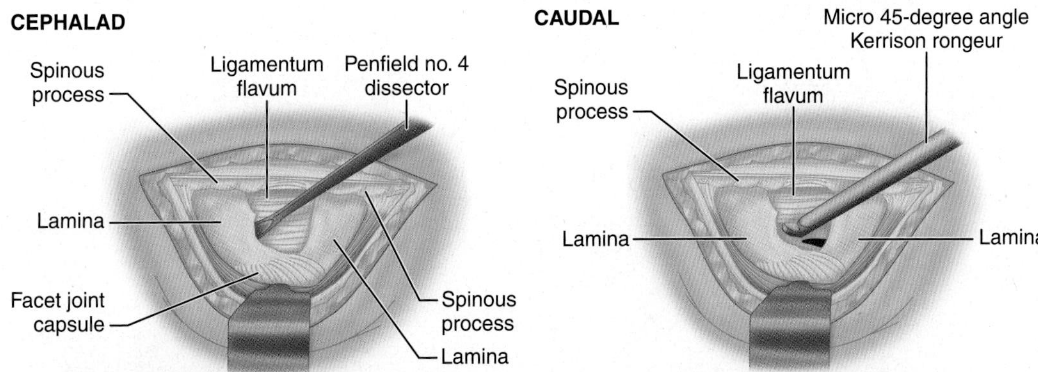

FIGURE 3.27 **Entrance to epidural space by detachment of ligamentum flavum.** (From Gardocki RG: Microscopic lumbar discectomy. In Canale ST, Beaty JH, Azar FM, editors: *Campbell's Core procedures,* Philadelphia, Elsevier, 2016.) **SEE TECHNIQUE 3.16.**

will be used to define the center of the tubular approach. Typically it is best to place the needle in line with the superior endplate of the caudal vertebral body, but that depends on the type of herniation and its location.

- Infiltrate the operative field (paraspinous muscle, subcutaneous tissue, and skin) with 10 mL of 0.25% bupivacaine with epinephrine for preemptive analgesia and hemostasis.
- Make a 20-mm long incision centered on the needle stick and place the blunt end of the guidewire just through the lumbodorsal fascia. The younger and more fit the patient, the more force necessary to pop the blunt end of the guidewire through the fascia. Do not use the sharp end of the guidewire or advance the guidewire down to bone because it is very easy to pierce the interlaminar space and dural sac with the guidewire.
- Once the guidewire is through the fascia, advance the first pencil-shaped dilator through the fascia over the guidewire and use it to gently probe for the trailing edge of the cephalad lamina, which should feel like a bump at the end of the dilator. The guidewire can be removed as soon as the lumbodorsal fascia is pierced with the first dilator.
- Sequentially dilate down to bone with enlarging tubular retractors to expose the interlaminar space. Each dilator can be used as a curet to remove soft-tissue attachments from the interlaminar space.
- Mount the final tubular retractor to a stationary arm attached to the table and obtain a final fluoroscopic image to confirm the location of the retractor orthogonal with the target disc space before bringing in the microscope and adjusting the field of view. We prefer 14- to 16-mm diameter tubular retractors for this approach, depending on the size of the patient and the level of surgical experience with this technique. Tubular retractors in the 18- to 24-mm diameter range can be used when first becoming familiar with this approach. From this point on, the surgical technique is essentially the same for both approaches.
- Identify the ligamentum flavum and lamina. Use a curet to elevate the superficial leaf of the ligamentum flavum from the leading edge of the caudal lamina.
- Use a Kerrison rongeur to resect the superficial leaf of the ligamentum flavum to allow identification of the critical angle, which is junction of the leading edge of the caudal lamina and the medial edge of the superior articular process. Identifying the critical angle is essential in primary microlumbar discectomy because it has a constant relationship to the corresponding pedicle, traversing nerve root, and target disc. The pedicle is always just lateral to the critical angle, the traversing nerve is always just medial to the pedicle, and the disc of interest is always just cephalad to the critical angle and pedicle. It sometimes is necessary to drill the medial aspect of the inferior articular process to allow adequate visualization of the critical angle.
- Use a high-speed drill to remove the trailing edge of the cephalad lamina up to the insertion of the ligamentum flavum to allow easier and more complete removal of the ligament, keeping in mind that the ligament attaches to the lamina as you move medially. This makes initially detaching the ligament from the undersurface of the cephalad lamina with an angled curet much easier toward the midline.
- After the lateral portion of the ligamentum flavum has been detached from the caudal edge of the superior lamina and the cephalad edge of the inferior lamina with a curet, use a blunt dissector to lift the edge of the ligamentum flavum so that it can be excised with a Kerrison rongeur. Take care to orient the rongeur parallel to the nerve root as much as possible. The goal when resecting the ligamentum flavum should be removal in one piece, which prevents nibbling away at it while trying to grab and mop end with the rongeur. En bloc removal is made easier by using the rongeur to remove some bone along with the lateral edge of the ligamentum flavum from caudal to cephalad, starting at the critical angle and working up the medial edge of the superior articular process where the ligamentum flavum attaches (Fig. 3.27).
- Once the ligamentum flavum is removed, the medial wall of the corresponding pedicle should be palpable with a nerve hook or angled dissector. If not, more bone may need to be removed lateral to the critical angle. Once the medial wall of the corresponding pedicle is identified, the traversing nerve can be found just medial to it and the target disc can be found just cephalad to it.

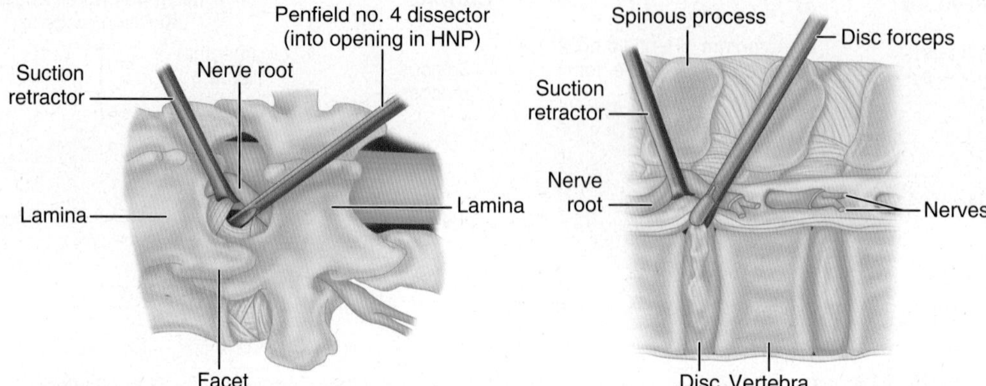

FIGURE 3.28 **Dilation of annular defect to facilitate disc fragment removal.** (From Gardocki RG: Microscopic lumbar discectomy. HNP, herniated nucleus pulposus. In Canale ST, Beaty JH, Azar FM, editors: *Campbell's core procedures*, Philadelphia, Elsevier, 2016.) **SEE TECHNIQUE 3.16.**

- When the nerve root is identified, carefully mobilize the root medially. Gently dissect the nerve free from the disc fragment to avoid excessive traction on the root. Bipolar cautery for hemostasis is helpful. When mobilized, retract the root medially. If the root is difficult to mobilize, consider that a conjoined root may be present.
- Make a gentle extradural exploration beneath the nerve with a 90-degree blunt hook, taking care not to tear the dura. The small opening and magnification can make the edge of the dural sac appear to be the nerve root.
- When using bipolar cautery, ensure that only one side is in contact with the nerve root to avoid thermal injury to the nerve. Epidural fat is not removed in this procedure.
- Insert the suction/nerve root retractor with its tip turned medially under the nerve root and hold the manifold between the thumb and index finger. With the nerve root retracted, the disc is now visible as a white, fibrous, avascular structure. Under magnification, small tears may be visible in the annulus.
- Enlarge the annular tear with a Penfield no. 4 dissector and remove the disc material with the appropriate-sized pituitary rongeur. Do not insert the instrument into the disc space beyond the angle of the jaws, usually about 15 mm, to minimize the risk of anterior perforation and vascular injury. Downward pressure on the adjacent intact annulus can sometimes help express loose disc fragments from the subannular space (Fig. 3.28).
- Remove the exposed disc material. Remove additional loose disc or cartilage fragments. Inspect the root and adjacent dura for disc fragments. Forcefully irrigate the disc space using a Luer-Lok syringe and an unused no. 8 suction tip inserted into the disc space. Maintain meticulous hemostasis.
- The discectomy is complete when (1) the lateral recess is adequately decompressed; (2) the 90-degree dissection can be probed to the back of the cephalad vertebral body, the disc space, and the back of the caudal vertebral body out to the midline without any protrusions into the canal; (3) the 90-degree dissector can be spun (helicopter maneuver) beneath the traversing nerve root without any restrictions; and (4) the traversing nerve root is freely retractable both medially and laterally. It is comforting to see the dura pulsate with the heartbeat and expand and contract with respiration, but these findings alone do not indicate an adequate discectomy and decompression.
- If the expected pathologic process is not found, review preoperative imaging studies for the correct level and side. Also obtain a repeat radiograph or fluoroscopic image with a metallic marker at the disc level to verify the level. Be aware of bony anomalies that may alter the numbering of the vertebrae on imaging studies.
- Close the fascia and the skin in the usual fashion using absorbable sutures if using the McCulloch retractor. When using a tubular retraction, it can simply be removed and the skin closed subcutaneously because the lumbodorsal fascia will seal itself like Chinese finger cuffs when the paraspinous muscles contract, because the lumbodorsal fascia was only dilated between its fibers and not incised.

POSTOPERATIVE CARE Postoperative care is similar to that after standard open disc surgery. Typically this procedure is done on an outpatient basis. Injecting the paraspinal muscles on the involved side with bupivacaine 0.25% with epinephrine at the beginning of the procedure and additional bupivacaine at the conclusion aids patient mobilization immediately postoperatively. We prefer to use a skin glue product for final skin closure without the use of dressing and allow the patient to shower the day of surgery. Activity can be allowed as tolerated once the skin incision is healed.

ENDOSCOPIC TECHNIQUES

TRANSFORAMINAL AND INTERLAMINAR ENDOSCOPIC LUMBAR DISCECTOMY

A combination of transforaminal and interlaminar endoscopic approaches to the lumbar spine allows access to any disc herniation from L1 to S1 without significant bone resection while maintaining direct light-based visualization of the anatomy and pathology. Iatrogenic instability is minimized because the zygapophyseal joint is not violated. These approaches can be used with the patient prone or in the lateral decubitus position and without the need for general anesthesia. The transforaminal approach requires a uniportal technique with a single working channel within the endoscope, while the interlaminar technique can be performed with uniportal or biportal approaches. One study has shown lower levels of C-reactive protein and interleukin 6 in the postoperative period after endoscopic lumbar discectomy when compared to traditional microdiscectomy, confirming the less invasive nature of the endoscopic technique. With endoscopic lumbar discectomy, the underlying degenerative pathology is what limits recovery, not the surgical approach.

TRANSFORAMINAL ENDOSCOPIC LUMBAR DISCECTOMY

TECHNIQUE 3.17

- This technique can be used for any herniation that is central, posterolateral, foraminal, or extraforaminal from L1-L4 and sometimes at L5-S1 if anatomy allows.
- We prefer patients in the prone position for uniformity of room setup and orientation of anatomy, but this can be done with the patient in the lateral decubitus position with the affected side up, which allows intraoperative straight-leg-raise testing.
- Use monitored anesthesia care with intermittent doses of propofol for painful portions of the procedure. The patient should be able to respond to questions and communicate throughout most of the procedure.
- The angulation of the approach depends on the offending pathology. It is critical that the pathology be targeted with the angle of approach.
- Place a diagnostic transforaminal epidural injection into Kambin's triangle at the site of the herniation to confirm the diagnosis and the space available in the foramen for the endoscopic approach. If the patient gets profound relief from the transforaminal epidural, it is a good predictor of surgical outcome, and endoscopic surgery can be planned if the pain from the lumbar disc herniation returns.
- Plan the approach to the appropriate foramen on preoperative imaging.
- Place the patient prone on a radiolucent table.
- Advance an 18- to 20-gauge needle into the foramen obliquely at the level of the herniation based on the preoperative imaging plan.
- Place a guidewire through the needle and remove the needle.
- Anesthetize the skin, subcutaneous tissue, and lumbar fascia with 10 mL of 1% lidocaine with epinephrine and use a no. 11 blade to make a 1-cm incision.
- Place dilators over the guidewire and advance them into the foramen under fluoroscopic guidance.
- Some systems allow reaming of the foramen with percutaneous reamers under fluoroscopic guidance. Alternatively, the operative cannula can be advanced into the foramen and the foramen opened with a diamond burr under direct light-based endoscopic visualization for surgeons who are more comfortable with bone resection under direct visualization (author's preferred technique). Enough room must be created in the foramen for the working cannula to pass through the full excursion required by the herniation.
- Adjust fluid pressure and flow through the endoscope by the fluid pump to control epidural bleeding, but not to exceed diastolic blood pressure.
- After the bony anatomy of the arch formed by the inferior pedicle and superior articular process is visualized (Wagner arch), identify the herniation.
- Use instruments to remove disc material from under the nerve root using direct light-based visualization through the endoscope; probes can be used to feel for central fragments ventral to the dura.
- Decompression is complete once the affected nerve root is seen pulsating to heartbeat without deformity and the patient notes resolution of the typical radicular pain.
- Suction excess fluid from the wound and infiltrate the epidural space with 1 mL of steroid and 2 mL 0.25% Marcaine.
- Remove the operative cannula, close the skin with a single subcuticular stitch, and close the wound with a dab of skin glue.
- Ask the patient to transfer himself or herself to the gurney.

POSTOPERATIVE CARE The patient is limited in bending, lifting, and twisting but may shower the day of the procedure. Patients typically are discharged from the surgery center as soon as they can ambulate independently and empty their bladder. Driving is delayed until postoperative day 2 or until narcotics are discontinued, but this procedure typically is done with only NSAIDS for postoperative pain control. Patients are allowed to begin a trunk stabilization therapy program and advance to activities as tolerated 2 weeks after surgery.

INTERLAMINAR ENDOSCOPIC LUMBAR DISCECTOMY

This technique typically is used for posterolateral herniations at L5-S1 but can be used at higher levels if the interlaminar window is wide enough to accommodate the operative cannula. This is the facet-sparing technique used when there is no need for lateral recess decompression.

TECHNIQUE 3.18

- Place the patient prone on the operating room table. Because of our anesthesiologist's preference, we perform this procedure with the patient under general anesthesia on an open-top frame (abdomen hanging free), but it can be done under monitored anesthesia care with local anesthetic.
- Mark the laminae, medial pedicular line, and midline on the skin with fluoroscopy to aid in placing the incision targeting the pathology.
- Place an 18-gauge needle to the trailing edge of the L5 lamina at the desired trajectory based on preoperative

imaging plans. Use a more medial-to-lateral approach for more lateral herniations and a more lateral-to-medial approach for more central herniations.

- Inject 8 mL of 1% lidocaine with epinephrine at the trailing edge of the L5 lamina to allow easier dissection of the soft tissue overlying the ligamentum flavum.
- Make a 1-cm incision with a no. 11 blade at the needle insertion site.
- Place a guidewire through the needle and remove the needle, taking great care not to puncture the ligamentum flavum.
- Advance dilators over the wire and dock them on the trailing edge of the L5 lamina.
- Dock the working cannula on the trailing edge of the L5 lamina and remove the dilators.
- A 15-degree or 30-degree scope can be used based on surgeon preference, but the cannula should be no larger than 8 mm to prevent undue tension on the nerve root while retracting.
- Clear soft tissue off the trailing edge of the L5 lamina and superficial ligamentum flavum.
- Use an endoscopic punch to fenestrate the ligamentum flavum just medial to the superior articular process of S1. Do not violate the L5-S1 facet joint. The fenestration in the ligamentum needs to be only 3 to 4 mm in length. The tang on the operative cannula can be used to stretch the pliable ligamentum and advance the cannula into the spinal canal.
- Use a pituitary rongeur to carefully remove epidural fat and the Hoffman epidural ligaments.
- Turn the tang of the cannula laterally and advance it into the canal lateral to traversing S1 nerve root for a posterolateral herniation. Advance it to the floor of the canal in the axilla of the S1 nerve root between the root and dural sac in the case of an axillary herniation.
- Once the tang on the working cannula is docked on the floor of the canal or the disc herniation, release the ventral Trolard epidural ligaments with a pituitary rongeur to allow retraction of the affected nerve root with the tang of the cannula.
- With the root retracted behind the tang of the working cannula, there is a safe working zone to remove the disc herniation within the working cannula.
- Once the disc is decompressed, the nerve should be freely retractable medially and laterally; it should be round and plump, the dura should pulsate to heartbeat, and there should be no protrusions into the canal when probing under the root and dural sac to the midline.
- Suction excess fluid from the wound and infiltrate the epidural space with 1 mL of steroid and 2 mL of 0.25% Marcaine.
- Remove the operative cannula, close the skin with a single subcuticular stitch, and close the wound with a dab of skin glue.

POSTOPERATIVE CARE The patient is limited in bending, lifting, and twisting but may shower the day of the procedure. Patients typically are discharged from the surgery center as soon as they can ambulate independently and empty their bladder. Driving is delayed until postoperative day 2 or until narcotics are discontinued, but this procedure typically is done with only NSAIDS for postoperative pain control. Patients are allowed to begin a trunk stabilization therapy program and advance to activities as tolerated 2 weeks postoperatively.

ADDITIONAL EXPOSURE TECHNIQUES

A large disc herniation or other pathologic condition, such as lateral recess stenosis or foraminal stenosis, may require a greater exposure of the nerve root. The additional pathologic condition usually can be identified before surgery. If the extent of the lesion is known before surgery, the proper approach can be planned. Additional exposure includes hemilaminectomy, total laminectomy, and facetectomy. Hemilaminectomy usually is required when identifying the root as a problem. This may occur with a conjoined root. Total laminectomy usually is reserved for patients with spinal stenoses that are central, which occur typically in cauda equina syndrome. Facetectomy usually is reserved for foraminal stenosis or severe lateral recess stenosis. If more than one facet is removed, a fusion should be considered in addition. This is especially true in the removal of facets and the disc at the same interspace in a young, active individual with a normal disc height at that level.

Rarely, disc herniation has been reported to be intradural. An extremely large disc that cannot be dissected from the dura or the persistence of an intradural mass after dissection of the disc should alert one to this potential problem. Excision of an intradural disc may require a transdural approach, which increases the risk of complications from CSF leak and intradural scarring.

A disc that is far lateral may require exposure outside the spinal canal (Fig. 3.29). This area is approached by removing the intertransverse ligament between the superior and inferior transverse processes lateral to the spinal canal. The disc hernia usually is anterior to the nerve root that is found in a mass of fat below the intertransverse ligament. A microsurgical approach is a good method for dealing with this problem. A long tubular retractor is especially useful for the far lateral approach if the tube is inserted at the proper

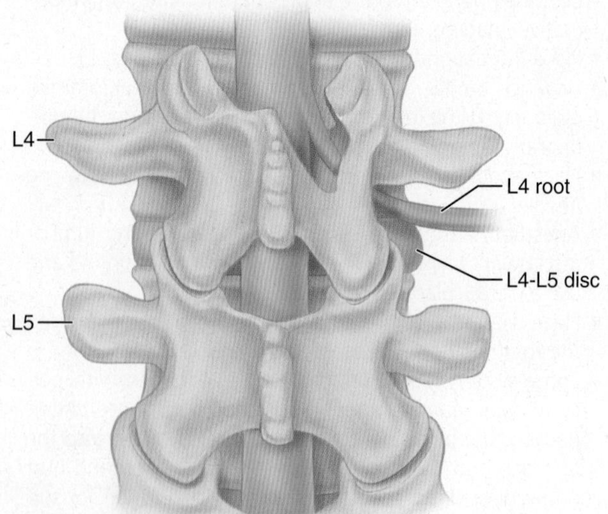

FIGURE 3.29 Lateral approach for discectomy. L4 foraminotomy allows exposure of root.

trajectory to treat pathology in or lateral to the foramen. If the facet is not hypertrophic and the plane between the facet joint capsule and intertransverse ligament can be identified, foraminal and far lateral disc herniations can sometimes be removed without bony resection above the L5 level. The least invasive approach to a far lateral lumbar disc herniation is a transforaminal endoscopic approach with a slightly steeper angle than would be used for pathology inside the spinal canal. This minimizes bleeding and eliminates the need for bony resection but is a more advanced endoscopic technique because of the lack of bony anatomy in the extraforaminal zone.

LUMBAR ROOT ANOMALIES

Several different types of nerve root anomalies are relatively common in anatomic studies but less common with imaging studies, which suggest they are underrecognized clinically. These congenital anomalies may account for a portion of the poor results from lumbar disc surgery because the abnormal and unrecognized roots may be injured. This is of even more concern with some minimally invasive techniques with less direct nerve visualization.

Conjoined nerve roots are the most common type of anomaly. Various anatomic studies show some type of conjoined root in 14% to 17% of cadavers. Clinical studies using advanced imaging, such as myelography or MRI, show conjoined roots in only 2% to 5% of patients. Conjoined roots have been classified anatomically (Figs. 3.30 to 3.33). There are three classes, the first two of which are subdivided. Type 1 occurs when two roots exit the dura with one common sheath. With type 1A anomalies, the cephalad root departs the conjoined stalk at an acute angle to exit below the appropriate pedicle, and the caudal root travels within the canal to exit also below the appropriate pedicle. If the cephalad root exits at 90 degrees from the conjoined portion, this is a type 1B anomaly. Type 2 anomalies occur when two roots exit through a single foramen. Type 2A anomalies have one vacant foramen; type 2B anomalies have a portion of one of the roots exiting via the other foramen, which may be cephalad to the foramen occupied by the two nerve roots. Type 3 anomalies occur when there is an anastomosing branch between two adjacent nerve roots. This branch crosses the disc space and can easily be injured during discectomy.

These root anomalies can cause false-positive interpretations of imaging studies and can be confused with disc bulges or herniations. Particularly if the herniation appears in an atypical location, such as near the pedicle, or if the signal intensity is different from disc material, a diagnosis of a conjoined root should be considered. Also, if a patient presents with a history of failed disc surgery, this diagnosis should be considered. The anomalous roots not only can be divided inadvertently but also can be injured by excessive tension because the conjoined roots usually are less mobile than normal roots. The most common location for conjoined roots involves the L5 and S1 levels. A second type of anomaly that may be as common as conjoined roots is a furcal nerve root (Fig. 3.32); this refers to a bifurcation of a single nerve root. Often furcal roots are bilateral and can occur at multiple levels. Increased awareness of these anomalies is important to reduce the risk of nerve injury and to avoid surgery with an incorrect diagnosis of disc herniations. Surgical outcomes in patients with conjoined roots tend to be significantly worse than in the general population.

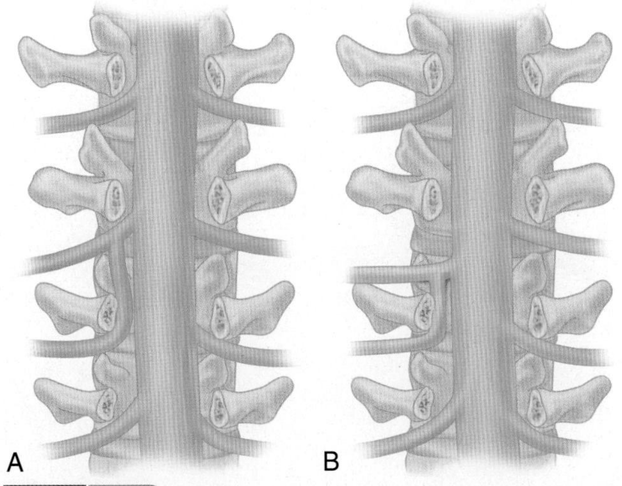

FIGURE 3.30 **A,** Type 1A conjoined nerve root. **B,** Type 1B conjoined nerve root.

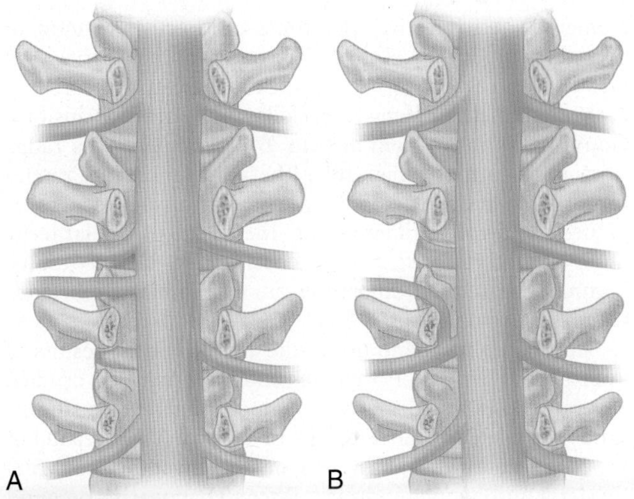

FIGURE 3.31 **A,** Type 2A conjoined nerve root. **B,** Type 2B conjoined nerve root.

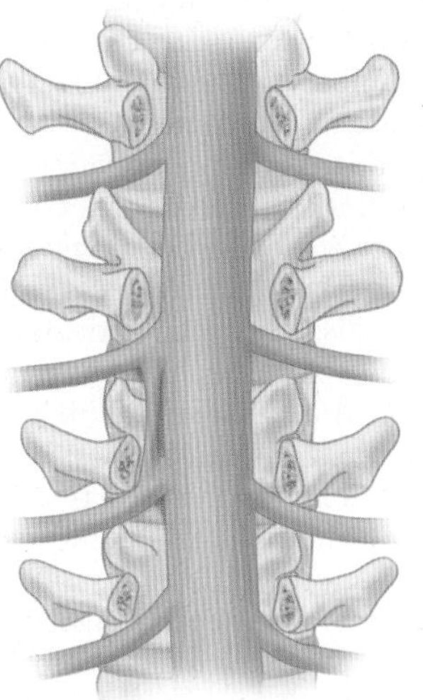

FIGURE 3.32 Type 3 conjoined nerve root.

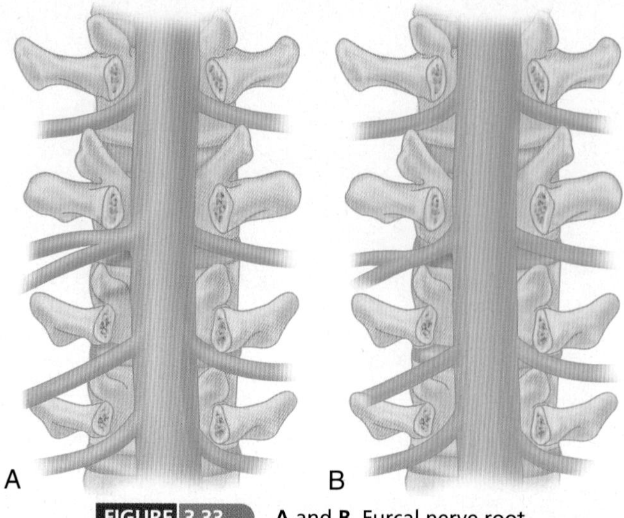

FIGURE 3.33 A and B, Furcal nerve root.

RESULTS OF SURGERY FOR DISC HERNIATION

Numerous retrospective and some prospective reviews of open disc surgery are available. The results of these series vary greatly with respect to patient selection, treatment method, evaluation method, length of follow-up, and conclusions. Good results range from 46% to 97%. Complications range from none to more than 10%. The reoperation rate ranges from 4% to more than 20%. A comparison between techniques also reveals similar results. There is no particular technique of discectomy that yields consistently superior results. Technical procedural differences are of minimal importance with regard to outcome.

Several points stand out in the analysis of the results of lumbar disc surgery. Patient selection seems to be crucial. Several studies noted that a low educational level is significantly correlated to poor results of surgery. Valid results of the Minnesota Multiphasic Personality Inventory (MMPI) (hysteria and hypochondriasis T-scores) appear to be good indicators of surgical outcome regardless of the degree of the pathologic condition. The duration of the current episode, the age of the patient, the presence or absence of predominant back pain, the number of previous hospitalizations, and the presence or absence of compensation for a work injury have been identified as factors affecting final outcome. In the latest report on lumbar disc herniation (2008) from the multicenter Spine Patient Outcomes Research Trial (SPORT), operative was compared with nonoperative treatment in 501 patients and additional observational cohorts (743 participants). The results were overwhelmingly in favor of surgery: patients treated operatively had far less pain, better physical function, and less disability than patients who did not have surgery. The validity of the conclusions generated by SPORT has been questioned because of the high crossover rates in the randomized intent-to-treat studies and the variability of the patient population, nonoperative treatments, and operative procedures. The finding of durability of operative results (4-year follow-up), however, is important. In a later study of patients with degenerative spondylolisthesis and spinal stenosis who had operative treatment, those with predominant leg pain had a better prognosis than those with predominant back pain.

TABLE 3.2

Complications of Lumbar Disc Surgery

COMPLICATION	INCIDENCE (%)
Cauda equina syndrome	0.2
Thrombophlebitis	1
Pulmonary embolism	0.4
Wound infection	2.2
Pyogenic spondylitis	0.07
Postoperative discitis	2 (1122 patients)
Dural tears	1.6
Nerve root injury	0.5
Cerebrospinal fluid fistula	*
Laceration of abdominal vessels	*
Injury to abdominal viscera	*

*Rare occurrence (nos. 10 and 11 not identified in Spangfort's study, but reported elsewhere).
Modified from Spangfort EV: The lumbar disc herniation: a computer-aided analysis of 2504 operations, *Acta Orthop Scand Suppl* 142:1–99, 1972.

COMPLICATIONS OF DISC EXCISION

The complications associated with standard disc excision and micro lumbar disc excision are similar. One large series (Table 3.2) of 2503 open disc excisions listed a postoperative mortality of 0.1%, a thromboembolism rate of 1%, a postoperative infection rate of 3.2%, and a deep disc space infection rate of 1.1%. Postoperative cauda equina lesions developed in five patients. Laceration of the major vascular structures also has been described as a rare complication of this operation. Dural tears with CSF leaks, pseudomeningocele formation, CSF fistula formation, and meningitis also are possible but are more likely after reoperation. The complications of micro lumbar disc excision seem to be less than with standard laminectomy.

In a retrospective review of 1326 patients who had spinal surgery, 51 dural tears (4%) were identified; 48 of these occurred with a posterior thoracolumbar approach. The presence of a dural tear or leak results in the potentially serious problems of pseudomeningocele, CSF leak, and meningitis. Eismont, Wiesel, and Rothman suggested five basic principles in the repair of these leaks (Fig. 3.34):

1. The operative field must be unobstructed, dry, and well exposed.
2. Dural suture of a 4-0 or 6-0 gauge with a tapered or reverse cutting needle is used in a simple or a running locking stitch. If the leak is large or inaccessible, a free fat graft or fascial graft can be sutured to the dura. Fibrin glue applied to the repair also is helpful but used alone does not seal a significant leak.
3. All repairs should be tested by using the reverse Trendelenburg position and Valsalva maneuvers.
4. Paraspinous muscles and overlying fascia should be closed in two layers with nonabsorbable suture used in a watertight fashion. Drains should not be used.
5. Bed rest in the supine position should be maintained for 4 to 7 days after the repair of lumbar dural defects. A lumbar drain should be placed if the integrity of the closure is questionable. The development of headaches on standing and a stormy postoperative period should alert one to the possibility of an undetected CSF leak. This can be confirmed by MRI.

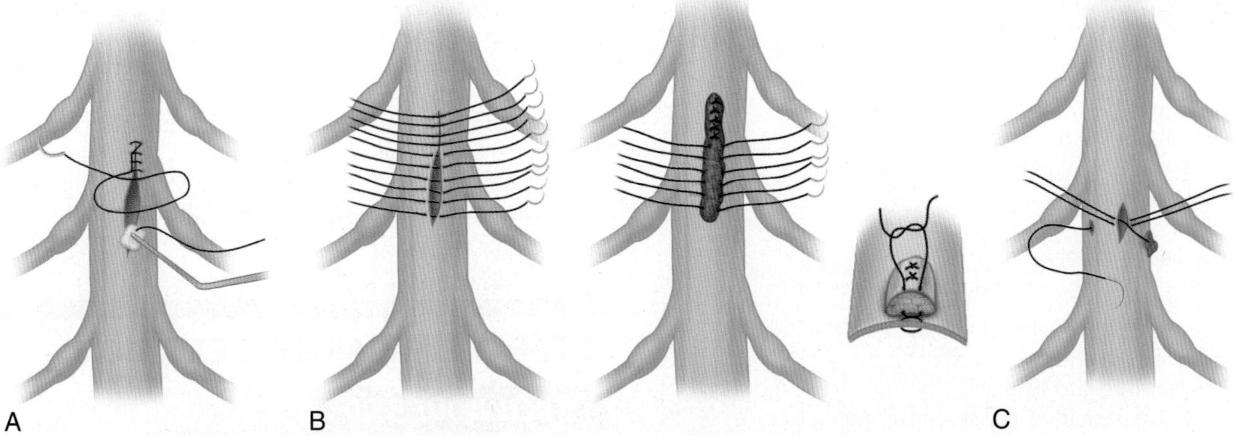

FIGURE 3.34 **A,** Dural repair using running-locking dural suture on taper or reverse-cutting, one-half-circle needle. Smaller-sized suture should be used. Use of suction with sucker and small cotton pledgets is essential to protect nerve roots while operative field is kept dry of cerebrospinal fluid. **B,** Single dural stitches can be used to achieve closure, each suture end being left long. Second needle is attached to free suture end, and ends of suture are passed through piece of muscle or fat, which is tied down over repaired tear to help achieve watertight closure. Whenever dural material is inadequate to allow closure without placing excessive pressure on underlying neural tissues, free graft of fascia or fascia lata or freeze-dried dural graft should be secured to margins of dural tear using simple sutures of appropriate size. **C,** For small dural defects in relatively inaccessible areas, transdural approach can be used to pull small piece of muscle or fat into defect from inside out, sealing cerebrospinal fluid leak. Central durotomy should be large enough to expose defect from dural sac. Durotomy is closed in standard watertight fashion.

The presence of glucose in drainage fluid is an unreliable diagnostic test. Rarely, a pseudomeningocele has been implicated as a cause of persistent pain from pressure on a nerve root by the cystic mass. In our experience, these principles are valid with the exception of maintaining bed rest. With good closure, patients can be mobilized the day after surgery. If closure is not watertight, extended bed rest with a drain may be helpful.

One of the advantages of endoscopic lumbar discectomy and tubular lumbar discectomy with an 18-mm or smaller diameter tube is in the treatment of small dural tears. Because the dead space is so small, these tears usually can be treated simply with fibrin glue when there is no root herniation. We follow the usual postoperative course in patients who have endoscopic or tubular discectomy with dural repair using fibrin glue as long as there are no postoperative headaches or symptoms of meningeal irritation. A 3-day course of acetazolamide (Diamox) is prescribed, which acts as a chemical drain by decreasing CSF production in the choroid plexus by inhibiting carbonic anhydrase. This is the same course of Diamox prescribed for acute mountain (altitude) sickness. Patients are advised to lie flat for 72 hours after surgery only if they have positional headaches. If the spinal headache does not respond, it usually can be immediately resolved with a blood patch.

DURAL REPAIR AUGMENTED WITH FIBRIN GLUE

Dural repair can be augmented with fibrin glue. Pressure testing of a dural repair without fibrin glue reveals that the dura is able to withstand 10 mm of pressure on day 1 and 28 mm on day 7. With fibrin glue, the dura is able to withstand 28 mm on day 1 and 31 mm on day 7. Fibrin glue also can be used in areas of troublesome bleeding or difficult access for closure, such as the ventral aspect of the dura. Fibrin glue is an adjunct for closure, and every effort should be made for primary closure, even if fibrin glue is to be used. However, fibrin glue tends to be sufficient in the setting of a transmuscular approach using a tubular retractor or fully endoscopic technique because the amount of dead space is significantly limited and dural leaks can be tamponaded with fibrin glue alone.

TECHNIQUE 3.19

- Mix 20,000 U of topical thrombin and 10 mL of calcium chloride and draw the mixture up into a syringe.
- In another syringe, draw 5 U of cryoprecipitate, and simultaneously inject equal quantities of each onto the dural repair or tear.
- Allow the glue to set to the consistency of "Jell-O" (Box 3.5). Commercially available kits also are available.

FREE FAT GRAFTING

Fat grafting for the prevention of postoperative epidural scarring has been shown to be superior to Gelfoam in the prevention of postoperative scarring. The current rationale for free fat grafting seems to be the possibility of making any reoperation easier. Neither the benefit of reduced scarring and its relationship to the prevention of postoperative pain nor the increased ease of reoperation in patients in whom fat grafting

BOX 3.5

Fibrin Glue

Ingredients

Two vials of topical thrombin, 10,000 U each
10 mL of calcium chloride
5 U of cryoprecipitate
Two 5-mL syringes
Two 22-gauge spinal needles

Instructions

1. Do not use saline that comes with thrombin.
2. Mix thrombin and calcium chloride.
3. Draw mixture into syringe.
4. Draw cryoprecipitate into second syringe.
5. Apply equal amounts to area of need.
6. Allow to set to a "Jell-O" consistency.

was performed has been established. Caution should be taken in applying a fat graft to a large laminar defect because this has been reported to result in an acute cauda equina syndrome in the early postoperative period. We currently reserve the use of a fat graft (or fascial grafts) for dural repairs and small laminar defects where the graft is supported by the bone. A study by Jensen et al. found that fat grafts decreased dural scarring but not radicular scar formation. The clinical outcome was not improved.

The technique of free fat grafting is straightforward. At the end of the procedure, just before the incision is closed, a large piece of subcutaneous fat is inserted over the laminectomy defect. If the patient is thin, a separate incision over the buttock may be required to obtain sufficient fat to fill the defect.

REPEAT LUMBAR DISC SURGERY

Making the diagnosis of recurrent disc herniation is significantly more difficult than that of primary disc herniation. The clinical presentation may be identical to that of primary herniation but usually has a larger component of axial pain. Most recurrences happen in the relatively early postoperative period, primarily the first 6 months after surgery. To date, no operative technique has been shown to reduce the incidence of recurrent disc herniations, which is reported in 3% to 7% of patients. Specifically, more aggressive disc removal does not reduce this complication and may be detrimental to the function of the motion segment. MRI with intravascular contrast material has been helpful in identifying recurrent herniations. It is difficult, however, to distinguish a peridural scar from a small recurrent herniation. For patients with a history of no or minimal improvement after disc excision, the diagnostic difficulties are even greater. A possible incorrect original diagnosis, incorrect level, root anomaly, root injury, CSF leak, and infection must be considered in addition to recurrent disc herniation.

With regard to surgery for recurrent herniation, the principles of identifying and protecting the nerve root and then removing the herniation are the same as for a primary discectomy. The area of exposure generally should be larger, although usually the procedure still can be done on an outpatient basis.

Treatment of recurrent disc herniation is one of the advantages of the transforaminal endoscopic approach. The technique can be used for recurrence after a traditional microdiscectomy. The surgery is very similar to a primary transforaminal endoscopic approach. If both the primary and recurrence approaches are transforaminal, the total level of invasiveness typically is still less than a primary microscopic approach, since there is no violation of the facet joint.

REPEAT LUMBAR DISC EXCISION

TECHNIQUE 3.20

This procedure is most often used for recurrent herniation but can be used in primary disc excisions.

- After thoroughly preparing the back, identify the spinous processes of L3, L4, L5, and S1 by palpation. Inject 25 mL of 0.25% bupivacaine with epinephrine into the paraspinal muscles on the involved side.
- Make a midline incision 4 cm long, centered over the interspace where the disc herniation is located. Incise the supraspinous ligament; by subperiosteal dissection, strip the muscles from the spinous processes and laminae of these vertebrae on the side of the lesion.
- Retract the muscles with a self-retaining retractor, or with the help of an assistant, and expose one interspace at a time.
- Verify the location with a radiograph so that no mistake is made regarding the interspaces explored.
- Secure hemostasis with electrocautery, bone wax, and packs. Leave a portion of each pack completely outside the wound for ready identification.
- Identify normal tissue first. Use a curet to remove scar from the edges of the laminae carefully. Remove additional bone as necessary to expose normal dura.
- Identify the pedicles superiorly and inferiorly if there is any question of position and status of the root. Carry the dissection from the pedicles to identify each root; this may allow the development of a normal plane between the dura and scar. This requires patience, and small curets or Penfield dissectors work best. Maintain meticulous hemostasis with bipolar cautery.
- Once the lateral edge of the root is identified, it is often helpful to mobilize the root and epidural scar as a single mass off the floor of the canal using a curet, which will sometimes uncover the underlying disc herniation.
- Remove the disc herniation and explore the axilla of the root and the subligamentous space for retained fragments. Also, ensure that the nerve root is well decompressed in the lateral recess.
- Spinal fusion is not done unless an unstable spine is created by the dissection or was identified preoperatively as a correctable and symptomatic problem.
- If the initial procedure was done using the tubular retractor technique (see Technique 3.16), a tubular retractor is used for recurrent disc herniations.

POSTOPERATIVE CARE Postoperative care is the same as after disc excision (see Technique 3.16).

DISC EXCISION AND FUSION

The necessity of lumbar fusion at the same time as disc excision was first suggested by Mixter and Barr. In the first 20 years after their discovery the combination of disc excision and lumbar fusion was common. More recent data comparing disc excision alone with the combination of disc excision and fusion indicate that there is little, if any, advantage to the addition of a spinal fusion to the treatment of simple disc herniation. These studies indicate that spinal fusion increases the complication rate and lengthens recovery. The indications for lumbar fusion should be independent of the indications for disc excision for radiculopathy.

THORACIC AND LUMBAR SPINE ARTHRODESIS

Arthrodesis of the lumbosacral region is done for degenerative, traumatic, and congenital lesions. Indications for and techniques of spinal fusion and care after surgery vary from one orthopaedic center to another. Many orthopaedists prefer posterior arthrodesis, usually some modification of the intertransverse process type fusion, using a large quantity of autogenous iliac bone. Internal fixation can be used with posterior arthrodesis. Before the use of instrumentation, the current status of the implant—its risks and indications and approval by the FDA—should be reviewed carefully and completely with the patient. Posterolateral or intertransverse process fusions are used most frequently, either alone or occasionally in combination with an anterior fusion and with or without posterior internal fixation. Interbody fusions from posterior, anterior, retroperitoneal, or transperitoneal approaches are preferred by other orthopaedic surgeons.

For lumbar fusion, the best technique for a particular patient remains controversial. The decision should be based on the pathologic entity being treated, expected applicable biomechanics and healing potential of different constructs, and the surgeon's experience. With regard to the pathologic entity, consideration must be given to the spinal column and the neural elements. In this way the proper balance can be obtained between the need for possible increased instability from neural decompression and strategies to increase stability to promote fusion. After determining the optimal operative plan for a particular patient, additional controversy exists regarding the best technique to execute the plan, that is, an open technique versus a minimally invasive approach.

ANTERIOR ARTHRODESIS

TRANSTHORACIC APPROACH TO THE THORACIC SPINE

For anterior arthrodesis of the thoracic spine, a transthoracic approach provides direct access to the vertebral bodies T2 to T12. The midthoracic vertebral bodies are best exposed by this approach, whereas views of the upper and lower extremes of the spine are more limited.

TECHNIQUE 3.21

- Approach the involved vertebra as described in chapter 1.
- Remove the disc material at the confirmed level with sharp dissection in the outer two thirds of the disc.
- Carefully remove the remaining disc material with Kerrison rongeurs and curets using magnification.
- With the disc removed and the canal free of all obstructions, prepare the endplates by removing the cartilage without penetrating the cortical bone.
- Insert tricortical bone graft, prepared structural allograft, or a bone cage as desired.
- Internal fixation may be added as necessary.
- Close the chest cavity in layers over a chest tube.

POSTOPERATIVE CARE The patient is allowed to ambulate rapidly after the procedure. The chest tube is removed once drainage is minimal and there is no air leak. Initially a removable brace such as a Jewett brace or thoracolumbosacral orthosis can be used for ambulation. The brace can be discontinued as pain relief improves and radiographic union is noted.

Numerous indications for anterior arthrodesis of the lumbar spine are reported in the literature. At this clinic the indications include debridement of infection, tuberculosis, excision of tumors, correction of kyphosis, scoliosis, neural decompression after fracture, and to achieve stability when posterior arthrodesis is not feasible. Less frequently, we have used this technique in the treatment of spondylolisthesis or internal intervertebral disc derangements. The surgical approach used in tuberculosis by Hodgson and Stock should be applicable in most instances (see chapter 6).

■ ANTERIOR DISC EXCISION AND INTERBODY FUSION OF THE LUMBAR SPINE

The rationale of management of lower back pain must be based on an accurate diagnosis. The pain syndromes in this area are many, and diagnostic pitfalls are ever present. Treatment varies according to the physical and emotional profile of the patient and the experience of the surgeon involved. Hemilaminectomy and decompression of nerve roots still constitute the most widely used surgical procedure for unremitting lower back pain. With continued instability of the anterior and posterior elements, supplemental posterior or posterolateral fusion usually proves satisfactory.

There is a group of patients for whom standard surgical procedures are unsuccessful. The following causes of persistent symptoms after disc surgery have been identified:

- Mistaken original diagnosis
- Recurrent herniation of disc material (also incomplete removal)
- Herniation of disc at another level
- Bony compression of nerve root
- Perineural adhesions
- Instability of vertebral segments
- Psychoneurosis

In this group, improved diagnostic accuracy currently can be obtained with the use of electromyography, a psychologic profile assessment, postmyelographic CT, MRI with and without gadolinium contrast, and possibly discography. Finally, differential spinal anesthesia is helpful in discriminating between the various pain types.

As a rule, failure of the usual posterior methods of fusion to relieve pain in the presence of a solid arthrodesis and in the absence of other pathology as listed earlier dictates consideration of anterior intervertebral disc excision and interbody spinal fusion. The reported outcomes of anterior interbody fusion have been variable, with success rates ranging from 36% to 90%. Although reports of long-term results are inconclusive, pain relief appears to be obtained in 80% to 90% of patients.

Suggested indications include (1) instability causing backache and sciatica, (2) spondylolisthesis of all types, (3) pain after multiple posterior explorations, and (4) failed posterior fusions. Good results have been reported with the use of three iliac wedge grafts for degenerative disease and a block graft for spondylolisthesis (Fig. 3.35).

ANTERIOR INTERBODY FUSION OF THE LUMBAR SPINE

TECHNIQUE 3.22

(GOLDNER ET AL.)

- Administer general anesthesia and place the patient in the Trendelenburg position.
- Develop the retroperitoneal approach to the vertebral bodies and identify the psoas muscle, the iliac artery and vein, and the left ureter. If more than three interspaces are to be fused, retract the ureter toward the left.
- Identify the sacral promontory by palpation.
- Inject saline solution under the prevertebral fascia over the lumbar vertebra and lift the sympathetic chain for easier dissection.
- Expose the lumbosacral disc space by retracting the left iliac artery and vein to the left.
- In exposing the fourth lumbar interspace, displace the left artery and vein and ureter to the right side.
- Elevate the anterior longitudinal ligament as a flap with the base toward the left.
- Tag the flap with sutures and retract it to give additional protection to the vessels.
- Separate the intervertebral disc and annulus from the cartilaginous endplates of the vertebrae with a thin osteotome and remove them with pituitary rongeurs and large curets.
- Clean the space thoroughly back to the posterior longitudinal ligament without removing bone, thereby keeping bleeding to a minimum until the site is ready for grafting.
- Remove the cartilaginous endplates from the vertebral bodies with an osteotome until bleeding bone is encountered.
- Cut shallow notches in the opposing surfaces of the vertebrae and measure the dimensions of the notches carefully with a caliper.
- Cut grafts from the iliac wing, making them larger than the notches for later firm impaction (Fig. 3.36).
- Hyperextend the spine, insert multiple grafts, and relieve the hyperextension.
- Bipolar electrocautery is useful in obtaining hemostasis, but take care not to coagulate the sympathetic fibers over the anterior aspect of the lumbosacral joint. Use of silver clips in this area is preferred.
- After completion of the fusion, close all layers with absorbable sutures.

POSTOPERATIVE CARE Nasogastric suction may be necessary for gastric decompression for about 36 hours. Attention must be paid to mobilization of the lower extremities to prevent dependency and blood pooling.

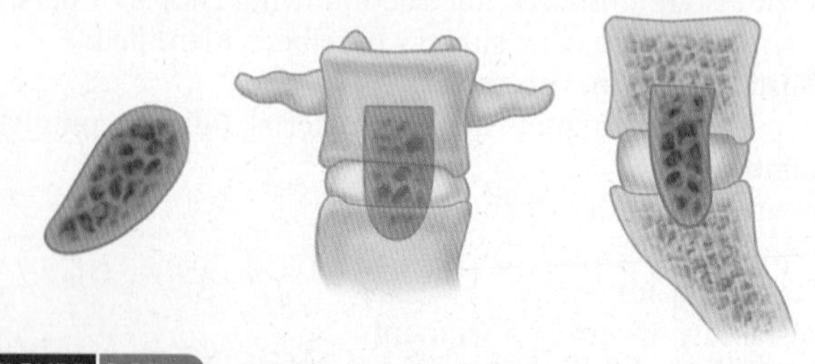

FIGURE 3.35 Anterior interbody fusion in lower lumbar spine.

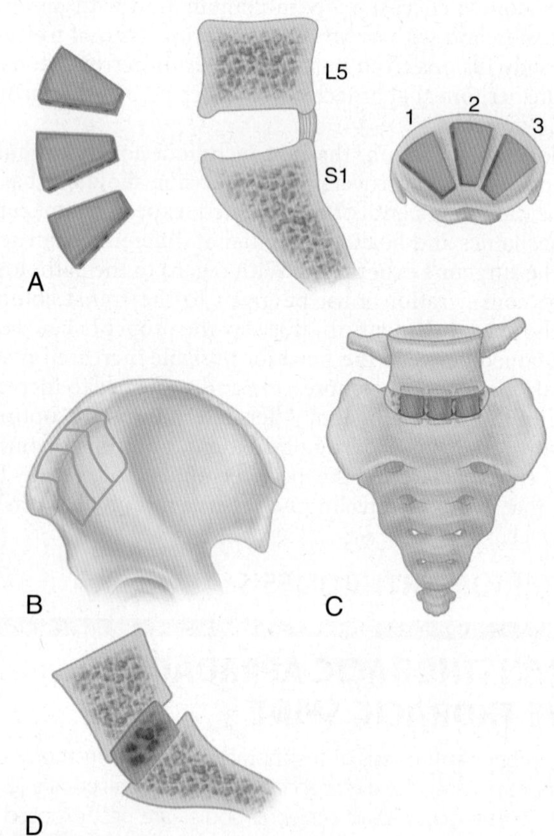

FIGURE 3.36 Technique of Goldner et al. for anterior interbody fusion of lumbosacral joint. **SEE TECHNIQUE 3.22.**

Thigh-length hose for prevention of thromboembolic disease, intermittent compression boots, and low-molecular-weight heparin all are used for deep vein thrombosis prophylaxis. In-bed exercises with straight-leg raising are started on the first postoperative day and continued indefinitely. The patient is allowed to sit and walk with a low back corset used for postoperative immobilization as tolerated. Postoperative radiographs are made before discharge from the hospital to serve as a baseline for judging graft appearance. Three months later, side-bending and flexion and extension radiographs are made in the standing position to provide information about the success of arthrodesis. Radiographs are then repeated at 6 and 12 months after surgery, with the solid fusion not confirmed until 1 year after surgery. Tomograms may be useful in evaluating suspected pseudarthrosis.

We have used a retroperitoneal approach to L2, L3, L4, and L5 discs. For the L5 or lumbosacral disc, some prefer a transperitoneal approach if good anterior access is needed. The incidence of deep venous thrombosis after these approaches, especially the midline transperitoneal approach, is much higher than after ordinary spinal surgery. Suitable prophylaxis is indicated, even though it may not be successful in preventing this complication.

MINIMALLY INVASIVE ANTERIOR FUSION OF THE LUMBAR SPINE

Laparoscopic and VATS techniques have been applied to anterior spine surgery with significant improvements in these same areas. We have limited experience with this technique; currently it is seldom used because of the risk of catastrophic complications.

Laparoscopic transperitoneal lumbar instrumentation and fusion also has been developed, and several systems are currently available. These systems allow disc removal and insertion of threaded cylindrical devices, as well as trapezoidal cages packed with autogenous bone into the disc spaces, typically at the L5-S1 and the L4-L5 levels. Although these techniques provide an effective means of achieving anterior interbody fusion with maintenance of disc space distraction, they appear to require a significant learning curve. Both the VATS and laparoscopic techniques should be performed by surgeons experienced in these techniques to minimize potentially catastrophic complications. The ultimate success of the procedure depends on the proper diagnosis and patient selection. Each device has a technique guide specific to it, and the reader is referred to these guides for specific device use.

PERCUTANEOUS ANTERIOR LUMBAR ARTHRODESIS—LATERAL APPROACH TO L1 TO L4-5

Direct lateral anterior lumbar fusion and extreme lateral interbody fusion can be done through a minimally invasive direct lateral approach (see Technique 1.15); however, there is a definite learning curve for disc excision and fusion techniques done through the small access provided by the dilating retractor systems. Complications, primarily related to nerve root injury or irritation, have been reported in 22% of patients after a minimally invasive direct lateral anterior lumbar fusion and extreme lateral interbody fusion. Knowledge of "safe zones" for this approach and familiarity with the dilating retractor systems are essential for avoiding these complications.

TECHNIQUE 3.23

- After confirmation of the correct position of the retractor (see Technique 1.19) with anteroposterior and lateral fluoroscopy, center the anterior annulotomy window in the anterior half of the disc.
- Make the window opening wide enough to accommodate the implant.
- Remove the disc with standard instruments.
- Leave the posterior annulus intact.
- Release the contralateral annulus using a Cobb dissector to allow distraction of the disc space to insert the implant.
- Insert an implant that will rest on both lateral margins of the epiphyseal ring.
- Irrigate the cavity copiously.
- Carefully remove the retractor while observing the psoas muscle covering the defect and watching for bleeding.
- Close the fascial and subcutaneous layers.
- The skin can be closed with a subcuticular method.
- Supplementary posterior instrumentation must be used to maintain stability.

POSTERIOR ARTHRODESIS

Posterior arthrodeses of the lumbar and thoracic spine generally are based on the principles originated by Hibbs in 1911. In the Hibbs operation, fusion of the neural arches is induced by overlapping numerous small osseous flaps from contiguous laminae, spinous processes, and articular facets. In the thoracic spine, the arthrodesis is generally extended laterally out to the tips of the transverse processes so that the posterior cortex and cancellous bone of these portions of the vertebrae are used to widen the fusion mass. Accurate visual identification of a specific vertebral level is always difficult except when the sacrum can be exposed and thus identified. At any other level, despite the fact that identification of a given vertebra may be possible because of the anatomic peculiarities of spinous processes, laminae, and articular facets, it is always advisable to make marker radiographs at surgery. Marker films occasionally are made before surgery, using a metal marker on the skin with a scratch on the skin to identify the level. We recommend a method consisting of the radiographic identification of a marker of adequate size clamped to a spinous process within the operative field. The closer to the base of the spinous process the marker can be inserted, the more accurate and easier the identification. Cross-table lateral or anteroposterior radiographs taken on the operating table to compare with good-quality preoperative radiographs usually are sufficient for accurate identification of the vertebral level, although the quality of the portable radiographs may at times make this difficult. Patient positioning to maintain lumbar lordosis also is important.

HIBBS FUSION

With the Hibbs technique, fusion is attempted at four different points—the laminae and articular processes on each side. The procedure has been modified slightly over the years.

TECHNIQUE 3.24

(HIBBS, AS DESCRIBED BY HOWORTH)

- Incise the skin and subcutaneous tissues in the midline along the spinous processes and attach towels to the skin edges with clips or use an adhesive plastic drape. Divide the deep fascia and supraspinous ligament in line with the skin incision. With a Kirmisson or Cobb elevator, remove the supraspinous ligament from the tips of the spines.
- Strip the periosteum from the sides of the spines and the dorsal surface of the laminae with a curved elevator. Control bleeding with long thin sponge packs (Hibbs sponges).
- Incise the interspinous ligaments in the direction of their length, making a continuous longitudinal exposure.
- Elevate the muscles from the ligamentum flavum and expose the fossa distal to the lateral articulation overlying the pars interarticularis and transverse process base. Excise the fat pad in the fossa with a scalpel or curet.
- Thoroughly denude the spinous processes of periosteum and ligament with an elevator and curet, split them longitudinally and transversely with an osteotome, and remove them with the Hibbs biting forceps.
- Using a thick chisel elevator, strip away the capsules of the lateral articulations.
- Free with a curet the posterior layer (about two thirds) of the ligamentum flavum from the margins of the distal and proximal laminae in succession and peel it off the anterior layer; leave the latter to cover the dura.
- Excise the articular cartilage and cortical bone from the lateral articulations with special thin osteotomes, either straight or angled at 30, 45, or 60 degrees as required. A.D. Smith emphasized that the lateral articulations of the vertebra above the area of fusion must not be disturbed, because this may cause pain later. However, it is important to include the lateral articulations within the fusion area, because if they are not obliterated, the entire fusion is jeopardized. After curetting the lateral articulations in the fusion area, he narrowed the remaining defect by making small cuts into the articular processes parallel with the joint line so that these thin slices of bone separate slightly and fill the space. This, he believed, is preferable to packing the joint spaces with cancellous bone chips.
- Using a gouge, cut chips from the fossa below each lateral articulation and turn them into the gap left by the removal of the articular cartilage or insert a fragment of spinous process into the gap.
- Denude the fossa of cortical bone and pack it fully with chips.
- Also with a gouge, remove chips from the laminae and place them in the interlaminar space in contact with raw bone on each side. Use fragments from the spinous processes to bridge the laminae. Also use additional bone from the ilium near the posterosuperior spine or from the spinous processes beyond the fusion area.
- When large or extensive grafts are taken from the posterior ilium, postoperative pain or sensitivity of the area may be marked. Care should be taken to avoid injury to the cluneal nerves with subsequent neuroma formation. Bone from the bone bank can be used, especially if the bone available locally is scant because of spina bifida.
- The bone grafts should not extend beyond the laminae of the end vertebrae because the projecting ends of the grafts can cause irritation and pain.
- If the nucleus pulposus is to be removed, the chips are cut before exposure of the nucleus and are kept until needed. The remaining layer of the ligamentum flavum is freed as a flap with its base at the midline, is retracted for exposure of the nerve root and nucleus, and after removal of the nucleus is replaced to protect the dura.
- Suture the periosteum, ligaments, and muscles snugly over the chips with interrupted sutures. Then suture the subcutaneous tissue carefully to eliminate dead space and close the skin either with a subcuticular suture or nonabsorbable skin suture technique.

At this clinic we routinely use an adhesive plastic film material to isolate the skin surface from the wound rather than attaching towels to skin edges with clips, because clips have an unfortunate tendency to become displaced and can get lost within the wound. We routinely use modified Cobb elevators, which when sharp are efficient in stripping away the capsules of the lateral articulations. The most important single project at the time of surgery is preparing an extensive fresh cancellous bed to receive the grafts. This means denuding the facet joints, articular processes, pars interarticularis, laminae, and spinous processes. Subcuticular wound closure is used routinely to improve patient comfort.

POSTOPERATIVE CARE We routinely use closed-wound suction for 12 to 36 hours, with removal of the suction device mandatory by 48 hours. Depending on the level of the arthrodesis, the age of the patient, and the presence or absence of internal fixation, walking is allowed in 24 to 48 hours when pain permits. For obese patients, all types of external fixation or support likely will be inadequate and limitation of activity may be the only reasonable alternative. The appropriateness of bracing remains controversial. Generally, for fusions with marked preoperative instability (e.g., burst fractures), rigid bracing is continued for 12 weeks. For fusions without marked instability (e.g., degenerative spondylolisthesis), bracing generally, if used, is less rigid and of shorter duration.

POSTEROLATERAL OR INTERTRANSVERSE FUSIONS

In 1948 Cleveland, Bosworth, and Thompson described a technique for repair of pseudarthrosis after spinal fusion in which grafts are placed posteriorly on one side over the laminae, lateral margins of the articular facets, and base of the transverse processes. Watkins described what he called a posterolateral fusion of the lumbar and lumbosacral spine in which the facets, pars interarticularis, and bases of the transverse processes are fused with chip grafts and a large graft is placed posteriorly on the transverse processes. When the lumbosacral joint is included, the grafts extend to the posterior aspect of the first sacral segment.

We, like many others, use this operation and its modifications for primary lumbar and lumbosacral fusions and in patients with pseudarthrosis, laminar defects either congenital or surgical, or spondylolisthesis with chronic pain from instability. The operation may be unilateral or bilateral but usually is bilateral, covering one or more joints depending on the stability of the area to be fused. The retraction instruments designed by McElroy and others are useful. However, one should be mindful of the ischemia caused by retractors, and they should be periodically released to allow perfusion of the paraspinal musculature. When placing the retractors, minimal retractor bulk and tension should be used. The technique described by Watkins allows exposure for a posterolateral fusion without much need for soft-tissue retraction.

POSTEROLATERAL LUMBAR FUSION

TECHNIQUE 3.25

(WATKINS)

- Make a longitudinal skin incision along the lateral border of the paraspinal muscles, curving it medially at the distal end across the posterior crest of the ilium (Fig. 3.37A). Alternatively, a single midline skin incision can be used with bilateral fascial incisions.
- Divide the lumbodorsal fascia and establish the plane of cleavage between the border of the paraspinal muscles and the fascia overlying the transversus abdominis muscle. The tips of the transverse processes can now be palpated in the depths of the wound (Fig. 3.37B).
- Release the iliac attachment of the muscles with an osteotome, taking a thin layer of ilium.
- Continue the exposure of the posterior crest of the ilium by subperiosteal dissection and remove the crest almost flush with the sacroiliac joint, taking enough bone to provide one or two grafts. Removal of the iliac crest increases exposure of the spine.
- Retract the sacrospinalis muscle toward the midline and denude the transverse processes of the dorsal muscle and ligamentous attachments; expose the articular facets by excising the joint capsule.
- Remove the cartilage from the facets with an osteotome and level the area down to allow the graft to fit snugly against the facets, pars interarticularis, and base of the transverse process at each level.
- Comminute the facets with a small gouge or osteotome and turn bone chips up and down from the facet area, upper sacral area, and transverse processes.
- Split the resected iliac crest longitudinally into two grafts. Shape one to fit into the prepared bed and impact it firmly in place with its cut surface against the spine (Fig. 3.37B). Preserve the remaining graft for use on the opposite side with or without additional bone from the other iliac crest.
- Pack additional ribbons and chips of cancellous bone from the ilium about the graft.
- Allow the paraspinal muscles to fall in position over the fusion area and close the wound.

POSTOPERATIVE CARE Postoperative care is the same as that described for posterior arthrodesis (see Technique 3.24). Modifications of the Watkins technique include splitting of the sacrospinalis muscle longitudinally; inclusion of the laminae, as well as the articular facets and transverse processes, in the fusion (Figs. 3.38 and 3.39); and combining posterolateral fusion using a midline approach with a modified Hibbs type fusion in routine lumbar and lumbosacral fusions (Fig. 3.40). Adkins used an intertransverse or alar transverse fusion in which tibial grafts are inserted between the transverse processes of L4 and L5 and between that of L5 and the ala of the sacrum on one or both sides.

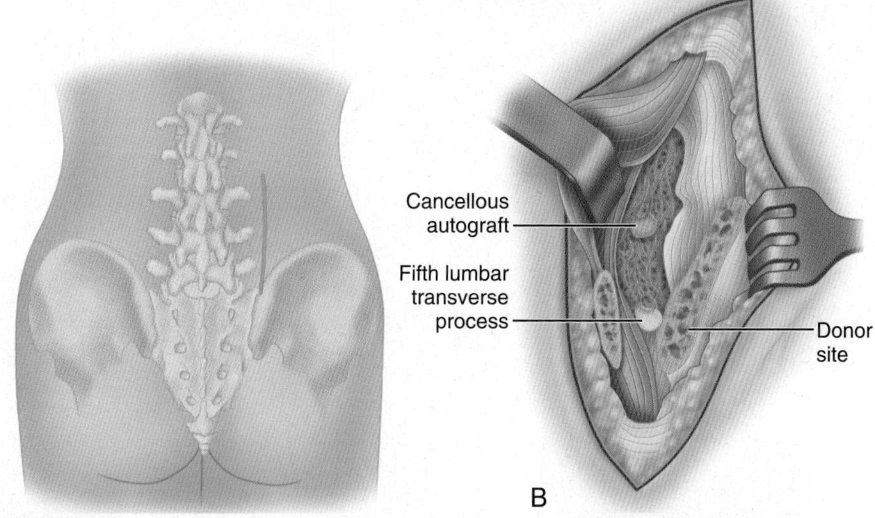

FIGURE 3.37 Watkins posterolateral fusion. **A,** Incision. **B,** Lumbothoracic fascia has been incised, paraspinal muscles have been retracted medially, and tips of transverse processes are now palpable. Split iliac crest and smaller grafts have been placed against spine. **SEE TECHNIQUE 3.25.**

INTERTRANSVERSE LUMBAR FUSION

TECHNIQUE 3.26

(ADKINS)

- Dissect the erector spinae muscles laterally from the pedicles, exposing the transverse processes and ala of the sacrum. This is easier when the facets have been removed, but if these are intact, exposure can be obtained without disturbing them.
- Cut a groove in the upper or lower border of each transverse process with a sharp gouge or forceps. Take care not to fracture the transverse process.
- In the ala of the sacrum, first make parallel cuts in its posterosuperior border with an osteotome. Then drive a gouge across the ends of these cuts and lever the intervening bone out of the slot so made.
- For fusions of the fourth to the fifth lumbar vertebra, cut a tibial graft with V-shaped ends; insert it obliquely between the transverse processes and then rotate it into position so that it causes slight distraction of the processes and becomes firmly impacted between them.
- For the lumbosacral joint, cut the graft so that it is V-shaped at its upper end and straight but slightly oblique at its lower end. Insert one arm of the V in front of the transverse process and punch the lower end into the slot in the sacrum. If only one side is grafted, arrange the patient so that there is a slight convex curve of the spine on the operated side; thus, firm impaction occurs when the spine is straightened. Bilateral grafts are preferred. The grafts should be placed as far laterally as possible to avoid the nerve roots and to gain maximal stability.
- Alternatively, strips of iliac wing cortex no more than 2 to 3 mm thick are placed anterior to the transverse processes of L4 and L5 to bridge the gap and lie on the intertransverse fascia. Similarly, another strip is placed between the ala of the sacrum and L5 by wedging it into the space after the ala has been slotted and decorticated. Care must be taken that these grafts do not protrude too far anterior to the plane of the transverse processes. This modification does not require a tibial graft and is recommended.

POSTOPERATIVE CARE Postoperative care is the same as that described for posterior arthrodesis (see Technique 3.24).

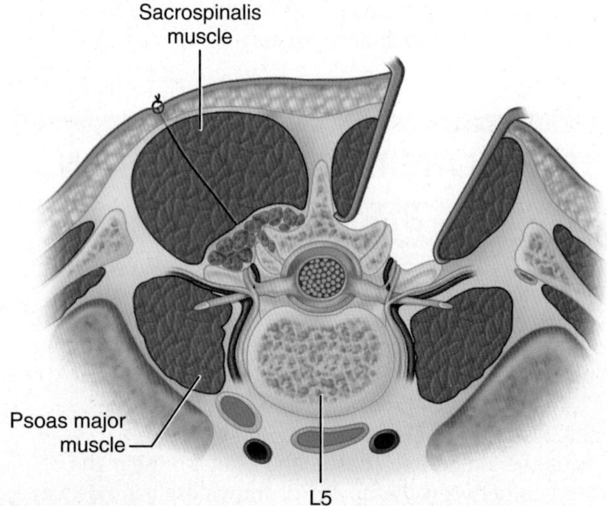

FIGURE 3.38 Technique of posterolateral fusion in which sacrospinalis muscle is split longitudinally and laminae, articular facets, and transverse processes are all included in fusion.

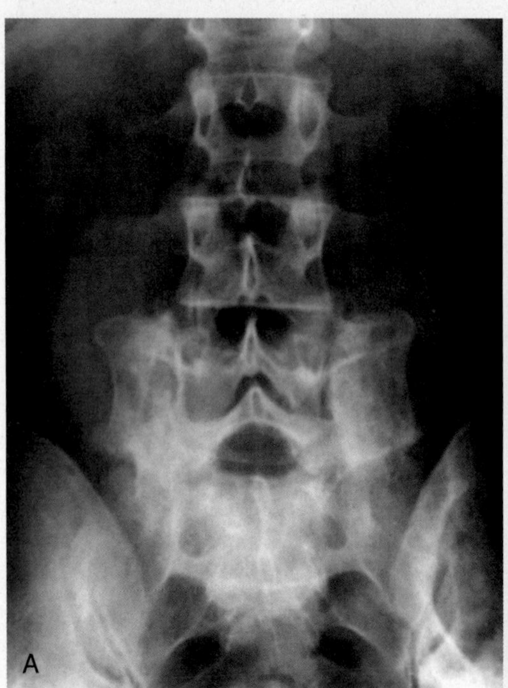

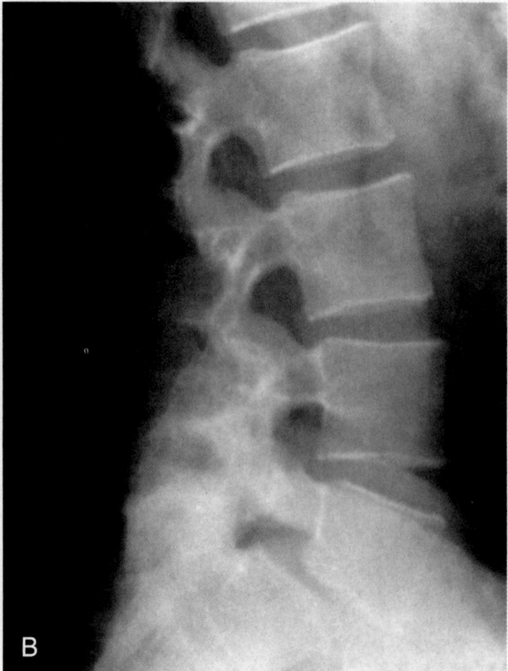

FIGURE 3.39 Bilateral posterolateral fusion for spondylolisthesis in adult. Anteroposterior **(A)** and lateral **(B)** radiographs 6 months after surgery.

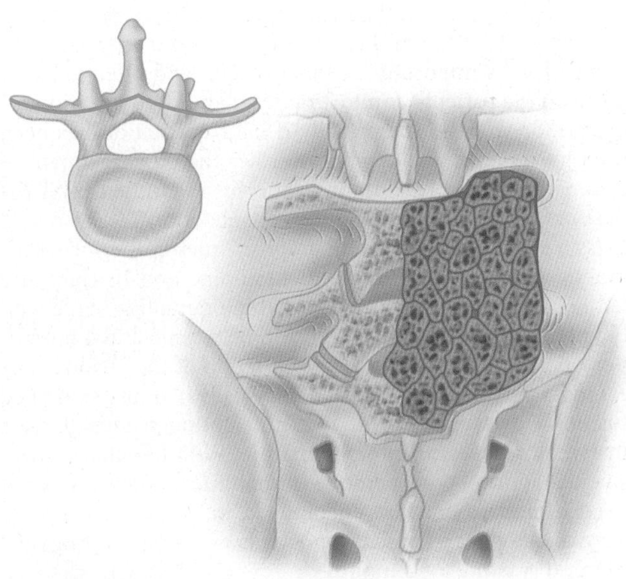

FIGURE 3.40 Slocum technique combining posterior (modified Hibbs) and posterolateral fusions. Midline incision is used. *Inset,* All bone posterior to *blue line* is removed.

MINIMALLY INVASIVE TRANSFORAMINAL LUMBAR INTERBODY FUSION

A microscope and tubular retractors allow minimally invasive transforaminal lumbar interbody fusions to achieve decompression and stabilization while safely performing the procedure with less collateral damage to surrounding structures and the posterior dynamic stabilizers of the spine than with open procedures. Because the surgical corridor required is minimal, tubular retractors eliminate the need for traditional muscle-stripping techniques and preserve the form and function of the paraspinous musculature, which allows more normal physiologic function of the spine and sparing of the dynamic posterior stabilizers. Other advantages include reduced blood loss, less postoperative back pain, shorter time to ambulation, shorter hospital stay, and shorter duration of narcotic usage postoperatively compared with open approaches as well as lower infection rates. Minimally invasive techniques also have been reported to result in significant reductions in total hospital costs compared with standard open techniques, and there is early evidence that adjacent segment degeneration may be decreased compared with open surgery.

TECHNIQUE 3.27

(GARDOCKI)

- After induction of general endotracheal anesthesia, position the patient prone on a radiolucent table.
- Obtain lateral and anteroposterior C-arm fluoroscopic images to ensure that the pedicles can be adequately imaged.
- Insert a spinal needle into the paraspinal musculature at the interspace of interest, 40 to 60 mm lateral to the midline depending on patient depth and confirm its position with lateral fluoroscopy.
- The trajectory should approach the anterior and middle third of the disc space.
- Remove the needle and make a 20-mm vertical incision at the puncture site.
- Insert the blunt end of a guidewire through the incision and direct it toward the appropriate anatomy under fluoroscopic guidance. Advance the guidewire only through the lumbodorsal fascia, taking care not to penetrate the ligamentum flavum and to avoid inadvertent dural puncture.
- Insert the cannulated soft-tissue dilator over the guidewire with a twisting motion.
- Once the fascia is penetrated, remove the guidewire and use progressively larger dilators to create a muscle-sparing surgical corridor down to the appropriate interlaminar space while remaining orthogonal to the disc.
- Dock the appropriate-length 16- or 18-mm tubular retractor on the facet joint complex and interlaminar space.
- With the use of an operating microscope or loupe magnification, carry out a total facetectomy with a high-speed drill (preferred) or osteotomes. The osteotomy is L-shaped and should connect the interlaminar space at the base of the spinous process with the pars interarticularis just above the disc space but below the pedicle.
- Denude all removed bone of soft tissue and morcellize it for later use as interbody graft material.
- Perform a conventional discectomy by incising the anulus with a no. 15 scalpel blade lateral to the dural sac while retracting the traversing nerve root. There is no need to retract the exiting root. All cartilage should be removed from the disc space up to the outer anulus.
- Sequentially distract the disc space until the original disc space height is obtained and the normal foraminal opening is restored. This can be done with shavers, trials, or mechanical distractors depending on the system being used.
- Remove soft tissue and the cartilaginous endplate covering with scraping or curettage. Scrape medially under the midline and gradually work laterally in a sweeping motion until both caudal and cephalad endplates are cleared of soft tissue, exposing the compressed cancellous endplate of both vertebrae.
- Insert an appropriately sized graft based on the distractors or trials. The graft material can be bone, polymer, or metal. Do not place a graft that is too long because it may increase the risk of later posterior displacement.
- Countersink the graft until it is 4 to 5 mm below the posterior margin of the disc space.
- Probe the extradural space and foramina to ensure adequate decompression of the neural elements.
- Once the graft is in place, confirm positioning on anteroposterior and lateral fluoroscopic images. If positioned adequately with adequate restoration of disc height and lordosis, place bilateral percutaneous pedicle screws to allow a stable environment for fusion across the disc space.
- Use anteroposterior and lateral images of the pedicle for cannulation with an appropriately sized Jamshidi needle

using a "pencil-in-cup" technique. The remaining technique varies depending on the implant manufacturer.

- Once all implants have been adequately placed, close the incisions subcutaneously with 2-0 Vicryl and use skin glue (e.g., Dermabond or Histoacryl) for final skin closure. When a 20-mm or smaller tube is used there is no need for fascial closure.

POSTOPERATIVE CARE Patients are encouraged to walk as much as possible immediately after surgery. Bending, lifting, and twisting are restricted for a period of 3 months. All restrictions are lifted at 3 months if radiographs show appropriate progression of fusion. Hospital stay is seldom longer than 24 hours, and this procedure can sometimes be done in the outpatient setting in carefully selected patients. When there is no contraindication, we suggest supplementation with calcium and vitamin D for 2 weeks before and 3 months after fusion surgery to encourage bone healing.

INTERNAL FIXATION IN LUMBAR SPINAL FUSION

Various types of internal fixation have been used in lumbar spinal fusion. The object is to immobilize the joints during fusion and thus hasten consolidation and reduce pain and disability after surgery. Additionally, the instrumentation maintains correction of deformity and normal contours during the consolidation of the fusion mass. For many years, surgeons fixed the spinous processes of the lumbar spine with heavy wire loops, as described by Rogers for fracture- dislocation of the cervical spine.

Early methods of fixing the articular facets used bone blocks or cylindrical bone grafts to transfix the facets, particularly at the lumbosacral joint. In one bone grafting technique (McBride), soft-tissue attachments to the spinous processes and laminae were elevated, the spinous processes of L4, L5, and S1 were removed at their bases, and special trephine cutting tools were used to cut mortise bone grafts from them. The laminae were then spread forcibly with laminae distractors, and, again with the use of special trephine cutting tools, a round hole was made across each facet joint into the underlying pedicle. The bone grafts were then impacted firmly across each joint into the pedicle, and the distractors were removed. H-shaped grafts between the spinous processes also have been described for articular facet fixation.

Internal fixation (such as pedicle screws and plates) is described in chapter 5. Again, however, before using these techniques the indications and current status of the use of these implants as approved by the FDA should be reviewed carefully with the patient. A special consent form should be signed by the patient if these devices are being used for anything other than the strictly approved indications.

TREATMENT AFTER POSTERIOR ARTHRODESIS

Opinions vary as to the proper treatment after spinal fusion. Usually the patient is placed on bed rest for a period of 12 to 24 hours; mobilization is then begun. No clear consensus exists on the duration of bed rest or the type of external support that should be used or even whether external support should be used. This depends on the pathologic condition being treated and on the location and extent of the fusion. Surgeon preference also is important in this decision and often is based more on the patient's comfort rather than immobilization for promotion of fusion, especially if instrumentation has been used for a degenerative process rather than for treatment of traumatic instability. Immobilization is continued until the patient is comfortable or until consolidation of the fusion mass occurs as seen on radiographs. Anteroposterior radiographs are made with the patient supine and in right and left bending positions, and a lateral radiograph is made with the patient in flexion and extension between 3 and 4 months postoperatively to confirm consolidation of the fusion mass. A longer period may be needed, especially in uninstrumented fusions. However, even with instrumentation, the fusion mass may require a year or more to mature. With newer, less invasive techniques, postoperative immobilization usually is not needed and patients are encouraged to gradually return to normal activities as much as possible, avoiding bending, lifting, and twisting for 3 months.

PSEUDARTHROSIS AFTER SPINAL FUSION

The possibility of pseudarthrosis after spinal arthrodesis should be remembered from the time the operation is proposed until the fusion mass is solid. A frank discussion of this problem with each patient before operation is important. The reported pseudarthrosis rate ranges from 9% to 30%. Some authors have correlated higher pseudarthrosis rates with a greater number of levels fused, but multiple studies have reported single-level pseudarthrosis rates as high as 30%. A critical analysis of the literature determined that instrumentation, fusion location, graft type, and brace type all affected lumbar fusion rates (Table 3.3). Careful patient selection and meticulous surgical technique in preparing the recipient site and in harvesting and preparing bone grafts are required to optimize fusion rates regardless of any other techniques that may be used.

It has been estimated that 50% of patients with pseudarthrosis have no symptoms. Persistent pain after spinal fusion with no other identifiable cause is presumed to be caused by pseudarthrosis when this condition is present. Yet, in some patients pain continues after a successful repair. Although pain can persist, repair of a pseudarthrosis is indicated when disabling pain persists; repair is contraindicated when pain is slight or absent.

The following findings are helpful in making a diagnosis of pseudarthrosis: (1) discretely localized pain and tenderness over the fusion area, (2) progression of the deformity or disease, (3) localized motion in the fusion mass, as found in biplane bending radiographs, and (4) motion in the fusion mass found on exploration. The amount of motion on flexion-extension radiographs that is consistent with solid fusion is controversial, ranging from no motion to 5 degrees of motion. When rigid instrumentation has been used, lack of motion does not necessarily indicate solid fusion; the presence of broken spinal implants does imply pseudarthrosis. Thin-cut CT scans appear to be more reliable than radiographs in evaluating fusion: a prospective study comparing imaging findings to intraoperative findings showed that CT most closely agreed with intraoperative findings compared with plain radiographs and MRI. The expense of MRI and its susceptibility to metallic artifact from instrumentation remain disadvantages to its routine use in the assessment of spinal fusion. Unfortunately exploration is the only way to be absolutely certain that a fusion mass is completely solid.

Treatment of a patient with a painful pseudarthrosis involves a second attempt at fusion and may require a different approach from that used in the original fusion surgery, as well as the use of additional instrumentation, bone graft, and osteobiologic agents.

PSEUDARTHROSIS REPAIR

TECHNIQUE 3.28

(RALSTON AND THOMPSON)

- Expose the entire fusion plate subperiosteally through the old incision; if the defect is wide and filled with dense fibrous tissue, subperiosteal stripping in that area can be difficult. A narrow defect often is difficult to locate because the surface of the plate usually is irregular and the line of pseudarthrosis may be sinuous in the coronal and sagittal planes. In our experience, adherence of the overlying fibrous tissue has been the key factor that aids in identifying a pseudarthrosis. The characteristic smooth cortical surface and easily stripped fibrous "periosteum" of a solid, mature fusion mass are quite different from the adherent fibrous tissue overlying a pseudarthrosis. Meticulous inspection of the region of the facet joint is needed. Often a mature and solid fusion mass extends across the transverse processes, but motion is detectable at the facet joint, indicating the fusion mass did not incorporate to the fusion bed (i.e., the transverse processes).
- Thoroughly clean the fibrous tissue from the fusion mass in the vicinity of the pseudarthrosis. The adjacent superior and inferior borders of the fusion mass on either side of the pseudarthrosis usually will be seen to move when pressure is applied with a blunt instrument, such as a curet.
- As the defect is followed across the fusion mass, it will be found to extend into the lateral articulations on each side. Carefully explore these articulations and excise all fibrous tissue and any remaining articular cartilage down to bleeding bone.
- If the defect is wide, excise the fibrous tissue that fills it to a depth of 3 to 6 mm across the entire mass and protect the underlying spinal dura.
- Thoroughly freshen the exposed edges of the defect.
- When the defect is narrow and motion is minimal, limit the excision of the interposed soft tissue to avoid loss of fixation.
- Fashion a trough 6 mm wide and 6 mm deep on each side of the midline, extending longitudinally both well above and well below the defect.
- "Fish scale" the entire fusion mass on both sides of the defect, with the bases of the bone chips raised being away from the defect.
- Obtain both strip and chip bone grafts either from the fusion mass above or below or from the ilium, preferably the latter.
- Pack these grafts tightly into the lateral articulations, into the pseudarthrosis defect, and into the longitudinal troughs.
- Place small grafts across the pseudarthrosis line and wedge the edge of each transplant beneath the fish-scaled cortical bone chips. Use all remaining graft material to pack neatly in and about the grafts.
- Internal fixation (see chapter 5) can be used to improve the rate of healing after pseudarthrosis repair but often is not necessary, and removal of loose implants improves postoperative imaging capability.

TABLE 3.3

Factors Affecting Fusion Rates in Lumbar Spine Surgery

	SUCCESSFUL FUSION (%)
INSTRUMENTATION TYPE	
None	84
Any	89
Semirigid	91
Rigid	88
FUSION LOCATION	
Posterolateral	85
Posterior interbody	89
Anterior interbody	86
Circumferential (360 degrees)	91
GRAFT TYPE	
Autogenous bone alone	87
Allograft alone	86
Autogenous bone + interbody cage	90
Allograft/autogenous bone mix	86
BRACE TYPE	
None	89
Any	88
Semirigid or nonrigid	87
Rigid	88

From Raizman NM, O'Brien JR, Poehling-Monaghan KL, et al: Pseudarthrosis of the spine, *J Am Acad Orthop Surg* 17:494–503, 2009.

DEGENERATIVE DISC DISEASE AND INTERNAL DISC DERANGEMENT

As has already been discussed, the degenerative process is fundamental to the development of disc herniations. Current research shows that genetic factors are more important than the mechanical stresses that have long been emphasized. The development of a disc herniation is only one of the pathways that the degenerative disc may follow. Alternatively, the disc may become the primary source of pain, rather than the nerve root, as is the case with herniations. This discogenic type of pain is most attributable to the internal disc derangement

(IDD) that accompanies the degenerative process. Correct diagnosis and treatment of painful degenerative discs are difficult and controversial.

There are many different treatment options for this diagnosis, including fusions, disc arthroplasty, nucleoplasty, and dynamic stabilization procedures. The number of fusion operations in the United States has consistently increased since the 1970s and is significantly higher than in other developed countries. The indication for most of these procedures is IDD. Currently there are three lumbar disc replacement prostheses approved by the FDA, but several designs are under investigation. The sole indication for these devices currently is to treat symptomatic degenerative disc disease. Likewise, the implants currently in development for nucleoplasty also are ultimately for treatment of the same process. There are multiple devices and models for "dynamic stabilization," only some of which are for the treatment of IDD. There is no shortage of treatment options. Treatment is controversial because no consensus of diagnostic criteria exists with regard to symptom type or severity, physical examination, or diagnostic imaging criteria. In addition to lack of consensus with regard to diagnosis, few prospective randomized data exist on outcomes for the numerous operative or nonoperative treatment options.

More recent research has helped considerably in understanding the anatomic basis for discogenic pain with nociceptive receptors and the innervation of the disc by the sinuvertebral nerves and basivertebral nerves being shown, as discussed earlier. Anatomic studies also are beginning to give insight into the complexities of normal disc structure and function. The understanding of pain and mechanisms that lead to inflammatory and mechanical pain is continually improving. These studies focus on the molecular structure of the matrix, the mechanical properties of the matrix, the cellular activities within the matrix, and the complexities of pain modulation (Fig. 3.41). Understanding the interplay between these processes and the complex psychosocial issues involved and instruments necessary for diagnosis allows for much more precise and rational treatment.

Current understanding of IDD defines this as a pathologic condition resulting in axial spine pain with no or minimal deformation of spinal alignment or disc contour. This is to be distinguished from measurable instability as can occur with fractures, traumatic ligamentous disruptions, degenerative listhesis, scoliosis, or other conditions. Although these conditions can be a source of pain, they are fundamentally different in that there are definite defined anatomic alterations and imaging abnormalities associated with each of these circumstances. There are no defined criteria for IDD, however.

Because there are no pathognomonic findings for IDD, the diagnosis requires a compilation of findings consistent with IDD and elimination of other diagnostic possibilities. Foremost among the consistent findings is the history. Patients usually are relatively young, in the third to sixth decades of life. Pain usually is chronic with symptoms present for several years, although the pain may have become constant or very frequent only in the previous several months.

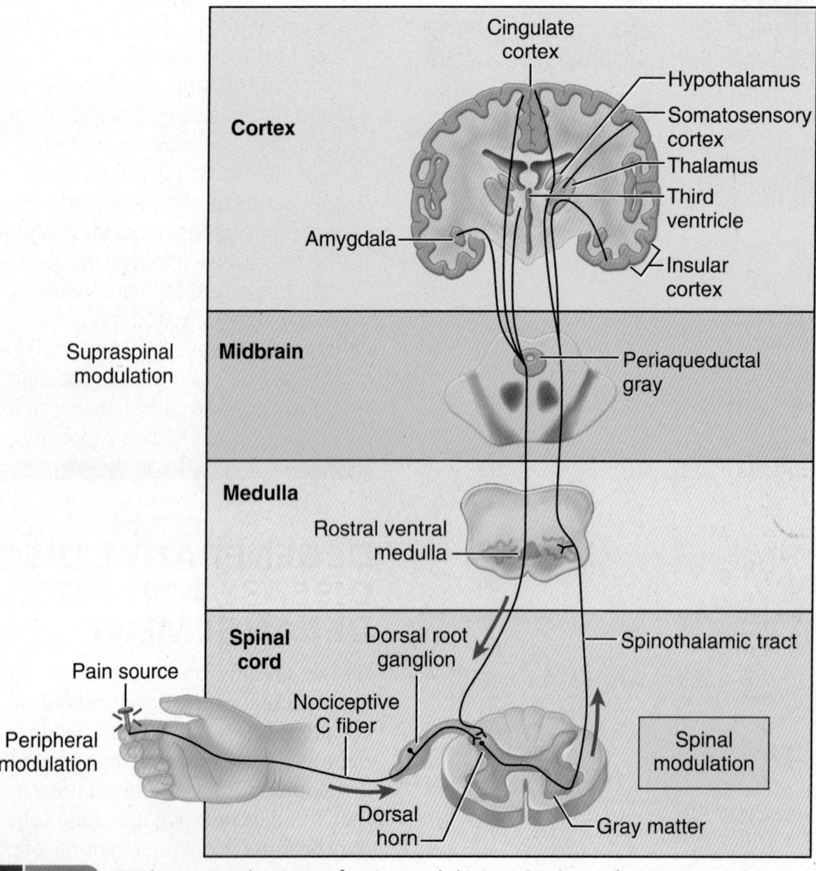

FIGURE 3.41 **Main anatomic areas of pain modulation.** (Redrawn from DeLeo JA: Basic science of pain, *J Bone Joint Surg* 88A:58–62, 2006.)

The pain is axial primarily, often with buttock and posterior thigh (sclerotomal) pain. Pain distal to the knee indicates either different or coexistent pathology. Positions and activities that increase intradiscal pressure, such as sitting or flexion, should exacerbate the symptoms. Likewise, recumbency, especially in the fetal position, often decreases the pain. This pattern of variable pain intensity is constant. Pain that is constant but has little or no variation in intensity or only random fluctuations probably is not caused by IDD.

Examination reveals no weakness or reflex changes if IDD is the only diagnosis. Lumbar range of motion is mildly limited, especially in flexion, and limitation is caused by lumbosacral pain or tightness. Straight-leg raising typically causes back and buttock pain but no pain distal to the knee. There is no spasm in the paraspinal musculature, and extension usually gives some relief temporarily. The patient often has a depressed mood and should be questioned about changes or stresses at work and at home. If the patient has identified significant stresses, anger, or anxiety, the diagnosis of IDD is in question. Also, examination for Waddell signs should be included (Table 3.4), and if three or more are present, an alternative diagnosis is more likely. The examination must include the hip joints as a possible cause of buttock and thigh pain.

Imaging studies should include a lumbar spine series and dynamic films to assess deformities, measurable instability, or destructive lesions. Additional diagnostic studies should be obtained to evaluate abdominal or intrapelvic pathology that may have been suggested by the patient's history and physical examination. Additionally, MRI of the lumbar spine should show diminished water content in the nucleus of one or more lumbar discs (Fig. 3.42). This may or may not be associated with a loss of disc height and broad-based disc bulging. Decreased water content leads to decreased signal intensity best seen on T2-weighted sagittal images. This finding alone has no diagnostic value unless the appropriate history and physical examination also are present and there is no other discernible diagnosis.

The clinical diagnosis of IDD requires a careful and methodical assessment of many different factors. When the diagnosis is established, treatment options can be considered. Most patients can be treated without operative intervention, especially if they are educated as to the nature of the process causing their pain, specifically that it is not relentlessly progressive generally and that continued pain does not equate with progressive deterioration or disability. Often this understanding and instruction on moderate activity modification, aerobic conditioning such as walking, and core muscle strengthening allow these patients to manage their symptoms long term without undue worry or resource consumption.

A small group of patients with persistent and debilitating symptoms may benefit from operative intervention. Before proceeding with any operative treatment, the patient should be informed that surgery leads to improvement in only 65%, leaving about 35% no better or possibly worse with respect to axial spine pain. Also, patients should understand that those who improve still have some activity limitations caused by pain or stiffness. This discussion must be very frank. For patients who still are considering surgery, a consistent and comprehensive assessment leads to the best overall outcomes. This approach is used for treating IDD, which is a diagnosis of exclusion and is separate from the treatment of measurable instability, spinal stenosis, disc herniations, spondylolisthesis, fractures, and other more objective diagnoses. The question

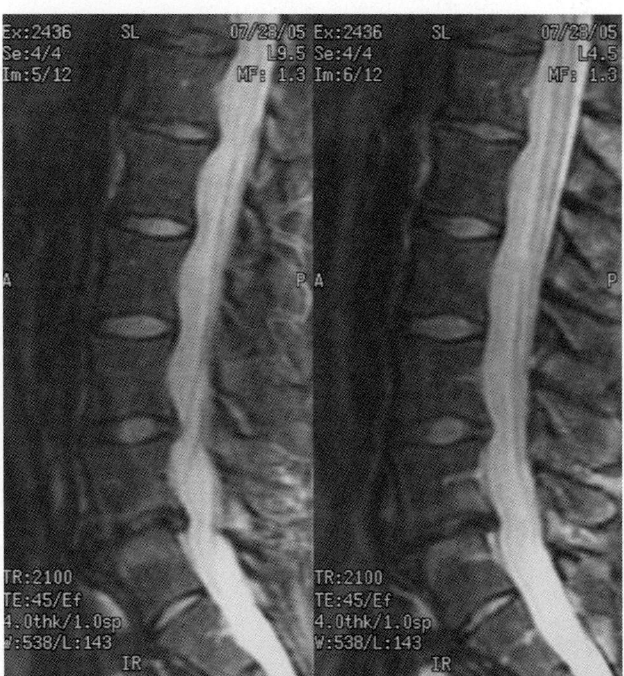

FIGURE 3.42 A 51-year-old patient with chronic axial spine pain without neurologic deficits that did not respond to nonoperative treatments.

becomes: of patients who have severe and debilitating axial spine pain that is not adequately improved with nonoperative methods and who have no objective diagnosis to explain their symptoms, which are likely to improve with surgery? Treatment of the other diagnoses is covered elsewhere.

PATIENT SELECTION PROCESS

Given that any other objective diagnosis has already been ruled out, the primary consideration in patient selection revolves around nonanatomic or psychosocial causes for disabling axial spine pain. For many years, patients with workers' compensation claims have been considered high risk for psychosocial causes of their pain, but more recent studies that independently assess this variable do not support this assertion. It has been found by several studies independently that being off work more than 8 weeks before surgery is an independent predictor of poorer outcome.

Many authors have tried to develop instruments to measure "abnormal illness behaviors." Waddell et al. defined this as "maladaptive overt illness related behavior, which is out of proportion to the underlying physical disease (including IDD) and more readily attributable to associated cognitive and affective disturbances." Waddell et al. also developed clinical tools designed to detect the presence of abnormal illness behavior by identifying physical signs or symptoms and descriptions that were nonorganic. Five nonorganic signs and seven nonorganic symptom descriptions have been identified (see Table 3.4). This group initially described these for use in patients with chronic pain and suggested that the presence of three or more was required to show abnormal illness behavior. Although these signs and symptoms cannot be used to predict return to work, the presence of multiple Waddell signs correlates with poor operative outcome and may temper the decision to offer a particular patient operative consideration.

TABLE 3.4

Signs and Symptoms for Diagnosis of Abnormal Illness Behavior

NONORGANIC SIGNS	DESCRIPTION
Regional disturbances	Widespread region of sensory changes or weakness that is divergent from accepted neuroanatomy
Superficial/ nonanatomic tenderness	Tenderness of skin to light touch (superficial) or depth tenderness felt over a widespread area not localized to one structure (nonanatomic)
SIMULATION	
Axial loading	Low back pain reported with pressure on the patient's head while standing
Rotation	Low back pain reported when shoulders and pelvis are rotated in the same plane as the patient stands
DISTRACTION	
Straight-leg raising	Inconsistent limitation of straight-leg raising in supine and seated positions
Overreaction	Disproportionate verbalization, facial expression, muscle tension, collapsing, sweating during examination
NONORGANIC SYMPTOM DESCRIPTORS	
Do you get pain in your tailbone?	
Do you have numbness in your entire leg (front, side, and back of leg at the same time)? Do you have pain in your entire leg (front, side, and back of leg at the same time)? Does your whole leg ever give way?	
Have you had to go to the emergency department because of back pain?	
Has all treatment for your back made your pain worse?	

From Fritz JM, Wainner RS, Hicks GE: The use of nonorganic signs and symptoms as a screening tool for return-to-work in patients with acute low back pain, *Spine* 25:1925–1931, 2000.

The first formal step in patient selection for operative treatment for IDD is the Minnesota Multiphasic Personality Inventory (MMPI). This study is done before any invasive studies to assess specifically for IDD. This instrument has been used in many studies and has been shown to be a predictor of operative outcomes, regardless of the spinal pathologic condition that is present. Riley et al. investigated the MMPI-2 and found that the results replicated the older MMPI. Patients with MMPI and MMPI-2 findings of depressed-pathologic profile and a conversion V profile reported greater dissatisfaction with operative outcomes. The MMPI is lengthy and difficult to administer in an orthopaedic clinical setting. An independent assessment by an experienced psychologist or psychiatrist who also administers the MMPI is best. By comparison, the Distress and Risk Assessment Method (DRAM) is relatively easily administered and scored and has been validated in clinical settings with regard to patients with back pain. The DRAM consists of the Modified Somatic Perception Questionnaire and the Zung Depression Index. With this simplified method, patients identified as psychologically distressed are three to four times more likely to have a poor outcome after any form of treatment.

We recommend that patients being considered for operative treatment with the working diagnosis of IDD have formal psychologic testing, which at our clinic consists of the MMPI. The current version of this test has predictive value for failure of operative treatment but has no predictive value for successful operative treatment. If the scoring and assessment from the psychologist administering the MMPI do not indicate the patient is at increased risk for failure, the second step in the assessment is taken.

DIFFERENTIAL SPINAL ANESTHETIC

The second formal step is the administration of a differential spinal anesthetic. This technique has been well reviewed by Raj, and the reader is referred to that work for a more complete description. Briefly, this technique, which is based anatomically on the relationship between nerve fiber size, conduction velocity, and fiber function, is shown in Table 3.5. The fiber diameter is the most critical physical dimension. The type A fibers are myelinated and subdivided into alpha, beta, gamma, and delta subtypes, each with different functions. Also, the unmyelinated B and C fibers serve different functions. The basic concept of the differential spinal is that by sequentially administering a local anesthetic agent, a predictable sequence of functional loss, beginning with sympathetic, then sensory, and finally motor blockade, is seen. The conventional technique (Table 3.6) is administered as a series of four solutions, each given in an identical fashion. The patient is questioned regarding his or her pain, and a series of observations is made by the physician to evaluate strength by dermatome, light touch, sharp and dull discrimination by dermatome, and reflexes (Table 3.7). The solutions should be referred to as "A" through "D" to avoid the term "*placebo*" in front of the patient. Also, the patient is not told ahead of time of the expected sequential changes to avoid bias. The four solutions are given as follows:

Solution A: contains no local anesthetic and serves as placebo.

Solution B: contains 0.25% procaine, which is known to represent the mean sympatholytic concentration of procaine in the subarachnoid space that is the concentration sufficient to block B fibers but usually insufficient to block A delta and C fibers

Solution C: contains 0.5% procaine, the mean sensory blocking concentration of procaine, that is, the concentration that usually is sufficient to block (in addition to B fibers) A delta and C fibers, but insufficient to block A alpha, A beta, and A gamma fibers

Solution D: contains 5% procaine and is used to provide complete blockade of all fibers. Each solution is given at 5-minute intervals for appropriate patient examination with documentation of findings. The interpretation of this differential spinal anesthetic is as follows.

PSYCHOGENIC PAIN

If solution A relieves the patient's pain, the pain should tentatively be considered as "psychogenic." Between 30% and 35% of all patients with true organic pain obtain relief from an inactive agent. Relief after the normal saline solution may represent a "placebo reaction," but it also may represent a true psychogenic mechanism that is subserving the patient's pain. Clinically, these two usually can be differentiated because the placebo reaction is short lived and self-limiting, whereas pain

TABLE 3.5

Classification of Nerve Fibers on the Basis of Fiber Size (Relating Fiber Size to Fiber Function and Sensitivity to Local Anesthetics)

FIBER GROUP/ SUBGROUP	DIAMETER (μM)	CONDUCTION VELOCITY (M/S)	MODALITY SUBSERVED	SENSITIVITY TO LOCAL ANESTHETICS (%)
A (MYELINATED)				
A alpha	15-20	80-120	Large motor, proprioception	1
A beta	8-15	30-70	Small motor, touch, and pressure	↓
A gamma	4-8	30-70	Muscle spindle, reflex	
A delta	3-4	10-30	Temperature, sharp pain, nociception	0.5
B (unmyelinated)	3-4	10-15	Preganglionic autonomic	0.25
C (unmyelinated)	1-2	1-2	Dull pain, temperature, nociception	0.5

↓ Indicates intermediate values in descending order.
From Raj PP, editor: *Practical management of pain*, ed 3, St. Louis, 2000, Mosby.

TABLE 3.6

Preparation of Solutions for Conventional Sequential Differential Spinal Blockade

SOLUTION	PREPARATION OF SOLUTION	YIELD	BLOCKADE
D	To 2 mL of 10% procaine, add 2 mL of normal saline	4 mL of 5% procaine	Motor
C	To 1 mL of 5% procaine, add 9 mL of normal saline	10 mL of 0.5% procaine	Sensory
B	To 5 mL of 0.5% procaine, add 5 mL of normal saline	10 mL of 0.25% procaine	Sympathetic
A	Draw up 10 mL of normal saline	10 mL of normal saline	

From Raj PP, editor: *Practical management of pain*, ed 3, St. Louis, 2000, Mosby.

TABLE 3.7

Observations after Each Injection

SEQUENCE	OBSERVATION
1	Blood pressure and pulse rate
2	Patient's subjective evaluation of the pain at rest
3	Reproduction of patient's pain by movement
4	Signs of sympathetic block (temperature change, psychogalvanic reflex)
5	Signs of sensory block (response to pin prick)
6	Signs of motor block (inability to move toes, feet, legs)

From Raj PP, editor: *Practical management of pain*, ed 3, St. Louis, 2000, Mosby.

relief provided by an inactive agent in a patient with true psychogenic pain usually is long lasting, if not permanent.

SYMPATHETIC PAIN

If the patient does not obtain relief with the placebo dose but does obtain relief from solution B, the mechanism causing pain tentatively is classified as sympathetic, provided that concomitant with the onset of pain relief there are signs of sympathetic blockade, without signs of sensory block. Although this is the mean sympatholytic dose, in some patients (who may have an increased sensitivity for A delta and C fibers) relief may be a result of the production of hypoalgesia, analgesia, or anesthesia. The diagnosis of a sympathetic mechanism is fortunate for the patient because it may be treatable with sympathetic blocks, especially if diagnosis and treatment are started early.

SOMATIC PAIN

If 0.25% procaine (solution B) does not produce pain relief, but the 0.5% concentration (solution C) does, this usually indicates the pain is subserved by A delta and C type fibers, and the pain is classified as somatic, provided that the patient did show signs of sympathetic blockade with the previous 0.25% concentration, and the onset of pain relief is accompanied by the onset of analgesia and anesthesia. This is important because if the patient had a decreased sensitivity for B fibers, pain relief at the 0.5% concentration is from delayed sympathetic block rather than sensory block.

CENTRAL PAIN

If pain relief is not obtained by any of the preceding injections, the 5% procaine (solution D) is injected to block all fiber types. If the 5% dose gives pain relief, the mechanism is still considered somatic and it is presumed that the patient has a decreased sensitivity for A delta and C fibers. If the patient fails to obtain relief despite complete blockade, the pain is classified as "central" in origin. This is not a specific diagnosis and may indicate one of four possibilities, including (1) a central lesion, (2) psychogenic pain, (3) encephalization, or (4) malingering (see Table 3.8 for more complete information).

TABLE 3.8

Diagnostic Possibilities of Central Mechanism

DIAGNOSIS	EXPLANATION/BASIS OF DIAGNOSIS
Central lesion	The patient may have a lesion in the central nervous system that is above the level of the subarachnoid sensory block. We have seen two patients who had a metastatic lesion in the precentral gyrus, which was the central origin of the patient's peripheral pain.
Psychogenic pain	The patient may have true psychogenic pain, and it is not going to respond to any level of block. This is an even more uncommon response in patients with psychogenic pain than a positive response to placebo.
Encephalization	The patient's pain may have undergone "encephalization," a poorly understood phenomenon in which persistent, severe, agonizing pain, originally of peripheral origin, becomes self-sustaining at a central level. This usually does not occur until severe pain has been endured for a prolonged period; when it has occurred, removal or blockade of the original peripheral mechanism fails to provide relief.
Malingering	The patient may be malingering. One cannot prove or disprove this with differential blocks. If a patient is involved in litigation concerning the cause of pain and anticipates financial benefit, it is unlikely that any therapeutic modality would relieve the pain. Empirically, however, we believe that a previous placebo reaction from solution A followed by no relief from solution D strongly suggests that a patient who ultimately appears to have a central mechanism is not malingering because the placebo reaction, depending as it does on a positive motivation to obtain relief, is unlikely in a malingerer. There is no way to document the validity of this theory, but it does suggest a greater motivation to obtain pain relief than to obtain financial gain.

From Raj PP, editor: *Practical management of pain*, ed 3, St. Louis, 2000, Mosby.

Although this technique was used for many years, more recently, a "modified" technique has been used. This modified technique allows more rapid recovery of the patient and eliminates some ambiguities. Also, the spinal needle can be removed after a shorter time, which may reduce infection risk, and patient position can be changed more easily to recreate better the usual painful position for the patient.

MODIFIED TECHNIQUE

The modified technique requires only two solutions: normal saline and 5% procaine (Table 3.9). As with the conventional technique after informed consent (but being careful to avoid bias), a small-bore needle is placed into the subarachnoid space. At that time, 2 mL of normal saline is injected and the same observations are made. If the patient has no or only partial relief from the placebo injection, 2 mL of 5% procaine is injected, the needle is withdrawn, and the patient is placed supine. The same observations are made at 5-minute intervals, as outlined earlier (see Table 3.7).

INTERPRETATION

If the pain is relieved with the saline injection, the interpretation is the same as described earlier (i.e., consider the pain psychogenic). If the patient does not obtain relief with the 5% procaine, the diagnosis is considered the same as when no pain relief occurs in the conventional technique (i.e., mechanism is central). If the patient obtains complete pain relief after the 5% procaine, the pain is considered organic. If the pain returns when the patient again appreciates pinprick as sharp (recovered from analgesia), the mechanism is considered somatic (i.e., subserved by A delta or C fibers or both). If pain relief persists for a prolonged time after recovery from analgesia, the mechanism is considered sympathetic.

In our experience, the primary benefit of this procedure is to distinguish patients with psychogenic or central pain mechanisms from the group with somatic pain. It is unusual to find a sympathetic etiology in this group of patients who have had extensive evaluations and trial therapies before the current evaluation was undertaken. Identification of a patient with true psychogenic or central mechanism of pain and avoiding any further operative interventions is very advantageous to a patient who is highly likely to have a poor outcome and to the conscientious surgeon who is treating this patient. If a patient has a somatic mechanism responsible for pain, the third component to the evaluation is discography.

TABLE 3.9

Preparation of Solutions for Modified Differential Spinal Blockade

SOLUTION	PREPARATION	YIELD
D	To 1 mL of 10% procaine, add 1 mL of cerebrospinal fluid	2 mL of 5% procaine (hyperbaric)
A	Draw up 2 mL of normal saline	2 mL of normal saline

From Raj PP, editor: *Practical management of pain*, ed 3, St. Louis, 2000, Mosby.

Discography was described earlier in this chapter, and the reader is referred there for the details of the procedure (see Techniques 3.9 and 3.10). Although the technique of discography generates some controversy, the interpretation and utility of the procedure generate even more controversy. In our practice, low-pressure discography is used. To be considered positive, there must be concordant pain above a minimal threshold that is similar, if not identical, to a patient's usual axial pain. Also, there must be radiographic abnormalities with annular disruption. If the examiner determines that the patient has one or more positive discogram levels and at least one normal control level, operative treatment is offered. The type of operative treatment can be subdivided into arthrodesis or disc replacement, but even with confirmatory imaging and specific concordant discogram results, the results of surgery for axial back pain are mediocre at best. The specific procedure that best fits each patient requires careful consideration of each available option and must involve the patient substantially in the decision-making process. With regard to arthrodesis, there are multiple options, including anterior lumbar interbody, direct lateral interbody, oblique lateral interbody, posterolateral, posterior interbody, and combined anterior and posterior fusion techniques. There are a variety of stabilization alternatives involving interbody devices, pedicle screw fixation, and combinations of these strategies. The ultimate goal in each type of surgery is a solid arthrodesis. Also, the arthrodesis may use autologous iliac bone graft, which is considered the standard, although bone morphogenetic proteins (BMPs) seem to have a role. At this time, no particular approach and no particular technique of stabilization have been shown to be superior to others, and there are several good studies that show statistical equivalency between anterior lumbar interbody fusion (ALIF), posterior lumbar interbody fusion (PLIF), and posterolateral fusion with instrumentation (Fig. 3.43). Also, there has been no superiority proved for the various minimally invasive options. Likewise, there is no study showing BMP superior to autogenous bone when used posteriorly in this setting. When used with ALIF, BMP-2 has been shown to be equal to autologous bone. Long-term questions remain, however, about use of BMP-2 in women of reproductive age. The use of BMP in anterior cervical fusions has been associated with an increased incidence of complications, especially wound infections; its use in thoracolumbar and posterior cervical fusions does not seem to be associated with more complications.

At this time, there is no commercially available prosthesis for nucleoplasty, so this remains only a potential treatment. Multiple dynamic stabilization-type devices are available. There are, however, no biomechanical or clinical data to support the use of this strategy for treatment of IDD.

THORACIC/LUMBAR DISC ARTHROPLASTY (TOTAL DISC REPLACEMENT)

A technique that has garnered greater attention in the past is lumbar total disc replacement (TDR) (Fig. 3.44). The reason for the interest is the belief by many experts that this motion-preserving technique reduces adjacent motion segment degeneration, which remains problematic. There is some evidence that genetics may be more important than mechanical factors in IDD. Serious questions remain in regard to this technology, however:

1. Is motion preserved over long periods of time with TDR?
2. Does motion preservation decrease adjacent segment disease, or is this primarily determined by genetic factors?
3. What are the long-term results for TDR with issues such as wear, subsidence, or aseptic loosening?
4. What are the optimal revision strategies for TDR?

At this time, there are only three lumbar disc prostheses with FDA approval: the INMOTION, which is a modification of the Charité (DePuy Spine, Raynham, MA), the ProDisc-L (DePuy Synthes), and the activL (Aesculap, Center Valley, PA). All are approved only for single-level disc replacement. Several other lumbar disc prostheses are currently in the approval process.

The patient should be informed of the current expected or possible benefits and the current uncertainties involved with TDR. Also, from an anatomic standpoint, the condition of the facets should be essentially normal because TDR treats only one of the three joints at each motion segment. If there is significant disc space narrowing with facet overload and facet degeneration noted on CT, then TDR at this time cannot be recommended. Also, as with virtually any spine implant, the quality of the patient's bone may preclude TDR if osteoporosis is present. The specific technique for TDR is similar to ALIF in principle. The mobilization of vascular structures needs to be slightly greater, especially at the L4 disc level. Also, proper sizing of the implant to optimize surface area of contact has been shown to reduce the risk for subsidence. Proper implant position is crucial to the function and possible catastrophic failure of each device. The reader is referred to the specific technique guides for these parameters. Our experience with these devices is limited at this time, and their ultimate value for patient care has not been determined.

FAILED SPINE SURGERY

One of the greatest problems in orthopaedic surgery and neurosurgery is the treatment of failed spine surgery. Numerous reasons for the failures have been advanced. Results from repeat surgery for disc problems seem to be best with the discovery of a new problem or identification of a previously undiagnosed or untreated problem. The best results from repeat surgery have been reported to occur in patients who have experienced 6 months or more of complete pain relief after the first procedure, when leg pain exceeds back pain, and when a definite recurrent disc can be identified. Adverse factors include scarring, previous infection, repair of pseudarthrosis, and adverse psychologic factors. Satisfactory results from reoperation have been reported to be 31% to 80%, and complications have been reported to be three to five times higher than for primary surgeries. Patients should expect improvement in the severity of symptoms rather than complete relief of pain. As the frequency of repeat back surgeries increases, the chance of a satisfactory result decreases precipitously.

The recurrence or intensification of pain in the subacute or late period after disc surgery should be treated with the usual conservative methods initially. If these methods fail to relieve the pain, the patient should be completely reevaluated. Frequently, a repeat history and physical examination give some indication of the problem. Additional testing should include psychologic testing, myelography, MRI to check for tumors or a higher disc herniation, and reformatted CT scans to check for areas of foraminal stenosis or for lateral herniation. The use of the differential spinal, root blocks, facet blocks, and discograms also can help identify the source of pain. The presence of abnormal psychologic test results or an abnormal differential spinal should serve as a modifier to any suggested treatment indicated by the other testing. Satisfactory nonoperative treatment of this problem should be attempted before additional surgery is performed. A distinct, operatively correctable, anatomic problem should be identified before surgery is contemplated. Pseudarthrosis, instability, and recurrent herniations are the diagnoses most likely to respond to further operative intervention after failed

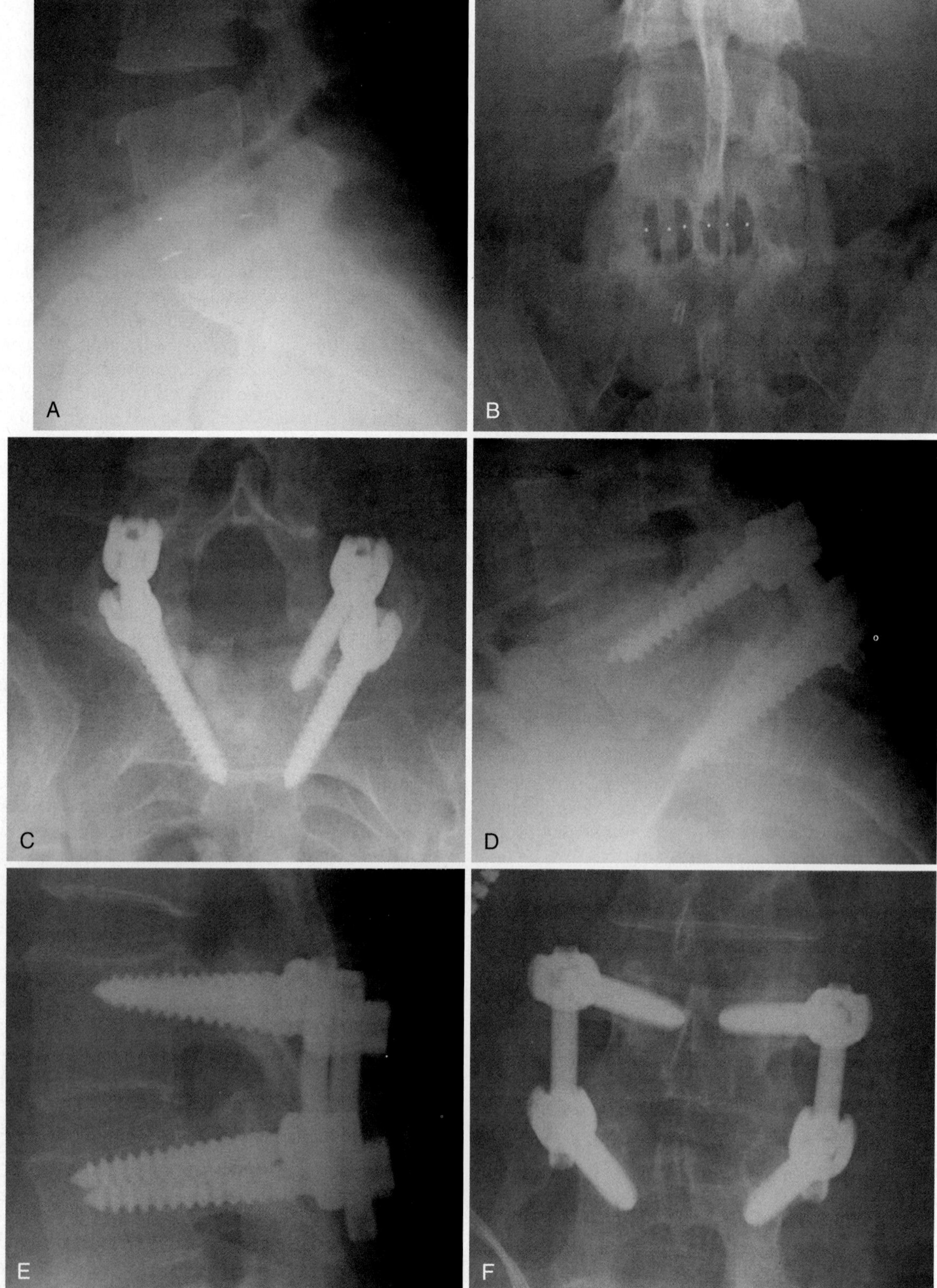

FIGURE 3.43 **A** and **B,** Solid arthrodesis after anterior lumbar antibody fusion with radiolucent threaded cages with bone morphogenetic protein type 2. **C** and **D,** Pedicle screw instrumentation with posterolateral autologous bone and transforaminal lumbar interbody fusion with allograft bone. **E** and **F,** Posterolateral fusion with autologous bone and pedicle screw instrumentation extending previous fusion.

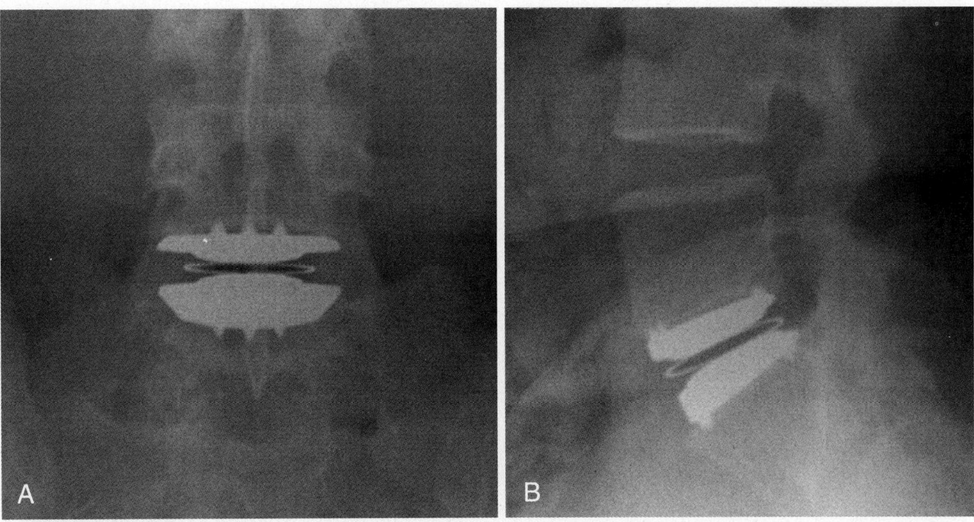

FIGURE 3.44 A and B, Anteroposterior and lateral views of patient with internal disc derangement treated with Charité total disc replacement.

spine surgery. The operative procedure should be tailored specifically to the anatomic problem identified.

STENOSIS OF THE THORACIC AND LUMBAR SPINE

Degenerative spinal stenosis is a progressive disorder that involves the entire spinal motion segment as described by Kirkaldy-Willis. Degeneration of the intervertebral disc results in initial relative instability and hypermobility of the facet joints. An increase in pressure on the facet joints with disc space narrowing and increasing angles of extension occurs and can lead to hypertrophy of the facet joint, particularly the superior articular process. As joint destruction progresses, the hypertrophic process ultimately may result in local ankylosis. Calcification and hypertrophy of the ligamentum flavum commonly are contributing factors. The end result anatomically is reduced spinal canal dimensions and compression of the neural elements. The resultant venous congestion and hypertension likely are responsible for the symptom-complex known as *intermittent neurogenic claudication.* Mild trauma and occupational activity do not seem to affect significantly the development of this disease, but they may exacerbate a preexisting condition.

ANATOMY

Spinal stenosis can be categorized according to the anatomic area of the spine affected, the region of each vertebral segment affected, and the specific pathologic entity involved (Table 3.10). Stenosis can be generalized or localized to specific anatomic areas of the cervical, thoracic, or lumbar spine. It is most common in the lumbar region, but cervical stenosis also occurs frequently. It has been rarely reported in the thoracic spine. Spinal stenosis can be localized or diffuse, affecting multiple levels, as in congenital stenosis. Degeneration of the disc occurs with disc narrowing and subsequent ligamentous redundancy, which compromises the spinal canal area. Instability may ensue. This relative hypermobility precipitates the formation of facet overgrowth and ligamentous hypertrophy. The ligamentum flavum may be markedly thickened into the lateral recess where it attaches to the facet capsule, causing nerve root compression. These phenomena occur alone or in combination to create the symptom-complex characteristic of spinal stenosis.

A description of spinal stenosis requires an understanding of the anatomy affected and the use of consistent terminology (Fig. 3.45). *Central spinal stenosis* denotes involvement of the area between the facet joints, which is occupied by the dura and its contents. Stenosis in this region usually is caused by protrusion of a disc, bulging anulus, osteophyte formation, or buckled or thickened ligamentum flavum. Symptomatic central spinal stenosis results in neurogenic claudication with generalized leg pain. Lateral to the dura is the lateral canal, which contains the nerve roots; compression in this region results in radiculopathy. The *lateral recess,* also known as "Lee's entrance zone," begins at the medial border of the superior articular process and extends to the medial border of the pedicle. This is where the nerve root exits the dura and courses distally and laterally under the superior articular facet (Fig. 3.46). The borders of the lateral recess are the pedicle laterally, the superior articular facet dorsally, the posterior ligamentous complex to disc and floor of the canal, and the central canal medially. Facet arthritis most frequently causes stenosis in this zone, along with vertebral body spurring and disc or anulus pathology. "Lee's midzone" describes the *foraminal region,* which lies ventral to the pars. Its borders are the lateral recess medially, the posterior vertebral body and disc ventrally, the pars and intertransverse ligament dorsally, and the lateral border of the pedicle laterally. The foramen is essentially the area between the cephalad and caudal pedicles. The dorsal root ganglion and ventral motor root occupy 30% of this space. This also is the point where the dura becomes confluent with the nerve root as epineurium. Causes of stenosis in this area are pars fracture with proliferative fibrocartilage or a lateral disc herniation. Thickening of the ligamentum flavum sometimes extends into the foramen and can be associated with a spur from the undersurface of the pars, especially if foraminal height is less than 15 mm and posterior intervertebral disc height is less than 4 mm. The *exit zone* is identified as the area lateral to the facet joint. The nerve root is present in this location and can be compressed by a "far lateral" disc, spondylolisthesis and associated subluxation, or facet arthritis.

TABLE 3.10

Classification of Spinal Stenosis

ANATOMIC	ANATOMIC REGION (LOCAL SEGMENT)
Cervical	Central Foraminal
Thoracic	Central Lateral recess Foraminal Extraforaminal (far-out)
PATHOLOGIC	**TYPE**
Congenital	Achondroplastic (dwarfism) Congenital forms of spondylolisthesis Scoliosis Kyphosis
Idiopathic	
Degenerative and inflammatory	Osteoarthritis Inflammatory arthritis Diffuse idiopathic skeletal hyperostosis Scoliosis Kyphosis Degenerative forms of spondylolisthesis
Metabolic	Paget disease Fluorosis

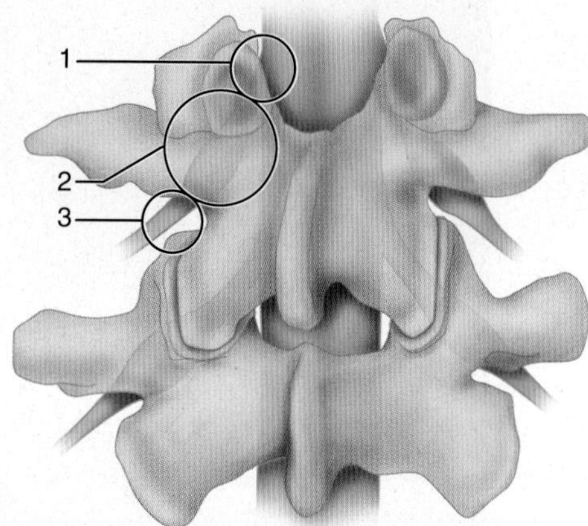

FIGURE 3.45 Zones of lateral canal as described by Lee. Entrance zone *(1)* is composed of cephalad and medial aspects of lateral recess, which begins at lateral aspect of thecal sac and runs obliquely down and laterally toward intervertebral foramen. Midzone *(2)* is located beneath pars interarticularis and just inferior to pedicle and is bound anteriorly by posterior aspect of vertebral body and posteriorly by pars; medial boundary is open to central spinal canal. Exit zone *(3)* is formed by intervertebral foramen.

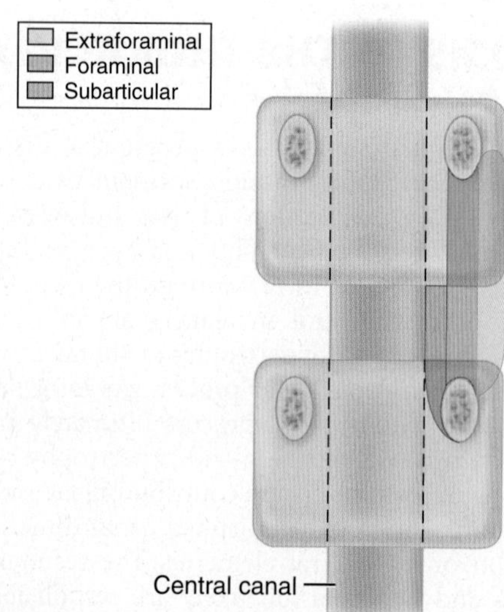

FIGURE 3.46 Central and lateral canal zones showing subarticular, foraminal, and extraforaminal divisions.

The most common type of spinal stenosis is caused by degenerative arthritis of the spine, including Forestier disease, and is characterized by hyperostosis and spinal rigidity in elderly patients. Other processes, such as Paget disease, fluorosis, kyphosis, scoliosis, and fracture with canal narrowing, may result in spinal stenosis. Hypertrophy and ossification of the posterior longitudinal ligament, which usually are confined to the cervical spine, and diffuse idiopathic skeletal hyperostosis (DISH) syndrome also may result in an acquired form of spinal stenosis. Congenital forms caused by disorders such as achondroplasia and dysplastic spondylolisthesis are much less common.

Congenital spinal stenosis usually is central and is evident on imaging studies. Idiopathic congenital narrowing usually involves the anteroposterior dimension of the canal secondary to short pedicles; the patient otherwise is normal. In contrast, in achondroplasia the canal is narrowed in the anteroposterior plane owing to shortened pedicles and in lateral diameter because of diminished interpedicular distance. These findings occur in addition to the other characteristic features of achondroplasia.

Acquired forms of spinal stenosis usually are degenerative (Box 3.6). This process is most commonly localized to the facet joints and ligamentum flavum, with the resultant arthritic changes in the joints visible on radiographic studies. Frequently, these abnormalities are symmetric bilaterally. The L4-5 level is the most commonly involved, followed by L5-S1 and L3-4. Disc herniation and spondylolisthesis may exacerbate the narrowing further. Spondylolisthesis and spondylolysis rarely cause spinal stenosis in young patients. The combination of degenerative change, aging, and spondylolisthesis or spondylolysis in patients 50 years old or older frequently results in lateral recess or foraminal stenosis. Paget disease and fluorosis have been reported to result in central or lateral spinal stenosis. Paget disease is one form of spinal stenosis that responds well to medical treatment with calcitonin.

NATURAL HISTORY

Although symptoms may arise from narrowing of the spinal canal, not all patients with narrowing develop symptoms. One study found no significant association between clinical symptoms and anteroposterior spinal canal diameter. In general, the natural history of most forms of spinal stenosis is the insidious development of symptoms. Occasionally, there can be an acute onset of symptoms precipitated by trauma or heavy activity. Many patients have significant radiographic findings

BOX 3.6

Types of Spinal Stenosis

Congenital
Idiopathic
Achondroplastic

Acquired
Degenerative
- Central canal
- Lateral recess, foramen
- Degenerative spondylolisthesis
- Degenerative scoliosis
- Combination of congenital and degenerative stenosis

Iatrogenic
- Postlaminectomy
- Postfusion
- Postchemonucleolysis
- Spondylolytic
- Posttraumatic

Miscellaneous
- Paget disease
- Fluorosis
- Diffuse idiopathic skeletal hyperostosis syndrome
- Hyperostotic lumbar spinal stenosis
- Oxalosis
- Pseudogout

with minimal complaints or physical findings. About 50% of patients treated nonoperatively report improved back and leg pain after 8 to 10 years, although functional ability after decompressive surgery has been shown in multiple studies to surpass that obtained after nonoperative treatment. A prospective, randomized study of 100 patients with symptomatic spinal stenosis treated operatively or nonoperatively found that pain relief occurred after 3 months in most patients regardless of treatment, although it took 12 months in a few patients. Results in patients treated nonoperatively deteriorated over time; however, at 4 years they were excellent or fair in 50%; 80% of patients treated operatively had good results at 4 years.

Reported studies suggest that for most patients with spinal stenosis, a stable course can be predicted, with 15% to 50% showing some improvement with nonoperative treatment. Worsening of symptoms despite adequate conservative treatment is an indication for operative treatment. Weinstein et al. showed significantly more improvement in all primary outcomes in patients treated operatively compared with those treated nonoperatively.

CLINICAL EVALUATION

In patients with spinal stenosis, symptoms include back pain (95%), sciatica (91%), sensory disturbance in the legs (70%), motor weakness (33%), and urinary disturbance (12%). In patients with central spinal stenosis, symptoms usually are bilateral and involve the buttocks and posterior thighs in a nondermatomal distribution. With lateral recess stenosis, symptoms usually are dermatomal because they are related to a specific nerve being compressed. Patients with lateral recess stenosis may have more pain during rest and at night but more walking tolerance than patients with central stenosis.

Differentiation of symptoms of vascular claudication from symptoms of neurogenic claudication is important (Table 3.11). Vascular symptoms typically are felt in the upper calf, are relieved after a short rest (5 minutes) while still standing, do not require sitting or bending, and worsen despite walking uphill or riding a stationary bicycle. Neurogenic claudication improves with trunk flexion, stooping, or lying but may require 20 minutes to improve. Patients often report better endurance walking uphill or up steps and tolerate riding a bicycle better than walking on a treadmill because of the flexed posture that occurs. Pushing a grocery cart also allows spinal flexion, which enhances endurance and decreases discomfort in most patients with neurogenic claudication (positive "shopping cart" sign).

Generally, physical findings with all forms of spinal stenosis are inconsistent. Distal pulses should be felt and confirmed to be strong, and internal and external rotation of the hips in extension should be full, symmetric, and painless. Straight-leg raising and sciatic tension tests usually are normal. The neurologic examination usually is normal, but some abnormality may be detected if the patient is allowed to walk to the limit of pain and is then reexamined. The gait and posture after walking may reveal a positive "stoop test." This test is done by asking the patient to walk briskly. As the pain intensifies, the patient may complain of sensory symptoms followed by motor symptoms. If the patient is asked to continue to walk, he or she may assume a stooped posture and the symptoms may be eased, or if the patient sits in a chair bent forward, the same resolution of symptoms occurs.

DIAGNOSTIC IMAGING

RADIOGRAPHY

Although plain radiography cannot confirm spinal stenosis, findings such as short pedicles on the lateral view, narrowing between the pedicles on the anteroposterior view, ligament ossification, narrowing of the foramen, and hypertrophy of the posterior articular facets can be helpful hints. Leroux et al. outlined hypertrophic radiographic changes associated with hyperostosis on plain tomography and CT (Box 3.7).

The radiographic identification and confirmation of lumbar spinal stenosis have improved with the development of new imaging techniques. Initially, only central spinal stenosis was recognized, with canal narrowing to 10 mm considered absolute stenosis. This could be measured using radiographs or, preferably, myelography. Schönström, Bolender, and Spengler compared two methods of identifying central spinal stenosis: (1) anteroposterior canal measurement by CT and (2) measurement of the dural sac with myelography in patients undergoing surgery for spinal stenosis. They found no correlation between the transverse area of the bony canal in normal patients and patients with spinal stenosis. A dural sac transverse area of 100 mm^2 or less correlated with symptomatic spinal stenosis. This method allows the inclusion of soft tissue in the determination of spinal stenosis. The analysis of this area can be calculated relatively easily using standard CT software.

Currently, axial imaging has supplanted standard radiographs in the diagnosis of spinal stenosis, although radiographs are important in the initial evaluation of patients with persistent pain of more than 6 weeks' duration or of patients with "red flags" of other disease, including recent trauma, history of cancer, immunosuppression, age older than 50 years or younger than 20 years, neurologic deficit, or previous surgery.

TABLE 3.11

Differentiation of Symptoms of Vascular Claudication From Symptoms of Neurogenic Claudication

EVALUATION	VASCULAR	NEUROGENIC
Walking distance	Fixed	Variable
Palliative factors	Standing	Sitting/bending
Provocative factors	Walking	Walking/standing
Walking uphill	Painful	Painless
Bicycle test	Positive (painful)	Negative
Pulses	Absent	Present
Skin	Loss of hair; shiny	Normal
Weakness	Rarely	Occasionally
Back pain	Occasionally	Commonly
Back motion	Normal	Limited
Pain character	Cramping—distal to proximal	Numbness, aching—proximal to distal
Atrophy	Uncommon	Occasional

Flexion and extension views are useful to identify preexisting instability before laminectomy and may be useful in determining the need for subsequent fusion. Translation of 4 mm or more or rotation of more than 10 to 15 degrees indicates instability. A reversal of the normal trapezoidal disc geometry with widening posteriorly and narrowing anteriorly also may indicate instability.

MAGNETIC RESONANCE IMAGING

MRI is helpful in identifying disease processes, such as tumors and infections, and is a good noninvasive study for patients with persistent lower extremity complaints after radiographic screening evaluation. MRI should be confirmatory in patients with a consistent history of neurogenic claudication or radiculopathy, but it should not be used as a screening examination because of the high rate of asymptomatic disease. Morphologic changes have been correlated with preoperative findings, such as pain and function, however, only to a limited extent. Sagittal T2-weighted MR images are a good starting point because they give a myelogram-like image. Sagittal T1-weighted images are evaluated with particular attention focused on the foramen. An absence of normal fat around the root indicates foraminal stenosis. Axial images provide a good view of the central spinal canal and its contents on T1- and T2-weighted images. Far lateral disc protrusions are identified on axial T1-weighted images by obliteration of the normal interval of fat between the disc and nerve root (Fig. 3.47). The foraminal zone is better evaluated with sagittal T1-weighted sequences, which illustrates the presence of fat around the nerve root. Foraminal disc herniations should be confirmed on both sagittal and axial MRI images. Absolute anatomic measures also can be used, as previously discussed. Spinal deformity, including scoliosis and significant spondylolisthesis, can result in suboptimal imaging by MRI. This is secondary to the curvature of the spine in and out of the plane of the scanner on sagittal sequences and difficulty obtaining true axial cuts. Another disadvantage of MRI is the cost; nonetheless, MRI has become a useful, noninvasive diagnostic tool for the evaluation of patients with extremity complaints.

BOX 3.7

Hypertrophic Radiographic Changes Associated With Hyperostosis

Plain Radiographs

Dorsal Level

1. Intervertebral osseous bridge
2. "Lobster claw"

Cervical Level

1. Exuberant osteophytosis
2. Narrow cervical canal

Lumbar Level

1. Marginal somatic osseous proliferation
2. "Candle flame"
3. "Lobster claw"
4. Intervertebral osseous bridge
5. Disc arthrosis
6. Acquired vertebral block
7. Hypertrophy of posterior articular processes
8. "Bulb" appearance of posterior articular hypertrophy
9. Anterior subluxation
10. Posterior subluxation

Lumbar Computed Tomography

1. Herniated disc
2. Disc protrusion
3. Vacuum disc sign
4. Hypertrophy of posterior articular processes
5. Osteoarthritis of apophyseal joints
6. Osseous proliferations of nonarticular aspects of superior apophyseal joint
7. Osseous proliferations of nonarticular aspects of inferior apophyseal joint
8. C/O of posterior longitudinal ligament
9. C/O of yellow ligament
10. C/O of supraspinal ligament
11. Anterior C/O of posterior articular capsule
12. Posterior C/O of posterior articular capsule
13. Anteroposterior diameter of spinal canal
14. Transverse diameters of spinal canal

C/O, Calcification or ossification or both.
Modified from Leroux JL, Legeron P, Moulinier L, et al: Stenosis of the lumbar spinal canal in vertebral ankylosing hyperostosis, *Spine* 17:1213–1218, 1992.

COMPUTED TOMOGRAPHIC MYELOGRAPHY

Despite the prevalence of MRI, myelography followed by CT is still accepted and widely used for operative planning in patients with spinal stenosis; it has a diagnostic accuracy of 91% but also involves significant radiation exposure. The addition of CT after a myelogram allows detection of 30% more abnormalities than with myelography alone. Because of the dynamic nature of the study, stenosis not visible on MRI with the patient recumbent may be identified on standing flexion and extension lateral views. CT after myelography

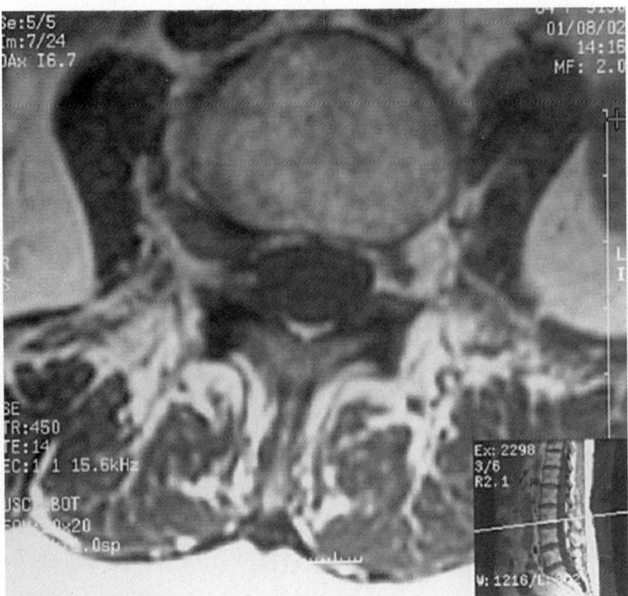

FIGURE 3.47 T1-weighted MR image showing far-lateral disc protrusion. Note obliteration of normal interval of fat between disc and root.

characterizes the bony anatomy better than MRI, which helps the surgeon plan decompression surgery. However, imaging of the nerve roots in the foraminal region lateral to the pedicle is impossible because of the confluence of the dura with the epineurium at this point. There also is additional morbidity associated with the lumbar puncture required for myelography as well as radiation exposure. Myelography followed by CT is best suited for patients with dynamic stenosis, postoperative leg pain, severe scoliosis or spondylolisthesis, metallic implants, contraindications to MRI, and lower extremity symptoms in the absence of findings on MRI.

Abnormal findings occur in 24% to 34% of asymptomatic individuals evaluated with CT myelography, just as with MRI, so clinical correlation is a must.

CT has been used to further define lateral recess stenosis and foraminal stenosis. These types of stenosis rarely are identified with myelography. The lateral recess is anatomically the area bordered laterally by the pedicle, posteriorly by the superior articular facet, and anteriorly by the posterolateral surface of the vertebral body and the adjacent intervertebral disc. The superior border of the corresponding pedicle is the narrowest portion of the lateral recess. Measurement of the recess in this area using the tomographic cross-section usually is 5 mm or greater in normal patients, but in symptomatic patients the diagnosis is confirmed if the height is 2 mm or less. The foramen is the area of the spine bordered by the inferior edge of the pedicle cephalad, the pars interarticularis with the associated inferior articular facet and the superior articular facet from the lower segment posteriorly, the superior edge of the pedicle of the next lower vertebra caudally, and the vertebral body and disc anteriorly. This area rarely can be seen with myelography. A standard CT in the cross-sectional mode suggests narrowing if the foraminal space immediately after the pedicle cut is present for only one or two more cuts (provided that the cuts are close together). The best way to appreciate foraminal narrowing is to reformat the lumbar scan, which can create sagittal views through the pedicles and structures situated laterally.

Wiltse et al. described a far-out compression of the root that occurs predominantly in spondylolisthesis when the root is compressed by a large L5 transverse process subluxed below the root and pressing the root against the ala of the sacrum. This "far our syndrome" is best confirmed with a reformatted CT scan with coronal cuts (Fig. 3.48).

Some studies have attempted to correlate clinical outcomes with pathologic findings on myelography and CT. A retrospective review found that patients who had a block on myelogram had a better chance of obtaining a good outcome. Another study confirmed postoperative stenosis in 64% of 191 patients at 4-year follow-up. Slight differences were noted in the Oswestry questionnaire between patients with and without stenosis but not in walking distances, and instability was present in 21% without demonstrable clinical effect. The degree of decompression on CT myelography did not correlate at all with outcomes, and regardless of the number of levels that had decompression, the results were similar. Nonetheless, decompression of all symptomatic levels with evidence of compression is recommended to enhance neural circulation and function and to avoid reoperation for recurrent spinal stenosis.

■ OTHER DIAGNOSTIC STUDIES

Electrodiagnostic studies should be used if the diagnosis of neuropathy is uncertain, especially in patients with diabetes mellitus. Needle electromyographic study was shown to have a lower false-positive rate than MRI in asymptomatic patients. The diagnostic use of such studies, including somatosensory evoked potentials, is limited by the lack of prospective studies to determine sensitivity or specificity. Vascular Doppler examinations are useful to identify inflow problems into the lower extremities and should be accompanied by a vascular surgery consultation when indicated. Differential diagnosis also can be aided by the use of exercise testing. Tenhula et al. described a bicycle-treadmill test that stresses the patient in an upright position on an exercise treadmill and subsequently in a seated position on an exercise bicycle that allows spinal flexion. Earlier onset of leg symptoms with level walking and delayed onset of symptoms with inclined treadmill walking were significantly associated with stenosis. Exercise treadmill testing also is useful to help determine baseline function for quantitative evaluation of functional status after surgery. This study showed significant postoperative improvement in treadmill walking and bicycling duration (88% preoperatively and 9% postoperatively for walking; 41% preoperatively and 17% postoperatively for bicycling), lower visual analogue scale pain scores, and a later onset of pain.

NONOPERATIVE TREATMENT

Symptoms of spinal stenosis usually respond favorably to nonoperative management (satisfactory results in 69% at 3 years according to Simotas et al.). Despite symptoms of back pain, radiculopathy, or neurogenic claudication, conservative management is successful in most patients. Patients with radicular type pain respond well to nonoperative treatment, but those with scoliosis tend to have worse results. Conservative measures should include rest not exceeding 2 days, pain management with antiinflammatory medications or acetaminophen, and participation in a trunk-stabilization exercise program,

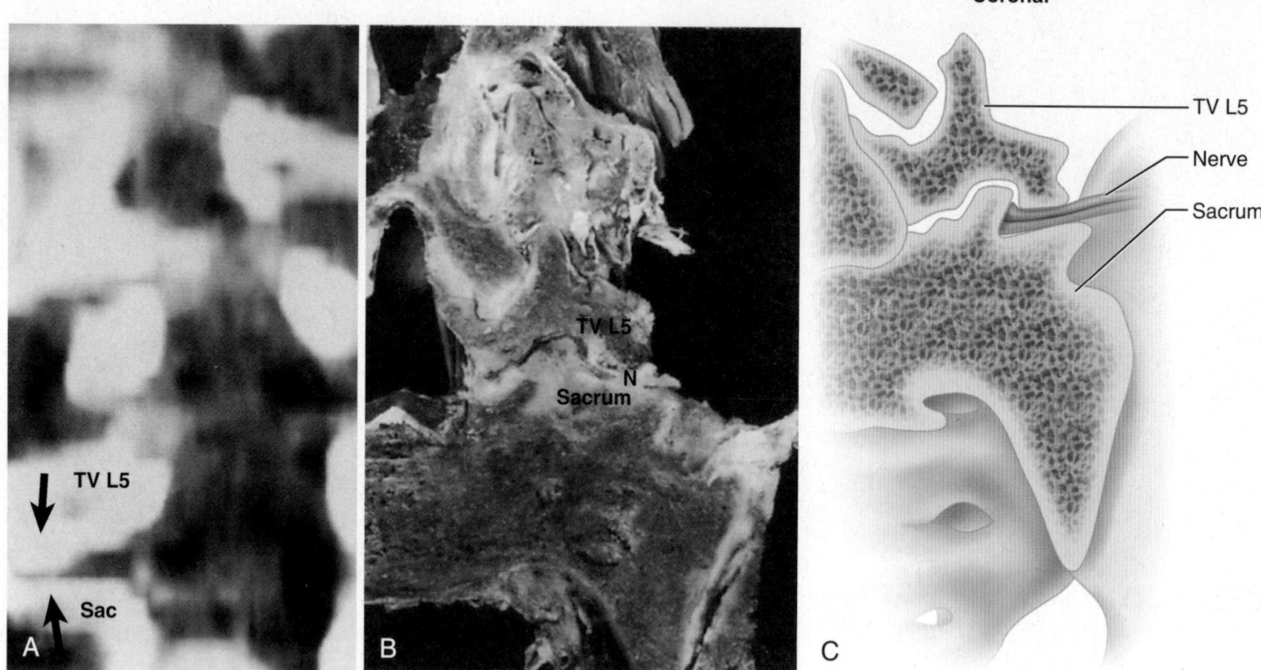

FIGURE 3.48 **A,** Coronal view of CT scan showing impingement of transverse process of L5 on sacrum. **B,** Coronal section showing right transverse process. **C,** Drawing of coronal section. (From Wiltse LL, Guyer RD, Spencer CW, et al: Alar transverse process impingement of the L5 spinal nerve: the far-out syndrome, *Spine* 9:31–41, 1984.)

along with good aerobic fitness. Other methods should be reserved for patients who are limited by pain and should be used to maximize participation in the exercise program. Traction has no proven benefit in the adult lumbar spine. For a patient with unremitting symptoms of radiculopathy or neurogenic claudication, epidural steroid injections may be useful in alleviating symptoms to allow better participation in physical therapy. Epidural steroids can give significant symptomatic relief, although no scientific study has documented long-term efficacy.

Manchikanti et al. reported significant pain relief in 76% of 25 patients who had percutaneous adhesiolysis with injection of lidocaine, hypertonic sodium chloride solution, and nonparticulate betamethasone. If spinal stenosis is present with coexistent degenerative arthritis in the hips or knees, some permanent limitation in activity may be necessary regardless of treatment.

EPIDURAL STEROID INJECTION

Spinal stenosis and the resultant mechanical compression of neural elements can cause structural and chemical injury to the nerve roots. Edema and venous congestion of the nerve roots can lead to further compression and ischemic neuritis. This may result in the leakage of neurotoxins, such as phospholipase and leukotriene B, which can lead to increased inflammation and edema. Steroids are potent antiinflammatory medications and result in a decrease in leukocyte migration, the inhibition of cytokines, and membrane stabilization. These actions coupled with their ability to reduce edema provide the rationale for the use of epidural steroid injections in spinal stenosis. Epidural steroid injections have been used in the treatment of spinal stenosis for many years, and no validated long-term outcomes have been reported to substantiate their use. Significant improvement in pain scores, however, has been reported at 3 months. Patients with a healthier emotional status and those with a higher body mass index reportedly experience more pain relief. A prospective, randomized study found caudal epidural injections (lidocaine 0.5%) with or without steroids to be effective in approximately 60% of patients in the short term.

The technique of placement—caudal, translaminar, or transforaminal—also is debated, as is whether fluoroscopy should be used. Lee et al. reported improvement in 87.5% of 216 patients using fluoroscopically guided caudal epidural steroid injection; however, they included minimal improvement in these results. Although one study reported no difference between interlaminar and transforaminal injection, Lee et al. noted that bilateral transforaminal epidural injection allowed delivery of a higher concentration of injectate. Using anatomic landmarks for caudal injections, Stitz et al. reported accurate placement in 65% to 74% of patients, with intravascular placement in 4%. Accurate placement of translaminar injections seems to be equally difficult, with successful placement reported in 70%.

Spinal canal dimension has not been shown to be predictive of success or failure of epidural steroid injection. Complications are infrequent but can occur and include hypercorticism, epidural hematoma, temporary paralysis, retinal hemorrhage, epidural abscess, chemical meningitis, and intracranial air. A 5% incidence of dural puncture has been reported, and, if it occurs, subarachnoid injection of steroids or local anesthetic should be avoided to prevent mechanical or chemical nerve root irritation. Headaches occur in 1% to 5% of patients and are related to dural puncture or the use of the caudal injection route. In patients with headaches associated with caudal injections, the cause has not been determined because dural puncture should not occur at this level, because the dural sleeve has terminated at midsacrum.

The ideal candidate for epidural steroid injection seems to be a patient who has acute radicular symptoms or neurogenic claudication unresponsive to traditional analgesics and rest, with significant impairment in activities of daily living. We have used this technique successfully in our treatment algorithm for neurogenic claudication and radiculopathy both as a diagnostic and therapeutic procedure. The authors prefer transforaminal injections because they allow more ventral placement of injectate in the foramen and lateral recess and also seem to reasonably predict surgical outcomes at the same anatomic level.

OPERATIVE TREATMENT

The primary indication for surgery in patients with spinal stenosis is increasing pain that is resistant to conservative measures. Because the primary complaint often is back pain and some leg pain, pain relief after surgery may not be complete. Operative intervention should be expected to give good relief of claudicatory leg pain with variable response to back pain. Most series report a 64% to 91% rate of improvement, with 42% in patients with diabetes, but most patients still have some minor complaints, usually referable to the preexisting degenerative arthritis of the spine. Neurologic findings, if present, improve inconsistently after surgery. Pearson et al. noted that patients whose predominant complaint was leg pain improved significantly more with operative treatment than those whose predominant complaint was low back pain. Both, however, improved significantly with operative treatment compared with conservative treatment. Reoperation rates vary from 6% to 23%. Prognostic factors include better results with a disc herniation, stenosis at a single level, weakness of less than 6 weeks' duration, monoradiculopathy, and age younger than 65 years. Depression, psychiatric disease, cardiovascular disease, higher body mass index, scoliosis, and disorders affecting ambulation have been associated with a poorer prognosis. Reversal of neurologic consequences of spinal stenosis seems to be a relative indication for surgery unless the symptoms are acute.

Radiographic findings alone are never an indication for surgery. Factors predicting outcome vary, and correlation of imaging with symptoms seems to be the best guarantee of improvement after surgery. Localized lesions on radiograph without general involvement respond best. Ganz reported a 96% success rate in patients whose preoperative symptoms were relieved by postural change.

A patient's inability to tolerate the restricted lifestyle necessitated by the disease and the failure of a good conservative treatment regimen should be the primary determining factors for surgery in a well-informed patient. The patient should understand the potential for the operation to fail to relieve pain or to worsen it, especially in regard to the axial component of the symptoms. In addition to the general risks of spinal surgery, the severity of symptoms and lifestyle modifications should be considered. Lumbar spinal stenosis does not result in paralysis, only decreased ambulatory capacity, and conservative management is warranted indefinitely in a patient with good function and manageable symptoms. Delaying surgical treatment for a trial of nonoperative treatment has not been shown to affect outcome; however, one study reported less favorable results in patients who had symptoms for more than 33 months.

Cervical and thoracic spinal stenoses are associated with painless paralysis in the form of cervical and thoracic myelopathy and require closer attention and follow-up.

PRINCIPLES OF SPINAL STENOSIS SURGERY

Decompression by laminectomy or a fenestration procedure is the treatment of choice for lumbar spinal stenosis (Fig. 3.49). Fusion is required if excessive bony resection compromises stability or if isthmic or degenerative spondylolisthesis, scoliosis, or kyphosis is present. Other important indications for fusion include adjacent segment degeneration after prior fusion and recurrent stenosis or herniated disc after decompression. Laminectomy may be preferable in older patients with severe, multilevel stenosis, whereas fenestration procedures, consisting of bilateral laminotomies and partial facetectomies that preserve the midline structures, are an alternative in younger patients with intact discs. This is an especially attractive procedure when performed through a minimally invasive approach because injury to the dynamic spinal stabilizers is minimized. In one study, fewer complications and less postoperative instability were reported after bilateral laminotomies than after laminectomy.

Whenever possible, the source of pain should be localized with selective root blocks preoperatively to allow a more focal decompression. At surgery, specific attention should be directed to the symptomatic area, which may result in less extensive decompression than would normally be done with the pain source unconfirmed. If radical decompression of only one root is necessary, additional stabilization by fusion with or without instrumentation is usually unnecessary. The removal of more than one complete facet joint may require instrumented fusion. It is advisable to prepare the patient for fusion in case the findings at surgery require a more radical approach than anticipated. When both an ipsilateral lateral recess decompression and foraminal decompressions are necessary, a transforaminal lumbar interbody fusion (TLIF) can be used without risking subsequent instability at the level. Positioning the patient with the abdomen hanging free minimizes bleeding. If fusion is likely, the hips should remain extended to prevent positional kyphosis. We do not recommend the use of a kyphosing frame when a fusion is performed. As in disc surgery, a microscope or magnifying loupes and a headlamp are helpful. The microscope allows for a smaller incision with less damage while maintaining binocular vision and depth perception caused by the smaller interocular distance of the microscope. When proceeding with the decompression, care should be taken to watch for adhesions that can result in dural tears, even if no previous surgery has been done. Frequently, the narrowing in the lateral recess and foramen is so great that a Kerrison rongeur cannot be used without damaging the root. Alternatively, dissection in the lateral recess and foramen may require a small, sharp osteotome or a high-speed burr, which allows the surgeon to thin the bone sufficiently to allow removal with angled curets. In contrast to disc surgery, for decompression the lateral recess is best seen from the opposite side of the table. During open procedures, the operating surgeon may find it necessary to switch sides during the operation to view the pathology and nerve roots better. Blunt probes with increasing diameters also are useful for determining adequate foraminal enlargement. Disc herniation should be treated at the same time as the spinal stenosis. A good approach is to start the decompression at a point of lesser stenosis and work toward the area of most severe stenosis. This often frees the neural structures enough to make the final decompression simpler and decreases the risk of damage to dura or nerve roots. This approach is especially useful when a minimally invasive undercutting laminoplasty technique is used to operatively treat spinal stenosis.

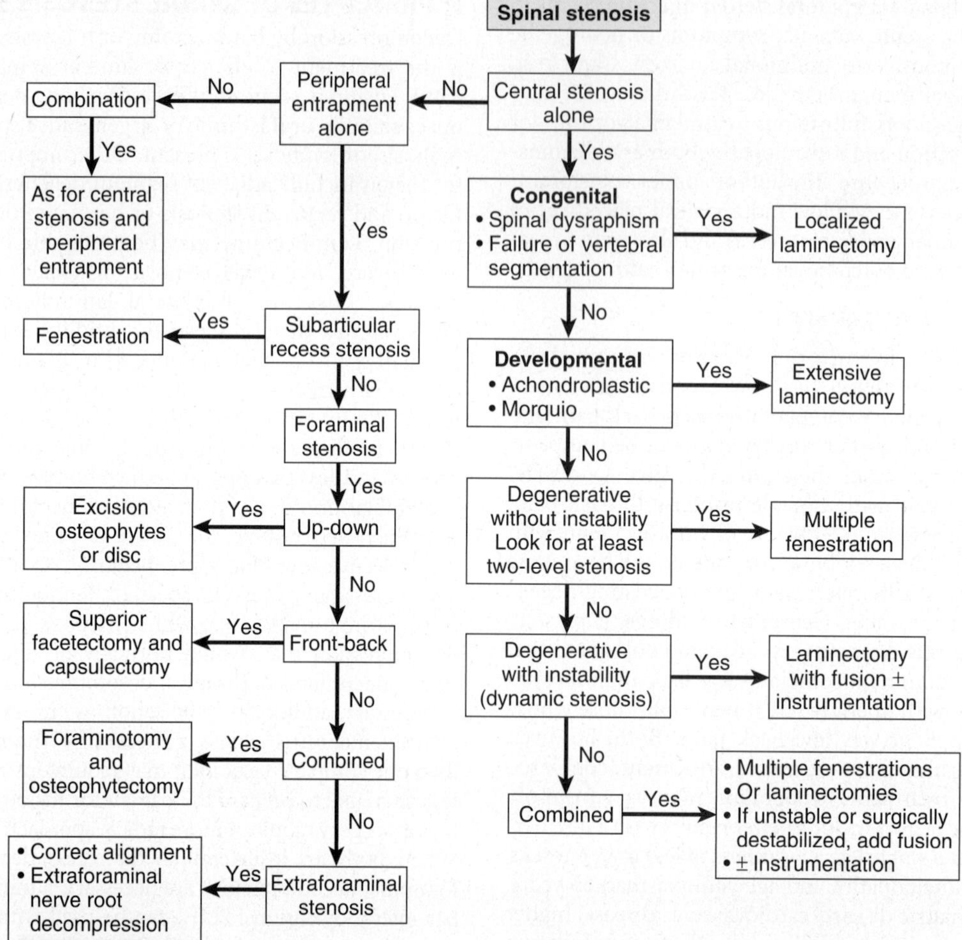

FIGURE 3.49 **Algorithm for treatment of spinal stenosis.** (From Hadjipavlou AG, Simmons JW, Pope MH: An algorithmic approach to the investigation, treatment, and complications of surgery for low back pain, *Semin Spine Surg* 10:193, 1998.)

ADJACENT SEGMENT DEGENERATION

Adjacent disc degeneration and stenosis, or the transition syndrome, deserves special mention. It is known that disc degeneration occurs adjacent to a fusion in 35% to 45% of patients because of the ensuing hypermobility of the unfused joint, usually above the fusion mass. Adjacent segment stenosis below the fusion mass, although less frequent, always occurred along with stenosis above the fusion in a study by Lehmann et al.

Adjacent segment breakdown may cause symptoms that require surgery in 30% of patients. Pathology, including spinal stenosis, herniated nucleus pulposus, and instability, may require treatment years after successful surgery. Breakdown is possible one or two levels above lumbosacral fusions and above or below thoracolumbar and "floating" lumbar fusions. Schlegel et al. reported 58 patients who developed spinal stenosis, disc herniation, or instability at a segment adjacent to a previously asymptomatic fusion that was done an average of 13.1 years earlier, although 70% had good or excellent results. These clinical findings have been substantiated by subsequent biomechanical studies that confirmed kinematic changes in segments adjacent to spinal fusions. Simple malalignment that occurs during patient positioning when the hips are not extended may result in hypolordosis and increase the load across implants and increase posterior shear and laminar strain at adjacent levels. These changes may help to explain the cause of adjacent segment breakdown. Posterior lumbar interbody fusion (PLIF) also resulted in adjacent segment changes in all patients, but this did not affect results at 5 years in the series of Miyakoshi et al. In a study comparing patients with spondylolytic spondylolisthesis, degenerative spondylolisthesis, and spinal stenosis, Yu et al. found no significant differences in superior adjacent segment degeneration, instability, or clinical outcome after partial or total laminectomy and single-level PLIF.

Rigidity of instrumentation has been hypothesized to correlate with motion at adjacent segments. Studies have fueled interest in less rigid and dynamic stabilization constructs. In a prospective study with 4-year radiographic follow-up comparing rigid, semirigid, and dynamic instrumentation devices, Korovessis et al. found no differences in adjacent segment degeneration among the three groups. It is undetermined whether more rigid fusion increases the likelihood of adjacent segment changes. There is some evidence that maintaining the function of the posterior dynamic stabilizing paraspinous musculature, including the multifidus, may lead to decreased rates of adjacent segment degeneration after lumbar fusion.

Fusion is more difficult as the number of levels fused increases, with L4-5 being the most frequent site of pseudarthrosis. The addition of a second level of fusion should be avoided if possible, and fusing a degenerative disc as a prophylactic measure does not seem to be supported by the data available. The actual source of transition syndromes is unknown; however, postoperative hypolordosis and rigidity of the fused segment probably contribute to the problem along with disruption of the posterior dynamic muscular stabilizers damaged during open posterior approaches. Surgery should attempt to maintain normal segmental lordosis and global sagittal balance, in addition to fusing the fewest segments possible while minimizing collateral damage to the paraspinous musculature and lumbodorsal fascia.

Complications are relatively infrequent after decompression for spinal stenosis and occur more often in patients with multiple comorbid conditions, especially diabetes. Comorbidities also contribute to poorer patient satisfaction and increased operative complications. Previous reports have cited increased morbidity and mortality associated with stenosis surgery in the elderly, although one study found that advanced age did not decrease patient satisfaction or return to activities, and there was no increase in morbidity associated with surgery for stenosis in the elderly.

Deep venous thrombosis also must be considered in patients after decompression. The incidence of this complication varies but is likely higher than reported. Pulmonary emboli are exceedingly rare, however. Prophylaxis is best limited to pneumatic compression devices of the foot or calf and early ambulation because the risk of epidural hematoma from pharmacologic agents is greater than the risk of a significant pulmonary event or deep venous thrombosis. Reoperation is necessary in 9% to 23% of patients with spinal stenosis.

DECOMPRESSION

There are no universal indicators of outcome after decompression. The number of levels requiring decompression have not been shown to affect the surgical results. Factors associated with poorer outcomes have included questionable radiographic confirmation of stenosis, female sex, litigation, previous failed surgery, and the presence of spondylolisthesis. A patient's self- assessment of health may be the best predictor of satisfaction. Cardiac comorbidity also may be predictive. Yukawa et al. found that the severity of central canal narrowing at a single level did not affect postoperative improvement in either functional ability, as determined by treadmill and bicycle testing, or patient self-assessment. Patients with multilevel stenosis had similar improvements in postoperative assessment scores.

Jönsson reported successful results after operative treatment in 62% to 67% of patients, although they noted deterioration at 5 years, with 18% requiring reoperation. Patients with a 6-mm or less anteroposterior canal diameter preoperatively had better results. Patients with hip arthritis, diabetes mellitus, previous surgery, vertebral fracture, or a postoperative complication had worse results. Although most are satisfied with the results of decompression, continued severe back pain and the inability to walk a distance have been reported. The Maine Lumbar Spine Group found that long-term (8 to 10 years) results were better after operative than nonoperative treatment. However, approximately half of the patients reported improvement in their back pain, leg pain, or both and were satisfied with their current status regardless of whether they were treated operatively or nonoperatively.

The cost of spinal stenosis surgery (decompressive laminectomy) at 2 years compared favorably with other treatment modalities in one SPORT study.

Progressive instability after decompression does not predict poor results. It appears that normal walking, sensory deficits, and ability to perform activities of daily living improved despite instability. Some further anterolisthesis is tolerated well after decompression, and it is appropriate to observe these patients for further symptoms before recommending fusion because 30% of patients develop anterolisthesis after decompression.

MIDLINE DECOMPRESSION (NEURAL ARCH RESECTION)

TECHNIQUE 3.29

- Perform the procedure with the patient under general endotracheal anesthesia. Position the patient prone using the frame of choice.
- Make the incision in the midline centered over the level of stenosis. Localizing radiographs should be taken to verify the level of surgery. Carry the incision in the midline to the fascia.
- Strip the fascia and muscle subperiosteally from the spinous processes and laminae to the facet joints to expose the pars interarticularis. Avoid damaging facet joints that are not involved in the bony dissection.
- Identify and remove the spinous processes of the levels to be decompressed. Clear the soft tissue with a sharp curet.
- Remove the lamina with a Kerrison rongeur or high-speed burr up to the insertion of the ligamentum flavum. If the lamina is extremely thick, a high-speed drill with a diamond or side-cutting burr can be used to thin the outer cortex to allow easier removal of the inner portion with a Kerrison rongeur. The lamina can be removed with impunity up to the insertion of the ligamentum flavum. Once the ligamentum insertion is identified, the ligamentum can be detached from the lamina with a curet. Take special care in removal of the lamina after the ligamentum flavum is released. The neural structures will be found compressed, and the usual space for instrument insertion may be unavailable. Remove the lamina until the pedicles can be felt. It can be helpful to begin the lateral recess decompression with the high-speed burr before removal of the ligamentum flavum to avoid having to place a rongeur into an already stenotic canal.
- Using the pedicle as a guide, identify the nerve root and trace it out to the foramen.
- With a chisel or rongeur, carefully remove the medial portion of the superior facet that forms the upper portion of the lateral recess (Fig. 3.50). Check the foramen for patency with an angled dural elevator or graduated probes. If there is further restriction, carry the dissection laterally and open the foramen; do not remove more than half of the pars. Undercutting into the foramen is especially helpful in this regard.

- Inspect the disc and remove gross herniations unilaterally, but try to avoid bilateral annulotomy because this compromises stability. Usually the disc is bulging, and the anulus is firm. Remove the anulus and bony ridge ventrally if it is kinking the nerve. This procedure involves some risk of nerve injury and requires a bloodless field. If safety is a concern, a complete facetectomy may be better.
- Complete the dissection at all symptomatic levels. Decompression should be from the caudal aspect of the most proximal pedicle to the cephalad aspect of the most distal pedicle, allowing observation of the lateral margins of the dura in the lateral recesses. This can be done with preservation of the proximal portion of the lamina and the intervening ligamentum flavum at the level above and below. Many failed decompressions are the result of inadequate decompression of the foraminal region, so probing the foramen is mandatory to determine if the decompression is adequate.
- If no obstructions are noted and all areas have been decompressed adequately, ensure hemostasis with bipolar cautery and the temporary use of thrombin-soaked absorbable gelatin sponge (Gelfoam). Inspect for cerebrospinal fluid (CSF) leakage. If desired, take a large fat graft from the incision or buttock and place it over the laminectomy defect. A ⅛-inch diameter drain can be placed deep in the wound, exiting through a separate stab incision. Close the wound in layers.

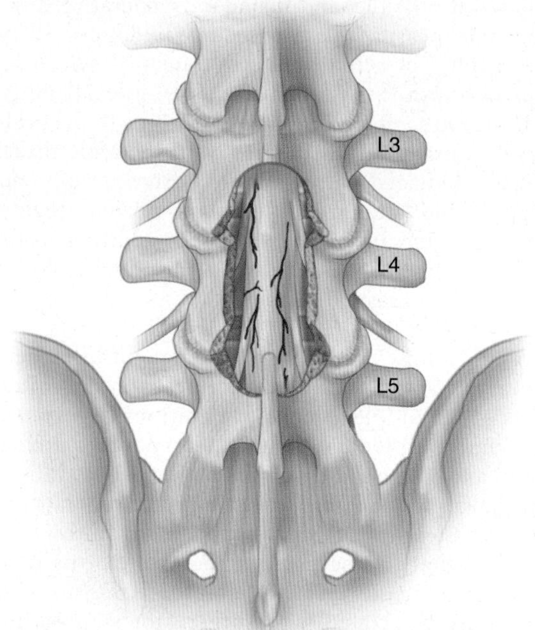

FIGURE 3.50 Typical midline decompression for spinal stenosis. Note medial facetectomy and foraminotomy with preservation of the pars. Decompression is from inferior border of L3 pedicle to superior border of L5 pedicle, exposing both lateral borders of dura in lateral recess. **SEE TECHNIQUE 3.29.**

LESS-INVASIVE DECOMPRESSION

The consequences of bone and ligament removal must be considered when performing decompression for spinal stenosis. Removal of the spinous processes, laminae, variable portions of the facets and pars, supraspinous and interspinous ligaments, ligamentum flavum, and portions of facet capsules is routine during these operative procedures. Denervation of the paraspinal musculature occurs with wide exposures, which results in altered muscle function. A minimally invasive technique allows decompression of the significant compressing anatomy while preserving paraspinal muscles, the spinous processes, and intervening supraspinous and interspinous ligaments. Results with full-endoscopic techniques have been shown to be equal to those of conventional procedures, with the advantages of fewer complications. Although Kelleher et al. noted that minimally invasive decompression is effective in most patients, including those with degenerative spondylolisthesis, patients with scoliosis, especially with listhesis, have a significantly higher revision rate, and this must be considered when making treatment decisions.

SPINOUS PROCESS OSTEOTOMY (DECOMPRESSION)

Weiner et al. reported a 47% improvement in the Low Back Outcome Score and a 66% improvement in average pain level in 46 of 50 patients evaluated 9 months after surgery. Spinous process osteotomy was done at one to four levels; the only complications were dural tears in four patients. Although three patients died of unrelated causes, 38 of the 46 remaining patients were satisfied or very satisfied with their operative results. On reexploration or postoperative CT scans, spinous processes usually united with the remaining lamina in patients with short decompressions, although nonunion did not correlate with poor results. Complete laminectomy may be necessary if adequate decompression is impossible through the limited laminotomy in patients with severe involvement.

TECHNIQUE 3.30

(WEINER ET AL.)

- Patient positioning and localization of spinal levels are as described in Technique 3.29.
- Make a midline incision to expose the dorsolumbar fascia. Make a paramedian incision in the fascia, preserving the supraspinous and interspinous ligaments with subperiosteal dissection of the paraspinal muscles from the spinous process and laminae. Avoid lifting the multifidus muscles beyond the medial aspect of the facet joint to preserve their innervation.
- With a curved osteotome, free each spinous process from the lamina at its base. Release only the levels shown to be affected on preoperative imaging.
- When the spinous process is freed, retract it to one side with the paraspinal muscles beneath the retractor and the other blade of the retractor beneath the multifidus muscles to expose the midline (Fig. 3.51A). Resect approximately half of the cephalad lamina and one fourth of the caudal lamina along with the underlying ligamentum flavum.

- Using a loupe or microscope for magnification, undercut the lateral recess and open the foraminal zone (Fig. 3.51B). Complete laminectomy is recommended for severe stenosis or congenital stenosis involving all anatomic zones (central, lateral recess, and foraminal zones).
- Close the incision in routine fashion, allowing the spinous process to return to its normal position with suture of the fascia (Fig. 3.51C).

MICRODECOMPRESSION

Microdecompression can be done in patients without disc herniations or instability, including degenerative spondylolisthesis with a risk of worsening instability. This is a technically demanding procedure and is not recommended for patients with severe stenosis or congenital stenosis, which require complete laminectomy. McCulloch reported that decompressions were done at one to five levels without intraoperative complications in 30 patients treated for neurogenic claudication unresponsive to nonoperative measures. One superficial wound infection occurred. Of the 30 patients, 26 were very satisfied or fairly satisfied with their results; all but one stated that they would recommend the procedure to a friend with a similar problem. Good to excellent results also have been reported (Orpen et al.) in 82 of 100 patients using a slightly modified microdecompression technique that allows decompression on both sides of the spine through a unilateral approach with bilateral decompression.

TECHNIQUE 3.31

(MCCULLOCH)

- Place the patient in a kneeling position to increase interlaminar distance and identify the operative level on standard radiographs.
- Make a midline incision centered over the affected levels documented on preoperative imaging studies. Make a paramedian fascial incision on the most symptomatic side 1 cm from the midline.
- Elevate the multifidus muscles subperiosteally from the spinous process and laminae, but do not retract them beyond the medial aspect of the facet joint. Obtain unilateral interlaminar exposure and maintain it with a discectomy retractor.
- Under microscopic magnification, perform laminotomy cephalad until the origin of the ligamentum flavum is encountered. Use undercutting to preserve as much dorsal bone as possible; angle the microscope to accomplish this.
- In a similar fashion, resect the proximal one fourth of the caudal lamina, completing removal of the ligamentum flavum from origin to insertion. Angling of the microscope into the lateral recess allows further decompression of the cephalad and caudal nerve roots and lateral dura.
- When decompression is completed on one side, angle the microscope toward the midline for contralateral decompression (Fig. 3.52A). Rotation of the operative table allows better viewing of the contralateral structures (Fig. 3.52B).
- Use a no. 4 Penfield elevator or similar instrument to release adhesions between the dura and opposite ligamentum flavum, which is resected in a similar fashion.
- Remove the bone at the base of the spinous processes of the cephalad and caudal levels to provide adequate vision of the opposite side (Fig. 3.52C). Some removal of the deepest portions of the interspinous ligament also is necessary to view the structures across the midline adequately.
- For surgeons comfortable with minimally invasive techniques, the same laminoplasty procedure can be performed through a fixed tubular retractor using a transmuscular approach with less damage to the paraspinous musculature. This minimizes the need to dissect the multifidus attachment from the spinous process and lamina. Maintaining the dynamic stabilizers may lead to decreased rates of adjacent segment instability.
- The same procedure can be done through a spinal endoscope with a working channel using a uniportal or biportal approach.

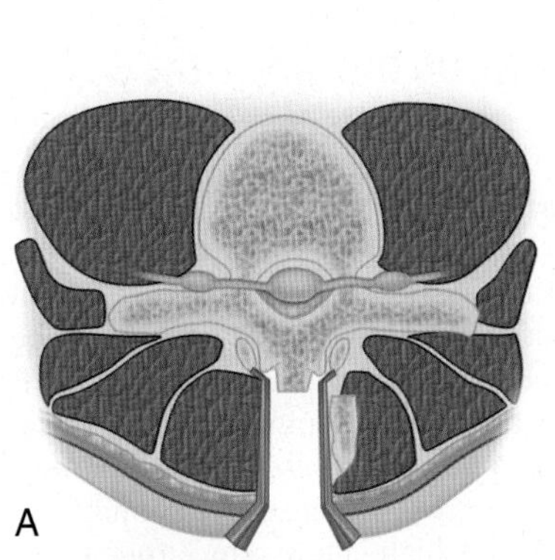

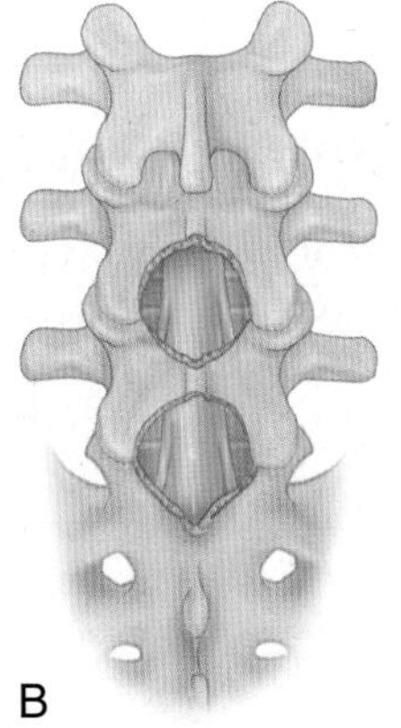

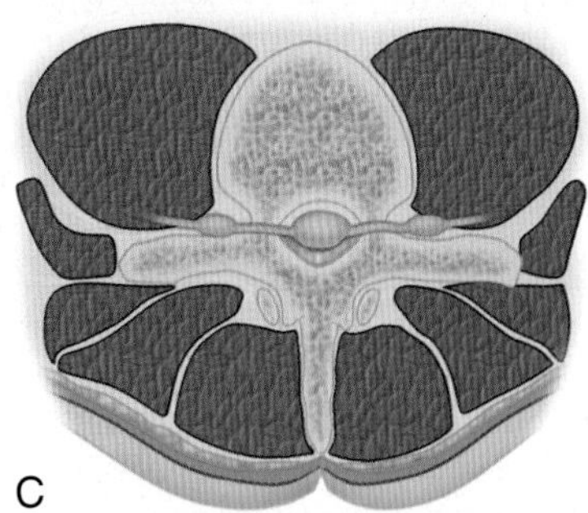

FIGURE 3.51 Spinous process osteotomy described by Weiner et al. **A,** Muscle is taken down on only one side and only to medial facet border. **B,** Decompression is performed under microscopic magnification. **C,** After closure, spine returns to normal position. **SEE TECHNIQUE 3.30.**

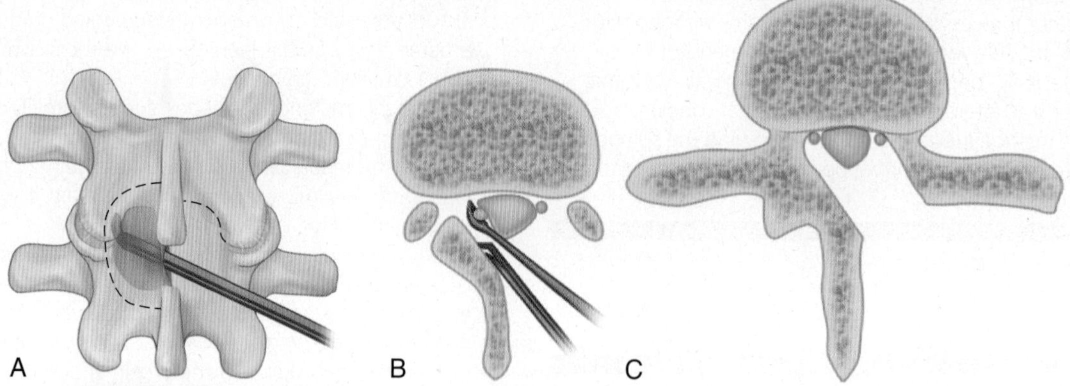

FIGURE 3.52 Microdecompression. **A,** Muscle is taken down on only one side, and ipsilateral decompressive hemilaminotomy is done; contralateral side is accessed under midline structures. **B,** Sac and root are gently retracted for contralateral decompression. **C,** End result is complete decompression with preservation of paraspinal musculature and interspinous and supraspinous ligaments, limited dead space, and excellent cosmetic result. **SEE TECHNIQUE 3.31.**

POSTOPERATIVE CARE There are no special considerations after a simple decompression. The patient should be examined carefully for the first few days for new neurologic changes that may indicate the formation of an epidural hematoma. The patient is encouraged to walk on the first day. Sutures are removed at 14 days if nonabsorbable sutures have been used. We prefer the use of absorbable subcutaneous sutures with a glue-type product for the final skin closure. The same limitations as after disc surgery apply to decompressions without fusion. For patients engaged in heavy manual labor, a permanent job change may be required. Return to work also is similar to return after disc surgery.

DECOMPRESSION WITH FUSION

The indications for spinal fusion with decompression for spinal stenosis are becoming more clearly defined. Preoperative and intraoperative factors must be carefully considered when decompression and fusion surgery are contemplated. Serious thought should be given to performing arthrodesis in addition to decompression in patients with preoperative degenerative spondylolisthesis, scoliosis, kyphosis, stenosis at a previously decompressed level, or stenosis adjacent to a previously fused lumbar segment. The finding of a synovial facet joint cyst radiographically or intraoperatively is important because these have been associated with development or progression of slipping postoperatively. Because cysts reflect derangement of the facet joint, fusion should at least be considered after decompression and excision of synovial cysts in patients with spinal stenosis with and possibly without preoperative instability.

The prevalence of postoperative problems related to instability varies, possibly because of the great variations in the extent of the operative decompression, but the likelihood of iatrogenic instability remains low if established principles of decompression are followed. White and Wiltse noted subluxation after decompression in 66% of patients with degenerative spondylolisthesis. They suggested that a fusion be done in conjunction with decompression in (1) patients younger than 60 years old with instability caused by the loss of an articular process on one side, (2) patients younger than 55 years old with a midline decompression for degenerative spondylolisthesis that preserves the facets, and (3) patients younger than 50 years old with isthmic spondylolisthesis. The complete removal of one facet, or more than 50% resection of both facets, may result in instability. In addition, generalized spinal stenosis that requires extensive decompression with the loss of multiple articular processes may require fusion. When complete bilateral facetectomies are necessary, the addition of a lateral fusion may be difficult and the bone graft may impinge on the exposed nerve roots. In this instance, an anterior interbody fusion is warranted to prevent postoperative instability. Posterior segmental instrumentation for posterior spinal fusion has decreased the high incidence of pseudarthrosis after long lumbar fusions.

The complications of this procedure are similar to the complications of disc surgery; however, the risk of nerve root damage and dural laceration is greater. The rates of infection, thrombophlebitis, and pulmonary embolism also are slightly higher. When a facet has been partially resected, later facet or pars fracture may account for a recurrence of symptoms, although the most important cause of failure to relieve symptoms has been found to be inadequate decompression. Bone regrowth has been noted in 88% of patients after total laminectomy and in all patients with associated spondylolisthesis.

INTERSPINOUS DISTRACTION

A distraction technique has been described as an alternative to decompression surgery. A spacer is inserted into the interspinous space as far anteriorly and as close to the posterior aspect of the lamina as possible. This procedure requires no ligamentous or bony resection, and the spinal canal is not breached, eliminating the risk of neural damage. Symptomatic benefit has been reported in 54% at 1 year in one study and in 78% at 4.2 years in another for degenerative spinal stenosis. Verhoof et al., however, did not recommend its use for the treatment of spinal stenosis in the presence of degenerative spondylolisthesis because of the unacceptably high failure rate. Fifty-eight percent of their patients required decompression and posterolateral fusion within 24 months. Long-term follow-up data are still lacking.

ANKYLOSING SPONDYLITIS

Ankylosing spondylitis is a chronic inflammatory disease of unknown etiology. It is a seronegative spondyloarthropathy that primarily affects the axial skeleton, sacroiliac joints, and pelvis. Less commonly, involvement of peripheral joints, eyes (iritis or uveitis), heart, and lungs can occur. Inflammation of the spinal joints and enthesopathies cause chronic pain and stiffness and can lead to progressive ankylosis of the spine in patients with long-standing disease. Ankylosing spondylitis typically affects young adults between the ages 20 and 40 years, with a male to female ratio of 3:1. The average onset of symptoms occurs at 23 years of age; there can be an 8.5- to 11.4-year delay from initial symptoms to diagnosis. There is a known association with the HLA-B27 antigen. Between 88% and 96% of patients who have ankylosing spondylitis are HLA-B27 positive, but only 5% of the HLA-B27 population develops ankylosing spondylitis.

Initially, morning stiffness is the primary symptom. Other early symptoms usually are chronic pain and stiffness in the middle and lower spine, as well as buttock pain from the sacroiliac joint. The symptoms are nonspecific for ankylosing spondylitis. As the disease progresses, ankylosis of the sacroiliac joints and spine can occur. Ankylosis usually progresses from caudal to cephalad. After ankylosis, however, pain symptoms often improve. Other symptoms may be related to hip arthritis, which occasionally progresses to spontaneous arthrodesis. Pulmonary cavitary lesions with fibrosis occur, as do aortic insufficiency and conduction defects. Amyloid deposition can cause renal failure. Uveitis requires special ophthalmologic care and follow-up to prevent permanent vision changes. Breathing may be restricted because of fusion of the costochondral and costovertebral articulations.

In the spine, ankylosis can lead to a loss of lumbar spinal lordosis and progressive kyphosis of the cervical and thoracic spine. This combined with hip flexion deformities can result in a loss of sagittal balance and disabling functional deficits, such as an inability to look above the horizon or to lie in bed. Furthermore, fused sections of the spine make it more susceptible to fracture, pseudarthrosis, or spondylodiscitis.

Radiographs initially show fusion of the sacroiliac joints, which characteristically occurs bilaterally. In the vertebral bodies, inflammatory resorption of bone at the enthesis causes periarticular osteopenia. This resorption initially is seen as a "squaring off" of the corners of the vertebral bodies. Subsequent ossification occurs in the anulus fibrosis, sparing the anterior longitudinal ligament and disc and giving the "bamboo spine" appearance on radiographs. The posterior elements are similarly affected, with ossification of the facet joints, interspinous and supraspinous ligaments, and ligamentum flavum. Atlantoaxial instability must be identified, especially in any patient having surgery for conditions associated with ankylosing spondylitis. Because of the stiff subaxial spine, instability occurs in 25% to 90% of patients with ankylosing spondylitis.

Treatment is directed at maintaining flexibility with stretching of the hip flexors and hamstrings and maintaining spinal alignment with exercises and posture. Sleeping supine on a firm mattress with one pillow may help maintain sagittal alignment and prevent hip flexion contractures. Medications used in the treatment of ankylosing spondylitis fall into three categories. The first includes NSAIDs that relieve pain by decreasing joint inflammation. The second group comprises disease-modifying antirheumatic drugs such as minocycline, sulfasalazine, and methotrexate. This is an unrelated group of drugs found to slow the disease process, but they do not provide a cure. Finally, tumor necrosis factor-α blockers have been shown to be effective.

Operative management in patients with ankylosing spondylitis is indicated to decrease pain and improve function. Total hip arthroplasties are the most common surgical interventions performed in this population followed by spinal osteotomies to correct sagittal imbalances.

Spinal fractures in patients with ankylosing spondylitis are always serious and frequently are life-threatening injuries. Spine osteopenia that is common in this population combined with fused segments make patients more vulnerable to fractures, especially from minor trauma. Furthermore, distorted anatomy from disc ossification, ectopic bone, and sclerosis can make the spinal fractures difficult to see on plain radiographs, and these injuries often are missed. It should be up to the treating physician to prove that the patient with ankylosis does not have a fracture after trauma. Spinal precautions and immobilization in a position accommodating the patient's posture is very important. Often CT or MRI studies are needed. Fractures usually occur in the lower cervical spine, frequently are unstable, and usually are discovered late. Persistent pain may be the only finding until late neurologic loss occurs. In patients with established kyphosis, the deformity may suddenly improve. The patient's previous deformity may be unknown to individuals providing emergency care. Any perceived change in spinal alignment, even if the result of trivial trauma, should be considered a fracture in a patient with ankylosing spondylitis. The standard procedure is to immobilize the patient in the position in which he or she is found because extension may result in sudden neurologic loss. A widened anterior disc space, which may be the only obvious radiographic finding, creates an unstable configuration that is prone to translation, late neurologic loss, and slow healing. Imaging with MRI, CT, or bone scan may be helpful in making the diagnosis.

Surgical stabilization of fractures in patients with ankylosing spondylitis can be challenging. For cervical fractures, anterior and posterior or long posterior constructs are recommended because of the poor bone quality. Thoracolumbar fractures can be stabilized with a long posterior construct across the fractured level. More recently, percutaneous techniques of long-segment stabilization are being used. The morbidity and mortality associated with these procedures in patients with ankylosing spondylitis are very high because of the comorbidities many of these patients have.

OSTEOTOMY OF THE LUMBAR SPINE

Smith-Petersen, Larson, and Aufranc in 1945 described an osteotomy of the spine to correct the flexion deformity that often develops in ankylosing spondylitis and sometimes in rheumatoid arthritis. Since then, others have reported similar procedures. The technique described by Smith-Petersen et al. is done in one stage. Others have described surgery done in two stages, consisting of division of the anterior longitudinal ligament under direct vision instead of allowing it to rupture when the deformity is corrected by gentle manipulation, as in the method of Smith-Petersen et al.

If the flexion deformity is severe, the patient's field of vision is limited to a small area near the feet and walking is extremely difficult. This is evident by looking at the chin-brow to vertical angle (Fig. 3.53). Respiration becomes almost completely diaphragmatic. Gastrointestinal symptoms resulting from pressure of the costal margin on the contents of the upper abdomen are common; dysphagia or choking may occur. In addition to improvement in function, the improvement in appearance made by correcting the deformity is important to the patient. If extreme, the deformity should be corrected in two or more stages because of contracture of soft tissues and the danger of damaging the aorta, the inferior vena cava, and the major nerves to the lower extremities. According to Law, 25 to 45 degrees of correction usually can be obtained, resulting in marked improvement functionally and cosmetically. Initially, mortality was about 10% with operative treatment; however, a later series reported no deaths or serious complications.

The safest and most efficient position for this procedure is with the patient lying on his or her side. This lateral position has several advantages: (1) it is easier to place the grossly deformed patient on the table; (2) the danger of injuring the ankylosed cervical spine by pressure of the forehead against the table is eliminated; (3) the anesthesia is easier to manage because maintaining a clear airway and free respiratory exchange is less difficult; and (4) the operation is easier because any blood would flow out from the depth of the wound rather than into it. Adams described hyperextending the spine with an ingenious three-point pressure apparatus, and Simmons described surgery with the patient on his or her side and under local anesthesia. When the osteotomy is complete, the patient is turned prone, carefully fracturing the anterior longitudinal ligament with the patient briefly under nitrous oxide and fentanyl anesthesia.

The osteotomy usually is made at the upper lumbar level because the spinal canal here is large, and the osteotomy is distal to the end of the cord. A lumbar lordosis is created to compensate for the thoracic kyphosis; motion of the spine is not increased. Osteotomy methods include resection of the spinous processes from the laminae to the pedicles, simple wedge resection of the spinous processes into the neural foramina (Fig. 3.54A and B), chevron excision of the laminae and spinous processes (Fig. 3.54C and D), and combined anterior opening wedge osteotomy after posterior resection of the spinous processes and laminae.

An average correction from 80 to 44 degrees has been reported after upper lumbar osteotomy, with correction maintained by internal fixation. Manual osteoclasis worked best in patients with calcified ligaments. Complications from this procedure include hypertension, gastrointestinal problems, neurologic defects, urinary tract infections, psychologic problems, dural tears with leakage, retrograde ejaculation, and, rarely, rupture of the aorta.

Spinal osteotomy is a demanding procedure for which proper training and experience are mandatory. The surgeon should be familiar with the several options available.

SMITH-PETERSEN OSTEOTOMY

The Smith-Petersen osteotomy is an excellent option for correction of smaller degrees of spinal deformity. Bone is removed through the pars and facet joints (Fig. 3.54C and D). If a previous fusion has been done, care should be taken to thin the fusion mass gradually until the ligamentum flavum or dura is exposed. Symmetric resection is necessary to prevent creating a coronal deformity. Removal of the underlying ligament also is helpful in preventing buckling of the dura or iatrogenic spinal stenosis. Approximately 10 degrees of correction can be obtained with each 10 mm of resection. Excessive resection should be avoided because it may result in foraminal stenosis. In patients with degenerative discs, decreased flexibility may limit the amount of correction that can be obtained. The osteotomy is closed with compression or with in situ rod contouring, and bone graft is applied.

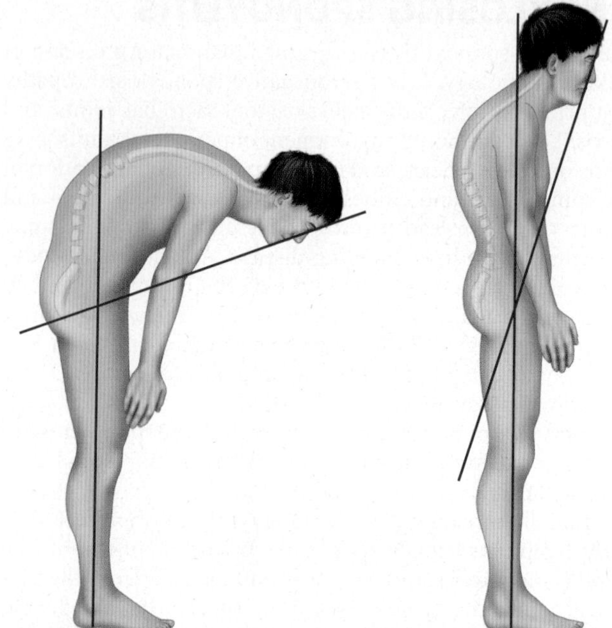

FIGURE 3.53 Chin-brow to vertical angle is measured from brow to chin to vertical while patient stands with hips and knees extended and neck in fixed or neutral position.

PEDICLE SUBTRACTION OSTEOTOMY

Pedicle subtraction osteotomy (Fig. 3.54A and B) is best suited for patients who have significant sagittal imbalance of 4 cm or more and immobile or fused discs. Pedicle subtraction osteotomy is inherently safer than the Smith-Petersen osteotomy because it avoids multiple osteotomies. Typically, 30 degrees or more of correction can be obtained with a single posterior osteotomy, preferably at the level of the deformity. If the deformity is at the spinal cord level, pedicle subtraction osteotomy can be used, but manipulation of the cord must be avoided. Thomasen and Thiranont and Netrawichien described the use of this osteotomy after laminectomy and pedicle resection. In their technique, compression instrumentation was used, along with simultaneous flexion of the head and foot of the operating table (Fig. 3.55). Care must be taken to avoid compression of the dura or creation of a coronal deformity. A wake-up test is done after correction and cancellous bone grafting have been completed.

EGGSHELL OSTEOTOMY

The eggshell osteotomy requires anterior and posterior approaches and usually is reserved for severe sagittal or coronal imbalance of more than 10 cm from the midline (Fig. 3.56). This is a spinal shortening procedure with anterior decancellization followed by removal of posterior elements, instrumentation, deformity correction, and fusion.

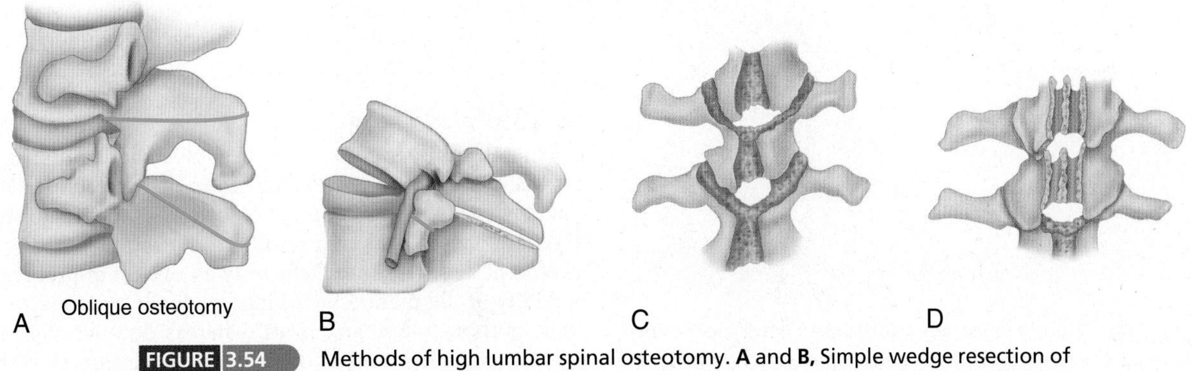

FIGURE 3.54 Methods of high lumbar spinal osteotomy. **A** and **B,** Simple wedge resection of spinous processes into neural foramina. **C** and **D,** Chevron excision of laminae and spinous processes.

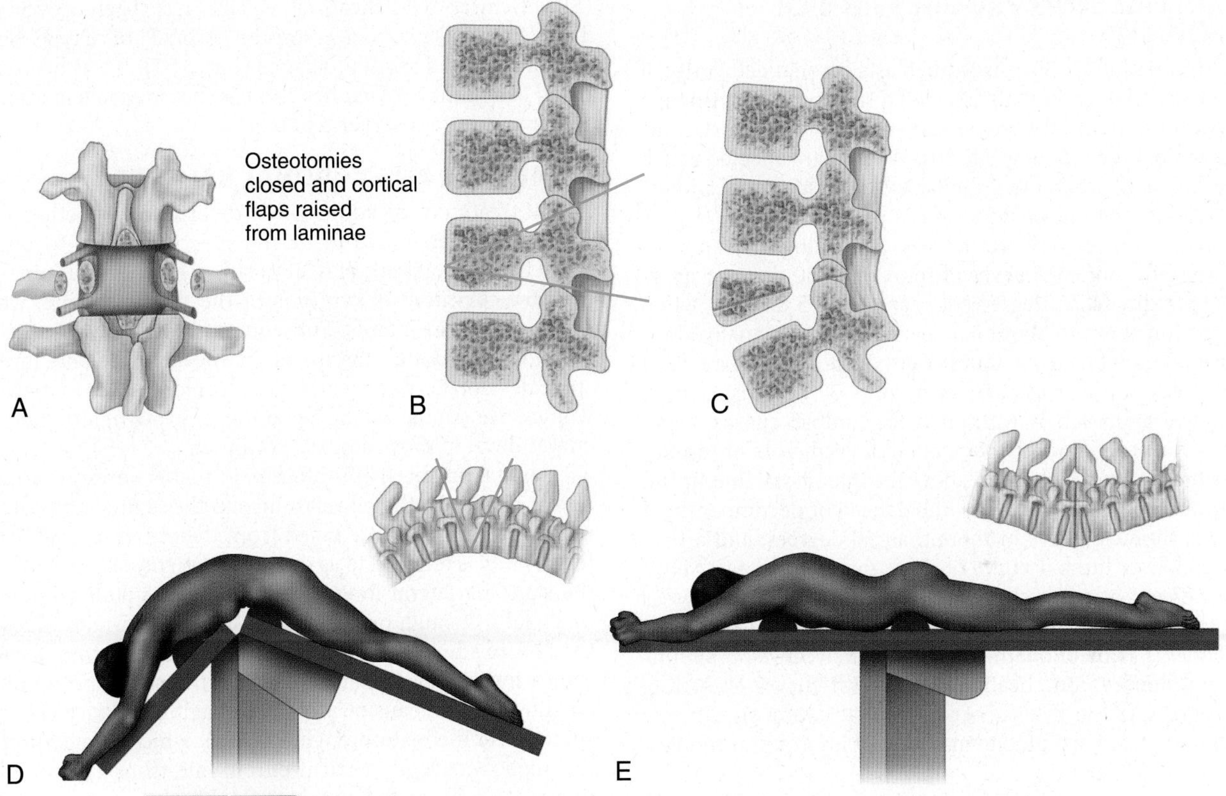

FIGURE 3.55 **A,** Total laminectomy. **B,** Rather than osteotomy with opening of disc in front, Thomasen used resection of posterior wedge and resection of pedicles **(C)**. Patient's position on operating table before **(D)** and after **(E)** reduction of osteotomy. Osteotomy gap is closed when table is brought from flexed to straight position.

ADULT SPINAL DEFORMITY

Although nearly 60% of the adult population has some form of spinal deformity, only approximately 6% are symptomatic. Most patients with symptoms from their spinal deformity are 70 years of age or older, and most report pain and impaired health-related quality of life. Approximately 60% of patients with late-onset degenerative scoliosis are female. Degenerative curves tend to be short segment, usually lumbar, and less severe than the curves in idiopathic scoliosis. Symptoms of spinal stenosis are more common in patients with degenerative scoliosis. The goal of treatment of degenerative scoliosis is to relieve back pain and the symptoms of spinal stenosis, whereas the treatment goals for adult idiopathic scoliosis usually are pain control and deformity correction. Treatment of adult idiopathic and degenerative scoliosis requires a different approach from that used for typical adolescent idiopathic scoliosis (AIS), is more challenging, and is more likely to have complications such as dural tears, nonunion, implant breakage, and wound infection. Adult spinal deformity curves tend to be more rigid than those in adolescents, and surgery is further complicated by the prevalence of medical comorbidities and osteopenia in these older patients.

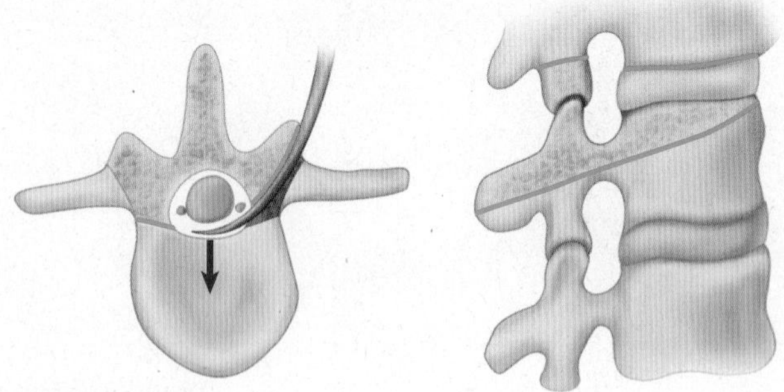

FIGURE 3.56 Heinig eggshell procedure. After posterior elements have been removed and pedicles have been collapsed outward, long, sharp curet is used to collapse "eggshell."

INCIDENCE AND PROGRESSION OF DEFORMITY

Adult idiopathic scoliosis is defined as a coronal deformity of more than 10 degrees with associated structural changes in a patient older than 20 years at time of diagnosis, most commonly in patients in their late 30s. Women are affected much more frequently than men, similar to the incidence of adolescent scoliosis. Studies have shown a prevalence of 2% to 4% for curves of more than 10 degrees. According to Weinstein and Ponseti, thoracic curves of more than 50 degrees progress approximately 1 degree per year up to 75 degrees, when progression slows to about 0.3 degrees per year, finally stopping at about 90 degrees. Lumbar curves progress at a rate of 0.4 degrees per year after reaching only 30 degrees; a more aggressive approach is warranted for lumbar curves, especially after progression is documented. Predictors of lumbar curve progression include L5 above the intercristal line, apical rotation of more than 30%, an unbalanced or decompensated curve, a thoracic curve of more than 50 degrees, and a thoracolumbar or lumbar curve of more than 30 degrees. Sixty-eight percent of adult curves progress more than 5 degrees over time.

Patients with idiopathic scoliosis rarely develop significant pulmonary complications, even with curves exceeding 100 degrees. In the absence of overt thoracic lordosis, surgery generally is not warranted to maintain or improve pulmonary function in adults.

Degenerative scoliosis develops in patients with previously straight spines after age 40 years, typically affecting the lumbar spine with an associated lumbar hypolordosis, lateral olisthesis, and spinal stenosis. Men and women are affected more equally than patients with idiopathic curves, with 60% to 70% of those affected being women. Degenerative scoliosis occurs in 6% to 30% of the elderly population, with most curves being minor, affecting fewer segments (two to five segments) than in adult idiopathic scoliosis (seven to 11 segments), with an equal distribution of right and left lumbar curves. Rotary subluxation varies and seems to be worse after decompression surgery without fusion. Curves can be progressive, but the natural history has not been elucidated conclusively. Progression of 1 to 6 degrees a year has been reported. Symptoms of spinal stenosis occur most often in degenerative curves that have defects in the convexity and concavity, possibly because significant degenerative changes preceded the development of the scoliosis. As a result, treatment of degenerative scoliosis often is necessary to relieve spinal stenosis by decompression, with instrumented fusion to prevent instability and further progression of deformity.

CLASSIFICATION

In general, adult scoliosis can be broadly divided into two categories: deformity due to progression of untreated or inadequately treated AIS or de novo scoliosis, which is primary degenerative scoliosis that results from asymmetric disc and facet joint degeneration. Deformity as a result of progression of AIS typically manifests as long, gradually progressive thoracic or thoracolumbar curves, whereas de novo deformity presents as sharp lumbar or thoracolumbar curves with an apex at L2-3 or L3-4. A third type of adult spinal deformity can be caused by an adjacent idiopathic curve or metabolic bone disease. More recently, the Scoliosis Research Society (SRS)-Schwab classification system has been developed. This system takes into account the coronal curve type, pelvic parameters, and sagittal balance (Fig. 3.57). It has been validated in a number of studies and has shown excellent interobserver and intraobserver reliability.

■ SAGITTAL AND CORONAL BALANCE

In the treatment of adult spinal deformities, whether idiopathic or degenerative in origin, it is important to understand the normal sagittal relationships. In a normal spine, the primary curvature is kyphosis of the thoracic spine, which develops first in infants. Subsequent to upright posture, the secondary lordotic curvatures in the cervical and lumbar spine develop between 5 and 15 years old. Curves in men and women are similar at the cessation of growth, although the curves develop more quickly in women.

Sagittal balance is the alignment that is necessary to center the head over the pelvis or hips in the sagittal and coronal planes. A plumb line dropped from the center of the C7 vertebral body is referred to as the *sagittal vertical axis* (SVA). On the standing lateral long-cassette view, the plumb line normally falls through or behind the sacrum. Normal values for the SVA in adults are from +48 mm to −48 mm, with negative values indicating a position behind the sacral promontory. An alternative means of measuring sagittal balance is the T1 spinopelvic inclination angle (T1SPI), which is measured as the angle between a vertical plumb line from T1 and a line drawn from T1 to the center of the bicoxofemoral axis (Fig. 3.57). The advantage of using T1SPI over the SVA is that it is not vulnerable to radiographic calibration errors. Another method of assessing sagittal balance is the T1 pelvic angle (TPA). Similar to the T1SPI, TPA is the angle formed by a line drawn from the center of T1 to the bicoxofemoral axis and then to the center of the S1 endplate. The two distinct advantages of TPA are that it does not require radiographic calibration and it integrates both T1SPI and pelvic tilt, both of which have been shown to correlate with outcome scores.

Coronal balance is quantified globally by the amount of offset between the C7 plumb line and the center-sacral vertical line (CSVL) and the offset between the apical vertebra from the CSVL. Any translation of the coronal vertical axis to either side of the midline is considered decompensation.

Sagittal and coronal vertical axes are used to evaluate and estimate global balance. Global balance is the result of segmental alignment of the functional spinal unit and regional alignment of the cervical, thoracic, and lumbar segments.

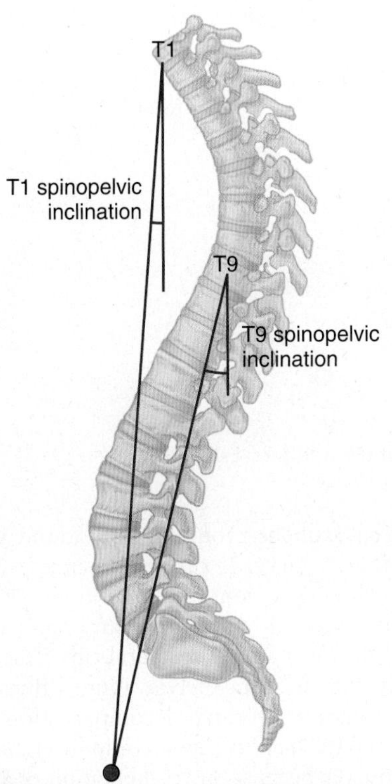

FIGURE 3.57 Measurement of the T1 spinopelvic inclination angle.

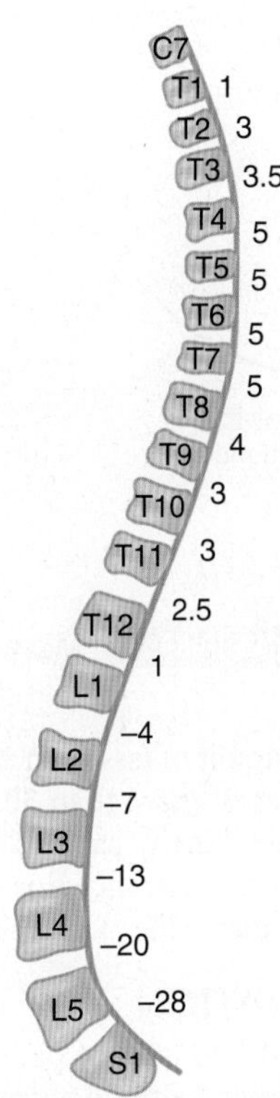

FIGURE 3.58 Bernhardt and Bridwell segmental sagittal measures of thoracic and lumbar spine. Note contribution of L4-5 and L5-S1 discs to overall lumbar lordosis (67%).

Bernhardt and Bridwell measured 102 radiographs of normal spines to determine normal sagittal plane alignment (Fig. 3.58). By convention, kyphosis is represented as a positive measurement and lordosis is represented as a negative value. In a normal adult spine, there is a small amount of kyphosis segmentally at each end of the thoracic kyphosis, reaching a maximum at the apical region (T6-7) of about +5 degrees. Apical discs or vertebrae are identified in the sagittal plane as those that are parallel to the floor. Considered independently, the thoracolumbar junction is a transition zone of force transmission and alignment. In this region, a shift occurs from the thoracic kyphosis to lumbar lordosis. The first lordotic disc is typically at L1-2, and normal thoracolumbar alignment as measured from the cephalad T12 endplate to the caudal L2 endplate is 0 to −10 degrees. The lumbar spine is a region of lordosis, reaching a maximal segmental lordosis at L4-5 and L5-S1. The sagittal apex of the lumbar spine usually is L3. Greater than 60% of lumbar lordosis is created by the discs at L4-5 and L5-S1, which contribute −20 degrees and −28 degrees to the regional lordotic measurement.

Because most lordosis is present in the distal lumbar spine, it is important to maintain normal segmental and regional interrelationships so that global balance is preserved. As a rule of thumb, on a lateral radiograph taken with the patient facing the surgeon's right, there is a "sagittal clock," as described by Bridwell. In a normal, standing patient, the apical L3 disc or endplate points at the 3-o'clock position, L4 points at the 4-o'clock position, and L5 points at the 5-o'clock position. If this regional alignment is maintained, the likelihood of a postoperative flatback deformity is minimized.

Achieving appropriate sagittal balance in adult spinal deformity correction is essential. The relationship between balanced SVA and health-related quality of life scores has been well established in the literature. Sagittal malalignment results in compensatory pelvic retroversion (increased pelvic tilt), which helps the patient maintain an upright posture; however, pelvic retroversion has been shown to increase energy expenditure and negatively affect ambulation. Some patients are limited in their ability to compensate with pelvic retroversion because of hip flexion contractures or stiffness. Schwab et al. listed as goals of surgical correction (1) SVA less than 50 mm, (2) T1SPI less than 0 degrees, (3) pelvic incidence–lumbar lordosis mismatch less than 9 degrees, and (4) pelvic tilt less than 20 degrees.

SPINOPELVIC ALIGNMENT

Research has established the importance of spinopelvic parameters—pelvic incidence, pelvic tilt, and sacral slope—in the evaluation of adult patients with spinal deformity (Fig. 3.59). Pelvic incidence is defined as the angle between a line perpendicular to the center of the sacral endplate and a line drawn from the center of the sacral endplate to the center of the bicoxofemoral axis (Fig. 3.59A). It is important to understand that pelvic incidence is a fixed morphologic parameter that does not change after skeletal maturity. Pelvic incidence can be considered the "take-off" degree of the lumbar spine; the higher this angle, the more lumbar lordosis required to maintain an upright posture. Average pelvic incidence in adults is 52 ± 10 degrees. Pelvic tilt, on the other hand, is a variable angle that represents the amount of compensatory pelvic retroversion the patient is using to maintain an upright posture (Fig. 3.59B). It is defined as the angle between a vertical reference line through the bicoxofemoral axis and a line from the center of the bicoxofemoral axis to the center of the

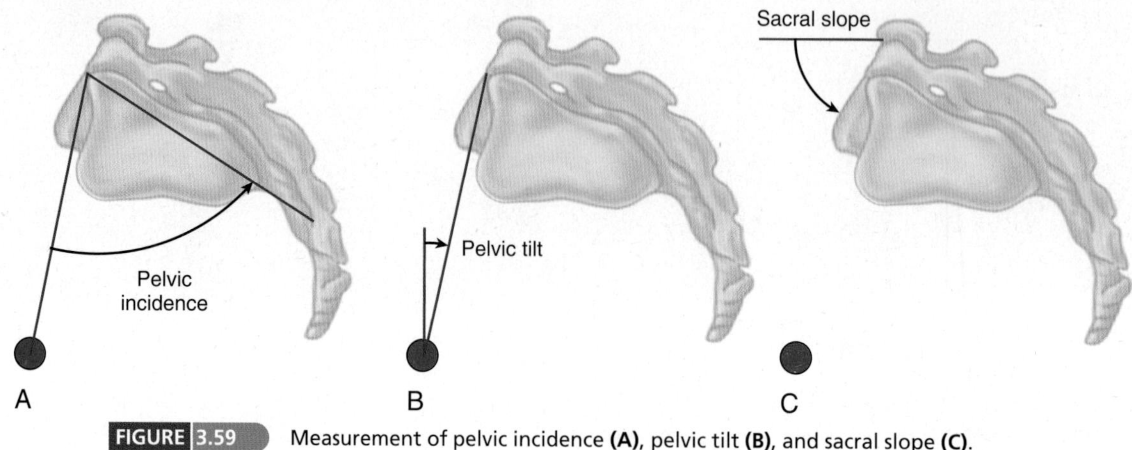

FIGURE 3.59 Measurement of pelvic incidence **(A)**, pelvic tilt **(B)**, and sacral slope **(C)**.

sacral endplate. A pelvic tilt of less than 20 degrees is considered normal, and values of more than 30 degrees are considered markedly increased. Finally, sacral slope is defined by the angle between a horizontal reference line and a line parallel to the superior sacral endplate (Fig. 3.59C).

CLINICAL EVALUATION

Back pain occurs in 60% to 80% of patients with idiopathic scoliosis, which is similar to the occurrence in the general population. Pain is the chief presenting complaint in 25% to 80% of patients with adult idiopathic curvatures. This can include mechanical back pain, buttock pain, and, occasionally, radiculopathy or neurogenic claudication. Neurogenic claudication occurs in 13% as a result of degenerative changes within or, more commonly, distal to the lumbar curve. Radiculopathy occurs in only 4%, with entrapment of nerve roots within the foramina of the concavity. In contrast to degenerative scoliosis, most adult patients with idiopathic scoliosis have more mechanical symptoms than neurologic complaints. Patients may relate symptoms of curve progression, such as a progressive lean or list to one side, changes in waistline symmetry, hip prominence, protuberant or flaccid abdomen, hemline changes, or a loss in height in the absence of fracture. Neurologic symptoms may include radiculopathy or neurogenic claudication, which usually is a result of degenerative changes in the distal fractional curve. Diminished pulmonary function in patients with curves of more than 60 degrees or cor pulmonale in patients with curves of more than 100 degrees occasionally is caused by the scoliosis and should be evaluated carefully to rule out other causes. Predictors of pain include curves of more than 45 degrees, lumbar curves, and thoracolumbar and lumbar curves of more than 45 degrees with apical rotation and coronal decompensation.

Physical examination findings usually are negative except for the spinal deformity. The skin should be examined for evidence of pathologic lesions and hair patches that suggest underlying intraspinal anomalies. If spinal cord anomalies exist, atrophy may be evident in the lower extremities or intrinsic atrophy of the foot may be present with pes cavus and clawing of the toes. Reflexes should be documented, as should the results of a comprehensive neurologic examination.

The deformity should be evaluated by looking for structural features of the rib and lumbar paraspinal prominence on forward bending while also recording flexibility. This test also helps to determine which curve is primary because more rotation and subsequent prominence is found in the more structural primary curve. If rib prominence exceeds 3 cm, thoracoplasty should be considered if surgery is performed. Trunk shift is identified by dropping an imaginary line perpendicular to the floor from the lateral ribs. This line should symmetrically intersect the pelvis. Plumb lines should be dropped to evaluate for coronal decompensation and to help in estimating sagittal balance. Special attention should be paid to the left shoulder because instrumentation of a curve with a structural upper thoracic curve must include this segment to avoid a high left shoulder postoperatively. Waistline asymmetry should be noted, and any limb-length inequality must be considered. Equalizing limb length with ¼-inch blocks sometimes is helpful if limb-length discrepancy is more than 1 inch. Placing the patient prone on the examination table often gives information regarding curve flexibility and the extent of deformity that will be found during intraoperative positioning. Some surgeons find traction and bending films useful to evaluate curve flexibility.

In degenerative scoliosis, symptoms of neurogenic claudication are present in 71% to 90% of patients and usually cause them to seek medical attention, with deformity incidentally noted. These symptoms often do not improve with forward bending, and to obtain relief patients support the trunk with the arms or assume a supine position. This is in contrast to the usual patient with spinal stenosis and neurogenic claudication. Radiculopathy from facet overgrowth, foraminal stenosis within the concavity of curvature, or nerve root tension along the curve convexity can occur, although neurologic deficits are rare, and back pain is ubiquitous. Primary treatment is directed at decompression of spinal stenosis, with fusion or instrumentation indicated based on the potential for increased instability.

Physical findings are nonspecific in most patients. Motion usually is preserved, but patients guard against hyperextension. Symptoms may be reproduced by this maneuver in the presence of spinal stenosis. Neurologic examination rarely identifies significant motor, sensory, or reflex deficits; however, any abnormal findings should be documented. Evaluation of distal pulses is necessary to help rule out peripheral vascular disease and vascular claudication. Bilateral absence of Achilles tendon reflexes may be an indicator of peripheral neuropathy. Flattening of the lumbar spine represents degenerative change, and a lumbar prominence on forward bending accentuates the convexity of a coronal deformity. Sagittal and coronal balance should be estimated clinically. When contemplating any decompressive or stabilizing procedure, correction of the entire degenerative scoliotic segment must be considered because of sagittal or coronal decompensation.

ANATOMY AND BIOMECHANICS

Adult scoliosis shares most of the anatomic features of idiopathic adolescent scoliosis. Unique to adult patients with scoliosis are the diminished elasticity of the ligamentous structures and the narrowing of disc spaces that combine to stiffen primary and secondary or compensatory curves. Osteopenia also must be considered in older patients, especially in patients with risk factors for osteoporosis, such as glucoid use, postmenopausal status, and a personal or family history of fragility fractures.

The biomechanics of the bone-implant interface must be considered if long instrumentation constructs are used, especially when extended to the sacrum. Because of the long lever arm produced in long deformity constructs and the relatively poor fixation obtained in the sacrum, S1 screws have a high likelihood of biomechanical failure if not protected. To obtain purchase anterior to the biomechanical pivot point at the anterior sacrum, many surgeons choose iliac instrumentation. The two most commonly used modern instrumentation options for protecting the S1 screws are iliac screws and S2-alar-iliac (SAI) screws. Iliac screws provide strong fixation and ease of insertion with the potential risk of implant prominence and the theoretical technical difficulty of rod alignment with the S1 screws. SAI screws somewhat mitigate the implant prominence and rod alignment issues of traditional iliac screws. Fixation can be augmented with a load-sharing structural interbody fusion device. The most significant biomechanical increase in posterior instrumentation strength is with the addition of the iliac screws. The superiority of any of these techniques has not been established, and the surgeon's experience and preference determine the choice.

Finally, osteoporosis is a significant consideration in the treatment of these patients. Although there is no cause-and-effect relationship between bone density and degenerative scoliosis, these patients usually are older and more predisposed to osteoporosis. Compression fractures and compromised operative fixation may complicate the treatment of patients with concomitant disease. Attention should be paid to the optimization of bone metabolism and bone density before any major spinal deformity surgery. If indicated, supplementary vitamin D and calcium should be started before surgery and continued afterward throughout the phases of bone healing.

DIAGNOSTIC IMAGING

RADIOGRAPHY

For both idiopathic and degenerative scoliosis, standing radiographs on 36-inch cassettes must be obtained and scrutinized for coronal and, more important, sagittal balance. It is critical for this to be conducted in a standardized fashion. Patients should be instructed to stand in a neutral upright position with the hips and knees comfortably extended and the fingers on the clavicles (shoulders at 45 degrees of forward elevation). Lateral bending radiographs over a foam fulcrum are ideal for assessing flexibility, although standard maximal effort bending films often suffice. Often, simple prone radiographs give a good estimate of sagittal and coronal alignment that can be found intraoperatively. For sagittal deformities, appropriate fulcrum bending films can be obtained to determine flexibility. Push prone views, as described by Kleinman et al. and Vedantam et al., are useful in determining the response of the lowest instrumented vertebra to instrumentation. With degenerative scoliosis, degenerative disc changes and flattening of the normal lumbar lordosis are present. With both degenerative and idiopathic scoliosis, rotary subluxation may be evident in some patients, with lateral olisthesis of varying degrees.

COMPUTED TOMOGRAPHIC MYELOGRAPHY AND MAGNETIC RESONANCE IMAGING

By providing information regarding central, lateral recess, and foraminal stenosis, MRI is very useful in the preoperative evaluation of adult patients with spinal deformity. In addition, disc hydration and excessive facet degeneration are useful pieces of information provided by T2-weighted sequences that may influence whether surgery stops at or includes a lower degenerative segment. The degree of desiccation of the L5-S1 disc should prompt extra consideration to end at the adjacent disc above or include the degenerative segment. Adjacent segment pathology is common, and in older patients it may be prudent to include such diseased discs.

CT myelogram can be used instead of MRI in patients with contraindications (such as a pacemaker); however, it is an invasive procedure and should not be used routinely. Nonmyelogram CT scans can be useful in patients with extreme deformity or prior surgery. Finally, DICOM images from CT scans can be used by 3D printers to create life-size, three-dimensional models, which occasionally can be useful for surgical planning in severe deformities.

NONOPERATIVE TREATMENT

Several studies have called into question the value of nonoperative care in adult scoliosis, given the high cost and lack of improvement in outcome measures. However, given the potential morbidity of surgical treatment, we believe that attempting traditional methods of nonoperative treatment of back and leg pain are appropriate in patients with adult scoliosis. Orthoses may be helpful for the relief of axial degenerative symptoms. Intermittent use of a soft thoracolumbosacral orthosis (TLSO) is better tolerated than use of a rigid TLSO by older, often endomorphic, patients. The orthosis should be worn during symptomatic periods and kept to a minimum otherwise. Correction of deformity or prevention of progression of these curves is impossible, and an orthosis is used only for the management of symptoms; the patient should be aware of the treatment goals. Physical therapy should be continued in addition to bracing, with the ultimate goal of paraspinal strengthening and subsequent core stabilization that allow the brace to be discarded. Cognitive behavioral therapy is another key aspect of the patient with chronic pain that should not be overlooked.

OPERATIVE TREATMENT

When adequate nonoperative treatment has failed in a patient with unremitting symptoms or radiographic progression, surgery should be considered. Curves of more than 50 degrees with documented progression, loss of pulmonary function (believed to be caused by the scoliosis when curves exceed 60 degrees), progressive neurologic changes, and significant coronal or sagittal decompensation are relative indications for surgery. Cosmetic considerations are a genuine concern for patients as well and may play a small role in operative decision-making. The goal of surgery is to maintain a balanced spine, with the head centered over the pelvis, while fusing the minimum number of segments possible.

Although improvement radiographically and clinically can be expected with operative treatment, the overall incidence of complications has been reported to be from 13% to 40% and the incidence of pseudarthrosis is 13% to 17%. Several authors have noted that although elderly patients have the greatest risk of complications, they show greater improvement in pain and disability compared with younger patients. Revision rates are relatively low.

A spinal implant should be used that allows segmental placement of screws and allows iliac fixation. If fusion of the lumbosacral joint is anticipated, interbody fusion has traditionally been obtained with allograft or fusion cages that are cut to maintain the normal segmental lordotic disc alignment. The use of cell-saver autotransfusion is encouraged. Spinal cord monitoring should include somatosensory and transcranial motor evoked potentials. If useful data are obtained and maintained with somatosensory and motor evoked potentials, wake-up testing is unnecessary until the conclusion of the surgery. If pedicle screws are used below T8, pedicle screw stimulation can be useful to confirm proper placement. Although we find free-hand pedicle screw technique to be safe and to reduce patient and surgical team radiation exposure, some surgeons may not be comfortable with this. Fluoroscopy or computer-aided navigation enhances the use of anatomic landmarks and is helpful for some surgeons, especially in the setting of deformity and prior fusion. Regardless, this surgery is complex and has an extended recuperation period, with a significant risk of complications, which the patient must understand when operative treatment is chosen.

DECOMPRESSION IN DEGENERATIVE SCOLIOSIS

Decompression alone is a viable option for a patient with symptomatic spinal stenosis and minimal kyphosis, a neutral SVA, and no instability on dynamic imaging. Attempts should be made to avoid destabilizing the spine during decompression, and fusion should be done if more than 50% of either facets or an entire facet is resected. Degenerative scoliosis should be considered the coronal variant of spondylolisthesis; if the ligamentous structures are violated and facet and disc resections are necessary, fusion should be considered. Decompression alone is inadequate if claudicatory leg symptoms originate from foraminal stenosis within the concavity of a degenerative curve. Transfeldt et al. found a higher complication rate in patients with full curve fusion and less improvement in the Oswestry Disability Index than in patients with decompression alone.

POSTERIOR INSTRUMENTATION AND FUSION

IDIOPATHIC SCOLIOSIS

Patients with flexible idiopathic curves of less than 70 degrees and no significant kyphosis or decompensation are candidates for posterior instrumentation and fusion alone. This can be done with numerous instrumentation systems and techniques (see chapter 8). The ideal candidate for a posterior procedure has a smaller, flexible curve; hypokyphosis; and a flexible compensatory lumbar curve. Posterior procedures also are an appropriate choice for a King type V or Lenke subclass 2 or 4 structural upper thoracic curve. Similar correction clinically and radiographically has been reported with posterior-only approaches compared with combined anterior and posterior procedures, with the advantages of decreased blood loss, anesthesia, and operative time.

Standard posterior approaches are used, and instrumentation may include hooks, wires, or screws for curve correction. The current trend involves the use of all-pedicle screw constructs for deformity correction because of the segmental fixation that is obtained and the three-column control that is provided by a pedicle screw placed into the vertebral body. With this fixation, derotation may be possible to some extent during the correction maneuver. Another benefit of the use of pedicle screws is the extraspinal placement of implants, which avoids the space-occupying phenomenon created by hooks or wires placed within the spinal canal. Finally, the cortical fixation of a screw through the pedicle is superior biomechanically to hook fixation, which makes this technique appealing for an osteoporotic adult spine. These benefits are not without risks, however, and the primary concern is pedicle screw malposition that affects the great vessels or the spinal cord, dura, or nerve roots. When done by surgeons with proper training, pedicle screw placement so far has been safe and effective for the treatment of adult scoliosis; however, it is wise to discuss procedures in detail with patients before surgery and to explain the inherent risks involved.

Selection of fusion levels is similar to that in adolescent scoliosis patients. The goal of surgery is a balanced spine with the head centered over the pelvis in the sagittal and coronal planes. Fusion should be from stable vertebra to stable vertebra, unless pedicle screw instrumentation is used, and fusion can safely be stopped short of the stable vertebra. For curves with features similar to King types II and V curves without severe kyphosis, pedicle screw fixation seems ideal. This technique allows fusion of the curve from end vertebra to end vertebra, which can save one to three fusion levels distally in some patients compared with typical hook constructs. In adults, flexibility of the compensatory curve must be considered more than in adolescents with scoliosis because overcorrection of the thoracic curve in a spine with a relatively inflexible lumbar curve results in decompensation and an unsatisfactory result. It is prudent to apply only a conservative amount of correction that can be accommodated by the compensatory curve so that normal balance is restored and further progression is halted. The amount of correction that can be obtained is estimated from preoperative bending films.

Avoiding a flatback deformity during posterior distraction is mandatory because this deformity is much easier to prevent than to treat. Nonetheless, because of pseudarthrosis, implant failure, transition syndromes, adjacent level fracture, patient positioning, and other technical reasons, flatback deformity can occur in some patients under the best of circumstances. Concave distraction of the lumbar spine, especially beyond L2, should be avoided because this maneuver is kyphogenic. Segmental instrumentation allows differential correction along the same rod, which is helpful in preventing flatback deformity and shoulder decompensation. Avoiding distraction, or even applying some convex compression, along with precontouring the rods into lordosis helps to maintain normal lumbar alignment.

DEGENERATIVE SCOLIOSIS

In a patient with a flexible spine and mild-to-moderate scoliosis, symptomatic spinal stenosis is treated with traditional decompression. Occasionally, facetectomy or partial pedicle resection is necessary to decompress symptomatic nerve roots. In this situation, posterior intertransverse fusion is recommended. If laxity is present, instrumentation should extend from neutral and stable vertebrae at each end of the construct. Ending the instrumented fusion at a level of kyphosis potentiates adjacent segment changes and may result in a proximal junctional kyphosis, which remains a particularly vexing problem for deformity surgeons. Rotary subluxation also can occur after decompression alone in the presence of unstable degenerative scoliosis. The fusion should end at a neutrally rotated, level, and stable end vertebra and should restore sagittal and coronal balance. Care should be taken to avoid stopping instrumentation and fusion at any apical segments or at the apex of a kyphosis or scoliosis because this creates deformity later.

ANTERIOR SPINAL INSTRUMENTATION AND FUSION

Deformity correction through an anterior approach is described in chapter 8, but it warrants mention here because anterior instrumentation and fusion with third-generation implants have given excellent deformity correction in adults and have not caused significant problems with kyphosis as did the early Zielke and Dwyer implants. With single-rod or double-rod implant systems and structural grafts, anterior deformity correction is a viable alternative for lumbar and thoracolumbar curves because it allows short segment correction of flexible curves. Primary thoracic curves with flexible and compensatory lumbar curves in adults also can be treated effectively with anterior fusion. Correction must be appropriate, however, for the ability of the lumbar curve to compensate; overcorrection in adults results in more decompensation than in the flexible spines of children with scoliosis. Also, as in pediatric deformities, strict attention must be paid to the upper thoracic spinal segment from T1 or T2 to T6 to prevent shoulder asymmetry owing to a structural upper thoracic curve. An upper thoracic curve is a relative contraindication for anterior spinal instrumentation and fusion unless measures are taken to allow persistent tilt of the cephalad end vertebra, which would allow the upper thoracic curve to remain balanced. Anterior interbody fusion, either from a direct anterior or far lateral approach, can be especially helpful in restoring lordosis and indirectly decompressing foraminal stenosis in degenerative scoliosis but usually requires additional posterior stabilization.

POSTOPERATIVE MANAGEMENT

Patients are commonly monitored overnight in the intensive care unit with frequent neurologic evaluations and observation to prevent complications associated with fluid shifts, which occur after such long procedures. Sitting is encouraged the day after surgery, and formal physical therapy is initiated. Walking as tolerated is encouraged with assistance until independent ambulation is achieved. With modern pedicle screw constructs, a thoracolumbar orthosis generally is not necessary. The Foley catheter is removed when the patient is able to get to a bedside commode with minimal assistance. Antibiotics can be discontinued when drains are pulled or at 24 hours postoperatively, depending on surgeon preference, and oral narcotic analgesics usually are well tolerated by the third day after surgery. Pneumatic leg compression devices are used as prophylaxis against deep vein thrombosis because of the possible risk of epidural hematoma associated with pharmacologic agents. These are discontinued when the patient is fully independent with ambulation. Nonsteroidal antiinflammatory medications are avoided for 3 months postoperatively because of their potential inhibitory effect on fusion.

COMBINED ANTERIOR AND POSTERIOR FUSIONS

For a rigid curve of more than 70 degrees or a curve that is decompensated sagittally or coronally, or for instrumentation that crosses the lumbosacral joint, a combined approach can be more powerful. For severe rigid thoracic deformities of more than 100 degrees, which often are associated with translation of the trunk of more than 4 to 6 cm anterior or lateral to the pelvis, Boachie-Adjei and Bradford showed that vertebrectomy, as a combined or staged procedure, was effective in achieving spinal balance. It is preferable to complete combined procedures, if possible, under a single anesthesia because this results in fewer complications and a shorter hospitalization; however, if any portion of the procedure is unexpectedly long, blood loss is excessive, or a patient is unable to tolerate continuation of the procedure, it is prudent to postpone the second stage of the procedure. Parenteral nutrition between stages is recommended because patients often develop a postoperative ileus and do not tolerate enteral nutrition.

When a combined procedure is used, the first stage usually includes anterior release, discectomy, and fusion of the primary curve. If instrumentation is extended to the lumbosacral joint, interbody fusion is advisable at L4-5 and L5-S1, with structural grafting of these discs to maintain lordosis, improve fusion rates, and decrease stresses on the posterior implants. Morselized bone graft is placed in the thoracic disc spaces and usually consists of the rib excised for the exposure. Supplemental bone graft can be obtained from the inner table of the anterior iliac crest if the rib is small or osteoporotic. Instrumentation may or may not be necessary during the anterior portion of the procedure and is placed at the surgeon's discretion.

After anterior release and fusion, posterior instrumentation and fusion are done, with segmental fixation from stable vertebra to stable vertebra. Care is taken to avoid ending an instrumentation construct at the apex of a curve in either the coronal or the sagittal plane because of the risk of later decompensation. It also is prudent to include any disc level with severe degenerative changes, especially in degenerative deformities.

Boachie-Adjei and Cunningham reported the use of a hybrid approach consisting of limited anterior and overlapping posterior instrumentation for adult thoracolumbar and lumbar scoliosis. They noted 59% and 68% correction in thoracolumbar and lumbar curves, respectively.

PEDICLE SUBTRACTION OSTEOTOMY

This is a very useful technique for correction of sagittal imbalance when performed below the level of the conus. It can achieve greater correction than Smith-Petersen type osteotomies alone and may be necessary in the setting of sagittal imbalance in a previously fused spine.

TECHNIQUE 3.32

(BRIDWELL ET AL.)

- Pedicle screws should be placed as the first step. We prefer using a freehand technique whenever possible to reduce radiation exposure to the operative team and patient.
- Extend the central laminectomy to include all posterior elements, using Leksell and Kerrison rongeurs and osteotomes as much as possible to save bone graft material. This posterior element resection is, in essence, a Smith-Petersen osteotomy above and below the pedicles that are to be resected (Fig. 3.60A).
- Use an osteotome to create the transverse process osteotomy.
- Resect the pedicle itself with a Leksell rongeur, high-speed burr, or both.
- Carefully dissect along the vertebral wall with a small Cobb or Penfield elevator to avoid injuring the segmental vessels. Place specialized spoon retractors along the lateral aspect of the vertebral body.
- To make the osteotomy, a decancellation or sharp osteotomy technique can be used. Using an osteotome provides better control of the geometry of the osteotomy, thereby affording more precise and greater correction. Commercial osteotomy guides can guide the amount of resection required to achieve the desired angular correction. It is critical during this step to avoid iatrogenic injury, via stretch or direct sharp injury, to the dural sac and nerve roots. This is best accomplished with a nerve root retractor and a no. 4 Penfield elevator.
- Before the osteotomy is completed, a temporary rod can be placed to allow for controlled closure.
- Once the posterior vertebral wall is sufficiently thinned, use specialized impactors to impact the posterior body wall into the defect. It is critical to ensure that the dural sac is free of adhesions at this point.
- With a high-speed drill, resect the lateral vertebral wall, taking care to avoid injury to the nerve roots and dural sac. Alternatively, a thin Leksell rongeur can be used.
- Close the osteotomy by applying compression or cantilever bending maneuvers to the spine. During this process, it is critical to make sure that the decompression is wide enough above and below to avoid injury or iatrogenic stenosis to the dural sac.

OTHER TECHNIQUES

The newest generation of implants can be used to treat most deformities, allowing instrumentation of all thoracic levels down to the sacrum and pelvis. Approaches and techniques generally have remained the same, however. Pedicle screw instrumentation has been used in all levels in the treatment of spinal deformities, with excellent clinical and radiographic results. For lumbar curves, pedicle screw instrumentation is applied to the convexity and compressed to create lordosis; for typical thoracic curves, the pedicle screws are applied to the concavity of the deformity and distracted to restore kyphosis. Any compensatory curves must be treated appropriately with compression where lordosis is required and with distraction where kyphosis is desired. Upper thoracic curves are controlled by compression of the convexity because most of these curves also are kyphotic.

Computer-navigation and robotic devices can be helpful in the placement of pedicle screws; however, given the additional setup time required and the safety and ease of freehand techniques, we typically reserve navigation or robotics for placement of pedicle screws across a fusion mass that has lost all anatomic landmarks or in severe deformities where anatomy is difficult to identify. These technologies can confirm anatomic relationships and, although expensive, are being used more frequently. Image guidance and robotics can facilitate instrumentation placement and correction while reducing radiation exposure to the surgeon and patient in less-invasive decompression and fusion procedures.

For skilled endoscopic spinal surgeons, VATS surgery provides excellent visualization through relatively small incisions with the potential to decrease blood loss, postoperative pain, periscapular winging, and pulmonary dysfunction. The learning curve is very steep, however, with initial procedures taking a good deal longer than a typical thoracotomy. This technique requires double lumen intubation and places increased demands on the anesthesia staff. Although VATS surgery continues to develop, the options for its use in anterior instrumentation are still limited. In adult patients with spinal deformity, in whom osteoporosis and osteopenia are prevalent, structural grafts may be more difficult to place endoscopically, limiting the application of VATS.

Direct lateral or far lateral approaches to the interbody space in the lumbar spine are especially useful for degenerative scoliosis. These techniques allow for complete disc

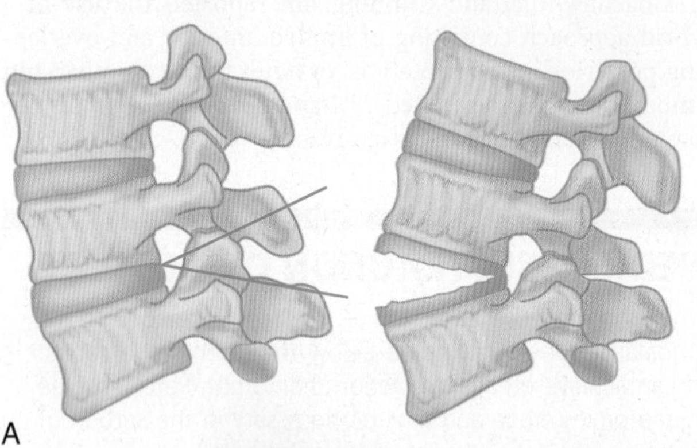

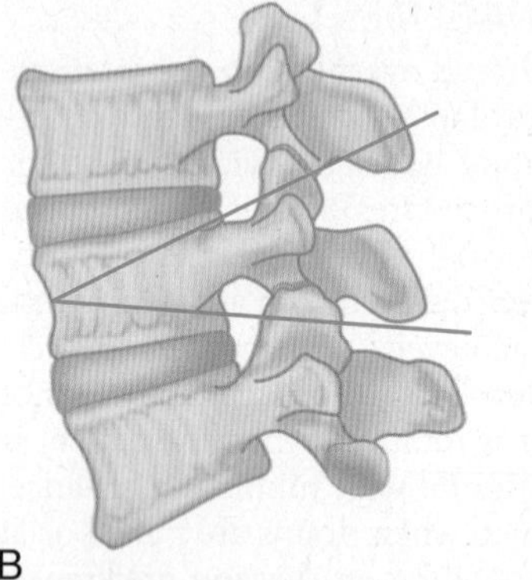

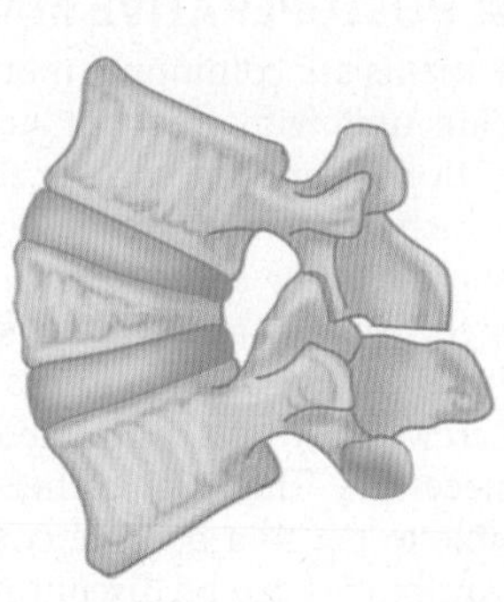

FIGURE 3.60 **A,** Smith-Petersen osteotomy. **B,** Pedicle subtraction osteotomy. **SEE TECHNIQUE 3.32.**

resection with a bony bed for fusion, excellent correction of coronal deformities, and very good indirect decompression of foraminal stenosis caused by degenerative changes and scoliotic foraminal compression. These are not typically done as stand-alone procedures and deformity corrections benefit from the addition of posterior pedicle screw instrumentation, which can be done posteriorly if the posterior fusion is omitted.

Anand et al. reported that minimally invasive multilevel percutaneous correction and fusion through a direct lateral transpsoas approach allowed multisegment correction with less blood loss and morbidity than an open approach. Reported complications of combined transpsoas extreme lateral interbody fusion and posterior pedicle screw instrumentation have included intraoperative bowel injury, motor radiculopathy, and postoperative thigh paresthesias or dysesthesias. The rate of major complications after a far lateral approach in one study, however, compared favorably to that of other procedures (12%). For these reasons, we commonly perform multilevel lateral interbody fusion and/or anterior interbody fusion as the first stage of adult deformity fusion surgery.

ILIAC FIXATION

Modern instrumentation techniques for correction of spinal deformity in adult patients often include iliac fixation. These large (>8.0 mm diameter) and very long (>80 mm) screws obtain purchase anterior to the lumbosacral pivot point. This creates a more rigid construct and unloads the S1 screws, which, even with tricortical purchase, can be prone to loosening and even fracture. Iliac fixation should be considered when fusion constructs extend proximally to L3 or beyond and when there is insufficient sacral fixation, significant sagittal or coronal imbalance that requires correction, L5 or S1 defects from tumor or infection, or an L5-S1 pseudarthrosis.

Although many iliac fixation techniques have been developed, currently the two most popular choices are iliac screws and S2-alar-iliac screws (S2AI). Traditional iliac screws involve placing a screw from the posterior superior iliac spine (PSIS) toward the anterior superior iliac spine (ASIS). This screw can be safely placed freehand or with the use of intraoperative fluoroscopy. However, there are two distinct disadvantages of this technique: (1) symptomatic screw prominence and (2) difficulty with aligning the iliac screw tulip with the S1 tulip without the use of an offset connector. Alternatively, the S2AI screw obviates both of these issues by starting more medially and distally, between the S1 and S2 foramen, extending through the SI joint, and obtaining purchase in the ilium. Early experience with the S2AI screws suggests they cause fewer symptomatic implant issues requiring removal. Adult deformity surgeons should be able to place both types of iliac fixation in case anatomic or implant issues preclude one option.

COCCYGEAL PAIN

Pain in the region of the coccyx is referred to as coccydynia or coccygodynia. Although the literature indicates that this is a rare disorder, physicians in our group who specialize in spine care evaluate and treat several cases of coccygeal pain every year.

The most common causes of coccydynia that we have observed in our practice are a single direct axial trauma, such as falling directly on the coccyx, and a subtle form of cumulative trauma that occurs as a result of long periods of sitting awkwardly. As with other musculoskeletal disorders, however, other causes need to be considered (Box 3.8). In the absence of any obvious pathologic changes involving the coccyx, coccygeal pain is classified as idiopathic and may actually be the result of spasticity or abnormalities affecting the musculature of the pelvic floor.

Body mass index appears to correlate with different coccygeal configurations (Table 3.12) and different coccygeal lesions. Obese patients have mainly posterior subluxation, normal- weight patients have mainly a hypermobile or radiographically normal coccyx, and thin patients have mainly anterior subluxation and spicules.

The most common presenting complaint is pain in and around the coccyx without significant low-back pain or radiation or referral of pain. Typically, the pain is associated with sitting and is exacerbated when rising from a seated position. Palpation in the region of the coccyx may reveal localized tenderness and swelling. Although coccydynia is a clinical diagnosis, imaging studies are helpful in the evaluation. Radiographs obtained with the patient sitting and standing are most useful because they allow measurement of the sagittal rotation of the pelvis and the coccygeal angle of incidence (Fig. 3.61). Advanced imaging studies, such as MRI and technetium-99 m bone scans, may demonstrate inflammation of the sacrococcygeal area, indicating coccygeal hypermobility, and are helpful to rule out some forms of underlying pathology such as chordoma.

BOX 3.8

Classification of Coccydynia

Based on Etiology

- Idiopathic
- Traumatic

Based on Pathology

- Degeneration of the sacrococcygeal and intercoccygeal disc and joints
- Morphology of the coccyx: types II, III, IV, presence of a bony spicule and coccygeal retroversion
- Mobility of the coccyx: hypermobile or posterior subluxation
- Referred pain: lumbar pathology or arachnoiditis of the sacral nerve roots, spasm of the pelvic floor muscles, inflammation of the pericoccygeal soft tissues
- Other: neoplasm, crystal deposits, infection, somatization or neurosis

Based on Coccygeal Morphology

- Type I—curved gently forward
- Type II—marked curve with apex pointing straight forward
- Type III—angled forward sharply between the first and second or second and third segments
- Type IV—anteriorly subluxed at the level of the sacrococcygeal joint or first or second intercoccygeal joint
- Type V—coccygeal retroversion with spicule
- Type VI—scoliotic deformity

Modified from Nathan ST, Fisher BE, Roberts CS: Coccydynia: a review of pathoanatomy, aetiology, treatment and outcome, *J Bone Joint Surg* 92B:1622–1627, 2010. Copyright British Editorial Society of Bone and Joint Surgery.

Nonsurgical methods such as NSAIDs and use of a donut cushion remain the standard initial treatment for coccydynia and are successful in approximately 90% of patients. When these methods fail to relieve pain, we have had success in reducing or eliminating coccygeal pain with the injection of a local anesthetic and corticosteroids under fluoroscopic guidance. Although there is no clear consensus in the literature regarding the exact site of injection, we generally target the vestigial disc at the point of maximal tenderness over the coccyx.

COCCYGEAL INJECTION

TECHNIQUE 3.33

- Place the patient prone on a pain management table, with the legs slightly abducted and the feet "pigeon-toed" in.
- Aseptically prepare the skin area from the lumbosacral junction to the coccyx with isopropyl alcohol and povidone-iodine. Drape the area in sterile fashion.
- Adjust the C-arm to an anteroposterior projection to visualize the coccyx. Insert a 22-gauge, 3.5-inch spinal needle with the bevel facing ventrally in the midline.
- A lateral fluoroscopic image can be used to confirm the depth of the needle. Great care must be taken to prevent overinsertion because of the proximity of the rectum to the ventral surface of the coccyx.
- The needle should be inserted down to the point of maximal tenderness on the coccyx, which will radiographically correlate with a vestigial disc segment. The goal is to dock the needle on the painful vestigial disc in the midline (Fig. 3.62).
- Once the needle is docked, remove the stylet and aspirate to check for blood. If blood is not evident, inject 0.5 mL of nonionic contract dye to confirm placement. When the correct contrast pattern is obtained, slowly inject a 5-mL volume consisting of 2 mL of 1 : 1 preservative-free lidocaine without epinephrine and 3 mL of 6 mg/mL Celestone Soluspan.

Excision of the mobile segment or total coccygectomy may be indicated for patients in whom conservative management fails, especially those with radiographic evidence of hypermobility or subluxation; success rates ranging from 60% to 91% have been reported in this group of patients. Outcomes of surgery are not as good in patients with normal coccygeal mobility. Excision is considered only if the patient gets relief of the coccygeal pain that corresponds to the duration of the local anesthetic at a minimum. If the local anesthetic yields no relief, then resection of the coccyx is unlikely to as well.

TABLE 3.12

Frequency of Different Coccygeal Lesions Correlated With Patient Body Mass Index

	POSTERIOR LUXATION	ANTERIOR LUXATION	HYPERMOBILITY	SPICULE	NORMAL COCCYX
Obese patients BMI >27.4	51%	4%	27%	2%	16%
Normal—weight patients BMI 19.5 to ≤27.4	15%	6%	30%	16%	33%
Thin patients BMI <19.5	4%	4%	15%	29%	48%

BMI, Body mass index.

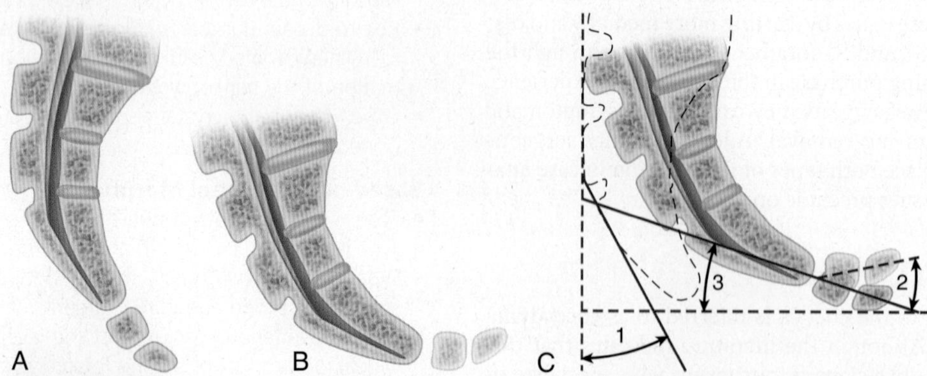

FIGURE 3.61 Evaluation of coccygeal mobility. **A,** Standing radiograph. **B,** Sitting radiograph shows flexion of the coccyx. **C,** Superimposition of sitting radiograph on standing radiograph, matching the sacrum by pivoting the sitting film through an angle representing sagittal pelvic rotation (angle *1* = angle of rotation). Coccygeal mobility is indicated by angle *2* (angle of mobility). Angle *3* is the angle at which the coccyx strikes the seat surface (angle of incidence).

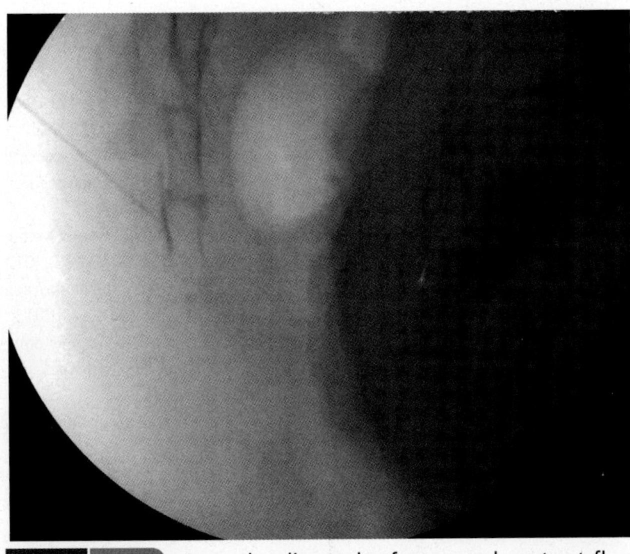

FIGURE 3.62 Lateral radiograph of coccygeal contrast flow pattern.

REFERENCES

OVERVIEW OF DISC DEGENERATION AND HERNIATION

Hughes SP, Freemont AJ, Hukins DW, et al.: The pathogenesis of degeneration of the intervertebral disc and emerging therapies in the management of back pain, *J Bone Joint Surg* 94A:1298, 2012.

Kadow T, Sowa G, Vo N, et al.: Molecular basis of intervertebral disc degeneration and herniations: what are the important translational questions? *Clin Orthop Relat Res* 473:1903, 2015.

Menezes-Reis R, Bonugli GP, Dalto VF, et al.: The association between lumbar spine sagittal alignment and L4-L5 disc degeneration among asymptomatic young adults, *Spine* 41:E1081, 2016.

Schroeder JE, Dettori JR, Brodt ED, Kaplan L: Disc degeneration after disc herniation: are we accelerating the process? *Evid Based Spine Care J* 3:33, 2012.

Weber KT, Jacobsen TD, Maidhof R, et al.: Developments in intervertebral disc disease research: pathophysiology, mechanobiology, and therapeutics, *Curr Ev Musculoskelet Med* 8:18, 2015.

DISC AND SPINE ANATOMY

Abuzayed B, Tuna Y, Gazioglu N: Thorascopic anatomy and approaches of the anterior thoracic spine: cadaver study, *Surg Radiol Anat* 34:539, 2012.

Morimoto T, Snonhata M, Kitajima M, et al.: The termination level of the conus medullaris and lumbosacral transitional vertebrae, *J Orthop Sci* 18:878, 2013.

Pattappa G, Li Z, Peroglio M, et al.: Diversity of intervertebral disc cells: phenotype and function, *J Anat* 221:480, 2012.

Teske W, Boudelal R, Zirke S, et al.: Anatomical study of preganglionic spinal nerve and discrelation at different lumbar levels: special aspect for microscopoic spine surgery, *Technol Health Care* 23:343, 2015.

Zhong W, Driscoll SJ, Wu M, et al.: In vivo morphological features of human lumbar discs, *Medicine (Baltimore)* 93:e333, 2014.

NATURAL HISTORY OF DISC DISEASE

Hutton MJ, Bayer JH, Powell J, Sharp DJ: Modic vertebral body changes: the natural history as assessed by consecutive magnetic resonance imaging, *Spine* 36:2304, 2011.

Kjaer P, Tunset A, Boyle E, Jensen TS: Progression of lumbar disc herniations over an eight- year period in a group of adult Danes from the general population—a longitudinal MRI study using quantitative measures, *BMC Musculoskelet Disord* 17:26, 2015.

Rahme R, Moussa R, Bou-Nassif R, et al.: What happens to Modic changes following lumbar discectomy? Analysis of a cohort of 41 patients with a 3- to 5-year follow-up period, *J Neurosurg Spine* 13:562, 2010.

Sharma A, Parsons M, Pilgram T: Temporal interactions of degenerative changes in individual components of the lumbar interbertebral discs: a sequential magnetic resonance imaging study in patients less than 40 years of age, *Spine* 36:1794, 2011.

Weiner BK, Vilendecic M, Ledic D, et al.: Endplate changes following discectomy: natural history and associations between imaging and clinical data, *Eur Spine J* 24:2449, 2015.

DIAGNOSTIC STUDIES

Eck JC, Sharan A, Resnick DK, et al.: Guideline update for the performance of fusion procedures for degenerative disease of the lumbar. Part 6: discography for patient selection, *J Neurosurg Spine* 21:37, 2014.

Reeves RS, Furman MB: Discography's role in low back pain management, *Pain Manag* 2:151, 2012.

Singh V, Manchikanti L, Onyewu O, et al.: An update of the appraisal of the accuracy of thoracic discography as a diagnostic test for chronic spinal pain, *Pain Physician* 15:E757, 2012.

Willems P: Decision making in surgical treatment of chronic low back pain: the performance of prognostic tests to select patients for lumbar pinal fusion, *Acta Orthop Suppl* 84:1, 2013.

Yu Y, Liu W, Song D, et al.: Diagnosis of discogenic low back pain in patients with probable symptoms but negative discography, *Arch Orthop Trauma Surg* 132:627, 2012.

INJECTION STUDIES

Benyamin RM, Wang VC, Vallejo R, et al.: A systematic evaluation of thoracic interlaminar epidural injections, *Pain Physician* 15:E497, 2012.

Bydon M, Macki M, De la Garza-Ramos R, et al.: The cost-effectiveness of CT-guided sacroiliac joint injections: a measure of QALY gained, *Neurol Res* 36:915, 2014.

Falco FJ, Manchikanti L, Datta S, et al.: An update of the effectiveness of therapeutic lumbar facet joint interventions, *Pain Physician* 15:E909, 2012.

Fekete T, Woernle C, Mannion AF, et al.: The effect of epidural steroid injection on postoperative outcome in patients from the lumbar spinal stenosis outcome study, *Spine* 40:1303, 2015.

Fotiadou A, Wojcik A, Shaju A: Management of low back pain with facet joint injections and nerve root blocks under computed tomography guidance. A prospective study, *Skeletal Radiol* 41:1081, 2012.

Gerszten PC, Smuck M, Rathmell JP, et al.: Plasma disc decompression compared with fluoroscopy-guided transforaminal epidural steroid injections for symptomatic contained lumbar disc herniation: a prospective, randomized, controlled trial, *J Neurosurg Spine* 12:357, 2010.

Hwang SY, Lee JW, Lee GY, Kang HS: Lumbar facet joint injection: feasibility as an alternative method in high-risk patients, *Eur Radiol* 23:3153, 2013.

Iversen T, Solberg TK, Romner B, et al.: Effect of caudal epidural steroid or saline injection in chronic lumbar radiculopathy: multicentre, blinded, randomised controlled trial, *BMJ* 343:d5278, 2011.

Kaufmann TJ, Geske JR, Murthy NS, et al.: Clinical effectiveness of single lumbar transforaminal epidural steroid injections, *Pain Med* 14:1126, 2013.

Kim M, Kim HS, Oh SW, et al.: Evolution of spinal endoscopic surgery, *Neurospine* 16:6, 2019.

Lee JH, An JH, Lee SH: Comparison of the effectiveness of interlaminar and bilateral transforaminal epidural steroid injections in treatment of patients with lumbosacral disc herniation and spinal stenosis, *Clin J Pain* 25:206, 2009.

Li K, Zhang T, Gao K, et al.: The utility of diagnostic transforaminal epidural injection in selective percutaneous endoscopic lumbar discectomy for multilevel disc herniation with monoradicular system: a prospective randomized control study, *World Neurosurg* 2019, Mar 2. [Epub ahead of print].

Manchikanti L, Benyamin RM, Falco FJ, et al.: Do epidural injections provide short- and long-term relief for lumbar disc herniation? A systematic review, *Clin Orthop Relat Res* 473:1940, 2015.

Manchikanti L, Cash KA, McManus CD, et al.: Preliminary results of a randomized, double- blind, controlled trial of fluoroscopic lumbar interlaminar epidural injections in managing chronic lumbar discogenic pain without disc herniation or radiculitis, *Pain Physician* 13:E279, 2010.

Manchikanti L, Kaye AD, Manchikanti K, et al.: Efficacy of epidural injections in the treatment of lumbar central spinal stenosis: a systematic review, *Anesth Pain Med* 5:e23139, 2015.

Manchikanti L, Malla Y, Wargo BW, et al.: A prospective evaluation of complications of 10,000 fluoroscopically directed epidural injections, *Pain Physician* 15:131, 2012.

Manchikanti L, Singh V, Falco FJ, et al.: Evaluation of the effectiveness of lumbar interlaminar epidural injections in managing chronic pain of lumbar disc herniation or radiculitis: a randomized, double-blind, controlled trial, *Pain Physician* 13:343, 2010.

Mandel S, Schilling J, Peterson E, et al.: A retrospective analysis of vertebral body fractures following epidural steroid injections, *J Bone Joint Surg* 95A:961, 2013.

McCormick Z, Cushman D, Casey E, et al.: Factors associated with pain reduction after transforaminal epidural steroid injection for lumbosacral radicular pain, *Arch Phys Med Rehabil* 95:2350, 2014.

Patel IJ, Davidson JK, Nikolic B, et al.: Consensus guidelines for periprocedural management of coagulation status and hemostasis risk in percutaneous image-guided interventions, *J Vasc Interv Radiol* 23(6):727, 2012.

Quraishi NA: Transforaminal injection of corticosteroids for lumbar radiculopathy: systemtic review and meta-analysis, *Eur Spine J* 21:214, 2012.

Rados I, Sakic K, Fingler M, Kapural L: Efficacy of interlaminar vs transforaminal epidural steroid injection for the treatment of chronic unilateral radicular pain: prospective, randomized study, *Pain Med* 12:1316, 2011.

Ribeiro LH, Furtado RN, Konai MS, et al.: Effect of facet joint injection versus systematic steroids in low back pain: a randomized controlled trial, *Spine* 38:1995, 2013.

Schilling LS, Markman JD: Corticosteroids for pain of spinal origin: epidural and intraarticular administration, *Rheum Dis Clin North Am* 42(1):137, 2016.

Schütz U, Cakir B, Dreinhöfer K, et al.: Diagnostic value of lumbar facet joint injection: a prospective triple cross-over study, *PLoS ONE* 6:e27991, 2011.

Shim E, Lee JW, Lee E, et al.: Flouroscopically guided epidural injections of the cervical and lumbar spine, *Radiographics* 37:537, 2017.

Zou YC, Li YK, Yu CF, et al.: A cadaveric study on sacroiliac joint injection, *Int Surg* 100:320, 2015.

THORACIC DISC DISEASE

Arnold PM, Johnson PL, Anderson KK: Surgical management of multiple thoracic disc herniations via a transfacet approach: a report of 15 cases, *J Neurosurg Spine* 15:76, 2011.

Arts MP, Bartels RH: Anterior or posterior approach of thoracic disc herniation? A comparative cohort of mini-transthoracic versus transpedicular discectomies, *Spine J* 14:1654, 2014.

Ayhan S, Nelson C, Gok B, et al.: Transthoracic surgical treatment for centrally located thoracic disc herniations presenting with myelopathy: a 5-year institutional experience, *J Spinal Disord Tech* 23:79, 2010.

Chandra SP, Ramdurg SR, Kurwale N, et al.: Extended costotransversectomy to achieve circumferential fusion for pathologies causing thoracic instability, *Spine J* 14:2094, 2014.

Choi KY, Eun SS, Lee SH, Lee HY: Percutaneous endoscopic thoracic discectomy: transforaminal approach, *Minim Invasive Neurosurg* 53:25, 2010.

Coppes MH, Bakker NA, Metzemaekers JD, Groen RJ: Posterior transdural disectomy: a new approach for the removal of a central thoracic disc herniation, *Eur Spine J* 21:623, 2011.

Cornips EM, Janssen ML, Beuls EA: Thoracic disc herniation and acute myelopathy: clinical presentation, neuroimaging findings, surgical considerations, and outcome, *J Neurosurg Spine* 14:520, 2011.

Elhadi AM, Zehri AH, Zaidi HA, et al.: Surgical efficacy of minimally invasive thoracic discectomy, *J Clin Neurosci* 22:1708, 2015.

Khoo LT, Smith ZA, Asgarzadie F, et al.: Minimally invasive extracavitary approach for thoracic discectomy and interbody fusion: 1-year-clinical and radiographic outcomes in 13 patients compared with a cohort of traditional anterior transthoracic approaches, *J Neurosurg Spine* 14:250, 2011.

Lubelski D, Abdullah KG, Steinmetz MP, et al.: Lateral extracavitary, costotransversectomy, and transthoracic thoracotomy approaches to the thoracic spine: review of techniques and complications, *J Spinal Disord Tech* 26:222, 2013.

Oppenlander ME, Clark JC, Kalyvas J, Dickman CA: Indications and techniques for spinal instrumentation in thoracic disk surgery, *Clin Spine Surg* 29:E99, 2016.

Snyder LA, Smith ZA, Dahdaleh NS, Fessler RG: Minimally invasive treatment of thoracic disc herniations, *Neurosurg Clin N Am* 25:271, 2014.

Wagner R, Telfeian AE, Iprenburg M, et al.: Transforaminal endoscopic foraminoplasty and discectomy for the treatment of a thoracic disc herniation, *World Neurosurg* 90:194, 2016.

Wait SD, Fox DJ, Kenny KJ, Dickman CA: Thoracoscopic resection of symptomatic herniated discs: clinical results in 121 patients, *Spine* 37:35, 2012.

Yamasaki R, Okuda S, Maeno T, et al.: Surgical outcomes of posterior thoracic interbody fusion for thoracic disc herniations, *Eur Spine J* 22:2496, 2013.

Yanni DS, Connery C, Perin NI: Video-assisted thoracoscopic surgery combined with a tubular retractor system for minimally invasive thoracic discectomy, *Neurosurgery* 68(1 Suppl Operative):138, 2011.

Yoshihara H: Surgical treatment for thoracic disc herniation: an update, *Spine* 39:E406, 2014.

Yoshihara H, Yoneoka D: Comparison of in-hospital morbidity and mortality rates between anterior and nonanterior approach procedures for thoracic disc herniation, *Spine* 39:E728, 2014.

LUMBAR DISC DISEASE

ETIOLOGY, DIAGNOSIS, AND CONSERVATIVE TREATMENT

Daffner SD, Hymanson HJ, Wang JC: Cost and use of conservative management of lumbar disc herniation before surgical discectomy, *Spine J* 10:463, 2010.

de Schepper EI, Damen J, van Meurs JB, et al.: The association between lumbar disc degeneration and low back pain: the influence of age, gender, and individual radiographic features, *Spine* 35:531, 2010.

Golinvaux NS, Bohl DD, Basques BA, et al.: Comparison of the lumbar disc herniation patients randomized in SPORT to 6,846 discectomy patients from NSQIP: demographic, perioperative variables, and complications correlate well, *Spine J* 15:685, 2015.

Hahne AJ, Ford JJ, McMeeken JM: Conservative management of lumbar disc herniation with associated radiculopathy: a systematic review, *Spine* 35:E488, 2010.

Jegede KA, Ndu A, Grauer JN: Contemporary management of symptomatic lumbar disc herniations, *Orthop Clin North Am* 41:217, 2010.

Jiang H, Deng Y, Wang T, et al: Interleukin-23 may contribute to the pathogenesis of lumbar

Kerr D, Zhao W, Lurie JD: What are the long-term predictors of outcomes for lumbar disc herniation? A randomized and observational study, *Clin Orthop Relat Res* 473:1920, 2015.

Kido T, Okuyama K, Chiba M, et al.: Clinical diagnosis of upper lumbar disc herniation: pain and/or numbness distribution are more useful for appropriate level diagnosis, *J Orthop Sci* 21:419, 2016.

Lee BH, Kim TH, Park MS, et al.: Comparison of effects of nonoperative treatment and decompression surgery on risk of patients with lumbar spinal stenosis falling: evaluation with functional mobility tests, *J Bone Joint Surg* 96A:e110, 2014.

Li Y, Fredrickson V, Resnick DK: How should we grade lumbar disc herniation and nerve root compression? A systematic review, *Clin Orthop Relat Res* 473:2015, 1986.

Malik KM, Cohen SP, Walega DR, Benzon HT: Diagnostic criteria and treatment of discogenic pain: a systematic review of recent clinical literature, *Spine J* 13:1675, 2013.

Oktay AB, Albayrak NB, Akgul YS: Computer aided diagnosis of degenerative intervertebral disc diseases from lumbar MR images, *Comput Med Imaging Graph* 38:613, 2014.

Pearson A, Blood E, Luire J, et al.: Predominant leg pain associated with better surgical outcomes in degenerative spondylolisthesis and spinal stenosis. Results from the Spine Patient Outcomes Research Trial (SPORT), *Spine* 36:219, 2011.

Siemionow K, An H, Masuda K, et al.: The effects of age, gender, ethnicity, and spinal level on the rate of intervertebral disc degeneration: a review of 1712 intervertebral discs, *Spine* 36:1333, 2011.

van der Windt DA, Simons E, Riphagen II , et al.: Physical examination for lumbar radiculopathy due to disc herniation in patients with low-back pain, *Cochrane Database Syst Rev* (2):CD007431, 2010.

Wade KR, Robertson PA, Thambyah A, Broom ND: How healthy discs herniate: a biomechanical and microstructural study investigating the combined effects of compression rate and flexion, *Spine* 39:1018, 2014.
Weinstein JN, Tosteson TD, Lurie JD, et al.: Surgical versus nonoperative treatment for lumbar spinal stenosis: four-year results for the Spine Patient Outcomes Research Trial (SPORT), *Spine* 35:1329, 2010.
Yu PF, Jiang FD, Liu JT, Jiang H: Outcomes of conservative treatment for ruptured lumbar disc herniation, *Acta Orthop Belg* 79:726, 2013.

OPERATIVE TREATMENT

Aichmair A, Du JY, Shue J, et al.: Microdiscectomy for the treatment of lumbar disc herniation: an evaluation of reoperations and long-term outcomes, *Evid Based Spine Care J* 5:77, 2014.
Banagan K, Gelb D, Poelstra K, Ludwig S: Anatomic mapping of lumbar nerve roots during a direct lateral transpsoas approach to the spine: a cadaveric study, *Spine* 36:E687, 2011.
Bydon M, De la Garza-Ramos R, et al.: Impact of smoking on complications and pseudarthrosis rates after single- and 2-level posterolateral fusion of the lumbar spine, *Spine* 39:1765, 2014.
Chen J, Li C, Jiang Y, et al.: Percutaneous endoscopic lumbar discectomy for L5-S1 lumbar disc herniation using a transforaminal approach versus an interlaminar approach: a systematic review and meta-analysis, *World Neurosurg* 116:412, 2018.
Dafford EE, Anerson PA: Comparison of dural repair techniques, *Spine J* 15:1099, 2015.
Dohrmann GJ, Mansour N: Long-term results of various operations for lumbar disc herniation: analysis of over 39,000 patients, *Med Princ Pract* 24:285, 2015.
Eun SS, Chachan S, Lee SH: Interlaminar percutaneous endoscopic lumbar discectomy: rotate and retract technique, *World Neurosurg* 118:188, 2018.
Fakouri B, Shetty NR, White TC: Is sequestrectomy a viable alternative to microdiscectomy? A systematic review of the literature, *Clin Orthop Relat Res* 473:1957, 2015.
Fakouri B, Stovell MG, Allom R: A comparative study of lumbar microdiscectomy in obese and non-obese patients, *J Spinal Disord Tech* 28:E352, 2015.
Fischer CR, Ducoffe AR, Errico TJ: Posterior lumbar fusion: choice of approach and adjunct techniques, *J Am Acad Orthop Surg* 22:503, 2014.
Guerin P, El Fegoun AB, Obeid I, et al.: Incidental durotomy during spine surgery: incidence, management and complications, A retrospective review, *Injury* 43:397, 2012.
Houten JK, Alexandre LC, Nasser R, Wollowick AL: Nerve injury during the transpsoas approach for lumbar fusion, *J Neurosurg Spine* 15:280, 2011.
Hsu WK, McCarthy KJ, Savage JW, et al.: The Professional Athlete Spine Initiative: outcomes after lumbar disc herniation in 342 elite professional athletes, *Spine J* 11:180, 2011.
Kamper SJ, Ostelo RW, Rubinstein SM, et al.: Minimally invasive surgery for lumbar disc herniation: a systematic review and meta-analysis, *Eur Spine J* 23:1021, 2014.
Kelly MP, Mok JM, Berven S: Dynamic constructs for spinal fusion: an evidence-based review, *Orthop Clin North Am* 41:203, 2010.
Kerr D, Zhao W, Lurie JD: What are long-term predictors of outcomes for lumbar disc herniation? A randomized and observational study, *Clin Orthop Relat Res* 473:1920, 2015.
Kim HS, Paudel B, Jang JS, et al.: Percutaneous endoscopic lumbar discectomy for all types of lumbar disc herniations (LDH) including severely difficult and extremely difficult LDH cases, *Pain Physician* 21:E401, 2018.
Lau D, Han SJ, Lee JG, et al.: Minimally invasive compared to open microdiscectomy for lumbar disc herniation, *J Clin Neurosci* 18:81, 2011.
Li X, Hu Z, Cui J, et al.: Percutaneous endoscopic lumbar discectomy for recurrent lumbar disc herniation, *Int J Surg* 27:8, 2016.
Lindley EM, McCullough MA, Burger EL, et al.: Complications of axial lumbar interbody fusion, *J Neurosurg Spine* 15:273, 2011.
Lurie JD, Tosteson TD, Tosteson AN, et al.: Surgical versus nonoperative treatment for lumbar disc herniation: eight-year results for the spine patient outcomes research trial, *Spine* 39:3, 2014.
Overley SC, McAnany SJ, Andelman S, et al.: Return to play in elite athletes after lumbar microdiscectomy: a meta-analysis, *Spine* 41:713, 2016.
Pan L, Zhang P, Yin Q: Comparison of tissue damages caused by endoscopic lumbar discectomy and traditional lumbar discectomy: a randomized controlled trial, *Int J Surg* 12:534, 2014.
Phan K, Rao PJ, Kam AC, Mobbs RJ: Minimally invasive versus open transforaminal lumbar interbody fusion for treatment of degenerative lumbar disease: systematic review and meta- analysis, *Eur Spine J* 24:1017, 2015.
Ran J, Hu Y, Zheng Z, et al.: Comparison of discectomy versus sequestrectomy in lumbar disc herniation: a meta-analysis of comparative studies, *PLoS ONE* 10:e0121816, 2015.
Sidhu GS, Henkelman E, Vaccaro AR, et al.: Minimally invasive versus open posterior lumbar interbody fusion: a systematic review, *Clin Orthop Relat Res* 472:1792, 2014.
Soliman J, Harvey A, Howes G, et al.: Limited microdiscectomy for lumbar disk herniation: a retrospective long-term outcome analysis, *J Spinal Disord Tech* 27:E8, 2014.
Strömqvist F, Strömqvist B, Jönsson B, et al.: Outcome of surgical treatment of lumbar disc herniation in young individuals, *Bone Joint J* 97B:1675, 2015.
Talia AJ, Wong ML, Lau HC, Kaye AH: Comparison of the different surgical approaches for lumbar interbody fusion, *J Clin Neurosci* 22:243, 2015.
Wang K, Hong X, Zhou BY, et al.: Evaluation of transforaminal endoscopic lumbar discectomy in the treatment of lumbar disc herniation, *Int Orthop* 39:1599, 2015.
Weistroffer JK, Hsu WK: Return-to-play rates in National Football League linemen after treatment for lumbar disk herniation, *Am J Sports Med* 39:632, 2011.
Wong AP, Smith ZA, Nixon AT, et al.: Intraoperative and perioperative complications in minimally invasive transforaminal lumbar interbody fusion: a review of 513 patients, *J Neurosurg Spine* 22:487, 2015.
Zhang B, Liu S, Liu J, et al.: Transforaminal endoscopic discectomy versus conventional microdiscectomy for lumbar disc hernation: a systematic review and meta-analysis, *J Orthop Surg Res* 13:169, 2018.

DEGENERATIVE DISC DISEASE AND INTERNAL DISC DERANGEMENT

Buttermann GR, Mullin WJ: Two-level circumferential lumbar fusion comparing midline and paraspinal posterior approach: 5-year interim outcomes of a randomized, blinded, prospspective study, *J Spinal Disord Tech* 28:E534, 2015.
Guyer RD, Shellock J, MacLennan B, et al.: Early failure of metal-on-metal artifical disc prostheses associated with lymphocytic reaction: diagnosis and treatment experience in four cases, *Spine* 36:E492, 2011.
Lao LF, Zhong GB, Li QY, Liu ZD: Kinetic magnetic resonance analysis of spinal degeneration: a systematic review, *Orthop Surg* 6:294, 2014.
Lee JC, Cha JG, Yoo JH, et al.: Radiographic grading of facet degeration, is it reliable? – a comparison of MR or CT grading with histologic grading in lumbar fusion candidates, *Spine J* 12:507, 2012.
Phan K, Rao PJ, Kam AC, Mobbs RJ: Minimally invasive versus open transforaminal lumbar interbody fusion for treatment of degenerative lumbar disease: systematic review and meta- analysis, *Eur Spine J* 24:1017, 2015.
Williams BJ, Smith JS, Fu KM, et al.: Does BMP increase the incidence of perioperative complications in spinal fusion? A comparison of 55,862 cases of spinal fusion with and without BMP, *Spine* 36:1685, 2011.

FAILED SPINE SURGERY

Adogwa O, Parker SL, Shau D, et al.: Long-term outcomes of revision fusion for lumbar pseudarthrosis, *J Neurosurg Spine* 15:393, 2011.
Bordoni B, Marelli F: Failed back surgery syndrome: review and new hypotheses, *J Pain Res* 9:17, 2016.
Bronson WH, Koehler SM, Qureshi SA, Hecht AC: The importance of pain radiography in the evaluation of radiculopathy after failed diskectomy, *Orthopedics* 33:358, 2010.
Chan CW, Peng P: Failed back syndrome, *Pain Med* 12:577, 2011.
Choi KC, Ahn Y, Kang BU, et al.: Failed anterior lumbar interbody fusion due to incomplete foraminal decompression, *Acta Neurochir (Wien)* 153:567, 2011.
Chun DS, Baker KC, Hsu WK: Lumbar pseudarthrosis: a review of current diagnosis and treatment, *Neurosurg Focus* 39:E10, 2015.

Czerwein Jr JK, Thakur N, Migliori SJ, et al.: Complications of anterior lumbar surgery, *J Am Acad Orthop Surg* 19:251, 2011.

Dede O, Thuillier D, Pekmezci M, et al.: Revision surgery for lumbar pseudarthrosis, *Spine J* 15:977, 2015.

Dickson DD, Lenke LG, Bridwell KH, Koester LA: Risk factors for and assessment of symptomatic pseudarthrosis after lumbar pedicle subtraction osteotomy in adult spinal deformity, *Spine* 39:1190, 2014.

Farjoodi P, Skolasky RL, Riley 3rd LH: The effects of hospital and surgeon volume on postoperative complications after lumbar spine surgery, *Spine* 36:2069, 2011.

Glenn JS, Yaker J, Guyer RD, Ohnmeiss DD: Anterior discectomy and total disc replacement for three patients with multiple recurrent lumbar disc herniations, *Spine J* 11:e1, 2011.

McCunniff PT, Young ES, Ahmadinia K, et al.: Smoking is associated with increased blood loss and transfusion use after lumbar spinal surgery, *Clin Orthop Relat Res* 474:1019, 2016.

Mobbs RJ, Phan K, Thayaparan GK, Rao PJ: Anterior lumbar interbody fusion as a salvage technique for pseudarthrosis following posterior lumbar fusion surgery, *Global Spine J* 6:14, 2016.

Rabb CH: Failed back syndrome and epidural fibrosis, *Spine J* 10:454, 2010.

Smith JS, Ogden AT, Shafizadeh S, et al.: Clinical outcomes after microendoscopic discectomy for recurrent lumbar disc herniation, *J Spinal Disord Tech* 23:30, 2010.

Tormenti MJ, Maserati MB, Bonfield CM, et al.: Perioperative surgical complications of transforaminal lumbar interbody fusion: a single-center experience, *J Neurosurg Spine* 16:44, 2012.

Turunen V, Nyyssönen T, Miettinen H, et al: Lumbar instrumented posterolateral fusion in spondylolisthetic and failed back patients: a long-term follow-up study spanning 11-13 years,

SPINAL STENOSIS

Ammendolia C, Stuber KJ, Rok E, et al.: Nonoperative treatment for lumbar spinal stenosis with neurogenic claudication, *Cochrane Database Syst Rev* (8):CD010712, 2013.

Athiviraham A, Wali ZA, Yen D: Predictive factors influencing clinical outcome with operative management of lumbar spinal stenosis, *Spine J* 11:613, 2011.

Briggs VG, Li W, Kaplan MS, et al.: Injection treatment and back pain associated with degenerative lumbar spinal stenosis in older adults, *Pain Physician* 13:E347, 2010.

Celik SE, Celik S, Göksu K, et al.: Microdecompressive laminotomy with a 5-year follow-up period for severe lumbar spinal stenosis, *J Spinal Disord Tech* 23:229, 2010.

Försth P, Michaëlsson K, Sandén B: Does fusion improve the outcome after decompressive surgery for lumbar spinal stenosis? A two-year follow-up study involving 5390 patients, *Bone Joint J* 95B:960, 2013.

Genevay S, Atlas SJ: Lumbar spinal stenosis, *Best Pract Res Clin Rheumatol* 24:253, 2010.

Harrop JS, Hilibrand A, Mihalovich KE, et al.: Cost-effectiveness of surgical treatment for degenerative spondylolisthesis and spinal stenosis, *Spine* 39(22 Suppl 1):S75, 2014.

He B, Yan L, Xu Z, et al.: Treatment strategies for the surgical complications of thoracic spinal stenosis: a retrospective analysis of two hundred and eighty three cases, *Int Orthop* 38:117, 2014.

Hong SW, Choi KY, Ahn Y, et al.: A comparison of unilateral and bilateral laminotomies for decompression of L4-L5 spinal stenosis, *Spine* 36:E172, 2011.

Hsieh MK, Chen LH, Niu CC, et al.: Combined anterior lumbar interbody fusion and instrumented posterolateral fusion for degenerative lumbar scoliosis: indication and surgical outcomes, *BMC Surg* 15:26, 2015.

Issack PS, Cunningham ME, Pumberger M, et al.: Degenerative lumbar spinal stenosis: evaluation and management, *J Am Acad Orthop Surg* 20:527, 2012.

Jalil Y, Carvalho C, Becker R: Long-term clinical and radiological postoperative outcomes after an interspinous microdecompression of degenerative lumbar spinal stenosis, *Spine* 39:368, 2014.

Kelleher MO, Timlin M, Persaud O, Rampersaud YR: Success and failure of minimally invasive decompression for focal lumbar spinal stenosis in patients with and without deformity, *Spine* 35:E981, 2010.

Komp M, Hahn P, Merk H, et al.: Bilateral operation of lumbar degenerative central spinal stenosis in full-endoscopic interlaminar technique with unilateral approach: prospective 2- year results of 74 patients, *J Spinal Disord Tech* 24:281, 2011.

Kovacs FM, Urrútia G, Alarcón JD: Surgery versus conservative treatment for symptomatic lumbar spinal stenosis: a systematic review of randomized controlled trials, *Spine* 36:E1335, 2011.

Lad SP, Babu R, Ugiliweneza B, et al.: Surgery for spinal stenosis: long-term reoperation rates, health care cost, and impact of instrumentation, *Spine* 39:978, 2014.

Lee JW, Myung JS, Park KW, et al.: Fluoroscopically guided caudal epidural steroid injection for management of degenerative lumbar spinal stenosis: short- and long-term results, *Skeletal Radiol* 39:691, 2010.

Lee JY, Whang PG, Lee JY, et al.: Lumbar spinal stenosis, *Instr Course Lect* 62:383, 2013.

Leonardi MA, Zanetti M, Min K: Extent of decompression and incidence of postoperative epidural hematoma among different techniques of spinal decompression in degenerative lumbar spinal stenosis, *J Spinal Disord Tech* 26:407, 2013.

Li C, He Q, Tang Y, Ruan D: The fate of adjacent segments with pre-existing degeneration after lumbar posterolateral fusion: the influence of degenerative grading, Eur Spine J

Minamide A, Yoshida M, Maio K: The natural clinical course of lumbar spinal stenosis: a longitudinal cohort study over a minimum of 10 years, *J Orthop Sci* 18:693, 2013.

Nemani VM, Aichmair A, Taher F, et al.: Rate of revision surgery after standalone lateral lumbar interbody fusion for lumbar spinal stenosis, *Spine* 39:E326, 2014.

Orpen NM, Corner JA, Shetty RR, Marshall R: Micro-decompression for lumbar spinal stenosis: the early outcome using a modified surgical technique, *J Bone Joint Surg* 92B:550, 2010.

Parker SL, Godil SS, Mendenhall SK, et al.: Two-year comprehensive medical management of degenerative lumbar spine disease (lumbar spondylolisthesis, stenosis, or disc herniation): a value analysis of cost, pain, disability, and quality of life: clinical article, *J Neurosurg Spine* 21:143, 2014.

Pearson A, Blood E, Lurie J, et al.: Predominant leg pain is associated with better surgical outcomes in degenerative spondylolisthesis and spinal stenosis: results from the Spine Patient Outcomes Research Trial (SPORT), *Spine* 36:219, 2011.

Pearson A, Blood E, Lurie J, et al.: Degenerative spondylolisthesis versus spinal stenosis: does a slip matter? Comparison of baseline characteristics and outcomes (SPORTS), *Spine* 35:298, 2010.

Pearson A, Lurie J, Tosteson T, et al.: Who should have surgery for spinal stenosis? Treatment effect predictors in SPORT, *Spine* 37:1791, 2012.

Resnick DK, Watters 3rd WC, Mummaneni PV, et al.: Guideline update for the performance of fusion procedures for degenerative disease of the lumbar spine. Part 10: lumbar fusion for stenosis without spondylolisthesis, *J Neurosurg Spine* 21:62, 2014.

Resnick DK, Watters 3rd WC, Mummaneni PV, et al.: Guideline update for the performance of fusion procedures for degenerative disease of the lumbar spine. Part 9: lumbar fusion for stenosis with spondylolisthesis, *J Neurosurg Spine* 21:54, 2014.

Sekiguchi M, Wakita T, Otani K, et al.: Lumbar spinal stenosis-specific symptom scale: validity and responsiveness, *Spine* 39:E1388, 2014.

Sigmundsson FG, Jönsson B, Strömqvist B: Preoperative pain pattern predicts surgical outcome more than type of surgery in patients with central spinal stenosis without concomitant spondylolisthesis: a register study of 9051 patients, *Spine* 39:E199, 2014.

Sigmundsson FG, Jönsson B, Strömqvist B: Outcome of decompression with and without fusion in spinal stenosis with degenerative spondylolisthesis in relation to preoperative pain pattern—a register study of 1,624 patients, *Spine J* 15:638, 2015.

Sigmundsson FG, Kang XP, Jönsson B, Strömqvist B: Correlation between disability and MRI findings in lumbar spinal stenosis: a prospective study of 109 patients operated on by decompression, *Acta Orthop* 82:204, 2011.

Slätis P, Malimivaara A, Heliövaara M, et al.: Long-term results of surgery for lumbar spinal stenosis: a randomised controlled trial, *Eur Spine J* 20:1174, 2011.

Smith CC, Booker T, Schaufele MK, Weiss P: Interlaminar versus transforaminal epidural steroid injections for the treatment of symptomatic lumbar spinal stenosis, *Pain Med* 11:1511, 2010.

Takahashi N, Kikuci S, Yabuki S, et al.: Diagnostic value of the lumbar-extension-loading test in patients with lumbar spinal stenosis: a cross-sectional study, *BMC Musculoskeletal Disord* 15:529, 2014.

Zhang L, Chen R, Xie P, et al: Diagnostic value of the nerve root sedimentation sign, a radiological sign using magnetic resonance imaging, for detecting lumbar spinal stenosis:

ADULT IDIOPATHIC AND DEGENERATIVE SCOLIOSIS

Bach K, Ahmadian A, Deukmedjian A, Uribe JS: Minimally invasive surgical techniques in adult degenerative spinal deformity: a systematic review, *Clin Orthop Relat Res* 472:1749, 2014.

Berven SH, Hohenstein NA, Savage JW, Tribus CB: Does the outcome of adult deformity surgery justify the complications in the elderly (above 70 y of age) patients? *J Spinal Disord Tech* 28:271, 2015.

Fu L, Chang MS, Crandall DG, Revella J: Does obesity affect surgical outcomes in degenerative scoliosis? *Spine* 39:2049, 2014.

Good CR, Lenke LG, Bridwell KH, et al: Can posterior-only surgery provide similar radiographic and clinical results as combined anterior (throacotomy/ thoracoabdominal)/

Graham RB, Sugrue PA, Koski TR: Adult degenerative scoliosis, *Clin Spine Surg* 29:95, 2016.

Ha KY, Jang WH, Kim YH, Park DC: Clinical relevance of the SRS-Schwab classification for degenerative lumbar scoliosis, *Spine* 41:E282, 2016.

Hallager DW, Hansen LV, Dragsted CR, et al.: A comprehensive analysis of the SRS-Schwab Adult Spinal Deformity Classification and confounding variables—a prospective, non-US cross-sectional study in 292 patients, *Spine* 41:E589, 2016.

Hassanzadeh H, Jain A, El Dafrawy MH, et al.: Clinical results and functional outcomes of primary and revision spinal deformity surgery in adults, *J Bone Joint Surg* 95A:1413, 2013.

Hong JY, Suh SW, Modi HN, et al.: Correlation of pelvic orientation with adult scoliosis, *J Spinal Disord Tech* 23:461, 2010.

Isaacs RE, Hyde J, Goodrich JA, et al.: A prospective, nonrandomized, multicenter evaluation of extreme lateral interbody fusion for the treatment of adult degenerative scoliosis: perioperative outcomes and complications, *Spine* 35:S322, 2010.

Lehman Jr RA, Kang DG, Lenke LG, et al.: Pulmonary function following adult spinal deformity surgery: minimum two-year follow-up, *J Bone Joint Surg* 97A:32, 2015.

Li M, Shen Y, Gao ZL, et al.: Surgical treatment of adult idiopathic scoliosis: long-term clinical radiographic outcomes, *Orthopedics* 34:180, 2011.

Liu S, Diebo BG, Henry JK, et al.: The benefit of nonoperative treatment for adult spinal deformity: identifying predictors for reaching a minimal clinically important difference, *Spine J* 16:210, 2016.

Manoharan SR, Baker DK, Pasara SM, et al.: Thirty-day readmissions following adult spinal deformity surgery: an analysis of the national surgical quality improvement program (NSQIP) database, *Spine J* 16:862, 2016.

Park P, Fu KM, Mummaneni PV, et al.: The impact of age on surgical goals for spinopelvic alignment in minimally invasive surgery for adult spinal deformity, *J Neurosurg Spine* 29:560, 2018.

Passias PG, Soroceanu A, Yang S, et al.: Predictors of revision surgical procedure excluding wound complications in adults spinal deformity and impact on patient-reported outcomes and satisfaction: a two-year follow-up, *J Bone Joint Surg* 98A:536, 2016.

Pichelmann MA, Lenke LG, Bridwell KH, et al.: Revision rates following primary adult spinal deformity surgery: six hundred forty-three consecutive patients followed-up to twenty- two years postoperative, *Spine* 35:219, 2010.

Riouallon G, Bouyer B, Wolff S: Risk of revision surgery for adult idiopathic scoliosis: a survival analysis of 517 cases over 25 years, *Eur Spine J* 25:2527, 2016.

Sansur CA, Smith JS, Coe JD, et al.: Scoliosis research society morbidity and mortality of adult scoliosis surgery, *Spine (Phila Pa 1976)* 36:E593, 2011.

Scheer JK, Khanna R, Lopez AJ, et al.: The concave versus convex approach for minimally invasive lateral lumbar interbody fusion for thoracolumbar degenerative scoliosis, *J Clin Neurosurg* 22:1588, 2015.

Scheer JK, Mundis GM, Klineberg E, et al.: Post-operative recovery following adult spinal deformity surgery: comparative analysis of age in 149 patients during 1-year follow up, *Spine* 40:1505, 2015.

Scheufler KM, Cyron D, Dohmen H, Eckardt A: Less invasive surgical correction of adult degenerative scoliosis, part 1: technique and radiographic results, *Neurosurgery* 67:697, 2010.

Scheufler KM, Cyron D, Dohmen H, Eckardt A: Less invasive surgical correction of adult degenerative scoliosis, part II: complications and clinical outcome, *Neurosurgery* 67:1609, 2010.

Shaw R, Skovrlj B, Cho SK: Association between age and complications in adult scoliosis surgery: an analysis of the Scoliosis Research Society Morbidity and Mortality database, *Spine* 41:508, 2016.

Smith JS, Klineberg E, Lafage V, et al.: Prospective multicenter assessment of perioperative and minimum 2-year postoperative complication rates associated with adult spinal deformity surgery, *J Neurosurg Spine* 26:1–14, 2016.

Smith JS, Lafage V, Shaffrey CI, et al: Outcomes of operative and nonoperative treatment for adult spinal deformity: a prospective, multicenter, propensity-matched cohort assessment

Smith JS, Shaffrey CI, Glassman SD, et al: Risk-benefit assessment of surgery for adult scoliosis: an analysis based on patient age, *Spine* 36:2011.

Soroceanu A, Burton DC, Diebo BG, et al.: Impact of obesity on complications, infection, and patient-reported outcomes in adult spinal deformity surgery, *J Neurosurg Spine* 23:656, 2015.

Soroceanu A, Diebo BG, Burton D, et al.: Radiographical and implant-related complications in adult spinal deformity surgery: incidence, patient risk factors, and impact on health-related quality of life, *Spine* 40:1414, 2015.

Tormenti MJ, Maserati MB, Bonfield CM, et al.: Complications and radiographic correction in adult scoliosis following combined transpsoas extreme lateral interbody fusion and posterior pedicle screw instrumentation, *Neurosurg Focus* 28:E7, 2010.

Transfeldt EE, Topp R, Mehbod AA, Winter RB: Surgical outcomes of decompression, decompression with limited fusion, and decompression with full curve fusion for degenerative scoliosis with radiculopathy, *Spine* 35:1872, 2010.

Verla T, Adogwa O, Toche U, et al.: Impact of increasing age on outcomes of spinal fusion in adult idiopathic scoliosis, *World Neurosurg* 87:591, 2016.

Wang G, Hu J, Liu X, Cao Y: Surgical treatments for degenerative lumbar scoliosis: a meta

Wollowick AL, Kang DG, Lehman Jr RA: Timing of surgical staging in adults spinal deformity surgery: is later better? *Spine J* 13:1723, 2013.

Worley N, Marascalchi B, Jalai CM, et al.: Predictors of inpatient morbidity and mortality in adult spinal deformity surgery, *Eur Spine J* 25:819, 2016.

Yadla S, Maltenfort MG, Ratliff JK, Harrop JS: Adult scoliosis surgery outcomes: a systematic review, *Neurosurg Focus* 28:E3, 2010.

Yagi M, Boachie-Adjei O, King AB: Characterization of osteopenia/osteoporosis in adult scoliosis. Does bone density affect surgical outcome? *Spine* 36:1652, 2011.

Yagi M, Ohne H, Kaneko S, et al.: Does corrective spine surgery improve the standing balance in patients with adult spinal deformity? *Spine J* 18:36, 2018.

Zhu F, Bao H, Liu Z, et al: Unanticipated revision surgery in adult spinal deformity: an

ANKYLOSING SPONDYLITIS

Arun R, Dabke HV, Mehdian H: Comparison of three types of lumbar osteotomy for ankylosing spondylitis: a case series and evolution of a safe technique for instrumented fusion, *Eur Spine J* 20:2252, 2011.

Baraliakos X, Listing J, von der Recke A, Braun J: The natural course of radiographic progression in ankylosing spondylitis: differences between genders and appearance of characteristic radiographic features, *Curr Rheum Rep* 13:383, 2011.

Park YS, Him HS, Baek SW: Spinal osteotomy in ankylosing spondylitis: radiological, clinical, and psychological results, *Spine J* 14:1921, 2014.

Park YS, Kim HS, Baek SW, Oh JH: Preoperative computer-based simulations for the

Ravinsky RA, Ouellet JA, Brodt ED, Dettori JR: Vertebral osteotomies in ankylosing spondylitis—comparison of outcomes following closing wedge osteotomy versus opening wedge osteotomy: a systematic review, *Evid Based Spine Care J* 4:18, 2013.

Zhang W, Zheng M: Operative strategy for different types of thoracolumbar stress fractures in ankylosing spondylitis, *J Spinal Disord Tech* 27:423, 2014.

Zheng GQ, Song K, Zhang YG, et al.: Two-level spinal osteotomy for severe thoracolumbar kyphosis in ankylosing spondylitis: experience with 48 patients, *Spine* 39:1055, 2014.

COCCYGEAL PAIN

Haddad B, Prasad V, Khan W, et al.: Favourable outcomes of coccygectomy for refractory coccygodynia, *Ann R Coll Surg Engl* 96:136, 2014.

Hanley EN, Ode G, Jackson BJ, Seymour R: Coccygectomy for patients with chronic coccydynia: a prospective, observational study of 98 patients, *Bone Joint J* 98B:526, 2016.

Hanley EN, Ode G, Jackson BJ, et al.: Coccygectomy for patients with chronic coccydynia: a prospective, observational study of 98 patients, *Bone Joint J* 98-B:526, 2016.

Karadimas EJ, Trypsiannis G, Giannoudis PV: Surgical treatment of coccygodynia: an analytic review of the literature, *Eur Spine J* 20:698, 2011.

Kerr EE, Benson D, Schrot RJ: Coccygectomy for chronic refractory coccygodynia: clinical case series and literature review, *J Neurosurg Spine* 14:654, 2011.

Lirette LS, Chaiban G, Tolba R, Eissa H: Coccydynia: an overview of the anatomy, etiology,

Maigne J, Pigeau I, Aguer N, et al.: Chronic coccydynia in adolescents: a series of 53 patients, *Eur J Phys Rehabi Med* 47:245, 2011.

Nathan ST, Fisher BE, Roberts CS: Coccydynia: a review of pathoanatomy, aetiology, treatment and outcome, *J Bone Joint Surg* 92B:1622, 2010.

Ramieri A, Domenicucci M, Cellocco P, et al.: Acute traumatic instability of the coccyx: results in 28 consecutive coccygectomies, *Eur Spine J* 22(Suppl 6):S939, 2013.

Sarmast AH Kirmani AR, Bhat AR: Coccygectomy for coccygodynia: a single center experience over 5 years, *Asian J Neurosurg* 13:277, 2018.

Trollegaard AM, Aarby NS, Hellberg S: Coccygectomy: an effective treatment option for chronic coccydynia: retrospective results in 41 consecutive patients, *J Bone Joint Surg* 92B:242, 2010.

Woon JT, Stringer MD: Clinical anatomy of the coccyx: a systematic review, *Clin Anat* 25:158, 2012.

Woon JT, Stringer MD: CT morphology of the normal human adult coccyx, *Anat Sci Int* 89:126, 2014.

The complete list of references is available online at Expert Consult.com.

CHAPTER 4

SPONDYLOLISTHESIS

Keith D. Williams

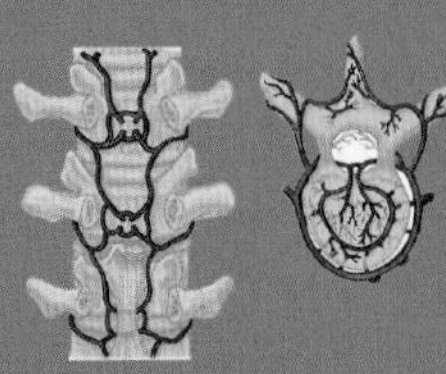

GENERAL INFORMATION

Spondylolisthesis is a descriptive term derived from the Greek *spondylo* (spine) and *olisthesis* (slip) and was first described by Herbinaux, an obstetrician, in 1782. The varied etiologies of spondylolisthesis were first classified by Wiltse, with other classifications of subtypes of spondylolisthesis added over the years. The common feature of the various types is anterior translation of the cephalad vertebra relative to the adjacent caudal segment. The biomechanical force causing this translation is the anteriorly directed vector created by the contraction of the posteriorly located erector spinae muscles, coupled with the force of gravity acting on the upper body mass through the lordotic lumbar spine and lumbosacral junction, which explains why this deformity is not seen in children before they are ambulatory. For spondylolisthesis of any type to occur there must be a failure of anatomic structure(s) that normally resist this anteriorly directed force. These structures include the facets, annulus fibrosus, posterior bony arch, and pedicles. Symptoms of spondylolisthesis include axial pain, neurogenic claudication, radiculopathy, and even cauda equina syndrome. In addition, the deformity associated with spondylolisthesis can range from not clinically apparent to severe with significant sagittal imbalance and associated truncal shortening. More recent literature has focused on the role that spinopelvic radiographic parameters may play in the development and progression of spondylolisthesis. Better understanding of the biomechanical forces and the radiographic parameters will result in better treatment decisions for spondylolisthesis.

DIAGNOSIS

In young patients with high-grade spondylolisthesis, truncal shortening and lumbar hyperlordosis may suggest the diagnosis. With less significant grades of listhesis a palpable step-off may be present associated with local tenderness. Axial pain associated with hyperextension of the lumbar spine is the most common complaint reported in young athletes.

In patients with degenerative spondylolisthesis, axial pain and a history of neurogenic claudication with reduced walking and standing tolerance are the most common features. Initial radiographic evaluation includes standing anteroposterior, lateral, and spot lateral images. Flexion/extension seated or standing lateral radiographs are helpful in identifying those with a dynamic component once the spondylolisthesis has been identified.

ETIOLOGY

Wiltse initially described five different etiologies of spondylolisthesis and later added iatrogenic instability as a sixth type. The most common types are dysplastic, isthmic, and degenerative. In a radiographic study over a 25-year period, Fredrickson et al. found that 92% of children with spondylolysis also had dysplastic features of the lumbar spine, specifically spina bifida occulta, which persisted into adulthood in 70%.

Congenital malformations of the posterior elements, especially elongation of the pars interarticularis and spina bifida occulta, can significantly compromise the ability of the posterior bony elements to resist the anteriorly directed forces applied to the spine that can lead to spondylolisthesis.

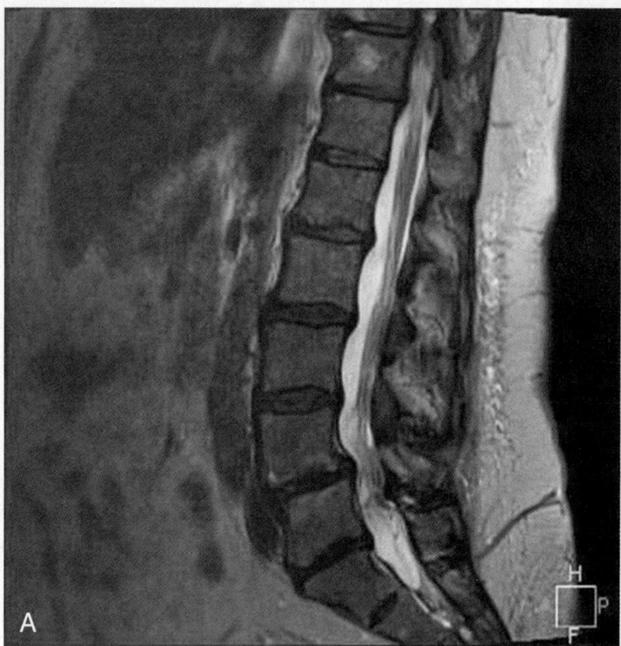

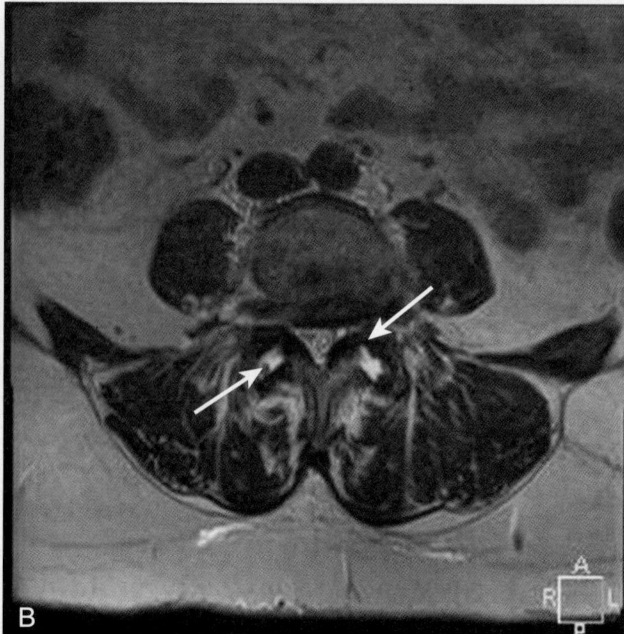

FIGURE 4.1 Degenerative spondylolisthesis with spinal stenosis. **A,** Sagittal CT. **B,** On axial view, note hypertrophic facet and ligamentum flavum *(right arrow)* and facet effusions *(left arrow)* indicating dynamic instability.

BOX 4.1

Classification of Spondylolisthesis by Wiltse et al.

Type I, dysplastic—Congenital abnormalities of the upper sacral facets or inferior facets of the fifth lumbar vertebra that allow slipping of L5-S1. No pars interarticularis defect is present in this type.

Type II, isthmic—Defect in pars interarticularis allows forward slipping of L5 on S1. Three types of isthmic spondylolistheses are recognized:

- Stress fracture of pars interarticularis (lytic)
- Elongated but intact pars interarticularis
- Acute fracture of pars interarticularis

Type III, degenerative—Intersegmental instability of long duration with subsequent remodeling of the articular processes at the level of involvement

Type IV, traumatic—Fractures in the area of the bony hook other than the pars interarticularis, such as the pedicle, lamina, or facet

Type V, pathologic—Generalized or localized bone disease and structural weakness of the bone, such as osteogenesis imperfecta

Even though these anomalies are present at birth the spondylolisthesis does not occur until after the child is able to ambulate, which causes the anteriorly directed force to be generated. As the forces increase with growth, the annulus is unable to restrain the caudal-ventral force, which leads to the development of the spondylolisthesis. As the anterior translation occurs progressively severe spinal stenosis can result with variable neurologic sequelae.

Fracture of the pars interarticularis results in an isthmic type of spondylolisthesis. Development of a pars interarticularis stress fracture is the most common reason for a spondylolysis. Less commonly, fatigue fracture with healing and resultant elongation of the pars or acute traumatic pars fracture can result in an isthmic spondylolisthesis. The incidence of spondylolysis is 0% at birth and increases to 7% by age 18. Most people with spondylolysis will develop a grade 1 slip over time. Longitudinal studies to evaluate the risk factors for developing a high-grade (greater than 50%) slip have identified several radiographic factors of importance, including disc degeneration, high slip angle, and increased pelvic incidence. It remains unclear which, if any, of these findings may actually cause slip progression and which may result from it.

Degenerative spondylolisthesis occurs as a result of the degenerative cascade as described by Kirkaldy-Willis. The loss of disc height allows the cephalad vertebra to translate anteriorly. The associated hypertrophic facet and ligamentous changes result in spinal stenosis centrally and in the lateral recess more so than in other types of spondylolisthesis (Fig. 4.1).

CLASSIFICATION

Two classification systems are most commonly used to describe spondylolisthesis. The Wiltse classification describes six types of spondylolisthesis based on the location of the deficiency of the posterior elements that allows the listhesis to occur (Box 4.1). The other classification system in common usage was developed by Marchetti and Bartolozzi and divides spondylolisthesis types into dysplastic and acquired types. In addition to classification systems based primarily on etiology, Meyerding devised a widely used grading system based on the amount of translation at the affected level that provides an easily determined metric for the severity of the slip. This grading system divides the superior endplate of the caudal vertebra into four equal portions. This allows for five possible grades, based on the position of the posterior inferior corner of the cephalad vertebral body relative to the four segments of the superior endplate below (Table 4.1 and Fig. 4.2).

WILTSE CLASSIFICATION OF SPONDYLOLISTHESIS

TYPE 1 DYSPLASTIC

Malformation or dysplasia of the posterior elements, particularly the pars or inferior facet of the cephalad vertebra or the superior facet of the caudal vertebra (or both), results in a loss of the normal buttressing effect to resist the anterior and caudally directed forces on the cephalad vertebra as a result of gravity and contraction of the erector spinae muscles. This dysplasia most often occurs at the lumbopelvic junction and affects the geometry of the sacrum and L5. In addition, congenital defects such as spina bifida or elongation of the pars can result in instability and resultant progressive slippage.

TYPE 2 ISTHMIC

The hallmark of this type is a defect in the pars interarticularis. This defect can be lytic, the result of a stress fracture (most common), or attributed to bone remodeling of microfractures resulting in an elongated pars, or an acute pars fracture. Isthmic spondylolisthesis often occurs in children, adolescents, and young adults but can occur into the fifth decade. Because of the cortical nature of the bone of the pars interarticularis, fracture healing potential is relatively poor.

TABLE 4.1

Meyerding Classification of Spondylolisthesis

GRADE	DISPLACEMENT*
I	0%-25%
II	26%-50%
III	51%-75%
IV	76%-100%
V (spondyloptosis)	>100%

*As measured on lateral radiograph, distance from the posterior edge of the superior vertebral body to the posterior edge of the adjacent inferior vertebral body; distance is reported as a percentage of the total superior vertebral body length.

TYPE 3 DEGENERATIVE

Degenerative spondylolisthesis is the most common type. It results from segmental instability as a result of disc degeneration and facet remodeling and thus occurs later in life. Patients with degenerative spondylolisthesis are more likely to have a dynamic component to their deformity, meaning the amount of translation is affected by their body position. This type of listhesis is most common at the L4-L5 level, usually in women over 50 years of age, particularly those of African descent. For patients with a dynamic component, it is important to obtain upright films, because the spondylolisthesis may not be visible on supine imaging such as MRI.

TYPE 4 TRAUMATIC

This is an uncommon type of spondylolisthesis. Unlike the isthmic type, the fracture is not through the pars. Rather, it is through any other part of the posterior elements, usually involving the pedicles or facets. These tend to be high-energy injuries.

TYPE 5 PATHOLOGIC

This also is an uncommon etiology involving a pathologic process that affects the posterior arch, such as infection or Paget disease, leading to instability at the affected segment.

TYPE 6 IATROGENIC

This type was added after the original description of the classification. Iatrogenic spondylolisthesis occurs when there has been surgical treatment at the involved segment and the instability is the result of the surgical intervention. Most commonly this is as a result of transection of the pars with facetectomy or excessive pars thinning and subsequent fracture of the pars leading to instability.

MARCHETTI-BARTOLOZZI CLASSIFICATION OF SPONDYLOLISTHESIS

Marchetti and Bartolozzi developed a classification based on etiology with acquired types and developmental types. Acquired types include traumatic (acute or stress fractures),

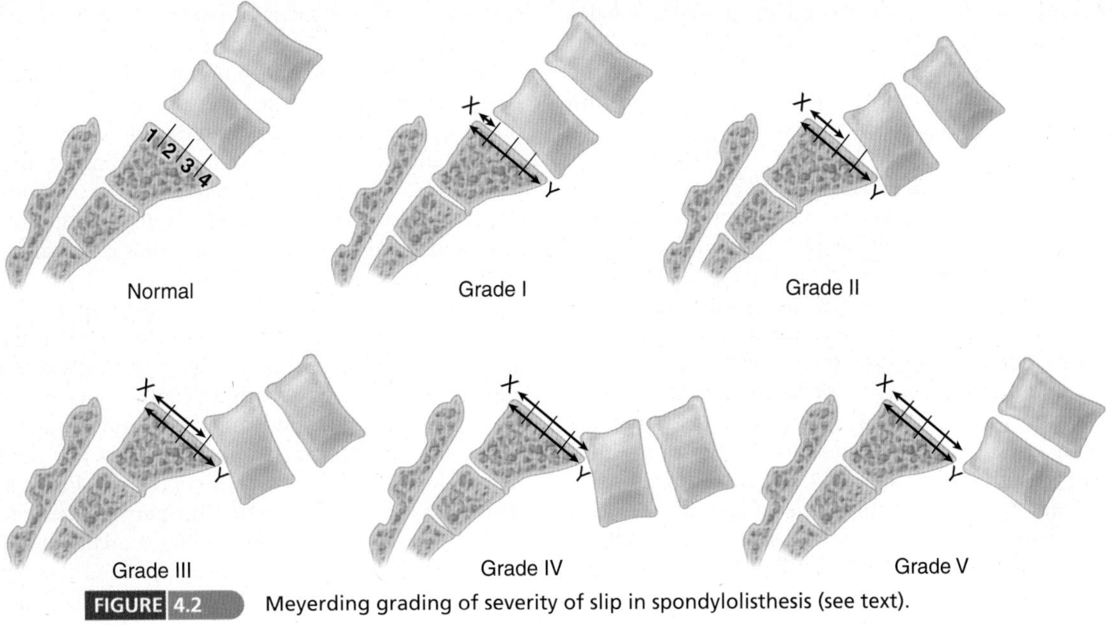

FIGURE 4.2 Meyerding grading of severity of slip in spondylolisthesis (see text).

BOX 4.2

Classification of Spondylolisthesis by Marchetti and Bartolozzi

Developmental

High Dysplastic
- With lysis
- With elongation

Low Dysplastic
- With lysis
- With elongation

Acquired

Traumatic
- Acute fracture
- Stress fracture

Post-Surgery
- Direct surgery
- Indirect surgery

Pathologic
- Local pathology
- Systemic pathology

Degenerative
- Primary
- Secondary

From deWald RL: Spondylolisthesis. In Bridwell KH, DeWald RL, editors: *The textbook of spinal surgery*, ed 3, Philadelphia, 2011, Lippincott Williams & Wilkins.

postsurgical (direct or indirect), pathologic (local or systemic), and degenerative (primary or secondary). Developmental types were subclassified into high dysplasia and low dysplasia (Box 4.2). In the low dysplasia type, the S1 endplate and the L5 vertebral body maintain a normal anatomic shape. In the high dysplasia type, the S1 endplate becomes rounded and the L5 body becomes more trapezoidal shaped. This system was first described in 1982 with a subsequent revision in 1994. The purpose of the classification was to determine what factors may predict progression of the spondylolisthesis and thereby direct treatment. This classification divides the presumed etiologies of spondylolisthesis into two categories: developmental, in which there is a morphologic abnormality of the anatomy, or acquired, in which the anatomy is normal and the deformity results from trauma, degeneration, or pathologic causes.

DEVELOPMENTAL SPONDYLOLISTHESIS

The cardinal feature of this group is that there is some degree of dysplasia of the posterior elements present. This category is further divided into low dysplasia and high dysplasia based on the severity of the anomalies present, as indicated by the degree of kyphosis at the affected level and the slip angle.

Developmental high dysplastic spondylolisthesis is characterized by major deficiencies of the posterior arches, intervertebral discs, upper endplate of S1 (which often is rounded), and the body of L5, which is trapezoidal. The pars is either elongated or lytic. In adolescents, the L5-S1 level is most commonly affected. Patients with this type of spondylolisthesis often have progression of the spondylolisthesis before adulthood. The risk of progression is directly proportional to the severity of dysplasia.

In *developmental low dysplastic spondylolisthesis*, the L4 and L5 bodies remain rectangular and the S1 endplate remains flat. Also there is no hyperlordosis and verticalization of the sacrum. Progression is less common and when present is a small increase in translation and not an increase in kyphosis and slip angle.

ACQUIRED SPONDYLOLISTHESIS

ACQUIRED TRAUMATIC SPONDYLOLISTHESIS

The acute type is rare and results from significant trauma with fracture of the pars or other portions of the posterior elements.

ACQUIRED POSTSURGICAL SPONDYLOLISTHESIS

This type is subdivided into direct and indirect types. In the direct type, the instability is at the level of surgical intervention because of fracture or bony resection such as facetectomy. The indirect type occurs at a level adjacent to prior surgery such as a fusion.

ACQUIRED PATHOLOGIC SPONDYLOLISTHESIS

This type results from pathologic processes affecting the integrity of the posterior elements such as infection or Paget disease.

ACQUIRED DEGENERATIVE SPONDYLOLISTHESIS

This occurs as a result of degenerative changes in the disc and facets without any disruption of the pars and occurs without a history of prior surgery.

The classification of Marchetti and Bartolozzi is most useful in evaluating patients who have developmental, high dysplastic spondylolisthesis. In this group, the relationship between pelvic incidence, sacral slope, and pelvic tilt is most relevant (see next section). The pelvis is either "balanced" or "unbalanced" (Fig. 4.3), and Hresko et al. developed a nomogram (Fig. 4.4) to help define each group based on the relation between pelvic tilt and sacral slope.

RADIOGRAPHIC PELVIC PARAMETERS AND SPINOPELVIC ALIGNMENT

In recent years numerous studies have demonstrated that spinopelvic alignment is important to maintain an energy-efficient posture. An understanding of the relationship between sacropelvic morphology and spinopelvic balance is particularly important in evaluating developmental dysplastic spondylolisthesis in adolescents and young adults. As understanding of this relationship improves, the ability to determine optimal treatment regimens should also increase. Patients with developmental dysplastic spondylolisthesis have abnormal sacropelvic morphology, which can result in abnormal sacropelvic orientation.

One of the most important radiographic parameters is *pelvic incidence* (PI). Other parameters remain under evaluation, as does the optimal method to measure each parameter. Pelvic incidence is significantly increased in patients with degenerative spondylolisthesis and dysplastic spondylolisthesis, and the relative increase in pelvic incidence correlates directly with the severity of the slip. Pelvic incidence is defined as the angle between a line perpendicular to the sacral endplate at its midpoint extending caudally and a line joining the midpoint of the sacral endplate to the hip axis (Fig. 4.5). It is important to understand that pelvic incidence is a

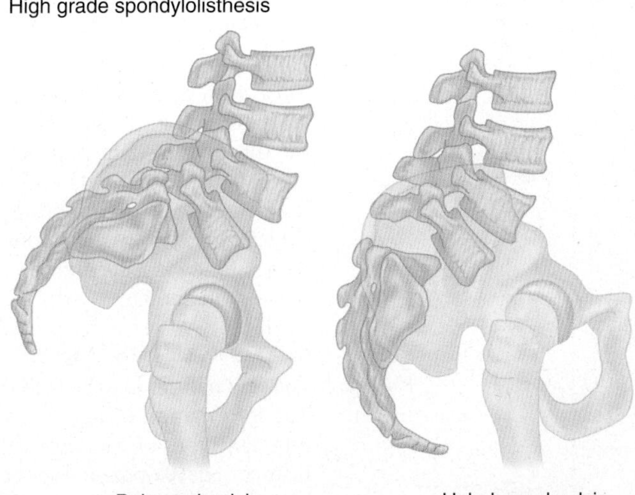

FIGURE 4.3 **Balanced and unbalanced pelvis as described by Hresko et al. Balanced pelvis has a high sacral slope and low pelvic tilt. Unbalanced pelvis has a low sacral slope and high pelvic tilt.** (Redrawn from Hresko MT, LaBelle H, Roussouly P, et al: Classification of high-grade spondylolistheses based on pelvic version and spine balance: Possible rational for reduction, *Spine* 32:2208, 2007.)

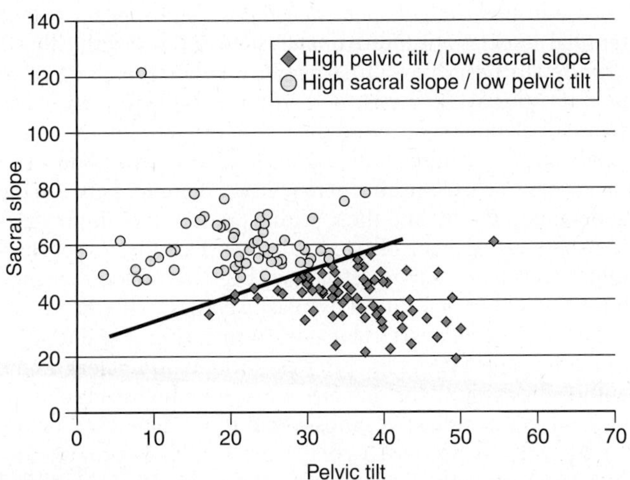

FIGURE 4.4 **Nomogram defining groups based on relation between pelvic tilt and sacral slope.** (From Hresko MT, Labelle H, Roussouly P, et al: Classification of high-grade spondylolistheses based on pelvic version and spine balance: Possible rational for reduction, *Spine* 32:2208, 2007.)

morphologic measurement, meaning it is determined by the individual anatomy and it is not affected by the position of the sacropelvis in space. The pelvic incidence does increase slightly with growth before stabilizing in adulthood. Patients with spondylolisthesis have higher than normal values and the higher the grade of the spondylolisthesis the higher the pelvic incidence. Huang et al. found, however, that pelvic incidence does not predict the probability of spondylolisthesis progression. This finding is in contrast to the findings of Enyo et al., who found that increased pelvic incidence was a relative risk factor for the development of degenerative spondylolisthesis in a 15-year longitudinal study of 200 patients.

Two other important radiographic parameters are the *sacral slope* (SS) and *pelvic tilt* (PT) (Fig. 4.6). Both of these measurements are determined by pelvic orientation on a

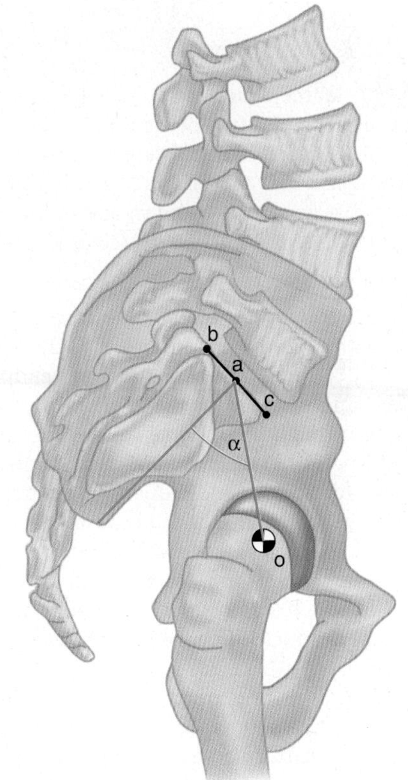

FIGURE 4.5 **Pelvic incidence (PI) is defined as an angle subtended by line oα, which is drawn from the center of the femoral head to the midpoint of the sacral endplate and a line perpendicular to the central of the sacral endplate (α). The sacral endplate is defined by the line segment *bc* constructed between the posterior superior corner of the sacrum and the anterior tip of the S1 endplate at the sacral promontory.** (Redrawn from Berthonnaud E, Dimnet J, Labelle H, et al: Spondylolisthesis. In O'Brien MF, Kuklo TR, Blanke KM, et al, editors: *Spinal Deformity Study Group radiographic measurement manual,* Memphis, TN, 2004, Medtronic Sofamor Danek.)

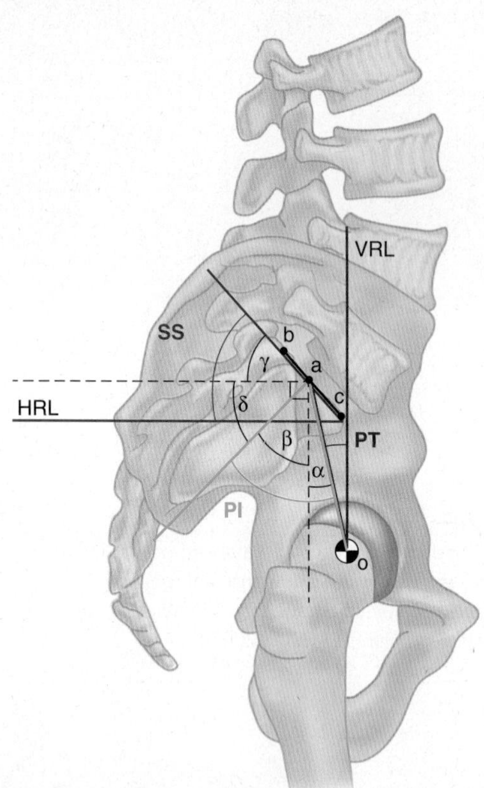

FIGURE 4.6 Mathematical relationship between pelvic incidence (PI), sacral slope (SS), and pelvic tilt (PT). *HRL*, Horizontal reference line; *VRL*, vertical reference line. (Redrawn from Berthonnaud E, Dimnet J, Labelle H, et al: Spondylolisthesis. In O'Brien MF, Kuklo TR, Blanke KM, et al, editors: *Spinal Deformity Study Group radiographic measurement manual,* Memphis, TN, 2004, Medtronic Sofamor Danek.)

standing lateral radiograph; their values are dependent on the position of the sacropelvis in space. Sacral slope is the angle formed by a line parallel to the sacral endplate and a horizontal line, and pelvic tilt is the angle formed by a vertical line passing through the hip axis and a line from the hip axis to the mid-point of the sacral endplate. The equation SS +PT=PI is true for a given individual in the standing position. Labelle et al. concluded that because pelvic incidence is a constant anatomic pelvic variable specific to each individual and strongly determines sacral slope, pelvic tilt, and lumbar lordosis, which are position-dependent variables, pelvic anatomy has a direct influence on the development of a spondylolisthesis.

The *slip angle* is a measure of the local kyphosis at the L5-S1 level (Fig. 4.7A). It is defined as the angle formed between a line perpendicular to the posterior aspect of the upper sacrum and a line parallel to the L5 inferior endplate. The slip angle has been found to have some predictive value for slip progression when it is larger than 30 degrees.

The *lumbosacral angle* is defined as the angle formed by the intersection of a line perpendicular to the upper sacrum and a line parallel to the upper endplate of the L5 vertebra (Fig. 4.7B and C). It has been found to have some predictive value for progression when it is larger than 10 degrees.

The relationship between spinopelvic alignment and spondylolisthesis has been an area of intense evaluation in recent years. This is true for dysplastic spondylolisthesis as well as other types of spondylolisthesis. Ferrero et al. compared 654 patients with degenerative spondylolisthesis with 709 asymptomatic matched volunteers and concluded that those with degenerative spondylolisthesis had increased pelvic incidence and that there were several subgroups based on C7 tilt, emphasizing the need to evaluate overall spinopelvic balance in patients with degenerative spondylolisthesis. Radovanovic et al. found that a sagittal vertical axis (SVA) of over 50 mm was associated with worse patient reported outcomes following decompression and fusion for degenerative spondylolisthesis.

NATURAL HISTORY

The few natural history studies that are available provide limited information in light of our current understanding of the different types of spondylolisthesis. It is clear that the natural history of developmental spondylolisthesis is different from that of acquired spondylolisthesis because of a lytic defect in an otherwise normal pars, and degenerative spondylolisthesis is different from both of these. Also, the association of spondylolysis and spondylolisthesis with clinically relevant low back pain is not clear. A recent systematic review by Andrade et al. failed to establish this link and suggested careful evaluation of the cause of low back pain even in patients with isthmic spondylolisthesis.

With *spondylolytic spondylolisthesis* there appears to be a familial association: approximately 26% of those with isthmic spondylolisthesis have a first-degree relative who also had an isthmic spondylolisthesis. A long-term follow-up study (45 years) by Beutler et al. found the risk of progression to be very small, and no children with a unilateral lytic defect had a slip that progressed. Clinically there was no difference between the general population and those with a grade I or II slip regarding the development of back pain. Most children (approximately 90%) with a lytic defect have been found to have spina bifida occulta, suggesting a dysplastic etiology. The incidence of lytic defects increases with age, from 4.4% at age 6 to 6.0% in adults. Risk factors for progression remain unclear. Some authors have found that females, those with higher grade slips (>50%) at the time of diagnosis, and those diagnosed before adolescent growth have a greater probability of progression. In a recent study by Eroglu et al., facet tropism was identified as a risk factor for isthmic spondylolisthesis in males.

Developmental spondylolisthesis with dysplasia is more likely to progress than the spondylolytic type. Dysplasia of the anterior sacrum correlates best with progression in the dysplastic group. Long-term follow-up of Meyerding types III and IV spondylolisthesis treated both operatively and nonoperatively found that most patients had done relatively well. None had severe neurologic sequelae, and only 45% had even mild neurologic symptoms. At 18-year follow-up, 36% of patients treated nonoperatively were asymptomatic. Yue et al. studied 27 patients with spondyloptosis and found pars defects in 89% and also spina bifida occulta in 89%. All of these patients had an abnormality of the proximal sacrum with rounding, suggesting that a physeal injury may have contributed to the deformity of the sacral endplate. In patients with doming or rounding of the S1 endplate the measurement of pelvic incidence is unreliable. Sebaaly et al. showed that a similar measurement using the L5 superior endplate rather than the S1 endplate, which is termed L5 incidence, was more reliable. In addition, they found that a value of 60 degrees was a threshold to define spinopelvic balance versus unbalance in high-grade developmental spondylolisthesis.

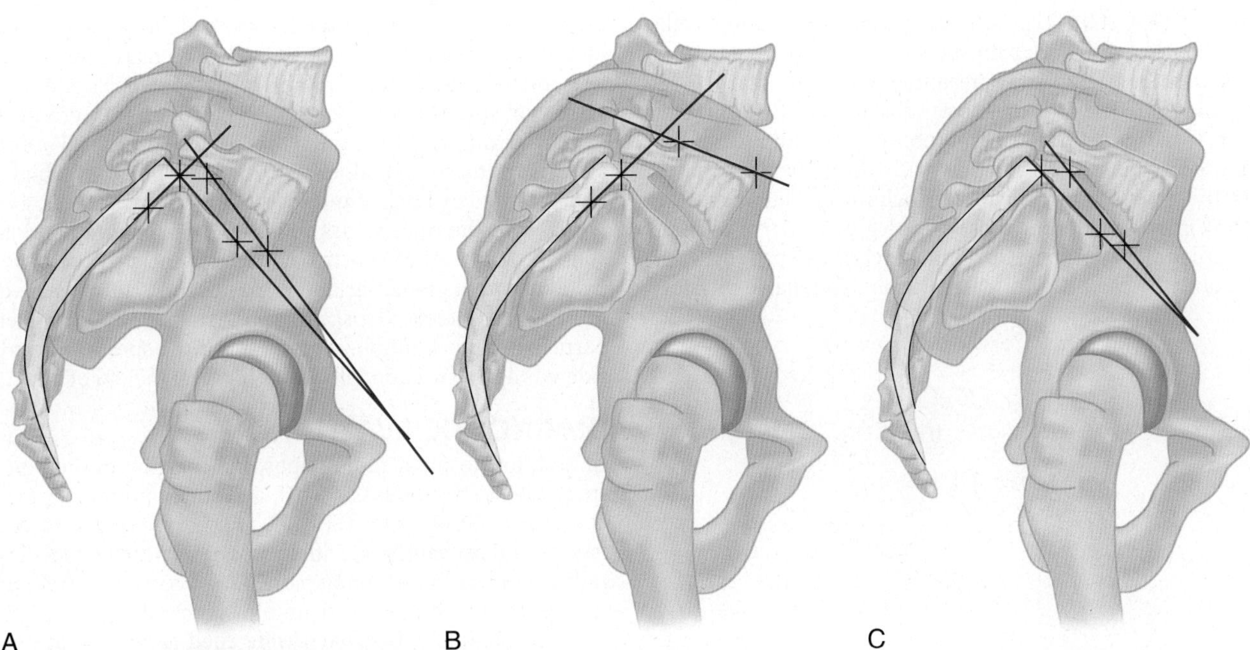

FIGURE 4.7 **A,** Slip angle. **B,** Lumbosacral angle (Dubousset). **C,** Lumbosacral angle (Spinal Deformity Study Group). (Redrawn from Glavas P, Mac-Thiong JM, Parent S, et al: Assessment of lumbosacral kyphosis in spondylolisthesis: A computer-assisted reliability study of six measurement techniques, *Eur Spine J* 18:212, 2009.)

Degenerative spondylolisthesis usually occurs at the L4-L5 level, primarily affects females over the age of 50, and is more frequent in people of African descent. Slip progression has been found to occur in about 30% of patients, but there usually is only mild progression. If neurologic symptoms are present, operative treatment is superior to nonoperative treatment. Matsunaga et al. found that 76% of patients without neurologic symptoms remained stable over long-term follow-up (10 to 18 years). A more recent study of 200 individuals by Enyo et al. found a baseline incidence of degenerative spondylolisthesis of 10% in those between the ages of 40 and 75 years. When the same group was radiographically re-examined 15 years later, the incidence had increased to 22.5%, with 14% of the previously normal population having developed a new degenerative spondylolisthesis. The presence of facet joint effusions at the listhetic level has been quantified as a risk factor for dynamic instability. Snoddy et al. were able to show that for each 1 mm of effusion on T2 MRI axial images there was a 42% probability of dynamic instability. However, the presence of an effusion was not diagnostic of instability, and 15% of patients with dynamic instability did not have facet effusions present on MRI. Factors associated with risk of progression were L4-L5 degenerative spondylolisthesis present before age 60, female sex, and facet sagittalization. Additional risk factors for progression of degenerative spondylolisthesis identified by Enyo et al. were increased pelvic incidence, smaller vertebral size, and increased L4 vertebral angle. Correction of pelvic balance defined by the relation between sacral slope and pelvic tilt described by Hresko (Fig. 4.4) has not been correlated with improved patient reported outcomes as shown by Maciejczak et al.

LUMBOSACRAL DYSPLASIA

The primary areas of posterior dysplasia include the facet joints, pars interarticularis, and spina bifida occulta. These dysplastic posterior changes lead to an inability of the L5 vertebra to resist the anterior and ventral forces created by the upright posture on the lordotic spine. This increases the anterior column stresses and can lead to growth related abnormalities and bone remodeling abnormalities that combine to cause anterior column dysplasia that can exacerbate the posterior deficiencies. As a result of these changes a progressive deformity consisting of kyphosis at the lumbosacral junction and translation of L5 on the rounded S1 endplate can occur, resulting in an unbalanced spinopelvic alignment. Evaluation of sacral "doming" is important because this has been identified as a risk factor for slip progression. The Spinal Deformity Study Group (SDSG) index (Fig. 4.8) has excellent intraobserver and interobserver reliability. An SDSG index of 25% has been suggested to be the threshold of significant sacral deformity.

As the L5 disc becomes more vertical on the standing lateral radiograph, the ability of the dysplastic posterior elements to resist the shear stresses progressively decreases. To correct the inability of the dysplastic L5 posterior elements to resist this shear force at the lumbosacral junction, the posterior tension band needs to be restored and anterior column support needs to be reestablished.

SPONDYLOLYSIS

PATIENT PRESENTATION

Spondylolysis without any spondylolisthesis is present in 2% to 5% of the population, but only a portion become symptomatic. An even smaller portion potentially require surgical treatment (Fig. 4.9). Typically the patient is an athletically active teenager with back pain and sometimes with leg pain as well. Often the back pain is presumed to be muscular in origin, which can delay the diagnosis substantially. Examination reveals localized pain, most commonly in the midline at the lumbosacral junction. Palpation with the patient prone to relax the extensor musculature is helpful to determine the level of involvement. For those with leg pain, nerve tension signs are present but somewhat muted relative to patients with radiculopathy caused by disc herniation. No reliable physical examination findings specific for spondylolisthesis have been identified. In a study by Selhorst et al. of teenage nonelite athletes, males were 1.5 times more likely than females to develop spondylolisthesis. The sports implicated in this group are somewhat different than the sports for elite athletes. For male athletes in the study cohort of 1025, baseball had the highest risk, followed by hockey and soccer. For female athletes, gymnastics had the highest risk followed by marching band and softball. Many other sports have been associated with spondylolysis and regional variations may occur. Selhorst et al. did not find an increased risk for spondylolisthesis for athletes participating in multiple sports, even if the sports were considered high risk. Spondylolysis is bilateral in 80% of cases.

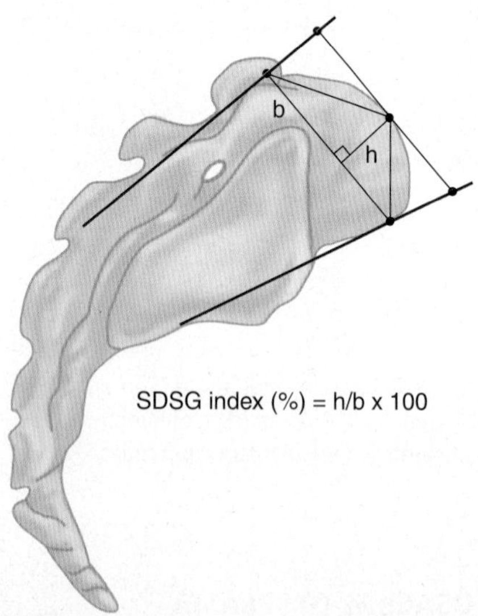

FIGURE 4.8 **Spinal Deformity Study Group (SDSG) index for assessment of sacral doming.** (Redrawn from Berthonnaud E, Dimnet J, Labelle H, et al: Spondylolisthesis. In O'Brien MF, Kuklo TR, Blanke KM, et al, editors: *Spinal Deformity Study Group radiographic measurement manual,* Memphis, TN, 2004, Medtronic Sofamor Danek.)

DIAGNOSTIC EVALUATION

In addition to plain radiographs, the imaging evaluation of spondylolysis includes CT, MRI, and single-photon emission computed tomography (SPECT). Each has relative advantages and disadvantages. Differences in sensitivity/specificity, radiation dose to the young patient, and cost are all relevant. In a review by Tofte et al., plain films, including standing lateral and oblique views, often were cited as the initial imaging. They found that SPECT had the highest sensitivity but also had more false-positives, requiring a confirmatory CT to distinguish stress reactions from true fractures. Also, SPECT may not detect chronic defects. CT was the second most sensitive and considered the gold standard for fracture recognition. MRI is less sensitive than SPECT and CT for fracture but can show stress reactions. A study by Miller et al. found that, relative to two plain radiographs, the radiation dose of a CT scan of four views was doubled. The radiation from a bone scan with SPECT was seven to nine times that of two plain radiographs. In a cost analysis, MRI was most expensive, followed by CT, SPECT, then plain radiographs. Tofte et al. recommended two radiographic views as the initial evaluation.

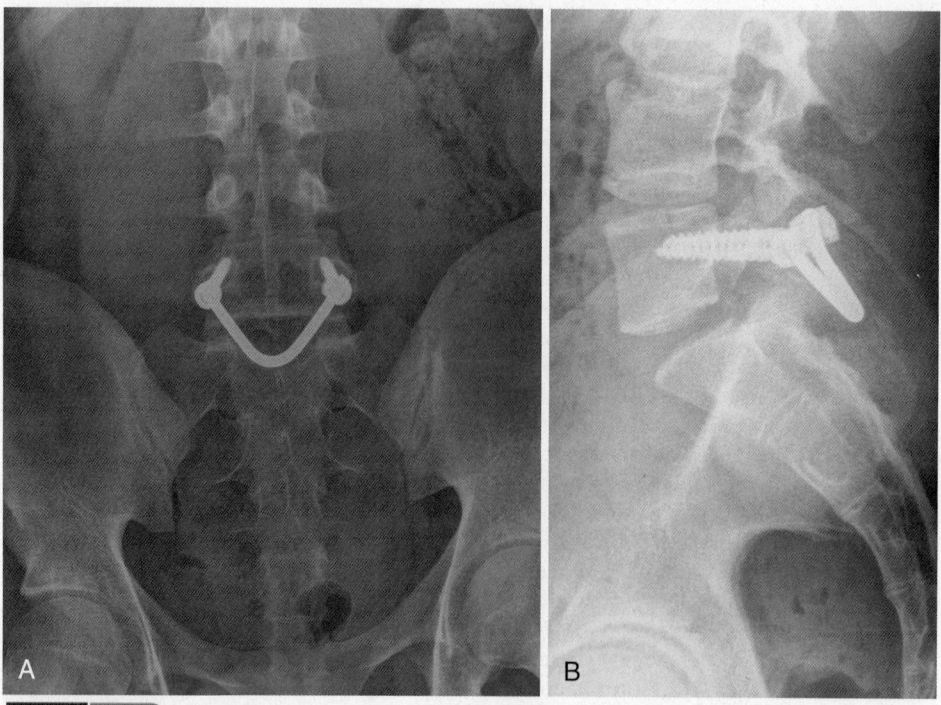

FIGURE 4.9 Anteroposterior **(A)** and spot lateral **(B)** views of direct pars repair in an adolescent patient.

If a patient fails to improve, CT is ordered for those with subacute to more chronic presentations, and MRI is obtained for more acute presentations. They did not recommend SPECT, despite the high sensitivity, because of the high radiation dose. Our preference is to establish the presence or absence of a fracture defect with the least radiation possible, as this determines treatment. For patients without a defect, a 6-week period of relative rest and sport avoidance usually is adequate. If a fracture line is present, a rigid orthosis for 6 to 10 weeks or until symptoms resolve is recommended.

There is no high-level evidence in the literature supporting the use of a rigid orthosis. In both those with healed fractures and those with fibrous unions a program of trunk and pelvic stabilization is initiated with a gradual return to full activities. Patients are allowed to return to full activity based on clinical outcome, not necessarily radiographic evidence of bony healing. Patients who remain symptomatic longer than 3 months with this treatment regimen require either more significant activity modifications or consideration for operative treatment depending on the severity of symptoms. Sakai et al. reported 63 consecutive pediatric patients with spondylolysis who were treated nonoperatively with rest, avoidance of sports, and a thoracolumbosacral orthosis (TLSO). MRI was repeated monthly until resolution of edema, and then CT was done to judge fracture healing. Fractures were categorized by age. Healing rates were 100% for the most acute and 80% for more chronic defects. Patients with recurrences typically healed as well with extended treatment.

Athletes treated with rest were found to be 16 times more likely to have a positive long-term outcome than those treated with surgery. It also has been shown that adolescents who have more than 30 consecutive days of low back pain are four times more likely to have chronic low back pain as adults than those with shorter durations of pain.

EVALUATION FOR OPERATIVE TREATMENT

For patients being considered for operative treatment, upright lateral flexion/extension radiographs are obtained. We prefer seated films, although others prefer standing lateral bending radiographs. This is necessary to detect the presence of a significant spondylolisthesis, which may not be evident even on an upright standing lateral radiograph. To be a candidate for repair of the pars interarticularis several radiographic criteria must be met: (1) absence of spondylolisthesis, (2) absence of degenerative change at the involved disc level (best determined by MRI), (3) absence of degenerative facet changes (best determined by high-resolution CT scan), and (4) absence of dysplastic changes such as spina bifida occulta, elongation of the pars interarticularis, or dysplastic facet morphology, which are all contraindications for direct pars repair (best evaluated by CT scan). In addition to these radiographic evaluations, it sometimes is helpful to use a diagnostic pars injection with a very small volume of local anesthetic. Typically, we use this when more than one level of spondylolysis is present or in other circumstances when the etiology of symptoms is not completely clear.

OPERATIVE TREATMENT

The original papers on posterior spinal fusion by Albee and Hibbs independently described the procedure for the treatment of spondylolysis and spondylolisthesis over 100 years ago. Later came descriptions of posterolateral fusions (PLFs) and still later the use of autogenous iliac bone graft for fusion. Buck described direct osteosynthesis of the pars fracture with a screw technique in 1970. Subsequently several different techniques have been described that use pedicle screw fixation at the involved level and various rod or hook constructs. Each construct is intended to allow compression across the lytic defect. No one technique has been shown to be superior. It is likely that the bone graft source and grafting technique are the most critical aspect of the procedure. We have used iliac crest bone graft in this setting, which can be harvested with minimal morbidity or risk of complication in this group of young patients.

In addition to direct fracture repair, single-level fusion is an accepted treatment option for patients in whom nonoperative treatment fails. The recommendation for direct fracture repair rather than fusion is based on several clinical factors. These criteria include a normal MRI appearance of the disc at the involved level, no abnormal motion at the involved level on upright flexion/extension radiographs, and normal facet morphology. Patients who do not meet these criteria tend to be older, and fusion typically is recommended. Validation of these or other criteria in a controlled trial is not currently available.

Translaminar screw fixation across the defect into the ipsilateral pedicle or a pedicle screw and rod construct, both with autologous iliac bone grafting, are well described. Both techniques have proven effective with equivalent positive patient reported outcomes, as shown in a study by Karatas et al. The V-rod technique has been shown to have good patient outcomes and is our preferred method. Various fusion techniques have been retrospectively compared as well and found to be equivalent in this patient population. Instrumented techniques that were found to be equivalent in a study by Gala et al. included transforaminal lumbar interbody fusion (TLIF), posterior spine fusion (PSF), anterior lumbar interbody fusion (ALIF), and 360-degree fusions. This study did not describe the bone graft source used. Fusion techniques are described in later sections.

REPAIR OF PARS INTERARTICULARIS DEFECT WITH V-ROD TECHNIQUE

TECHNIQUE 4.1

GILLET AND PETIT

PATIENT POSITIONING

- Position the patient prone on a Jackson table after induction of anesthesia. Proper positioning is important to avoid complications.
- Make sure the chest pad is just above the nipple line, with the hip pads centered at the anterior superior iliac spine.
- Support the face without pressure on the eyes and align the cervical spine in neutral to a flexed position.
- Cervical extension can be caused by some commercially available pillows for the Jackson frame and should be avoided.

- Place the hips in extension or in only slight flexion and flex the knees using pillows to decrease nerve tension.
- Confirm pedal pulses to ensure the femoral artery is not compressed by the anterior superior iliac spine pad.
- Position the upper extremities with the elbows at the level of the shoulders, placing the arm forward about 30 degrees and the elbow flexed less than 90 degrees to minimize ulnar nerve tension. Ensure that the elbows are well padded, as are all bony prominences. Administer prophylactic antibiotics and, after sterile preparation and draping are completed, complete the intraoperative "Time Out."

EXPOSURE AND GRAFT HARVEST

- Localize the involved level radiographically and make a midline incision overlying this location.
- Carry dissection down to the fascia and obtain a localization image with a clamp affixed to the spinous process, which is then marked with a rongeur confirming the level.
- Use Cobb elevators and electrocautery to expose the entire spinous process of the lytic level and the caudal portion of the spinous process cephalad to the lytic level.
- Expose the lamina at each level, taking care not to damage the capsule. Expose the L4-L5 facet capsule and lateral superior articular mass of L5 for repair of an L5 pars defect because the pedicle screw will be placed at the L5 level.
- Meticulously expose the pars at the involved level and expose the entire lamina of the lytic level bilaterally.
- Carefully curet the fibrocartilage out of the lytic defect to expose bone on both sides of the defect.
- Expose the base of the transverse process at the involved level.
- Use an awl to penetrate the cortex and advance a pedicle probe into the vertebral body, using fluoroscopy to assist in screw hole preparation.
- Take a slightly cranial orientation with the probe to move the ultimate position of the screw head away from the facet.
- Make a separate incision overlying the posterior superior iliac spine and carry dissection down to the fascia, which is divided along the lateral margin of the posterior superior iliac spine.
- Carefully elevate the fascia as a single layer to expose the iliac crest. There is no need to expose the outer table or inner table.
- Use an osteotome to reflect the cortex of the crest and expose the cancellous bone of the ilium between the cortices.
- Use a narrow gouge and a large curet to harvest multiple strips of cancellous bone. After harvesting the available bone, repair the fascia well and close the wound in layers.

PEDICLE SCREW INSERTION

- Use a high-speed burr to decorticate to bleeding bone the base of the transverse process, lateral superior articular mass, and the pars interarticularis on both sides of the defect. Carefully place the strips of cancellous bone onto the decorticated surfaces.
- Place a polyaxial pedicle screw at the appropriate level (e.g., L5). The screw chosen usually is a smaller diameter than would be chosen for a fusion as the stresses are less and a smaller screw is less likely to impinge on the facet capsule.
- Repeat pedicle screw placement on the contralateral side.
- With both defects grafted and both screws in place, use a sterile intubating stylet as a template to form a V shape with the caudal aspect of the L5 spinous process at the apex of the V and the upper ends engaging each of the pedicle screws (Fig. 4.10). Tubular benders will likely be needed to get the desired amount of rod contouring. It may be necessary to contour lordosis into the V-shaped rod to improve rod position relative to the lamina.
- Leave the rod long until after contouring is complete, because it is difficult to contour a short rod to the degree necessary. Cut the rod and place it caudal to the L5 spinous process at its base. Apply compression to the rod

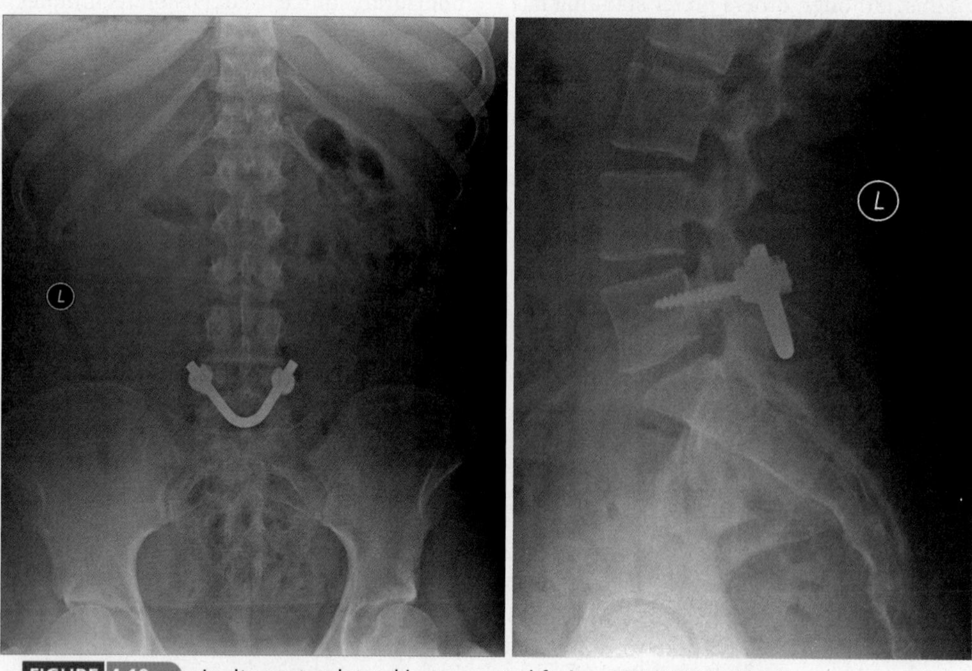

FIGURE 4.10 In situ posterolateral instrumented fusion. **SEE TECHNIQUE 4.1.**

and secure it with set screws. Torque the set screws to the manufacturer's specifications.
- Close the lumbodorsal fascia to bone to restore the normal resting length of the paraspinal musculature and close the subcutaneous and subcuticular layers.

POSTOPERATIVE CARE Postoperatively the patient receives analgesics and muscle relaxants and begins mobilization immediately. Typically these patients are independent and able to be discharged home within 2 days.

ADULT ISTHMIC SPONDYLOLISTHESIS

Patients with isthmic spondylolisthesis are the second largest group of patients with spondylolisthesis presenting to the spine surgeon. Only degenerative spondylolisthesis is more common. Most patients with isthmic spondylolisthesis (some prefer the term "acquired lytic spondylolisthesis") present with low-grade deformities (less than a 50% slip); 90% to 95% involve the L5-S1 level, with 5% to 8% at L4-L5, and very few at the more cephalad levels. Low-grade slips are much more common than those of more than 50% by a ratio of 10:1; however, the severity can range from spondylolysis (no slip) all the way to grade V. Fortunately, most cases of low-grade isthmic spondylolisthesis are not associated with significant kyphosis or spinal imbalance. The typical presentation is a patient with axial low-back pain that tends to be mechanical and radicular pain in an L5 distribution. Initial radiographic evaluation should consist of standing anteroposterior and lateral views, as well as a spot view at the L5-S1 level (Fig. 4.11). The spondylolisthesis generally is easily diagnosed, and upright lateral flexion/extension films are useful to diagnose dynamic instability, which is common at the L4-L5 level but less so at the L5-S1 level. The radiographic assessment must also include an evaluation of the regional and, if needed, global spinal balance. If significant imbalance is present, the treatment plan must correct this if surgery is indicated.

PATHOPHYSIOLOGY

The presence of an isthmic spondylolisthesis is not sufficient to identify the cause of the patient's symptoms because 7% of the population has spondylolysis, with or without spondylolisthesis, and most are asymptomatic. From retrospective long-term studies it has been found that about 80% of acquired lytic defects occur between the ages of 5 and 10 years, with the remaining 20% of fractures occurring before the age of 20 years. In most patients, spondylolisthesis is asymptomatic. Determining whether spondylolisthesis is the source of back pain requires a careful evaluation of the complaints. Mechanical back pain can originate from the pars defect but also from the disc, which often is more degenerative than would be expected for the patient's age because of the abnormal stresses applied to the disc as a result of the lack of stability. Adult isthmic spondylolisthesis at the L5 level can cause radicular complaints involving the L5 root; symptoms can be generated by several different pathologic processes. As the disc degenerates and loses height, the foraminal cross-sectional area is diminished, leaving less space available for the nerve root. The annulus remains attached to the inferior endplate of the cephalad vertebra. As this vertebra translates anteriorly, the annulus becomes located posterior to the vertebra (pseudoherniation) and occupies space within the foramen. In addition, the pseudarthrosis that forms at the pars defect consists of cartilage, bone, and fibrous tissue, all of which occupy space within the foramen. Thus, the cross-sectional area of the foramen is decreased in a cephalocaudal direction by the loss of disc height. The pseudoherniation and the fibrocartilage decrease the foramen in the anterior to posterior dimension. If there is translational instability at the involved level, this can cause traction on the nerve root

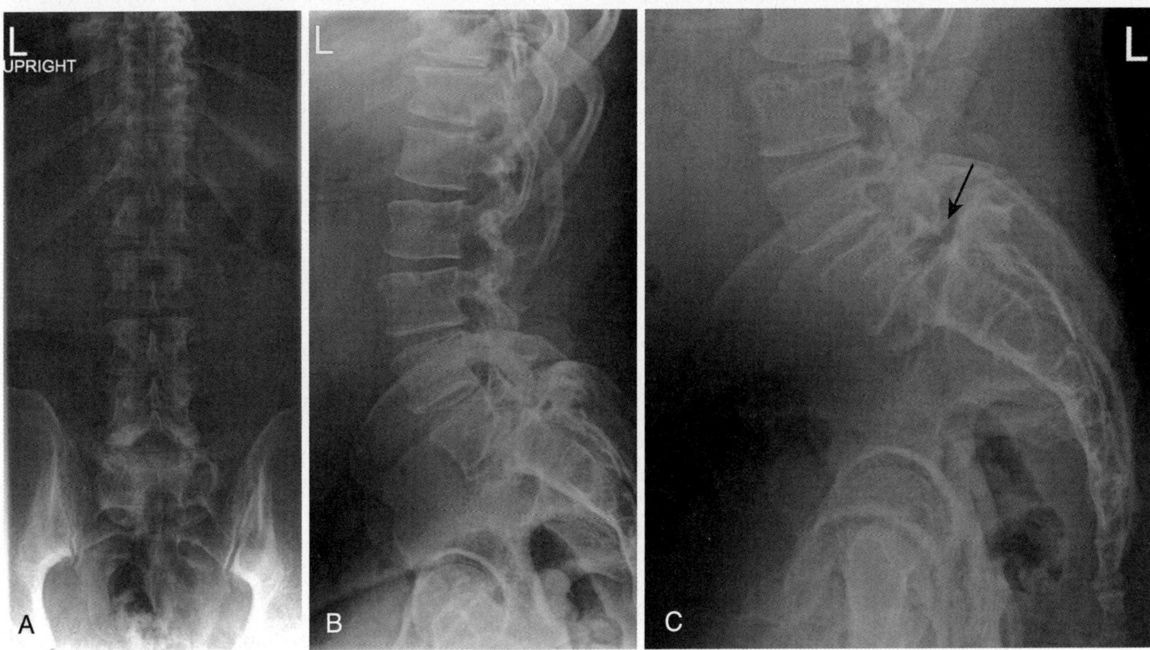

FIGURE 4.11 Initial radiographic evaluation of isthmic spondylolisthesis. **A,** Standing anteroposterior view. **B,** Standing lateral view. **C,** Spot view at L5-S1 level (*arrow* shows pars defect).

and produce radicular symptoms as well. In addition to these possibilities at the L5-S1 level, the L5 root can be compromised by lateral recess stenosis at the L4-L5 level or less commonly by a disc herniation at the L4 disc level. Determination of the patient's primary complaint (mechanical back pain or radicular pain) will have a significant impact on the type of treatment, including surgery that will be most appropriate if conservative treatment is not successful.

NONOPERATIVE TREATMENT

If an adolescent patient has a spondylolisthesis of more than 2 mm at presentation, an orthosis is not recommended, because fracture healing is unlikely with significant displacement. Most patients presenting with a spondylolisthesis are in the 20- to 45-year-old age range. In the absence of significant neurologic deficits, patients are initially treated with a brief period of rest, antiinflammatory medications, and muscle relaxers. Narcotics are used very sparingly, if at all, and the patient is mobilized as early as possible. Once the acute symptoms begin to subside, a program of low-impact aerobic exercise, trunk stabilization avoiding extension, and hamstring stretching is instituted. This often is successful in allowing the patient to return to full activity over a period of 8 to 12 weeks. Even with good resolution of mechanical symptoms, the patient needs to understand that trunk stabilization exercises will be necessary indefinitely to manage the expected episodic back pain.

Patients with a lytic defect of the pars have abnormal load sharing. Normally 20% of the axial load of the lumbar spine is transmitted through the posterior column, with 80% transmitted anteriorly. When a pars fracture is present, no load is carried posteriorly at the involved level and all the load is transferred to the anterior column, which leads to premature disc degeneration and potentially episodic back pain; however, with proper exercise and relatively minor activity modifications, most patients can be managed nonoperatively throughout their lives.

Neurologic symptoms are less common in younger patients and often develop as the patient enters the third to fourth decades. The presence of significant neurologic deficits is an indication that operative treatment may soon become necessary because the chronic changes causing the neurologic symptoms will not resolve, although they often can be mitigated in the short-to-intermediate (months) term but generally not the long term. For patients with significant neurologic symptoms or more than 6 months of persistent back pain not adequately controlled with the above treatment regimen, operative treatment is recommended.

OPERATIVE TREATMENT

SURGICAL OPTIONS

Patients with isthmic spondylolisthesis can be appropriately managed using a number of techniques; however, some surgical procedures generally should not be considered in this patient group. Because patients with spondylolisthesis have instability at the involved segment, by definition, a total laminectomy (Gill procedure) in isolation is contraindicated. Inserting a posterior device designed to apply a distractive force at the level of an isthmic spondylolisthesis is contraindicated because distraction cannot be applied through the lytic defect. Pars repair can be a good procedure in the right patient population (see Technique 4.1); however, adult patients with isthmic spondylolisthesis symptoms generally are not good candidates because of the associated disc degeneration and facet arthrosis that are almost always present in this older group of patients.

EVALUATION FOR OPERATIVE TREATMENT

To appropriately plan operative treatment, additional imaging is needed. Standing lateral and posteroanterior scoliosis radiographs should be obtained to adequately assess the patient's global balance and pelvic parameters. These images should include the skull and both proximal femoral heads so the hip axis can be determined. The slip angle is not likely to be significantly positive in patients with low-grade acquired lytic spondylolisthesis; however, when it is positive (kyphotic), anterior column support generally will be needed. Usually the sacral endplate morphology is relatively normal, indicating that the sacral buttress is maintained. The sacral table angle can be used to assess the sacral buttress (Fig. 4.12). Each L5 transverse process should have at least 2 cm^2 of surface area if PLF is considered. Given the high incidence of dysplastic changes in this group of patients, we obtain a high-resolution CT scan to evaluate pedicle morphology, adequacy of the L5 transverse process, sacral morphology, facet arthritis at adjacent levels, and the bony foraminal dimensions when more thorough anatomic evaluation is needed. If the patient has significant radicular symptoms, an MRI usually is obtained to determine the specific location and etiology of the nerve root symptoms, which usually are caused by nerve compression but traction on the nerve root caused by instability also is possible. Although a pseudoherniation is common and can be readily seen on the MRI and may explain L5 root symptoms, the L4 disc must also be assessed. Occasionally, a patient may have an L4 disc herniation causing the L5 root symptoms, and this generally can be managed more simply with a microdiscectomy at the L4 level rather than operative stabilization at the L5-S1 level if the patient has only mild axial back-pain complaints. Also the health of the adjacent disc levels can be assessed on MRI, which will influence how many levels may need to be fused and the method of fusion. Some authors have recommended provocative discography to evaluate adjacent levels, but we have not found this to be reliable. We have found that a pars injection with a small volume of long-acting local anesthetic is helpful as a diagnostic tool when evaluating patients with extensive degenerative changes at multiple levels in addition to isthmic spondylolisthesis.

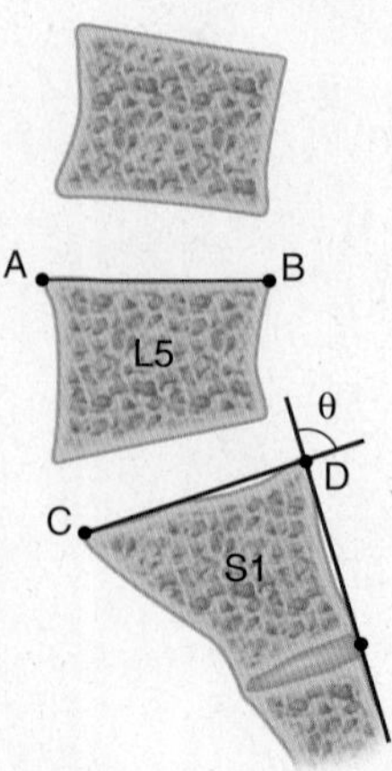

FIGURE 4.12 The sacral table angle is measured between a line along the sacral endplate and a line drawn along the posterior aspect of the S1 vertebral body.

OUTCOMES OF OPERATIVE TREATMENT

Seuk et al. evaluated improvement in patient-reported outcomes in patients with low-grade isthmic spondylolisthesis treated operatively. They defined the minimum clinically important difference (MCID) for VAS as 3 points and the MCID for Oswestry Disability Index (ODI) as a 12-point improvement over baseline. They included patients with ALIF and pedicle screw instrumentation and patients with TLIF for low-grade isthmic spondylolisthesis at L4-L5 and L5-S1. In a consecutive series of 105 patients followed for a minimum of 36 months and average follow-up of 77 months, the overall achievement of MCID for VAS back was 80% and for VAS leg, 73%; ODI MCID was obtained in 83%. They also evaluated radiographic parameters of pelvic incidence, lumbar lordosis, pelvic tilt, and sacral slope. These authors found that restoration of foraminal height was more important than overall lordosis and that patients with L4-L5 pathology responded better than those with L5-S1 spondylolisthesis.

Kwon and Albert showed in their literature review that using rigid pedicle screw constructs improved fusion rates in patients with acquired lytic spondylolisthesis. They found a 90% fusion rate with the use of rigid pedicle screw instrumentation and a 77% fusion rate in uninstrumented cases. A systematic review by Noorian et al. evaluating clinical outcomes in patients with low-grade spondylolisthesis treated with PLF, with or without pedicle screws; interbody fusions, including ALIF with pedicle screws; and circumferential fusions with pedicle screws did not find a clear advantage of any one technique over the others. The analysis included six randomized controlled trials and nine observational studies. Interbody fusions techniques tended to produce better outcomes with longer follow-up than did PLF with or without pedicle screws. Levin et al. had similar findings also in their systematic review, identifying a trend toward more improvement in back pain, ODI, and fusion rates with TLIF than with PLF; however, these differences did not reach significance. The PSF group had shorter operative times. There were no differences in blood loss, infection rate, leg pain improvement, or health-related quality of life (HRQOL) improvement.

High-quality studies comparing minimally invasive techniques to open techniques for operative treatment of low-grade isthmic spondylolisthesis are lacking. A systematic review of studies comparing minimally invasive and open procedures identified only 10 such studies, and all were either low or very low quality. The review by Lu et al. found no significant difference between minimally invasive and open surgery with regard to pain or functional outcomes. Subgroup analysis of the prospective studies revealed that minimally invasive techniques had longer operative times and slightly better final ODI scores (13.8 vs 16.1).

Open posterior fusions can be done using a midline approach or the muscle-splitting approach described by Wiltse and Spencer (see Technique 1.26), which uses the intermuscular plane between the multifidus and longissimus muscles. The latter approach is considered by most to have the advantage of being less traumatic to the musculature and producing less "fusion disease" attributable to muscle fibrosis postoperatively. The muscle-splitting approach is not recommended if a direct decompression is planned. Current minimally invasive techniques are an extension of this concept and are less traumatic to the soft tissues; however, so far it remains unclear if they will prove superior or equivalent with respect to fusion rates and clinical outcomes. For patients requiring direct decompression and interbody support, an open or minimally invasive TLIF is preferred. Steps are taken to minimize the muscle ischemia associated with this open approach in an effort to minimize the potential for persistent pain related to soft-tissue trauma.

Another finding by Kwon and Albert was that patients who had a laminectomy had a slightly lower fusion rate and slightly lower outcome scores than those without laminectomy, but neither of these reached statistical significance. These authors did find a statistically significant difference in fusion rates between circumferential fusions (anterior lumbar interbody or combined posterior lumbar interbody fusion or TLIF with posterior spinal fusion) and either anterior only or posterior only fusions. Patients with an interbody fusion and a posterior fusion had the highest fusion rate (98%) compared with anterior-only (75%) or posterior-only fusion (83%). Clinical success rates were similar: 86% for circumferential fusion, 79% for anterior fusion only, and 75% for posterior only fusion. An economic evaluation by Bydon et al. found that adding an interbody device increased the cost per quality-adjusted life-year (QALY) compared with a PLF alone initially; however, when the costs of reoperations were factored in, the addition of interbody fusion resulted in a modest cost savings compared with PLF alone. Lee et al. found that complication rates and fusion rates were similar in adult patients with PLF alone and those with posterolateral interbody fusion for isthmic spondylolisthesis. A more recent economic study by Fischer et al. found surgical treatment for spondylolisthesis to be cost-effective at 2 years with a cost/QALY of $89,065.

OPERATIVE PLANNING

It is important to realize that adult patients with low-grade isthmic spondylolisthesis and progressive complaints of lower back and hip pain may well have hip or knee pathology contributing to their symptoms. Before embarking on operative management of the spinal pathology, evaluation of these two areas is worthwhile. If the patient has significant degenerative changes of the hip, an intraarticular hip injection can be confirmatory as to whether the hip is the primary pathology. In patients with significant hip or knee degeneration, correction of these problems usually is recommended before spinal surgery. The mechanical lumbar complaints often improve with improvement in gait and aerobic activities made possible by pain reduction. When neurologic symptoms predominate, spinal surgery generally should be done first.

After clinical and imaging evaluations are complete, specific surgical procedures can be recommended based on the findings. For patients without significant neurologic complaints and with good spinal alignment, instrumented PLF can be recommended if there is sufficient surface area for fusion. In many patients, the L5 transverse process is hypoplastic and may be inadequate (less than 2 cm^2 of surface area). For patients with inadequate area for PLF, a posterior-only approach with circumferential fusion (posterior or TLIF) or an ALIF with posterior supplemental fixation provides a good alternative. An uninstrumented posterior-only fusion rarely is recommended in this patient population.

For patients with nerve root symptoms, direct or indirect decompression is a necessary part of the procedure. Indirect decompression is accomplished through realignment and reestablishment of the disc height using an interbody spacer device including allograft bone. Currently, a variety of devices are available for this purpose, including femoral cortical allografts, polyetheretherketone (PEEK) cages, titanium mesh cages, expandable cages, and carbon fiber devices. These devices are used in conjunction with autograft bone, allograft bone, and bone morphogenetic proteins (BMPs) in an off-label application. A recent randomized, controlled, multicenter trial showed that BMP-7 (OP-1) with a collagen carrier was not as effective as autologous iliac crest bone for obtaining fusion. Because of the higher fusion rate with autologous iliac crest grafts (74%) than with BMP (54%), these authors did not recommend the use of BMP in instrumented posterior lumbar fusion procedures. Wang et al. recently published a study using structural autografts from resected facets as interbody grafts. Results were equivalent to PEEK cages and local autograft.

Indirect reduction can be accomplished with a TLIF, which can be combined with an instrumented PLF. For patients who need a direct decompression in addition to the realignment and reduction, we generally prefer a TLIF coupled with an instrumented PLF. Minimally invasive techniques are described in chapter 3. Bai et al. performed a systematic review evaluating reduction of spondylolisthesis and found that reduction of a low-grade spondylolisthesis did not improve patient outcomes compared with fusion in situ.

IN SITU POSTEROLATERAL INSTRUMENTED FUSION: WILTSE AND SPENCER APPROACH

TECHNIQUE 4.2

- After induction of anesthesia, position the patient as described in Technique 4.1. Montgomery et al. demonstrated that proper positioning allows some reduction of the spondylolisthesis.
- Apply pneumatic compression devices and initiate neuromonitoring (see chapter 8) if it is to be used.
- Administer prophylactic antibiotics and tranexamic acid loading dose and begin continuous infusion. After sterile preparation and draping are completed, complete the intraoperative "Time Out."
- Make a midline skin incision at the L5-S1 level down to the fascia. Sharply dissect superficial to the fascia on both sides about 4 cm from the midline, for the length of the skin incision (see Technique 1.26).
- On each side of the midline make a 4 cm to 5 cm long fascial incision 3 cm off the midline at the approximate interval between the multifidus and longissimus muscles, curving the incisions slightly medially at the inferior end.
- Use blunt dissection to develop the plane down to the L5-S1 facet joint.
- Expose the L5 transverse process and the sacral ala subperiosteally.
- Verify the level radiographically with a metal instrument resting on the transverse process. Once the correct level is confirmed, make a generous facetectomy.
- Prepare the pedicle screw holes at the L5 level and the S1 level bilaterally, using fluoroscopy to assist in pedicle location and orientation.
- Prepare the S1 screw holes for a bicortical technique for enhanced screw purchase. Penetrate the sacral cortex medially at the promontory just caudal to the endplate.
- Sound each screw hole to ensure there are no cortical breaches and place a cottonoid for hemostasis.
- Removal of hypertrophic bone from the lateral aspect of the L5 superior articular mass may be needed to allow placement of the L5 screw, which also enlarges the area for bone graft incorporation.
- Place polyaxial pedicle screws bilaterally at L5 and S1 after thorough decortication and placement of bone graft under direct vision. Generally, a separate autologous iliac graft is harvested or local autograft is combined with allograft cancellous bone soaked in antibiotic solution at least 30 minutes before implantation. Some have recommended off-label use of BMP or demineralized bone matrix to augment local autograft.
- Contour the rods and affix them with the set screws, which are torqued according to the manufacturer's recommendation.
- Thoroughly irrigate the wound throughout the procedure and again before closure. Note that if BMP is used irrigation should not be done after BMP has been placed into the wound.
- Close the fascial wounds with interrupted sutures and place two subcutaneous drains. Minimize dead space by tacking the subcutaneous layer to the fascia bilaterally. Complete subcutaneous and subcuticular closure.
- This procedure can be done through a midline fascial incision (see Technique 1.25) rather than the Wiltse and Spencer approach (see Technique 1.26). If a midline incision is used, close the fascia over a drain and to the spinous processes to maintain proper muscle resting length in the lordotic spine.

POSTOPERATIVE CARE The patient is mobilized without a brace beginning the morning after surgery. Parenteral and oral analgesics and muscle relaxers are given to facilitate rest and mobilization. Generally patients are independent with activity and can be discharged the second or third postoperative day.

POSTERIOR INSTRUMENTED FUSION WITH INTERBODY FUSION (PLIF AND TLIF)

TLIF is the procedure we most commonly used for adult patients with low-grade isthmic spondylolisthesis. It is preferred because of the ability to better restore normal lumbosacral alignment parameters when necessary and restore disc height. Posterior and TLIF techniques are very similar and are described together. Each is combined with a PLF if done open to achieve a circumferential arthrodesis. Minimally invasive TLIF is described in chapter 3. A TLIF is preferred, and a complete laminectomy (Gill procedure) usually is done for direct decompression in these patients.

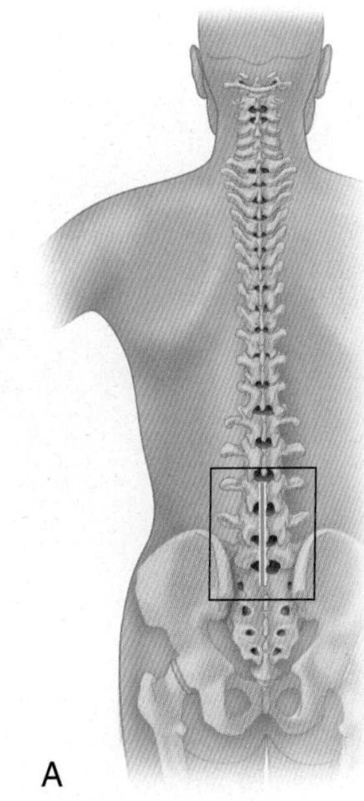

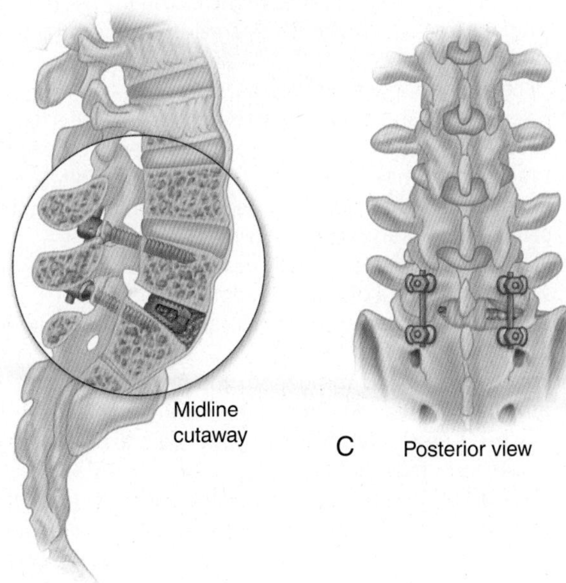

FIGURE 4.13 Posterior instrumented fusion with interbody fusion. **A**, Incision. **B**, Polyaxial screws inserted at S1 and expandable cage device placed. **C**, Rods inserted. **SEE TECHNIQUE 4.3.**

TECHNIQUE 4.3

- Position the patient as described in Technique 4.1 and complete sterile preparation and draping, followed by the intraoperative "Time Out."
- Administer prophylactic antibiotics. Initiate continuous infusion of tranexamic acid after a loading dose. Typical loading dose is 20 mg/kg, and the infusion is 2 mg/kg/hr.
- Make a midline incision centered at the L5-S1 level (Fig. 4.13A).
- Release the fascia and obtain a localization image with a clamp on the spinous process to confirm the operative level. Use a rongeur to mark the spinous process that had the clamp applied as a reference.
- Carry subperiosteal dissection laterally over the lamina at the L4, L5, and S1 levels.
- Remove the joint capsule at the L5-S1 level bilaterally, but preserve the capsule at the L4-L5 facet.
- Expose the transverse process of L5 and the sacral ala bilaterally and prepare pedicle screw holes at the L5 level and the S1 level bilaterally, using fluoroscopy to assist in pedicle location and orientation.
- Prepare the S1 screw holes for a bicortical technique for enhanced screw purchase. Penetrate the sacral cortex medially at the promontory just caudal to the endplate. Sound each screw hole to ensure there are no cortical breaches and place a cottonoid for hemostasis.
- Remove the posterior elements of the L5 vertebra (Gill fragment) piecemeal or en bloc. For en bloc removal, detach the ligamentum flavum from the caudal and cephalad margins using small angled curets. As the fragment is mobilized, advance the curet down to the pseudarthrosis site to release the fibrocartilaginous tissue around the L5 nerve root. Careful dissection is necessary here as the nerve root usually is already quite compressed and aggressive curetting may damage the root (Fig. 4.14).
- Once the lamina has been removed, remove additional fibrocartilage from around the nerve root with a Kerrison rongeur. The exiting L5 root should be visible all the way to the lateral aspect of the foramen. The operating microscope is very helpful during this dissection.
- Through the S1 foraminotomy identify the traversing S1 root. Remove the ligamentum attached to the L4 lamina to adequately decompress the L5 root in the L4-L5 lateral recess as well. Removal of the osteophyte from the medial aspect of the L5 facet may also be needed to decompress the S1 root.
- After the decompression is completed, decorticate the transverse processes and sacral alae and pack the lateral gutter with a local autograft from the Gill fragment and allograft cancellous bone.
- Insert the pedicle screws to allow distraction (if necessary) across the disc space to facilitate disc removal and reduction of the spondylolisthesis. Standard polyaxial screws and rod reduction tools usually can be used at L5 if the amount of translation desired is less than 1.5 cm. If more translation is needed, reduction screws with extended threaded portions are quite helpful. This is only necessary for high-grade spondylolisthesis.
- Insert standard polyaxial screws at the S1 level (Fig. 4.13B). Typically with sufficient decompression, the pedicles can be directly inspected for cortical breaches at the L5 and S1 locations. If neuromonitoring is used, screw resistance can be determined. We use an impedance of 10 mA as a threshold for a safe screw. Neuromonitoring is most useful to detect deficits caused by tension during reduction of the spondylolisthesis, which is not routine.
- If more than 15 mm of reduction is planned, cut a working rod and contour it to allow rod placement if temporary distraction will be used. Secure this working rod to the S1 screw and then gradually reduce it into the L5 screw while maintaining a distractive force between the two screws (Fig. 4.13C). Reduce the rods bilaterally in a gradual alternating fashion, taking care not to apply so much force that the L5 screw pulls out. Monitor the translation of the L5 vertebra fluoroscopically. This type

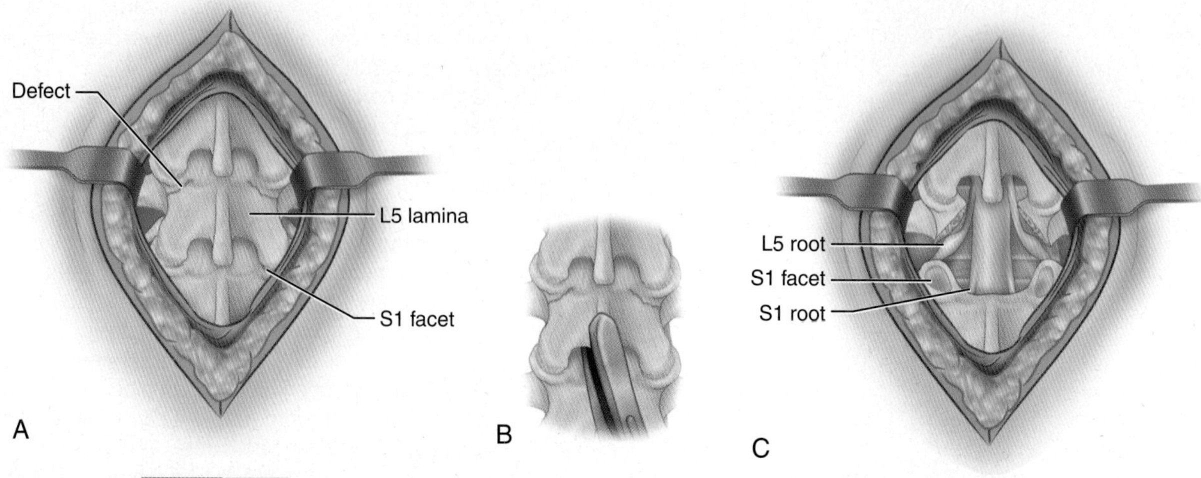

FIGURE 4.14 Gill-Manning-White laminectomy for decompression. **SEE TECHNIQUE 4.3.**

of formal reduction is not commonly needed; usually the spondylolisthesis adequately reduces with positioning and exposure.

- Release of the posterior annulus and disc space preparation are the next phase of the procedure. Often there is a leash of epidural veins in the axilla of the L5 nerve root that cross the disc. Coagulate these vessels with bipolar cautery, if possible, before annulotomy. They can be difficult to control otherwise, but Gelfoam and thrombin usually are effective.
- Make a wide annulotomy by gently retracting the thecal sac medially. Extend the annulotomy into the foramen if the nerve position allows. This can be done bilaterally if two cages are planned or unilaterally if one of the elongated designs is to be used. In either case, the posterior osteophyte extending from L5 may need to be removed with a Kerrison rongeur to adequately open the annulotomy and access the disc space. Remove the cephalad half of the S1 facet to allow access to the disc space.
- Use intervertebral reamers/sizers and curets to prepare the endplates, with fluoroscopic monitoring of instrument position within the disc space to avoid anterior annulus violation and potential vascular injury.
- Once the endplates are prepared and the reduction is satisfactory, thoroughly irrigate the disc space to remove any residual soft tissue.
- Pack allograft cancellous bone against the anterior annulus and morselized local autograft bone in behind this. Submerge the allograft cancellous bone in antibiotic irrigation solution at the beginning of the case and maintain it there until implantation. This has decreased postoperative deep wound infections associated with allograft bone usage. Take care to leave adequate space to allow placement of the interbody device no more posteriorly than the anterior 20% of the disc space so lordosis can be achieved.
- The goals of cage placement are to restore disc height and improve alignment with sufficient lordosis through the segment. Biomechanically, coverage of 35% of the endplate is desirable for stability. This can be achieved with two or more smaller devices, such as mesh cages packed with bone, or a larger footprint single device. We prefer a lordotic, titanium cage device packed with local autograft placed just anterior to the midbody. The subchondral bone is strongest around the perimeter of the endplate and weakest centrally, increasing the risk of cage subsidence if the device is too small or only centrally located.
- Place the device as transversely as possible.
- Release the distraction from the working rods, which may need to be cut or exchanged because they likely will be too long and may impinge on the L4-L5 facet joint.
- If temporary distraction is not required, complete decortication and grafting before screw insertion.
- Place the final rods and apply mild compression for lordosis, being mindful of the L5 foramina dimensions.
- Torque the set screws to specifications of the manufacturer.
- Irrigate the wound throughout the procedure and thoroughly at the conclusion of the instrumentation. If BMP has been used, irrigation should not be done after it is placed into the wound.
- Place a fluted drain (because of the exposed dura) and close the fascia to the remaining spinous processes with interrupted sutures to restore the normal resting length of the muscle. Close the subcutaneous and subcuticular layers individually. The procedure for a TLIF is very similar to the PLIF as just described when done through a midline approach. When indirect decompression through the spinal implants is sufficient, TLIF may be preferred and can be done without the need for the Gill laminectomy. The discectomy and annulus removal are not as complete with this approach and the ability to translate the vertebra is more limited. Indirect decompression can be accomplished through a Wiltse approach or with minimally invasive techniques in patients with less severe pathology.

POSTOPERATIVE CARE The patient is mobilized without a brace beginning the morning after surgery. Parenteral and oral analgesics and muscle relaxers are given to facilitate rest and mobilization. Generally patients are independent with activity and can be discharged the second or third postoperative day with open techniques and somewhat sooner with minimally invasive methods.

L5-S1 ANTERIOR LUMBAR INTERBODY FUSION

There are certain advantages to ALIF, particularly for high-grade spondylolisthesis, because of the soft-tissue release than can be obtained to allow reduction; however, this usually is not the first choice for treatment of low-grade isthmic spondylolisthesis. The two general circumstances in which this technique is most commonly used are (1) patients appropriate for posterolateral in situ fusion with prohibitively small transverse processes and (2) as a salvage procedure in patients who had an in situ PLF but developed a nonunion. In the first instance, supplemental posterior instrumentation normally is used, as well as the anterior surgery, to restore the posterior tension band. In the second case, the anterior procedure should be done before the previously placed posterior instrumentation has failed. This approach is often done with the assistance of an experienced approach surgeon. The risks of the approach need to be clearly discussed with the patient, particularly the risk of retrograde ejaculation in young male patients, as well as other risks.

TECHNIQUE 4.4

- Position the patient supine on a radiolucent table, such as the OSI flat top. After induction of anesthesia, fold the patient's arms across the chest on pillows and secure them in place. Place a pillow behind the knees to flex the hips and knees slightly.
- Apply pneumatic compressive devices and affix an O_2 saturation monitor to the left great toe.
- Place a bolster under the patient at the lumbosacral junction; this can be an inflatable pressure bag or rolled towels.
- Sterilely prepare and drape the infraumbilical area and administer prophylactic antibiotics. Complete the intraoperative "Time Out."
- Image the operative level fluoroscopically and determine the level of the incision.
- Make a low transverse incision down to the rectus sheath. Open the rectus sheath and mobilize the left rectus muscle toward the midline.
- Open the posterior sheath distal to the arcuate line and enter the preperitoneal space. Mobilize the peritoneal contents to the patient's right.
- After the ureter has been positively identified, set up a table-mounted retractor with several retractor blades.
- Identify the aortic bifurcation and carefully expose the anterior spine. Usually the aortic bifurcation is located at the L4 disc level, but this is variable and a fluoroscopic lateral view is used to definitively confirm the level.
- When the L5 disc level is located caudal to the bifurcation, divide the middle lumbar vessels and mobilize the left iliac vein and artery to the left.
- The dissection at the level of the disc space should be done gently and without the use of electrocautery, only bipolar cautery. The oxygen sensor on the hallux allows monitoring of the level of retraction on the artery.
- Once the disc is sufficiently exposed, make a wide annulotomy and carry out the disc excision with curets and Kerrison rongeurs.
- Use lateral image intensifier views as the posterior disc preparation is completed, which can be taken back all the way to the posterior longitudinal ligament. The most common error is inadequate posterior release.
- If the sacrum is rounded, use an osteotome to reshape it to provide a flat surface for the interbody device. A variety of cage devices are available, including titanium cages and mesh cylinders, PEEK devices with fixation capabilities, femoral allograft bone, and carbon fiber implants. The commercially available systems have trial sizes with varying degrees of lordosis. Determine the optimal size and footprint. Usually by this point the spondylolisthesis has been substantially if not completely reduced.
- To obtain a fusion, harvest autograft bone or use BMP to fill the chamber within the implant. Take care if BMP is placed posteriorly and the annulus has been violated because bone can form in the canal or BMP-induced radiculitis may affect the nerve root.
- Once the interbody device is implanted (Fig. 4.15), close the wound in the usual fashion.

This same technique can be used at the L4 disc level or L3. Exposure at the L4 level is often difficult and usually requires sacrifice of the iliolumbar vein, which ascends from the left common iliac vein and must be identified and divided before the vein can be sufficiently mobilized. Excess traction on the iliac veins also can lead to deep venous thrombosis in the postoperative period.

POSTOPERATIVE CARE The patient is allowed a clear liquid diet the next day, and mobilization is started on the first postoperative day, usually without a brace. Patients usually can be discharged home the second or third postoperative day. If aggressive disc space mobilization was needed, these patients usually complain of significant lumbar pain when ambulation is initiated.

DEGENERATIVE SPONDYLOLISTHESIS

Degenerative spondylolisthesis is the most common form of spondylolisthesis seen in adults. It is more homogeneous with respect to pathoanatomy than the acquired lytic type because there usually is no contributory congenital or developmental dysplasia. Degenerative spondylolisthesis is most frequent in women over the age of 50 years, especially those of African descent, and typically occurs at the L4-L5 level. It is believed to result from the degenerative cascade, as originally described by Kirkaldy-Willis. The L4-L5 level is affected six times more often than other levels, and spondylolisthesis is four times more likely above a sacralized L5 segment. Degenerative spondylolisthesis is present in 10% of women over 60 years of

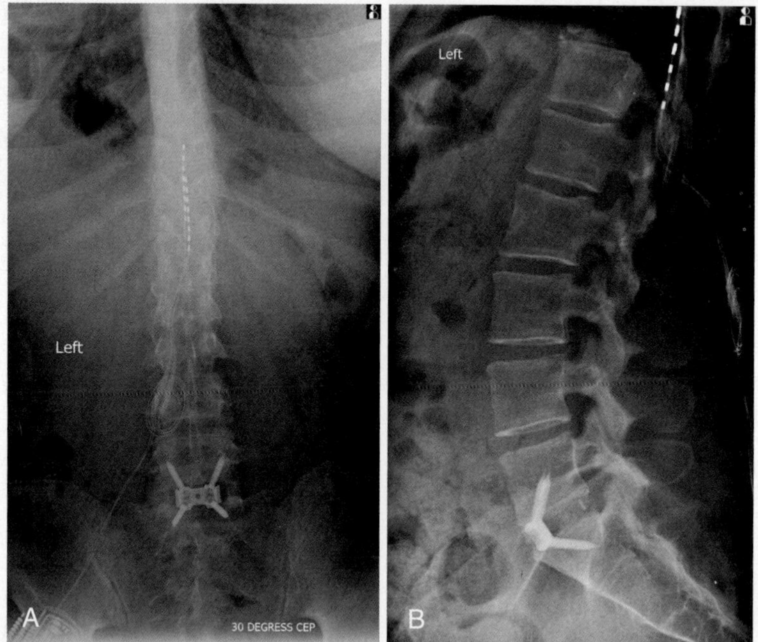

FIGURE 4.15 Ferguson (**A**) and lateral spot view (**B**) of anterior lumbar interbody fusion. **SEE TECHNIQUE 4.4.**

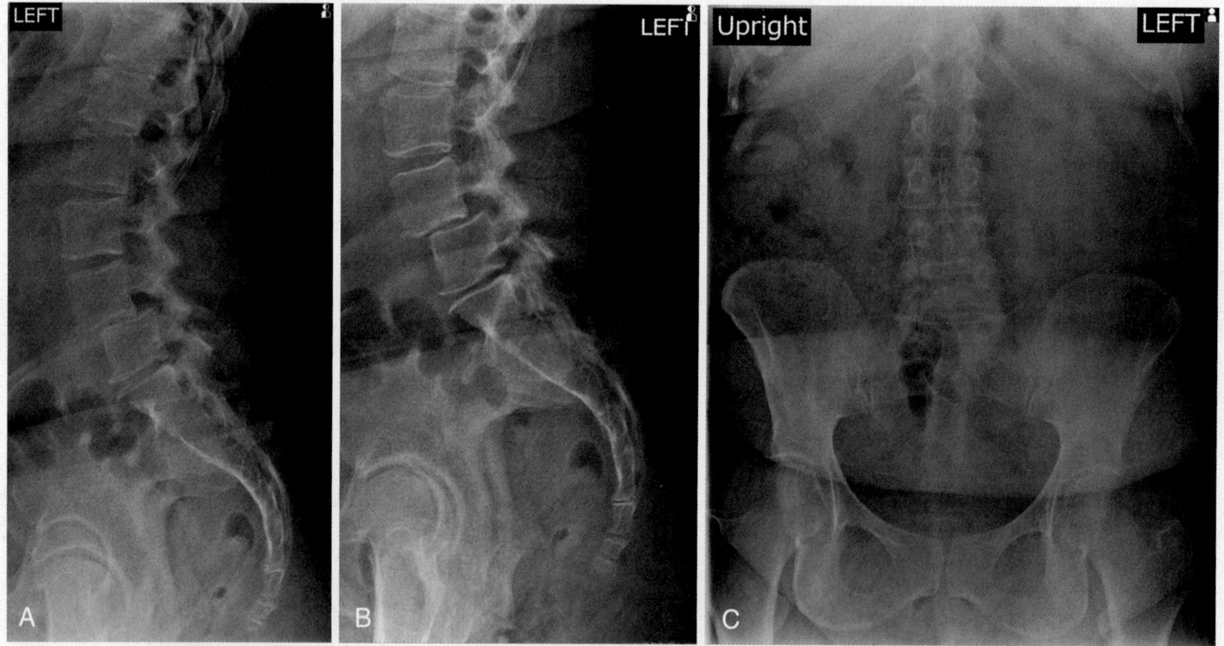

FIGURE 4.16 Degenerative spondylolisthesis at L4-L5. Degenerative spondylolisthesis can be differentiated from isthmic spondylolisthesis by the presence of an intact pars.

age, many of whom are asymptomatic. Diabetes has been present in a disproportionate number of study patients, and Imada et al. found that patients who had undergone oophorectomy had a three times greater rate of degenerative spondylolisthesis than did patients who had not undergone oophorectomy.

PATHOPHYSIOLOGY

Degenerative spondylolisthesis is differentiated from isthmic spondylolisthesis by the presence of an intact pars (Fig. 4.16). Because the arch is intact and moves forward with the L4 vertebral body, progressive spinal stenosis occurs in addition to facet degenerative changes. The true deformity of degenerative spondylolisthesis does not seem to be pure translation, but rather a rotary deformity that may distort the dura and its contents and exaggerate the appearance of spinal stenosis. Existing theories to explain the development of degenerative spondylolisthesis include the primary occurrence of sagittal facets and disc degeneration, with secondary facet changes accounting for anterolisthesis. The sagittal facet theory suggests a predilection for slippage because of facet orientation that does not resist anterior translation forces and, over time, results in degenerative spondylolisthesis. The disc degenerative theory proposes that the disc narrows first, and subsequent overloading of the facets results in accelerated arthritic changes, secondary remodeling, and anterolisthesis. Facet arthritic changes seem to be more severe than disc space narrowing, with the most advanced anterolisthesis present when disc narrowing is more pronounced. A continuum seems to exist as degeneration progresses. In addition, facets that are aligned in a more sagittal orientation provide less stability at the involved level, but whether these changes result from chronic instability or from a primary anatomic variant is debatable. Boden et al. showed that sagittal facet angles of more than 45 degrees at L4-L5 predicted a 25 times greater likelihood of degenerative spondylolisthesis. Despite the increased frequency of degenerative spondylolisthesis in women, there seems to be no sex-specific difference in facet orientation, which calls into question the theory that sagittal facet joints are a primary cause of degenerative spondylolisthesis. Sagittal facet orientation has been correlated with disc space narrowing, suggesting that disc narrowing increases loading of the facet, resulting in secondary facet changes. Regardless of the exact nature of the first inciting event, this instability causes facet arthritis, disc degeneration, and ligamentous hypertrophy, which all contribute to produce symptoms. Facet orientation may be part of the consideration of potential instability when evaluating a patient for surgery, especially decompression alone.

Most of the literature describing natural history concerns spinal stenosis rather than degenerative spondylolisthesis. Matsunaga et al. reported that in 145 patients examined annually for a minimum of 10 years, progressive spondylolisthesis occurred in 34% and further disc space narrowing continued in the patients without further slip. Patients with disc space narrowing, spur formation, and ligamentous ossification did not develop an increased amount of slip. There was no correlation between radiographic findings and a patient's clinical picture. Low back pain improved in patients with continued disc space narrowing, which may imply autostabilization. Of the 145 patients, 76% remained without neurologic deficits; however, 83% of patients with neurologic symptoms, including claudication and vesicorectal disorder, experienced a deterioration in their disorder and had a poor prognosis. This finding is in agreement with an earlier study by Matsunaga et al., which showed that, over 60 to 176 months, progressive slipping occurred in 30% of patients without significant effect on clinical outcome. A more recent prospective study with a cohort of 160 patients by Cushnie et al. found that over 5 years only 32% had slip progression. Many patients improved over a 5-year period with regard to ODI and SF-12 Physical Health Composite scores, even in those with slip progression. However, back pain improved only in the group without slip progression.

NONOPERATIVE TREATMENT

The symptoms attributed to degenerative spondylolisthesis tend to be stable over time or progress rather slowly. The typical complaints related to degenerative spondylolisthesis include lower back pain and lower extremity pain and weakness that are claudicatory in nature, meaning they progress in severity and distribution in a dermatomal pattern with ambulation and standing. The neurologic symptoms are related to spinal stenosis, which may exist not only at the level of the spondylolisthesis but at other degenerative levels.

The back pain may respond to physical therapy for core strengthening with avoidance of extension exercises, although there is no clear optimal regimen. Aerobic conditioning also has a role in reducing symptoms and maintaining cardiac fitness. Activities such as stationary bike, swimming, elliptical machines, and walking as tolerated are all reasonable to try. Antiinflammatory drugs also are helpful for some patients. All of these measures must be used over the long term because of the chronic nature of this problem. Due to the chronic nature of this process opioids should be used judiciously if at all. Most patients remain stable with regard to symptoms over long periods, with intermittent periods of exacerbation and do not need surgery.

Adogwa et al. reviewed a large insurance database to evaluate the costs of nonoperative care in a group of 4133 patients who ultimately had spinal fusion for degenerative spondylolisthesis. They did not include an analysis of these costs for patients with degenerative spondylolisthesis who did not have subsequent surgery. They found that 67% used nonsteroidal antiinflammatory drugs (NSAIDs), 84% used opioids, 66% had lumbar epidural steroid injections, 67% had at least one physical therapy session, 21% had emergency department visit, and 25% received chiropractic care. The average cost of care per patient in the study was $2177. The use of opioids doubled relative to a similar earlier study by the same authors.

For patients with worsening symptoms, 12 weeks of directed treatment is reasonable before recommending operative intervention unless the patient develops a progressive neurologic deficit. Patients with neurologic symptoms, particularly radiculopathy or neurogenic claudication, may benefit from epidural steroid injections, although the benefit may only be temporary. No literature exists to support the use of a series of two or three epidural steroid injections unless symptoms improve partially after the first injection. If the first injection is done without fluoroscopy and is ineffective, a second injection can be done with fluoroscopy to ensure proper placement and dispersion of the steroid. Further injections are not warranted if there is not a favorable response after a single well-placed injection. There is some evidence that response to injections can be used to diagnostically confirm the anatomic origin of the symptoms (when done under fluoroscopy) and that the short-term response to injections may correlate well with operative outcomes. If epidural steroid injection is successful, physical therapy should be instituted.

A level II study by Passias et al. evaluated patient crossover from the nonoperative arm to the operative arm of the Spine Patient Outcomes Research Trial (SPORT) study for degenerative spondylolisthesis and stenosis. They found that the decision by patients to cross over and have surgery was influenced by the severity of their symptoms measured by ODI, but also by their age, attitude toward surgery, marital status, and absence of other major joint pathology. Factors that did not correlate with choosing surgery included levels of stenosis, radiographic severity of stenosis, and neurologic deficits.

OPERATIVE TREATMENT AND OUTCOMES

The decision to consider operative treatment is based primarily on the degree of disability and the severity of pain experienced by the patient. If the symptoms significantly limit the patient's necessary activities or those the patient enjoys, even after a reasonable trial of nonoperative care, operative treatment should be considered. Only 10% to 15% of patients with degenerative spondylolisthesis require surgery. In general, patients complaining primarily of neurogenic claudication or radiculopathy tend to have more improvement than those experiencing primarily axial low back pain. This is because many of the patients with primarily axial pain have degenerative levels other than the spondylolisthetic level contributing to their symptoms. The SPORT study demonstrated a significant benefit for patients with degenerative spondylolisthesis treated with decompression and fusion (type of fusion was not controlled) at the 2- and 4-year time frame compared with nonoperatively treated patients. This prospective, randomized, multicenter study has provided the highest level of evidence to date supporting the benefit of operative treatment in this group of patients. In a study by Golinvaux et al., the SPORT findings were determined to be generalizable to a larger group of patients in the National Surgical Quality Improvement Program (NSQIP) database. Additional economic studies have found the cost per QALY for operative treatment of degenerative spondylolisthesis to be $64,000 per QALY at 4 years, which is substantially less than the cost at 2 years. Multiple studies have found patient satisfaction rates of 85% to 90% in the operatively treated patients, with successful fusion being a key factor. In addition, Schulte et al. found "good" evidence in a literature review that operative treatment for degenerative spondylolisthesis is superior to nonoperative treatment in appropriately selected patients.

Hendrickson et al., in a literature review of operative treatment for degenerative spondylolisthesis, found that there is level II evidence showing sustained superior outcomes after decompressive surgical procedures with regard to pain, physical function, and disability compared with nonoperative treatment. Almost 95% of patients in the United States have spinal fusion at the time of decompression for degenerative spondylolisthesis, most with instrumentation. Numerous studies have documented improved outcomes with fusion, beginning with Herkowitz and Kurz. Instrumentation increases fusion rates, which have been correlated with better patient outcomes. Instrumentation also increases costs and length of hospital stay. There is no high-level evidence indicating which patients should or should not have fusion at the time of decompression. Likewise, there is no high-level evidence indicating an optimal technique of arthrodesis. An 8-year subgroup analysis of the SPORT study by Gerling et al. found that patients who had reoperations were significantly more likely to have had an uninstrumented fusion rather than with instrumentation. A study by Ikuta et al. suggests that improvement in lumbopelvic parameters, such as pelvic incidence and lumbar lordosis mismatch and SVA may be important in relieving back pain symptoms in these patients.

A more recent classification for degenerative spondylolisthesis has been proposed to replace the Meyerding system. The rationale for the new system, termed the Clinical and Radiographic Degenerative Spondylolisthesis classification (CARDS), has to do with varied and sometimes conflicting results of studies of this group of patients. Most patients with degenerative spondylolisthesis are Meyerding class I or II, and further description of these patients is not possible with the Meyerding system. The CARDS system classifies patients into four categories based on degree of slip, disc height, and kyphosis (Fig. 4.17). Type

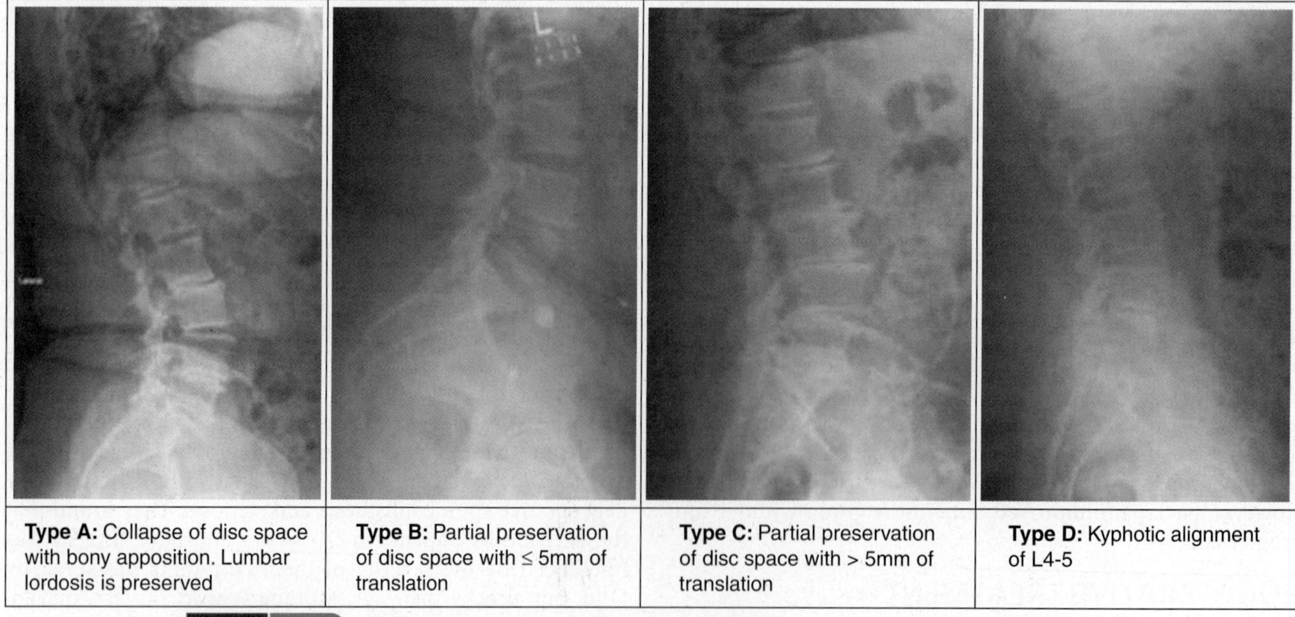

FIGURE 4.17 Clinical and Radiographic Degenerative Spondylolisthesis (CARDS) classification. (From Sobol GL, Hilibrand A, Davis A, et al: Reliability and clinical utility of the CARDS classification for degenerative spondylolisthesis, *Clin Spine Surg* 31:E69, 2018.)

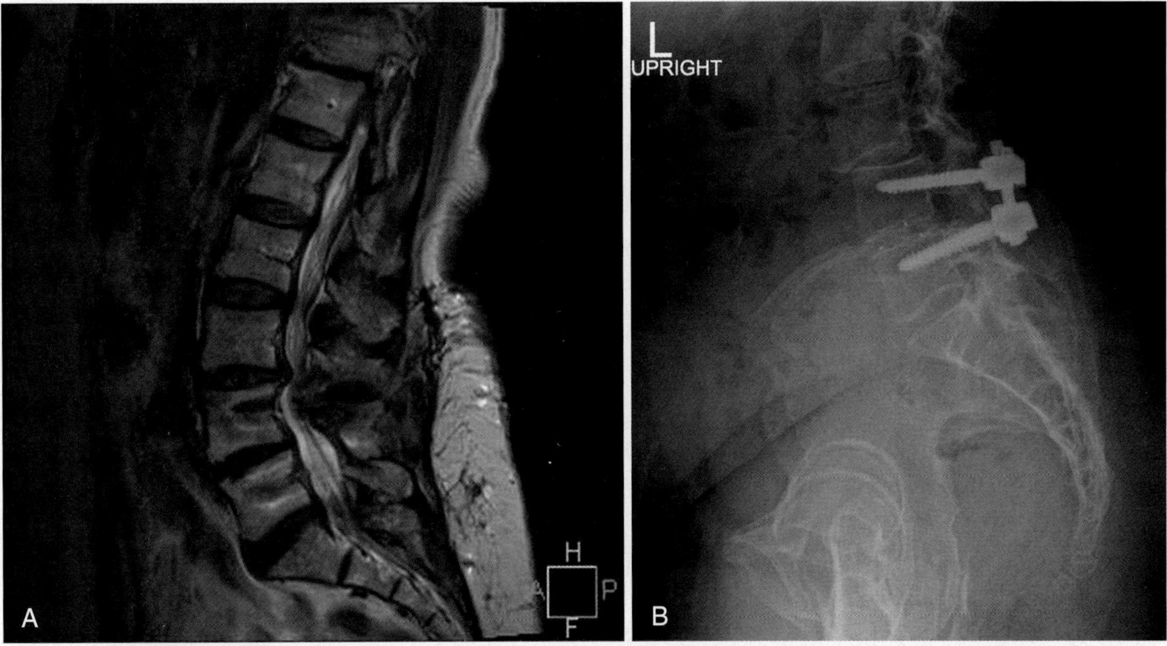

FIGURE 4.18 Evaluation of instability in degenerative spondylolisthesis. **A,** L3-L4 spondylolisthesis appears reduced on supine MRI. **B,** L3-L4 spondylolisthesis is visible on standing lateral radiographic spot view.

A is "bone-on-bone" apposition, which can be symmetric through the disc space or just the posterior endplates in contact. Type B is defined as partial disc space preservation with less than 5 mm of translation on all lateral views, including flexion/extension views. Type C has partial disc preservation with more than 5 mm of translation on any lateral view, and type D has kyphotic alignment on at least one lateral view. The description of the system by Sobol et al. showed clinical differences in the different types and reasonable interobserver reliability of the classification. The clinical utility remains to be determined.

OPERATIVE PLANNING

There should be an awareness that other pathologies can mimic or overlap the signs and symptoms of degenerative spondylolisthesis and the associated spinal stenosis. Primary among these conditions are vascular claudication, degenerative hip arthritis, and peripheral neuropathy. If the history and physical examination findings are inconsistent with degenerative spondylolisthesis, evaluation for these problems should be considered. At a minimum hip range of motion and irritability should be evaluated as well as peripheral pulses in the feet and proprioception.

Once the decision to recommend operative treatment has been made, a determination as to what type of operation is most appropriate for an individual patient also must be made. Given the findings of Hendrickson et al. just cited, a least aggressive surgical approach is appropriate, with regard to the type of surgery selected. This determination is based on the patient's primary complaints and imaging findings. Standing lateral, seated or standing flexion/extension laterals, and anteroposterior radiographs are imperative because 15% of deformities spontaneously reduce on supine imaging such as an MRI (Fig. 4.18). Instability is considered to be present when 4 mm of translation or 10 degrees of sagittal rotation greater than the adjacent level is identified. Disc space narrowing indicates degenerative changes. Upright flexion-extension lateral views may reveal translational motion, indicating a more unstable motion segment. The Ferguson anteroposterior view shows any significant degenerative changes in the lumbosacral joint and allows a better view of the transverse processes of L5. Hypoplastic transverse processes also should prompt consideration for interbody fusion because of the paucity of bony substrate for fusion, especially for lumbosacral fusions. Dynamically unstable spondylolisthesis also may benefit from interbody fusions that improve stability through annular tension and decrease shear stress on posterior instrumentation by sharing load through the disc space. The presence of retrolisthesis, scoliosis, or lateral listhesis also should be noted. In addition to plain radiographs, advanced neuroimaging is necessary to appropriately evaluate these patients. MRI generally is satisfactory, but a significant subset of patients cannot have an MRI because of the presence of a pacemaker or cardiac stents for example. In this case, lumbar myelography and post-myelogram high-resolution CT scans are quite satisfactory and often demonstrate the bony pathology better than MRI. Post-myelogram CT scans do not show pathology as well in the mid and lateral foramen because the subarachnoid space is not present out to the dorsal root ganglion and, thus, there is no contrast present in this area. Intraforaminal stenosis is relatively common, affecting the L4 nerve root, which is compressed against the inferior aspect of the L4 pedicle by annulus from a pseudoherniation due to the spondylolisthesis. The most severe stenosis usually is located at the level of the spondylolisthesis, but the entire course of each symptomatic nerve root must be thoroughly assessed. Usually the L5 root is compressed in the L4-L5 lateral recess, but there may be other pathology, such as a synovial cyst or disc herniation, affecting the same root or a different root level. The presence of a facet joint effusion more than 2 mm in width is highly suggestive of instability at that level and should prompt close inspection of the upright dynamic radiographs. As noted previously Snoddy et al. found a 42% probability of dynamic instability for each 1 mm of facet join effusion.

The most common procedure performed for degenerative spondylolisthesis is bilateral decompression and fusion. We typically use an interbody technique with instrumentation. A meta-analysis evaluating patients with degenerative spondylolisthesis treated with decompression alone or decompression with PLF, with or without instrumentation, found similar fusion rates (93% and 86%) and satisfaction rates (86% and 90%) with or without instrumentation. The nonfused group had a 69% satisfaction rate and 31% had slip progression. Other studies have found that patients with a solid fusion have better clinical outcomes than those who develop nonunions. Instrumentation and interbody stabilization both have been found to improve fusion rates but also to increase cost and potential risk. In a longitudinal study with minimum 10-year follow-up after PLIF, Okuda et al. found the rates of radiographic adjacent segment degeneration (ASD), symptomatic ASD, and operative ASD to be 75%, 31%, and 15%, respectively. Conversely, several studies, including a randomized controlled trial by Ghogawala et al. comparing laminectomy to PLF with instrumentation, found that 34% of patients with decompression only required reoperation within 4 years compared with 14% of those with fusion. They also found more improvement in the SF-36 physical component score at each time interval in the fusion group compared with the laminectomy group. A systematic review of articles comparing interbody fusion and instrumented PLF by McAnany et al. found no significant differences in outcomes, fusion rates, or other measures. Only length of hospital stay was different between the groups, with PLF being favored. Other studies with longer follow-up showed a slight benefit for interbody fusion, but patient numbers are too small to make any definitive conclusions.

The operative procedure chosen should aim to correct the identified sources of symptoms, not merely radiographic abnormalities. Fusion generally is recommended at the level of the spondylolisthesis but usually is not necessary at other stenotic levels without instability. These levels can be treated with decompression without fusion. Many patients with degenerative spondylolisthesis at the L4-L5 level have some degenerative disc changes at the L5-S1 disc level as well. There remains some controversy of how best to manage the L5 degenerative disc changes in the absence of instability at that level. Choi et al. in a retrospective study found that the presence of L5 disc degeneration which was not treated at the time of L4-L5 anterior fusion with posterior instrumentation did not affect the clinical or radiographic outcome. Although fusion for axial pain attributable only to degenerative change is very controversial and not well supported in the literature, fusion in the setting of instability is much more accepted and there is substantial literature support. The fusion can be done posterolaterally, with or without instrumentation. Fusions with interbody implants (PLIF or TLIF) are commonly used to treat patients with degenerative spondylolisthesis. Less commonly, anterior fusions are performed in this patient population. There is, however, also evidence to support decompression alone for the treatment of degenerative spondylolisthesis. Decompression alone can be the most appropriate procedure in some elderly patients or those with significant comorbidities who may not tolerate the added morbidity of a fusion, especially with instrumentation. Kim and Mortaz showed that decompression alone in patients with leg pain predominantly and no dynamic instability is significantly more cost-effective than instrumented fusion. Minimally invasive decompression does not appear inferior to open decompression in most studies. There are no recent high-level studies comparing minimally invasive decompression to open laminectomy in degenerative spondylolisthesis.

The procedure we use most often for degenerative spondylolisthesis is posterior decompression and fusion with interbody support and instrumentation which can be combined with a PLF. The primary advantage of this approach is that it allows optimal decompression and has a higher fusion rate than posterolateral instrumented fusion or interbody fusion alone. Higher fusion rates in general correlate with better patient outcomes. One potential drawback of this approach is that biomechanically the interbody fusion increases the stiffness of the fused segment and this may increase the rate of ASD. Minimally invasive posterior decompression and fusion techniques are described in chapter 3. ALIF is less commonly used as a first choice in treating degenerative spondylolisthesis because of the need for direct decompression in almost all of these patients. For patients with previous adequate decompression and persistent instability or failed PLF, ALIF can be a reasonable option (see Technique 4.4).

LUMBAR DECOMPRESSION

TECHNIQUE 4.5

- Position the patient, prepare and drape the operative area, and administer prophylactic antibiotics as described in Technique 4.1. Keeping the hips relatively extended is important to simulate the anatomy in the standing position to allow adequate assessment of the decompression. If a frame is used that flexes the lumbar spine to open the interlaminar space, this must be taken into account to avoid an inadequate decompression. Complete the intraoperative "Time Out."
- Make a midline incision centered at the level to be decompressed.
- Carry dissection down to the fascia and obtain a localization image with a clamp affixed to the spinous process to confirm the level. Mark this spinous process with a rongeur.
- Use Cobb elevators and electrocautery to subperiosteally expose the spinous processes and laminae of the levels to be decompressed bilaterally, taking care to preserve the facet capsule at each level.
- Expose the pars interarticularis so it is fully visible to avoid inadvertent excessive thinning of the pars, predisposing to pars fracture in the postoperative period.
- For a complete laminectomy, use a rongeur to remove the entire spinous process of the laminectomy level and the caudal one third of the cephalad level. For L4-L5 decompression this would mean removal of the caudal portion of L3 and the entire spinous process of L4. This will allow adequate access to the L4 and the L5 nerve roots.

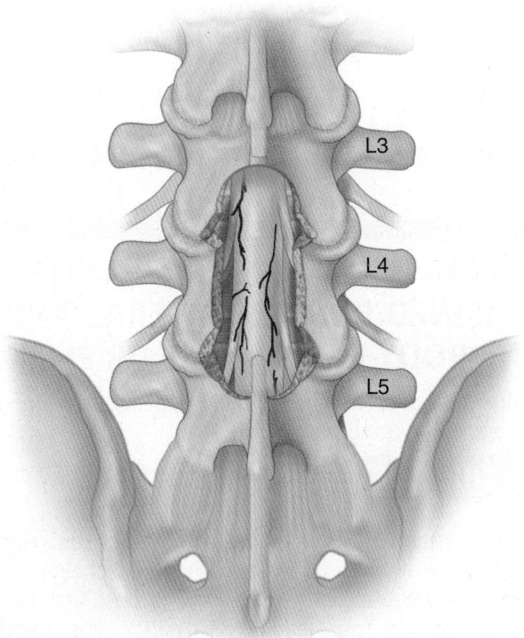

FIGURE 4.19 Typical midline decompression for spinal stenosis. Note medial facetectomy and foraminotomy with preservation of the pars. Decompression is from inferior border of L3 pedicle to superior border of L5 pedicle, exposing both lateral borders of dura in lateral recess. **SEE TECHNIQUE 4.5.**

- Once the bone at the base of the spinous process has been thinned with the rongeur or with the use of a high-speed burr, identify the midline cleft in the ligamentum flavum.
- Use a small curet to detach the ligamentum flavum from the caudal margin of the cephalad (L4) level. Use of the operating microscope or loupe magnification is very helpful.
- Remove the thinned lamina with a Kerrison rongeur proceeding from caudal to cephalad to have better protection of the dura by the ligamentum flavum.
- Carry the decompression up to the caudal margin of the L3 lamina, focusing initially on the central canal stenosis.
- Once the central decompression is complete, turn attention to the lateral recess and foraminal stenosis as demonstrated by the imaging studies. It generally is easier for the surgeon to work on the side of the patient opposite the side on which he or she is standing. This allows Kerrison placement parallel with the course of the nerve root.
- With the dura gently retracted with a Penfield #4 dissector, undercut the medial portion of the L3 inferior facet with a Kerrison rongeur. Identify the L4 nerve root and follow it into the foramen.
- Complete the foraminotomy with curets and Kerrison rongeurs such that a Murphy ball hook can pass easily between the root and the inferior aspect of the pedicle (ensuring an adequate cephalocaudal dimension) and posterior to the root ventral to the L4 pars (ensuring an adequate anteroposterior dimension) (Fig. 4.19).
- Pay careful attention to the amount of bony removal from the L4 pars so as not to risk fracture.

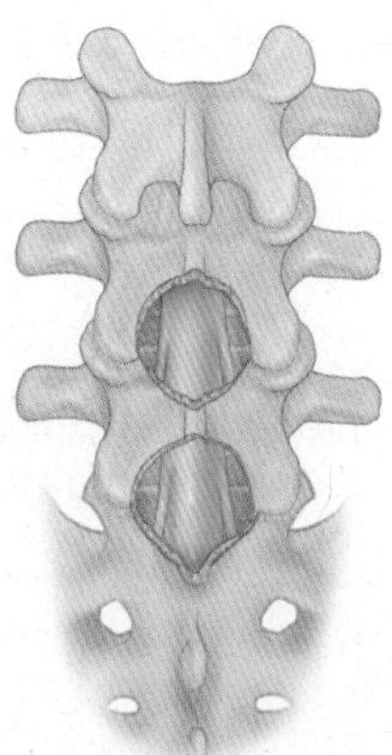

FIGURE 4.20 Decompression completed under microscopic magnification. **SEE TECHNIQUE 4.5.**

- After the L3 medial facetectomy and L4 foraminotomy are complete, decompress the L5 root in the L4-L5 lateral recess. Again, gently retract the dura and remove the osteophyte extending from the medial aspect of the L5 superior articular mass and ligamentum flavum. Remove the bone to the level of the medial aspect of the L5 pedicle, which marks the lateral extent of the canal. Complete the foraminotomy at the L5 level as described above for the L4 root.
- At this point the decompression is complete. If it was necessary to perform a complete facetectomy or if extensive bone removal was needed to adequately decompress the L4 nerve root, a fusion should be added.
- An alternative technique is a laminoforaminotomy (Fig. 4.20), which can be unilateral or bilateral. Achieving an adequate decompression is the primary goal, and usually this can be accomplished without a complete laminectomy.
- After achieving thorough hemostasis, irrigate the wound and close it over a fluted drain because of the exposed dura. Close the fascia to the spinous process where possible to better restore the normal resting length of the paraspinal musculature. Close the subcutaneous and subcuticular layers.

POSTOPERATIVE CARE Patients are started on oral analgesics and scheduled muscle relaxers. Mobilization is started either the evening of surgery or the next morning. Most patients are independent with mobility and can be discharged home the same day or at least by the second postoperative day.

LUMBAR DECOMPRESSION AND POSTEROLATERAL FUSION WITH OR WITHOUT INSTRUMENTATION

TECHNIQUE 4.6

- Position the patient, prepare and drape the operative area, and carry out preoperative tasks as described in Technique 4.1.

- Make a midline incision centered at the level to be decompressed.
- Carry dissection down to the fascia and obtain a localization image with a clamp affixed to the spinous process to confirm the level. Mark this spinous process with a rongeur.
- Use Cobb elevators and electrocautery to subperiosteally expose the spinous processes and laminae of the levels to be decompressed bilaterally, taking care to preserve the facet capsule at the cephalad level (L3-L4) level that is not to be fused.
- Use a Cobb elevator to sweep the musculature off the capsule and carry the exposure down the lateral aspect of the superior articular mass onto the transverse process which is fully exposed subperiosteally.
- At the caudal facet (L4-L5) level, remove the capsule and expose the transverse process.
- Expose the intertransverse membrane, taking care not to violate this membrane to avoid a hematoma or nerve injury.
- Completely expose the transverse processes at both levels bilaterally.
- At this point, prepare the screw holes in the following manner if pedicle screw instrumentation is to be used. Use a bone awl to penetrate the cortex at the junction of the transverse process and the superior articular mass. It is often necessary to remove the laterally overhanging bone particularly at the caudal screw level in order to start medially enough. Advance a pedicle probe into the pedicle using fluoroscopic control. Use a sound to ensure there are no cortical breaches, although after the laminectomy the pedicles can be inspected visually as well. After the screw holes are prepared, place cottonoids for hemostasis while the decompression is completed. Use fluoroscopy to facilitate advancement of the pedicle probe.
- Complete the laminectomy and foraminotomy as described in Technique 4.5 and proceed with fusion.
- Decorticate the transverse process of L4 and L5, the lateral surface of the articular masses, and the pars with a high-speed drill, and carefully pack bone graft into the lateral gutter. Use the local bone from the decompression to augment other graft material.
- In addition, decorticate the L4-L5 facet joint and pack it with bone.
- If instrumentation is to be used, insert the screws at each level after the bone graft is placed. Otherwise the screws make decortication and graft placement more difficult.
- Cut and contour the rods and secure them with set screws which are tightened to the manufacturer's recommended torque. Take care to make sure the rods do not impinge on the cephalad joint.
- After achieving thorough hemostasis, irrigate the wound and close it over a fluted drain because of the exposed dura. Close the fascia to the spinous process where possible to better restore the normal resting length of the paraspinal musculature. Close the subcutaneous and subcuticular layers.

POSTOPERATIVE CARE Patients are started on oral analgesics and scheduled muscle relaxers. A single dose of 5 mg epidural preservative-free morphine gives excellent postoperative pain relief but does require close monitoring for respiratory depression postoperatively. Mobilization is started the next morning. Most patients are independent with mobility and can be discharged home by the third postoperative day.

LUMBAR DECOMPRESSION AND COMBINED POSTEROLATERAL AND INTERBODY FUSION (TLIF OR PLIF)

The preferred procedure for treating degenerative spondylolisthesis is PLF combined with TLIF.

TECHNIQUE 4.7

- Patient positioning, approach, decompression, and placement of screw holes are as described in Technique 4.6. Complete the tranexamic acid loading dose and begin the infusion. The usual loading dose is 20 mg/kg, and the infusion is 2 mg/kg/hr.
- Place the interbody device from the side with the most severe nerve root compression and patient complaints. Thin the inferior facet on the selected side with a rongeur and keep the bone for later use.
- Use a small curet to detach the ligamentum flavum from the caudal lamina and remove the remaining inferior facet (of L4) and pars unilaterally with a Kerrison rongeur; preserve the bone for later use.
- Using the operating microscope, identify the exiting L4 root and decompress it to the lateral aspect of the foramen.
- Use a large rongeur to remove the cephalad 50% of the L5 superior articular mass to allow the desired transforaminal trajectory for insertion of the interbody device.
- Decompress the L5 nerve root to the medial border of the L5 pedicle and into the L5 foramen so that a Murphy ball hook will pass cephalad and posterior to the L5 root, indicating satisfactory decompression.
- Contralateral decompression is done at this point if desired. In some patients the indirect decompression from the interbody device placement will be sufficient.
- Next, prepare the disc space. Coagulate the epidural veins crossing the disc space with bipolar cautery. Once they begin to bleed they are harder to control.
- Incise the annulus in the axilla of the L4 nerve root and extending into the foramen, retracting the thecal sac slightly medially and the L4 root laterally. Extend the annulotomy laterally to the lateral edge of the pedicle.
- Introduce disc reamer distractors into the disc space, monitoring the depth of penetration on lateral fluoroscopic views.
- Use ring and cup curets to scrape the endplates after the desired implant height is determined with the reamer distractor.
- Complete careful disc removal to prepare the disc space and to mobilize the segment.
- Once the endplates are prepared, thoroughly irrigate the disc space to remove any residual soft tissue.
- Pack allograft cancellous bone against the anterior annulus and morselized local autograft bone behind this. This allograft cancellous bone is submerged in antibiotic irriga-

tion solution at the beginning of the case and maintained there until implantation. This has decreased deep wound infections postoperatively associated with allograft bone usage.

- Take care to leave adequate space to allow placement of the interbody device no more posteriorly than the anterior 25% of the disc space so lordosis can be achieved. The goals of interbody spacer device placement are to restore disc height and improve alignment with sufficient lordosis through the segment. Biomechanically coverage of 35% of the endplate is desirable for stability. We prefer a single cage device packed with local autograft placed just anterior to the midbody. The subchondral bone is strongest around the perimeter of the endplate and weakest centrally, increasing the risk of cage subsidence if the device is too small or only centrally located.
- Once the device is transversely positioned, expand it to the predetermined height if an expandable device is used; verify device position with orthogonal fluoroscopic views.
- To proceed with the fusion, decorticate the transverse process of L4 and L5, the lateral surface of the articular mass, and the pars opposite the TLIF with a high-speed drill, and carefully pack bone graft into the lateral gutter.
- Decorticate the remaining L4-L5 facet joint and pack with bone.
- Insert pedicle screws at each level after the bone graft is placed. Otherwise the screws make decortication and graft placement more difficult. Verify the position of each screw fluoroscopically.
- Cut and contour the rods and secure them with set screws which are tightened to the manufacturer's recommended torque. Take care to make sure the rods do not impinge on the cephalad joint.
- After achieving thorough hemostasis, irrigate the wound and close it over a fluted drain because of the exposed dura. Close the fascia to the spinous process where possible to better restore the normal resting length of the paraspinal musculature. Close the subcutaneous and subcuticular layers. Administer a second dose of tranexamic acid as wound closure is begun.

POSTOPERATIVE CARE Postoperative management is the same as after Technique 4.6.

PERIOPERATIVE MANAGEMENT AND COMPLICATIONS

PREOPERATIVE MANAGEMENT

The best way to manage complications is to avoid them wherever possible. This begins with an understanding of the risks associated with a particular surgical technique and the particular needs and pathology of a given patient. Having a candid preoperative discussion with the patient and his or her family about the specific and relative risks of different treatment options is an important step in limiting the risks of complications that are most unacceptable to that patient. A detailed description of potential procedures should be provided to the patient in lay terms. Additionally, printed material or a list of web sites, such as those sponsored by the American Academy of Orthopaedic Surgeons, the Scoliosis Research Society, and the Pediatric Orthopaedic Society of North America, with reliable patient information is helpful. The surgeon should discuss any planned "off label" uses of implants and disclose any financial benefit from industry that may be derived from the procedure. In this way, the patient can make an informed decision as to his or her choice of procedure.

The surgeon also should carefully evaluate the patient and document any medical conditions or circumstances that may increase the risk of complications. A careful neurologic examination to detect even subtle abnormalities that may indicate a greater risk of nerve root injury during or after surgery should be documented. If the patient has a history of diabetes, prior deep vein thrombosis, previous surgical infection, or osteoporosis, or is a current nicotine user, this should be documented and addressed preoperatively to enhance postoperative results. In adult patients, particularly those with degenerative spondylolisthesis, assessment of vitamin D levels preoperatively and correction where indicated are warranted. Diabetic patients should have HgA1c corrected to less than 0.4. All nicotine exposure should be eliminated before any fusion procedure. Baseline information should be obtained from the patient using the patient-reported outcome instrument to be used at follow-up.

INTRAOPERATIVE MANAGEMENT

The surgical treatment of spondylolisthesis is complex, ranging from a single-level decompression to a combined anterior and posterior procedure involving direct deformity correction and instrumentation involving multiple levels. Intraoperatively, the surgeon can affect the risk of infection, excessive hemorrhage, deep vein thrombosis (DVT), neurologic deficits both in and out of the surgical field, and development of pseudarthrosis by the choices that are made and techniques used.

Some actions should be routine, such as careful patient positioning to decrease neurologic risk, administration of prophylactic antibiotics, administration of agents to decrease excessive bleeding, and use of appropriate neuromonitoring in selected cases. The use of careful and precise surgical techniques also is important, including careful soft-tissue management, particularly in patients with significant dysplasia; bone graft bed preparation; type of bone graft selected; choice of implants; accurate instrumentation placement; and careful manipulations of the spine with the instrumentation.

The list of possible complications and the management of each is beyond the scope of this chapter. The most common complications after surgery for spondylolisthesis (of any etiology) are pseudarthrosis, instrumentation failure, neurologic deficits, thromboembolism, and infection.

PSEUDARTHROSIS

The most frequent serious complication after surgery for spondylolisthesis in most series is pseudarthrosis, although infection is more common in some series. The development of pseudarthrosis is linked to other complications, such as progression of deformity and instrumentation failure as well. Eliminating nicotine use and correcting vitamin D deficiency preoperatively have been shown to reduce the risk of pseudarthrosis in spinal fusion in general although not specifically in fusion for spondylolisthesis. Much of the spondylolisthesis literature deals with children and adolescents, and these issues are likely most relevant to older patients with degenerative spondylolisthesis. For large slip angles with sagittal imbalance and high-grade translational deformities, several studies have shown that correcting the segmental kyphosis appears to reduce the risk of pseudarthrosis more than reducing the translation. A finite analysis study by Chen et al. found that increased sacral slope caused higher loads on the posterior portion of the S1 screw. They also found that the S1 screw loads were higher in PLF than in PLIF. Careful preparation of the fusion bed (posteriorly and anteriorly) is important. The transverse processes should each have a surface area of at least 2 cm^2, and decorticating the pars (when present) and the lateral superior articular mass is necessary. There is good evidence that having adequate anterior column support is an important factor to reduce the risk of pseudarthrosis, and usually this is accomplished with the use of an anteriorly placed graft or device, but this is not universally required.

The diagnosis of pseudarthrosis often is difficult unless there is obvious and rapid loss of fixation or progression of deformity, both of which necessitate early surgical correction. Persistent complaints of back pain beyond 4 to 6 months, return of pain after initial resolution of back pain, worsening or new neurologic complaints, or persistent gait abnormality should prompt consideration of the diagnosis of pseudarthrosis. Evaluation involves standing plain radiographs, upright dynamic radiographs, and usually CT scans to try to detect the nonunion (Fig. 4.21). Generally, a pseudarthrosis is not diagnosed until a year after surgery because of the slow nature of fusion consolidation and incorporation. Findings such as a persistent lucent line at the fusion site (best seen on sagittal and coronal CT reconstructions) and visible motion on dynamic radiographs are most diagnostic. Findings such as broken hardware or lucencies around screws are suggestive but not always

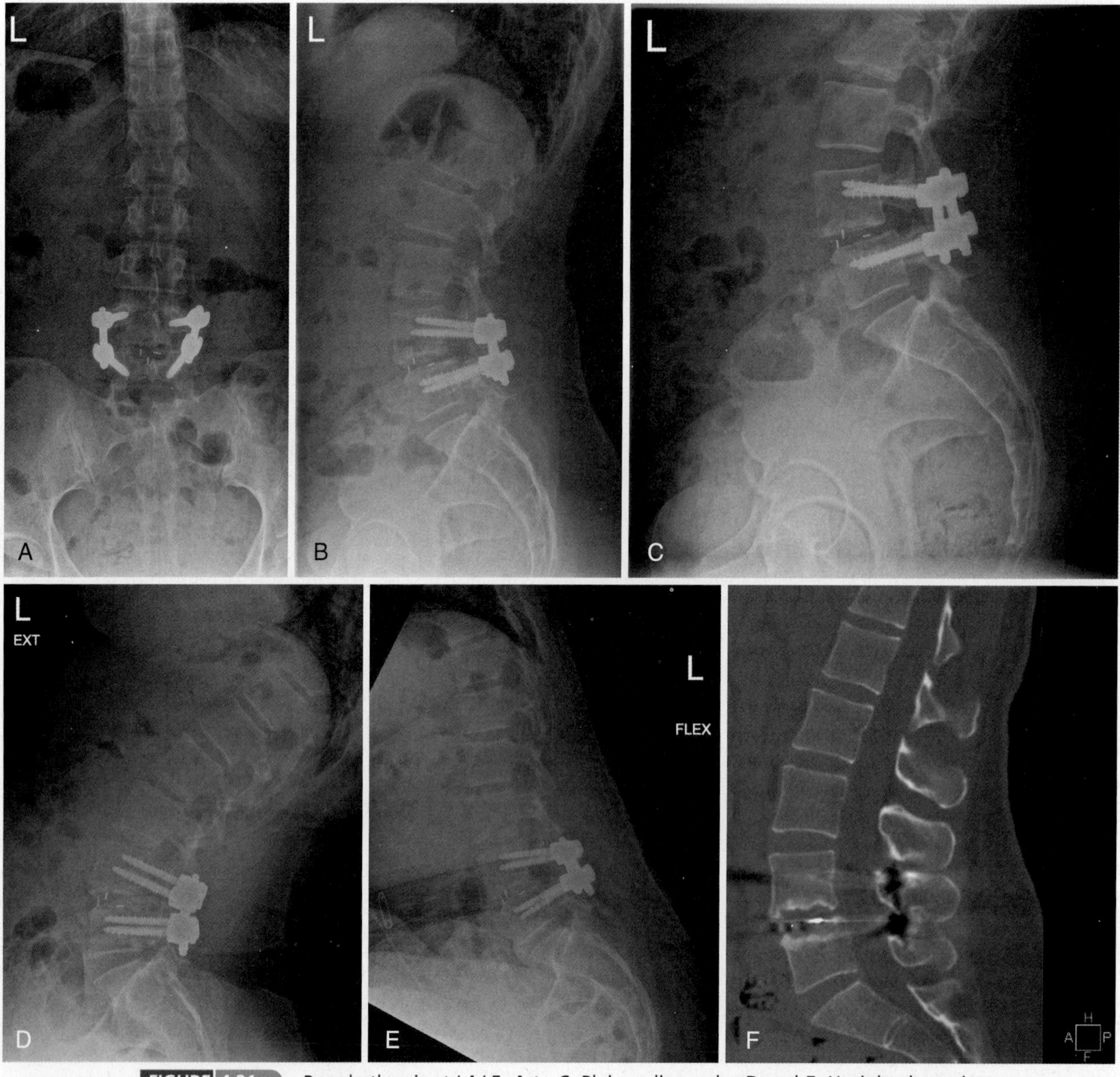

FIGURE 4.21 Pseudarthrosis at L4-L5. **A** to **C**, Plain radiographs. **D** and **E**, Upright dynamic radiographs. **F**, CT scan.

conclusive evidence of nonunion. In addition, it is important to realize that the mere presence of a pseudarthrosis, even when diagnostically not in doubt, is not an indication for revision surgery. If symptoms warrant revision surgery, a careful assessment of the potential reason for failure of the index procedure is important. Making the effort to determine if the failure is, for example, host related, is a biomechanical failure caused by the construct chosen, or resulted from poor execution of an appropriate construct is warranted to avoid the same outcome.

NEUROLOGIC DEFICITS

The avoidance of neurologic deficits begins with patient positioning. Taking care to pad all bony prominences, particularly the ulnar nerve at the elbow and the peroneal nerve at the knee, avoids palsies at these sites indirectly related to the surgery. In addition, keeping the knees flexed can decrease tension, particularly on the L5 root which is most at risk. The selective use of neuromonitoring, including motor evoked potentials, electromyography, somatosensory evoked potentials, impedance testing of pedicle screws, and even direct nerve stimulation of the L5 root, can all be useful techniques. Any intraoperative change in neuromonitoring parameters should be promptly evaluated. Technical issues and those related to anesthesia should be assessed, and if no clear cause is evident, the surgeon should suspect an actual neurologic injury. The anatomy and applied forces should be evaluated, and distractive or translational forces should be decreased until there is no tension on any of the neural structures. Caution should be used when applying corrective forces, particularly if the maneuver will cause tension on the L5 root. A cadaver study demonstrated that in spondylolisthesis reduction only 21% of the nerve strain occurs with the first 50% of the reduction and the remaining 79% of the measured nerve strain occurs when the final 50% of the reduction is accomplished.

Neurologic deficits also can occur from dissection around compromised neural structures. Decompression of the L5 root in particular should be cautiously undertaken to remove the fibrocartilaginous tissue in the foramen. If a developmental dysplastic spondylolisthesis is being reduced, careful dissection to release the nerve all the way out to the ala is necessary.

Malpositioned hardware is another potential cause for neurologic deficits. The anatomy can be quite abnormal with dysplastic type deformities, and careful preoperative planning and intraoperative fluoroscopy, and potentially image guided navigation, can be helpful in achieving proper and safe implant placement.

With anterior exposures of the lower lumbar spine, there is a small risk of retrograde ejaculation attributed to autonomic nerve injury. If this approach is selected, some patients may want to use a sperm bank preoperatively. Intraoperatively, limiting the use of electrocautery and gently dissecting only the area needed to access the disc space reduces this risk.

Cauda equina syndrome can occur in the immediate postoperative period. This may be attributed to a hematoma, which should be immediately decompressed, and if the segment was not instrumented initially, it should be at that time.

VASCULAR COMPLICATIONS

Preoperative positioning is important to decrease the risk of certain vascular complications. Postoperative blindness is a rare (1/60,000 to 1/100,000) post-anesthetic complication that occurs more often in spine surgery than in other types of orthopaedic surgery, particularly if the patient is prone. It seems to be related to hypotension with ischemia in the distribution of the central retinal artery. There is some evidence that external pressure on the globe in the prone position may contribute, but the evidence is unclear. In any case attention to the eyes in a prone patient is warranted.

Pressure can also be placed on the femoral artery by the pad at the level of the anterior superior iliac spine of a prone patient. Verifying the presence of the pedal pulses once the patient is prone will mitigate this risk.

Direct vascular injury can occur with anterior or posterior spinal surgery. With anterior surgery, exposing and gaining control of the vascular injury are more direct. A vascular injury occurring from a posterior procedure may not be immediately apparent if it is a venous or a small arterial injury. The type of injury may not be immediately apparent. After a period of time, the patient may show signs of hypovolemia, and attention should move to urgent vascular repair.

Postoperative vascular complications occur primarily in the form of DVT and very rarely pulmonary embolism. In patients undergoing postoperative venography without mechanical prophylaxis, some studies have reported a DVT rate of 10% to 15%, but this is decreased in similar studies using mechanical prophylaxis to 0.3% to 2%. However, in a study by Yoshioka et al., patients undergoing posterior single-level interbody fusion had a 10% rate of DVT even with mechanical prophylaxis.

INFECTION

An infection in a patient with spinal instrumentation in place is always a serious concern. Postoperative infections can manifest in the first few days after surgery or months later. Several factors are associated with infections, such as blood loss and operative time, which can be surrogates for the complexity of the procedure. However, it is incumbent on the surgeon to have a well-conceived operative plan and execute it efficiently. Adequate control of serum glucose preoperatively (HgbA1c less than 7.4) and perioperatively has been shown to improve infection rates. If a patient develops a pseudarthrosis, the possibility of infection should be considered and appropriately evaluated. In the immediate postoperative period, the presence of increasing pain, fever, wound drainage, wound erythema, or elevated C-reactive protein levels should raise suspicion of infection. The incidence of infection in the literature in instrumented lumbar spinal fusions is as high as 21%. In our experience, the infection rate for one- and two-level lumbar fusions with instrumentation should be less than 1%. The most common organisms include *Staphylococcus*, both coagulase negative and positive, including methicillin-resistant *Staphylococcus aureus* (MRSA), *Escherichia coli*, *Pseudomonas*, and *Enterobacter*. In the presence of wound drainage, it is prudent to presume infection and to wash out the wound to determine if the infection is deep to the fascia or not. Appropriate antibiotic therapy should be administered. Factors shown to increase infection risk include smoking, diabetes, and obesity.

REFERENCES

ADULT ISTHMIC SPONDYLOLISTHESIS

Alhammoud A, Schroeder G, Aldahamsheh O, et al.: Functional and radiological outcomes of combined anterior-posterior approach versus posterior alone in management of isthmic spondylolisthesis: a systematic review and meta-analysis, *Int J Spine Surg* 13:230, 2019.

Andrade NS, Ashton CM, Wray NP, et al.: Systematic review of observational studies reveals no association between low back pain and lumbar spondylolysis with or without isthmic spondylolisthesis, *Eur Spine J* 24:1289, 2015.

Chang HS: Microsurgical posterolateral foraminotomy on patients with adult isthmic spondylolisthesis, *World Neurosurg* 100:434, 2017.

Chen L, Feng Y, Che CQ, et al.: Influence of sacral slope on the loading of pedicle screws in postoperative L5/S1 isthmic spondylolisthesis patient: a finite element analysis, *Spine* 41:E1388, 2016.

Collados-Maestre I, Lizaur-Utrilla A, Bas-Hermida T, et al.: Transdiscal screw versus pedicle screw fixation for high-grade L5-S1 isthmic spondylolisthesis in patients younger than 60 years: a case-control study, *Eur Spine J* 25:1806, 2016.

Endler P, Ekman P, Ljungqvist H, et al.: Long-term outcome after spinal fusion for isthmic spondylolisthesis in adults, *Spine J* 19:501, 2019.

Endler P, Ekman P, Möller H, et al.: Outcomes of posterolateral fusion with and without instrumentation and of interbody fusion for isthmic spondylolisthesis: a prospective study, *J Bone Joint Surg Am* 99:743, 2017.

Eroglu A, Carli BA, Pusat S, et al.: The role of the features of the facet joint angle in the development of isthmic spondylolisthesis in young male patients with L5-S1 isthmic spondylolisthesis, *World Neurosurg* 104:709, 2017.

Fischer CR, Cassilly R, Dyrszka M, et al.: Cost-effectiveness of lumbar spondylolisthesis surgery at 2-year follow-up, *Spine Def* 4:48, 2016.

Kreiner DS, Baisden J, Mazanec DJ, et al.: Guideline summary review: an evidence-based clinical guideline for the diagnosis and treatment of adult isthmic spondylolisthesis, *Spine J* 16:1478, 2016.

Lee GW, Lee SM, Ahn MW, et al.: Comparison of posterolateral lumbar fusion and posterior lumbar interbody fusion for patients younger than 60 years with isthmic spondylolisthesis, *Spine* 39:E1475, 2014.

Maciejczak A, Jablonska-Sudol K: Correlation between correction of pelvic balance and clinical outcomes in mid- and low-grade adult isthmic spondylolisthesis, *Eur Spine J* 26:3112, 2017.

Macki M, Bydon M, Weingart R, et al.: Posterolateral fusion with interbody for lumbar spondylolisthesis is associated with less repeat surgery than posterolateral fusion alone, *Clin Neurol Neurosurg* 138:117, 2015.

McGuire KJ, Khaleel MA, Rihn JA, et al.: The effect of high obesity on outcomes of treatment for lumbar spinal conditions: subgroup analysis of the spine patient outcomes research trial, *Spine* 39:1975, 2014.

Mehta VA, Amin A, Omeis I, et al.: Implications of spinoplevic alignment for the spine surgeon, *Neurosurgery* 76(Suppl 1):S42, 2015.

Musacchio MJ, Lauryssen C, Davis RJ, et al.: Evaluation of decompression and interlaminar stabilization compared with decompression and fusion for the treatment of lumbar spinal stenosis: 5-year follow-up of a prospective, randomized, controlled trial, *Int J Spine Surg* 10:6, 2016.

Noorian S, Sorensen K, Cho W: A systematic review of clinical outcomes in surgical treatment of adult isthmic spondylolisthesis, *Spine J* 18:1441, 2018.

Schär RT, Sutter M, Mannion AF, et al.: Outcome of L5 radiculopathy after reduction and instrumented transforaminal lumbar interbody fusion of high-grade L5-S1 isthmic spondylolisthesis and the role of intraoperative neurophysiological monitoring, *Eur Spine J* 26:679, 2017.

Schulte TL, Ringel F, Quante M, et al.: Surgery for adult spondylolisthesis: a systematic review of the evidence, *Eur Spine J* 25:2359, 2016.

Seuk JW, Bae J, Shin SH, et al.: Long-term minimum clinically important difference in health-related quality of life scores after instrumented lumbar interbody fusion for low-grade isthmic spondylolisthesis, *World Neurosurg* 177:E493, 2018.

Tamburrelli FC, Meluzio MC, Burrofato A, et al.: Minimally invasive surgery procedure in isthmic spondylolisthesis, *Eur Spine J* 27(Suppl 2):S237, 2018.

Thakar S, Sivaraju L, Aryan S, et al.: Lumbar paraspinal muscle morphometry and its correlations with demographic and radiological factors in adult isthic spomdylolisthesis: a retrospective review of 120 surgically managed cases, *J Neurosurg Spine* 24:679, 2016.

Tye EY, Tanenbaum JE, Alonso AS, et al.: Circumferential fusion: a comparative analysis between anterior lumbar interbody fusion with posterior pedicle screw fixation and transforaminal lumbar interbody fusion for L5-S1 isthmic spondylolisthesis, *Spine J* 18:464, 2018.

Wang G, Han D, Cao Z, et al.: Outcomes of autograft alone versus PEEK + autograft interbody fusion in the treatment of adult lumbar isthmic spondylolisthesis, *Clin Neurol Neurosurg* 155:1, 2017.

DEGENERATIVE SPONDYLOLISTHESIS

Abdu WA, Sacks OA, Tosteson ANA, et al.: Long-term results of surgery compared with nonoperative treatment for lumbar degenerative spondylolisthesis in the Spine Patient Outcomes Research Trial (SPORT), *Spine* 43:1619, 2018.

Adogwa O, Davison MA, Vuong VD, et al.: Long term costs of maximum non-operative treatments in patients with symptomatic lumbar stenosis or sponylolisthesis that ultimately required surgery: a five-year cost analysis, *Spine* 44:424, 2019.

Ahmad S, Hamad A, Bhalla A, et al.: The outcome of decompression alone for lumbar spinal stenosis with degenerative spondylolisthesis, *Eur Spine J* 26:414, 2017.

Bai X, Chen J, Liu L, et al.: Is reduction better than arthrodesis in situ in surgical management of low-grade spondylolisthesis? A systematic review and meta analysis, *Eur Spine J* 26:606, 2017.

Bydon M, Macki M, Abt NB, et al.: The cost-effectiveness of interbody fusions versus posterolateral fusions in 137 patients with lumbar spondylolisthesis, *Spine J* 15:492, 2015.

Buyuk AF, Shafa E, Dawson JM, et al.: Complications with minimally invasive transforaminal lumbar interbody fusion for degenerative spondylolisthesis in the obese population, *Spine* 44:E1401, 2019.

Challier V, Boissiere L, Obeid I, et al.: One-level lumbar degenerative spondylolisthesis and posterior approach: is transforaminal lateral interbody fusion mandatory? A randomized controlled trial with 2-year follow-up, *Spine* 42:531, 2017.

Chan AK, Bisson EF, Bydon M, et al.: Laminectomy alone versus fusion fro grade 1 lumbar spondylolisthesis in 426 patients from the prospective Quality Outcomes Database, *J Neurosurg Spine* 30:234, 2018.

Chan AK, Shaqrma V, Robinson LC, et al.: Summary of guidelines for the treatment of lumbar spondylolisthesis, *Neurosurg Clin N Am* 30:353, 2019.

Choi KC, Shim HK, Kim JS, Lee SH: Does pre-existing L5-S1 degeneration affect outcomes after isolated L4-5 fusion for spondylolisthesis? *J Orthop Surg Res* 10:39, 2015.

Cuéllar JM, Field JS, Bae HW: Distraction laminoplasty with interlaminar lumbar instrumented fusion (ILIF) for lumbar stenosis with or without grade 1 spondylolisthesis: technique and 2-year outcomes, *Spine* 41:S97, 2016.

Cushnie D, Johnston R, Urquhart JC, et al.: Quality of life and slip progression in degenerative spondylolisthesis treated nonoperatively, *Spine* 43:E574, 2018.

de Kunder SL, van Kuijk SMJ, Rijkers K, et al.: Transforaminal lumbar interbody fusion (TLIF) versus posterior lumbar interbody fusion (PLIF) in lumbar spondylolisthesis: a systematic review and meta-analysis, *Spine J* 17:1712, 2017.

Delawi D, Jacobs W, van Susante JL, et al.: OP-1 compared with iliac crest autograft in instrumented posterolateral fusion: a randomized, multicenter non-inferiority trial, *J Bone Joint Surg* 98:441, 2016.

Dijkerman ML, Overdevest GM, Moojen WA, et al.: Decompression with or without concomitant fusion in lumbar stenosis due to degenerative spondylolisthesis: a systematic review, *Eur Spine J* 27:1629, 2018.

Enyo Y, Yoshimura N, Yamada H, et al.: Radiographic natural course of lumbar degenerative spondylolisthesis and its risk factors related to the progression and onset in a 15-year community-based cohort study: the Miyama study, *J Orthop Sci* 20:978, 2015.

Ferrero E, Illharreborde B, Mas V, et al.: Radiological and functional outcomes of high-grade spondylolisthesis treated by intrasacral fixation, dome resection and circumferential fusion: a retrospective series of 20 consecutive cases with a minimum of 2 years follow-up, *Eur Spine J* 27:2940, 2018.

Ferrero E, Ould-Slimane M, Gille O, et al.: Sagittal spinopelvic alignment in 654 degenerative spondylolisthesis, *Eur Spine J* 24:1219, 2015.

Fleming J, Glassman SD, Miller A, et al.: The effect of symptom duration on outcomes after fusion for degenerative spondylolisthesis, *Global Spine J* 9:487, 2019.

Gavaskar AS, Achimuthu R: Transfacetal fusion for low-grade degenerative spondylolisthesis of the lumbar spine: results of a prospective single center study, *J Spinal Disord Tech* 23:162, 2010.

Gerling MC, Leven D, Passias PG, et al.: Risk factors for reoperation in patients treated surgically for degenerative spondylolisthesis: a subanalysis of the 8-year data from the SPORT trial, *Spine* 42:1559, 2017.

Ghogawala Z, Dziura J, Butler WE, et al.: Laminectomy plus fusion versus laminectomy alone for lumbar spondylolisthesis, *N Engl J Med* 374:1424, 2016.

Golinvaux NS, Basques BA, Bohl DD, et al.: Comparison of 368 patients undergoing surgery for lumbar degenerative spondylolisthesis from the SPORT trial with 955 from the NSQIP database, *Spine* 40:342, 2015.

Gottschalk MB, Premkumar A, Sweeney K, et al.: Posterolateral lumbar arthrodesis with and without interbody arthrodesis for L4-L5 degenerative spondylolisthesis, *Spine* 40:917, 2015.

Hendrickson NR, Kelly MP, Ghogawala Z, et al.: Operative management of degenerative spondylolisthesis: a critical analysis review, *JBJS Rev* 6:e4, 2018.

Hong SW, Lee HY, Kim KH, Lee SH: Interspinous ligamentoplasty in the treatment of degenerative spondylolisthesis: midterm clinical results, *J Neurosurg Spine* 13:27, 2010.

Hsieh MK, Kao FC, Chen WJ, et al.: The influence of spinopelvic parameters on adjacent-segment degeneration after short spinal fusion for degenerative spondylolisthesis, *J Neurosurg Spine* 29:407, 2018.

Hsu HT, Yang SS, Chen TY: The correlation between restoration of lumbar lordosis and surgical outcome in the treatment of low-grade lumbar degenerative spondylolisthesis with spinal fusion, *Clin Spine Surg* 29:E16, 2016.

Inose H, Kato T, Yuasa M, et al.: Comparison of decompression, decompression plus fusion, and decompression plus stabilization for degenerative spondylolisthesis: a prospective, randomized study, *Clin Spine Surg* 31:E347, 2018.

Kaner T, Dalbayrak S, Oktenoglu T, et al.: Comparison of posterior dynamic and posterior rigid transpedicular stabilization with fusion to treat degenerative spondylolisthesis, *Orthopedics* 12:33, 2010.

Karsy N, Bisson EF: Surgical versus nonsurgical treatment of lumbar spondylolisthesis, *Neurosurg Clin N Am* 30:333, 2019.

Kim KH, Lee SH, Shim CS, et al.: Adjacent segment disease after interbody fusion and pedicle screw fixations for isolated L4-L5 spondylolisthesis: a minimum five-year follow-up, *Spine* 35:625, 2010.

Kim S, Hedjri SM, Coyte PC, Rampersaud YR: Cost-utility of lumbar decompression with or without fusion for patients with symptomatic degenerative lumbar spondylolisthesis, *Spine J* 12(1):44, 2012.

Kong LD, Zhang YZ, Want F, et al.: Radiographic restoration of sagittal spinopelvic alignment after posterior lumbar interbody fusion in degenerative spondylolisthesis, *Clin Spine Surg* 29:E87, 2016.

Kuo CH, Huang WC, Wu JC, et al.: Radiological adjacent-segment degeneration in L4-5 spondylolisthesis: comparison between dynamic stabilization and minimally invasive transforaminal lumbar interbody fusion, *J Neurosurg Spine* 29:250, 2018.

Levin JM, Tanenbaum JE, Steinmetz MP, et al.: Posterolateral fusion (PLF) versus transforaminal lumbar interbody fusion (TLIF) for spondylolisthesis: a systematic review and meta-analysis, *Spine J* 18:1088, 2018.

Liao JC, Chen WJ, Chen LH, et al.: Surgical outcomes of degenerative spondylolisthesis with L5-S1 disc degeneration: comparison between lumbar floating fusion and lumbosacral fusion at a minimum five-year follow-up, *Spine* 36:1600, 2011.

Lu VM, Kerezoudis P, Gilder HE, et al.: Minimally invasive surgery versus open surgery spinal fusion for spondylolisthesis: a systematic review and meta-analysis, *Spine* 42:E177, 2017.

Lyons KW, Klare CM, Kunkel ST, et al.: A 5-year review of hospital costs and reimbursement in the surgical management of degenerative spondylolisthesis, *Int J Spine Surg* 13:378, 2019.

Ma Z, Zhao C, Zhang K, et al.: Modified lumbosacral angle and modified pelvic incidence as new parameters for management of pediatric high-grade spondylolisthesis, *Clin Spine Surg* 31:E133, 2018.

Matz PG, Meagher RJ, Lamer T, et al.: Guideline summary review: an evidence-based clinical guideline for the diagnosis and treatment of degenerative lumbar spondylolisthesis, *Spine J* 16:439, 2016.

McAnany SJ, Baird EO, Qureshi SA, et al.: Posterolateral fusion versus interbody fusion for degenerative spondylolisthesis: a systematic review and meta-analysis, *Spine* 41:E1408, 2016.

Minamide A, Simpson AK, Okada M, et al.: Microscopic decompression for lumbar spinal stenosis with degenerative spondylolisthesis: the influence of spondylolisthesis stage (disc height and static and dynamic translation) on clinical outcomes, *Clin Spine Surg* 32:E20, 2019.

Minamide A, Yoshida M, Simpson AK, et al.: Minimally invasive spinal decompression for degenerative lumbar spondylolisthesis and stenosis maintains stability and may avoid the need for fusion, *Bone Joint Lett J* 100-B:499, 2018.

Mori G, Mikami Y, Aarai Y, et al.: Outcomes in cases of lumbar degenerative spondylolisthesis more than 5 years after treatment with minimally invasive decompression: examination of pre- and postoperative slippage, intervertebral disc changes, and clinical results, *J Neurosurg Spine* 24:367, 2016.

Okuda S, Nagamoto Y, Matsumoto T, et al.: Adjacent segment disease after single segment posterior lumbar interbody fusion for degenerative spondylolisthesis: minimum 10 years followup, *Spine* 43:E1384, 2018.

Passias PG, Poorman G, Lurie J, et al.: Patient profiling can identify spondylolisthesis patients at risk for conversion from nonoperative to operative treatment, *JB JS Open Access* 3:e0051, 2018.

Pateder DB, Benzel E: Noninstrumented facet fusion in patients undergoing lumbar laminectomy for degenerative spondylolisthesis, *J Surg Orthop Adv* 19:153, 2010.

Radovanovic I, Urquhart JC, Ganapathy V, et al.: Influence of postoperative sagittal balance and spinopelvic parameters on the outcome of patients surgically treated for degenerative lumbar spondylolisthesis, *J Neurosurg Spine* 26:448, 2017.

Rihn JA, Hilibrand AS, Zhao W, et al.: Effectiveness of surgery for lumbar stenosis and degenerative spondylolisthesis in the octogenarian population: analysis of the Spine Patient Outcomes Research Trial (SPORT) data, *J Bone Joint Surg* 97:177, 2015.

Sansur CA, Reames DL, Smith JS, et al.: Morbidity and mortality in the surgical treatment of 10,242 adults with spondylolisthesis, *J Neurosurg Spine* 13:589, 2010.

Sato S, Yagi M, Machida M, et al.: Reoperation rate and risk factors of elective spinal surgery for degenerative spondylolisthesis: minimum 5-year follow-up, *Spine J* 15:1536, 2015.

Schär RT, Kiebach S, Raabe A, et al.: Reoperation rate after microsurgical uni- or bilateral laminotomy for lumbar spinal stenosis with and without low-grade spondylolisthesis, *Spine* 44:E245, 2018.

Schöller K, Alimi M, Cong GT, et al.: Lumbar spinal stenosis associated with degenerative lumbar spondylolisthesis: a systematic review and meta-analysis of secondary fusion rates following open vs minimally invasive decompression, *Neurosurgery* 80:355, 2017.

Schroeder GD, Hsu WK, Kepler CK, et al.: Use of recombinant human bone morphogenetic protein-2 in the treatment of degenerative spondylolisthesis, *Spine* 41:445, 2016.

Sebaaly A, El Rachkidi R, Grobost P, et al.: L5 incidence: an important parameter for spinopelvic balance evaluation in high-grade spondylolisthesis, *Spine J* 18:1417, 2018.

Sembrano JN, Tomeh A, Isaacs R: Two-year comparative outcomes of MIS lateral and MIS transforaminal interbody fusion in the treatment of degenerative spondylolisthesis. Part I: clinical findings, *Spine* 41:S123, 2016.

Sigmundsson FG, Jönsson B, Strömqvist B: Outcome of decompression with and without fusion in spinal stenosis with degenerative spondylolisthesis in relation to preoperative pain pattern: a register study of 1,624 patients, *Spine J* 15:638, 2015.

Snoddy MC, Sielatycki JA, Divaganesan A, et al.: Can facet joint fluid on MRI and dynamic instability be a predictor of improvement in back pain following lumbar fusion for degenerative spondylolisthesis? *Eur Spine J* 25(8):2408, 2016.

Sobol GL, Hilibrand A, Davis A, et al.: Reliability and clinical utility of the CARDS classification for degenerative spondylolisthesis, *Clin Spine Surg* 31:E69, 2018.

Tay KS, Bassi A, Yeo W, et al.: Intraoperative reduction does not result in better outcomes in low-grade lumbar spondylolisthesis with neurogenic symptoms after minimally invasive transforaminal lumbar interbody fusion—a 5-year follow-up study, *Spine J* 16:182, 2016.

Turcotte JJ, Patton CM: Predictors of postoperative complications after surgery for lumbar spinal stenosis and degenerative lumbar spondylolisthesis, *JAAOS Glob Res Rev* 2:e085, 2018.

Vorhies JS, Hernandez-Boussard T, Alamin T: Treatment of degenerative lumbar spondylolisthesis with fusion or decompression alone results in similar rates of reoperation at 5 years, *Clin Spine Surg* 31:E74, 2018.

Wu MH, Dubey NK, Li YY, et al.: Comparison of minimally invasive spine surgery using intraoperative tomography integrated navigation, fluoroscopy, and conventional open surgery for lumbar spondylolisthesis: a prospective registry-based cohort study, *Spine J* 17:1082, 2017.

Yoshioka K, Murakami H, Demura S, et al.: Prevalence and risk factors for development of venous thromboembolism after degenerative spinal surgery, *Spine* 40:E301, 2015.

Yu CH, Lee JE, Yang JJ, et al.: Adjacent segment degeneration after single-level PLIF: comparison between spondylolytic spondylolisthesis, degenerative spondylolisthesis and spinal stenosis, *Asian Spine J* 5:82, 2011.

SPONDYLOLYSIS

Boyd ED, Mundluru SN, Feldman DS: Outcome of conservative management in the treatment of symptomatic spondylolysis and grade I spondylolisthesis, *Bull Hosp Jt Dis* 77:172, 2013, 2019.

Gala RJ, Bovonratwet P, Webb ML, et al.: Different fusion approaches for single-level lumbar spondylolysis have similar perioperative outcomes, *Spine* 43:E111, 2017.

Goda Y, Sakai T, Harada T, et al.: Degenerative changes of the facet joints in adults with lumbar spondylolysis, *Clin Spine Surg* 30:E738, 2017.

Grazina R, Andrade R, Santos FL, et al.: Return to play after conservative and surgical treatment in athletes with spondylolysis: a systematic review, *Phys Ther Sport* 37:34, 2019.

Hanke LF, Tuakli-Wosornu YA, Harrison JR, et al.: The relationship between sacral slope and symptomatic isthmic spondylolysis in a cohort of high school athletes: a retrospective analysis, *PM R* 10:501, 2018.

Kang WY, Lee JW, Lee E, et al.: Efficacy and outcome predictors of fluoroscopy-guided facet joint injection for spondylolysis, *Skeletal Radiol* 47:1137, 2018.

Karatas AF, Dede O, Atanda AA, et al.: Comparison of direct pars repair techniques of spondylolysis in pediatric and adolescent patients: pars compression screw versus pedicle screw-rod hook, *Clin Spine Surg* 29:272, 2016.

Lemoine T, Fournier J, Odent T, et al.: The prevalence of lumbar spondylolysis in young children: a retrospective analysis using CT, *Eur Spine J* 27:1067, 2018.

Linhares D, Cacho Rodrigues P, Ribeiro da Silva M, et al.: Minimum of 10-year follow-up of V-rod technique in lumbar spondylolysis, *Eur Spine J* 28:1743, 2019.

Miller R, Beck NA, Sampson NR, et al.: Imaging modalities for low back pain in children: a review of spondylolysis and undiagnosed mechanical back pain, *J Pediatr Orthop* 33(3):282, 2013.

Mohammed N, Patra DP, Narayan V, et al.: A comparison of the techniques of direct paqrs interarticularis repair for spondylolysis and low-grade spondylolisthesis: a meta-analysis, *Neurosurg Focus* 44:E10, 2018.

Sakai T, Tezuka F, Yamashita K, et al.: Conservative treatment for bony healing in pediatric lumbar spondylolysis, *Spine* 42:E716, 2017.

Selhorst M, Fischer A, MacDonald J: Prevalence of spondylolysis in symptomatic adolescent athletes: an assessment of sport risk in nonelite athletes, *Clin J Sport Med* 29:421, 2019.

Sterba M, Arnoux PJ, Labelle H, et al.: Biomechanical analysis of spino-pelvic postural configurations in spondylolysis subjected to various sport-related dynamic loading conditions, *Eur Spine J* 27:2044, 2018.

Tofte JN, CarlLee TY, Holte AJ, et al.: Imaging pediatric spondylolysis: a systematic review, *Spine* 42:777, 2017.

Warner Jr WC, de Mendonca RGM: Adolescent spondylolysis: management and return to play, *Instr Course Lect* 66:409, 2017.

West AM, d'Hemecourt PA, Bono OJ, et al.: Diagnostic accuracy of magnetic resonance imaging and computed tomography scan in young athletes with spondylolysis, *Clin Pediatr (Phila)* 58:671, 2019.

Wren PAL, Ponrartana S, Aggabao PC, et al.: Increased lumbar lordosis and small cross-sectional area are associated with spondylolysis, *Spine* 43:833, 2018.

Xing R, Dou Q, Li X, et al.: Posterior dynamic stabilization with direct pars repair via Wiltse approach for the treatment of lumbar spondylolysis: the application of a novel surgery, *Spine* 41:E494, 2016.

The complete list of references is available online at ExpertConsult.com.

CHAPTER 5

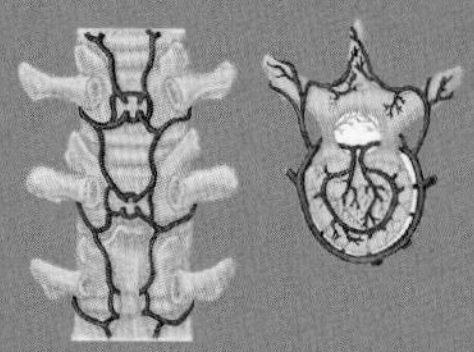

FRACTURES, DISLOCATIONS, AND FRACTURE-DISLOCATIONS OF THE SPINE

Keith D. Williams

Many factors make assessing and treating patients with injuries to the spinal column and spinal cord demanding. The most critical responsibilities are early recognition of the injuries, prevention of neurologic deterioration, optimization of initial medical management, correct interpretation of all the diagnostic evaluations, and delivery of the most appropriate definitive care.

The cervical spine is functionally the most important region of the spine. The complex anatomy, spinal biomechanics, and the common traumatic mechanisms involved make the cervical spine also the most difficult to assess. Careful evaluation of each region is necessary. No definitive level I or II evidence studies exist to guide clinicians through much of this process, and errors can have devastating consequences for patients. The process is made even more difficult by coexisting injuries and comorbidities that often are present in severely traumatized patients who are at risk for a significant spinal injury. An orderly and thoughtful approach that is based on the best available evidence gives patients the highest probability for an optimal outcome.

The scope of the problem is demonstrated by information from the National Spinal Cord Injury Statistical Center in Birmingham, Alabama (www.nscisc.uab.edu). The estimated annual incidence of spinal cord injury is approximately 17,730 new cases per year. Significant spinal column injuries are about twice as common as those causing spinal cord injury. Additionally, an estimated 249,000 to 363,000 people in the United States are living with the sequelae of spinal cord injury. The most common causes of these injuries are motor vehicle accidents (38%), falls (30%), violence (14%, primarily gunshot wounds), and sports mishaps (9%). Over the past few decades the average age at the time of injury has increased from 28.7 to 40.7 years, and the causes have shifted slightly toward falls and away from motor vehicle accidents and violence. Most patients with spinal cord injuries are men (80.7%). African-Americans are overrepresented based on general population trends and represent 24% of all spinal cord injuries, although 63% of patients are Caucasian. The most common neurologic category since 2005 has been incomplete tetraplegia (45%), followed by incomplete paraplegia (21%), complete paraplegia (20%), and, least commonly, complete tetraplegia (14%). Complete injuries have decreased slightly in recent years.

INITIAL MANAGEMENT OF SPINAL INJURY

Evaluation and management of the patient begin at the scene of the injury, and proper transport of the patient is very important. A retrospective review has shown that as many as 26% of spinal cord injuries occurred during transport or the early stages of evaluation at the primary medical facility. The deterioration was attributed primarily to poor immobilization and improper initial handling of the patients. Standardized protocols among emergency medical personnel have improved the safety of transport, but some controversy still remains. Total spine immobilization is recommended for

TABLE 5.1

National Emergency X-Radiography Utilization Study (NEXUS) Low-Risk Criteria

CRITERION	COMMENT
No posterior midline cervical spine tenderness	Midline posterior tenderness is deemed to be present if the patient reports pain on palpation of the posterior midline neck from the nuchal ridge to the prominence of the T1 vertebra, or if the patient evinces pain with direct palpation of any cervical spinous process.
No evidence of intoxication	Patients should be considered intoxicated if they have either of the following: a recent history provided by the patient or an observer of intoxication or intoxicant ingestion or evidence of intoxication on physical examination such as an odor of alcohol, slurred speech, ataxia, dysmetria, or other cerebellar findings or any behavior consistent with intoxication. Patients also may be considered to be intoxicated if tests of body fluids are positive for alcohol above 0.08 mg/dL or other drugs that affect the level of alertness.
A normal level of alertness	An altered level of alertness can include any of the following: a Glasgow Coma Scale score of 14 or less; disorientation to person, place, time, or events; inability to remember three objects at 5 minutes; a delayed or inappropriate response to external stimuli; or other findings.
No focal neurologic deficit	A focal neurologic deficit is any focal neurologic finding on motor or sensory examination.
No painful distracting injuries	No precise definition of painful distracting injury is possible. This category includes any condition thought by the clinician to be producing pain sufficient to distract the patient from a second cervical injury. Such injuries may include, but are not limited to, any long-bone fracture; visceral injury requiring surgical consultation; large laceration; degloving injury; crush injury; large burns; or any other injury causing acute functional impairment. Physicians may also classify any injury as distracting if it is thought to have the potential to impair the patient's ability to appreciate other injuries.

Adapted from Stiell IG, Clement CM, McKnight RD: The Canadian C-spine rule versus the NEXUS low-risk criteria in patients with trauma, *N Engl J Med* 349:2510, 2003.

all patients with a potential spinal injury. For patients who meet the NEXUS criteria (see below), cervical immobilization is not recommended. For all other patients, a hard collar with block supports (not sandbags) on a spine board appropriately sized for the age of the patient is used. This allows the patient to be moved and tilted as needed for transport. A 2- to 3-cm occipital pad is used in adults to avoid relative extension. In children, a spine board with an occipital recess is used to avoid relative flexion. Several studies have questioned whether all patients with potential injury need this form of immobilization because of the risk of pressure sores from the backboard. Also, studies have revealed that intracranial pressure can be elevated by an average of 25 mm of water by the use of a rigid cervical collar. The clinical importance of this in a patient with a head injury has not been determined. At the present time, this type of immobilization with the head taped to the board and the torso secured remains the most accepted method for patient transport. This recommendation is based on level III evidence, and it is unlikely there will be better evidence developed because of ethical limitations and practical issues of moving injured patients. The patient should be moved from a spine board and have the cervical spine cleared as soon as is safely possible. This is best done after the patient reaches a facility able to fully assess and treat all injuries that are present.

INITIAL SPINE ASSESSMENT

After the ABC (airway, breathing, and circulation) of the Advanced Trauma Life Support (ATLS) protocol has been completed, a thorough orthopaedic history should be obtained and full physical examination should be done. Important information includes the injury mechanism, preinjury functional level of the patient, patient report of weakness or sensory changes, signs of blunt head trauma, spine tenderness, spinal step offs, and interspinous widening. Findings of flaccidity in the extremities, incontinence, or penile erection may indicate spinal cord injury. A detailed neurologic examination, which includes motor function, sensory function, and rectal tone, recorded on the American Spinal Injury Association (ASIA) form and an assessment of mental status are part of this examination. The diagnostic imaging of a patient is inextricably linked to the neurologic examination. The initial spinal assessment of a trauma patient is to determine if the patient has a spinal cord injury. If an injury is found, all initial CT imaging, including that of the spine, is completed as rapidly as possible and treatment initiated. If a patient does not have a spinal cord injury, it should be determined if he or she meets the criteria to be considered asymptomatic with respect to the cervical spine. If the patient is found to be asymptomatic, then the cervical spine can be cleared clinically without the need for radiography. There are five specific criteria described in the National Emergency X-Radiography Utilization Study (NEXUS) that must be fulfilled to classify a patient as asymptomatic. The purpose of the study was to develop a decision rule that would reduce the number of radiographic examinations in trauma patients without missing significant injuries. The five specific criteria are noted in Table 5.1.

Using these criteria, one third of the trauma patients evaluated in the 21 community emergency departments or level 1 trauma centers were found to be asymptomatic (range 14% to 58%). The determination of a patient's level of alertness is the first step in the workup specifically for a spinal injury, which should begin immediately after the ABCs have been evaluated. If the patient is asymptomatic by the criteria of the NEXUS trial, no radiographs of the cervical spine are needed and the cervical spine may be "cleared" on clinical grounds, which significantly expedites care. Patients who are not alert or who do not meet the NEXUS trial criteria for other reasons require radiographic evaluation. The patient's motor and sensory examination should be documented thoroughly; the International Spinal Cord Society (ISCoS) form is the accepted instrument that best serves this important function. For patients who are found to have a neurologic deficit, serial neurologic examinations are recorded using this form, which has proven to be useful in detecting clinical deterioration and guiding decisions on additional imaging or other interventions that may become necessary. For patients with neurologic deficits, ISCoS forms are completed every 4 to 6 hours usually for the first 24 hours after arrival, but this varies based on the patient's course. If a patient is found to have a cervical spinal cord injury, then medical management and imaging workup will need to address this injury as the first priority in all but the most critically injured patients. In some patients immediate reduction of fractures or dislocations may be most appropriate, whereas other patients may benefit from MRI before proceeding with treatment.

Controversy persists about the optimal diagnostic imaging protocol for trauma patients as it relates to the spine. Our protocol is outlined in Figure 5.1. There are several objectives for which there is general consensus among trauma surgeons and spine surgeons. First is the detection of any significant spinal injury that places the patient at risk for neurologic deterioration. This may be an osseous injury, a soft-tissue injury, including posterior ligament complex injuries and other important injuries such as disc disruptions, or a combination of the two. Second, make a determination that there is no significant injury as early as possible to allow discontinuation of cervical immobilization and lifting of spine precautions. This will help avoid the recognized morbidities of immobilization and to facilitate other aspects of the patient's care. Rose et al. found that patients meeting the NEXUS criteria who had a "distracting injury" were correctly assessed on clinical grounds alone with 99% sensitivity and 99% negative predictive value. They concluded that the number of CT scans in this cohort of patients could be reduced by 61% and suggested that radiographic evaluation is unnecessary for safe clearance of the asymptomatic cervical spine in awake and alert blunt trauma patients with "distracting injuries." Additionally, the imaging should assess for associated injuries, including vertebral artery injuries in the cervical region or visceral injuries involving the chest, abdomen, and pelvic areas when evaluating the thoracic, lumbar, and sacral spine regions. The initial evaluation of the noncervical spine (thoracic to sacrum) is best done using multidetector computed tomography (MDCT) with both sagittal and coronal reformatted images.

SPINE PRECAUTIONS

Spinal precautions often are mentioned but rarely described in publications regarding trauma to the spine. The following protocol is derived from our experience. Spinal immobilization has already been described as it pertains to transport of an injured patient, but, as mentioned, one of the goals of the initial assessment is to be able to remove the patient from the backboard quickly once hemodynamic stability has been obtained and CT evaluation completed. Even if a significant spinal injury at any level is found, the patient can be moved to a bed but maintained with a cervical collar in place on a pillow as needed to avoid cervical extension. Patients with ankylosing spondylitis may require several pillows to keep them more upright because of their rigid cervicothoracic kyphosis (see chapter 2). If a patient is to be placed in cervical traction, the crossmember for the traction pulley is fixed to the bed frame such that the traction vector maintains neutral alignment and adjusts if the bed position is altered. With this level of precaution, a patient can be placed head up using the reverse Trendelenburg function of the bed. If the cervical CT is negative for injury and cervical immobilization is to be continued pending further evaluation, then the patient is allowed to be fully upright in a properly fitted rigid cervical orthosis until spinal clearance is possible unless other injuries prevent this. Prasarn et al. demonstrated in a cadaver study that a kinetic bed caused less cervical displacement through an injured segment than the traditional log roll maneuver.

Patients with unstable thoracic or lumbar injuries, such as fracture-dislocation or other injuries that will be treated with internal stabilization, are maintained flat in bed (using the reverse-Trendelenburg position to elevate the head) and log-rolled side-back-side every 2 hours while awake until the spine is stabilized. For patients with spinal cord injuries in whom operative stabilization will be delayed more than 24 to 48 hours a Roto-Rest (KCI, San Antonio, TX) type bed is preferred (also used in patients with cervical injuries). Once the thoracolumbar fracture is stabilized, or for those patients being treated in an orthosis, elevating the head of the bed 0 to 30 degrees is allowed without donning the orthosis. The orthosis is required when the head of the bed is above 30 degrees.

Keeping the head of the bed elevated is strongly encouraged if blood pressure, intracranial pressure, and other vital parameters permit, to reduce the risk of aspiration and to assist with pulmonary toilet. Once spinal stability is achieved, continued frequent turning of the patient or the use of a therapeutic air mattress is preferred as long as mobility is severely limited for any reason.

DIAGNOSTIC IMAGING

Injuries that involve the thoracic, lumbar, or sacral regions of the spine generally can be diagnosed using CT, which has been established as the diagnostic imaging modality of choice in these areas. It usually is obtained as part of the primary workup by the trauma surgeons or the physicians in the emergency department. Additional evaluation with MRI in these areas or use of other modalities typically is not necessary, although there are circumstances in which obtaining an MRI is appropriate. Because CT studies are obtained routinely for other reasons, the specific indications for radiographic evaluations of the thoracic and lumbar spines and the sacrum have not been extensively studied. Additional attention is given to this topic in later sections dealing specifically with injuries to these areas.

Patients who have cervical spine symptoms require imaging evaluation, and the recommendations for this process have changed in recent years. The standard radiographic evaluation of the cervical spine for trauma patients until relatively recently has been anteroposterior, lateral, and open-mouth odontoid radiographs. This three-view protocol has proven reliable when technically adequate images are obtained but has been documented to fail in demonstrating a small

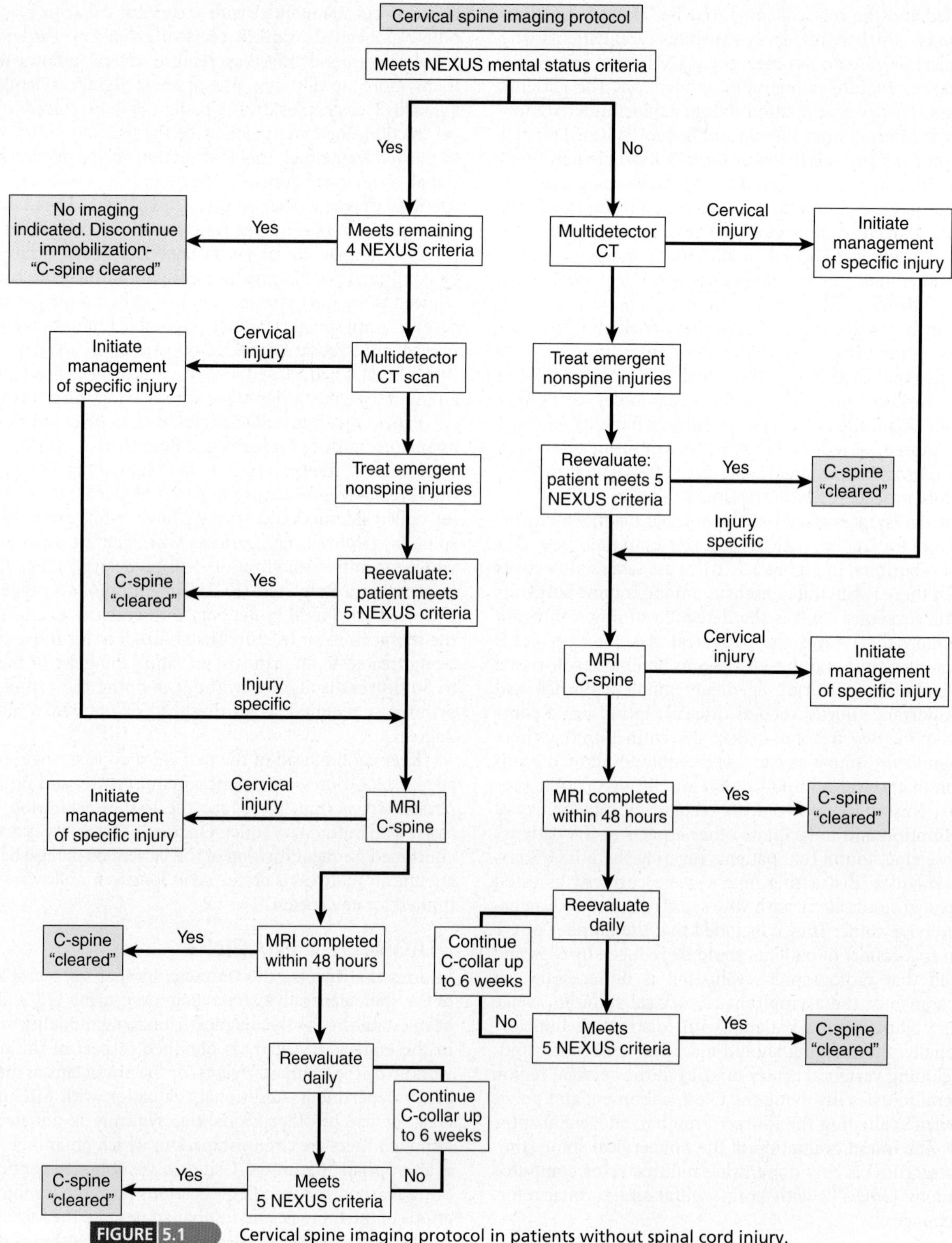

FIGURE 5.1 Cervical spine imaging protocol in patients without spinal cord injury.

number of significant cervical injuries. Because the incidence of cervical injury in trauma patients is between 2% and 6%, a very high sensitivity is required to optimally evaluate symptomatic patients. In a series of 32,117 patients, Davis found 34 missed injuries. As has also been documented in numerous other studies, the most common reason the injury was missed in Davis' series was failure to obtain adequate radiographs of the injured level (23 patients). Eight patients in the series had incorrect readings of adequate films, and only one patient was documented to have adequate radiographs that did not demonstrate the injury even in retrospect. Most studies on this topic have found that the occipitocervical junction and the cervicothoracic junction are the areas where injuries are most likely to be missed. Several studies have provided level I evidence that the negative predictive value of an adequate three-view series is from 93% to 98%; however, in these same studies the sensitivity was only 62% to 84%. Assuming a series of 100 patients, 6% of whom have cervical injury, five of six cervical injuries could be detected as abnormal on a three-view radiographic series and one truly injured patient would not be distinguished radiographically from the 94 correctly identified true negative series. This deficiency of plain radiographs is not improved with the addition of oblique films for a five-view series.

With greater availability of MDCT there has been a transition to using this modality for the primary evaluation of the cervical spine in trauma patients. In a large multicenter, level II study of patients failing to meet NEXUS criteria, Inaba et al. found that the sensitivity of CT was 98.5%, specificity was 91.0%, and negative predictive value was 99.97% for clinically significant injury. They also found that, for patients with neurologic injuries, CT alone missed a small number of clinically significant injuries and therefore recommended MRI in this group. Combining the cervical CT scan with the head-chest, abdomen, and pelvic scan, which often is ordered for these patients, has resulted in a lower cost than if the cervical study is done separately. Also, because the patient is already in the scanner and the scan times are much faster with MDCT compared with conventional CT, it actually takes less time to obtain an MDCT than it would for a three-view series of plain radiographs. When the relatively high proportions of technically inadequate studies that require CT are factored in, the MDCT has been found to be cost effective relative to plain radiographs. Despite these advantages, the higher radiation dose to the patient remains a concern with MDCT. Although comparisons between MDCT with coronal plane and sagittal plane reconstructions and plain radiographs have found higher sensitivity in detecting injuries with MDCT, several studies comparing autopsy findings with injuries noted on CT before death found that not all injuries present at autopsy were demonstrated by CT. Molina et al. found significant injuries in a small number of patients that were not demonstrated on the CT images. This indicates that CT may not be the "gold standard" by which to judge all other diagnostic imaging techniques. The role of MRI in the evaluation of the cervical spine in symptomatic patients to supplement MDCT continues to develop as the deficiencies of MDCT are better understood. A significant number of studies demonstrate improved diagnostic sensitivity with the use of MRI. Sarani et al. retrospectively found injuries on MRI in 42 of 164 (26%) trauma patients. All 164 patients had negative CT scans, and treatment was altered in 74% of these patients either with surgery or continuation of immobilization. In the subset of patients who could not be examined because of altered mental status, Sarani et al. found injuries on MRI in 5 of 46 (11%) patients who had negative CT scans, and 80% of these patients required surgery. Pourtaheri et al. found in a subset of patients with cervical fractures and altered mental status that MRI was very useful; MRI found additional injuries in 48% that changed treatment for 39%. This treatment change was from nonoperative to operative treatment 24% of the time. The clearest indication for MRI in a trauma patient is for the evaluation of an unexplained neurologic deficit at any spinal level. MRI has a higher sensitivity for detecting soft-tissue injuries, which are not well demonstrated on CT. MRI can detect a missed spinal column injury or neural compressive pathologic processes, such as disc fragments, epidural hematoma, or the presence of significant canal stenosis from other causes. For patients with a demonstrated injury and neurologic deficit at a corresponding level, MRI usually offers little additional information for that injury. However, noncontiguous injuries occur in up to 15% of patients. Because of this high rate of additional injuries, patients with cervical injuries demonstrated on MDCT at our institution are evaluated with MRI primarily to assess for soft-tissue injuries. This practice has resulted in alteration of the treatment plan for a significant percentage of patients when additional injuries are detected. Using MRI to assist in the "clearance" of the cervical spine remains controversial at this time. Although many of these additional injuries are significant and do alter treatment, some of the injuries are not clinically significant, so specific indications for obtaining MRI need to be defined. Determining which MRI findings correlate with clinical instability also needs to be better defined. Schoenfeld et al. found in a propensity-matched cohort that the addition of MRI to CT identified 8% more injuries than CT alone. Only 1% required surgery. The number needed to treat (NNT) in order to change patient management was 50 and the NNT for surgery was 167. Clearly MRI is not needed as a routine imaging modality. If a patient has abnormal findings on CT suggesting soft-tissue injury, such as soft-tissue density anterior to the midbody of C3 greater than 5 mm, a widened disc space (>1 to 2 mm) at one level relative to adjacent disc levels particularly if there is an anterior osteophyte avulsion at that level (Fig. 5.2), or excessive widening of the interspinous distance posteriorly, MRI should be obtained. An additional confounding issue is the timing of the MRI. Because MRI is most effective for evaluating soft-tissue injury, either by showing discontinuity of anatomic structures such as the ligamentum flavum and annulus fibrosus or hemorrhage and edema associated with tissue disruption, the timing of the study is very important. If the MRI is obtained within the first 48 hours after injury, the sensitivity for hemorrhage and edema is optimal. The ability of MRI to identify injury after 48 hours is dependent on the direct demonstration of tissue disruption or subluxation of the spine. Emery et al. found that MRI done an average of 11 days from injury failed to demonstrate known soft-tissue injuries in 2 of 19 patients. Evaluation of the available literature revealed level III evidence to support the "clearance" of the cervical spine in a symptomatic patient if CT and MRI done within 48 hours of injury are found to be normal. Our process is to obtain an MRI in the obtunded patient within this 48-hour window if the patient is stable enough to undergo the study. A patient is not considered obtunded if the mental status is altered because of the presence of substances that will only transiently impair the patient. In this case the patient has CT examination and remains in a rigid orthosis with repeat examinations until the impairment has resolved and a determination is made to either "clear" the cervical spine on clinical grounds or proceed with MRI within 48 hours. If the condition of the patient does not allow the MRI to be completed within 48 hours and the patient remains obtunded, an MRI is obtained as soon as the patient can safely undergo the study and any identified injuries are treated. However, if the delayed MRI does not directly demonstrate an injury, the patient is kept in a rigid orthosis for up to 6 weeks as treatment for presumed soft-tissue injury or until his or her mental status improves and he or she can be cleared on clinical grounds by meeting the NEXUS criteria. This protocol has been effective in avoiding neurologic deterioration because of missed injuries. Although there has been occasional morbidity such as decubitus ulcers attributable to the orthosis, this is very rare. Skin breakdown on the

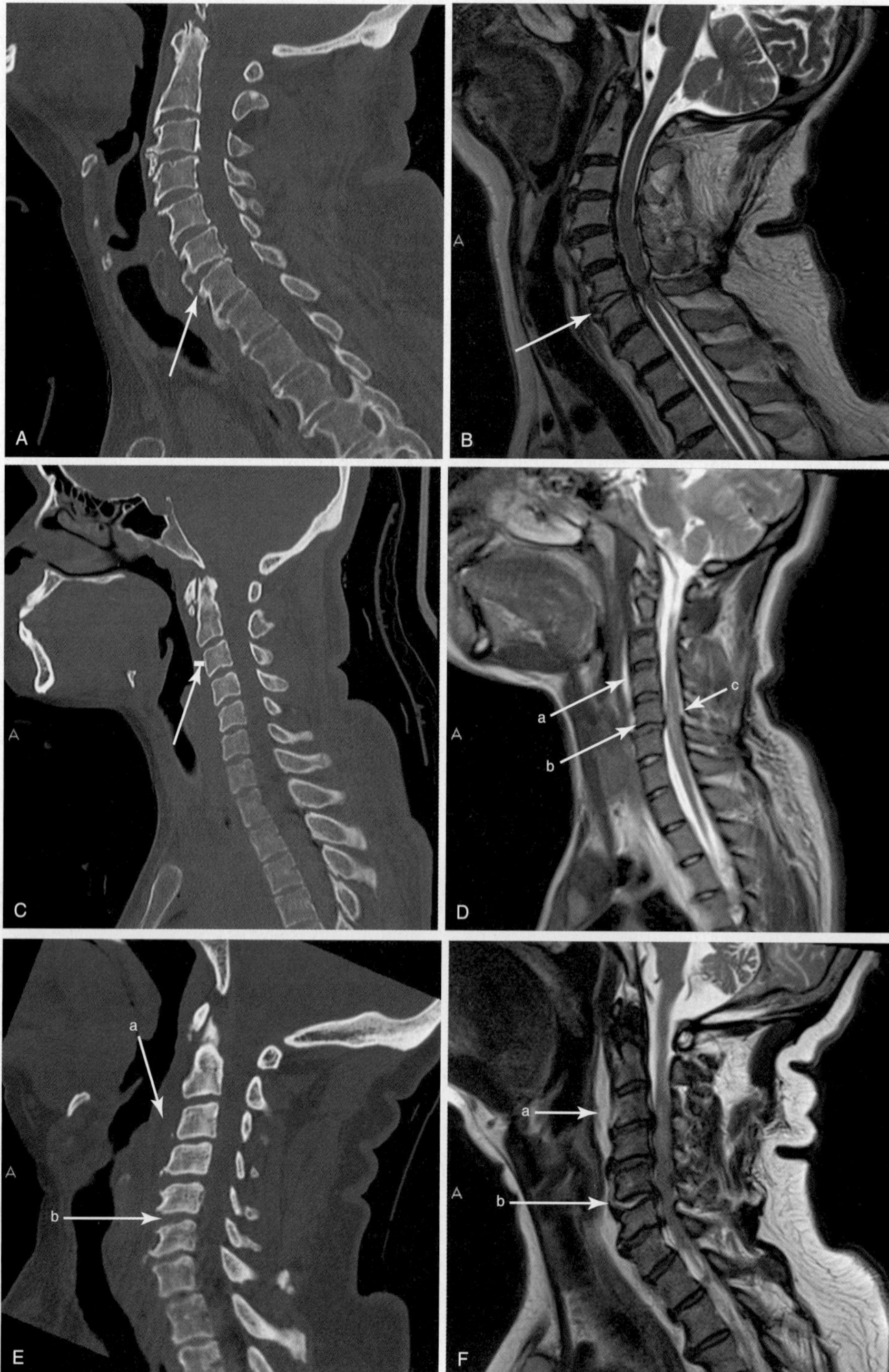

FIGURE 5.2 **A,** Disruption of C6 osteophyte suggesting disruption through disc *(arrow)*. **B,** Increased signal through C6 disc indicates disruption of disc *(arrow)*. **C,** Retropharyngeal soft tissue more than 5 mm on midsagittal image *(arrow)*. **D,** *Arrow a* indicates hemorrhage causing widening of soft-tissue density at C3 level. *Arrow b* indicates anterior annulus disruption. *Arrow c* indicates disruption of ligamentum flavum. Also note cord edema and swelling. **E,** *Arrow a* indicates more than 5 mm of soft-tissue density at C3 level. *Arrow b* indicates subtle angulation through C5 disc level. **F,** *Arrow a* indicates hemorrhage at C3 level. *Arrow b* indicates disruption through anterior annulus and through disc space.

posterior scalp above the orthosis results from improper fit of the orthosis, not keeping the patient upright, and not turning the patient adequately. No more serious morbidities from immobilization have occurred, although nursing care, especially tracheostomy care, is somewhat more difficult. Thus, the primary indications for cervical MRI are unexplained neurologic deficit, identified cervical injury, CT findings suggestive of soft-tissue injury, or a patient with altered mental status after intoxicants are metabolized. When possible, MRI is performed within 48 hours.

ADDITIONAL IMAGING

It is unusual for additional imaging to be required beyond that described. We have not found dynamic studies to be useful acutely to evaluate the cervical spine. There is a high rate of inadequate studies for a variety of reasons, foremost of which is inadequate range of motion. In obtunded patients, there have been reports of major neurologic injury caused by obtaining dynamic images. If a nonobtunded patient has adequate motion for flexion and extension lateral radiographs, typically clearance can be done on clinical grounds using the NEXUS criteria without further imaging.

On rare occasions a patient may have findings on MDCT suggestive but not definitive of a soft-tissue injury. Typically, an MRI study would be obtained, but in certain patients this is contraindicated (e.g., if the patient has a pacemaker). In these instances a "stretch test" as described by White, Southwick, and Panjabi is done to more completely assess the stability of the spine. This test allows measurement of the displacement within a motion segment under controlled conditions to identify soft-tissue injuries. Gardner-Wells tongs are applied before this test is performed. A head halter can be used but is less desirable because of the amount of weight that potentially may be used. The possible end points for the test are a change in neurologic status, an increase of 1.7 mm between adjacent vertebrae at any level, an angulatory change of 7.5 degrees at any disc level, or reaching one third of body weight or 65 lb, whichever is less. A prerequisite to performing a "stretch test" is that the patient must be alert and able to provide a consistent feedback for neurologic examination (Box 5.1). Resuscitation should be complete, and the patient should be hemodynamically stable. Head CT should confirm no fracture near the planned cranial pin sites.

STRETCH TEST

This test must always be done with direct supervision by the attending orthopaedic surgeon.

TECHNIQUE 5.1

- Apply traction through secured cranial skeletal traction (see Technique 5.2). Use of a head halter may be considered only if a small amount of weight is expected to be used. If a head halter is used, place a small piece of gauze sponge between the molars for patient comfort. Carefully place a rolled towel or sheet under the patient's head or neck as needed to maintain neutral alignment.
- Place the radiographic film as close as possible to the patient's neck, position the x-ray tube 72 inches from the film, and make a lateral exposure. This will serve as the baseline image.
- Begin with 10 lb of weight and increase traction in 3- to 5-lb increments. Complete a full neurologic examination and obtain a lateral radiograph before adding the next weight increment.
- The test is considered positive and should be discontinued and traction removed if any neurologic changes occur or if any abnormal separation or angulation occurs. The radiographic criterion is an increase of 1.7 mm between adjacent vertebrae or a change of 7.5 degrees at an intervertebral disc level relative to the baseline image that was obtained.
- By completing a neurologic examination and allowing the radiographic image to be processed, an adequate time of at least 5 minutes elapses between weight increases to overcome any muscle spasm that may occur.
- Be certain to compare measurements on each new radiograph to the baseline image, *not* the previous image.
- The test is considered negative for instability if traction equal to one third of body weight or 65 lb is reached without radiographic or neurologic change.

BOX 5.1

End Points for Stretch Test

- Change in neurologic status
- Increase of 1.7 mm between adjacent vertebrae at any level
- Angulatory change of 7.5 degrees at any disc level
- Reaching one third of body weight or weight limit for tongs, whichever is less

NEUROLOGIC ASSESSMENT

To properly direct the diagnostic imaging necessary for a patient, the neurologic examination findings play a key role. Assessment of mental status using the Glasgow Coma Scale (GCS) (Table 5.2) determines the level of consciousness. If the GCS score is not 15, then imaging will be required as outlined earlier. Clearly document the motor and sensory examination, including the function of the rectal sphincter and the presence of perianal sensation. We have used the ASIA form from ISCoS. Using the ISCoS form, sensation is recorded for light touch and pinprick in 28 dermatomal distributions on each side of the body (Fig. 5.3). Pinprick testing is done using a sterile needle rather than a pinwheel. A score of 2 (normal), 1 (altered), or 0 (absent) is determined for each dermatome, and specific "key" areas are identified on the diagram within each dermatome as optimal test locations. In addition, the presence of sensation for deep anal pressure is made to help determine if a spinal cord injury is complete or incomplete. Important dermatomal landmarks are the nipple line (T4), xiphoid process (T7), umbilicus (T10), inguinal region (T12, L1), and perianal region (S4 and S5). Motor function is scored 0/5 to 5/5 in each of 10 specific myotomes per side (Table 5.3). Also, the presence or absence of voluntary anal sphincter contraction is

TABLE 5.2

Glasgow Coma Scale

RESPONSE	SCORE	SIGNIFICANCE
EYE OPENING		
Spontaneously	4	Reticular activating system intact; patient may not be aware
To verbal command	3	Opens eyes when told to do so
To pain	2	Opens eyes in response to pain
No eye opening	1	Does not open eyes to any stimuli
VERBAL STIMULI		
Oriented, converses	5	Relatively intact CNS, aware of self and environment
Disoriented, converses	4	Well-articulated, organized, but disoriented
Inappropriate words	3	Random exclamatory words
Incomprehensible	2	Moaning, no recognizable words
No verbal response	1	No response or intubated
MOTOR RESPONSE		
Obeys verbal commands	6	Readily moves limbs when told to
Localizes to painful stimuli	5	Moves limb in an effort to remove painful stimuli
Flexion withdrawal	4	Pulls away from pain in flexion
Abnormal flexion	3	Decorticate rigidity
Extension	2	Decerebrate rigidity
No motor response	1	Hypotonia, flaccid—suggests loss of medullary function or concomitant spinal cord injury

CNS, Central nervous system.
From Papa L, Goldberg SA: *Rosen's emergency medicine: concepts and clinical practice,* ed 9, Philadelphia, PA, 2018, Elsevier, Table 34.2.

recorded. In some circumstances, the designation of "NT" for not testable or 5*/5 (weakness as expected, considered normal strength because of inhibiting factors such as fractures) are most appropriate. Before making a definitive determination of injury type the patient must be out of spinal shock. This usually occurs within 24 to 48 hours but can take substantially longer and is indicated by the return of the bulbocavernosus reflex and anal wink (Figs. 5.4 and 5.5). The ISCoS document lists the requirements for each motor grade along with the definitions of the ASIA Impairment Scale and a flow chart to properly interpret it. Using the AIS, a neurologic level of injury (NLI) determination is made to classify the spinal cord–injured patient.

The NLS is defined by the most caudal myotome with at least 3/5 function and 5/5 function at all higher levels that also has normal sensory function and normal sensation at all higher levels. At levels without key myotomes, the level is determined by the sensory level. Type A patients are motor complete and sensory complete, with no motor or sensory function more than three segments caudal to the named injury level. Function within the zone of partial preservation should be recorded because a change by even a single level can be very significant, especially in the cervical region. Type B patients are motor complete but sensory incomplete (incomplete sensory loss but complete motor loss with *no* motor function more than three segments caudal to the named injury level); sensory sparing may be only light touch, pinprick in the perianal segments, or deep anal pressure. Type C patients have either voluntary sphincter contraction *or* voluntary motor function more than three segments below the named injury level with sacral sensory sparing. This motor sparing can be in non-key myotomes according to the standard at this time. More than half of functioning key myotomes are graded *less* than 3/5. Type D patients have *at least* half of functioning key myotomes greater than or equal to grade 3/5. Type E patients have a spinal cord injury that improves to normal. This type is not used to describe a patient without a spinal cord injury initially. This examination should allow the clinician to distinguish spinal cord injuries from isolated nerve root or nerve plexus type injuries.

The initial neurologic examination should be completed as soon as possible after the arrival of the patient to establish the correct baseline for the patient to which all subsequent examinations will be compared. It is our practice to complete serial neurologic assessments on patients with spinal cord injuries or unstable spinal column injuries every 4 to 6 hours for at least the first 24 hours and continue less frequent reassessments thereafter based on the patient's clinical course. This regimen is derived from experience in a busy level I trauma center but is not evidence based, and it is unlikely that evidence-based practices could be used to examine how frequently optimal evaluations should be done. In addition to the motor and sensory examinations, it is important to include examination of the deep tendon reflexes. Acute spinal cord injury results in flaccid paralysis and areflexia. The presence of pathologic reflexes such as a Babinski or Hoffmann reflex or clonus indicates a more chronic process, which may be acutely worsened by trauma such as a central cord injury in the setting of chronic cervical stenosis. The purpose for serial examinations is to detect any neurologic change and institute management changes to improve the patient's ultimate neurologic outcome. Deterioration of neurologic

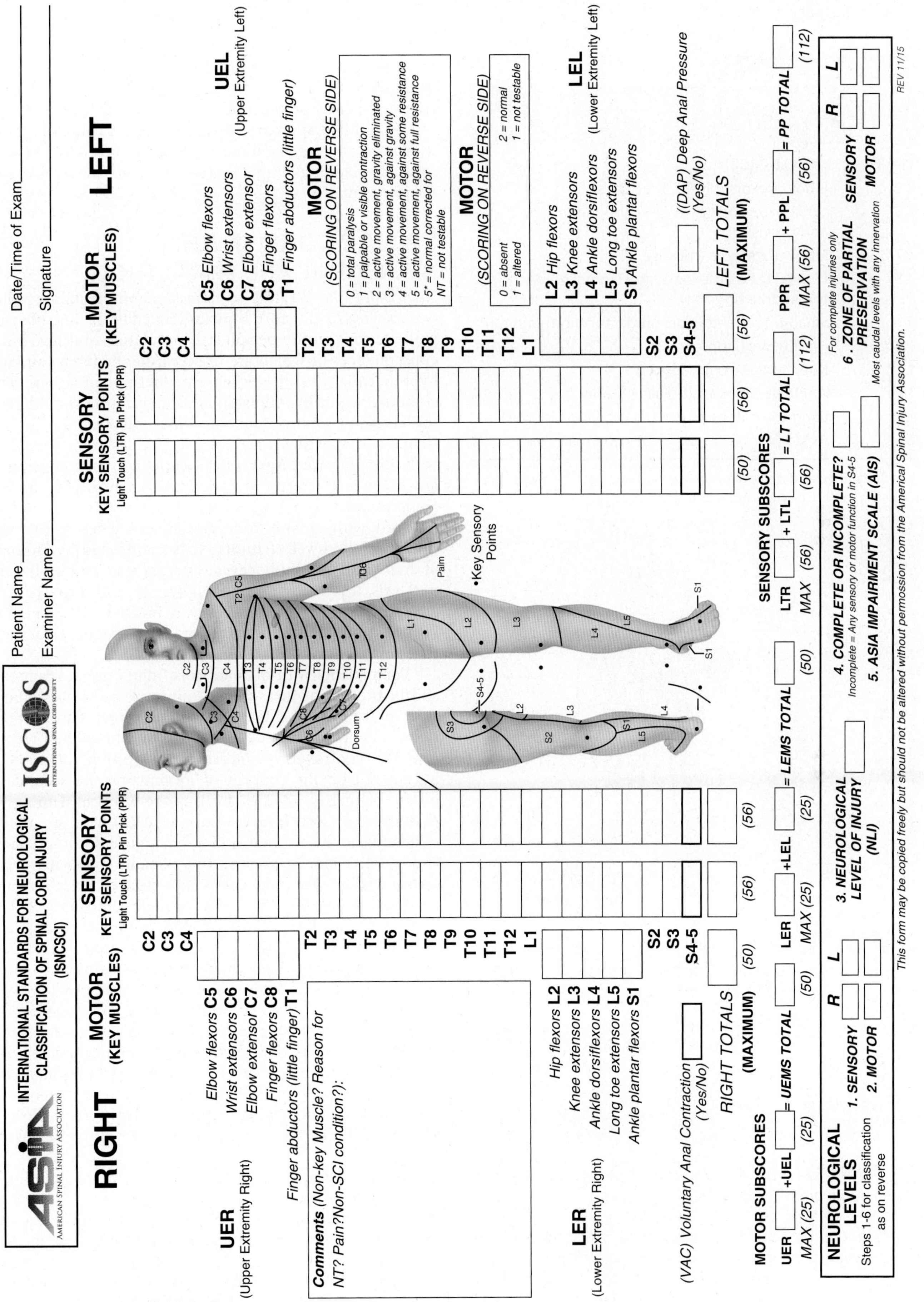

INTERNATIONAL STANDARDS FOR NEUROLOGICAL CLASSIFICATION OF SPINAL CORD INJURY (ISNCSCI)

ASIA — American Spinal Injury Association | ISCOS — International Spinal Cord Society

Patient Name ______________ Date/Time of Exam ______________

Examiner Name ______________ Signature ______________

RIGHT

MOTOR (KEY MUSCLES) | **SENSORY — KEY SENSORY POINTS** Light Touch (LTR) Pin Prick (PPR)

C2
C3
C4

UER (Upper Extremity Right)

- *Elbow flexors* **C5**
- *Wrist extensors* **C6**
- *Elbow extensor* **C7**
- *Finger flexors* **C8**
- *Finger abductors (little finger)* **T1**

T2 T3 T4 T5 T6 T7 T8 T9 T10 T11 T12 L1

Comments *(Non-key Muscle? Reason for NT? Pain?Non-SCI condition?):*

LER (Lower Extremity Right)

- *Hip flexors* **L2**
- *Knee extensors* **L3**
- *Ankle dorsiflexors* **L4**
- *Long toe extensors* **L5**
- *Ankle plantar flexors* **S1**

S2
S3
S4-5

(VAC) Voluntary Anal Contraction (Yes/No)

RIGHT TOTALS **(MAXIMUM)** *(50) (56) (56)*

LEFT

SENSORY — KEY SENSORY POINTS Light Touch (LTR) Pin Prick (PPR) | **MOTOR (KEY MUSCLES)**

C2
C3
C4

UEL (Upper Extremity Left)

- **C5** *Elbow flexors*
- **C6** *Wrist extensors*
- **C7** *Elbow extensor*
- **C8** *Finger flexors*
- **T1** *Finger abductors (little finger)*

T2 T3 T4 T5 T6 T7 T8 T9 T10 T11 T12 L1

MOTOR
(SCORING ON REVERSE SIDE)

0 = total paralysis
1 = palpable or visible contraction
2 = active movement, gravity eliminated
3 = active movement, against gravity
4 = active movement, against some resistance
5 = active movement, against full resistance
5 = normal corrected for*
NT = not testable

MOTOR
(SCORING ON REVERSE SIDE)

0 = absent *2 = normal*
1 = altered *1 = not testable*

LEL (Lower Extremity Left)

- **L2** *Hip flexors*
- **L3** *Knee extensors*
- **L4** *Ankle dorsiflexors*
- **L5** *Long toe extensors*
- **S1** *Ankle plantar flexors*

S2
S3
S4-5

((DAP) Deep Anal Pressure (Yes/No)

LEFT TOTALS **(MAXIMUM)** *(50) (56) (56)*

MOTOR SUBSCORES

UER ___ +UEL ___ = *UEMS TOTAL* ___ LER ___ +LEL ___ = *LEMS TOTAL* ___

MAX (25) (25) (50) MAX (25) (25) (50)

SENSORY SUBSCORES

LTR ___ + LTL ___ = *LT TOTAL* ___ PPR ___ + PPL ___ = *PP TOTAL* ___

MAX (56) (56) (112) MAX (56) (56) (112)

NEUROLOGICAL LEVELS
Steps 1-6 for classification as on reverse

R L
1. SENSORY
2. MOTOR

3. NEUROLOGICAL LEVEL OF INJURY (NLI)

4. COMPLETE OR INCOMPLETE?
Incomplete = Any sensory or motor function in S4-5

5. ASIA IMPAIRMENT SCALE (AIS)

For complete injuries only
6. ZONE OF PARTIAL PRESERVATION
Most caudal levels with any innervation

R L
SENSORY
MOTOR

REV 11/15

FIGURE 5.3 Standard neurologic classification of spinal cord injury from the American Spinal Injury Association (ASIA). For information on the use of the ASIA impairment scale, including grading of muscle and sensory function, testing of non-key muscles, and determining the steps in classification, download the full form at https://asia-spinalinjury.org/international-standards-neurological-classification-sci-isncsci-worksheet/.

TABLE 5.3

Key Muscle Groups Used in Motor Source Evaluation of Spinal Cord Injury

LEVEL	MUSCLE GROUP
C5	Elbow flexors (biceps, brachialis)
C6	Wrist extensors (extensor carpi radialis longus and brevis)
C7	Elbow extensors (triceps)
C8	Finger flexors (flexor digitorum profundus to the middle finger)
T1	Small finger abductors (abductor digiti minimi)
L2	Hip flexors (iliopsoas)
L3	Knee extensors (quadriceps)
L4	Ankle dorsiflexors (tibialis anterior)
L5	Long toe extensors (extensor hallucis longus)
S1	Ankle plantar flexors (gastrocnemius, soleus)

From Beaty JH, editor: *Orthopaedic knowledge update, home study syllabus 6*, Rosemont, IL, 1999, American Academy of Orthopaedic Surgeons, p 654.

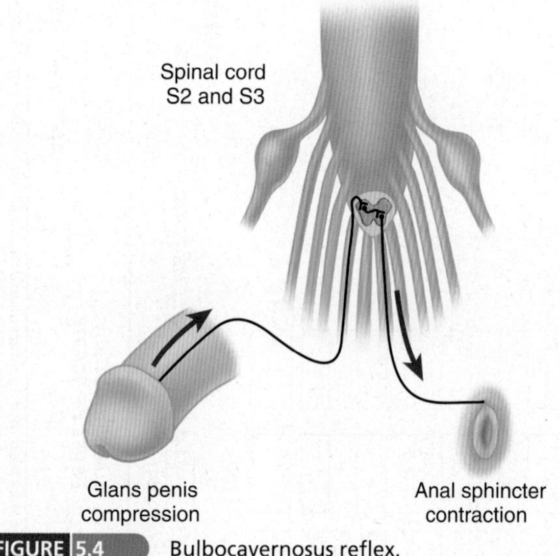

FIGURE 5.4 Bulbocavernosus reflex.

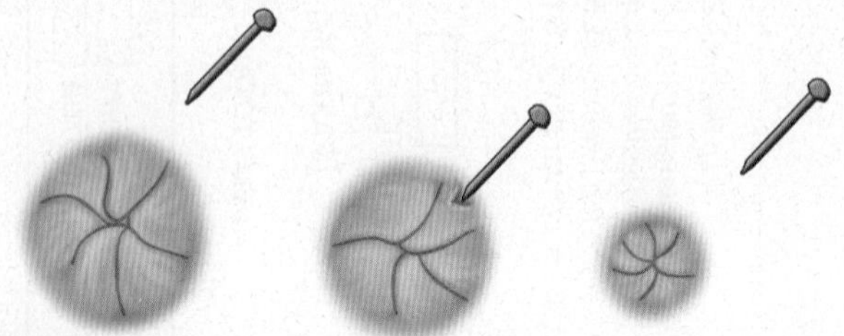

FIGURE 5.5 Anal wink. Contracture of external sphincter caused by pin prick.

function can be caused by intracranial processes such as hemorrhage, metabolic processes such as acidosis, or spinal pathologic processes. Bony malalignment causing spinal cord compression, hypotension, expanding epidural hematoma, spinal cord infarction, inadequate immobilization, or improper movement of a patient are some of the reasons for deterioration that must be considered by the orthopaedic surgeon in collaboration with other consultants so treatment can be adjusted appropriately. Likewise, if a patient is noted to improve, management may need to be altered as well with regard to planning of spinal stabilization or nonoperative spinal interventions.

SPINAL CORD INJURY

NEUROGENIC AND SPINAL SHOCK

Neurogenic shock refers to hemodynamic instability that occurs with rostral cord injuries related to the loss of sympathetic tone to the peripheral vasculature and heart, the consequences of which are bradycardia, hypotension, and hypothermia caused by absent thermoregulation. The combination of hypotension and bradycardia should alert the clinician to this cause of shock rather than hemorrhagic shock, which may coexist, particularly in patients with other injuries. Aggressive treatment of hypotension of any cause is a priority in patients with spinal cord injury. *Spinal shock* refers to a temporary dysfunction of the spinal cord, with a loss of reflexes and sensorimotor function caudal to the level of injury. It is manifested by absence of anal wink and bulbocavernosus reflexes and by flaccid paralysis. It is a temporary phenomenon and recovers usually in 24 to 48 hours even in severe injuries but can persist for weeks or rarely, months. There is no specific treatment for spinal shock.

For patients with a spinal cord injury, rapid diagnosis and institution of measures to minimize secondary spinal cord injury may be the most important interventions possible to improve ultimate neurologic and functional recovery. The controversy concerning the timing of surgery is centered on the concept of minimizing the secondary injury. Numerous studies such as the Surgical Timing in Acute Spinal Cord Injury Study (STACIS) have attempted to determine the optimal timing of surgical decompression and stabilization. At present, this remains somewhat of an open question, but evidence is mounting in favor of early decompression to enhance neurologic outcomes. Often this decompression is most rapidly accomplished by placing the patient in skeletal traction. This maneuver can be done much more quickly than operative treatment in most circumstances. In addition, multiple studies provide level III evidence that earlier decompression and stabilization are associated with shorter hospital stays and lower overall treatment costs for these patients. In a clinical study with direct measurements of spinal cord pressure and spinal cord perfusion, Werndle et al. found that spinal realignment and stabilization did not lead to improved spinal cord perfusion. This was attributed to spinal cord swelling within the inelastic dura mater.

The secondary injury cascade refers to the additional neurologic injury that results from cord ischemia, leading to electrolyte shifts with cell membrane alterations and accumulation of neurotransmitters and inflammatory mediators including free radicals that further injure neural tissue. A detailed discussion of these mechanisms is beyond the scope of this text; however, it must be recognized that proper medical management of a patient with a spinal cord injury is an important component in the overall care. The secondary mechanisms follow the initial or primary mechanical injury caused by compression, distraction, shear, or laceration of the spinal cord. The secondary injury cascade occurs over a period of hours to days, depending on the severity of injury and other injuries that may be present. Based on a number of animal models and level III evidence, it appears that the injury caused by ischemia of the spinal cord is the central feature of this secondary injury process. Avoiding or minimizing ischemia of the spinal cord appears to improve neurologic outcome. Spinal cord ischemia results in changes locally, with loss of autoregulation of spinal cord blood flow and changes to the systemic vasculature. These systemic alterations include cardiac rhythm irregularities, bradycardia, decreased mean arterial pressure (MAP), decreased cardiac output, and decreased peripheral vascular resistance. All of these abnormalities have the effect of a positive feedback loop to worsen the cord ischemia and thus worsen hemodynamic parameters. All of these hemodynamic parameters tend to be worse with more severe and more rostral injuries. Respiratory insufficiency or failure often accompanies spinal cord injury because of weakness of the respiratory muscles resulting in hypoxemia, which, in turn, worsens the spinal cord ischemia. Early detection and treatment of cardiopulmonary dysfunction does reduce the morbidity and mortality caused by these mechanisms. The goal for optimal blood pressure management is a MAP of 85 to 90 mm Hg with maintenance of 100% oxygen saturation. This is based on clinical observations and level III evidence, which remains the best guidance available to date. To properly treat these patients, arterial lines and central venous access or even Swan-Ganz catheters may be needed. Initially, hypotension should be treated as hemorrhagic in origin and fluid resuscitation should be with a balanced solution (e.g., lactated Ringer solution). After adequate crystalloid volume replacement, blood transfusion may be needed. If hypotension has not responded after fluid resuscitation and transfusion with normal central venous pressure, pressor agents should be administered to maintain the MAP in the desired range. Agents such as dobutamine, dopamine, or norepinephrine, with both alpha- and beta-agonist properties, are preferred over pure alpha agonists such as phenylephrine that can lead to reflex bradycardia. The duration of pressure support to maintain the median arterial pressure has been somewhat arbitrarily stated to be 7 days, but there is no evidence to support either a longer or shorter period of time. Supplemental oxygen should be administered and ventilator settings adjusted to keep oxygenation at or near 100% during this period as well.

IMMEDIATE CERVICAL SPINAL REDUCTION

The primary objective for rapid cervical reduction and stabilization is to improve spinal cord blood flow and thus minimize the harmful effects of ischemia. In animal models, rapidly relieving spinal cord compression has been shown to be beneficial. The short period of time from injury to decompression determined in these studies to be optimal has not been clinically achievable. One intervention that can be accomplished in some patients to relieve spinal cord compression and improve cord blood flow is to reduce fractures and dislocations using skeletal traction. If the injury is recognized and the patient is emergently taken to the radiology suite, often the reduction can be achieved within the first 1 to 2 hours after the patient arrives at the hospital. To be effective this must be done absolutely as soon as possible even if the initial workup has not been completed. However, limited evidence exists as to how beneficial this may be, and there is some risk from other undetected injuries in this setting. Closed reduction usually can be accomplished significantly faster than can be achieved by operative means, and completion of the evaluation in a hemodynamically stable patient can usually safely follow the reduction. Closed reduction is not always possible and is not appropriate to attempt, for example, in patients with distraction type injuries at other levels, in obtunded patients, in patients with certain cranial fractures, or if the patient becomes hemodynamically unstable.

A great deal of controversy exists regarding timing of cervical reductions and the need for cervical MRI, particularly in the context of a patient with unilateral or bilateral facet fractures or dislocations. The controversy has been centered on whether there is a need to obtain prereduction MRI to determine if there is a disc herniation. The value of this information compared with the risk of the increased time to reduction has not been established. Consideration must be given to several pieces of information when treating these patients. The first is that dislocation of the spine with spinal cord compression is definitely associated with neurologic injury. Rizzolo et al. reported that in 55% of patients with facet injuries, disc herniations or disruptions occurred and that often the disc material displaced into the canal. The importance of this is not clear as it relates to spinal reduction. Vaccaro et al. documented by MRI that more disc herniations were present after reduction than before reduction, but disc displacement did not correlate with neurologic deterioration in a small series of patients. Grauer et al. noted the significant variability of using MRI in the setting of cervical dislocations among spine surgeons based on their primary specialty. The second important fact is that only rarely has closed spinal reduction been associated with neurologic worsening if the patient is awake and alert at the time of reduction. Although there is no level I evidence on this topic, it appears that the important issue is whether the patient is awake and alert at the time of reduction, not the presence of a disc injury. Many clinical series that were reported over a period of decades found only 11 of 1200 awake patients (<1%) who developed permanent neurologic worsening after closed reduction. At least two were root level injuries. Additionally, one or two patients had transient worsening that returned to baseline. Reduction was accomplished in 80% of patients, which should allow for better spinal cord perfusion. Thus, the risk of causing additional harm in an awake and alert patient with a cervical facet fracture or dislocation and a significant neurologic deficit is very low. In an awake and alert patient with a cervical fracture or dislocation with a significant neurologic deficit, we recommend expeditious reduction without obtaining an MRI.

Significant neurologic injury in our protocol has been determined to mean less than grade 3/5 in more than one half of the key myotomes caudal to the level of injury (ASIA Impairment Scale A, B, or C). By using this regimen, most awake and alert patients have reductions before obtaining an MRI. These patients do have MRI after reduction but before definitive treatment to assist in surgical planning. For the rare patient with a bilateral facet injury, or more likely a unilateral facet injury, and more than half of the key myotomes caudal to the injury level grade 3/5 or higher, an MRI is obtained before reduction even if the patient is awake and alert. The rationale is that if a patient's neurologic function is grade 3/5 or higher initially, there is more potential for harm with immediate reduction and less benefit. If during the process of reduction worsening of neurologic deficit occurs, the attempt at reduction is terminated. Immediate MRI is obtained, and operative treatment is undertaken, depending on the pathologic process present. If the patient is obtunded, closed reduction cannot be undertaken safely and immediate reduction is not attempted. For patients in whom closed reduction is attempted but not successful, MRI is completed to help guide the surgical approach.

APPLICATION OF GARDNER-WELLS TONGS

TECHNIQUE 5.2

- Stabilize the patient's neck with a rigid cervical orthosis. A small bolster may be needed under the occiput or shoulders to maintain neutral cervical alignment.
- Identify a point 1 to 2 cm above the top of the ear and 0 to 2 cm posterior to the auditory meatus bilaterally. Pull the hair back over this area. If necessary, remove a small amount of hair to expose the skin.
- If slight extension is desired, place the pins in line with the auditory meatus but no farther forward to avoid injury to the temporal artery. Placing the pins more posteriorly will result in slight flexion. Flexion or extension also can be accomplished by adjusting the level of the traction pulley or by placing a bolster under the shoulders as needed.
- Clean the pin sites with an antiseptic soap and antiseptic solution.
- Infiltrate the pin sites with 1% or 2% lidocaine down to the periosteum.
- Check the tongs to ensure that the central pin is recessed, the pin points are not damaged, and the S hook is in place to attach the weight.
- Gently place the tongs over the patient's head and advance the pins toward the skin. Put the pins in a symmetric position.
- To avoid rotation, center the tongs by observing the patient's nose in the middle of the tongs.
- Advance the pins until the central pin protrudes by 1 mm. This will occur on one side only. Tighten the locking nuts securely after the pins are seated.
- The tongs are now set and traction can be applied. The other restraints can be removed. No dressing is needed.
- Place the pulley for the traction rope at a level to achieve in-line traction for the cervical spine (Fig. 5.6).

CLOSED REDUCTION OF THE CERVICAL SPINE

TECHNIQUE 5.3

- Before adding weight, configure the bed and traction so that the head of the bed is elevated 30 to 40 degrees and obtain a baseline radiograph.
- Apply initial weight equal to 8 to 10 lb. for the head and 3 to 5 lb per cervical level above the injury level, based on body habitus.
- Complete and document a neurologic examination.
- Administer medication for analgesia and muscle relaxation without decreasing patient's level of consciousness or cooperation.
- Obtain a lateral radiograph and assess for reduction of fracture or dislocation.
- Continue to incrementally add weight, assess neurologic examination, and repeat lateral radiograph until reduction is achieved or reduction must be terminated. By following this process, there should be 5 minutes between each weight addition to allow the traction to overcome any muscle spasm before adding more weight.
- The reasons closed reduction can fail are maximal weight reached, neurologic examination deterioration, and radiographic distraction of injury level more than 2 mm relative to normal adjacent disc. Be sure to compare most recent radiograph to the initial radiograph to determine if excessive distraction has occurred.
- After reduction is achieved or terminated, decrease traction to 10 to 15 lb based on body habitus.
- Repeat radiographs and examination. Further reduce weight if neurologic examination has not returned to baseline.
- Maintain patient in traction until definitive stabilization is done.

As noted previously, a small bolster may be needed under the patient's head or shoulders to achieve a neutral alignment in traction. Closed reduction should be successful in approximately 80% of patients. Further treatment after successful or failed reduction is discussed in the section regarding subaxial injuries.

SPINAL CORD INJURY TREATMENT

At this time there remains no effective treatment to reverse spinal cord injury that has been established by level I evidence. Many patients do improve neurologically, and in some the improvement is very dramatic. The measures that have been established to date are those detailed earlier that reduce the secondary injury. These include rapid realignment of the spine when appropriate, maintaining MAP at 85 to 90 mm Hg, and maintaining 100% oxygen saturation. The use of maintaining MAP in the range of 85 to 90 mm Hg continues to be evaluated. Hawryluk et al. evaluated minute-by-minute data on 100 patients with spinal cord injuries and found a correlation between maintaining a MAP of 85 to 90 mm Hg and better neurologic outcomes; intermittent lapses below the target

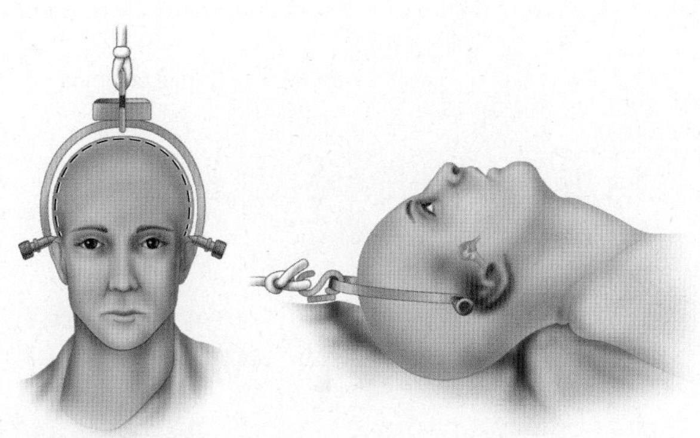

FIGURE 5.6 Gardner-Wells tongs placed just above ears, below greatest diameter of skull. **SEE TECHNIQUE 5.2.**

range negatively affected outcomes. Also, the effect appeared most important during the first 3 days after injury. An extensive literature review of cervical spinal cord injuries by the Congress of Neurological Surgeons also recommends maintaining MAP between 85 and 90 mm Hg during the first 7 days after injury. There has been extensive research into various interventions to discover any possible clinical benefit that may aid patients with spinal cord injury. One such intervention that initially gained clinical acceptance was the use of high-dose methylprednisolone using the National Acute Spinal Cord Injury Study (NASCIS) II and then the NASCIS III protocols. Subsequent evaluations of these studies found significant flaws in the data analysis, and the claimed benefits of corticosteroid use have not been realized. There is now level I and level II evidence showing that these high-dose protocols do not improve SCI recovery and are associated with significant harm. These protocols are generally not recommended as treatment options to patients because significant complications are associated with these very high corticosteroid doses, which outweigh any benefit.

SPINAL CORD SYNDROMES

When evaluating patients with spinal cord injuries, incomplete injuries must be distinguished from those that are complete because treatment decisions are based in part on this determination. If a complete spinal cord injury exists, the patient may regain some function within the zone of partial preservation but needs to understand that functional recovery at a more caudal level is not to be expected. This determination cannot be made until spinal shock has resolved and a reliable detailed neurologic examination is possible. In the case of an incomplete spinal cord injury, there are several recognized syndromes. If the injury can be categorized as one of these syndromes, prognostic information can be provided to the patient in general terms, but determination of specific functional recovery remains impossible at this time. There are, however, some generalizations that help inform the patient: (1) the greater the sparing of motor and sensory function is caudal to the injury, the greater is the expected recovery; (2) the earlier that recovery appears and the more rapidly it progresses, the greater is the expected recovery; (3) patients younger than 50 years have a better prognosis than older patients with the same deficit; and (4) recovery can occur over 12 to 15 months, but once progress ceases further recovery should not be expected. The most recognized syndromes are central cord syndrome, Brown-Séquard syndrome, anterior cord syndrome, posterior cord syndrome, conus medullaris syndrome, and cauda equina syndrome. There are some injuries that do not fit well into these described syndromes, and prognostic information cannot be given for these mixed syndromes.

Central cord syndrome is the most common. It consists of injury to the central area of the spinal cord, including gray and white matter (Fig. 5.7B). The centrally located upper extremity motor neurons in the corticospinal tracts are the most severely affected, and the lower extremity tracts are affected to a lesser extent. Generally, patients have a tetraparesis involving the upper extremities to a greater degree than the lower extremities with greater dysfunction distally in the extremities than proximally. Sensory sparing varies, but usually sacral pinprick sensation is preserved. These patients frequently show early partial recovery and may have preexisting cord compression and may not have spinal instability. Prognosis varies, but more than 50% of patients have return of bowel and bladder control, become ambulatory, and have improved hand function. This syndrome usually results from a hyperextension injury in an older individual with preexisting osteoarthritis of the spine. The spinal cord is pinched between the vertebral body anteriorly and the buckling ligamentum flavum and lamina posteriorly (Fig. 5.7A). It also may occur in younger patients with flexion injuries.

Management of acute traumatic central cord syndrome (ATCCS) remains controversial with regard to operative or nonoperative treatment superiority. A recent systematic review by the Spinal Cord Society and the Spine Trauma Study Group found important questions have not been answered. The study by Karthik Yelamarthy et al. did find evidence indicating that for ATCCS patients with instability caused by fractures, disc disruptions, or dislocations and persistent cord compression, outcomes are improved with early surgery (within 24 hours). For ATCCS patients without instability, there is no clear evidence that surgery or conservative treatment is superior. Both groups generally improve, and 70% to 80% of patients can expect to regain bladder control and the ability to ambulate with improvement in hand function relative to immediately after injury, although full recovery is not common. Because of the clinical ambiguity, our approach in these patients is initially to manage the spinal cord injury medically and monitor neurologic improvement. Once improvement plateaus after several weeks, a decision is made regarding surgery based on the functional level of the patient. For patients with instability, early surgery to achieve stability and relieve residual compression is recommended.

Brown-Séquard syndrome is an injury to either side of the spinal cord (Fig. 5.7C) and usually is the result of a unilateral laminar or pedicle fracture, penetrating injury, or rotational injury resulting in a subluxation. It is characterized by motor weakness with loss of proprioception on the side of the lesion and the contralateral loss of pain and temperature sensation. Prognosis for recovery is good, with significant neurologic improvement often occurring. Most of the recovery occurs in the first few months after injury, but improvement can occur over 2 years. Gait usually recovers within 6 months. Pollard and Apple noted that only central cord and Brown-Séquard

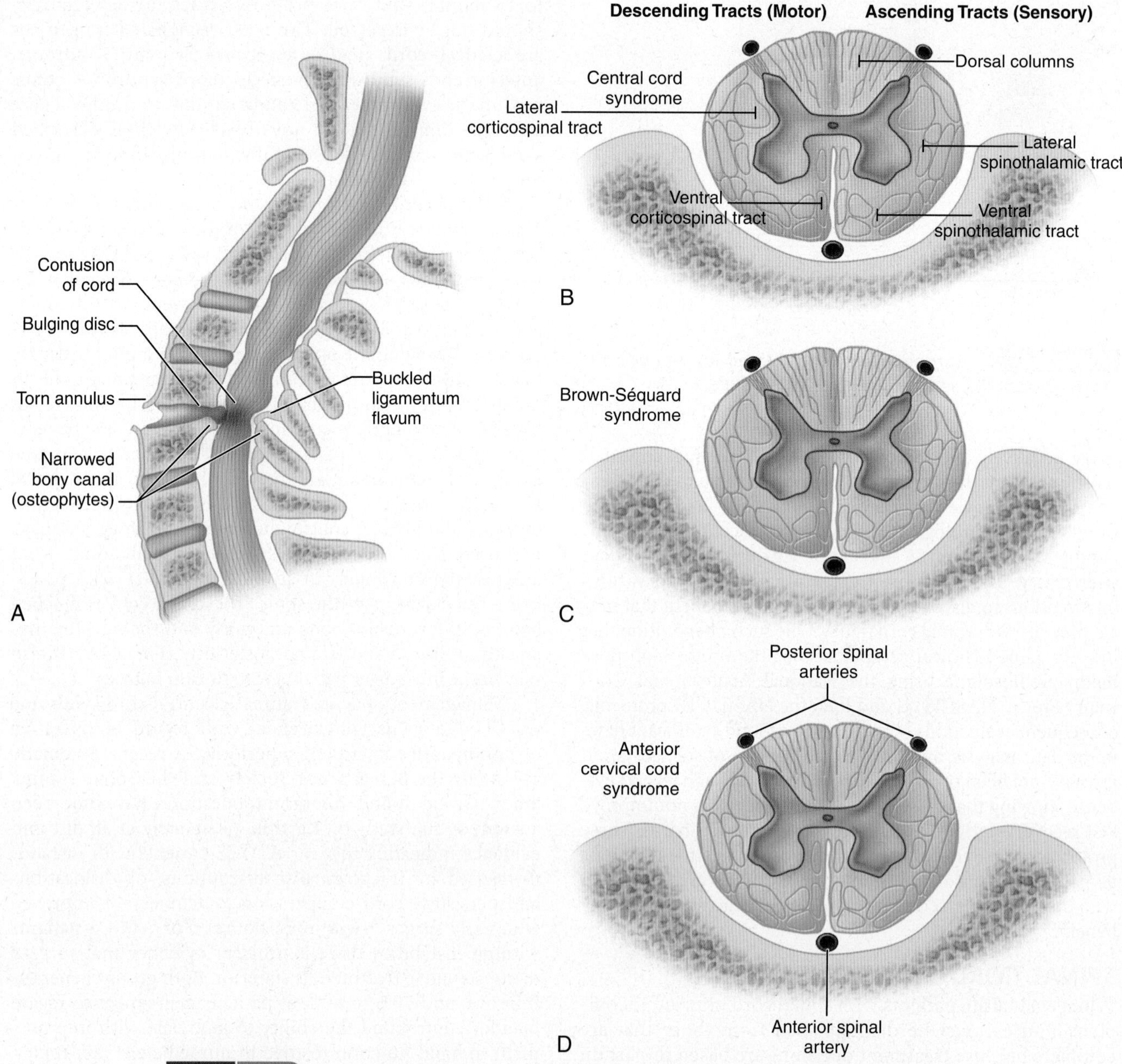

FIGURE 5.7 Spinal cord lesions. **A** and **B,** Central cord syndrome: spinal cord is pinned between vertebral body and buckling ligamentum flavum. **C,** Brown-Séquard syndrome. **D,** Anterior cervical cord syndrome.

syndromes were statistically associated with improved recovery at 2 years after injury. In carefully selected patients, nerve transfers may be of benefit.

Anterior cord syndrome usually is caused by a hyperflexion injury in which bone or disc fragments compress the anterior spinal artery and cord. It is characterized by complete motor loss and loss of pain and temperature discrimination below the level of injury. The posterior columns are spared to varying degrees (Fig. 5.7D), resulting in preservation of deep touch, position sense, and vibratory sensation. Prognosis for significant recovery in this injury is poor. Posterior cord syndrome involves the dorsal columns of the spinal cord and produces loss of proprioception and vibratory sense while preserving other sensory and motor functions. This syndrome is rare and usually is caused by tumors but can occur with an extension injury.

Conus medullaris syndrome, or injury of the sacral cord (conus) and lumbar nerve roots within the spinal canal, usually results in areflexic bladder, with urinary retention with overflow incontinence, areflexic bowel with fecal incontinence, and lower extremity weakness with increased tone that initially may be flaccid. Most of these injuries occur between T11 and L2 and result in flaccid paralysis in the lower extremities and loss of all bladder and perianal muscle control. The irreversible nature of this injury to the sacral segments is evidenced by the persistent absence of the bulbocavernosus reflex and the perianal wink. Motor function in the lower extremities between L1 and L4 may be present if nerve root sparing occurs.

Cauda equina syndrome, or injury between the conus and the lumbosacral nerve roots within the spinal canal, also can result in an areflexic bladder, bowel, and lower limbs.

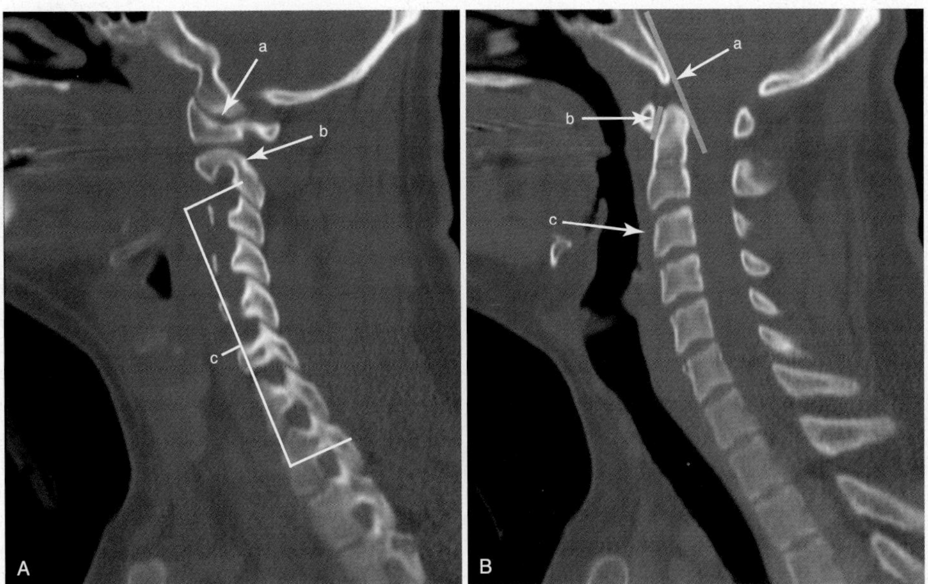

FIGURE 5.8 **A,** *Arrow a* indicates normal occiput-C1 joint congruity. *Arrow b* indicates intact C2 isthmus. *Bracket c* indicates normal facet relationships throughout cervical spine. **B,** *Arrow a* indicates Wackenheim's line with normal relationship between clivus and posterior dens. *Arrow b* indicates atlantodens interval, which is normal in width. *Arrow c* indicates normal soft-tissue density width less than 5 mm at C3 midbody.

With a complete cauda equina injury, all peripheral nerves to the bowel, bladder, perianal area, and lower extremities are lost and the bulbocavernosus reflex, anal wink, and all reflex activity in the lower extremities are absent, indicating absence of any function in the cauda equina. The cauda equina injuries are lower motor neuron injuries, and there is a possibility of return of function of the nerve rootlets if they have not been completely transected or destroyed. Most often, cauda equina syndrome manifests as a neurologically incomplete lesion.

CERVICAL SPINE INJURIES

RADIOGRAPHIC EVALUATION PROTOCOL

The helical CT scan is the imaging modality of choice for the diagnosis of cervical fractures and dislocations. Axial images, sagittal reconstructions, and coronal plane reconstructions each provide optimal visualization for particular injuries. Having a systematic and methodical routine for viewing these series is required to detect injuries. Beginning with the sagittal reconstructions, three images are of particular value. These are the midline image and each of the parasagittal plane images through the occipital condyle-C1 joint and the facet joints on each side. These parasagittal images should be evaluated specifically for (1) congruity of the occipital condyle-C1 joint, which should be concentric and should not be more than 2 mm wide laterally, (2) intact isthmus at the C2 level, and (3) a normal relationship at each facet joint and intact lateral masses. The midline image should be evaluated specifically for (1) relation of Wackenheim's line to the dens (normally tangential to the posterior aspect of the dens), (2) widening of the atlantodens interval (normal <3 mm; abnormal >5 mm), (3) soft-tissue swelling at the C3 midbody (normal <5 mm), (4) bony integrity of the dens, (5) anterior vertebral body alignment; (6) posterior vertebral body alignment, (7) alignment of the spinolaminar line, and (8) assessment for excess angulation or widening of each disc space.

The coronal reconstructions are best for evaluating the occiput-C1 joints, the C1-C2 joints, and the bony integrity of the dens.

The continuity of the posterior bony arch at each cervical level and the occiput is best determined on the axial images. Fractures involving the body, pedicle, foramen transversarium, lateral mass, lamina, and spinous process can be seen at individual levels (Fig. 5.8).

HALO VEST IMMOBILIZATION AND CERVICAL ORTHOSES

Cervical immobilization is a mainstay of treatment for many cervical injuries. There is extensive clinical experience covered in the orthopaedic literature over many years regarding cervical immobilization. This literature base is mostly level III and level IV evidence studies. Unfortunately, controlled randomized prospectively collected data on specific means of immobilization for specific injuries are not available. It is unlikely such data will become available given the difficulty of devising an ethical study that could appropriately collect this information. A cadaver study of various spinal orthoses, including rigid collar, sternal occipital mandibular immobilizer (SOMI), and halo vest, by Holla et al. found that generally the reduction in flexion/extension occurred at C0-C1 level and the reduction in rotation occurred at C1-C2. Additionally, they found that restriction in motion was progressively increased in order from rigid collar to SOMI to halo vest.

The first modern halo vest was developed at Ranchos Los Amigos and described by Perry and Nickel in 1959. Numerous modifications have been made to the halo vest, and other orthoses for the cervical spine have been developed. These orthoses generally have been designed to serve one of two purposes: immobilization during extrication and transport procedures or adjunctive or definitive treatment for unstable cervical injuries. The adjunctive role is either as temporary immobilization preoperatively or to provide immobilization after surgical stabilization. The goals of stable fixation and early mobilization are appropriate with spinal injuries, but often a short period of external support is recommended after surgery.

Extrication-type collars are not appropriate for treatment because they are too restrictive and would cause skin breakdown with prolonged use. They should be exchanged or removed if immobilization is not needed after initial assessment of the patient. The most commonly used types of orthoses for the cervical spine include a soft collar, a two-piece "rigid" collar, a SOMI, a Minerva (similar to a SOMI with some forehead control), and a halo vest. Several authors have compared the relative ability of these devices to limit motion in the cervical spine. Studies comparing limitation of motion in normal volunteers using devices of the same basic type usually have not found statistically significant differences between devices within the same class. These studies generally have shown progressively more limitation of motion by the orthosis type in the sequence they are listed above. These studies usually measure global motion of the cervical region and are limited in that the study participants do not have cervical injuries and as such their spinal biomechanics may be different than patients. Other authors have used cadaver models to assess the effectiveness of different orthoses in limiting motion after instability is created at a specific cervical level. Richter et al. studied an odontoid fracture model and found the halo vest to be more effective than a two-piece collar or a Minerva type brace. In another cadaver study, Horodyski et al. found that a two-piece rigid collar did not limit motion effectively after severe C5-C6 instability was created. Other studies have found atypical motion, such as "snaking," at individual levels that is caused by orthoses, especially the more restrictive types, during activities of daily living. Further studies are needed to evaluate the effect of these devices with mastication, swallowing, and oral hygiene, although these devices have been shown to affect these activities.

The halo vest has been studied more than other types of braces, and several findings have been determined. The halo vest is the most effective brace for limiting motion within the cervical spine. This appears true for the craniocervical junction, subaxial region, and cervicothoracic junction. Motion is allowed to a greater extent in the junctional areas than in the midcervical region in the halo vest. However, it is clear that motion remains throughout the cervical spine even with a halo vest properly applied. Despite this persistent motion, the halo vest has proven effective in the management of many types of cervical injuries, especially bony injuries involving the craniocervical junction. As surgical methods have improved, the halo vest has remained useful in part because for many upper cervical injuries normal motion can be preserved after fracture union. This region is responsible for a large portion of the normal cervical spine, and this motion is often permanently sacrificed with operative stabilization.

The use of halo vest immobilization does have significant associated complications. Recently, several studies have examined the morbidity and mortality associated with immobilization in a halo vest in elderly blunt trauma victims; however, no high-quality studies have prospectively evaluated this subgroup of patients. Retrospective studies in the trauma literature have noted an increased mortality rate in elderly trauma patients with cervical fractures treated with immobilization with a halo vest compared with those treated operatively or with a collar.

In institutions with higher death rates in patients with cervical spine injuries, higher rates of respiratory complications and deep vein thrombosis also were noted, suggesting that this group may not have been mobilized as well as the other subgroups evaluated. In a more thorough but still retrospective evaluation, Bransford et al. did not find an increased death rate associated with use of a halo vest. This study, which was a retrospective review of all patients at a level I trauma center for 8 years, evaluated treatment outcomes, complications, injury type, and patient age. Successful treatment was reported in 85% of patients treated with halo vest immobilization, although 11% of patients had the time in a halo vest shortened because of complications such as pin site infections. Treatment success was defined as healing of the injury in satisfactory alignment without additional intervention or secondary neurologic deterioration. The adverse events encountered in this study included death, pin site problems, pulmonary deterioration, skin breakdown, dysphagia, neurologic deterioration, and other miscellaneous complications. Twenty-two of 311 patients died after halo vest immobilization was initiated, and 19 of these deaths were within 21 days of starting halo vest immobilization. Review by a seven-member panel as to the cause of death, contributing comorbidities, and specifically whether the halo vest immobilization was a contributing cause of death was done in each case. It was determined that all 22 patients died for reasons that were not attributable to halo vest immobilization. The most common region treated with halo vest immobilization was the occiput to C2, especially odontoid fractures, although about a third of patients had subaxial injuries. Also, there were a significant proportion of study patients with more than one injury.

Complications of halo vest immobilization are frequent, with some studies having complication rates as high as 59%, although most studies identify complications in about 35% of patients. The most common type of complication involves pin site infection or loosening, which accounts for about 40% of all complications. Most pin site infections respond well to oral antibiotics if started early. Local pin cleaning daily and close follow-up of these patients allow early detection of these problems. Occasionally, infections are more serious and require pin site change or early discontinuation of halo vest immobilization. The most serious infections, which rarely occur, can lead to intracranial abscess requiring debridement and possibly result in death. Other less common pin-related complications include dural penetration, loosening without infection, or even skull fracture at or near the pin site. Another common complication of halo vest immobilization is failure to maintain adequate fracture reduction and spinal alignment. Rates of persistent instability with halo vest immobilization are 30% to 35% in most series. Most of these complications are detected in the first 7 to 10 days if radiographic imaging at the time halo vest immobilization is started is compared with imaging obtained after mobilization has been accomplished. Conversion to an alternative treatment may be necessary if alignment is not maintained because of the increased probability of nonunion. Nonunion detected after adequate halo vest immobilization for 12 to 16 weeks also may require surgical stabilization. Neurologic deterioration secondary to persistent instability also is a concern, although this is not common with halo vest immobilization. More serious complications, such as pneumonia or respiratory insufficiency, can occur but most often are related to inadequate mobilization of the patient. If a determination is made that adequate stability will not be attained with halo vest immobilization to allow mobilization to the full extent that the patient's other injuries would allow, then other treatment should be undertaken if possible. In this way, most of the serious complications can be avoided. Most of the later but less serious complications related to the pins are avoided by using care in applying the halo vest immobilization and by having appropriate follow-up.

HALO VEST APPLICATION

There are a variety of halo vest designs available. We typically have used a carbon-graphite composite horseshoe ring and four titanium pins. In patients younger than the age of 10 years, either six or eight pins may be used (see chapter 7). Proper sizing and location of the ring are important to reduce pin loosening or ring migration. The ring selected should be the smallest diameter that can be placed below the equator of the cranium and allow at least 1 cm of clearance circumferentially. A larger ring that is farther from the bone will increase motion at the pin-bone interface, as occurs with other external fixation components when placed farther from the bone. Planned pin locations also must be carefully evaluated on CT for possible fracture.

TECHNIQUE 5.4

- Select the smallest ring that allows at least 1 cm skin clearance when placed below the largest diameter of the skull.
- The anterior pins should be above the lateral third of the eyebrow. This position avoids the supraorbital and supratrochlear nerves and the temporalis muscle. The posterior pins usually are slightly lower than the anterior pins and posterior to the ear (Fig. 5.9).
- Position the posterior piece of the vest under the patient so that the shoulder strap is properly located.
- Shave hair if needed and cleanse each pin site with antiseptic solution three times.
- Using the ring positioning pins, set the ring position and have an assistant hold the ring in this position.
- Place a needle through the pin location in the ring to be used and inject 0.5 mL of local anesthetic subperiosteally. Avoid raising a large skin wheal when injecting because this leads to traction on the skin after pin placement.
- Have the patient gently close his eyes and maintain this during ring placement to make sure the upper lids can be closed after placement of the pins.
- Place each pin down to the skin surface.
- Tighten by hand one opposing pair of pins (e.g., right anterior with left posterior) one full turn and then tighten the other pair; repeat until all pins are as tight as possible by hand. This avoids translating the ring in one direction while tightening the pins.
- Using a torque-limiting screwdriver set at 8 in/lb, tighten the pins in a figure-of-eight sequence one full rotation each until all four are at 8 in/lb. Lower torque will increase pin loosening, and higher torque increases the risk of skull penetration.
- Securely tighten the locking nut on each pin.
- Apply the anterior vest piece and secure the shoulder and abdominal straps.
- Engage the four supports from the vest into the ring and adjust the position to allow unrestricted movement of the xiphoid hinge if necessary. Tighten all set screws to the manufacturer's suggested torque.
- Radiographically verify that the fracture reduction and spinal alignment are acceptable.
- In 24 hours, retighten the pins to 8 in/lb of torque.
- Begin daily pin cleaning with H_2O_2 or povidone-iodine solution.

POSTOPERATIVE CARE Daily pin cleaning is continued and, depending on how active the patient is, the superstructure of the halo vest is tightened every 2 to 4 weeks. The patient is mobilized as completely as the noncervical injuries will allow, and the cervical spine is imaged to verify that fracture reduction and overall alignment are stable. After the period of halo vest immobilization is completed and the pins are removed, the pin sites should be cleaned. Manually mobilizing the skin to prevent scar tethering to the periosteum allows for more normal facial expression and less noticeable scars.

OCCIPITOCERVICAL DISSOCIATION INJURY PATTERNS

Injuries to the craniocervical junction can occur at a variety of locations. Atlantooccipital dislocations, C1-C2 dislocations, or combinations of fractures and dislocations involving the occiput, atlas, and the axis also can disrupt soft tissues, such as the tectorial membrane, alar and apical ligaments, transverse atlantal ligament (TAL), and joint capsules at occiput-C1 or C1-C2 joints. Some injuries such as fracture of the occipital condyle or isolated joint capsule injuries may be stable. However, these injuries may occur as components of a more complex injury with occipital cervical instability, which can be fatal if not treated. Often these injuries result in fatalities before the patient is transported. The diagnosis of craniocervical junction injuries requires awareness of and suspicion for the expected injury patterns. The presence of cranial nerve (CN) VI, CN X, or CN XII palsies, subarachnoid hemorrhage at the craniocervical junction, or soft-tissue swelling anterior to the upper cervical spine should increase suspicion of a craniocervical injury. More severe deficits, including monoparesis, hemiparesis, tetraparesis, apnea, or other high cord symptoms, also have been reported with these injuries. Careful evaluation of the CT images, particularly the reconstruction images, is needed because these injuries often are dislocations and only the relative position of one bony structure to another may be abnormal without the presence of a fracture. Atlantooccipital dislocation has become recognized more frequently as awareness of the injury has increased and initial patient care has improved. The best method for the diagnosis of atlantooccipital dislocation has not been definitively determined.

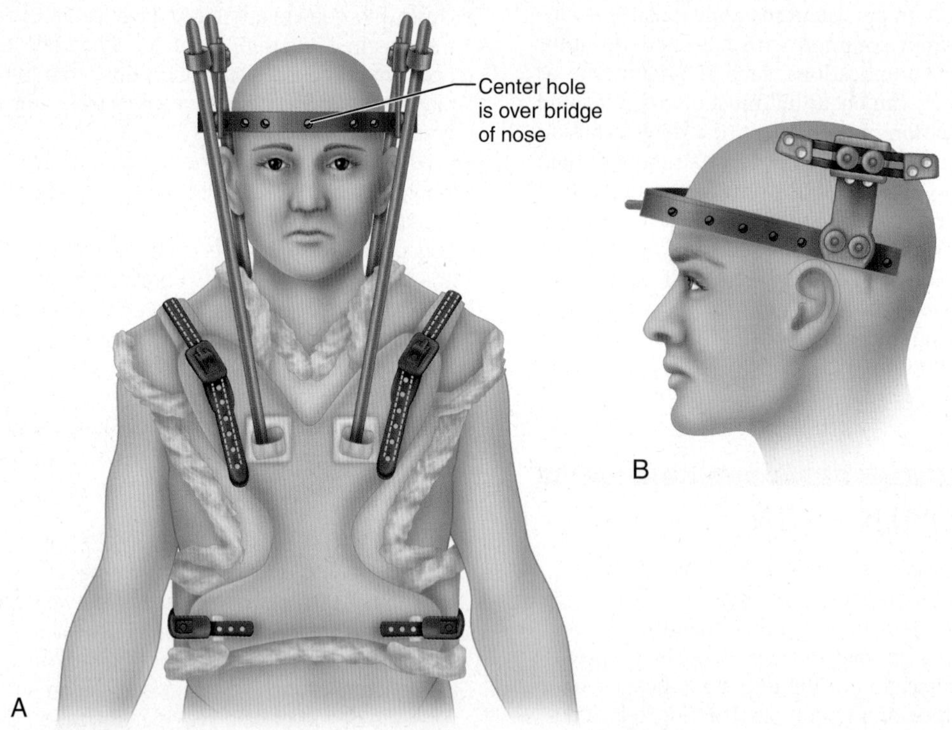

FIGURE 5.9 When applying halo ring, pin sites should be 1 cm above lateral one third of eyebrows and same distance above tops of ears in occipital area (mastoid area). **SEE TECHNIQUE 5.4.**

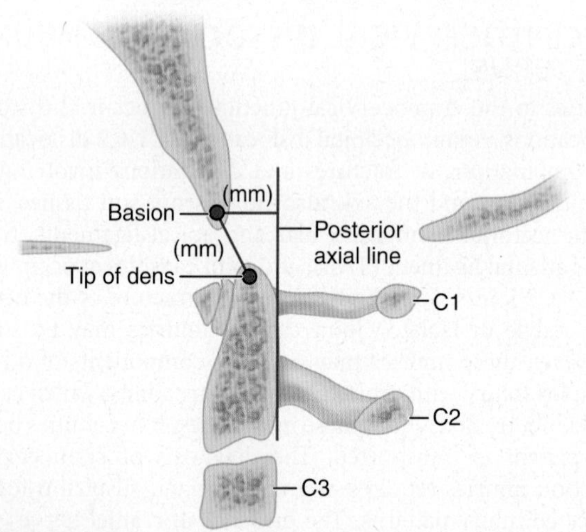

FIGURE 5.10 Measurement technique for basion dens interval and basion-axial interval described by Harris et al.

Older methods based on lateral radiographs such as the Power's ratio (basion to posterior arch distance/opisthion to anterior arch distance) have been described. Harris et al. described measuring the basion atlas interval and the basion dens interval (BAI-BDI), both of which should be less than 12 mm (Fig. 5.10). The BAI-BDI method as described by Harris et al. is the most reliable method using lateral radiographs. With the use of helical CT scans, more detailed analysis of the bony relationships is possible. The method that we have used to diagnose the presence of atlantooccipital dislocation is the Harris method, and we evaluate each of the occipital condyle-C1 joints for congruity and concentricity. Normally, these joints measure 0.5 to 1 mm and should be concentric. In a radiographic study by Martinez del Campo et al., a joint space of 1.5 mm or more was highly sensitive for atlantooccipital dislocation type of injury. If both joints are normal, there is no atlantooccipital dislocation. In addition, the relationship of Wackenheim's line to the dens is evaluated. If this relationship also is normal, there is no distraction injury between C1 and C2. The most commonly used classification system for atlantooccipital dislocation is the Traynelis system, which is described by direction of displacement, but it lacks treatment guidance. The Traynelis classification includes type I (anterior); type II (longitudinal); type III (posterior); and "other," which includes lateral or multidirectional displacement. Review of the literature revealed that patients with occipitocervical displacement who were not initially diagnosed had neurologic worsening 73% of the time before the diagnosis was recognized and about half did not improve even to their baseline neurologic examination after treatment. Ten percent of patients placed in traction had neurologic worsening in a small number of reported cases. Also, patients treated definitively with external immobilization excluding traction had a 40% rate of neurologic worsening that necessitated stabilization. Another 27% who did not worsen neurologically failed to achieve stability even after up to 22 weeks of immobilization. Patients treated with halo vest immobilization temporarily while awaiting operative stabilization had 0% neurologic worsening preoperatively. This evidence is level III but has led us to recommend operative stabilization

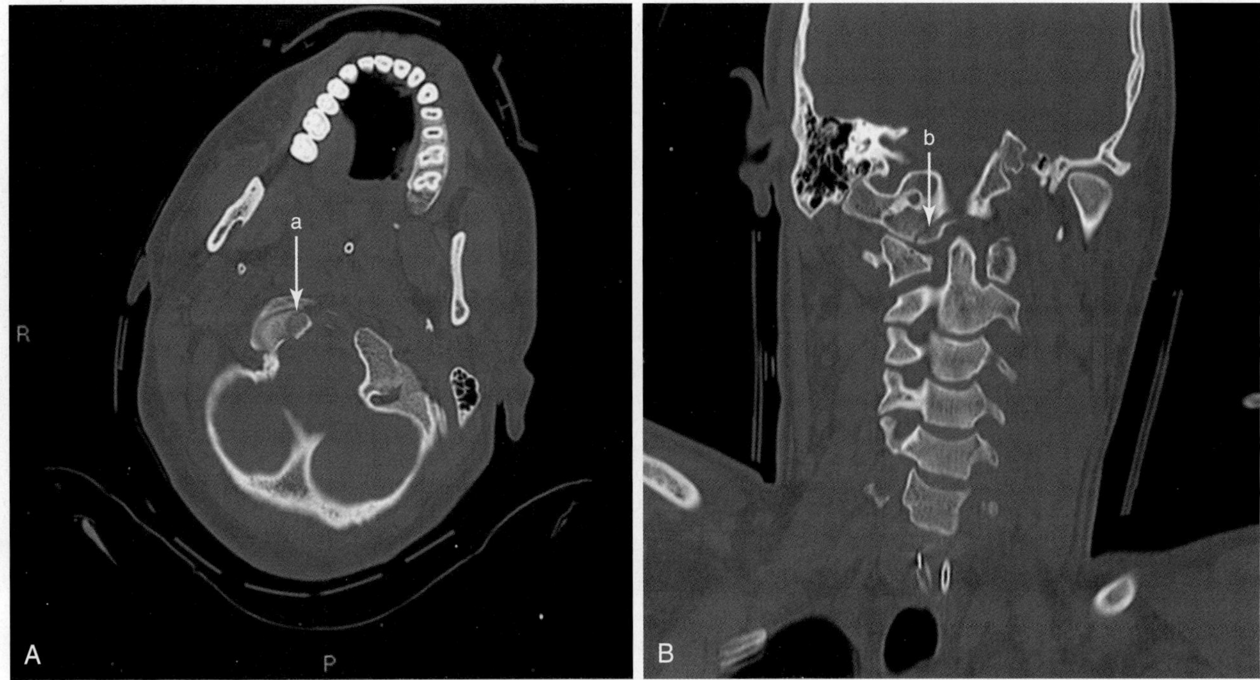

FIGURE 5.11 A and B, Right occipital condyle fracture *(arrows)*.

for all patients with unstable occipitocervical dislocations. Initial management is in a halo vest to provide provisional stabilization until the patient can undergo posterior occipitocervical fusion. Traction is not used under usual circumstances. Typically, fusion is from the occiput to C2 or C3, with multiple points of skull fixation and C1 lateral mass screws, C2 isthmus screws, and, when needed, C3 or lower lateral mass screws with autologous bone grafting. Some injuries to individual craniocervical structures without dislocation can be treated without operative stabilization.

OCCIPITAL CONDYLE FRACTURES

Fractures of the occipital condyle are recognized more often now with increased use of screening CT with reformatted images (Fig. 5.11). They occur in association with traumatic brain injuries in over half the cases, and frequently patients have additional cervical fractures. Dysfunction of cranial nerves is uncommon, but involvement of CN VI, CN IX, CN X, CN XI, and CN XII has been reported. Cranial nerve palsies most often are reported when fractures of the occipital condyle are untreated. These fractures do occur as isolated injuries but are most significant when they occur as part of a more severe craniocervical injury, such as occipital cervical dislocation. The occipital condyles articulate with the C1 lateral masses and are attached to the dens by the paired alar ligaments. The alar ligaments function to limit rotation of the occiput and atlas with respect to C2. The mechanisms for fractures of the occipital condyle usually are axial loading and lateral bending. Anderson and Montesano described the classification that is most commonly used: type I, impaction; type II, basilar skull fracture; and type III, avulsion fracture. Type I and type II fractures are usually stable and can be treated with a rigid orthosis for 6 to 12 weeks. About 6 to 8 weeks of immobilization in a rigid orthosis is usually recommended; there is no good evidence to support a specific treatment period. If instability is detected after a period of adequate immobilization, occiput to C2 fusion may be indicated. Type III fractures are potentially unstable, especially if displaced more than 2 mm, because of the avulsion of the alar ligament, which may be bilateral. Treatment in a halo vest for 12 weeks or surgical management may be needed for the rare unstable occipital condyle fracture. Occipital condyle fractures are most significant as indicators of high-energy blunt trauma to the head and neck. A large retrospective study by West et al. found the incidence to be 0.3% of the study population, but 30% of patients had associated intracranial injuries and 43.5% had significant other cervical injuries. Most were treated in a rigid orthosis, some with observation, and none required surgery.

TRANSVERSE ATLANTAL LIGAMENT RUPTURE

Rupture of the TAL or cruciform ligament usually occurs from a force applied to the back of the head, such as occurs in a fall. Thus, injuries involving the TAL can be a purely ligamentous midsubstance tear of the ligament or can occur as the result of an avulsion of the insertion into the C1 lateral mass. Dickman et al. classified these injuries as type I, disruptions of the substance of the ligament, and type II, fractures and avulsions involving the tubercle insertion of the TAL on the lateral mass of C1. Treatment is based on classification type. According to Dickman et al., type I injuries are incapable of healing without internal fixation and they should be treated with early surgery. Type II injuries, which render the transverse ligament physiologically incompetent even if the ligament substance is not torn, should be treated initially with a rigid cervical orthosis. Dickman et al. had a 74% success rate with nonoperative treatment of type II injuries, reserving surgery for patients who had a nonunion and persistent instability after 3 to 4 months of immobilization. Conversely,

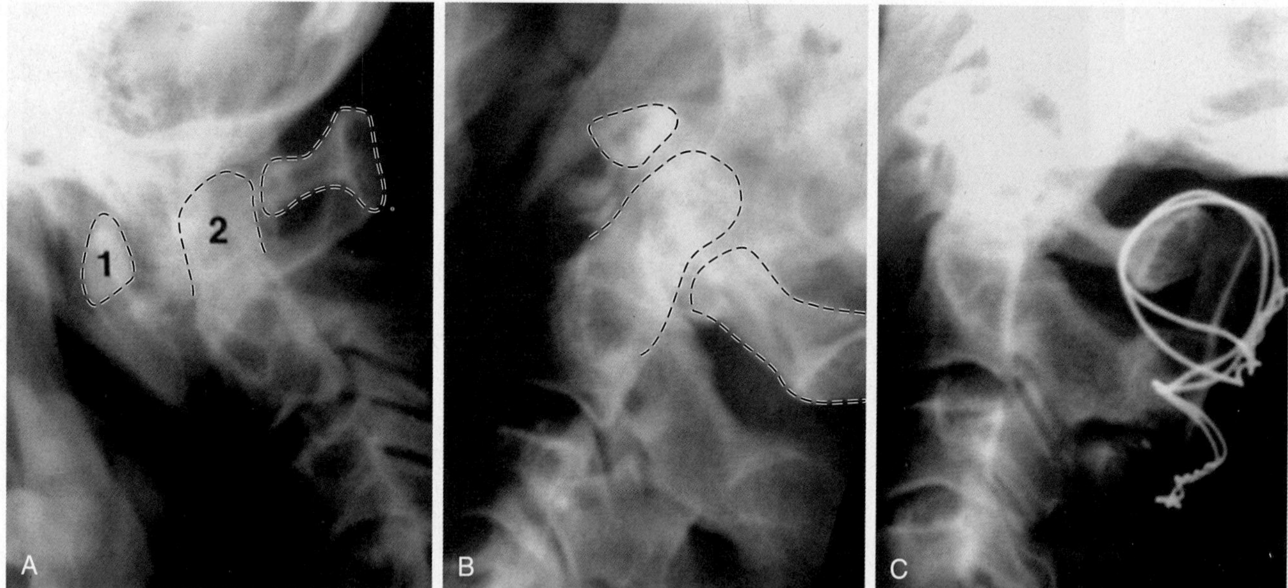

FIGURE 5.12 Patient sustained severe blow to back of head, resulting in instability of C1-C2 complex because of torn transverse ligament. **A** and **B**, Note widening of atlantodens interval in flexion **(A)** and reduction in extension **(B)**. **C**, After Gallie wiring.

26% of type II injuries in this study failed to heal after immobilization, suggesting that close follow-up is needed to determine which patients require delayed operative intervention. Usually the anterior subluxation of the ring of C1 can be detected on flexion films and the instability can be reduced in extension (Fig. 5.12). Sagittal midline reformatted CT views should be checked carefully for retropharyngeal swelling, which suggests an acute injury, and for small flecks of bone avulsed off the lateral masses of C1, which may indicate avulsion of the ligament. These avulsed fragments are best seen on coronal reformatted views. The primary indication of this injury is instability at C1-C2 on flexion and extension films. Anterior widening of the atlantodens interval of more than 3 mm on the midsagittal CT reconstruction or on a flexion view suggests that the transverse ligament is incompetent. MRI has become the standard imaging modality to evaluate the integrity of the TAL. Flexion and extension views should be made under the supervision of the physician, and the patient must be monitored closely for alterations in neurologic or respiratory function. As described by Dickman et al., mid-substance injury of the TAL will not heal with immobilization, and operative treatment is indicated. Posterior C1-C2 fusion using the fixation technique described by Harms with autologous bone graft is preferred. This technique is more rigid than wiring and has an advantage over wiring methods in that it can be used in the presence of fractures of the posterior ring of C1. An alternative fixation method is the Gallie method of wiring that creates a posteriorly directed force on C1 to reduce any atlantodens interval widening (see Fig. 5.12C). An intact dens will prevent over-reduction of C1. A Brooks-Jenkins bone block technique should not be used because it cannot maintain the reduction as well. In 12 patients with ruptures of the transverse ligament, Levine and Edwards found an average loss of correction of 4 mm after bone block techniques and 1 mm after Gallie wiring. Isolated TAL injuries without associated atlas fractures are rare.

OCCIPITOCERVICAL FUSION USING MODULAR PLATE AND ROD CONSTRUCT, SEGMENTAL FIXATION WITH OCCIPITAL PLATING, C1 LATERAL MASS SCREW, C2 ISTHMIC (PARS) SCREWS, AND LATERAL MASS FIXATION

The preferred method of occiput to cervical fusion uses a modular plate and rod system that incorporates multiple skull fixation points and multiple fixation points to the upper cervical spine. If the injury is soft tissue only at the occiput-C1 level, the construct usually can stop at the C2 level. If fixation is compromised by injury at the C1 or C2 level, fixation should be extended caudally to C3 or lower depending on the injury pattern.

The awake patient is moved to the turning frame and placed supine. After induction of anesthesia, the patient is secured between the two operating room tabletops and the entire bed is rotated to position the patient prone on the open frame. Typically, the patient will be in a halo vest on arrival to the operating room. A Mayfield head positioner is directly attached to the halo ring, and the anterior vest and supports are removed. If the patient is not in a halo vest, the Mayfield pinion head holder is used. After turning the bed, the posterior portion of the vest is removed. Fluoroscopic images are obtained to verify reduction of the injury and to make sure the position of the head is satisfactory for fusion. A position of slight occipitocervical flexion is preferred to allow the patient to potentially ambulate and perform daily activities with less difficulty (Fig. 5.13).

TECHNIQUE 5.5

- Position the patient prone on the rotating frame as described above.
- Shave the head several centimeters above the inion (posterior occipital protuberance).
- Prepare and drape the posterior head and neck, as well as the posterior iliac crest donor site.
- Score the skin sharply from the inion to the planned caudal level and inject dilute epinephrine solution (1 mg in 500 mL normal saline) through the score incision into the dermis and paraspinal musculature.
- Complete the skin incision sharply and then use electrocautery to dissect to the skull and spinous processes to at least the C3 level (if construct is planned to C2 level).
- Using Cobb elevators and electrocautery, subperiosteally expose the occiput from the inion to the foramen magnum.
- Expose the posterior ring of C1 laterally a distance of 15 mm from the midline or to the vertebral artery sulcus, whichever is less. Take care to keep the electrocautery on the ring of C1 and do not cauterize the atlantooccipital membrane, which is thin.
- Expose the bifid portion of the C2 spinous process and elevate the muscular attachments subperiosteally so that at closure the two sides can be sutured through bone to the spinous process of C2.
- Expose the spinous process, laminae, and entire lateral mass bilaterally at each level as needed, preserving the facet capsule at levels not to be included in the fusion.
- The C2 spinal nerve (greater occipital nerve) crosses posterior to the C2 isthmus in a dense venous plexus. Using bipolar cautery and a Penfield No. 4 elevator, gently mobilize this plexus cephalad, beginning at the upper lateral margin of the C2 lamina until the medial border of the C2 isthmus is visible. Expect bleeding during this step and control it with bipolar cautery, Gelfoam or Surgicel, and cottonoids. Placing the patient in a reverse Trendelenburg position helps control this bleeding.
- In a similar fashion, expose only the caudal edge of the ring of C1 laterally to a point even with the C2 isthmus and mobilize the venous plexus and C2 nerve caudally to allow exposure of the C1 lateral mass inferior to the posterior ring and vertebral artery.
- Using an image intensifier, verify that cervical alignment and injury reduction are satisfactory.
- The C1 screw is placed as described by Goel and subsequently refined by Harms and Melcher. Using a hand drill placed just caudal to the ring of C1 and 3 to 4 mm lateral to the medial edge of the lateral mass, advance the drill at an angle of 10 degrees medially and slightly cephalad to a point just posterior to the anterior margin of the dens on a lateral image intensifier view. This allows for unicortical screw placement and lowers the risk of injury to the internal carotid artery and hypoglossal nerve anterior to the C1 lateral mass.
- Place a polyaxial screw with a 10-mm smooth shank extension to the drilled depth.
- Place the C2 isthmic screw in a method similar to that described by Magerl and Seeman (see Technique 5.9). Place a Penfield No. 4 elevator to palpate and, if possible, view the isthmus medial cortex and determine the line of entry points on the inferior facet of C2 that will allow the medially directed drill to enter the isthmus. Using the lateral image intensifier view, select the point on this line that will orient the drill up the center of the isthmus. Use a high-speed burr to penetrate only the cortex at that point. Typically, the drill will be directed 25 degrees medially and 20 to 30 degrees cephalad, but anatomy varies considerably, and careful review of the CT scan is required. Direct the hand drill up the isthmus under fluoroscopic control to a point at the posterior margin of the C2 foramen transversarium as seen on the lateral image intensifier view.
- Place the appropriate length polyaxial screw to stop at the posterior foramen transversarium. In our experience this provides excellent fixation without placing the vertebral artery at risk by crossing the foramen transversarium into the C2 body.
- If additional lateral mass screws are to be used, they are placed using Anderson's modification of the technique of Magerl. Identify the four boundaries of the lateral mass and determine the geometric center of the rectangle defined by these boundaries. Penetrate the cortex 1 mm medial to the center point using a high-speed burr. Using this starting point, orient the hand drill laterally and cephalad by resting the drill sleeve at the margin of the tip of the spinous process of the next most caudal level (C4 spinous process for a C3 screw). Advance the drill in 2-mm increments until the far cortex is breached. Use a depth gauge to palpate for bone penetration after each 2 mm of drill advancement. Place the appropriate length screw bicortically. Unicortical 14-mm screws have been shown to provide satisfactory fixation and can be used if desired.
- After placement of these screws, the rod position at the skull can be determined. Some modular systems allow for either a single midline plate or two unilateral plates to be used. The occipital bone is thicker along the midline ridge, and screw purchase is enhanced if this bone can be used. However, if the midline plate does not align well with the screws as placed, bilateral plates are preferred. If two plates will be used, contour and place them to engage the thickest bone possible.
- For each occipital screw placed through the plate, use a hand drill for bicortical screw placement. Advance the hand drill in 2-mm increments, taking particular care during drilling of the occipital bone if the plate position requires drilling outside of the safe zone described above. The sagittal sinus and the transverse sinus are deep to the inner cortex of the occipital bone in this area. Unicortical screws can be placed in the thicker midline bone.
- After affixing the plate component to the occiput, contour, cut, and connect the rod to the cervical screws and plate on each side. If two plates are used, it is often easier to attach the contoured rod to the plate. Engage the rod into the cervical screws and then place the screws through the plate after it is in position.
- Tighten all connections securely.
- Harvest iliac bone graft as described in Technique 1.7.
- Decorticate the occipital bone and the posterior elements of the exposed levels using a high-speed burr.
- Carefully place morselized autologous bone graft over the decorticated areas. Avoid packing the bone over the atlantooccipital membrane because compression here may result in apnea from brainstem compression. For this reason, final hemostasis should be meticulous.
- Check final alignment and reduction.

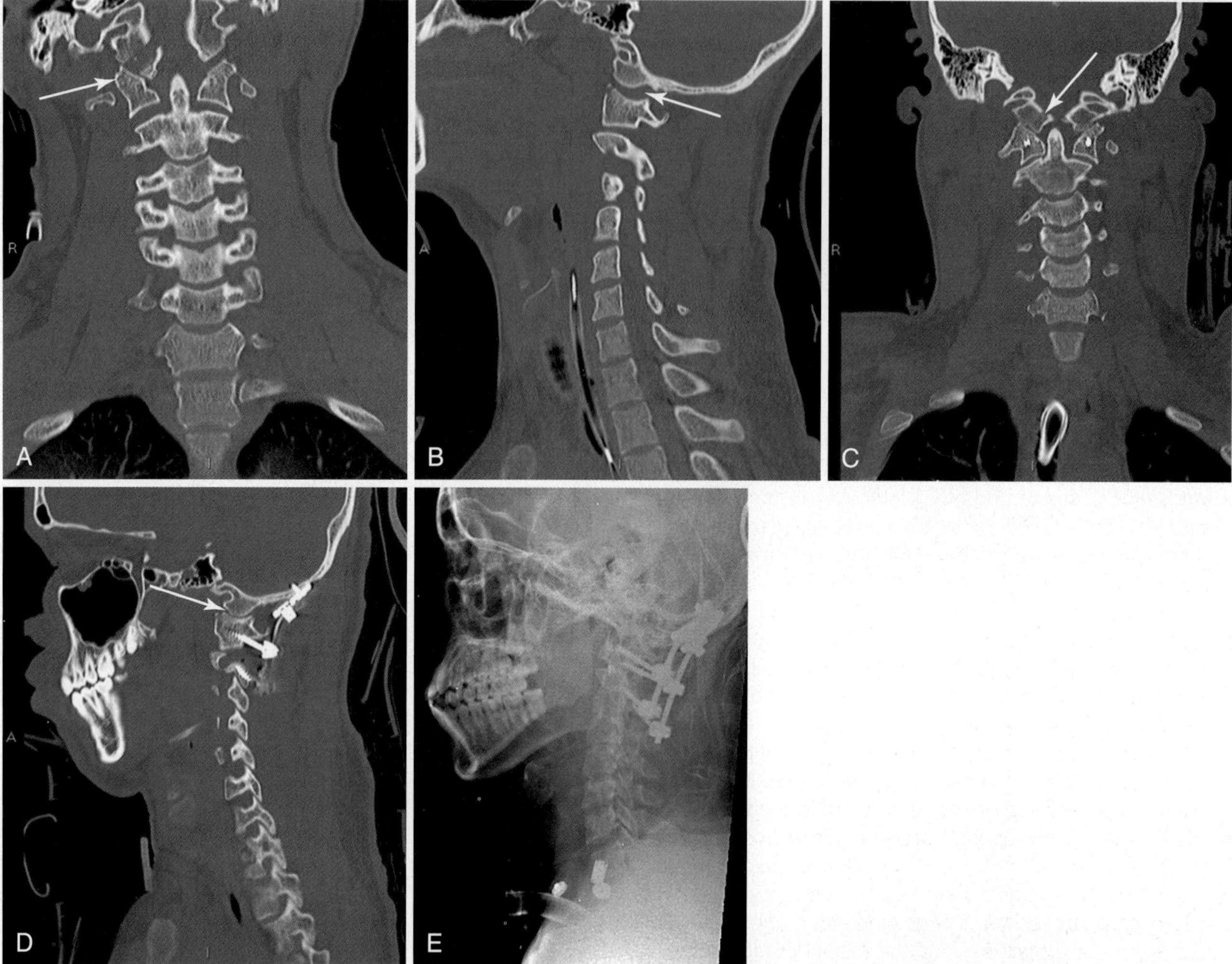

FIGURE 5.13 **A,** *Arrow* indicates fracture of right occipital condyle in patient with occipital-cervical dissociation injury. **B,** *Arrow* indicates widened and incongruous occipital condyle-C1 joint. **C,** *Arrow* indicates the right occipital condyle fracture has been reduced. *Arrow* indicates left occipital condyle-C1 joint is congruous. **D,** Anatomic alignment with fixation to skull, C1 lateral mass, and C2 isthmus. **E,** Lateral radiograph of occipitocervical plate-rod construct. **SEE TECHNIQUE 5.5.**

- Close the fascial layer over a drain back to bone when possible with particular attention to the C2 level.
- Close the wound in layers with a subcuticular skin closure.

ALTERNATIVE C2 PEDICLE SCREW TECHNIQUE A C2 pedicle screw is placed using a very similar technique to that described earlier for the isthmic screw. The primary difference is that the pedicle screw is longer and passes into the C2 body. In so doing, the course of the vertebral artery is traversed and therefore the artery is at higher risk for injury. The other difference is that with pedicle screws the trajectory is less medially oriented. Careful preoperative planning is needed because at least 8% to 10% of patients do not have anatomy that allows safe pedicle screw placement. This is especially true in women. The biomechanical advantage of the longer pedicle screw does not seem clinically important, and in general little is gained for the patient for the added risk. The isthmic screw technique is our preferred method. Several studies recently evaluated the safety and accuracy of C2 pedicle screw placement using either intraoperative CT or navigation systems, both of which were found to improve screw placement.

POSTOPERATIVE CARE The patient is maintained in a cervical collar for 8 to 12 weeks postoperatively until healing of the fusion has progressed satisfactorily. The drain is removed on the first postoperative day.

OCCIPITOCERVICAL FUSION USING WIRES AND BONE GRAFT

TECHNIQUE 5.6

(WERTHEIM AND BOHLMAN)

- The initial positioning, induction of anesthesia, preparation, neuromonitoring, and exposure are as described in Technique 5.5.

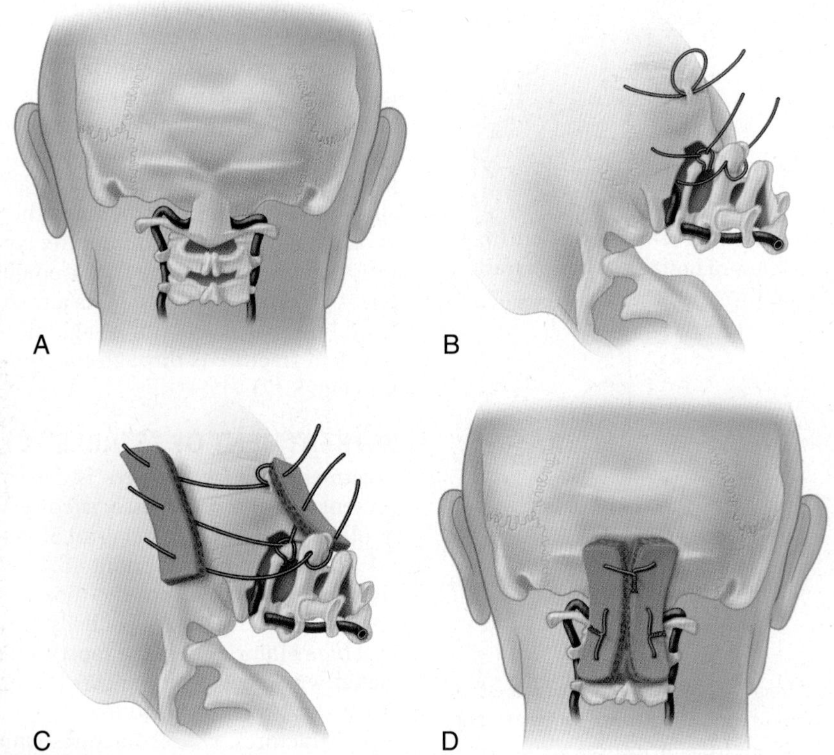

FIGURE 5.14 Wertheim and Bohlman method of occipitocervical fusion. **A,** Burr is used to create ridge in external occipital protuberance, and hole is made in ridge. **B,** Wires are passed through outer table of occiput, under arch of atlas, and through spinous process of axis. **C,** Grafts are placed on wires. **D,** Wires are tightened to secure grafts in place. **SEE TECHNIQUE 5.6.**

- Use a high-speed burr to penetrate the cortex on each side of the midline ridge of bone that extends from the inion to the foramen magnum (Fig. 5.14A). The thickest area of bone is an inverted triangle that extends 2 cm to either side of the inion and caudally 2 cm from the center of the inion. Use a towel clip to form a connection between the two openings in the cortex. Take care not to penetrate the inner cortex of the occipital bone.
- Make a hole through the base of the spinous process of C2 using a towel clip or bone tenaculum.
- Pass a 20-gauge wire through, around, and back through the hole in the spinous process of C2 to encircle the caudal portion of the C2 process and a second wire through the channel in the occipital bone in similar fashion.
- Use a small angled curet to dissect the ventral side of the C1 lamina bilaterally to allow for midline sublaminar wire passage.
- Cut a 24-inch length of 20-gauge wire and bend it tightly back on itself at its midpoint to create a loop. Contour the loop of wire into a "C" shape.
- Pass the loop of 20-gauge wire from caudal to rostral sublaminarly at the C1 level. Flatten the curve in the wire as needed to minimize intrusion of the wire into the spinal canal. A small blunt hook passed from the rostral side can be used to engage the loop of wire and pull the wire so that intrusion of the wire is minimized as it is advanced rostrally (Fig. 5.14B). Alternatively, pass a suture to tie to the wire and use this to pull the wire rostrally.
- Pass the free ends of the sublaminar wire through the looped portion and tighten the wire around the C1 lamina in the midline.
- Measure the distance from the occipital wire to the wire through the C2 spinous process and harvest a corticocancellous bone graft from the ilium outer table that can be divided into two 1.5-cm wide grafts that are long enough to span this distance with all wires passing through the graft.
- Decorticate the occiput and the laminae at C1 and C2 with a high-speed burr.
- Drill through each slab of bone graft to allow the wire to come through at each level (Fig. 5.14C).
- Tighten the occipital wire ends in the midline until the luster of the wire dulls slightly and turn down the cut end of the wires between the two grafts.
- Tighten the C1 and C2 wires together over the bone graft in a similar way. The grafts should be very secure (Fig. 5.14D).
- Close the fascial layer over a drain back to bone where possible with particular attention to the C2 level.
- Close the remaining wound in layers and the skin with a subcuticular closure. Reapply the halo vest.

POSTOPERATIVE CARE Halo vest immobilization is continued until graft consolidation, which usually occurs in 12 to 16 weeks. The drain is removed on the first postoperative day.

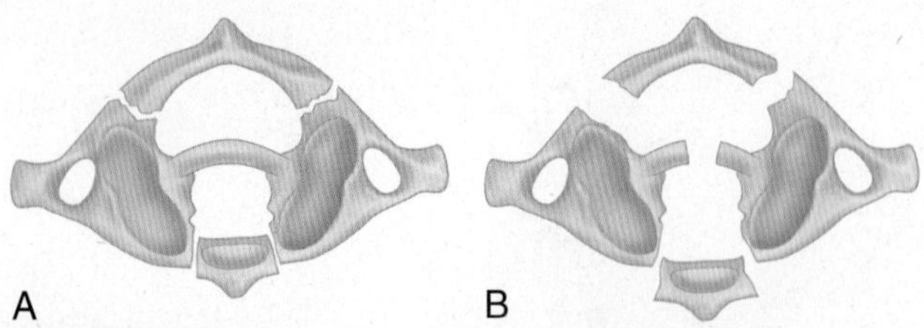

FIGURE 5.15 **A,** Axial view of stable Jefferson fracture (transverse ligament intact). **B,** Axial view of unstable Jefferson fracture (transverse ligament ruptured).

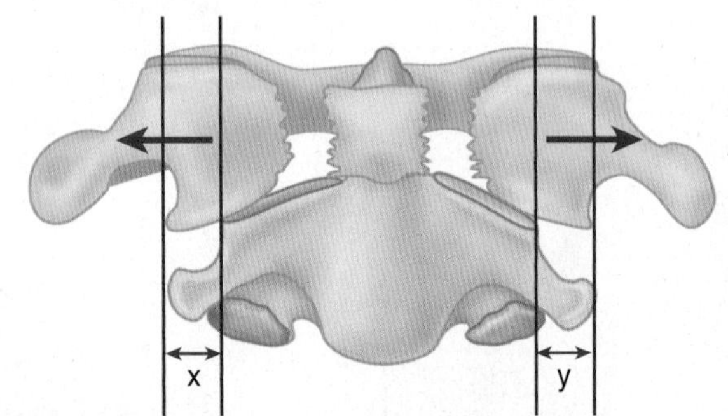

FIGURE 5.16 Displaced fractures with widening of more than 6.9 mm overhang on open-mouth odontoid views suggests injury of the transverse atlantal ligament (rule of Spence).

ATLAS FRACTURES

The first description of a C1 fracture was by Cooper in 1822, and Jefferson published his case review adding four new cases in 1920. This paper contained his classification system, which has subsequently been revised by multiple authors, but his description of a burst fracture of the ring of C1 continues to carry the label of a "Jefferson fracture" (Fig. 5.15). Spence et al. published their work in 1970 on injuries to the transverse ligament in association with C1 fractures in 10 cadaver specimens. They found that if the total lateral displacement of the lateral masses was 6.9 mm or more, then the transverse ligament was likely incompetent (Fig. 5.16). This determination based on plain radiographs is referred to as the rule of Spence. Later, this was revised to 8.1 mm to account for magnification on plain radiographs. Dickman et al. studied 39 patients with injuries to the TAL with plain radiographs, thin-cut CT, and high-resolution MRI. MRI was found to be very sensitive in detecting rupture of the transverse ligament, and their classification of these injuries was described previously. These authors found that applying the rule of Spence would have missed 61% of the transverse ligament injuries.

Biomechanical studies by Panjabi et al. and Oda et al. have shown that axial loading is the primary force that leads to C1 fractures. Because the C1 lateral masses are wedge shaped, axial loading creates a hoop stress and bone failure occurs at the weakest points that are just anterior and posterior to the lateral masses. Less force is required if the head is in extension when force is applied. Even when the TAL is injured, the alar ligaments, joint capsules, and tectorial membrane are spared with axial-loading injuries. This is an important difference for TAL injuries associated with C1 fractures and those associated with more complex injuries of the craniocervical junction. Landells and Van Peteghem modified Jefferson's classification into three fracture types, which is useful for treatment. Type I injuries include isolated anterior or posterior arch fractures, type II injuries involve the anterior and posterior portion of the ring, and type III injuries involve the lateral mass with or without a fracture of the ring. Gehweiler et al. also described a classification system that is perhaps the most useful. Type I is an isolated anterior arch fracture, type II is an isolated posterior arch fracture, type III is a combined anterior and posterior arch fracture, type IV is a fracture involving only the lateral mass usually with a sagittally oriented fracture, and a type V fracture is through the foramen transversarium of C1 (Fig. 5.17).

■ TREATMENT OF "STABLE" C1 FRACTURES

Treatment of atlas fractures is determined primarily by the presence or absence of associated cervical injuries. Fractures at other cervical levels occur in 30% to 70% of patients with C1 fractures. By far, odontoid fractures and C2 isthmic (hangman) fractures are the most common injuries associated with C1 fractures. Landells and Van Peteghem found that type I injuries were the most common and were not associated with neurologic injuries. Our treatment regimen for isolated C1 fractures is to use a rigid collar for nondisplaced type I fractures, type II fractures with 0 to 7 mm combined lateral mass displacement, and type III fractures of the lateral mass with less than 2 mm of displacement. Immobilization is maintained for 6 to 8 weeks if the ring is intact (some type III) and for 10 to 12 weeks if the ring is disrupted. Halo vest immobilization usually is reserved for C1 fractures with the associated injuries. It is rare to operatively stabilize isolated atlas fractures even if the transverse atlantal ligament (TAL) is disrupted. Stability after immobilization is demonstrated on flexion-extension radiographs if the atlantodens interval is maintained at less than 3 mm. If this distance is greater than 5 mm, posterior C1-C2 fusion is recommended. If a wiring technique is planned, the posterior C1 ring must be healed. Some authors recommend the use of a crosslink with the screw and rod method to help maintain the C1 reduction. Appropriate external immobilization has been shown in many level III and IV studies to result in stable unions in a high percentage of patients, but outcome measures for range of motion and persistent pain have not been widely studied. In their literature review, Lewkonia et al. found that after nonoperative management of isolated C1 fractures, 8% to 20% of patients had stiffness, 14% to 80% had mild pain, and 34% had limitation of activities.

Treatment of atlas fractures that occur with TAL injuries or other fractures is based primarily on the concomitant injuries. The additional fractures increase the level of instability, but external immobilization with a halo vest for 12 to 16 weeks has proven sufficient in the vast majority of cases that usually involve the axis. If the halo vest does not maintain alignment sufficiently when the patient is mobilized, operative stabilization is indicated. Traction can be used to reduce the lateral mass displacement before halo vest treatment, but the halo cannot maintain the distractive force, and 3 weeks of traction may be needed to allow healing adequate to prevent loss of reduction once halo vest immobilization is initiated.

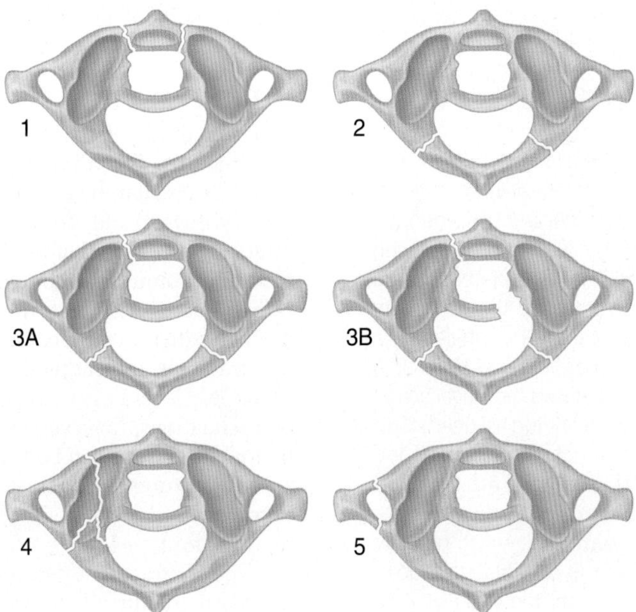

FIGURE 5.17 Gehweiler classification of atlas fractures. A type 1 atlas fracture is isolated fracture of the anterior arch; type 2 fracture is isolated, predominately bilateral, fracture of posterior atlas ring; type 3 fracture is combined injury of anterior and posterior arch of the atlas, the "classic Jefferson-fracture." In stable injuries, the transverse atlantal ligament is intact (type 3a); in type 3b these fractures are associated with lesion of transverse atlantal ligament and are classified as unstable (type 3b). Type 4 fractures are fractures of lateral mass, and type 5 fractures are isolated fractures of C1 transverse process.

TREATMENT OF "UNSTABLE" C1 FRACTURES

Hein defined an unstable fracture of C1 as a fracture of the anterior and posterior arches of the atlas associated with rupture of the TAL and an incongruence of the atlantooccipital and atlantoaxial facet joints. While this definition has been accepted for decades, it has been reexamined recently. Injuries causing failure of the TAL without a C1 fracture are caused by flexion with distraction. C1 fractures can have TAL injuries, but these are caused by axial loading mechanisms, as shown by Oda et al. TAL injuries from axial load mechanisms have been shown to have preservation of the joint capsules and alar ligaments, which is an important difference from TAL injuries caused by flexion as described by Dickman (see above) in which the alar ligaments, C0-C1 facet capsules, and other ligaments also are disrupted. This explains why lateral mass displacement reduces with traction and why external immobilization can be successful in achieving stability when TAL injuries are present by MRI in association with Jefferson fractures. The characterization of C1 fractures as "unstable" based on the presence of TAL disruption is based on an oversimplification of the anatomy and may not be an adequate criterion for operative intervention. Studies by Shatsky et al. and Kandziora et al. describe their experience with primary C1 osteosynthesis in patients with wide displacement of the C1 lateral mass with or without associated TAL failure. Ruf et al. described a transoral technique for primary fracture stabilization without fusion, but the indication for this technique remains to be determined at this time given reliable outcomes with immobilization. For the rare patient who requires operative stabilization as primary treatment or after failed immobilization, posterior C1-C2 fusion is done (see Technique 5.6); however, primary C1 osteosynthesis also is used.

POSTERIOR PRIMARY OSTEOSYNTHESIS OF C1

TECHNIQUE 5.7

SHATSKY ET AL.

- Move the awake patient to the rotating frame table and place him or her supine for induction of general anesthesia. Use a Mayfield pinion head holder to avoid pressure on the eyes, and rotate the patient prone. Open the mouth widely with dressing sponges to allow an open-mouth anteroposterior view and rotate the table.
- Shave the head to the level of the inion (posterior occipital protuberance).
- Place the table in a reverse Trendelenburg position and tape the patient's shoulders to apply traction to the fracture and reduce it by ligamentotaxis.
- Prepare and drape the posterior head and neck.
- Score the skin sharply from foramen magnum to the C2 level and inject dilute epinephrine solution (1 mg in 500 mL injectable saline) through the score incision into the dermis and paraspinal musculature.
- Complete the skin incision sharply and then use electrocautery to dissect to the spinous processes of the C1 level.
- Expose the posterior ring of C1 laterally a distance of 15 mm from the midline or to the vertebral artery sulcus, whichever is less. Take care to keep the electrocautery on the ring of C1 and do not cauterize the atlantooccipital membrane, which is thin.

- Expose only the caudal edge of the ring of C1 laterally to the point where the posterior arch meets the lateral mass. Then gently mobilize the venous plexus and C2 nerve caudally to allow exposure of the C1 lateral mass inferior to the posterior ring and vertebral artery.
- Using an image intensifier, verify that injury reduction is satisfactory on the open mouth and lateral views.
- Place the C1 screw as described by Goel and subsequently refined by Harms and Melcher. Using a hand drill placed just caudal to the ring of C1 and 3 to 4 mm lateral to the medial edge of the lateral mass, advance the drill at an angle of 10 degrees medially and slightly cephalad to a point just anterior to the anterior margin of the dens on a lateral image intensifier view. This allows bicortical screw placement. Careful preoperative planning is needed to lower the risk of injury to the internal carotid artery and hypoglossal nerve anterior to the C1 lateral mass.
- Place a polyaxial screw with a 10-mm smooth shank extension to the drilled depth. A monoaxial screw can be used and aids the reduction. Repeat on the contralateral side.
- Cut a rod and contour a slight bow into the rod. Place the rod between the 2 screws and tighten the blockers slightly. Compress the screws on the rod to better reduce the fracture if needed. Direct pressure to the neck by an unscrubbed assistant may also be helpful to reduce the fracture.
- Check final alignment and reduction on the open mouth and lateral views and complete final tightening of the blockers.
- Close the fascial layer over a drain.
- Close the wound in layers with a subcuticular skin closure.

POSTOPERATIVE CARE The patient is maintained in a rigid cervical orthosis for 8 to 12 weeks. The patient's clinical course and flexion and extension radiographs are used to verify stability and fusion progression. The drain is removed on the first postoperative day. Postoperative CT is used to evaluate adequacy of the reduction and screw placement.

AXIS FRACTURES

The most common fractures of the axis are those involving the odontoid process. The remaining fractures are those involving the isthmus (hangman fracture), which are the next most common fracture patterns of the axis body. Although any of these fracture types can occur with concomitant cervical injuries, they frequently occur as isolated fractures and are discussed separately. Odontoid fractures are especially common in the elderly, and in this patient group the most common mechanism is a low-energy fall.

ODONTOID FRACTURES

The classification of odontoid fractures described by Anderson and D'Alonzo in 1974 remains the most widely used system. Their scheme has three fracture types: type I, avulsion of the tip of the odontoid; type II, fracture through the base or waist of the odontoid process; and type III, originally described as fractures of the body below the base of the odontoid (Fig. 5.18). Additional fracture characteristics have been studied in numerous publications, including degree of initial fracture displacement, angulation through the fracture, patient age, fracture orientation, and smoking history of the patient. With respect to treatment outcomes, the primary factors that have been shown to be significant are fracture type, initial fracture displacement of 6 mm, and age (progressively worse outcomes are noted when patients are stratified by age).

TREATMENT

Many methods of treatment have been described for odontoid fractures, including no treatment, traction to reduce, followed by a collar, halo vest immobilization, anterior primary osteosynthesis, and posterior fusion of the C1-C2 joint. A multicenter review that included patients who did not receive treatment found that none of these patients went on to fracture union. Older literature described delayed myelopathy and death in patients with a history of untreated or nonunited odontoid fractures, indicating the importance of achieving fracture union. No level I evidence is available to make treatment recommendations; however, there is level III evidence on which treatment options can be based. Julien et al. found that type I and III fractures can be treated with rigid external immobilization such as a halo vest. One hundred percent union rates were reported for type I fractures, 65% for type II fractures, and 84% for type III fractures. Greene et al. noted an 80% union rate in type II fractures with immobilization, although in a small number the immobilization was extended beyond 13 weeks. The higher rate of success with immobilization in Greene et al.'s study may be because of early surgical treatment in 20 patients who had greater than 6 mm of displacement or more comminuted fractures that were not stable after initial halo placement. Again, this study found 100% union rates for type I fractures and 98.5% union rates for type III fractures treated with immobilization. Type III fractures treated with collars had substantially lower healing rates of 50% to 65% compared with union rates using halo vest immobilization. Collar immobilization has been found effective in type I fractures in several small series because this pattern is very infrequent.

There has been a clear trend in the United States away from use of the halo vest and toward surgical treatment of type II fractures, especially if they are displaced more than 5 mm and in elderly patients. There are conflicting reports as to whether surgical treatment improves or worsens outcomes, particularly in the elderly. In a multicenter retrospective study of 147 patients comparing nonoperative with various operative treatment options, De Bonis et al. found that surgery did not improve functional outcomes. Charles et al. found that age and comorbidities were the determinates of outcomes rather than treatment type. Robinson et al. reviewed registry information and found improved survival in surgically treated patients.

Our treatment regimen has been to use rigid immobilization for isolated type I and type III fractures. Most often halo vest immobilization is used, but rigid collars are an option especially for the rare type I fractures. For treatment of type II fractures that are minimally displaced, immobilization is recommended because it preserves motion at the highly mobile C1-C2 joint. If anatomic reduction is achieved and there is no loss of reduction after mobilization, fracture healing with preservation of motion can be expected in 80%. All patients treated with halo vest immobilization should be aggressively mobilized and made ambulatory if at all possible, especially elderly patients. Mortality rates as high as 42% have been reported in patients with halo vest immobilization who are nonambulatory and not mobilized. Schoenfeld et al. found that the mortality was the same at various time points whether patients were treated in a collar or with halo vest immobilization, suggesting that factors other than simply treatment with halo vest immobilization result in the high mortality rates

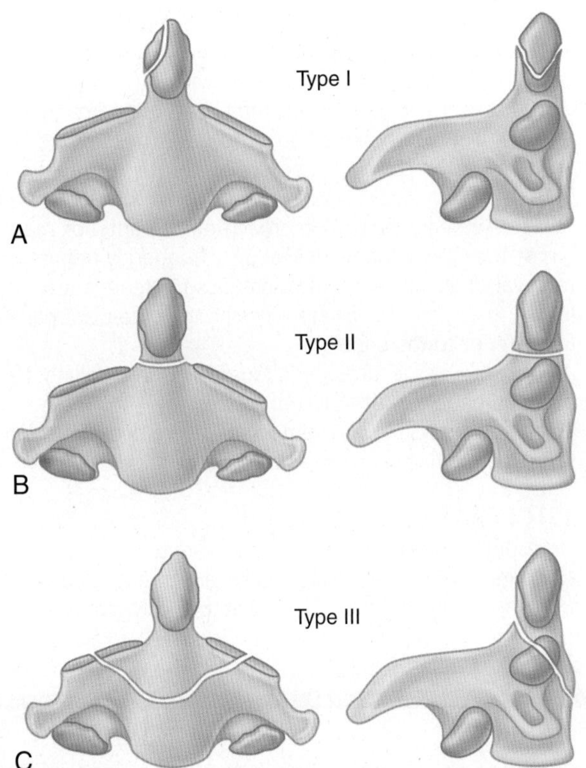

FIGURE 5.18 **A** to **C,** Three types of odontoid process fractures as seen in anteroposterior and lateral planes. Type I is oblique fracture through upper part of odontoid process. Type II is fracture at junction of odontoid process and body of second cervical vertebra. Type III is fracture through upper body of vertebra.

seen in elderly patients. More recently, DePasse et al. reported similar findings. In their study, Schoenfeld et al. found that patients with type II fractures treated operatively had lower mortality than those treated nonoperatively. Schoenfeld et al. did find a progressively higher mortality in both the operative and nonoperative treatment groups with age, and the benefits of surgery were in those age 74 years and younger. Wood et al. also found that operative benefits were greater in those under the age of 75 years. They also found that aspiration pneumonia was the most common cause of death in both operatively (55%) and nonoperatively (64%) treated patients. Vaccaro et al. showed in a level II study that neither operatively nor nonoperatively treated geriatric patients returned to their preinjury functional levels. The surgically treated patients had a smaller loss than those treated nonoperatively, but the study was not randomized. Graffeo et al. found no survival advantage for operative over nonoperative care at any time point. They reported a 41% 1-year mortality in 111 patients with an average age of 87 years.

We generally reserve operative treatment for type II fractures in patients in whom anatomic reduction cannot be achieved in traction or is not maintained with a rigid collar or halo vest after the patient is fully mobilized. Operative treatment also is recommended if initial fracture translation is 6 mm or more and in patients who are not expected to be able to mobilize because of other injuries and comorbidities. Several studies have noted a trend toward operative treatment of type II fractures in the elderly in particular. This recommendation is based on level III evidence. In these patients, posterior C1-C2 fusion or anterior primary osteosynthesis may be recommended. The primary advantage of anterior fracture fixation is maintenance of motion at C1-C2, which accounts for 50% of cervical rotation, and expected acute fracture union rates of 80% to 95%. Posterior fusion of C1-C2 sacrifices this motion but can reliably achieve stability in 85% to 98% of patients and is preferred by some authors. Anterior screw fixation is not appropriate for nonunions that are treated with posterior fusion. Ni et al. described a technique of posterior instrumentation without fusion as a salvage method when anterior osteosynthesis is not possible; instrumentation is removed once fracture healing is complete. The Neck Disability Index (NDI) scores were improved, as was range of motion after hardware removal. The C1 screw was placed using the Resnick modification for screw entry point.

ANTERIOR ODONTOID SCREW FIXATION

Anterior screw fixation can be accomplished with a single-screw or two-screw technique. Comparable union rates of 81% and 85% for the single-screw and two-screw techniques, respectively, have been reported. More important than the number of screws used is the orientation of the fracture and proper technique to achieve a lag-screw effect with compression across the fracture. Fractures that are transverse or oblique from anterosuperior to posteroinferior are best suited for this technique because the compression from the screw(s) will be applied perpendicular to the fracture line. This technique is challenging because obtaining an anatomic reduction requires visualization on anteroposterior and lateral dual image intensifiers that are both draped into the operative field simultaneously (Fig. 5.19).

TECHNIQUE 5.8

(ETTER)

- Position the patient supine on the operating table and induce general anesthesia.
- Use an adjustable or a removable head support to allow cervical extension in traction. This usually will reduce even posteriorly displaced fractures. Apply traction with either a head halter, Gardner-Wells tongs, or a halo ring.
- Anatomic reduction must be obtained before internal fixation with the cannulated screw system.
- A nasogastric tube can be inserted to allow localization of the esophagus to help prevent perforation.
- Use a padded occipital ring attached to the operating table to stabilize the patient's head. The head and neck must be positioned to allow maximal access to the anterior cervical spine. A large vertical mandibular-sternal distance is required because of the size of the instrumentation and the steep inferior angle of approach necessary for screw placement. With traction applied even posteriorly displaced fractures will usually reduce in maximal cervical extension. This position improves access to the C2 level. High-resolution fluoroscopic image intensification in the anteroposterior and lateral planes using two

machines is necessary for insertion of the screws. Place cotton sponges in the mouth to maximally open the jaw for an adequate open-mouth view (Fig. 5.19A).

- Before beginning the surgical procedure, confirm a free working path for the instrumentation by placing a long Kirschner wire along the side of the neck in the direction of the intended screw placement and confirm safe trajectory on the lateral image intensifier view. If clearance of the sternum is inadequate, modify the patient's position (Fig. 5.19B–D).
- Prepare and drape the operative field in a sterile fashion, with sterile draping of both the image intensifiers into the field.
- Make an anteromedial approach to the cervical spine through a transverse skin incision 6 to 7 cm long at the level of the C5-C6 disc space as determined using the Kirschner wire.
- Because of the steep angle of inclination required relative to the anterior plane of the neck, undermine the subcutaneous fat superficial to the platysma 1 to 2 cm cephalad to the skin incision. Divide the platysma muscle vertically in line with its fibers 2 to 3 cm lateral to the midline.
- Bluntly dissect the pretracheal fascia and develop an interval between the carotid sheath laterally and the strap muscles overlying the trachea and esophagus medially.
- Bluntly develop the prevertebral space anteriorly along the front of the cervical spine until the anteroinferior margin of the C2 body is reached.
- Place a radiolucent retractor on the anterior body of C2, gently retracting the trachea and esophagus to allow direct visualization of the C2 disc. Delineate the C2-C3 intervertebral disc space and vertically incise the anterior longitudinal ligament at this level, confirming the desired entry point on the anteroposterior view for the screw(s). Ligation of the superior thyroid artery may be necessary for exposure of the C2-C3 level.
- Identify with lateral image intensification the entry site through the C2 endplate and *not* through the body at the anterior margin just proximal to the endplate (Fig. 5.19E).
- Using a long drill sleeve, insert one or two 1.2-mm Kirschner wires. If one screw is planned it should be placed midline on the anteroposterior view. If using two screws, the guidewires should converge slightly but remain separated enough to allow both to fully penetrate the tip of the odontoid. On the lateral view, wire entry is at the anterior edge of the endplate and oriented to exit just posterior to the tip of the odontoid. Check advancement of the wire frequently to confirm proper trajectory. Redirecting these wires after incorrect placement is difficult.
- Verify penetration of the dens cortex and appropriate wire alignment by image intensification in two planes.
- Measure directly the guidewire insertion depth. Insert the cannulated drill bit for the cannulated 3.5-mm screw over each guidewire and drill the length of the wire to penetrate the tip of the odontoid. Monitor frequently on image intensifier views to avoid advancing the guidewire toward the brainstem. Also make certain the drill is perfectly aligned in both planes with the wire to avoid wire fracture attributed to binding with the drill bit.
- Insert self-tapping, partially threaded 3.5-mm screws of appropriate length over each guidewire and advance them with the cannulated screwdriver until the opposing apical cortical bone is secured again, using image intensifier views to make sure not to advance the wire as the screw advances, which occurs easily after drilling (Fig. 5.19F).
- The screw heads tend to encroach on the anterior margin of the C2-C3 intervertebral disc, frequently requiring removal of a small amount of annulus to create a recess. Ideally, the screw heads are recessed into the disc space just inferior to the endplate.
- Always use tissue protection guards during drilling to avoid damage to soft-tissue structures.
- Close the platysma and remaining layers over a fluted style drain, which is removed the following day.

POSTOPERATIVE CARE The patient is observed closely for respiratory status in the intensive care unit for the first 24 hours after surgery. A rigid cervical orthosis is applied and is worn for 6 to 8 weeks. The orthosis may be removed for eating. Clinical and radiographic evaluations are performed at 6, 12, and 24 weeks.

POSTERIOR C1-C2 FUSION TECHNIQUES

The preferred method for C1-C2 fusion for most injuries is to use a polyaxial screw placed in the C1 lateral mass and an isthmic screw placed at C2 with autologous iliac bone graft (Fig. 5.20). This is a stable construct and can be used in the presence of a posterior ring fracture of C1. Wiring techniques are less rigid but have proven effective for many years when done properly and in the appropriate setting. The Gallie technique creates a posteriorly directed force on C1 and can be used with TAL injuries and other injuries that require a posterior force vector to maintain the reduction. The Gallie technique does not resist rotational forces well because the fixation is midline. The Brooks bone-block technique does resist rotation forces but does not create the posteriorly directed vector.

POSTERIOR C1-C2 FUSION USING ROD AND SCREW CONSTRUCT WITH C1 LATERAL MASS SCREWS

TECHNIQUE 5.9

(HARMS)

- Move the awake supine patient to the rotating frame table and induce general anesthesia. Use a Mayfield pinion head holder to avoid pressure on the eyes and rotate the patient prone.
- Shave the head to the level of the inion (posterior occipital protuberance).
- Prepare and drape the posterior head and neck, as well as the posterior iliac crest donor site.

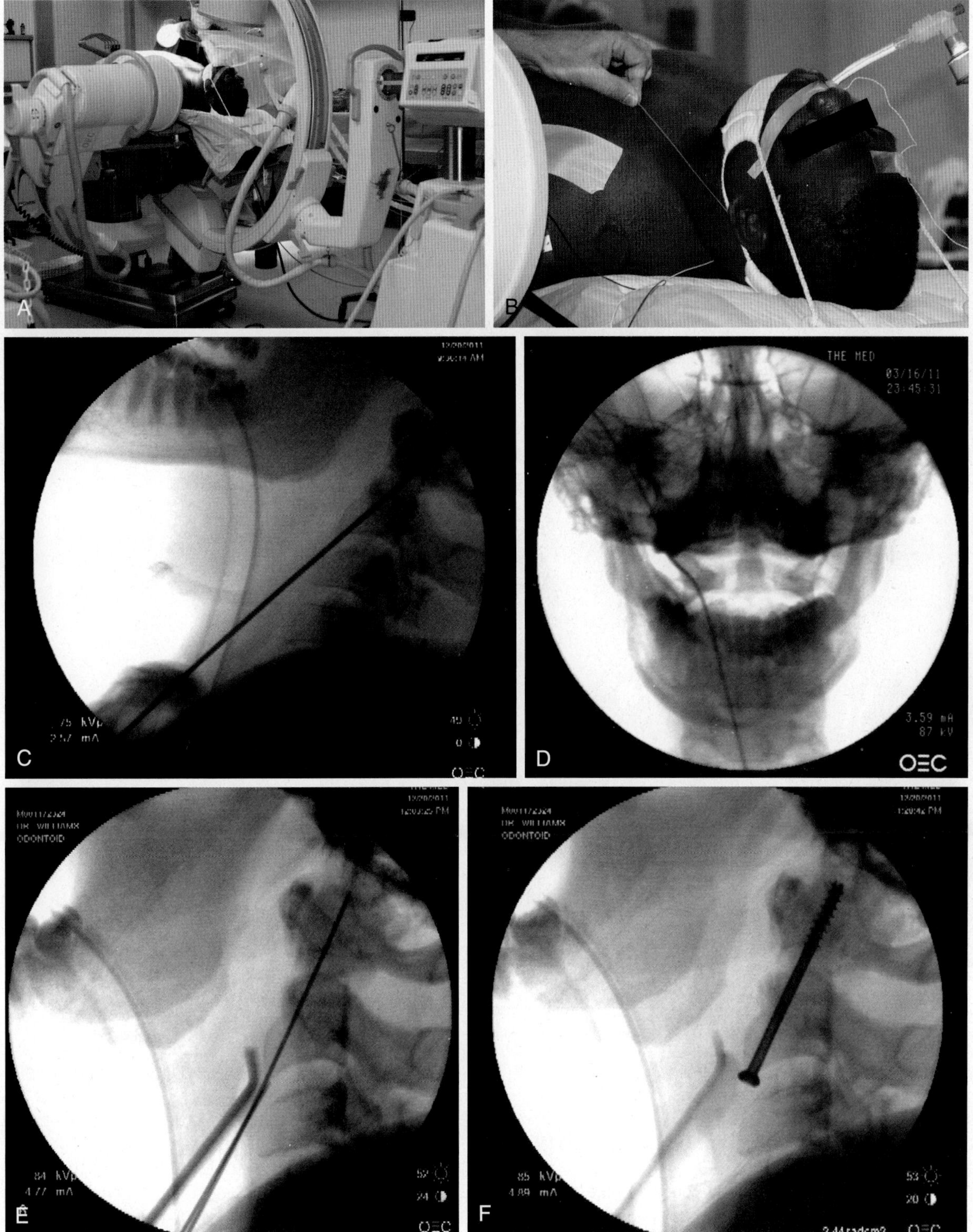

FIGURE 5.19 Odontoid fracture. **A,** Patient positioned with traction applied and image intensifiers for open-mouth and lateral images in position. **B,** Wire held in place while lateral view is obtained to indicate level of incision placement. **C,** Image with wire held in place. **D,** Open-mouth view. **E,** Lateral view after placement of first guidewire. **F,** Bicortical screw placement. **SEE TECHNIQUE 5.8.**

- Score the skin sharply from the foramen magnum to the C3 level and inject dilute epinephrine solution (1 mg in 500 mL normal saline) through the score incision into the dermis and paraspinal musculature.
- Complete the skin incision sharply and then use electrocautery to dissect to the skull and spinous processes to the C3 level.
- Using Cobb elevators and electrocautery subperiosteally, expose the occiput just above the foramen magnum bilaterally.

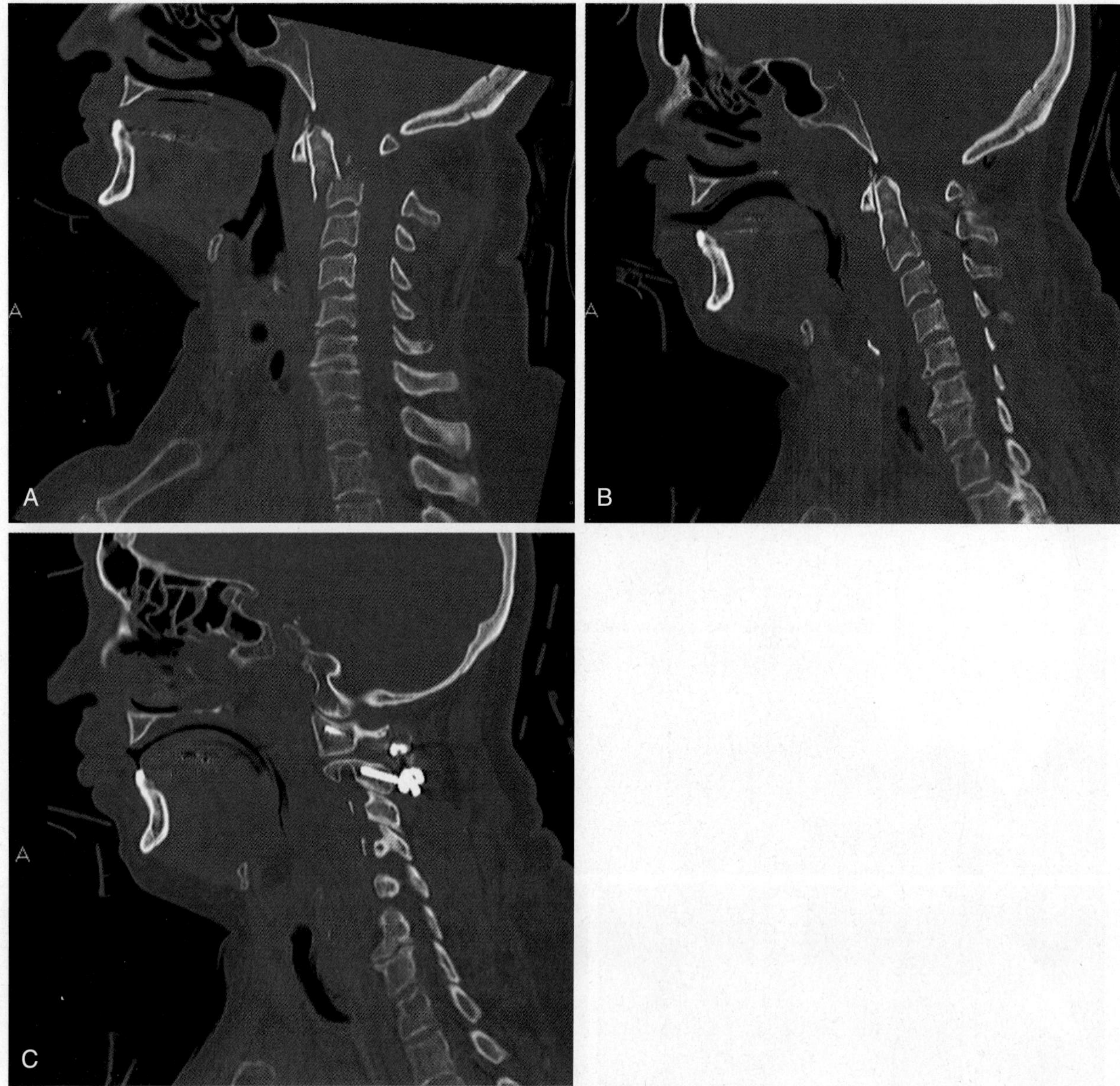

FIGURE 5.20 **A,** Anterior displaced odontoid fracture. **B,** Anatomic reduction achieved. **C,** C1 lateral mass screw and C2 isthmus screw in good position.

- Expose the posterior ring of C1 laterally a distance of 15 mm from the midline or to the vertebral artery sulcus, whichever is less. Take care to keep the electrocautery on the ring of C1 and do not cauterize the atlantooccipital membrane, which is thin.
- Expose the bifid portion of the C2 spinous process and elevate the muscular attachments subperiosteally so that at closure the two sides can be sutured through bone to the spinous process of C2.
- Expose the C2 spinous process, laminae, and entire lateral mass bilaterally, preserving the facet capsule at C2-C3.
- The C2 spinal nerve (greater occipital nerve) crosses posterior to the C2 isthmus in a dense venous plexus. Using bipolar cautery and a small angled curet, gently mobilize this plexus cephalad beginning at the upper lateral margin of the C2 lamina until the medial border of the C2 isthmus is visible. Expect bleeding during this step, which can be significant and can be controlled with Gelfoam or Surgicel and cottonoids. Positioning the patient in a reverse Trendelenburg also helps reduce this venous bleeding. Some authors advocate sacrificing the nerve, but in our experience this is unnecessary.
- In similar fashion, expose only the caudal edge of the ring of C1 laterally to a point even with the C2 isthmus and then mobilize the venous plexus and C2 nerve caudally to allow exposure of the C1 lateral mass inferior to the posterior ring and vertebral artery.
- Using an image intensifier, verify that injury reduction is satisfactory.
- The C1 screw is placed as described by Goel and subsequently refined by Harms and Melcher. Using a hand drill placed just caudal to the ring of C1 and 3 to 4 mm lateral to the medial edge of the lateral mass, advance the drill at an angle of 10 degrees medially and slightly cephalad to a point just posterior to the anterior margin of the dens on a lateral image intensifier view. This allows for unicorti-

cal screw placement and lowers the risk of injury to the internal carotid artery and hypoglossal nerve anterior to the C1 lateral mass.

- Place a polyaxial screw with a 10-mm smooth shank extension to the drilled depth.
- The C2 isthmic screw is placed in a method similar to that described by Magerl. Place a Penfield No. 4 elevator to allow a view of the isthmus medial cortex and determine the line of entry points on the inferior facet of C2 that will allow the medially directed drill to enter the isthmus. Using the lateral image intensifier view, select the point on this line that will orient the drill up the center of the isthmus. A high-speed burr is used to penetrate only the cortex at that point. Typically, the drill will be directed 25 degrees medially and 20 to 30 degrees cephalad, but anatomy varies considerably and careful review of the CT scan is required. Direct the hand drill up the isthmus under fluoroscopic control to a point at the posterior margin of the C2 foramen transversarium as seen on the lateral image intensifier view (see Technique 5.4).
- Place the appropriate length polyaxial screw to stop at the posterior foramen transversarium. In our experience, this gives excellent fixation without placing the vertebral artery at risk by crossing the foramen transversarium into the C2 body.
- Cut and contour the rod as desired. Place the rod and tighten the blocker screws securely.
- Harvest iliac bone graft as described in Technique 1.7.
- Decorticate the laminae of C1 and C2 using a high-speed burr.
- Carefully place morselized autologous bone graft over the decorticated areas. Avoid packing the bone over the atlantooccipital membrane because compression here may result in apnea from brainstem compression. For this same reason, final hemostasis should be meticulous. Decorticating and packing the facet significantly increases bleeding risk and with autograft usually is not necessary.
- Check final alignment and reduction.
- Close the fascial layer over a drain, securely incorporating bone at the C2 spinous process level.
- Close the wound in layers with a subcuticular skin closure.

POSTOPERATIVE CARE The patient is maintained in a rigid cervical orthosis for 8 to 12 weeks. The patient's clinical course and flexion and extension radiographs are used to verify stability and fusion progression. The drain is removed on the first postoperative day.

POSTERIOR C1-C2 FUSION WITH C2 TRANSLAMINAR SCREWS

This technique was described in 2004 as an alternative technique with less risk for vertebral artery injury, although there are other risks such as dural or spinal cord injuries. When the procedure is done properly, these are small risks. The technique employs two crossing screws inserted through the base of the C2 spinous process and contained within the lamina on the contralateral side. The screws must be placed with one slightly more caudal on one side and directed cephalad at a steeper angle than the other screw. The translaminar screws are then connected to the C1 lateral mass screws. Biomechanically, this method has equivalence to the Harms technique for C1-C2 fusion but not for occiput-C2 fusion. If the construct is to extend below C2, rod contouring can be problematic because the translaminar screws are not as well aligned with the lateral mass screws. Generally, this method is used if anatomic constraints preclude C2 isthmic screw placement, such as with known vertebral artery injuries preoperatively.

TECHNIQUE 5.10

(WRIGHT)

- Patient preparation, positioning, and administration of anesthesia are as described in Technique 5.7.
- Use lateral image intensification to check the reduction of the C1-C2 complex.
- Perform posterior midline exposure of the cervical spine from the occiput to C2 as described in Technique 5.7.
- Place the C1 lateral mass screws as described in Technique 5.6.
- Fully expose the caudal edge of the C2 lamina at the midline and extend it laterally.
- Use an angled curet to detach the ligamentum flavum from the ventral surface and the cephalad and caudal margin of C2 so that a Penfield No. 4 dissector or other blunt instrument can be used to palpate the anterior C2 lamina during screw placement.
- With a Penfield No. 4 dissector or blunt hook ventral to the lamina, use the drill to penetrate the cortex at the base of the C2 spinous process contralateral to the Penfield dissector at the location determined preoperatively to allow room for both screws. Using the Penfield dissector as a guide, maintain the drill posterior to the canal and advance it laterally into the C2 inferior articular mass. The drill should not penetrate the posterior or anterior cortex as it is advanced. Screw lengths usually are 25 to 35 mm.
- Place the contralateral screw similarly.
- Contour the rod to engage the C1 lateral mass screws and secure the connections.
- Decorticate and place autologous bone graft as described in Technique 5.6.
- Close the wound in layers over a drain, taking care to reattach the fascia to bone at the C2 level. Use a subcuticular skin closure.

POSTOPERATIVE CARE Postoperative immobilization with a halo vest usually is unnecessary. A cervical collar may be worn for 8 to 12 weeks. The drain is removed on the first postoperative day.

POSTERIOR C1-C2 TRANSARTICULAR SCREWS

The use of C1-C2 transarticular screw fixation as described by Magerl and Seemann preceded the Harms method and provides more rigid fixation than traditional posterior wiring methods, such as the Gallie or Brooks-Jenkins method. Transarticular screw placement is technically difficult, and there are clearly some patients who cannot be treated with this method because of anatomic constraints that are present in as many as 23% of patients. A properly placed transarticular screw passes through the C2 isthmus and crosses the C1-C2 facet joint and into the anterior portion of the C1 lateral mass (Fig. 5.21). Careful review of the C2 anatomy is required because in some people the vertebral artery is too medial to allow screw placement or the isthmus is too small to accept the screw. Other structures at risk include the internal carotid artery and hypoglossal nerve, which typically lie less than 3 mm anterior to the C1 lateral mass and can be injured if the screw is too long. Additionally, the patient's body habitus can make the necessary approach angle difficult if there is excessive cervicothoracic kyphosis.

TECHNIQUE 5.11

(MAGERL AND SEEMANN)

- Careful preoperative planning is needed to assess safety of screw placement.
- Patient preparation, positioning, and administration of anesthesia are as described in Technique 5.6.
- Use lateral image intensification to check the reduction of the C1-C2 complex and fracture reduction.
- Perform midline posterior cervical exposure from occiput to C3 as described in Technique 5.6. The exposure should be to the lateral edge of the C2 lateral mass.
- Expose the medial wall of the isthmus up to the C1-C2 joint. If possible, curet or burr the joint. The area around the greater occipital nerve is highly vascular.
- Place intraarticular bone graft if desired; however, expect significant venous bleeding. With posterior autograft, the intraarticular graft is not required.
- Identify the landmarks for the entry portal of the transarticular screw at the lower medial edge of the inferior articular process of C2 (Fig. 5.21A). Determine the proper trajectory of the screw and make a stab incision in the skin if needed to attain the correct trajectory, which may be at C7.
- Using a 2-mm bit, incrementally drill through the isthmus near its posteromedial surface, exiting from the articular surface of C2 at the posterior aspect of the superior articular surface and entering the lateral mass of the atlas through the articular surface. If the isthmus is oriented too medially, the exiting drill will miss the C1 lateral mass or the drill will exit the isthmus laterally and risk injuring the vertebral artery. The drill bit should just perforate the anterior cortex of the lateral mass of C1 (Fig. 5.21B).
- Determine the appropriate screw length (Fig. 5.21C). Use a 3.5-mm cortical tap to cut threads in the drill hole and insert the appropriate 3.5-mm cortical screw across the C1-C2 joint. Typically, screws are 34 to 43 mm in length. Take care not to extend more than 1 mm anterior to the C1 lateral mass to reduce the risk to the internal carotid artery and hypoglossal nerve. Cannulated screws can be used.
- After placing the C1-C2 transarticular screws, perform a traditional posterior C1-C2 fusion using either the Gallie or the Brooks technique if intraarticular grafting was not possible (Fig. 5.21D).
- Close the wound in layers over a drain, taking care to reattach the fascia to bone at the C2 level. Use a subcuticular skin closure.

POSTOPERATIVE CARE Because this technique provides excellent rotational stability, postoperative immobilization with a halo vest usually is unnecessary. A cervical collar may be worn for 8 to 12 weeks. The drain is removed on the first postoperative day.

POSTERIOR C1-C2 FUSION USING THE MODIFIED GALLIE POSTERIOR WIRING TECHNIQUE

TECHNIQUE 5.12

(GALLIE, MODIFIED)

- Patient positioning, administration of anesthesia, preparation, and exposure are as described in Technique 5.6.
- After exposing the C2 spinous process, laminae, and entire lateral mass bilaterally, and preserving the facet capsule at C2-C3, use a small angled curet to dissect the ventral side of the C1 lamina to allow for midline sublaminar wire passage.
- Cut a 24-inch length of 20-gauge wire and bend it tightly back onto itself at its midpoint to create a loop. Contour the loop of wire into a "C" shape.
- Pass the loop of 20-gauge wire from caudal to rostral sublaminarly at the C1 level. Flatten the curve in the wire as needed to minimize intrusion of the wire into the spinal canal. A small blunt hook passed from the rostral side can be used to engage the loop of wire and pull the wire so that intrusion of the wire is minimized as it is advanced rostrally. Alternatively, pass a suture to tie to the wire and use this to pull the wire rostrally.
- Pass the free ends of the sublaminar wire through the looped portion and tighten the wire around the C1 lamina in the midline at the rostral margin of the C1 ring.
- Make a hole through the base of the spinous process of C2 using a towel clip or bone tenaculum.
- Harvest a corticocancellous bone graft and notch it on one side to fit over the rostral edge of the C2 spinous process. Decorticate the C1 and C2 laminae and place the graft as an onlay type graft.
- There are a number of variations described for using a single wire or two wires to secure the only graft (Fig 5.22).

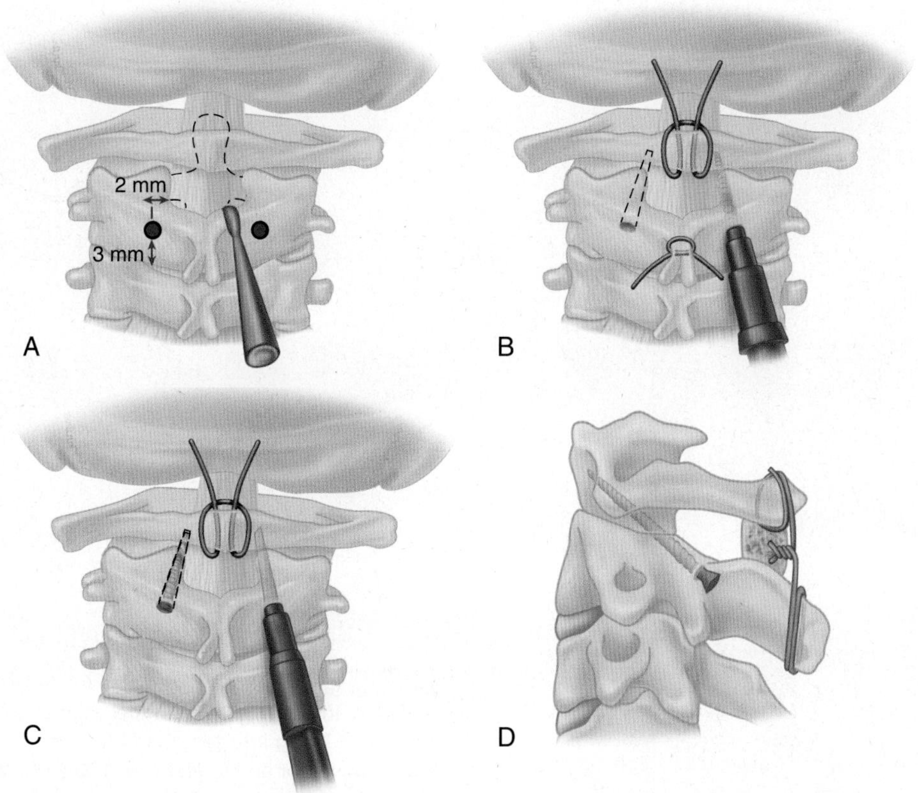

FIGURE 5.21 C1-C2 transarticular screw fixation (Magerl and Seemann). **A,** Landmarks for entry point of transarticular screw. **B,** Wires are brought around arch of C1 and spinous process of C2 to manipulate these two vertebrae. Screw holes are drilled through isthmus near its posterior and medial surface of C2 and outer lateral mass of atlas. **C,** Measuring screw length and tapping with 3.5-mm cortical tap. **D,** Proper screw placement for C1-C2 fusion. **SEE TECHNIQUE 5.11.**

With any of the wiring techniques, use a wire twister and tighten until the wire just begins to change luster.
- Check final alignment and reduction.
- Close the fascial layer securely over a drain, incorporating bone at the C2 spinous process level.
- Close the wound in layers with a subcuticular skin closure.

POSTOPERATIVE CARE The patient is maintained in a halo vest for 10 to 12 weeks. The patient's clinical course and flexion and extension radiographs are used to verify stability and fusion progression. The drain is removed on the first postoperative day.

POSTERIOR C1-C2 WIRING

Wiring techniques are seldom used as the primary method of stabilization, but they remain useful for adjunctive stabilization and to maintain corticocancellous grafts in position. The Brooks and Jenkins method provides a bone block between the arch of C1 and the C2 lamina. The wires are located laterally and provide more rotational stability than is provided by the midline Gallie wiring.

TECHNIQUE 5.13

(BROOKS AND JENKINS)
- Patient preparation, positioning, and administration of anesthesia are as described in Technique 5.7.
- Expose the C1-C2 level through a midline incision.
- Use a small-angled curet to clear the ventral surface of the C1 and C2 lamina.
- Use an aneurysm needle to pass a No. 2 Mersilene suture on each side of the midline in a cephalad to caudal direction, first under the arch of the atlas and then under the lamina of the axis (Fig. 5.23A). These sutures serve tethers to pull two doubled 20-gauge stainless steel wires into place. Cut the wire to a 24-inch length and fold it back on itself at the midpoint to create a loop. Alternatively, braided cables can be passed in place of the wires to increase flexibility and strength significantly. The suture is tied to the wire or cable, which is then pulled, using the suture to maintain tension on the wire or cable to minimize canal intrusion as it is passed.

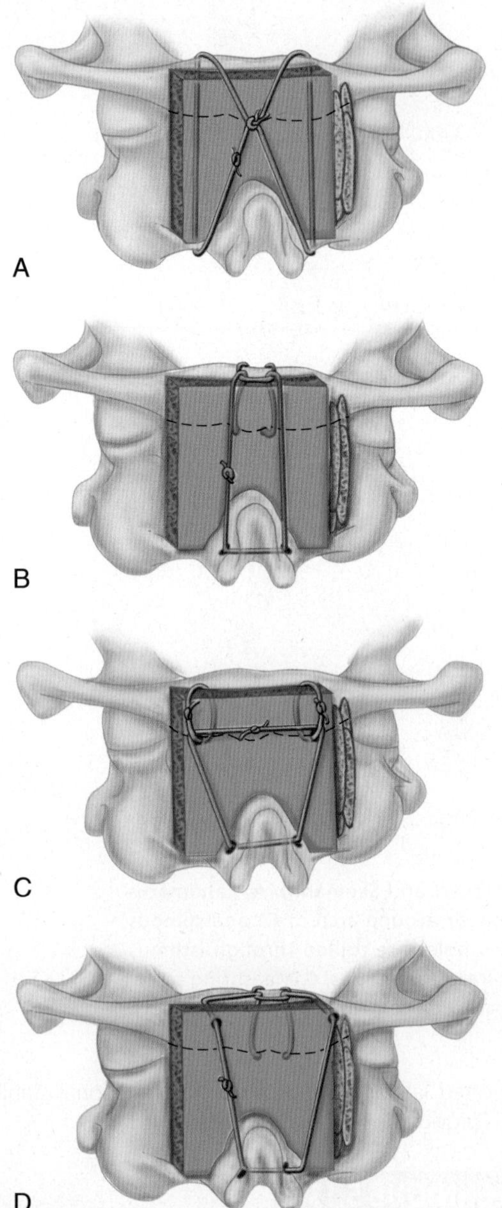

FIGURE 5.22 Modified Gallie method of using wires to hold graft in place. **A,** Wire passes under lamina of atlas and axis and is tied over graft. **B,** Wire passes under lamina of atlas and through the spinous process of axis and is tied over graft. **C,** Wire passes through holes drilled in lamina of atlas and through spine of axis; holes are drilled through graft. **D,** Wire passes under lamina of atlas and through spine of axis; holes are drilled through graft. **SEE TECHNIQUE 5.12.**

- Obtain a thick corticocancellous rectangular bone graft approximately 1.5 × 4.0 cm from the iliac crest. Divide the graft in half along the short axis. Bevel the grafts to fit snugly into the interval between the arch of the atlas and each lamina of the axis with the cancellous portion of the graft in contact with the decorticated portion of the ring of C1 and the lamina of C2 (Fig. 5.23B).
- While holding the grafts in position on each side of the midline and maintaining the width of the interlaminar space, tighten the doubled wires over them and twist and tie the wires to secure the grafts (Fig. 5.23C and D).
- Irrigate and close the wound in layers over suction drain.

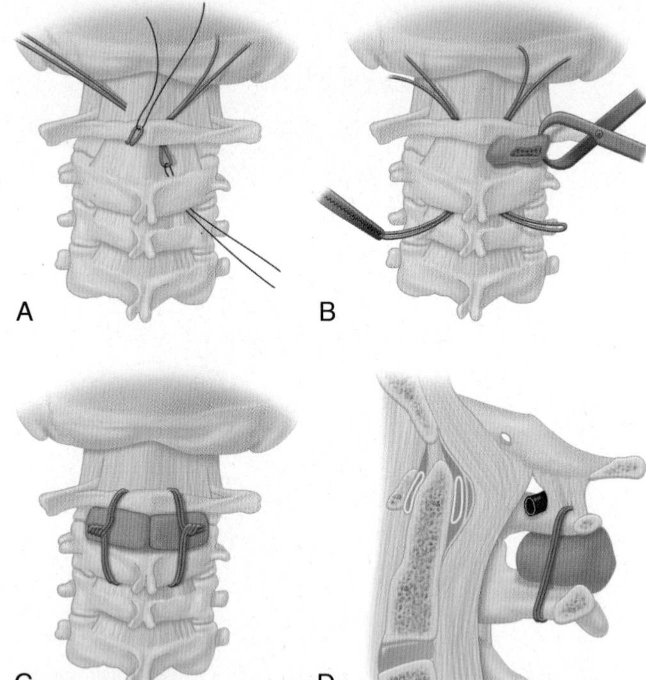

FIGURE 5.23 Brooks and Jenkins technique of atlantoaxial fusion. **A,** Insertion of wires under atlas and axis. **B,** Wires in place with graft being inserted. **C** and **D,** Bone grafts secured by wires (anteroposterior and lateral views). **SEE TECHNIQUE 5.23.**

POSTOPERATIVE CARE When used as a primary fusion method, halo vest immobilization is continued for 10 to 12 weeks. If wiring is adjunctive, immobilization is based on the primary stabilization method.

TRAUMATIC SPONDYLOLISTHESIS OF THE AXIS (HANGMAN FRACTURE)

Fractures of the posterior elements of the axis through the isthmic portion or pars interarticularis are relatively common. The usual mechanism causing this fracture pattern is hyperextension and axial loading, although some injury patterns involve flexion as well. Effendi et al. classified the injury into three types based on the apparent mechanism of injury and the radiographic characteristics. Type I injury is caused by hyperextension and is minimally displaced (0 to 2 mm of translation of the C2 body relative to C3) with no kyphosis through the disc space. Type II injury is caused by hyperextension and axial loading followed by flexion. The fracture line is relatively vertical in orientation with at least 3 mm of translation through the C2 disc. Levine and Edwards modified the Effendi type II fracture to include a flexion-distraction injury that has a relatively horizontal fracture line and significant kyphosis through the C2 disc with posterior annulus disruption but minimal translation of C2 on C3 (Fig. 5.24). Type III fractures are flexion-compression injuries, and in addition to the traumatic spondylolisthesis, dislocation of the C2-C3

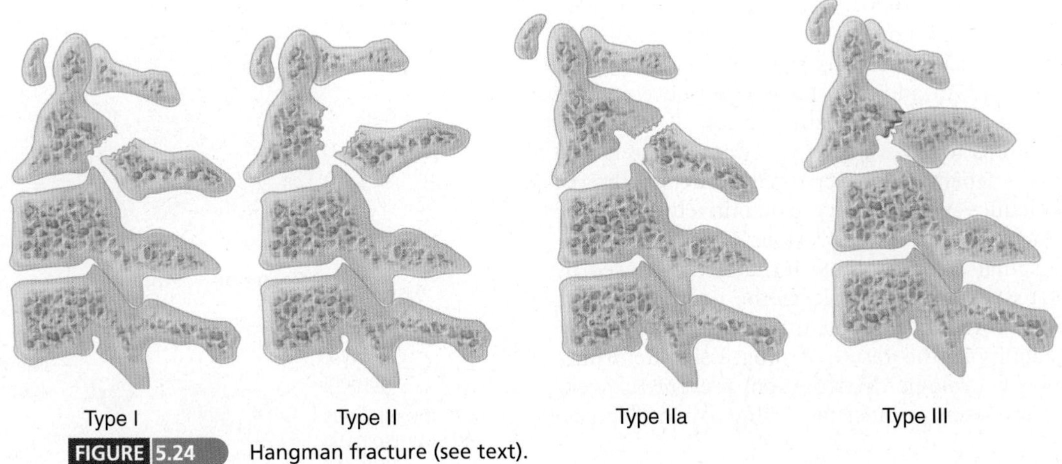

FIGURE 5.24 Hangman fracture (see text).

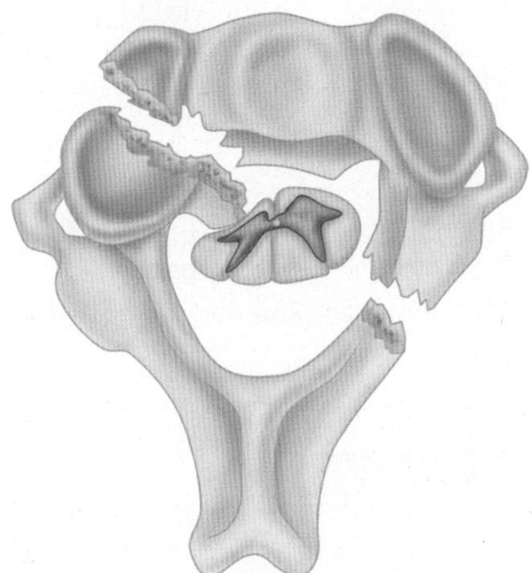

FIGURE 5.25 Atypical hangman fracture with cord impingement described by Starr and Eismont.

facet joints occurs. One additional fracture pattern of note, reported by Starr and Eismont, occurs when the fracture extends into the posterior body of the axis on one or both sides. This variant is important because it is associated with a higher rate of neurologic injury (Fig. 5.25).

TREATMENT

Treatment of traumatic spondylolisthesis of the axis is based on fracture type, and immobilization of the fracture usually is adequate. Francis et al. reported that 95 of 123 patients healed satisfactorily with immobilization. In most series, operative treatment was performed for patients with radiographic instability despite appropriate external bracing, for patients with type III injuries, and for patients demonstrating instability after immobilization. A recent systematic review by Murphy et al. concluded that union rates were slightly higher (99% vs. 94%) with a variety of surgical treatments compared to a variety of nonoperative treatments. Mortality was not significantly different between the two groups. No specific recommendations could be made.

Type I injuries generally do not have associated ligamentous injuries, given the mechanism, and can be treated with a rigid collar. Type II and IIa injuries must be distinguished from one another because treatment is quite different. Type II injury usually can be reduced with traction if necessary, and then the patient is placed in a halo vest for 12 weeks. The patient with a type IIa fracture should not be placed in traction because of the posterior discal disruption, which allows for overdistraction and potential neurologic injury. Type IIa injuries should be reduced with gentle manual extension and slight compression, and the patient is maintained in a halo vest for 12 weeks. Type III fracture-dislocations require open reduction of the dislocation because the arch fragment cannot be controlled with traction because of the fracture. In some patients, direct stabilization of the fracture with C2 pedicle screws placed as described earlier is possible as definitive treatment. More commonly, these screws are combined with C3 lateral mass screws and a rod construct to accomplish fusion at the C2-C3 level. If the C2 level cannot be stabilized with screw placement, a C1-C3 fusion with lateral mass screws at each level is recommended. Anterior C2-C3 stabilization is an option. The Starr and Eismont variant is treated in traction initially and then halo vest immobilization for 12 weeks. If reduction cannot be maintained, posterior fusion using C2 isthmic or pedicle screws and C3 lateral mass screws with a rod construct is most appropriate. This posterior fixation is biomechanically more stable than anterior C2-C3 stabilization. Placement of this instrumentation is described in Technique 5.9 and placement of lateral mass screws is described below.

SUBAXIAL CERVICAL SPINE INJURY (C3-T1)

CLASSIFICATION

Although the axis is the individual vertebra most commonly injured, the subaxial region of the cervical spine accounts for about 65% of all cervical spine injuries and most cervical spinal cord injuries. Despite the relatively high incidence of subaxial injuries (C3-T1), the optimal management often is not clear from existing medical literature. There are several reasons for this, including development of improved surgical methods and options with improved outcomes and lower morbidities. Also, no ideal classification system exists that allows reproducible and valid characterization of specific injuries that are required to compare treatments and outcomes. There have been many efforts to classify these injuries, and improvements continue to be made. Central to any classification is the concept of spinal stability, which classically has been defined by White and Panjabi as "the ability of the spine under physiologic loads to maintain an association between vertebral segments in such a way that there is neither damage nor subsequent irritation of the spinal cord or nerve roots, and, in addition, there is no development of incapacitating deformity or pain because of structural changes." The ability to make a determination of current and future stability is dependent on a complete understanding of spinal biomechanics and the ability to definitively determine the presence of injury to all the various anatomic components of the spinal column. Acute instability is caused by bone or soft-tissue injury that places the neural elements at risk of injury with any subsequent loading or deformity. Chronic instability is the result of progressive deformity that may cause neurologic deterioration, prevent recovery of injured neural tissue, or cause increasing pain or decreasing function.

In a series of cadaver studies, White and Panjabi systematically cut the various supporting structures and noted the resulting instabilities of the spine. The supporting structures of the subaxial spine can be divided into two groups: anterior and posterior (Fig. 5.26). A motion segment is made up of two adjacent vertebrae and the intervening soft tissues connected directly to each vertebra. If a motion segment has all the anterior elements and one posterior element, or all the posterior elements and one anterior element, it remains stable under physiologic loads. White, Southwick, and Panjabi developed a checklist for the diagnosis of clinical instability of the subaxial cervical spine (Box 5.2). This checklist includes radiographic criteria to consider in determination of clinical instability. Each criterion is assigned a point value, and if a total of 5 points is reached, clinical instability is likely. These criteria include sagittal translation of 3.5 mm on a lateral view (Fig. 5.27). An additional criterion is more than 11 degrees of difference in sagittal rotation between two adjacent motion segments (2 points) as measured on a lateral radiograph (Fig. 5.28).

This body of information and imaging capabilities continue to improve. The classification system described by Allen and Ferguson remains the most widely used, although several alternative systems have been described. The Allen and Ferguson system is based on a mechanistic description of the injury based on the radiographic appearance of the cervical spine. These authors reviewed 165 subaxial injuries and categorized them into six common patterns and then further subdivided each pattern into stages of severity of osseous and ligamentous injury (Table 5.4).

The terminology of this system has become familiar to spine surgeons and is accepted to describe injuries, but precise definitions of each stage are lacking, and the number of stages in the system make it difficult to use precisely in clinical practice. An alternative classification system was proposed by Moore et al. and subsequently modified by Vaccaro et al. and presented as the Subaxial Injury Classification (SLIC) scoring system. This particular system has three categories that are scored and summed. The authors proposed that the numerical value obtained can then be used to determine whether nonoperative or operative treatment should be performed. The categories that are scored are morphology, discoligamentous complex integrity, and neurologic status of the patient. An increasing score within each category is intended to reflect increasingly severe injury (Table 5.5). The primary improvement of this severity scoring system is the reincorporation of the neurologic status of the patient, which is integral to the determination of spinal stability. This severity score was compared with the Allen and Ferguson system among a group of experienced spine surgeons, and the two systems had similar reliability for treatment recommendations. With continued improvements in imaging, particularly of the soft-tissue components of the spine,

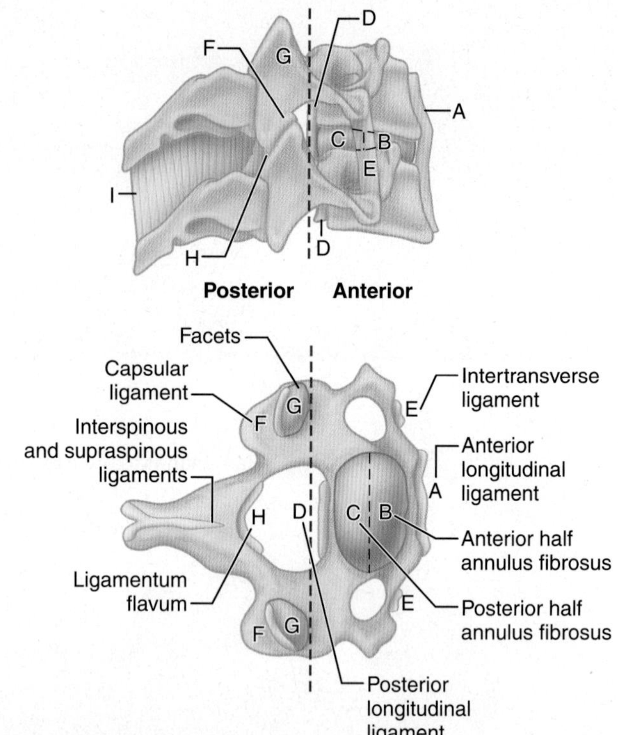

FIGURE 5.26 Important anterior and posterior supporting structures of spine.

BOX 5.2

Checklist for Diagnosis of Clinical Instability in Lower Cervical Spine*

Element	Point value
Anterior elements destroyed or unable to function	2
Posterior elements destroyed or unable to function	2
Relative sagittal plane translation >3.5 mm	2
Relative sagittal plane rotation >11 degrees	2
Positive stretch test	2
Medullary (cord) damage	2
Root damage	1
Abnormal disc narrowing	1
Dangerous loading anticipated	1

*Total of 5 or more = unstable.

From White AA, Southwick WO, Panjabi MM: Clinical instability in the lower cervical spine: a review of past and current concepts, *Spine* 1:15, 1976.

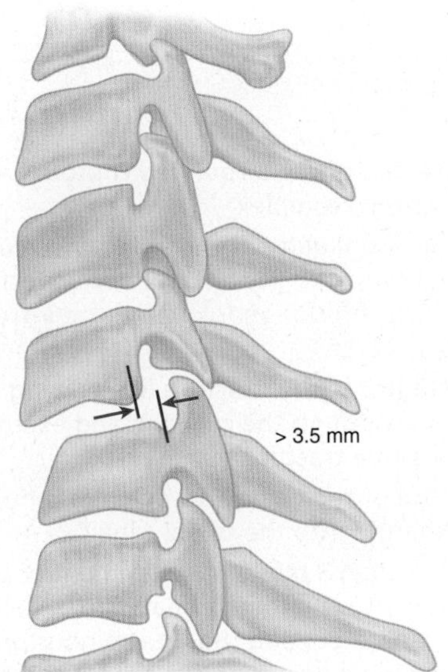

FIGURE 5.27 **Sagittal plane translation of more than 3.5 mm suggests clinical instability.** (Redrawn from White AA, Johnson RM, Panjabi MM: Biomechanical analysis of clinical stability in the cervical spine, *Clin Orthop Relat Res* 109:85, 1975.)

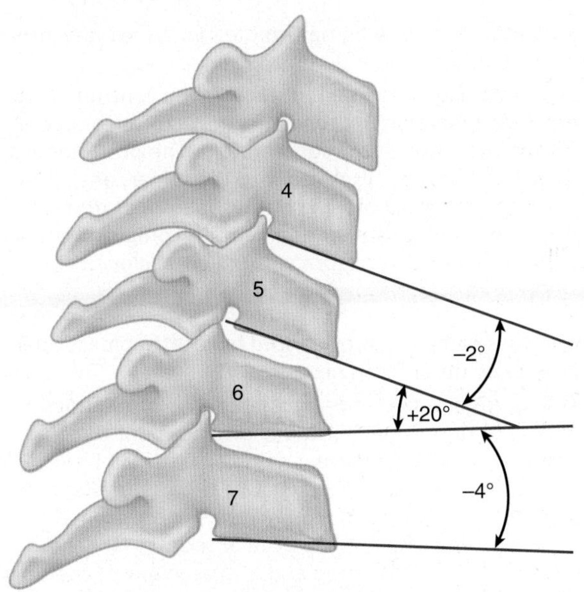

FIGURE 5.28 **Significant sagittal plane rotation (>11 degrees) suggests instability.** (Redrawn from White AA, Johnson RM, Panjabi MM: Biomechanical analysis of clinical stability in the cervical spine, *Clin Orthop Relat Res* 109:85, 1975.)

determination of the optimal classification of or treatment for a particular injury can be decided with certainty. A third classification system has been developed by the AO Spine Group. This system has three main injury types based on the type of primary injuring force, with subtypes based on progressive severity with a separate rating for facet injuries. The most recent version also includes a grading of neurologic injury and modifiers for comorbidities such as ankylosing spondylitis or vertebral artery injuries.

TREATMENT

Until there is a validated classification system that substantially improves on the available systems, spine surgeons will continue to use the best information available coupled with experience to determine treatments. A systematic approach as discussed earlier in this chapter is necessary when determining treatment. After the imaging has been obtained and any emergent closed reduction attempt completed, a decision for definitive treatment is necessary.

Most cervical injuries do not disrupt the structural integrity of the spine sufficiently to require operative intervention. Evaluation of individual injuries based on the injury patterns of the Ferguson-Allen system and the patient's neurologic examination has been the basis for our treatment rationale in each region of the spine. This mechanistic description is considered using the three-column model described by Denis to determine which structures are injured and make a determination of stability. The anterior column consists of the anterior longitudinal ligament and the anterior half of the vertebral body and disc, the middle column consists of the posterior half of the body and disc and the posterior longitudinal ligament, and the posterior column includes the pedicles and all posterior osseous and ligamentous structures. The controlling principle is that single-column injuries without neurologic deficit will, in general, be stable without progressive deformity, neurologic injury, or postinjury pain, although care must be taken to evaluate ligamentous structures, including discal disruption, which often accompany facet fractures. This has been consistent with our practice experience, and these patients do well with immobilization. In contrast, injuries that involve three columns are considered unstable even when there is no neurologic deficit (rare) and typically require operative stabilization. This, of course, leaves the two-column injuries, which are considered unstable. These tend to be treated operatively, but some of these injuries can be treated with immobilization. In our experience, immobilization has a low morbidity when the patient is able to mobilize immediately. In patients with two-column injuries, the neurologic status often is the determining factor as to whether operative treatment is recommended. Patients with incomplete injuries or complete injuries generally are treated operatively, whereas those with normal results of examination or possibly isolated root injuries may be treated with immobilization. Other injuries, comorbidities, congenital anomalies, and degenerative conditions can influence the treatment decision.

The goals of stabilization are to realign the spine, prevent further loss of neurologic function, enhance neurologic recovery, restore biomechanical integrity to the spine, and promote early functional recovery. Operative treatment for subaxial spine injuries can be from an anterior, posterior, or combined (360-degree) approach. There are a variety of acceptable treatment options that can achieve these goals in a given patient. The simplest and most direct strategy is to base the approach on the area of greatest structural injury: injuries to the anterior or middle columns usually are approached anteriorly, and three-column injuries and those requiring direct reduction usually are approached posteriorly.

The primary advantages of anterior surgery include decompression of the neural elements and restoration of the axial load-bearing support function with use of a strut graft and anterior plating, particularly over one to two motion

TABLE 5.4

Allen and Ferguson Classification of Subaxial Cervical Spine Fractures

COMPRESSIVE FLEXION—FIVE STAGES	
Compressive flexion stage 1	Blunting of the anterosuperior vertebral margin to a rounded contour, with no evidence of failure of the posterior ligamentous complex
Compressive flexion stage 2	In addition to the changes seen in stage 1, obliquity of the anterior vertebral body with loss of some anterior height of the centrum. The anteroinferior vertebral body has a "beak" appearance, concavity of the inferior endplate may be increased, and the vertebral body may have a vertical fracture.
Compressive flexion stage 3	In addition to the characteristics of a stage 2 injury, fracture line passing obliquely from the anterior surface of the vertebra through the centrum and extending through the inferior subchondral plate and a fracture of the beak.
Compressive flexion stage 4	Deformation of the centrum and fracture of the beak with mild (<3 mm) displacement of the inferoposterior vertebral margin into the spinal canal
Compressive flexion stage 5	Bony injuries as in stage 3 but with more than 3 mm of displacement of the posterior portion of the vertebral body posteriorly into the spinal canal. The vertebral arch remains intact, the articular facets are separated, and the interspinous process space is increased at the level of injury, suggesting a posterior ligamentous disruption in a tension mode.
VERTICAL COMPRESSION—THREE STAGES	
Vertical compression stage 1	Fracture of the superior or inferior endplate with a "cupping" deformity. Failure of the endplate is central rather than anterior, and posterior ligamentous failure is not evident.
Vertical compression stage 2	Fracture of both vertebral endplates with cupping deformities. Fracture lines through the centrum may be present, but displacement is minimal.
Vertical compression stage 3	Progression of the vertebral body damage described in stage 2. The centrum is fragmented, and the displacement is peripheral in multiple directions. Most commonly, the centrum fails, with significant impaction and fragmentation. The posterior aspect of the vertebral body is fractured and may be displaced into the spinal canal. The vertebral arch may be intact with no evidence of ligamentous failure, or it may be comminuted with significant failure of the posterior ligamentous complex; the ligamentous disruption is between the fractured vertebra and the one below it.
DISTRACTIVE FLEXION—FOUR STAGES	
Distractive flexion stage 1	Failure of the posterior ligamentous complex, as evidenced by facet subluxation in flexion, with abnormal divergence of the spinous process.
Distractive flexion stage 2	Unilateral facet dislocation (the degree of posterior ligamentous failure ranges from partial failure sufficient only to permit the abnormal displacement to complete failure of the anterior and posterior ligamentous complexes, which is uncommon). Subluxation of the facet on the side opposite the dislocation suggests severe ligamentous injury. In addition, a small fleck of bone may be displaced from the posterior surface of the articular process, which is displaced anteriorly. Widening of the uncovertebral joint on the side of the dislocation and displacement of the tip of the spinous process toward the side of the dislocation may be seen. Beatson serially divided the posterior interspinous ligaments, facet capsule, posterior longitudinal ligament, annulus fibrosus, and anterior longitudinal ligament and found that unilateral facet dislocation can occur with rupture of only the posterior interspinous ligament and the facet capsule.
Distractive flexion stage 3	Bilateral facet dislocations, with approximately 50% anterior subluxation of the vertebral body. Blunting of the anterosuperior margin of the inferior vertebra to a rounded corner may or may not be present. Beatson showed that rupture of the interspinous ligament, the capsules of both facet joints, the posterior longitudinal ligament, and the annulus fibrosus of the intervertebral disc was necessary to create this lesion.
Distractive flexion stage 4	Full vertebral body width displacement anteriorly or a grossly unstable motion segment, giving the appearance of a "floating" vertebra
COMPRESSIVE EXTENSION—FIVE STAGES	
Compressive extension stage 1	Unilateral vertebral arch fracture with or without anterior rotatory vertebral displacement. Posterior element failure may consist of a linear fracture through the articular process, impaction of the articular process, and ipsilateral pedicle and lamina fractures, resulting in the "transverse facet" appearance on anteroposterior radiographs, or a combination of ipsilateral pedicle and articular process fractures.

TABLE 5.4

Allen and Ferguson Classification of Subaxial Cervical Spine Fractures—cont'd

Compressive extension stage 2	Bilaminar fractures without evidence of other tissue failure. Typically, the laminar fractures occur at multiple contiguous levels.
Compressive extension stage 3	Bilateral vertebral arch fractures with fracture of the articular processes, pedicles, lamina, or some bilateral combination, without vertebral body displacement
Compressive extension stage 4	Bilateral vertebral arch fractures with partial vertebral body width displacement anteriorly
Compressive extension stage 5	Bilateral vertebral arch fracture with full vertebral body width displacement anteriorly. The posterior portion of the vertebral arch of the fractured vertebra does not displace, and the anterior portion of the arch remains with the centrum. Ligament failure occurs at two levels: posteriorly between the fractured vertebra and the one above it and anteriorly between the fractured vertebra and the one below it. Characteristically, the anterosuperior portion of the vertebra below is sheared off by the anteriorly displaced centrum.
DISTRACTIVE EXTENSION—TWO STAGES	
Distractive extension stage 1	Either failure of the anterior ligamentous complex or a transverse fracture of the centrum. The injury usually is ligamentous, and there may be a fracture of the adjacent anterior vertebral margin. The radiographic clue to this injury is abnormal widening of the disc space.
Distractive extension stage 2	Evidence of failure of the posterior ligamentous complex, with displacement of the upper vertebral body posteriorly into the spinal canal, in addition to the changes seen in stage 1 injuries. Because displacement of this type tends to reduce spontaneously when the head is placed in a neutral position, radiographic evidence of the displacement may be minimal, rarely greater than 3 mm on initial films with the patient supine.
LATERAL FLEXION—TWO STAGES	
Lateral flexion stage 1	Asymmetric compression fracture of the centrum and ipsilateral vertebral arch fracture, without displacement of the arch on the anteroposterior view. Compression of the articular process or comminution of the corner of the vertebral arch may be present.
Lateral flexion stage 2	Lateral asymmetric compression of the centrum and either ipsilateral displaced vertebral arch fracture or ligamentous failure on the contralateral side with separation of the articular processes. Ipsilateral and compressive and contralateral disruptive vertebral arch injuries may be present.

segments. Maintaining the patient supine rather than prone during surgery also is an advantage if the patient has significant pulmonary dysfunction from blunt trauma or infection. Wound complications are infrequent with anterior surgery, although dysphagia has been recognized more frequently in recent years. Access to any level from the C2 disc to the C7 disc is possible in most patients but can be quite challenging in obese patients or those with short necks. Adequate decompression often can be accomplished with a discectomy. In a trauma setting, this is preferred to a corpectomy, which is inherently less stable. At times, such as with a burst fracture, a corpectomy is needed, and adequate stability is achieved with careful fitting and placement of the strut graft or cage and use of unicortical screws and a fixed-angle locking type plate. The dynamic type plates are of questionable benefit in degenerative indications but really do not have a place in the management of trauma patients because of the greater level of instability. Preservation of intact endplates and careful sizing of the strut graft without overdistracting the facets posteriorly also are critical to achieving enough stability to allow primary bone healing at the graft-host interface. There are multiple series in the literature demonstrating good outcomes with this type of anterior-only construct even with posterior ligamentous injuries. Postoperative immobilization in an orthosis generally is adequate with satisfactory plating. If fixation is compromised because of the injury pattern or bone quality, consideration should be given to posterior fixation or halo vest immobilization that may be advantageous for the patient rather than additional surgery. Anterior reconstruction and plating has been shown by Johnson et al. to have a high failure rate if the endplates are not intact, especially if there are associated facet fractures at the level treated with discectomy and reconstruction. Corpectomies at more than two levels are rare for trauma indications but if required may need to be supplemented with posterior instrumentation. Combined approaches rarely are needed for a good outcome except as discussed.

TABLE 5.5

Subaxial Injury Classification Scale

MORPHOLOGY	POINTS
No abnormality	0
Compression + burst	1 + 1 = 2
Distraction (e.g., facet perch, hyperextension)	3
Rotation or translation (e.g., facet dislocation, unstable teardrop, or advanced stage flexion compression injury)	4
DISCOLIGAMENTOUS COMPLEX	
Intact	0
Indeterminate (e.g., isolated interspinous widening, magnetic resonance imaging signal change only)	1
Disrupted (e.g., widening of anterior disc space, facet perch, or dislocation)	2
NEUROLOGIC STATUS	
Intact	0
Root injury	1
Complete cord injury	2
Incomplete cord injury	3
Continuous cord compression (neuro-modifier in the setting of a neurologic deficit)	+1

From Dorak M, Fisher CG, Fehlings MG, et al: The surgical approach to subaxial cervical spine injuries, *Spine* 32:2620, 2007.

Posterior fixation with current segmental fixation systems allows treatment of the most unstable injuries, even those that extend across the craniocervical or cervicothoracic junctions. These constructs use rods with lateral mass fixation from C3-C6 and pedicle screw placement at C2 to C7, and in the upper thoracic region. Pedicle screws can be placed at C7 and are biomechanically superior to C7 lateral mass screws. Pedicle screws are technically more difficult to place than lateral mass screws at C3 to C6 and usually offer no significant benefit. When necessary, fixation can be extended above C3 as has already been discussed. Because posterior fixation restores the posterior tension band and segmental fixation is possible, these constructs are stiffer than anterior constructs in flexion and torsion, so fusion rates are superior for multilevel fusions treated posteriorly than for similar length anterior constructs. Decompression done posteriorly is not associated with quite the same level of neurologic improvement in some studies, probably because of less effective restoration of blood flow to the anterior cord as was shown by Brodke et al. If posterior decompression is done, it should always be accompanied by stabilization and fusion in the setting of trauma. Because of the more extensive dissection required posteriorly, there has been a higher incidence of wound infection and greater blood loss relative to anterior procedures. However, for limited posterior approaches, such as for direct reduction of facet dislocations and fusion, wound-related complications are rare. Patients who are designated as poor hosts are more likely to be osteoporotic, and, in general, posterior methods are preferred because segmental fixation is possible.

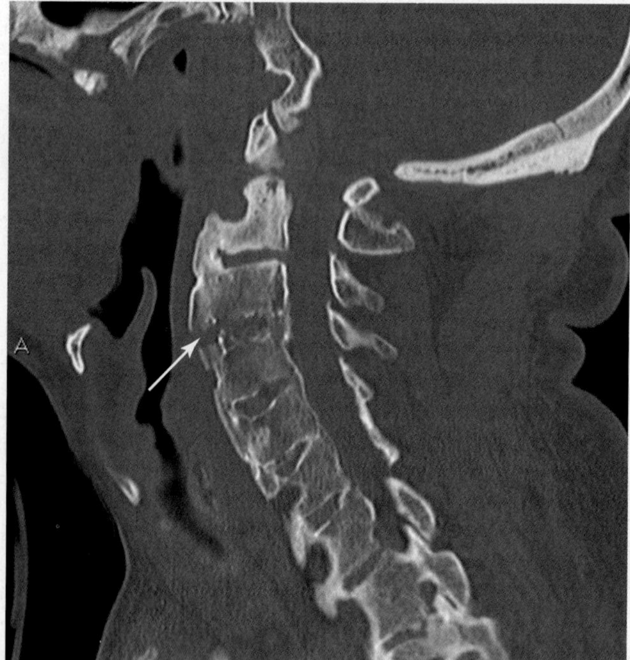

FIGURE 5.29 Extension fracture through C3 disc level in patient with diffuse idiopathic skeletal hyperostosis.

EXTENSION INJURIES

An extension injury is the result of hyperextension of the cervical spine (Fig. 5.29). Often the patient is older and had a relatively low-energy mechanism of injury such as a same level fall. The injury occurs in part from a loss of motion in the cervical spine, which is unable to dissipate the energy without failure. The patient may have diffuse idiopathic skeletal hyperostosis (DISH) or ankylosing spondylitis that predisposes to this injury pattern. Patients with ankylosing

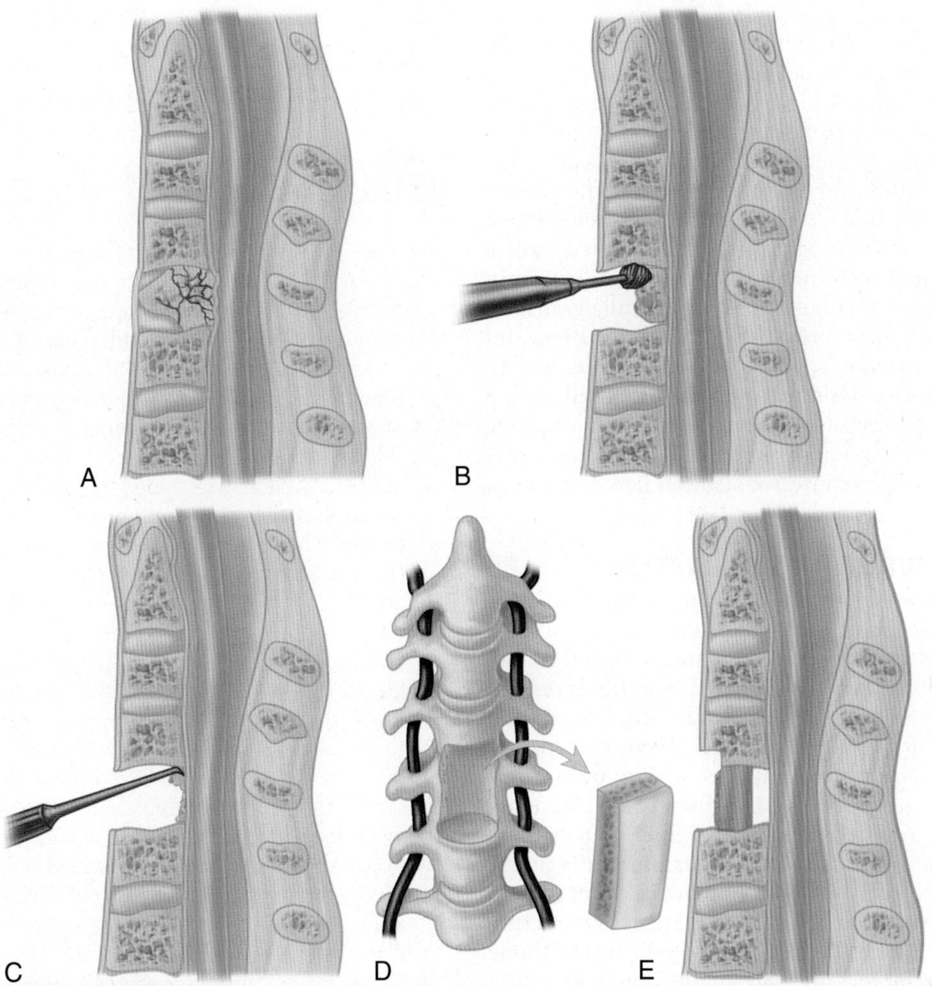

FIGURE 5.30 **A,** Typical burst fracture at C5 with retropulsed bone and disc fragments in spinal canal compressing neural elements. **B,** Disc material above and below fractured vertebra has been removed, and high-speed power burr is used to remove bone back to level of posterior longitudinal ligament. **C,** Residual posterior vertebral margin is removed with small curet to decompress neural elements. **D,** Extent of anterior cervical corpectomy. **E,** Placement of tricortical iliac crest graft or fibular allograft after adequate cervical decompression. **SEE TECHNIQUE 5.14.**

spondylitis actually have a fracture through the disc space and are treated somewhat differently (see later section). Patients with an incomplete disc disruption determined by acute MRI usually can be treated with immobilization. Patients with an annulus disruption that extends through the anterior and posterior margins of the annulus fibrosus are treated with anterior discectomy and fusion with bone graft and an anterior locking plate.

BURST FRACTURES

This injury is exemplified by shortening of the vertebral body, with comminution and retropulsion of the vertebral body into the canal (Fig. 5.30). Burst fractures with comminution extending to both endplates usually are treated with corpectomy and anterior reconstruction with a tricortical iliac bone graft, fibular allograft, or cylindrical mesh cage packed with the resected vertebral body and anterior plating. The endplates are prepared to maintain intact subchondral bone as a secure footing for the chosen strut type. Usually, these patients are relatively young and do not have preexisting disease of the posterior longitudinal ligament, which is not injured by axial loading. The posterior longitudinal ligament should be preserved and will provide a counterforce for the implanted strut unless decompression cannot be satisfactorily accomplished without posterior longitudinal ligament resection. An anterior locking plate is then applied.

FACET DISLOCATIONS

Facet dislocations should be distinguished from facet fractures with subluxation. Bilateral facet dislocations are severe pure soft-tissue injuries with disruption of the facet capsules, which are the most important posterior ligamentous stabilizers. Additional injury occurs to the interspinous ligaments, ligamentum flavum, and posterior longitudinal ligament, and there is discal disruption with possible herniation. Anterior translation of up to 50% of the vertebral body dimension occurs. The algorithm for imaging and reduction as previously described should be followed. After failed or successful closed reduction, MRI is obtained. If there is a significant disc herniation present, anterior cervical discectomy with fusion and bone graft is done. If reduction was accomplished preoperatively or at the time of discectomy and fusion, an anterior locking plate is applied. This construct is stable with a reduced facet dislocation that has no bony injury. If reduction cannot be accomplished at the time of discectomy, the graft is placed and the anterior wound is closed, followed by open posterior reduction and fusion with instrumentation. If the closed reduction fails and MRI demonstrates no significant disc herniation, open posterior reduction with stabilization is the treatment of choice. Open reduction in an anesthetized patient is associated with a higher rate of spinal cord injury than closed reduction in an awake patient, as previously discussed. Unilateral facet dislocations usually have only about 25% translation, but the management scheme is similar. In some patients with unilateral facet dislocations with successful closed reduction, consideration to closed treatment is reasonable if there is no persistent neural compression, but close radiographic follow-up is essential because subluxation can recur even weeks later.

FACET FRACTURE WITH SUBLUXATION

Assessment of stability of facet fractures remains difficult. The AO Spine classification considers facet fractures in addition to the primary fracture pattern. Specter et al. studied a group of patients with isolated facet fractures and found that if the fracture measured more than 1 cm and more than 40% of the lateral mass length of the contralateral side, there was a significant probability of instability and failure of nonoperative treatment. More recently these parameters were confirmed by Pehler. When there is a facet fracture associated with subluxation, this injury usually will reduce easily with traction but may not remain reduced as the patient mobilizes. If there is no fracture of either endplate, anterior discectomy with fusion, bone grafting, and anterior locking plate application is an option but should be undertaken with caution. This construct is subject to shear forces because of the incompetent facet(s), and displacement can occur. Although neurologic worsening is unusual, it has certainly been reported. Loss of fixation will require revision. Careful follow-up is recommended, and the patient must be compliant with orthosis usage. Alternatively, posterior instrumentation and fusion provide more stability and will maintain alignment more consistently, but an additional level of fusion generally is needed because fixation usually is not possible at the fractured level.

FRACTURE-DISLOCATIONS

These are the most severe injuries usually with combined soft-tissue and osseous injuries, translational displacement in one or more planes, and often associated spinal cord injury. Closed reduction must be undertaken with caution to avoid overdistracting the injured segment and potentially worsening the spinal cord injury. In this injury group, combined anterior and posterior surgery may be the more conservative approach, although a combined approach is not always needed. The principle of treating the most severely injured area first is followed to reestablish spinal alignment and decompress the spinal cord. This usually is accomplished anteriorly first, and if necessary posterior supplemental stabilization and fusion are added at a second stage and may be delayed depending on the overall condition of the patient (Fig. 5.31).

ANTERIOR CERVICAL DISCECTOMY AND FUSION WITH PLATING

TECHNIQUE 5.14

- If the patient is already in traction, maintain traction and alignment. Coordinate with the anesthesiologist for an awake intubation or manually maintain head position and use a GlideScope (Verathon Inc., Bothell, WA). If the patient has a spinal cord injury, maintain a mean arterial pressure of 85 to 90 mm Hg during the procedure.
- Expose the spine through either a transverse or a longitudinal incision, depending on the surgeon's preference. We usually prefer a left-sided transverse incision (Fig. 5.32) because of the more constant anatomy of the recurrent laryngeal nerve and the lower risk of inadvertent injury.
- Make a 3-cm incision at the cricoid level for the C5 disc or adjust accordingly depending on the injury level. A transverse incision can be used even for an extensile exposure. Locate the skin incision with the midpoint on the lateral border of the trachea on the side of the approach.
- Incise the skin and dissect through the subcutaneous layer to the platysma. Sharply dissect the fat off the platysma fascia at least 10 mm in all directions from the skin incision to mobilize the incision and improve exposure.
- Incise the platysma muscle vertically in line with its fibers.
- In the lateral portion of the wound, identify the medial border of the sternocleidomastoid muscle and bluntly develop the plane to the carotid sheath. At the C5 disc level it will be covered by the omohyoid muscle.
- Sweep the omohyoid superiorly or inferiorly (at the C5 disc level) as needed and sharply incise the pretracheal fascia along the medial border of the carotid sheath. Open the pretracheal fascia generously with blunt dissection.
- With blunt finger dissection, develop the plane of the prevertebral space. Use a Kittner dissector to better define the anterior spine that is visible between the longus colli muscles.
- Radiographically identify the injured level with a metallic marker (22-gauge spinal needle) within the injured disc or bone and permanently store the image. Mark the confirmed level using a No. 11 blade scalpel to remove a small amount of anterior annulus that is easily visible.
- Using blunt retractors, mobilize the trachea and esophagus just enough to safely elevate the longus colli muscles bilaterally from the midbody of the superior end vertebra to the midbody of the inferior end vertebra but avoid unnecessary exposure that may lead to adjacent segment degeneration.
- Place a self-retaining retractor with the blade deep to the medial border of the longus colli on each side of the spine at the affected level.
- Incise the annulus at the injured disc level widely to the level of the uncinate process bilaterally. Use curets to remove most of the disc and clearly view the uncinate process bilaterally.
- Under the operating microscope, use a high-speed burr to remove the anteriormost portion of the inferior body of the cephalad vertebra. This bone removal is only to the level of the highest point of the concavity of the inferior

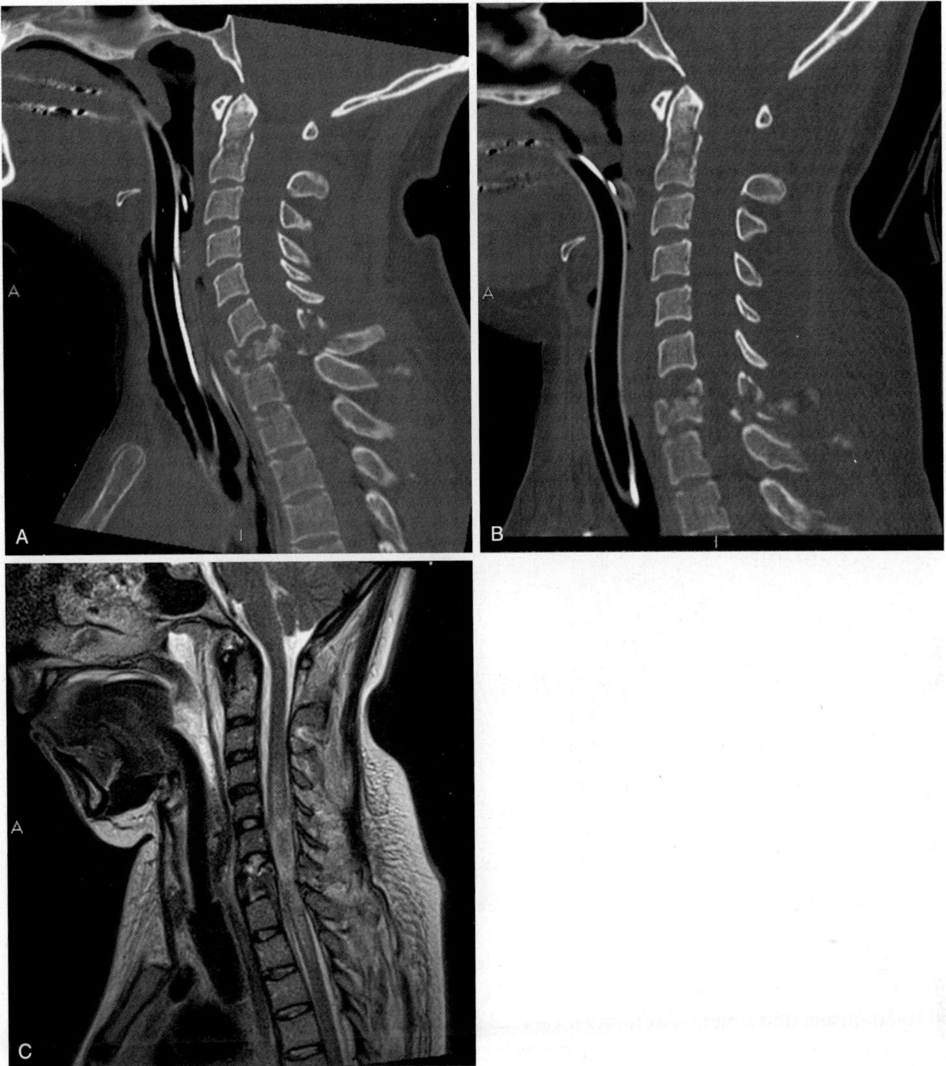

FIGURE 5.31 **A,** Fracture-dislocation involving C6 and C7 levels. Note C2 fracture. **B,** Alignment has been improved with skeletal traction. **C,** MR image after traction reveals severe spinal cord swelling and increased signal.

endplate. This allows the endplate to be flat, and it forms a right angle with the anterior and posterior body walls and preserves the subchondral bone (Fig. 5.30).

- Remove any anterior osteophyte as well. With this anterior bone resection, visibility is enhanced and the posterior disc material, posterior longitudinal ligament, and posterior osteophytes can be removed as needed. If the foramina are tight, perform foraminotomies.
- Contour the superior endplate of the inferior vertebra with a burr, preserving the subchondral bone and creating a flat surface parallel with the inferior endplate of the cephalad vertebra, anterior to posterior and side to side. The medial portion of the uncinates may need to be burred away so the defect is wide enough to accept the graft.
- Carefully measure the height of the disc space both with traction applied and without traction. Do not size the graft to maintain the traction interval if there is more than 1 mm difference between the measurements. The graft size should allow stable fit without being excessively tight.
- Either harvest tricortical iliac graft or select a composite corticocancellous allograft product. The graft typically is 12 to 13 mm in anterior to posterior dimension so it can be countersunk 2 mm and not intrude into the canal. Tamp the graft into place and verify radiographically or by direct vision that the posterior graft does not enter the canal. With traction removed the graft should be stable enough to resist being pulled easily from the disc space. Avoid making the fit excessively tight.
- Select the shortest locking plate possible to avoid impingement injury to the adjacent discs. The prepared endplates should be just visible through the screw holes of the plate when it is properly positioned (Fig. 5.33).
- Drill and place unicortical screws most commonly 14 mm in length, but this should be individualized. Make sure screws are placed at the correct angle to optimize locking of the screw and plate. Engage the antibackout mechanism of the plate after placing all four screws.
- Achieve meticulous hemostasis and close the platysma over a fluted style drain; close the remaining layers.

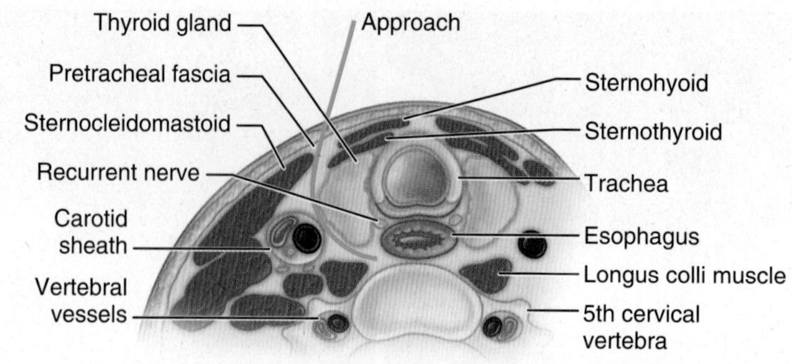

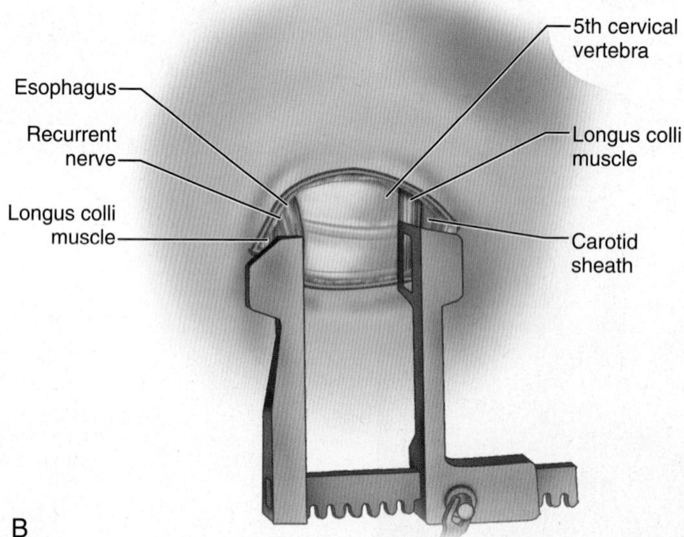

FIGURE 5.32 **A,** Anterior approach to middle and lower cervical spine through left-sided transverse incision is carried medially to carotid sheath and laterally to trachea and esophagus. **B,** Deep dissection to middle and lower cervical spine. Thorough knowledge of anatomic fascial planes is mandatory to gain adequate exposure of the anterior aspect of the cervical spine. **SEE TECHNIQUES 5.14 AND 5.15.**

POSTOPERATIVE CARE A rigid orthosis is worn for 4 to 6 weeks until there is radiographic evidence of healing at the graft interfaces. Flexion and extension radiographs are obtained to verify stability and to determine if the orthosis can be discontinued.

CERVICAL CORPECTOMY AND RECONSTRUCTION WITH PLATING

TECHNIQUE 5.15

- Preparation, positioning, and exposure are as described in Technique 5.14 with the exception being that a 4-cm incision is made at the cricoid level for C5 (see Fig. 5.32).
- Incise the disc widely to the level of the uncinate process bilaterally above and below the fractured vertebra. Use curets to remove most of the disc and clearly view the uncinate process bilaterally at each level. If a metal cage or fibular allograft is to be used, remove the injured body piecemeal and save it to fill the cage or graft. If structural autograft will be used, remove the body with a high-speed burr. This is our preferred method.
- Under the operating microscope, use a high-speed burr to make a vertical groove on each side of the body to be removed that begins above the uncinate process of the normal vertebra caudally to the uncinate process of the injured segment. These grooves define the area of bone to be removed. Using the burr, remove all the bone between the two grooves, deepening each groove as needed. This can be done very rapidly until the cancellous bone of the body gives way to cortical bone, indicating the posterior cortex has been reached. By staying medial to the uncinate the vertebral artery can be avoided, although rarely a tortuous artery can erode medial to the uncinate, and this should be detected on the CT during preoperative planning. Remove the posterior cortex with the burr as well.

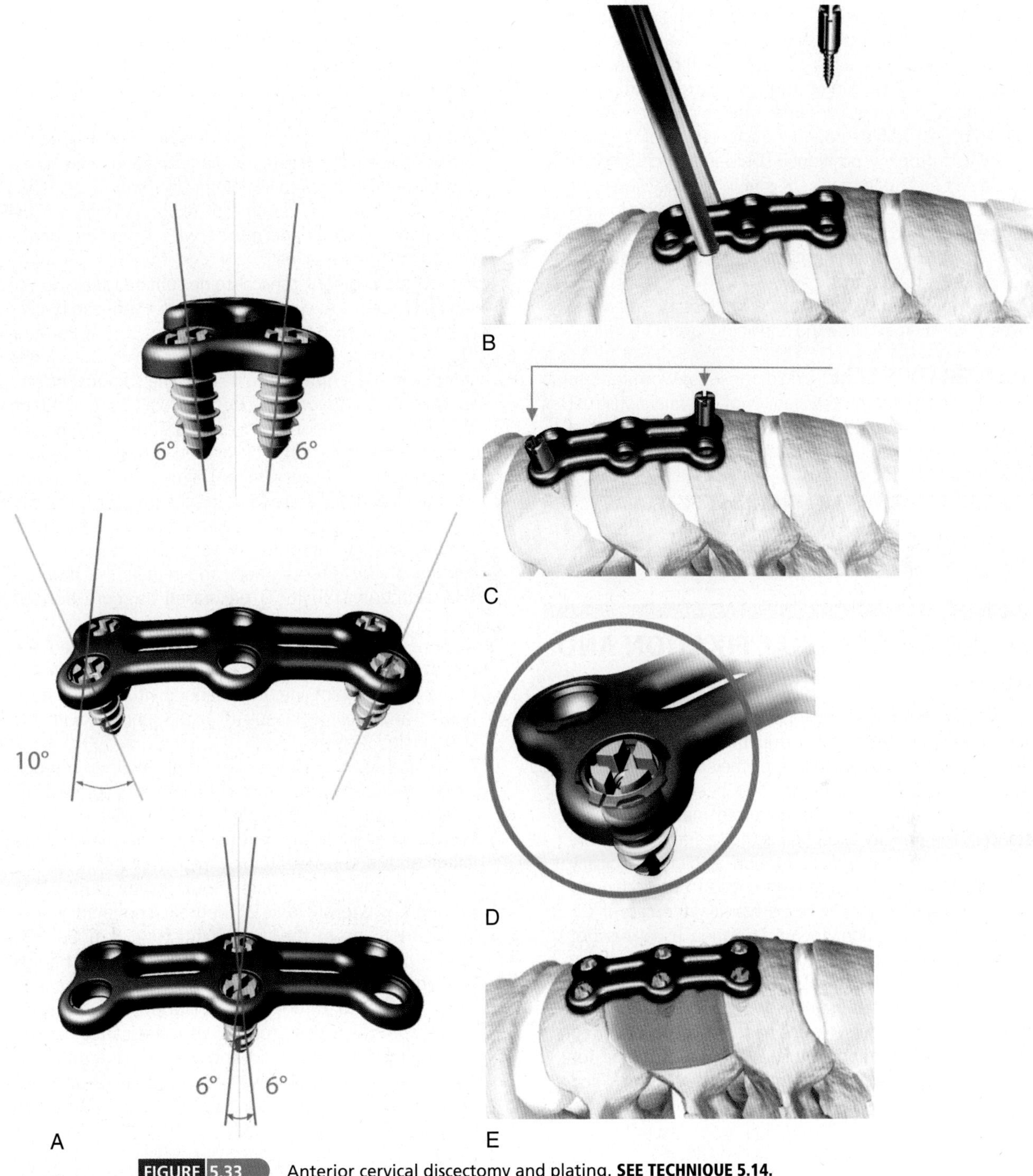

FIGURE 5.33 Anterior cervical discectomy and plating. **SEE TECHNIQUE 5.14.**

- Remove the posterior longitudinal ligament and posterior osteophytes as needed and perform foraminotomies as needed. Normally, the corpectomy defect is at least 17 mm in width. Remove the anterior portion of the cephalad end vertebra to leave a flat surface with preservation of the subchondral bone. Similarly, contour the superior endplate of the caudal end vertebra. The two endplates should each be flat and parallel to one another.
- Carefully measure the distance between the endplates with and without traction applied. When there is little to no movement when traction is discontinued, very careful sizing of the graft is required to avoid graft subsidence or displacement. This length can be easily measured by using a sterile cotton applicator stick cut to the desired length; this cut piece serves as a template for the cage or graft.
- Create an appropriate length autograft, fibular allograft, or cage filled with local bone.
- Reapply traction and increase slightly if needed to insert the strut and carefully tamp the strut into place. Because of the inclination of the endplates the graft will be more posterior at the caudal end than it is rostrally when it is resting squarely on each endplate. Verify radiographically or by direct vision that the strut does not extend into the

canal. With traction removed, the strut should be stable enough to resist being pulled easily from the corpectomy defect. Proper fit is critical for stability and bony union.

- Select the shortest locking plate possible to avoid impingement injury to the adjacent discs. The prepared endplates should be just visible through the screw holes of the plate when it is properly positioned. Drill and place unicortical screws most commonly 14 mm in length. Make sure screws are placed at the correct angle to optimize locking of the screw and plate. Engage the anti-backout mechanism of the plate after placing all four screws. Screws are not placed into the strut.
- Achieve meticulous hemostasis and close the platysma over a fluted drain; close the remaining layers.

POSTOPERATIVE CARE A rigid orthosis is worn for 6 to 8 weeks depending on the stability of the final construct and radiographic evidence of graft incorporation. Flexion and extension radiographs are obtained to verify stability and discontinue the orthosis.

POSTERIOR SUBAXIAL FIXATION AND FUSION

The instrumentation systems for posterior fixation are polyaxial screws that can be placed in the lateral mass with unicortical or bicortical purchase, or they can be placed in the pedicle. Lateral mass fixation has been shown to be effective and safe and is the preferred method in most instances. The primary exception is the lateral mass of C7, which is smaller, and where fixation is biomechanically inferior to other levels. If the construct is to be continued into the thoracic region, which is typically the case if C7 is included in the fusion, then C7 fixation usually is not included because there is insufficient space for the screw head of the T1 screw and a C7 screw on the rod because of the different orientation of the two screws. If C7 fixation is desirable, pedicle screw placement usually is preferred over lateral mass fixation at this level. The technique for lateral mass screw placement is that of Magerl, as modified by Anderson.

LATERAL MASS SCREW AND ROD FIXATION

TECHNIQUE 5.16

(MAGERL)

- If the patient is already in traction, maintain traction and alignment. Coordinate with the anesthesiologist for an awake intubation or manually maintain head position and use a GlideScope. If the patient has a spinal cord injury, maintain a mean arterial pressure of 85 to 90 mm Hg throughout the procedure. Use a turning frame such as the Jackson table to position the patient prone.
- Radiographically verify injury reduction; if pedicle screws are to be used, make sure imaging can adequately be accomplished before preparation and draping.
- Incise the skin over the area of exposure. Infiltrate the subcutaneous tissue and muscle with 1 mg epinephrine in 500 mL normal saline.
- Expose the posterior cervical spine subperiosteally to the lateral border of the lateral masses after verifying levels.
- If an unreduced dislocation is present, use a Penfield No. 4 dissector or Freer elevator to gently unlock the joint(s). Make a hole in the base of the spinous process of each of the involved vertebrae. Using a tenaculum through each spinous process, carefully distract and posteriorly translate the dislocated vertebra to reduce both facets while an assistant simultaneously uses a Penfield No. 4 dissector to guide the inferior facet into the reduced position. If this cannot be accomplished, remove a small amount of bone from the superior margin of the inferior facet and repeat the process. Postreduction stability is decreased as more bone is resected.
- Remove any facet capsules in the area to be fused and identify the boundaries of the lateral mass, which consist of the superior joint line, the inferior joint line, the lateral border, and the medial sulcus at the junction with the lamina (Fig. 5.34A).
- If a laminectomy or laminoplasty is planned, do not perform it until the screw holes are completed so the bony landmarks can be used for drilling screw holes.
- Select an entry portal 1 mm medial to the center of the lateral mass and penetrate only the cortex with a burr.
- Drilling of the lateral mass should be directed 25 to 35 degrees laterally and 25 degrees cephalad (parallel to the plane of the facet joint) for C3 to C6 (Fig. 5.34B). This trajectory can reliably be accomplished by placing the drill guide against the inferior aspect of the posterior tip (remove large osteophytes if present) of the spinous process of the vertebra caudal to the level being drilled. Use a hand drill set to a depth of 14 mm that will provide unicortical fixation in most patients. For example, rest the drill guide against the inferior C4 spinous process if drilling the C3 lateral mass.
- If bicortical fixation is planned, use a drill of preset length and drill in 2-mm increments. Use a ball-tipped wire or depth gauge to sound the drill hole after each advance of the drill and feel the far cortex. Ideally, the drill will exit just lateral to the vertebral artery, but the artery is at risk if the drill is too medially directed.
- If a cervical pedicle screw is to be placed, carefully review the CT preoperatively to measure the size and orientation of the pedicle. The entry point into the pedicle as described by Abumi and Kaneda is just lateral to the center point of the lateral mass. Penetrate the cortex and advance a probe into the pedicle. The direction of the probe is 30 to 40 degrees medially relative to the sagittal plane, which also has been found to be 90 degrees relative to

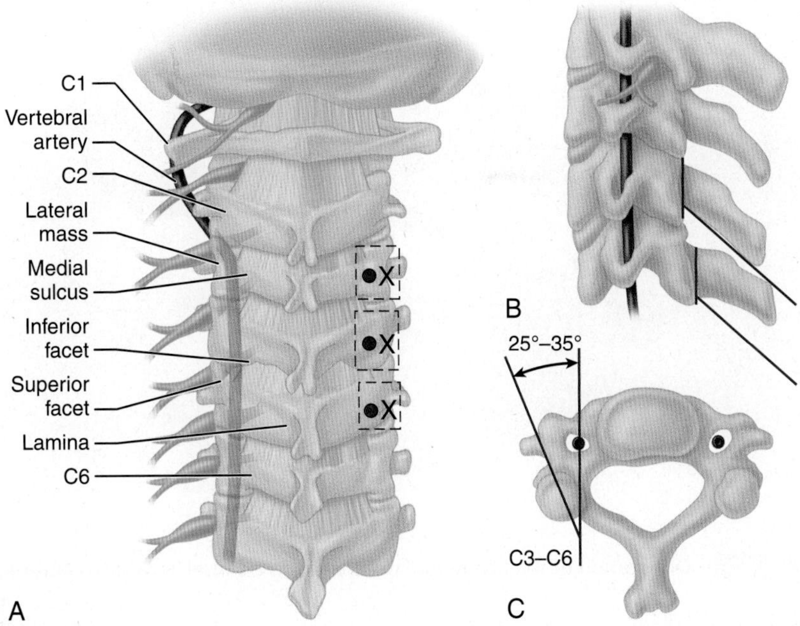

FIGURE 5.34 Posterior cervical plating. **A,** Landmarks used for identifying center of lateral mass and point for drilling. **B,** Relationship of facet joints, nerve root, and drill angle. **C,** Superior view of cervical vertebra showing relationship of drill angle, foramen transversarium, and vertebral artery. **SEE TECHNIQUE 5.15.**

the ipsilateral lamina. With regard to orientation in the cephalad to caudal direction, this varies by level and usually is slightly caudal at the C7 level and can be identified using image intensification. Ludwig et al. recommended making a laminoforaminotomy and directly palpating the superomedial pedicle to help orient the probe (Fig. 5.35).

- If a thoracic pedicle screw is to be placed, the technique described for all thoracic pedicle screws is used (see Technique 5.17).
- Place each screw. Decorticate the lateral mass and lamina and burr each joint. Cut and contour the rod and secure the rod to the screws with the blockers.
- Pack the bone graft into place.
- Close the wound in layers over a drain.

POSTOPERATIVE CARE A rigid orthosis is used for 6 weeks and is removed if reduction has been maintained and flexion and extension films indicate there is no motion at the stabilized level(s) after the immobilization period.

ANKYLOSING SPONDYLITIS

Patients with ankylosing spondylitis form a subgroup of patients who merit special consideration with regard to spinal injuries in general and cervical spine injuries in particular. These patients can present with injury from high-energy mechanisms, but often there is a relatively low-energy mechanism such as a same-level fall. If there is no neurologic deficit or obvious fracture, a high level of clinical suspicion must be maintained to avoid potentially serious harm to the patient. A systematic review by Rustagi et al. found a delay in diagnosis in up to 41% of patients. The injury mechanism is most often extension such as a blow to the face or head while falling. Because of the ossification of the outer portions of the disc, the spine is unable to absorb the energy imparted and a fracture occurs. The radiographic findings can be very subtle and often require CT or MRI to be appreciated. These fractures are most common in the C5 to T1 region, and noncontiguous injuries are reported in 10% of patients. Mortality in this patient group is 6% to 10% within the first 7 to 10 days of injury. Patients with a history of ankylosing spondylitis or those who have a characteristic kyphotic deformity at the cervicothoracic junction should be supported to maintain the kyphosis during the evaluation process and should not be laid flat. Instead, the head of the bed should be elevated and maintained at 30 to 40 degrees at all times. Even in this position, a bolster to support the head may be needed. If a fracture is identified, these patients almost always require operative treatment with posterior segmental fixation over relatively long spans because osteoporotic bone typically coexists with ankylosing spondylitis. Before stabilization, the patient should be moved as infrequently as possible to minimize risk of neurologic worsening. A rigid collar is not adequate for immobilization, and halo vest immobilization should be instituted early as a temporary measure. Halo vest immobilization also is helpful when moving the patient for surgery. Turning the patient into the prone position requires planning and considerable care. These patients are at risk for significant epidural bleeding; a decline in neurologic function requires immediate investigation and early decompression to optimize outcomes. Careful assessment of the entire spine is necessary because of the high incidence of noncontiguous injuries.

VERTEBRAL ARTERY INJURIES

Considerable controversy still remains regarding the optimal screening criteria and treatment of vertebral artery injuries associated with cervical fractures (Table 5.6)— 60 years after this relationship was first described by Carpenter in 1961.

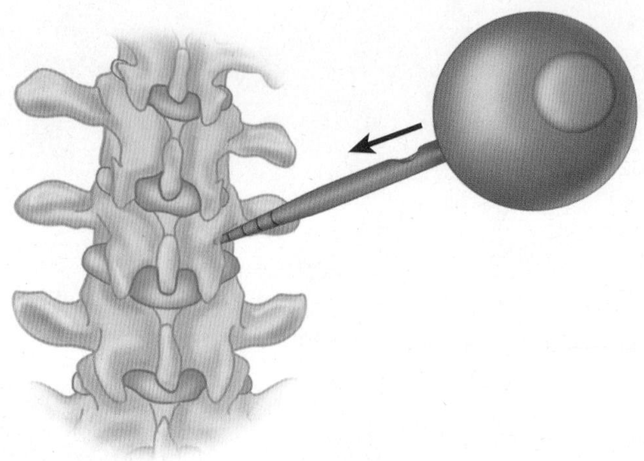

FIGURE 5.35 Orientation of the probe for lateral mass screw insertion. **SEE TECHNIQUE 5.16.**

TABLE 5.6

Screening Criteria for Blunt Cerebrovascular Injury (BCVI)

SCREENING CRITERIA	PATIENTS TO BE SCREENED	
	Signs and Symptoms of BCVI	*Risk Factors of BCVI*
Modified Denver Criteria	Arterial hemorrhage (from neck, nose, or mouth) Cervical bruit in patients <50 yr of age Expanding cervical hematoma Focal neurologic defect (transient ischemic attack, hemiparesis, vertebrobasilar symptoms, Horner syndrome) Stroke on CT or MRI Neurologic deficit inconsistent with head CT	High-energy transfer mechanism with the following: • Le Fort II or III fracture • Basilar skull fracture involving carotid canal • Cervical vertebral body or transverse foramen fracture, subluxation, or ligamentous injury at any level; any fracture at C1-C3 • Closed head injury consistent with diffuse axonal injury and with Glasgow Coma Scale score <6 • Near-hanging with anoxia • Clothesline-type injury or seat belt abrasion with significant swelling, pain, or altered mental status
Memphis Criteria	Cervical spine fracture Neurologic exam not explained by brain imaging Horner syndrome Le Fort II or III facial fractures Skull base fractures involving the foramen lacerum Neck soft-tissue injury (e.g., seat belt injury, hanging)	

There have been numerous studies with prospectively collected data primarily to establish the incidence and evaluate treatment options. Based on a literature review, Fassett et al. found a 0.5% incidence of vertebral artery injuries in trauma patients; however, 70% had associated cervical fractures. The fractures most commonly associated with vertebral artery injury are those involving the foramen transversarium, the C1 to C3 levels, and displaced fractures or dislocations. Other studies have found an association with type III occipital condyle fractures. The injury patterns associated with vertebral artery injury have been further characterized by Lebl et al., who showed an association of vertebral artery injury with foramen transversarium fractures displaced >1 mm, basilar skull fractures, ankylosing spondylitis, DISH, occipitocervical dislocations, and facet subluxations and dislocations. The clinical presentation of vertebral artery injury is highly variable. Patients can remain asymptomatic or develop signs of posterior circulation stroke with a reported mortality in some series as high as 33%, although in the study of Lebl et al. mortality was 4.8%. Foramen transversarium fractures at the level of entry of the vertebral artery are probably more significant than other levels, and although this usually is C6, in 5% of people the artery enters the C7 foramen transversarium. To date, the most reliable diagnostic method has been catheter cerebral angiography, although CT angiography and MR angiography continue to improve. Roberts et al. demonstrated the diagnostic accuracy of CT angiography in detecting vertebral artery injury. Diagnostic-associated complications do occur, which in some series include an iatrogenic stroke incidence of 1% related to cerebral angiography; thus, four-vessel angiography is limited to symptomatic vertebral artery injury and not screening. Treatment is anticoagulation with heparin acutely and may be maintained for 3 to 6 months; in some series, observation is recommended. Because no level I evidence guides treatment, careful coordinated treatment for each individual patient is indicated because it is not yet clear if current treatment improves patient outcomes. Other treatment protocols, including aspirin therapy, have been adopted depending on the severity of the vertebral artery injury.

Another important aspect of vertebral artery injury is the influence it may have on operative planning with regard to the cervical spine. Because the vertebral artery is at risk with certain instrumentation techniques, the presence of a vertebral artery injury must be factored into the treatment plan, as well as the effects of anticoagulation therapy if this is instituted.

THORACIC AND LUMBAR INJURIES

Thoracolumbar injuries usually are the result of high-energy trauma, and often associated visceral injuries are present in patients who have sustained significant injuries in this region. As was discussed for cervical injuries, patients with a suspected thoracolumbar injury need rapid evaluation in the trauma assessment area. This should follow the ATLS protocol with a secondary survey that includes inspection and palpation of the entire spine, noting skin condition, tenderness, step offs, mental status, motor and sensory examination in the extremities, and a rectal examination for tone and the presence or absence of the bulbocavernosus reflex. The ISCoS form is used to record the neurologic findings. The radiographic assessment should be completed as expeditiously as possible to allow the spine to be cleared and to remove the patient from the spine board or, if injury is present, to identify the injury so prompt treatment can be undertaken. To this end, CT has become the standard method for evaluation of the thoracic and lumbar regions. CT of the chest, abdomen, and pelvis with contrast enhancement is routinely obtained in the same population at risk for thoracic or lumbar spine fractures to assess for visceral injury. Several authors have shown that CT of the chest, abdomen, and pelvis has superior specificity and sensitivity for detecting injuries compared with plain radiographs. Additionally, CT of the chest, abdomen, and pelvis allows completion of the evaluation more quickly and with fewer transfers of the patient. Hauser et al. found that neither CT of the chest, abdomen, and pelvis nor plain radiographs failed to demonstrate any unstable thoracic or lumbar injuries in the 222 patients studied. Identification of additional injuries considered minor by CT of the chest, abdomen, and pelvis compared with plain radiographs was shown to change treatment with respect to pain management and how patients were mobilized. These minor injuries included spinous process and transverse process fractures without displacement.

BOX 5.3

Factors Related to Spinal Instability

Neurologic Function
- Degree of neurologic deficit
- Potential for additional neurologic injury

Structural Disruption
- Severity of overall structural damage
- Comminution of the vertebral body
- Degree of canal compromise
- Disruption of spinal ligaments
- Disruption of the facet joints, lamina, and pedicles
- Disruption of the intervertebral disc
- Presence of multiple contiguous injuries
- Effect of previous destabilizing procedures

Deformity
- Severity of deformity (kyphosis or scoliosis)
- Buckling of the spinal column (loss of height)
- Potential for progression of deformity
- Redisplacement after reduction
- Potential for late collapse

Anticipated Function
- Loss of stiffness
- Expected future physical exertion
- Potential for developing chronic pain
- Potential impact on future employment

From Mirza SK, Mirza MJ, Chapman JR, Anderson PA: Classifications of thoracic and lumbar fractures: rationale and supporting data, *J Am Acad Orthop Surg* 10:364, 2002.

CLASSIFICATION

The classification of thoracic and lumbar spine injuries is still evolving more than 80 years after the first published report of Böhler. The classification of these injuries remains difficult in part because the goals of classification, anatomic structures to consider, and definitions have not been agreed upon by the community of spine surgeons. Thus, some systems have been developed to direct treatment, whereas others are not intended for this purpose. Terminology, particularly relating to "stability" of the spine, does not have a universally agreed upon definition, which introduces conflicting meanings in different schemes (Box 5.3). Additionally, the concept of "instability" has progressed to include immediate instability and delayed instability, as described by Abbasi Fard et al. Nicoll et al. were the first to focus on patient outcomes and found that anatomic reduction was not crucial to good outcomes in a population of miners who were the basis of their studies. They also classified fractures as stable or unstable based on the probability of increasing deformity and spinal cord injury. Other systems use "instability" as a surrogate term for neurologic injury and consider injuries unstable if a neurologic injury is present without considering the fracture pattern. To classify fractures it is necessary to image the spine, but imaging has changed significantly over time; CT is now the modality of choice in most centers. The

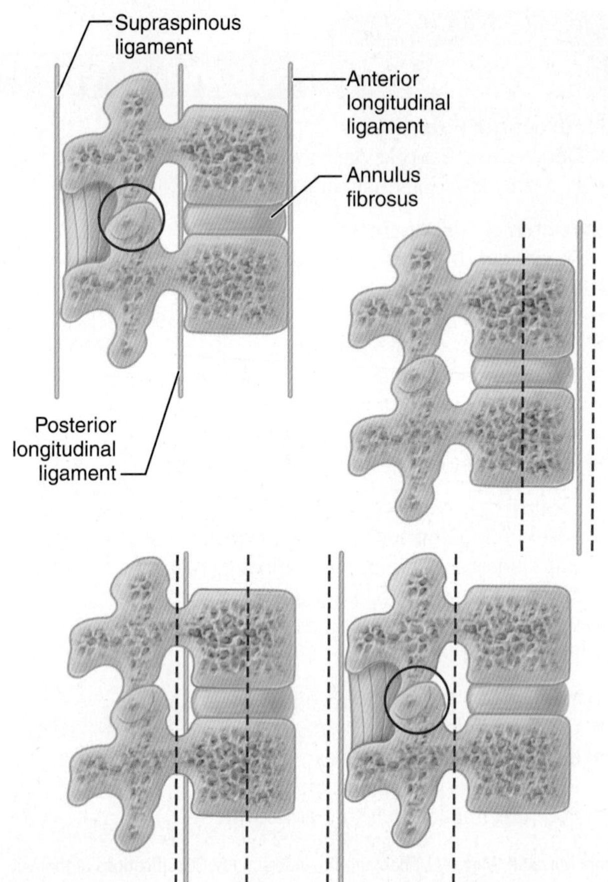

FIGURE 5.36 Three-column classification of spinal instability. Illustrations of anterior, middle, and posterior columns (see text).

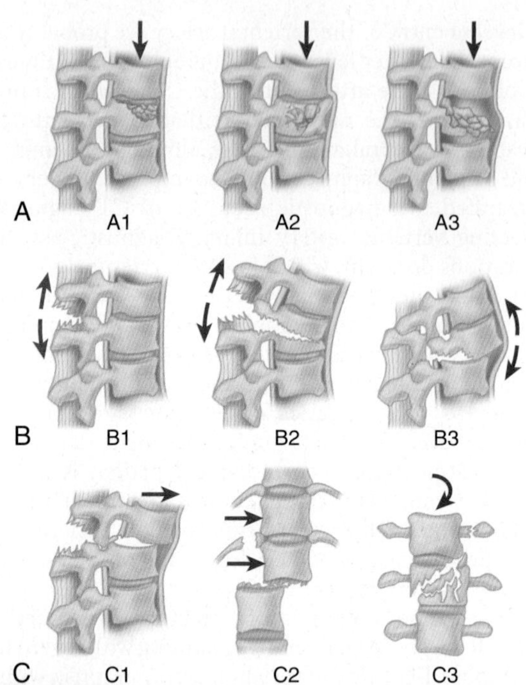

FIGURE 5.37 AO/Magerl classification of spinal injuries. **A,** Compression injuries: A1, impaction; A2, split; A3, burst. **B,** Distraction injuries: B1, posterior ligamentous; B2, posterior osseous; B3, anterior through disc. **C,** Torsion injuries: C1, type A with torsion; C2, type B with torsion; C3, torsion shear.

use of MRI remains controversial and has a limited role in the thoracic and lumbar regions. Khoury et al. found that MRI added very little to the management of patients with CT-proven thoracic and lumbar injuries. It was helpful only in a small group of patients with planned surgery based on the CT. Several recent studies have shown that the CT findings can be well correlated with MRI findings, negating the need for MRI in most thoracolumbar injuries.

Classification systems have followed treatment options that have become more diverse as instrumentation for posterior segmental fixation, anterior reconstruction and fixation, intraosseous techniques, and minimally invasive systems have been used in the trauma setting.

Most of the various classification systems currently in use are either based on a presumed mechanism of injury with specific injury patterns recognized or they are based on fracture morphology. The Denis classification, based on a three-column model of the spine (Fig. 5.36), is an example of a mechanistic system that remains in widespread use. The AO system (Fig. 5.37) is based on fracture morphology with more severe injuries progressing from type A to type C with subtypes 1 to 3 within each type of injury. These subtypes are further subdivided into 53 possible patterns. In 2005, a collaborative effort of the Spine Trauma Study Group produced the Thoracolumbar Injury Severity Score (TLISS) system. This system incorporates the neurologic examination of the patient in a more direct way than previous systems and uses this information with the fracture morphology and the integrity of the posterior ligamentous complex to derive a numeric score for a given injury. The numeric value is then used to guide treatment options, and these treatment options are based on consensus opinions. This system was subsequently modified to become the Thoracolumbar Injury Classification and Severity Score (TLICS) by the original author in an effort to improve the reliability of classifying injuries (Table 5.7). There have been numerous articles evaluating the reliability of various classification systems and comparing one system to another or comparing the results of the same surgeons classifying the same cases at different time points. Generally, these studies have not shown one classification system to be superior to another. The TLICS system is appealing because it incorporates the neurologic function of the patient, which is the single most important determinant of functional outcome for a patient with spine injury. Although the reliability of the system has been found to be equivalent to other systems, the validity of the criteria has not been demonstrated, which also is the case for the other classifications. Also, the treatment recommendations are level IV evidence as consensus opinion.

Denis developed the three-column model as an extension of the work of several other authors based on his review of 412 thoracolumbar injuries, only 53 of which had CT scans. His goal was to highlight the injury patterns resulting from specific injury mechanisms, and this system did not consider treatment or functional outcomes that have become increasingly important to demonstrate. Denis introduced the abstract idea of the "middle column," which is not a distinct anatomic structure but rather the posterior half of the vertebral body, posterior half of the intervertebral disc, and the posterior longitudinal ligament. The mode of failure of the

TABLE 5.7

Thoracolumbar Injury Classification and Severity Score

FRACTURE MECHANISM	POINTS
Compression fracture	1
Burst fracture	1
Translation/rotation	3
Distraction	4
NEUROLOGIC INVOLVEMENT	
Intact	0
Nerve root	2
Cord, conus medullaris, incomplete	3
Cord, conus medullaris, complete	2
Cauda equina	3
POSTERIOR LIGAMENTOUS COMPLEX INTEGRITY	
Intact	0
Injury suspected/indeterminate	2
Injured	3

Score of ≤3: nonoperative treatment; score of ≥5: operative treatment; score of 4: either nonoperative or operative treatment, depending on qualifiers such as comorbid medical conditions and other injuries.
From Vaccaro AR, Zeiller SC, Hulbert RJ, et al: The thoracolumbar injury severity score: a proposed treatment algorithm, *J Spinal Disord Tech* 18:209, 2005.

middle column was used to determine the injury type and the risk of neurologic injury. His description did not include a definition of stability. Injuries were designated as minor (e.g., transverse process, pars interarticularis, spinous process) or as major. The major injuries were divided into four categories based on the presumed mechanism of compression, burst, seat belt (Chance injury), or fracture-dislocation. In a CT study of 100 consecutive patients with potentially unstable fractures and fracture-dislocations, McAfee et al. determined the mechanisms of failure of the middle osteoligamentous complex and developed a new system based on these mechanisms. McAfee et al. categorized the failure of the middle osteoligamentous complex into one of three modes: axial compression, axial distraction, or translation. We have found their simplified system useful in classifying injuries of the thoracolumbar spine.

Wedge compression fractures cause isolated failure of the anterior column and result from forward flexion. They rarely are associated with neurologic deficit except when multiple adjacent vertebral levels are affected.

In stable burst fractures, the anterior and middle columns fail because of a compressive load, with no loss of integrity of the posterior elements.

In unstable burst fractures, the anterior and middle columns fail in compression and the posterior column is disrupted. The posterior column can fail in compression, lateral flexion, or rotation. There is a tendency for posttraumatic kyphosis and progressive neural symptoms because of instability. If the anterior and middle columns fail in compression, the posterior column cannot fail in distraction.

Chance fractures are flexion-distraction injuries and are horizontally oriented distraction injuries of a single vertebra or the osteoligamentous structures of a single motion segment caused by distraction and flexion around an axis of rotation anterior to the anterior longitudinal ligament. The entire vertebra is pulled apart by a strong tensile force. As a result, there is no comminution with these fractures.

In flexion-compression injuries, the flexion axis of rotation is posterior to the anterior longitudinal ligament. The anterior column fails in compression with comminution and shortening, whereas the middle and posterior columns fail in tension. This injury is unstable because the ligamentum flavum, interspinous ligaments, and supraspinous ligaments usually are disrupted.

Translational injuries are characterized by malalignment of the neural canal, which has been totally disrupted. Usually all three columns have failed in shear. At the affected level, one part of the spinal canal has been displaced in the transverse plane.

The AO system (see Fig. 5.37) is based on fracture morphology with more severe injuries progressing from type A to type C with subtypes 1 to 3 within each type of injury. These subtypes are further subdivided into 53 possible patterns. In 2005, a collaborative effort of the Spine Trauma Study Group produced the Thoracolumbar Injury Severity Score (TLISS) system. This system incorporates the neurologic examination of the patient in a more direct way than previous systems and uses this information with the fracture morphology and the integrity of the posterior ligamentous complex to derive a numeric score for a given injury. The numeric value is then used to guide treatment options, and these treatment options are based on consensus opinions. This system was subsequently modified to become the TLICS by the original author in an effort to improve the reliability of classifying injuries (see Table 5.7). There have been numerous articles evaluating the reliability of various classification systems and comparing one system to another or comparing the results of the same surgeons classifying the same cases at different time points. Generally, these studies have not shown one classification system to be superior to another. The TLICS system is appealing because it incorporates the neurologic function of the patient, which is the single most important determinant of functional outcome for a patient with spine injury. Although the reliability of the system has been found to be equivalent to other systems, the validity of the criteria has not been demonstrated, which also is the case for the other classifications. Also, the treatment recommendations are level IV evidence as consensus opinion. Schnake et al. reviewed the most current version of the AO Spine system based on the TLICS and AO/Magerl systems. This iteration has type A (compression) fractures with five subtypes, type B (anterior or posterior tension band failure) with three subtypes, and type C (fracture dislocations with translational displacement), which are not subdivided. In addition, there are five subtypes of neurologic examinations, from intact to indeterminate, as well as two subtypes of patient-specific modifiers. They found generally substantial reliability among surgeons in classifying injuries. Treatment recommendations remain based on expert consensus. Several studies have found the AO Spine system to have higher reliability than the TLICS system with regard to determining fracture morphology.

TREATMENT

The treatment of fractures that involve the thoracic and lumbar spine remains controversial for several reasons. The first is the determination of which injuries are truly best treated operatively and which are best treated nonoperatively; the second is the optimal approach for patients who will be treated operatively; and the third is whether operative treatment should include a direct decompression or if indirect decompression is sufficient. The optimal nonoperative treatment likewise is not settled with respect to whether a postural reduction should be performed, whether initial casting or a thoracolumbosacral orthosis (TLSO) should be used for the duration, or whether treatment should include a period of recumbency or if mobilization should be started quickly. To date, there are only two randomized controlled trials comparing operative with nonoperative treatment of thoracolumbar fractures. In the study of Wood et al. of 53 patients, there were no significant radiographic or functional outcome advantages to operative treatment. In addition, patients treated operatively had a much higher cost of care and higher complication rate than those treated nonoperatively. In a second study, however, Siebenga et al. did report outcome advantages of short-segment posterior fixation compared with nonoperative treatment. A larger series of patients was reported more recently with a novel methodology based on surgeon equipoise as an inclusion criterion to limit bias without the severe limitations of a prospective randomized controlled study. This study, by Stadhouder et al., retrospectively compared 190 patients treated at two different centers either operatively or nonoperatively for thoracolumbar injuries regardless of neurologic status, with the 190 patients selected from 636 total patients on the basis of discordant treatment recommendations from the two centers. The follow-up averaged 6.2 years with a 2-year minimum. Functional outcomes with respect to pain and return to work were determined for 137 of these patients. The authors concluded that with regard to functional recovery and return to work there was no significant difference in the two groups. The operative group had more patients with neurologic deficits and showed a trend toward more neurologic improvement, but this did not reach statistical significance. A systematic literature review by Bakhsheshian et al. confirmed these earlier findings in that functional outcomes after nonoperative treatment were equal to those after operative treatment in patients without neurologic deficits. They also noted that the optimal conservative management method has not been determined. In a review of 5748 patients, Verlaan et al. found that the admission AIS grade is the best predictor of neurologic recovery and that neurologic recovery is not predicted by operative or nonoperative care. To date, no clear benefit for neurologic recovery has been noted after operative treatment. Multiple studies have demonstrated that neurologic recovery does occur in patients with thoracolumbar fractures treated nonoperatively. Typically, incomplete injuries (ASIA B-D) will improve one grade with either form of treatment; several studies, including that of Wood et al., showed no benefit to surgery with respect to correcting spinal canal stenosis caused by retropulsion of bony fragments. Daniels et al., in a retrospective series of 24,098 patients with thoracolumbar injuries from 25 U.S. hospitals, found that 91.7% of patients had no neurologic injury. Nine percent of patients without a neurologic injury were treated operatively compared with 61.4% of patients who had a neurologic deficit. The type of hospital setting where treatment was rendered was a significant determinant of whether a patient received operative or nonoperative care. Patients, with or without neurologic injury, treated at an urban teaching hospital or a high-volume hospital were more likely to have surgery than at a nonteaching hospital. These numbers were significantly different. A Cochrane report on operative compared to nonoperative treatment of thoracolumbar fractures without neurologic deficits did not find enough data to make a determination, in part because of the heterogenous groups of fractures included in most studies without detailed classification of injuries. Numerous relatively small series have described percutaneous instrumentation, often in neurologically intact patients who have been found to do well with nonoperative treatment, and do not contain relevant patient-reported outcomes. The technique appears to be safe, but clinical benefit remains to be determined. Several reports have indicated that patients with instrumented thoracolumbar fractures without fusion have similar kyphosis progression over long-term follow-up as patients with instrumentation and fusion. Several recent studies have shown that implant removal after healing can restore some regional mobility.

The issues of approach and the need for decompression often are linked. Although there is no definitive literature proving the benefits of operative decompression in thoracolumbar fractures, most spine surgeons would not recommend allowing persistent neural compression in the presence of a neurologic deficit. This is based on numerous animal studies dating back several decades that have shown a correlation between neurologic recovery and decompression of neural tissue, which allows for restoration of regional blood flow. Also, a study done by Bohlman et al. demonstrated neurologic recovery occurring after a recovery plateau was reached when a late decompression was done. There is no absolute value for canal compromise that has been found to correlate with neurologic deficit. Panjabi et al. demonstrated with a dynamic injury model that the canal encroachment at the time of injury was 85% greater than was evident on static postinjury images. This explains why there is no correlation between canal compromise on static postinjury imaging studies and neurologic deficit. Direct decompression is not indicated if the patient has no neurologic deficit even with significant canal encroachment at presentation, because this is not related to the development of a subsequent deficit. An indirect decompression often is accomplished during operative stabilization for thoracolumbar injuries. The approach that affords the best opportunity for decompression is selected when a direct decompression is deemed warranted because fixation options have become more versatile, and stable fixation usually is possible with either anterior or posterior fixation, and rarely combined anterior and posterior fixation is necessary depending on which anatomic structures are injured.

In our practice, the treatment of thoracic and lumbar fractures is determined primarily by the neurologic status of a patient, a determination of spinal column functional integrity based on which specific structures are injured, and the type and magnitude of deformity present. Most patients with thoracic or lumbar injuries do not have neurologic compromise, and most of these patients are treated nonoperatively. A relatively small portion of these patients have injury patterns that necessitate operative treatment, and some patient factors, such as ankylosing spondylitis, may require surgical stabilization. Progressive neurologic deficit is one circumstance that results in a change to operative treatment. This occurs infrequently; in most studies the incidence is between 0% and 2% of patients, which is consistent with our experience. Patients who develop significant worsening of their deformity with global imbalance in the sagittal or coronal plane rather than regional deformity are treated operatively. There is poor correlation between regional kyphosis at the injured level and functional outcome, although injury to the posterior ligamentous complex is considered structurally important. To detect changes in overall alignment, upright radiographs are obtained after the patient has begun to mobilize, rather than relying on MRI to evaluate the posterior ligamentous complex to predict deformity progression in most patients.

Patients who have spinal cord, conus medullaris, or cauda equina injuries are most often treated operatively to facilitate rehabilitation, especially if the deficits are complete neurologic injuries. Short-segment posterior instrumentation is the most common construct used, but specific construct design is dictated by the injury pattern and the neurology of the patient. Anatomic fracture reduction, although desirable, has not been the primary treatment objective. The acceptable limits of residual deformity in the sagittal and coronal planes before functional outcome is compromised have not been determined. In his original series of patients, Nicoll et al. found that of the 50 patients who returned to full function, working as miners for at least 2 years, 24 (48%) had some residual deformity. What is not clear is whether these same patients would have reached functional recovery more quickly and with less difficulty had the deformity not been present.

Nonoperative treatment consists of a TLSO for most patients with injuries at or caudal to T7 to help control lateral bending, although Jewett-type braces also are used fairly frequently if lateral bending is less of a concern and if dictated by body habitus. Injuries that are rostral to T7 are difficult to brace, especially if there are rib fractures at the injured level. Many compression fractures and burst fractures with only partial vertebral body involvement are treated without an orthosis and close radiographic follow-up to monitor for deformity development. Comorbidities, concomitant injuries, and anticipated activity level of the patient are some of the individual factors considered when determining whether brace treatment is a reasonable option for a particular patient. Brace treatment is initiated as soon as possible to begin mobilization, and a postural reduction usually is not done. After the patient has mobilized sufficiently, upright radiographs centered at the injury level are reviewed to confirm adequate maintenance of alignment and full-length radiographs are obtained as soon as feasible. The orthosis is worn at all times when the patient is upright beyond 30 degrees from horizontal for 12 weeks or longer if clinical progress is not as rapid as expected. Progression of deformity is a reason to change treatment to operative stabilization.

COMPRESSION FRACTURES

Compression fractures are characterized by loss of vertebral height anteriorly, with no loss of posterior vertebral height and no posterior ligamentous or bony injury. MRI is not routinely indicated unless ligamentous injury is suspected because of more than 25 degrees of segmental kyphosis. Radiographs obtained after mobilization can be used to determine spinal stability rather than MRI assessment of posterior ligamentous structures. Compression fracture treatment is with a TLSO for 12 weeks with medical management of pain, which is significant, and graduated return to activity. The most severe pain usually improves after 3 to 6 weeks. Upright radiographs must be reviewed after mobilization to verify that there is no worsening of deformity. If the patient has a posterior ligamentous injury and an anterior body fracture, operative treatment is a consideration. Short-segment posterior tension band reconstruction that can be percutaneously placed has shown promise in this setting, but longer-term study is needed. Intraosseous procedures such as kyphoplasty should be reserved for low-energy pathologic fractures. Higher-energy fractures can have fracture lines not visible on CT scan that may extend through the posterior cortex, allowing ingress of bone cement into the spinal canal.

BURST FRACTURES

The key features of this injury are posterior vertebral body cortex fracture with retropulsion of bone into the canal and widening of the interpedicular distance relative to the adjacent levels. Multiple studies have shown that there is no reliable correlation between degree of canal compromise and neurologic function, so the percentage of canal compromise is not used as a stand-alone indication for surgery. It is very uncommon for a patient to develop a neurologic deficit with proper immobilization for a burst fracture even in the setting of severe canal compromise. Fractures of the laminae that are nondisplaced and vertically oriented do not significantly affect the ability of the spine to bear axial load forces, and the mere presence of such a fracture line does not require operative intervention. Such fractures can, however, entrap nerve rootlets, and if neurologic deficits necessitate decompression, then stabilization will be necessary after decompression. If the patient has a neurologic deficit involving more than a single root level, operative decompression and stabilization are recommended. The decompression can be indirect using distraction and ligamentotaxis through the intact posterior longitudinal ligament or a direct decompression that can be done either anteriorly or posteriorly. If there is a horizontally oriented injury posteriorly in the pars interarticularis, laminae, or a facet disruption, this would suggest a distractive force and not an axial load injury, and the posterior longitudinal ligament is likely to be disrupted, so ligamentotaxis should not be employed. For patients without neurologic deficit who are treated operatively, posterior indirect reduction is used. The terms *stable burst* and *unstable burst* are ambiguous and in our opinion should be avoided in favor of a structural assessment of each specific portion of vertebrae. This allows an overall assessment of the structural integrity of the spine and forms the most logical basis for treatment. If operative treatment is chosen, it also can help direct the anatomic approach and the extent of stabilization that is needed. If operative stabilization is undertaken, short-segment constructs to preserve motion segments are desirable, particularly in the mid and lower lumbar levels. The load-bearing fracture classification of McCormack et al. is helpful in determining if a short construct is likely to fail based on fracture characteristics

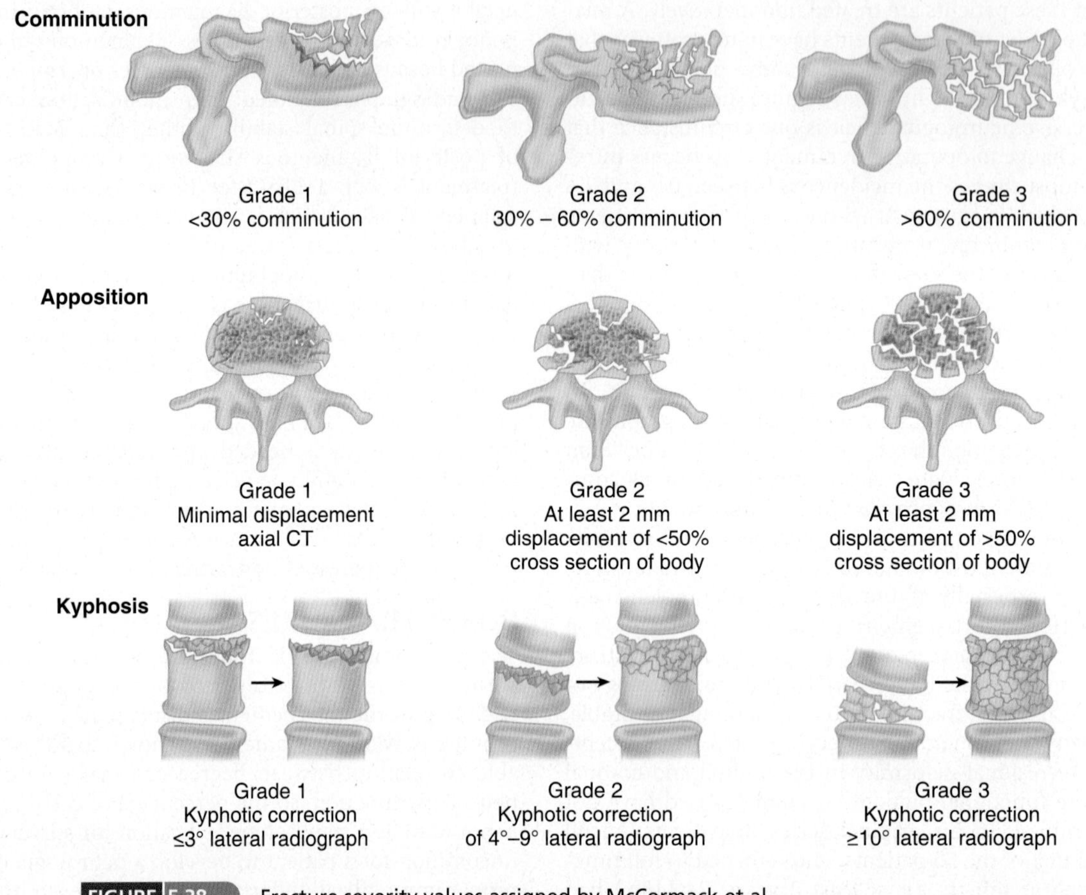

FIGURE 5.38 Fracture severity values assigned by McCormack et al.

(Fig. 5.38). For injuries that cannot be stabilized using short constructs, a longer construct can be used in the thoracic spine without sacrificing clinically important motion. In the lumbar spine, anterior decompression and reconstruction usually allow preservation of motion segments and rarely need supplemental posterior stabilization at the same levels. The patient's neurologic status and coexisting injuries must be considered in operative planning. Achieving adequate stability to allow fracture and fusion healing to progress to definitive stability is the objective. For patients requiring the most complete decompression of the spinal cord, direct anterior decompression is favored.

DISTRACTION INJURIES

The cardinal feature of this type of injury is lengthening of the posterior spine that extends into the middle column and anterior columns of the spine. Distractive forces are indicated on spine radiographs by a lack of comminution. It is important to distinguish between flexion-distraction injuries and flexion-compression injuries. Both injuries have posterior lengthening, indicating injury to the posterior osteoligamentous complex. The difference is where the instantaneous center of rotation is located at the time of injury. Flexion-distraction injuries are best represented by the "Chance" injury, described in 1948. This injury classically is located in the upper lumbar spine in people involved in motor vehicle collisions who were using two-point restraints across the lap. Upon impact, the lumbar spine flexes around the lap belt, and the injury occurs as the osseous structures, ligamentous structures, or both fail in tension around the center of rotation created by the seat belt, compressing the abdominal contents against the anterior spine. Because the rotation occurs around a point anterior to the spine, the lengthening occurs even though the anterior longitudinal ligament fails in tension, so there is no structure left intact. It is important to recognize this if operative treatment is to be undertaken. Posterior compression constructs are used to stabilize these injuries, and distraction should be avoided because there is no intact structure to prevent excessive lengthening of the spine and neural elements. Flexion-compression injuries occur when the center of rotation is located within the spine such that posterior structures fail in tension and anterior structures fail in compression. Compression is a failure mode for bone but not for ligamentous structures, so in this instance the anterior longitudinal ligament is preserved and can be used as a hinge point during operative stabilization. Operative stabilization can be achieved posteriorly, using careful and monitored distraction and a rod with slightly overcontoured lordosis. This allows better correction of the kyphosis that is present with this type of injury than a compression construct. Because the posterior bone injury occurs in distraction and there is minimal comminution once reduction is achieved, the injuries are able to withstand some axial loading, so short constructs generally are sufficient. Distraction injuries often are associated with neurologic deficits, and these injuries are treated operatively with short constructs and removal of the torn ligamentum flavum that can enfold into the canal, especially if a compression construct is used. If the injury is a true Chance bone injury with no neurologic deficit, satisfactory reduction can be obtained with a hyperextension TLSO for 12 weeks.

EXTENSION INJURIES

Extension injuries are identified by anterior spinal lengthening and most commonly occur in the thoracic spine. Unlike the cervical extension injuries, which can be purely ligamentous or include fractures, the injuries in the thoracic and lumbar regions are almost always fractures in patients with ankylosing spondylitis or disseminated idiopathic skeletal hyperostosis. For patients with a minimal neurologic deficit on presentation, the early recognition of this injury pattern is crucial to avoid iatrogenic injury associated with moving the patient for further evaluation or treatment of other injuries. These injuries can be very unstable, and translation, usually retrolisthesis, can cause spinal cord injury. It is critical to avoid placing the patient in a horizontal supine position if they have a significant kyphotic deformity. Early stabilization with a long posterior construct using segmental fixation is the recommended treatment for three-column injuries. In addition to neurologic deficits from translation of the spinal column, patients are at risk for development of epidural hematomas. If a patient has neurologic worsening, emergent MRI is indicated to assess the spinal canal alignment and for a hematoma. During the evaluation, the patient is supported in his or her native kyphosis.

FRACTURE-DISLOCATIONS

The pathognomonic feature for this type of injury is translational displacement in the axial plane. The displacement may be most evident on either the sagittal or the coronal reconstruction but may not be well demonstrated on the axial images unless two vertebral bodies happen to be imaged on the same axial slice. There also can be a rotational component (either flexion or extension) present; some injuries have distraction as a major component, but the translational displacement identifies the fracture-dislocation. This injury pattern is the most severe and is usually associated with a significant neurologic injury. These injuries are unstable in shear and require long constructs with segmental fixation. Fracture reduction and proper spinal alignment are more important goals in these injuries than decompression because many have complete neurologic injuries that will not be improved by decompression. Achieving spinal stability is dependent on achieving a solid fusion.

DECOMPRESSION

The role of surgical decompression is controversial. There are regional differences in cord blood flow and differences in susceptibility to neural injury by anatomic region, progressing from spinal cord to conus medullaris and cauda equina. The spinal canal in the thoracic area is small, and the cord blood supply is sparse; significant neurologic injury is common with severe fractures and dislocations in the thoracic spine. Fractures or fracture-dislocations in the lumbar region may result in marked displacement and still cause little or no neurologic deficit. Not only is the canal larger in this area, but also the spinal cord ends at approximately the first lumbar vertebra, and the cauda equina is less vulnerable than the cord to injury. Wilcox et al. in an in vitro dynamic model showed that maximal compression of the cord and narrowing of the spinal canal occur at the time of impact; both improved after recoil of the spine. The degree of final narrowing of the canal was poorly related to the CT obtained after injury. Krompinger et al. reported that late CT analysis of patients with burst fractures treated conservatively showed significant resolution of bony canal compromise. This finding also was demonstrated by Wood et al. The remodeling process seems to be age and time dependent and follows expected principles of bone remodeling to applied stress. Fontijne et al. showed that remodeling and reconstitution of the spinal canal occurs within the first 12 months after injury (50% of normal diameter at injury and 75% at 1-year follow-up). These authors concluded that conservative management of thoracolumbar burst fractures is followed by a marked degree of spontaneous redevelopment of the deformed spinal canal, which supports conservative management of thoracolumbar burst fractures in selected patients. Neurologic deficits have not developed in these patients. The treatment of thoracic and lumbar burst fractures must be individualized, and canal compromise from retropulsed bone fragments is not in itself an absolute indication for surgical decompression.

Canal compromise without ongoing residual neural tissue compression, which does not correlate with neurologic deficit, must be distinguished from ongoing neural compression, which does correlate with neurologic deficit. Compression of the neural elements by retropulsed bone fragments can be relieved indirectly by the application of distractive forces through posterior instrumentation or directly by exploration of the spinal canal through a posterolateral or anterior approach. There is no universal agreement as to indications for each of these. The indirect approach to decompression of the spinal canal using ligamentotaxis is a technique that uses the posterior instrumentation and a distraction force applied to the intact posterior longitudinal ligament to reduce the retropulsed bone from the spinal canal by tensioning the posterior longitudinal ligament. Numerous authors have documented excellent results with this technique, and it is a familiar technique to most orthopaedic surgeons. Problems with this technique occur if surgery is delayed for more than 10 to 14 days because indirect reduction of the spinal canal cannot be achieved after fracture healing begins. In addition, severely comminuted fractures with multiple pieces of bone pushed into the spinal canal may not be completely reduced by distraction instrumentation. If the reverse cortical sign is present, the posterior longitudinal ligament is likely not intact and ligamentotaxis will not occur.

The posterolateral technique for decompression of the spinal canal is effective at the thoracolumbar junction and in the lumbar spine. This procedure involves hemilaminectomy and removal of a pedicle with a high-speed burr to allow posterolateral decompression of the dura along its anterior aspect (Fig. 5.39). In the thoracic spine, where less room is available for the cord, this technique involves increased risk to the neural elements. The anterior approach allows direct decompression of the thecal sac but is a less familiar approach to many surgeons. Visceral and vascular structures may be injured, and this approach carries the greatest risk of potential morbidity. In addition, anterior decompression and placement of a strut graft or cage provides modest immediate stability to the fracture if the anterior longitudinal ligament is preserved. To have adequate stability, anterior fixation is needed if anterior decompression is done. The role of anterior internal fixation devices has evolved in recent years, and these devices

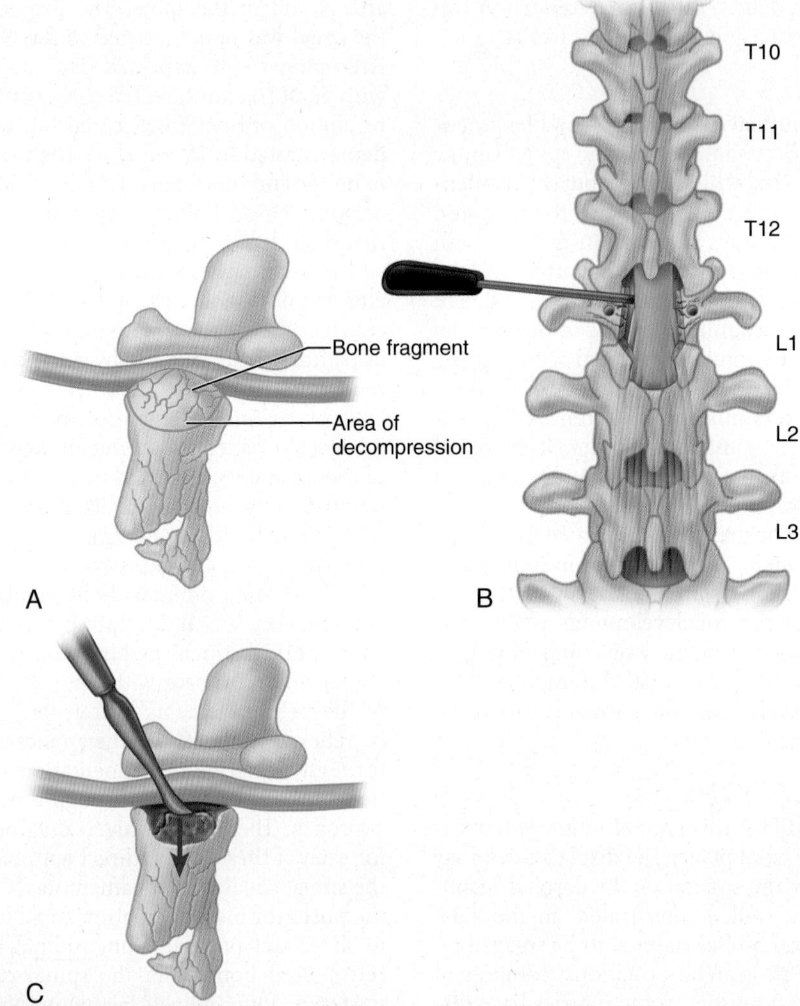

FIGURE 5.39 Posterolateral decompression technique. **A,** L1 burst fracture. **B,** Pedicle, transverse process, and lateral portions of T12-L1 facet are removed after L1 root has been isolated. **C,** After fragments have been undercut, they are reduced into vertebral body.

have proven to be safe and beneficial in achieving spinal stabilization. The need for additional posterior stabilization procedures has been eliminated in some patients. When anterior decompression and strut grafting or cage placement are performed in the presence of posterior instability, posterior instrumentation and fusion can be done to improve stability. This combined posterior and anterior fixation allows for shorter constructs.

At this time, we favor early posterior instrumentation with indirect or posterolateral direct decompression in most patients requiring operative treatment. If significant residual neural compression (not mere canal compromise) exists postoperatively in a patient with an incomplete spinal cord injury, an anterior decompression and reconstruction are done if no significant clinical improvement over a reasonable period of time is noted. Posterior decompression must be carefully considered in all patients with posterior vertical laminar fractures because of the increased frequency of dural tears with exposed nerve roots and the possibility of severe post-traumatic arachnoiditis. Careful neurologic examination is required to detect some deficits; however, in severely injured or obtunded patients, reliable neurologic examination may not be possible. Ozturk et al. found dural tears in 25% of 25 patients with thoracic and lumbar burst fractures in conjunction with vertical lamina fractures. They were more common at L2 to L4. For patients with severe but incomplete spinal cord injuries at the T12 to L3 levels, anterior decompression and reconstruction is the favored treatment. A minimally invasive approach is used when possible.

Postoperatively, a CT scan of the spine with sagittal reconstruction is obtained through the injured segment to evaluate further the adequacy of spinal cord decompression. In a retrospective review of 49 nonparaplegic patients who sustained an acute, unstable, thoracolumbar burst fracture, Danisa et al. concluded that patients treated with posterior surgery had a statistically significant lower operative time and blood loss. They noted no significant intergroup differences between those treated with anterior decompression and fusion, posterior decompression and fusion, and combined anteroposterior surgery when considering postoperative kyphotic correction, neurologic function, pain assessment, or the ability to return to work. Posterior surgery was found to be as effective as anterior or anteroposterior surgery when treating unstable thoracolumbar burst fractures. Of the three procedures, posterior surgery takes the least time, causes the least blood loss, and is the least expensive.

POSTERIOR STABILIZATION

THORACIC AND LUMBAR SEGMENTAL FIXATION WITH PEDICLE SCREWS

Pedicle screw and rod constructs have continued to increase in use for both thoracic and lumbar fractures over the past decade. By using segmental fixation, rod contouring, and compression and distraction forces as indicated on an individual rod, excellent fracture reduction is possible. Most current systems offer a variety of screw size options and a choice of rod material for the surgeon to tailor stabilization to the specific patient need. Minimally invasive techniques currently are not quite as versatile but do allow for corrective force application such as compression or distraction. The role of minimally invasive stabilization is not well established, and at this time we rarely use these techniques. We believe spinal implants should be used only by experienced spinal surgeons who have a thorough knowledge of spinal anatomy to reduce the incidence of complications, including pedicle fracture, dural tear, nerve root injury, spinal cord injury, and vascular injuries. Image intensification is routinely used to assist in screw placement; image-guided navigation has not been found useful except in unusual cases.

TECHNIQUE 5.17

- A fully radiolucent table is used. Position the patient to allow for postural reduction when placed prone using a four-post frame or chest rolls placed transversely or longitudinally, depending on the extent of postural support desired. If the patient is neurologically intact or incomplete, neuromonitoring is used if the spinal canal dimensions will be manipulated (e.g., distraction for ligamentotaxis and indirect fracture reduction) during the operation.
- Obtain images of the spine to confirm the degree of postural spinal reduction after positioning and determine the limits of the incision.
- Prepare and drape the thoracolumbar spine to be instrumented and the iliac crest if desired.
- Harvest morselized cancellous bone graft from the iliac crest.
- Make a score incision from one spinous process above the area to be instrumented to one spinous process below the area to be instrumented.
- Infiltrate the incision, subcutaneous tissue, and muscle with epinephrine solution (1 mg in 500 mL of injectable saline) and then complete the incision sharply.
- Continue the dissection with electrocautery to the fascia. Delineate the fascia for later closure. Continue the dissection through the fascia and subperiosteally expose the necessary levels after radiographically confirming the level.
- Use electrocautery to release the muscle from the bone carefully at the level of the fracture. Watch for evidence of a cerebrospinal fluid leak or the presence of free nerve roots.
- Continue to widen the dissection to the tips of the transverse processes in the thoracic and lumbar spine.
- Use image intensification to identify the upper level to be instrumented.

THORACIC PEDICLE SCREW PLACEMENT

- Obtain a true anteroposterior view of the vertebra. On this view the superior endplate should appear as a sharply defined line with the superiormost portion of the pedicle just rostral to the endplate. The pedicles should be symmetric with one another, and the tip of the spinous process should be superimposed in the midline of the vertebra. It is critical to adjust the image until such a view is acquired.
- Position a burr near the superior medial base of the transverse process such that it is superimposed at the 2 o'clock position on the right pedicle or the 10 o'clock position on the left pedicle on the anteroposterior view. Use the burr to penetrate the cortex in this location. Use this as the starting point for a pedicle probe.
- Advance the pedicle probe, monitoring the anteroposterior image and directing the probe medially such that it crosses from the lateral cortex of the pedicle to the medial cortex of the pedicle as it penetrates deeper into the pedicle. The trajectory of the probe should be chosen such that the tip of the probe rests at the medial border of the pedicle image after advancing to a depth of 18 mm. This will allow the probe to traverse the length of the pedicle and enter the posterior vertebral body in most patients before becoming medial to the medial margin of the pedicle. This can be confirmed on lateral image intensifier views if the anatomy is atypical. As the probe is advanced, direct it slightly caudally within the pedicle.
- With the probe confirmed in the vertebral body, advance it to the desired depth. It is not necessary to advance into the anterior third of the body.
- Use a small ball-tipped probe to sound the pedicle for cortical breaches in all four quadrants and to confirm the vertebral body was not penetrated anteriorly.
- Place the largest diameter screw that the pedicle will accept. This can be determined from the anteroposterior view of the pedicle. The most narrow pedicles are typically at the T4 to T6 levels. If the bone is very dense or the screw is very large in relation to the pedicle, a tap is used before screw placement.
- If the pedicle is too narrow to accept even the smallest diameter screw, this same technique will allow for safe screw placement with an "in-out-in" path of the pedicle probe. It will enter the bone and then exit the bone into the costovertebral joint and reenter through the lateral pedicle wall to enter the vertebral body. This allows for safe screw placement, although screw purchase is less than with an intact pedicle.
- Most commonly, polyaxial screws are used, although monoaxial screws are occasionally used if more rigidity is needed.
- Place all thoracic screws in a similar fashion (Fig. 5.40).

(Details of rod placement follow lumbar screw technique.)

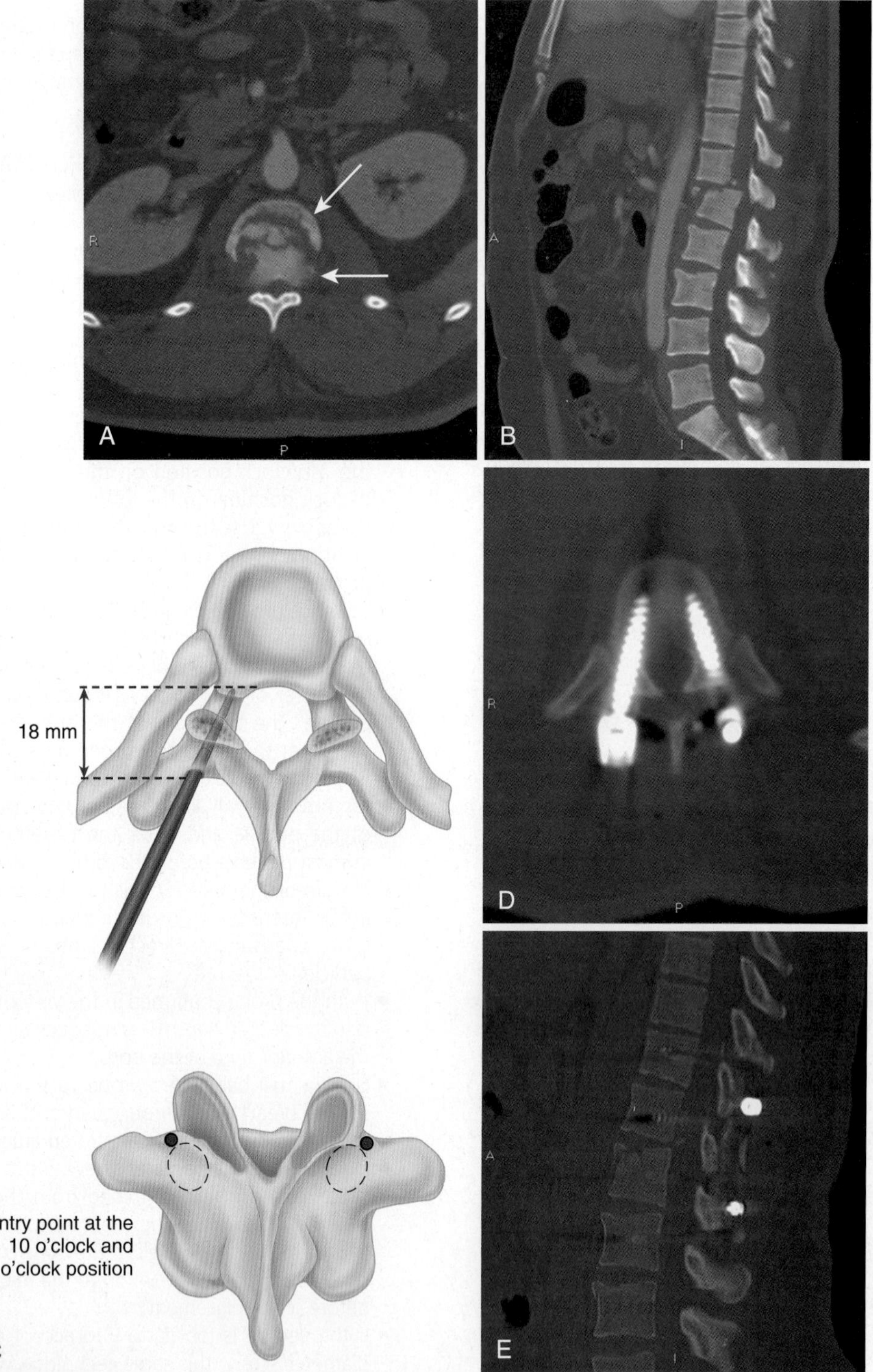

FIGURE 5.40 Axial (**A**) and sagittal (**B**) reformatted images in patient with T12-L1 fracture-dislocation. **C,** Pedicles are drilled to depth of 18 mm from entry points at 10 o'clock and 2 o'clock positions. **D** and **E,** Pedicle screws in place with restoration of anatomic alignment. **SEE TECHNIQUE 1.17.**

LUMBAR PEDICLE SCREW PLACEMENT

- In the upper lumbar segments, the same technique described for the thoracic spine is useful because these pedicles can be quite narrow, especially at L1 and L2. For the lower levels with larger pedicles, we usually prefer to place the lumbar screws using a lateral image of the vertebra being instrumented to help guide screw placement.
- Obtain a true lateral view of the vertebra as indicated by sharply defined endplates with perfectly superimposed pedicles. Adjust the image intensifier until this image is obtained.
- Place the burr just posterior to the junction of the transverse process and the superior articular mass in line with the bisector of the pedicle on the lateral image intensifier

view. Penetrate the cortex at this location, which is near the junction of the pars interarticularis and the superior articular mass. Decorticating the transverse process before screw insertion improves the effectiveness of decortication and enhances the fusion bed.

- Use the cortical opening as the starting point and advance a pedicle probe into the pedicle. The probe is advanced anteriorly and medially simultaneously. Direct the probe more medially at the lower lumbar levels (usually 20 to 30 degrees at L5 and 0 to 10 degrees at the L1 level). The cephalad to caudal orientation is guided by the image intensifier view. Advance the probe to the anterior third of the body.
- Use a small ball-tipped probe to sound the pedicle in all four quadrants and to palpate the vertebral body laterally and anteriorly to make sure there are no cortical breaches.
- The largest diameter screw the pedicle will accept (up to a 6.5-mm screw) is typically placed. Larger screws can be placed but little is usually gained, and the larger screws are more likely to cause pedicle fracture and loss of screw purchase. Polyaxial screws are most commonly used, but monoaxial screws can be useful when short constructs with a single level of fixation above or below the fracture is used. Using a tap will lower the risk of pedicle fracture in sclerotic bone.
- Place the screw after placing the bone graft onto the decorticated surface.
- Adjust the image intensifier to obtain an "end on" view of the screw to verify radiographically that the screw is within the pedicle.
- Place the remaining screws in the same fashion.

ROD PLACEMENT

- Direct decompression, if needed, is completed before rod placement. Costotransversectomy is not used as frequently as transpedicular decompression, but both are useful techniques.
- Cut the rod, allowing some excess length if distraction will be applied.
- Contour the rod to assist in achieving reduction. This usually means undercontouring the kyphosis to help reduce the kyphotic deformity as the rod is reduced into the screw "tulip."
- Reduce the rod to the screws, using multiple reduction instruments if needed to avoid excessive pull on any individual screw, and insert the blockers into the screw "tulip" loosely at each level.
- Apply distraction or compression as the injury dictates and complete in situ rod contouring if necessary to reduce the fracture. Apply final tightening to the blockers and place crosslinks if necessary.
- Confirm adequacy of the reduction on anteroposterior and lateral views.
- Decorticate the posterior elements and transverse processes at each instrumented level and place the bone graft onto the decorticated surface. In the lumbar spine, decortication and graft placement are best done before screw placement. Cancellous allograft can be used if additional bone is needed.
- Close the fascia over a drain with suture passed through the spinous processes.
- Close remaining layers using a subcuticular skin closure for fewer wound problems.

POSTOPERATIVE CARE Postoperatively a CT scan can be obtained to verify screw position and to determine if there is any residual neural compression in a patient with a neurologic deficit. The patient is mobilized on the first postoperative day with an orthosis unless other injuries preclude this. The orthosis is continued 8 to 12 weeks, depending on resolution of pain and radiographic follow-up for evidence of healing and maintenance of spinal alignment.

ANTERIOR STABILIZATION

Anterior reconstruction can provide satisfactory stability without necessarily requiring a posterior procedure. Sasso et al. reviewed a series of 40 patients with three-column injuries who were treated with anterior reconstruction and found that 91% of those with incomplete neurologic deficits improved one modified Frankel grade and 95% of patients had satisfactory healing with maintenance of alignment. The study was retrospective but included multiple surgeons and two sites.

The approach for anterior reconstruction varies considerably by level of injury (T4 to L3), and many centers have a joint approach using either a cardiovascular surgeon or general surgeon along with a spine surgeon. The primary advantages of an anterior approach are direct decompression and restoration of the axial load-bearing portion of the spine with a strut device. With restoration of some load bearing through the anterior spine, shorter constructs are possible that can allow preservation of more normal motion segments in some clinical settings. Correction of kyphosis also is enhanced with a direct anterior approach. The anterior construct can consist of bone graft or a metallic cage that may be adjustable with respect to length in conjunction with a plate or rod device with screw fixation. Additionally, with a direct anterior decompression of the spinal canal, it is possible to completely remove retropulsed fragments of bone or disc material. The morbidity of the standard thoracotomy and retroperitoneal approaches prohibits their use in many patients, making these advantages less attractive relative to the more common posterior approach. However, with advances in retractor systems and fixation devices, the approach is less morbid and adjunctive posterior fixation often is not necessary, so a larger proportion of injuries can now be operatively treated anteriorly. Also, the dimensions of the implants have decreased somewhat, allowing for safer implantation of the devices. Even with these advances, injuries with posterior ligamentous complex disruption should be considered very carefully before recommending anterior-only stabilization. Injuries with translational displacement usually are treated with posterior constructs. Anterior fixation devices consist of a plate or paired rods secured to the spine with bone screws or bolts that have a threaded portion extending through the plate and accepting a nut to capture the plate. Most systems have two fixation points at each vertebral level to better resist flexion. Construct stability is most dependent on the fit of the strut (bone or cage), followed by the integrity of the endplates the strut is in contact with, native bone quality, and the inherent

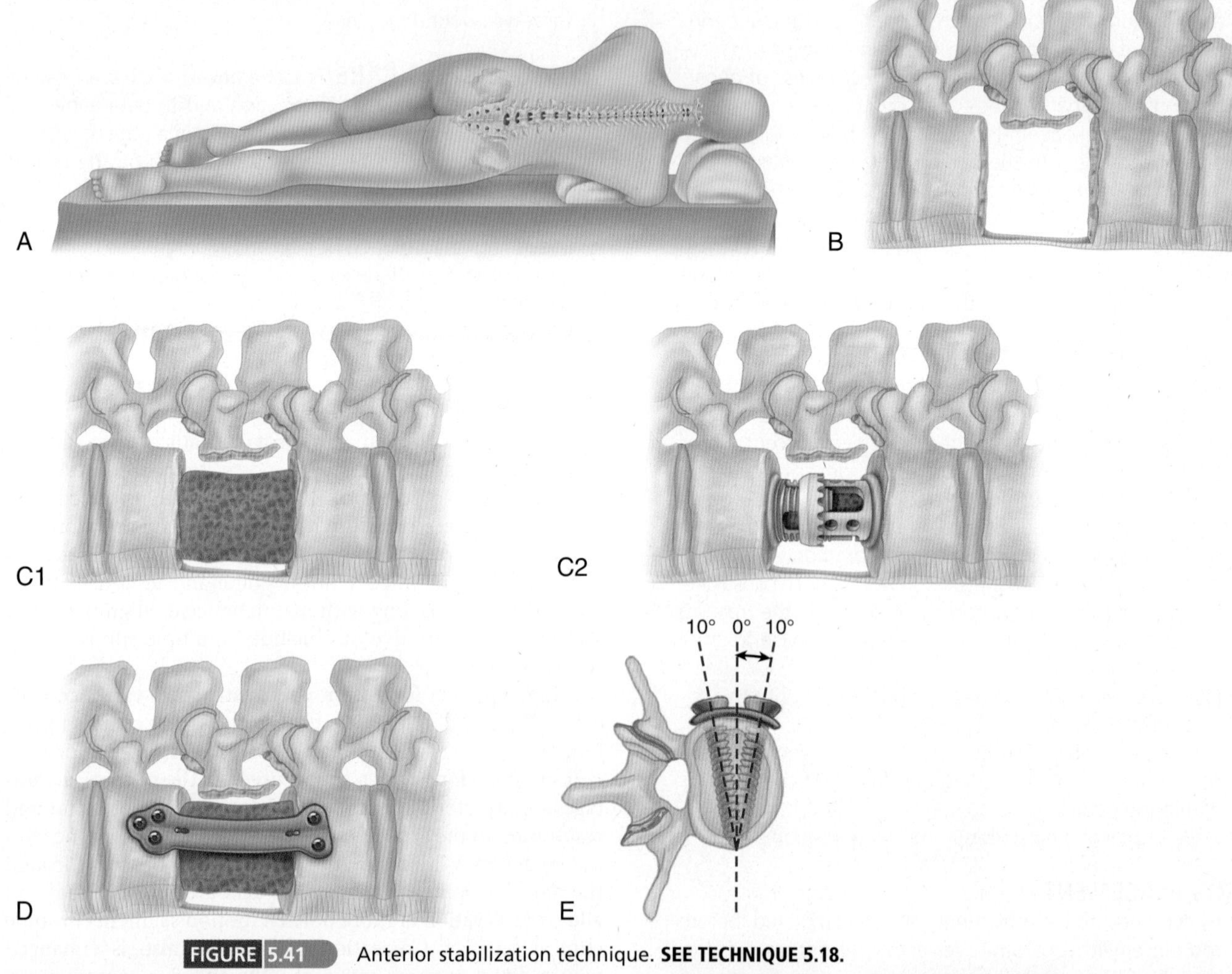

FIGURE 5.41 Anterior stabilization technique. SEE TECHNIQUE 5.18.

fixation device properties that can be decreased with technical errors in placement.

ANTERIOR PLATING

TECHNIQUE 5.18

- After induction of anesthesia, place the patient in a right lateral decubitus position, with appropriate padding to allow for a left-sided thoracic or retroperitoneal approach. Only rarely is a right-sided approach indicated. Secure the patient to the table to prevent him or her from rolling forward or backward during the procedure, which if undetected can lead to increased risk for neurologic or vascular injury. It is important that the patient remain in a true lateral position so screw trajectory can be correctly determined (Fig. 5.41A). Neuromonitoring generally is used when anterior thoracic or lumbar decompression is planned.
- Complete routine skin preparation including the iliac crest if this will be used as a graft.
- Use the image intensifier to locate the intended incision directly lateral to the injured segment. In the thoracic spine this is typically through the rib that is two levels above the injured level. For lumbar injuries a retroperitoneal approach through the 10th or 11th rib usually is used.
- Make an incision overlying the rib and dissect down to the rib periosteum with electrocautery. Elevate the periosteum circumferentially around the rib and elevate the neurovascular bundle from the inferior rib margin. Resect the portion of the rib necessary for access to the spine. Make sure to remove enough rib posteriorly. The rib can be used along with the resected vertebral body for bone graft and should be maintained.
- For a transthoracic approach (T4 to T10), enter the pleural space and retract the lung with a wet laparotomy sponge. Shape a malleable retractor to maintain the operative field. Some prefer to deflate the lung and use a double-lumen endotracheal tube, but we have not routinely found this to be necessary to maintain the lung out of the field. Identify the aorta by palpation and ligate the segmental vessels 1 cm from the aorta. Divide between ligatures at the injured level. It may be necessary to similarly divide the segmental arteries at the level and below the injured vertebra. Vascular clips can be used to supplement the

ligatures. Ligating the artery of Adamkiewicz, which has a variable location, is an inherent risk of this procedure.

- For a retroperitoneal approach (T11 to L3), maintain the pleura intact if possible and enter the retroperitoneal space, dissecting bluntly down to the iliopsoas. Use a wet laparotomy sponge and a malleable retractor to maintain the operative field. Ligate the segmental arteries at the injured level and the level above and below 1 cm from the aorta. It may be necessary to similarly divide the segmental arteries at the level above and below the injured segment. Divide between ligatures with supplemental vascular clips if needed. The artery of Adamkiewicz can be as low as L2. The crus of the diaphragm is taken down as needed, depending on the level of injury. Elevate the iliopsoas from the spine from the anterior margin, taking care to avoid the genitofemoral nerve and ureter.
- Incise the discs above and below the injured segment and remove most of the disc, leaving the anteriormost disc and anterior longitudinal ligament intact. Protect the aorta from sharp instruments with a malleable retractor placed gently between the aorta and the anterior spine.
- Using the space created by removing the discs, remove the vertebral body in its midportion with a rongeur, again leaving the anterior longitudinal ligament and anteriormost bone in place. An osteotome is useful to remove the posterior bone, which is preserved for graft. During bone removal ensure that the patient position has not changed to avoid inadvertent entry into the spinal canal (Fig. 5.41B).
- After creating a cavity in the midportion of the body, remove the posterior bone by progressively thinning the remaining bone and pulling it into the created defect across the canal to the level of the far pedicle medial wall to achieve a satisfactory decompression. If decompression of the posterior cortex is begun on the far side of the canal, troublesome bulging of the dura into the space created by removing the vertebral body is minimized and the surgeon's view is less obstructed.
- Take care throughout not to violate the endplates of the intact vertebra that will support the strut.
- Meticulously clean the two endplates of all cartilage and soft tissue. A surgical assistant should apply firm, anteriorly directed pressure over the spine to correct kyphosis. Measure the corpectomy defect for length of the strut in the corrected position. Additional anterior distraction with a lamina spreader can be applied but must not injure the endplates. Release of the anterior longitudinal ligament seldom is necessary in acute injuries. Modular expandable cage devices are well suited for this application and can be constructed to accommodate kyphosis if necessary.
- Obtain a bone graft or cage device of the desired length. Fill allograft humeral shaft or a metallic cage with the available bone from the operative field. With kyphosis correction maintained, impact the strut into place. The strut should be secure once it is in position, but avoid excessive length because it increases the risk of mechanical failure through subsidence. Image intensification views are used to verify spinal alignment and satisfactory placement of the strut (Fig. 5.41C and D).
- Determine the appropriate plate length and position the plate.
- Determine the transverse dimension of the intact vertebra so appropriate-length screws or bolts can be used for bicortical fixation, depending on the device used.
- Identify the entry points of screws as shown (Fig. 5.41E).
- Place the first screw or bolt in the posterior position of the caudal vertebra. Take care when determining placement of this screw to drill and place the screw parallel to the end plate and directed away from the spinal canal.
- Place the adjacent screw again parallel to the endplate and angled slightly posteriorly.
- Place the screws at the cephalad level similarly. Some devices allow for additional compression to be applied if desired.
- Once all screws are secured, obtain hemostasis and close the wound in a routine manner over suction drains or chest tube as appropriate.

POSTOPERATIVE CARE The patient is kept at bed rest until the chest tube is removed. The patient is then mobilized in a TLSO that is worn at all times when the spine is more vertical than 30 degrees from the horizontal plane. The TLSO is used for 12 to 16 weeks, depending on the clinical course.

SACRAL FRACTURES AND SPINOPELVIC DISSOCIATION INJURIES

The sacrum plays a central role in the stability of both the pelvis and the spinal column. The complex of ligaments that invest the sacrum anteriorly and posteriorly, the ligaments of the pelvic floor, and the osseous structure of the sacrum and pelvis all contribute to lumbopelvic stability and help prevent injury to the neurovascular structures in the region. The important neurologic structures at risk with sacral injuries include not only the L5 and S1 roots but also the lower sacral roots and autonomic nerves that are important for continence of the bowel and bladder and sexual function. Injuries to the sacrum are frequently missed at presentation because these patients often are involved in high-energy trauma and present with multiple injuries and may be hemodynamically unstable on arrival to the treating facility. Denis reported a large series of patients with sacral fractures, and 30% were identified late. This indicates how important a careful examination and a high index of suspicion are for detection of these injuries. As discussed earlier, the ATLS protocol should be followed for trauma patients, including palpation and inspection of the spine and posterior pelvis. Soft-tissue injuries are common in patients with sacral fractures, including Morel-Lavallée lesions that can significantly complicate the ultimate care for the patient. The neurologic evaluation must include a rectal examination to assess rectal tone and maximal contraction of the anal sphincter and rectal tears and anterior perineal lacerations. The ISCoS neurologic examination form should be completed to document possible L5 or S1 root injuries. The usual presence of a Foley catheter prevents assessment of bladder continence. Likewise, there is no clinical examination to detect injury to the anterior rami of S2 to S5, which contribute to the parasympathetic system and are important for sexual function and normal bladder and rectal function. Injuries to the sacrum also can damage the sympathetic ganglia of the inferior hypogastric plexus that are medial to the S2 to S4 foramina anteriorly. The L5 nerve is at risk at the anterior junction of the ala and the sacral promontory, and the S1 nerve root can be injured within the foramen. Extremity motor and sensory testing and rectal examination with pinprick and light touch examination in the perianal concentric dermatomes should be done to evaluate S2 to S5 function, as well as eliciting the anal wink and bulbocavernosus and cremasteric reflexes.

Plain radiographs have not proven sensitive in demonstrating injuries to the sacrum and lumbosacral region. CT of the chest, abdomen, and pelvis is the imaging modality of choice to screen for injuries to the pelvis and sacrum. If injuries are identified, a dedicated CT scan of the pelvis with 2-mm slices and sagittal and coronal reformatted images should be obtained. When there are associated neurologic deficits with displaced fractures, MRI also may be of value, but the best indications for MRI presently have not been fully delineated.

CLASSIFICATION

A discussion of all pelvic fractures is beyond the scope of this section; only the relatively rare injuries with subluxation or dislocation of the L5-S1 joint and fractures of the sacrum that are associated with lumbopelvic instability are covered.

Multiple classification schemes have been devised for these injuries over the past several decades, but there is no single system that encompasses sacral and lumbopelvic injuries. Denis et al. categorized 236 sacral fractures into three types based on three zones (Fig. 5.42). Zone 1 fractures are lateral to the neuroforamina and were the most common in the series, accounting for 50% of injuries with a 6% incidence of L5 and S1 injuries. Zone 2 injuries are through the neuroforamina and accounted for 34% of the injuries, and 28% of these patients had neurologic deficits unilaterally at the L5, S1, or S2 levels. Some zone 2 injuries have a shear component that increases the instability of the injury and increases the risk of nonunion. Zone 3 injuries are medial to the foramen and involve the spinal canal, comprising the remaining 16% of injuries. In the original study by Denis, 60% of patients had neurologic symptoms that involved bowel and bladder dysfunction, and 76% had sexual dysfunction. In a more recent study, Khan et al. reviewed a series of 683 consecutive patients and found much lower rates of neurologic injury and lower rates of the higher-level injuries. Their study revealed 453 (66%) zone I, 172 (25%) zone II, and 58 (9%) zone III injuries. Associated neurologic deficits occurred in only 3.5% of patients with 1.9% zone I, 6% zone II, and 9% of zone III injuries. They also found that patients with neurologic injuries were more likely to have displaced or comminuted fractures. Patients with spinopelvic dissociation (SPD) injuries had a 17% chance of neurologic injury.

Roy-Camille et al. and Strange-Vognsen and Lebech subclassified the Denis zone 3 injuries that have a transverse component that connects the zone 3 fracture to another fracture on the contralateral side in zone 1 or 2, which defines the SPD injury (Fig. 5.43). Isler developed a classification to describe injuries at the lumbosacral joint level with increasing probability of lumbosacral subluxation progressing from type 1 to type 3 injuries (Fig. 5.44).

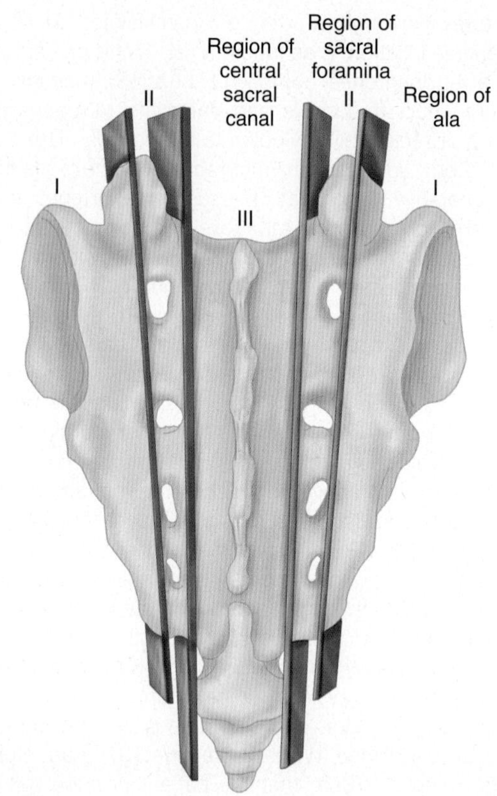

FIGURE 5.42 Three zones of sacrum described by Denis et al.: region of ala, region of sacral foramina, and region of central sacral canal.

TREATMENT

Many sacral fractures can be treated nonoperatively as well as some pelvic fractures, and a more complete discussion of these injuries is presented in other chapters. Fractures of the sacrum that are displaced and unstable or are associated with pelvic instability or spinal instability require operative treatment. Disruptions of the sacroiliac joint and some vertically unstable sacral fractures can be treated with percutaneous iliosacral screws (see p. 1895). The best trajectory is horizontal with purchase in the S1 body. For Denis zone 2 injuries, compression should be avoided to reduce risk of injury to the L5 root, which is at risk of being iatrogenically compressed within the fracture. If compression is not achieved, fracture stability is compromised.

Injuries with subluxation or dislocation at the lumbosacral joint or that involve spinopelvic dissociation can be treated with iliosacral or lumbopelvic fixation constructs. Nonoperative treatment of these injuries generally is not recommended because of the high nonunion rates, severe chronic pain, and neurologic worsening that can occur and can be very difficult to treat late (Table 5.8).

The operative approach we use to stabilize these injuries is similar to that described by Schildhauer et al. The goals of treatment are to decompress the sacral nerves, restore stability, and improve alignment. Lindahl et al. reviewed 36 cases to determine factors associated with neurologic recovery and late pain. The severity of translation through the fracture correlated with neurologic recovery, and the quality of reduction correlated with pelvic pain. The patients are initially resuscitated and stabilized with

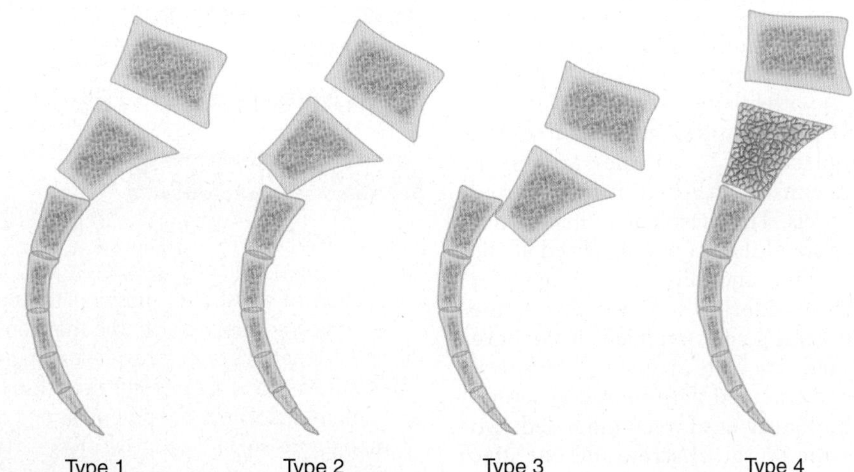

FIGURE 5.43 Roy-Camille and Strange-Vognsen and Lebech subclassifications of Denis zone 3 fractures. Type 1, angulation with no translation; type 2, angulation and translation; type 3, complete displacement of cephalad and caudal sacrum; type 4, segmental comminution. (Reproduced from Vaccaro AR, Kim DH, Brodke DS, et al: Diagnosis and management of sacral spine fractures, *Instr Course Lect* 53:375, 2004.)

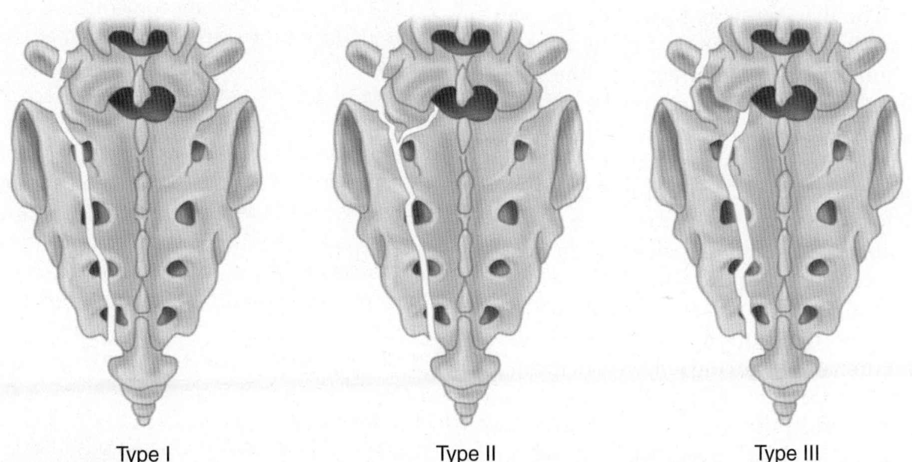

FIGURE 5.44 Isler classification for fractures of sacrum and lumbosacral junction. Type I, injury lateral to L5-S1 facet joint affecting pelvic ring stability; type II, injury through L5-S1 facet joint associated with displacement and neurologic symptoms; type III, injury involving spinal canal that is unstable. (From Vaccaro AR, Kim DH, Brodke DS, et al: Diagnosis and management of sacral spine fractures, *Instr Course Lect* 53:375, 2004.)

TABLE 5.8

Gibbons Classification of Cauda Equina Impairment

TYPE	NEUROLOGIC DEFICIT
1	None
2	Paresthesias only
3	Lower extremity motor deficit
4	Bowel/bladder dysfunction

From Shildhauer TA, Bellabarba C, Nork SE, et al: Decompression and lumbopelvic fixation for sacral fracture-dislocations with spino-pelvic dissociation, *J Orthop Trauma* 20:447, 2006.

respect to other injuries, and definitive spinopelvic fixation is completed as soon as the patient is able to tolerate the surgery. Ruatti et al. described a reduction maneuver that is done closed and as early as possible, even if definitive stabilization will be delayed. The technique involves strong and rapidly applied traction through femoral traction and countertraction applied to the torso with extension of the lumbosacral spine over a bolster. The average time to surgery reported by Schildhauer et al. was 6 days. If the patient has anterior pelvic instability, this is reconstructed first. Posterior stabilization is then done when the soft tissues are thought to be satisfactory. This stabilization is done through a midline approach, using pedicle screw fixation in the lower lumbar and S1 segments if possible and iliac screws. Because of the large forces being neutralized by the pedicle screws, we have used at least four points of fixation in the lumbar spine, and this was also the recommendation by Schildhauer et al. Typically, the construct begins at L4 with bilateral screws at this level and the L5 level. The S1 pedicles often are fractured and not available for screw placement, but if they are intact, L4 can be left out of the construct. Fusion is done across all instrumented spine levels. The sacroiliac joints are not fused. Iliac fixation consists of iliac screws inserted at the posterior superior iliac spine and directed through the sciatic buttress toward the anterior superior iliac spine and, when possible, iliosacral screws are placed. We have typically used a single iliac screw on each side (8.5 mm × 100 to 120 mm) and supplemented with iliosacral screws if reduction allows. Schildhauer et al. recommended two iliac screws per side or one iliosacral screw and one iliac screw per side. In either case, biomechanical data are not available. The prominence of the implants is an issue to consider because of the high wound complication rate. When placing the iliac screws, every effort is made not to elevate soft tissue unnecessarily, and the posterior superior iliac spine is instrumented using the "teardrop" (obturator outlet) view on image intensification with very minimal direct visualization. The iliac screw is started on the ventral portion of the posterior superior iliac spine near the sacroiliac joint to minimize the prominence of the screw head (Fig. 5.45). This also helps in connecting the rod. This usually can be done without a separate connecting rod and minimizes the hardware profile. A wide decompression of the sacral nerve roots is completed with removal of bone, which can be used for bone grafting at the L4 to S1 segments. Dural lacerations are directly repaired when possible and patched with dural graft and fibrin glue if primary closure cannot be obtained. Reduction often is difficult and using Schanz pins inserted into the S1 body to assist in disimpacting the fracture and restoring length is helpful, as is the use of a femoral distractor attached to a Schanz pin in the L5 pedicle and a pin in the ilium. Femoral traction also is useful. Once reduction is achieved, bilateral rods are contoured and secured to the screws. Contouring the rods before determining the site for the iliac screws is very helpful. After placing the rods bilaterally, they are compressed toward one another and a crosslink is applied (Fig. 5.46). Another reduction technique described by Starantzis involves a temporary rod on one side from L4 to the pelvis with a reduction screw placed at L4. A rod reduction tool is placed at L4, and distraction is applied to the reduction tower (persuader) until length has been restored. With the fracture out to length, the rod is reduced into the L4 screw and provisionally fixed. Fixation does allow mobilization without bracing, but persistent pain, neurologic dysfunction in the lower extremities, sexual dysfunction, and incontinence often remain problematic, and treatment recommendations must be individualized (Fig. 5.47).

For injuries that involve lumbosacral subluxation or dislocation without pelvic ring or vertical sacral fracture, stabilization is accomplished with pedicle screw fixation at L4 and L5 on the cephalic side of the injury and S1 and S2 fixation on the caudal side of the injury. Bone grafting is used posteriorly. If S1 fixation is not possible because of the injury pattern, fixation to the pelvis is used without fusion of the sacroiliac joint.

LUMBOPELVIC FIXATION (TRIANGULAR OSTEOSYNTHESIS)

TECHNIQUE 5.19

(SHILDHAUER)

- Bowel preparation is completed preoperatively. After induction of anesthesia, position the patient prone on a radiolucent four-poster frame that can accommodate an anterior pelvic fixator if needed, such as a Jackson frame. Femoral traction also may be helpful in fracture reduction. Somatosensory evoked potentials and electromyographic monitoring are initiated. Use image intensification to obtain a lateral view of the sacrum.
- After routine skin preparation and draping, make a midline incision extending caudally far enough to allow adequate decompression, without unnecessary skin tension.
- Divide tissue down to fascia with electrocautery and carefully elevate the soft tissue subperiosteally to expose the necessary lumbar segments and sacrum. Expose the transverse processes at each lumbar level and the intertransverse ligament. Subperiosteally expose the sacral ala at least 1.5 cm lateral to the lateral face of the sacral facet. Expose the posterior sacrum caudally to the fracture site and laterally as wide as the spinal canal. The posterior superior iliac spine will overhang this area, but it is not necessary to elevate the soft tissue from the sacroiliac joint and the posterior superior iliac spine, and this tissue should be left attached to the maximal extent possible. Only a small area of the ventral portion of the posterior superior iliac spine must be visible.
- Using Kerrison rongeurs and small curets, unroof the spinal canal and expect the nerves to be compressed or impaled by the bone. Repair the dural injury if possible. Mobilize the sacral roots and push the ventral bone anteriorly if needed to relieve tension on the roots.
- Reducing the fracture is difficult. Place a Schanz pin in the posterior body of S1 between the S1 and S2 foramen to manipulate the spine in relation to the pelvis. Femoral traction and a femoral distractor between the spine and ilium can be used to disimpact the fracture. Hyperextending the hips by raising the femoral traction outrigger can help reduce the kyphosis. If reduction can be adequately achieved, iliosacral screws can sometimes be placed as transfixation screws, taking care not to compress through the vertical foramina fractures. Individual anatomy and incomplete reduction may preclude safe placement of iliosacral screws.
- Correction of the angulation and some shortening through the fracture site improve the decompression.
- Decorticate the sacral ala and transverse processes and pack the lateral gutter for hemostasis. Decortication after pedicle screw placement is less effective and may limit fusion.
- Obtain a true lateral view of the vertebra, as indicated by sharply defined endplates with perfectly superimposed pedicles. Adjust the image intensifier until this image is obtained.

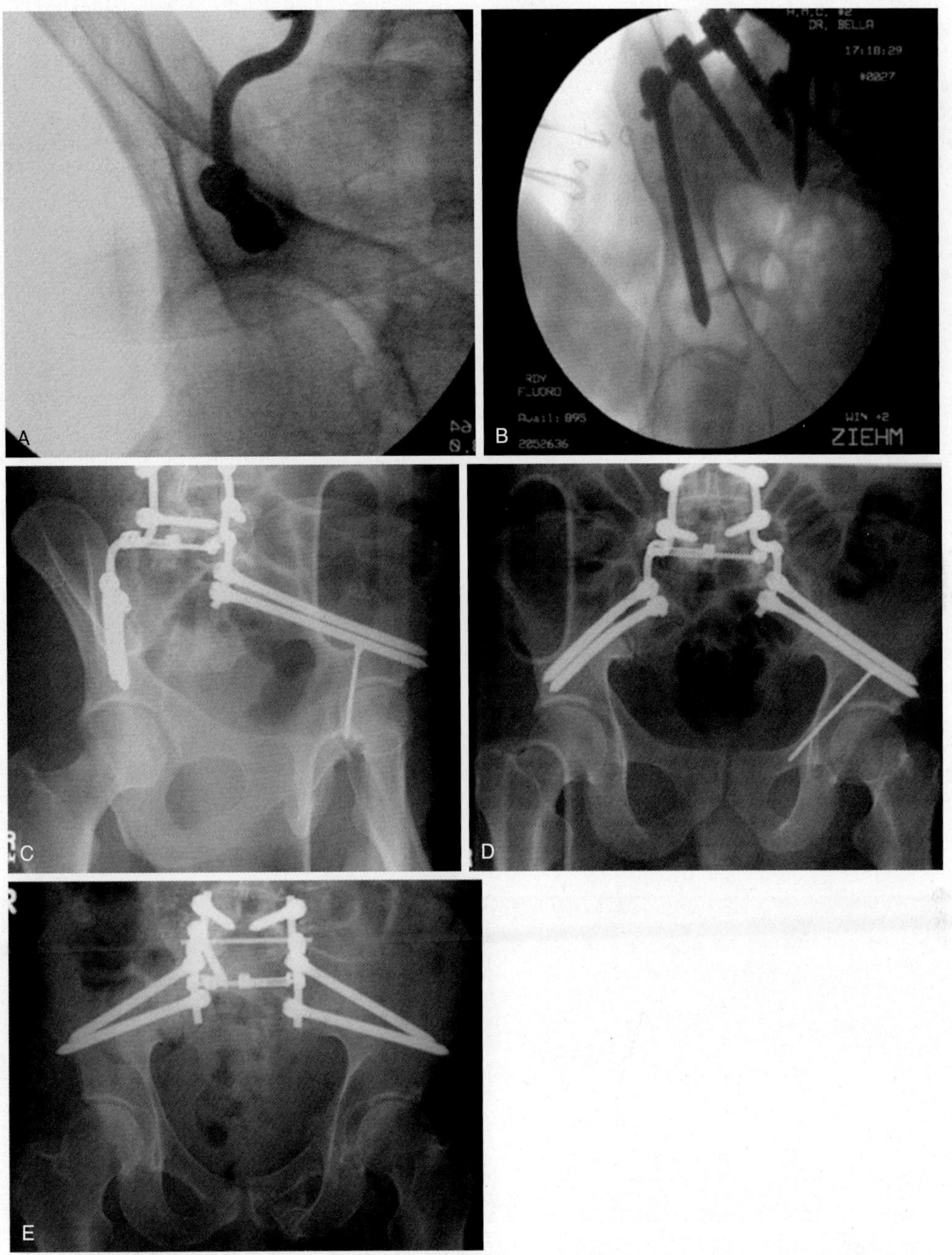

FIGURE 5.45 Obturator-outlet and obturator-inlet views and iliac oblique intraoperative views guide accurate screw insertion. **A,** Bone corridor between posterior superior iliac spine and anterior inferior iliac spine, in which iliac screws are ideally placed, projects as teardrop on combination obturator-outlet oblique image. **B,** Screw is extraosseous if it extends beyond cortical boundary of radiographic teardrop. Intraosseous screw placement between inner and outer tables of ilium can also be guided and confirmed with obturator-inlet oblique view. **C,** Iliac oblique image ensures accurate screw length and appropriate location above greater sciatic notch. **D,** Two iliac screws positioned parallel or more cephalad (**E**) can be used for placement of second iliac screw, yielding triangular configuration. (From Shildhauer TA, Bellabara C, Nork SE, et al: Decompression and lumbopelvic fixation for sacral fracture-dislocations with spino-pelvic dissociation, *J Orthop Trauma* 20:447, 2006.). **SEE TECHNIQUE 5.19.**

- Place the burr just posterior to the junction of the transverse process and the superior articular mass in line with the bisector of the pedicle on the lateral image intensifier view. Penetrate the cortex at this location, which will also be near the junction of the pars interarticularis and the superior articular mass.
- Use the cortical opening as the starting point and advance a pedicle awl into the pedicle. Advance the awl anteriorly and medially simultaneously. The pedicle awl must be advanced carefully owing to the mobility of the spine. If S1 screws will be placed, bicortical purchase is optimal with screws exiting the anterior promontory just caudal to the S1 endplate. The S1 screws should be medialized so the screw tips are at or near the midline.
- Use a small ball-tipped probe to sound the pedicle in all four quadrants and to palpate the vertebral body laterally and anteriorly to make sure there are no cortical breaches. The probe should exit anteriorly at S1 just below the endplate.
- The largest-diameter screw that the pedicle will accept (up to 6.5 mm) is typically placed. Larger screws can be placed, but little is usually gained, and the larger screws are more likely to cause pedicle fracture and loss of screw purchase. Polyaxial screws are used. Using a tap for the anterior S1 cortex and the pedicle will lower the risk of pedicle fracture in sclerotic bone. Place the bone graft onto the decorticated surface before screw insertion.
- Adjust the image intensifier to obtain an "end on" view of the screw to verify radiographically that the screw is within the pedicle.
- Place the remaining screws in the same fashion.
- Contour rods so they will be adjacent to the posterior superior iliac spine when connected to the lumbar screws. Adjust the image intensifier for the "teardrop" view after verifying that a true lateral view of the pelvis with superimposition of the sciatic notches can be obtained (see Fig. 5.45). Select the entry point into the posterior superior iliac spine on the teardrop view and advance the straight pedicle awl or 3.2-mm drill to a depth of 80 to 100 mm

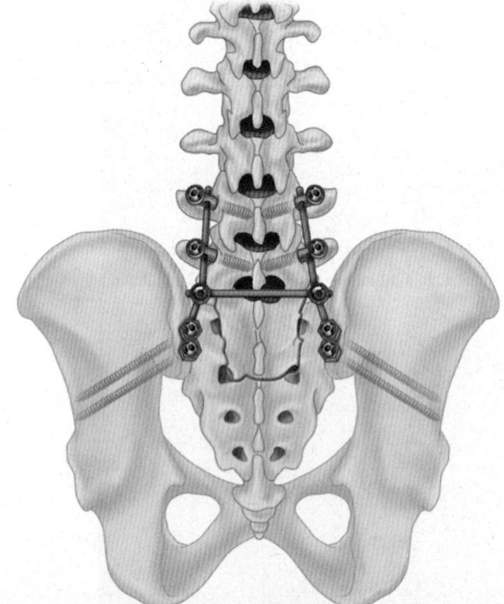

FIGURE 5.46 Lumbopelvic fixation for sacral fracture with spinopelvic dissociation. **SEE TECHNIQUE 5.19.**

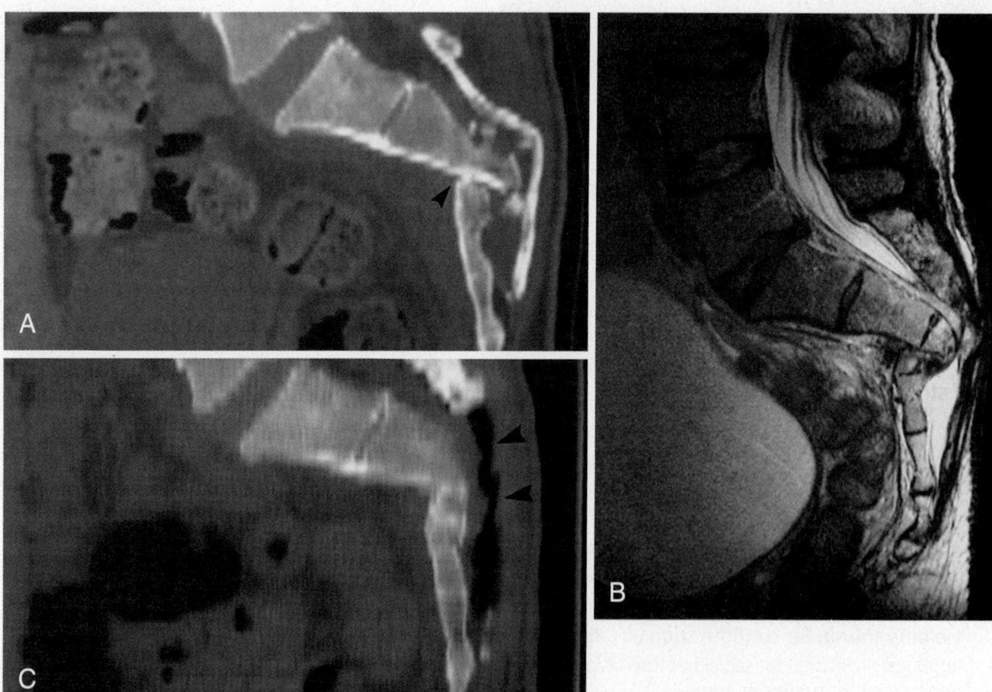

FIGURE 5.47 **A,** Sagittal CT scan of transverse fracture through S3 resulting in transection of sacral nerve roots *(arrowhead).* **B,** MR image of sacral fracture resulting in complete canal compromise. **C,** Postoperative CT scan shows decompression of sacral spinal canal after laminectomy *(arrowheads).*

remaining within the confines of the teardrop. Sound the hole for cortical defects and place a large caliber screw. We have used a single 8.5-mm screw even if iliosacral screws cannot be placed. Schildhauer et al. recommends two iliac screws that may need to be somewhat smaller depending on the teardrop size.

- Confirm that the iliac screws are intraosseous bilaterally, using obturator-outlet oblique and obturator-inlet oblique views, and confirm their length on the iliac oblique views.
- Secure the rods to the screws.
- Compress the rods toward one another and crosslink at the lumbosacral level to minimize hardware prominence.
- Decorticate the facet joints and pack with additional bone.
- Carefully close the fascia back to bone where possible over a suction drain.
- Close the thin subcutaneous layer and then the skin with subcuticular suture.

POSTOPERATIVE CARE The patient is maintained off the wound as much as possible for the first several days. The drain usually is removed on the first postoperative day, and mobilization without a brace is allowed. Full weight bearing is allowed unless precluded by pelvic or other injuries.

REFERENCES

GENERAL

Aarabi B, Alexander M, Mirvis ST, et al.: Predictors of outcome in acute traumatic central cord syndrome due to spinal stenosis, *J Neurosurg Spine* 14:122, 2011.

Aarabi B, Hadley MN, Dhall SS, et al.: Management of acute traumatic central cord syndrome (ATCCS), *Neurosurgery* 72(Suppl 2):195, 2013.

Ahuja CS, Schroeder GD, Vaccaro AR, Fehlings MG: Spinal cord injury – what are the controversies? *J Orthop Trauma* 31(Suppl 4):S7, 2017.

Alizadeh A, Dyck SM, Karimi-Abdolrezaee S: Traumatic spinal cord injury: an overview of pathophysiology, models and acute injury mechanisms, *Front Neurol* 10:282, 2019.

Antwi P, Grant R, Kuzmik G, Abbed K: "White Cord Syndrome" of acute hemiparesis after posterior cervical decompression and fusion for chronic cervical stenosis, *World Neurosurg* 113:33, 2018.

Arul K, Ge L, Ikpeze T, Baldwin A, Mesfin A: Traumatci spinal cord injuries in geriatric population: etiology, management, and complications, *J Spine Surg* 5(1):38, 2019.

Badhiwala JH, Ahuja CS, Fehlings MG: Time is spine: a review of translational advances in spinal cord injury, *J Neurosurg Spine* 30(1):1, 2018.

Battistuzzo CR, Armstrong A, Clark J, et al.: Early decompression following cervical spinal cord injury: examining the process of care from accident scene to surgery, *J Neurotrauma* 33(12):1161, 2016.

Bernstein MP, Young MG, Baxter AB: Imaging of spine rrauma, *Radiol Clini North Am* 57(4):767, 2019.

Boggenpoel B, Madasa V, Jeftha T, Joseph C: Systematic scoping review protocol for clinical prediction rules (CPRs) in the management of patients with spinal cord injuries, *BMJ Open* 9(1):e025076, 2019.

Bono CM, Heggeness M, Mich C, et al.: Commentary North American Spine Society. Newly released vertebroplasty randomized controlled trials: a tale of two trials, *Spine J* 10:238, 2010.

Botolin S, VanderHeiden TF, Moore EE, et al.: The role of pre-reduction MRI in the management of complex cervical spine fracture-dislocations: an ongoing controversy? *Patient Saf Surg* 11:23, 2017.

Brodell DW, Jain A, Elfar JC, Mesfin A: National trends in the management of central cord syndrome: an analysis of 16, 134 patients, *Spine J* 15(3):435, 2015.

Brooks NP: Central Cord Syndrome, *Neurosurg Clin N Am* 28(1):41, 2017.

Cahill CW, Radcliffe KE, Reitman C: Enhancing evaluation of cervical spine: thresholds for normal CT relationships in the subaxial cervical spine, *Int J Spine Surg* 11:36, 2017.

Carreon LY, Dimar JR: Early versus late stabilization of spine injuries: a systematic review, *Spine* 36:E727, 2011.

Casper DS, Zmistowski B, Schroeder GD, et al.: Preinjury patient characteristics and postinjury neurological status are associated with mortality following spinal cord injury, *Spine* 43(13):895, 2018.

Cooper K, Glenn CA, Martin M, et al.: Risk factors for surgical site infection after instrumented fixation in spine trauma, *J Clin Neurosci* 23:123, 2016.

Dahdaleh NS, Lawton CD, El Ahmadieh TY, et al.: Evidence-based management of central cord syndrome, *Neurosurg Focus* 35(1):E6, 2013.

Dakson A, Brandman D, Thibault-Halman G, Christie SD: Optimization of the mean arterial pressure and timing of surgical decompression in traumatic spinal cord injury: a retrospective study, *Spinal Cord* 55(11):1033, 2017.

Daly MC, Patel MS, Bhatia NN, Bederman SS: The influence of insurance status on the surgical treatment of acute spinal fractures, *Spine* 41:E37, 2016.

Dawodu ST, Cauda equina and conus medularris syndromes, *Medscape* https ://emedicine.medscape.com/article/1148690-print, August 6, 2019.

deAmeida RL, Rodrigues CC, Melo E Silva CA, et al.: Comparison of two pharmalogical prophylaxis strategies for venous thromboembolism in spinal cord injury patients: a retrospective study, *Spinal Cord* 57(10):890, 2019.

Decramer T, Wouters A, Kiekens C, Theys T: Froins syndrome after spinal cord injury, *World Neurosurg* 127:490, 2019.

Dhall SS, Hadley MN, Aarabi B, et al.: Nutritional support after spinal cord injury, *Neurosurgery* 72(Suppl 2):255, 2013.

Dinar JR, Carreon LY, Riina J, et al.: Early versus late stabilization of the spine in the polytrauma patient, *Spine* 21S:S187, 2010.

D'Souza MM, Choudhary A, Poonia M, et al.: Diffusion tensor MR imaging in spinal cord injury, *Injury* 48(4):880, 2017.

Du JP, Fan Y, Zhang JN, et al.: Early versus delayed decompression for traumatic cervical spinal cord injury: application of the AOSpine subaxial cervical spinal injury classification system to guide surgical timing, *Eur Spine J* 28(8):1855, 2019.

Dyas AR, Niemeier TE, Mcgwin G, Theiss SM: Ability of magnetic resonance imaging to accurately determine alar ligament integrity in patients with atlanto-occipital injuries, *J Craniovertebr Junction Spine* 9(4):241, 2018.

El Tecle NE, Dahdaleh NS, Bydon M, et al.: The natural history of complete spinal cord injury: a pooled analysis of 1162 patients and a meta-analysis of modern data, *J Neurosurg Spine* 28(4):436, 2018.

El Tecle NE, Dahdaleh NS, Hitchon PW: Timing of surgery in spinal cord injury, *Spine 41*(16):E995, 2016.

Fehlings MG, Rabin D, Sears W, et al.: Current practice in the timing of surgical intervention in spinal cord injury, *Spine* 35:S166, 2010.

Fehlings MG, Tetreault LA, Wilson Jr , et al.: A clinical practice guideline for the management of patients with acute spinal cord injury and central cord syndrome: recommendations on the timing (≤ 24 hours versus > 24 hours) of decompressive surgery, *Global Spine J* 7(3 Suppl):195S, 2017.

Fehlings MG, Wilson JR: Timing of surgical intervention of spinal trauma: what does the evidence indicate? *Spine* 35:S159, 2010.

Hachem LD, Ahuja CS, Fehlings MG: Assessment and management of acute spinal cord injury: from point of injury to rehabilitation, *J Spinal Cord Med* 40(6):665, 2017.

Harris AM, Vasu C, Kanthila M, et al.: Assessment of MRI as a modality for evaluation of soft tissue injuries of the spine as compared to intraoperative assessment, *J Clin Diagn Res* 10(3):TC01, 2016.

Harrop JS, Chi JH, Anderson PA, et al.: Congress of Neurological surgeons systematic review and evidence-based guidelines on the evaluation and treatment of patients with thoracolumbar spine trauma: neurological assessment, *Neurosurgery* 84(1):E32, 2019.

Hashmi SZ, Marra A, Jenis LG, Patel AA: Current concepts: central cord syndrome, *Clin Spine Surg* 31(10):407, 2018.

Hawryluk G, Whetstone W, Saigal R, et al.: Mean arterial blood pressure correlated with neurological recovery after human spinal cord injury: analysis of high frequency of physiologic data, *J Neurotrauma* 32:1958, 2015.

Huang P, Anissipour A, McGee W, Lemak L: Return-to-play recommendations after cervical, thoracic, and lumbar spine injuries: a comprehensive review, *Sports Health* 8:19, 2016.

Hurlbert RJ, Hadley MN, Walters BC, et al.: Pharmacological therapy for acute spinal cord injury, *Neurosurgery* 72(Suppl 2):93, 2013.

Inaba K, Byerly S, Bush LD, et al.: Cervical spinal clearance: a prospective western trauma association multi-institutional trial, *J Trauma Acute Care Surg* 81(6):1122, 2016.

Karthik Yelamarthy PK, Chhabra HS, Vaccaro A, et al.: Management and prognosis of acute traumatic cervical central cord syndrome: systematic review and Spinal Cord Society – Spine Trauma Study Group position statement, *Eur Spine J* 28(10):2390, 2019.

Kepler CK, Kong C, Schroeder GD, et al.: Early outcome and predictors of early outcome in patients treated surgically for central cord syndrome, *J Neurosurg Spine 23*(4):490, 2015.

Khorasanizadeh M, Yousefifard M, Eskian M, et al.: Neurological recovery following traumatic spinal cord injury: a systematic review and meta-analysis, *J Neurosurg Spine* 15:1, 2019.

Kim KD, Ament JD: Spinal cord injury treatment: what's on the horizon? *Spine 42*(Suppl7):S21, 2017.

Krappinger D, Lindtner RA, Zegg MJ, et al.: Spondylotic traumatic central cord syndrome: a hidden discoligamentous injury? *Eur Spine J* 28(2):434, 2019.

Kurpad S, Martin AR, Tetreault LA, et al.: Impact of baseline magnetic resonance imaging on neurologic, functional, and safety outcomes in patients with acute traumatic spinal cord injury, *Global Spine J* 7(3 Suppl):151S, 2017.

Lau BPH, Hey HWD, Lau ET, et al.: The utility of magnetic resonance imaging in addition to computed tomography scans in the evaluation of cervical spine injuries: a study of obtunded blunt trauma patients, *Eur Spine J* 27(5):1028, 2018.

Lenehan B, Fisher CG, Vaccaro A, et al.: The urgency of surgical decompression in acute central cord injuries with spondylolis and without instability, *Spine* 35:S180, 2010.

Li P, Qiu D, Shi H, et al.: Isolated decompression for transverse sacral fractures with cauda eqina syndrome, *Med Sci Monit* 25:3583, 2019.

Li Y, Zhou P, Cui W, et al.: Immediate anterior open reduction and plate fixation in the management of lower cervical dislocation with facet interlocking, *Sci Rep* 9(1):1286, 2019.

Loch-Wilkinson T, McNeil S, White C, et al.: Nerve transfers in patients with Brown-Séquard pattern of spinal cord injury: report of 2 cases, *World Neurosurg* 110:152, 2018.

Lubelski D, Tharin S. Como JJ, et al: Surgical timing for cervical and upper thoracic injuries in patients with polytrauma, J Neurosurg Spine 27(6):633, 2017.

Mac-Thiong JM, Feldman DE, Thompson C, et al.: Does timing of surgery affect hospitalization costs and length of stay for acute care following a traumatic spinal cord injury? *J Neurotrauma* 29:2816, 2012.

Martinez-Perez R, Munarriz PM, Paredes I, et al.: Cervical spinal cord injury without computed tomography evidence of trauma in adults: magnetic resonance imaging prognostic factors, *World Neurosurg* 99:192, 2017.

Mascarenhas D, Dreizin D, Bodanapally UK, Stein DM: Parsing the utility of CT and MRI in the subaxial cervical spine injury classification (SLIC) system: is CT SLIC enough? *AJR Am J Roentgenol* 206(6):1292, 2016.

Miao DC, Wang F, Shen Y: Immediate reduction under general anesthesia and combined anterior and posterior fusion in the treatment of distraction-flexion injury in the lower cervical spine, *J Orthop Surg Res* 13(1):126, 2018.

Nagata K, Inokuchi K, Chikuda H, et al.: Early versus delayed reduction of cervical spine dislocation with complete motor paralysis: a multicenter study, *Eur Spine J* 26(4):1272, 2017.

Nakajima H, Takahashi A, Kitade I, et al.: Prognostic factors and optimal management for patients with cervical spinal cord injury without major bone injury, *J Orthop Sci 24*(2):230, 2019.

Nwosu K, Eftekhary N, McCoy E, et al.: Surgical management of civilian gunshot-induced spinal cord injury: is it overutilized? *Spine* 42(2):E117, 2017.

Ouchida J, Yukawa Y, Ito K, et al.: Delayed magnetic resonance imaging in patients with cervical spinal cord injury without radiographic abnormality, *Spine 41*(16):E981, 2016.

Pakzad H, Roffey DM, Knight H, et al.: Delay in operative stabilization of spine fractures in multitrauma patients without neurologic injuries: effects on outcomes, *J Can Chir* 54:270, 2011.

Perez-Orribo L, Kalb S, Snyder LA, et al.: Comparison of CT versus MRI measurements of transverse atlantal ligament integrity in craniovertebral junction injuries, part 2: a new CT-based alternative for assessing transverse ligament integrity, *J Neurosurg Spine* 24(6):903, 2016.

Perez-Orribo L, Snyder LA, Kalb S, et al.: Comparison of CT versus MRI measurements of transverse atlantal ligament integrity in craniovertebral junction injuries, part 1: a clinical study, *J Neurosurg Spine 24*(6):897, 2016.

Phang I, Mada M, Kolias AG, et al.: Magnetic resonance imaging of the codman microsensor transducer used for intraspinal pressure monitoring: findings from the injured spinal cord pressure evaluation study, *Spine 41*(10):E605, 2016.

Phang I, Zoumprouli A, Saadoun S, Papadopoulos MC: Safety profile and probe placement accuracy of intraspinal pressure monitoring for traumatic spinal cord injury: injured spinal cord pressure evaluation study, *J Neurosurg Spine* 25(3):398, 2016.

Piazza M, Schuster J: Timing of surgery after spinal cord injury, *Neurosurg Clin N Am* 28(1):31, 2017.

Ploumis A, Ponnappan RK, Sarbello J, et al.: Thromboprophylaxis in traumatic and elective spinal surgery: analysis of questionnaire response and current practice of spine trauma surgeons, *Spine* 35:323, 2010.

Pronin S, Koh CH, Bulovaite E, et al.: Compressive pressure versus time in cauda equina syndrome: a systematic review and meta-analysis of experimental studies, *Spine* 10.1097/BRS.0000000000003045, 2019, [Epub ahead of print].

Rajasekaran S, Maheswaran A, Aiyer SN, et al.: Prediction of posterior ligamentous complex injury in thoracolumbar fractures using non-MRI imaging techniques, *Int Orthop* 40(6):1075, 2016.

Roberts DJ, Chaubey VP, Zygun DA, et al.: Diagnostic accuracy of computed tomographic angiography for blunt cerebrovascular injury detection in trauma patients: a systematic review and metaanalysis, *Ann Surg* 257:621, 2013.

Rodriguez-Romero V, Guizar-Sahagún G, Castañeda-Hernández G, et al.: *Spine* 43(15):E885, 2018.

Rozzelle CJ, Aarabi B, Dhall SS, et al.: Spinal cord injury without radiographic abnormality (SCIWORA), *Neurosurgery* 72(Suppl 2):227, 2013.

Ruiz IA, Squair JW, Phillips AA, et al.: Incidence and natural progression of neurogenic shock after traumatic spinal cord injury, *J Neurotrauma* 35(3):461, 2018.

Samuel AM, Grant RA, Bohl DD, et al.: Delayed surgery after acute traumatic central cord syndrome is associated with reduced mortality, *Spine* 40:349, 2015.

Schoenfeld AJ, Lehman RA, Hsu JR: Evaluation and management of combat-related spinal injuries: a review based on recent experiences, *Spine J* 12:817, 2012.

Schoenfeld AJ, Tobert DG, Le HV, et al.: Utility of adding magnetic resonance imaging to computed tomography alone in the evaluation of cervical spine injury: a propensity-matched analysis, *Spine 43*(3):179, 2018.

Segal DN, Grabel ZJ, Heller JG, et al.: Epidemiology and treatment of central cord syndrome in the United States, *J Spine Surg* 4(4):712, 2018.

Shibahashi K, Nishida M, Okura Y, Hamabe Y: Epidemiological state, predictors of early mortality, and predictive models from traumatic spinal cord: a multicenter nationwide cohort study, *Spine 44*(7):479, 2019.

Song KJ, Ko JH, Choi BW: Relationship between magnetic resonance imaging findings and spinal cord injury in extension injury of the cervical spine, *Eur J Orthop Surg Traumatol* 26(3):263, 2016.

Srikandarajah N, Wilby M, Clark S, et al.: Outcomes reported after surgery for cauda equine syndrome, *Spine* 43(17):E1005, 2018.

Stevenson CM, Dargan DP, Warnock J, et al.: Traumatic central cord syndrome: neurological and functional outcome at 3 years, *Spinal Cord* 54(11):1010, 2016.

Tsuji O, Suda K, Takahat-a M, et al.: Early surgical intervention may facilitate recovery of cervical spinal cord injury in DISH, *J Orthop Surg* 27(1):2309499019834783, 2019.

Vandenakker-Albanese C: Brown-Sequard syndrome, *Medscape* https://emedicine.medscape.com/article/321652-print, August 6, 2019.

van Middendorp JJ, Audigé L, Hanson B, et al.: What should an ideal spinal injury classification system consist of? A methodological review and conceptual proposal for future classifications, *Eur Spine J* 19:1238, 2010.

Vinodh VP, Rajapathy SK, Sellamuthu P, Kandasamy R: White cord syndrome: a devastating complication of spinal decompression surgery, *Surg Neurol Int* 9:136, 2018.

Wagner PJ, DiPaola CP, Connolly PJ, Stauff MP: Controversies in the management of central cord syndrome: the state of the art, *J Bone Joint Surg Am* 100(7):618, 2018.

Werndle MC, Saadoun S, Phang I, et al.: Monitoring of spinal cord perfusion pressure in acute spinal cord injury: initial findings of the Injured Spinal Cord Pressure Evaluation Study, *Crit Care Med* 42:646, 2014.

Yorkgitis BK, McCauley DM: Cervical spine clearance in adult trauma patients, *JAAPAI* 32(2):12, 2019.

Yoshihara H, Yoneoka D: Trends in the treatment for traumatic central cord syndrome without bone injury in the United States from 2000 to 2009, *J Trauma Acute Care Surg* 75(3):453, 2013.

CERVICAL SPINE

Aarabi B, Mirvis S, Shanmuganathan K, et al.: Comparative effectiveness of surgical versus nonoperative management of unilateral, nondisplaced, subaxial cervical spine facet fractures without evidence of spinal cord injury, *J Neurosurg Spine* 20:270, 2014.

Aarabi B, Walters BC, Dhall SS, et al.: Subaxial cervical spine injury classification systems, *Neurosurgery* 72(Suppl 2):170, 2013.

Alessandrino F, Bono CM, Potter CA, et al.: Spectrum of diagnostic errors in cervical spine trauma imaging and their clinical significance, *Emerg Radiol* 26(4):409, 2019.

Alhashash M, Shousha M, Gendy H, et al.: Percutaneous posterior transarticular atlantoaxial fixation for the treatment of odontoid fractures in the elderly: a prospective study, *Spine* 43(11):761, 2018.

Bajada S, Ved A, Dudhniwala AG, Ahuja S: Predictors of mortality following conservatively managed fractures of the odontoid in elderly patients, *Bone Joint J* 99-B(1):116, 2017.

Baogui L, Juwen C: Fusion rates for odontoid fractures after treatment by anterior odontoid screw versus posterior C1-C2 arthrodesis: a meta-analysis, *Arch Orthop Trauma Surg* 139(10):1329, 2019.

Barlow DR, Higgins BT, Ozanne EM, et al.: Cost effectiveness of operative versus non-operative treatment of geriatric type-II odontoid fracture, *Spine* 41(7):610, 2016.

Bayley E, Zia Z, Kerslake R, Boszczyk BM: The ipsilateral lamina-pedicle angle: can it be used to guide pedicle screw placement in the sub-axial cervical spine? *Eur Spine J* 19:458, 2010.

Bayley E, Zia Z, Kerslake R, et al.: Lamina-guided lateral mass screw placement in the sub-axial cervical spine, *Eur Spine J* 19:660, 2010.

Beaty N, Slavin J, Diaz C, et al.: Cervical spine injury from gunshot wounds, *J Neurosurg Spine* 21:442, 2014.

Bevevino AJ, Tee J, Ailon T, Dvorak M: Are Jefferson fractures with a transverse ligament avulsion potentially unstable? *Clin Spine Surg* 29(2):39, 2016.

Bhimani AD, Chiu RG, Esfahani DR, et al.: C1-C2 fusion versus occipito-cervical fusion for high cervical fractures: a multi-institutional database analysis and review of the literature, *World Neurosurg* 119:e459, 2018.

Biakto KT, Arifin J, Lett J, Benjamin M: Occipitocervical fusion and posterior fossa decompression in neglected Jefferson fracture-dislocation of atlas associated with odontoid peg fracture: a case report, *Int J Spine* 13(1):11, 2019.

Bodon G, Kiraly K, Tunyogi-Csapo M, et al.: Introducing the craniocervical Y-ligament, *Surg Radiol Anat* 41(2):197, 2019.

Botolin S, VanderHeiden TF, Moore EE, et al.: The role of pre-reduction MRI in the management of complex cervical spine fracture-dislocations: and ongoing controversy? *Patient Saf Surg* 11:23, 2017.

Bransford RJ, Lee MJ, Reis A: Posterior fixation of the upper cervical spine: contemporary techniques, *J Am Acad Orthop Surg* 19:63, 2011.

Burks JD, Conner AK, Briggs RG, et al.: Blunt vertebral artery injury in occipital condyle fractures, *J Neurosurg Spine* 29(5):500, 2018.

Cao BH, Wu ZM, Liang JW: Risk factors for poor prognosis of cervical spinal cord injury with subaxial cervical spine fracture-dislocation after surgical treatment: a consort study, *Med Sci Monit* 25:1970, 2019.

Chang YM, Kim G, Peri N, et al.: Diagnostic utility of increased STIR signal in the posterior atlanto-occipital and atlantoaxial membrane complex on MRI in acute C1-C2 fracture, *AJNR Am J Neuroradiol* 38(9):1820, 2017.

Charles YP, Ntilikina Y, Blondel B, et al.: Mortality, complication, and fusion rates of patients with odontoid fracture: the impact of age and comorbidities in 204 cases, *Arch Orthop Trauma Surg* 139(1):43, 2019.

Chun DH, Yoon DH, Kim KN, et al.: Biomechanical comparison of four different atlantoaxial posterior fixation constructs in adults: a finite element study, *Spine* 43(15):e891, 2018.

Clark S, Nash A, Shasti M, et al.: Mortality rates after posterior C1-2 fusion for displaced type II odontoid fractures in octogenarians, *Spine* 43(18):E1077, 2018.

Dagtekin A, Avci E, Hamzaoglu V, et al.: Management of occipitocervical junction and upper cervical trauma, *J Craniovertebr Junction Spine* 9(3):148, 2018.

De Bonis P, Iaccarino C, Musio A, et al.: Functional outcome of elderly patients treated for odontoid fracture: a multicenter study, *Spine*, 2019, https://doi.org/10.1097/BRS.0000000000002981, [Epub ahead of print].

Deepak AN, Salunke P, Sahoo SK, et al.: Revisiting the differences between irreducible and reducible atlantoaxial dislocation in the era of direct posterior approach and C1-2 joint manipulation, *J Neurosurg Spine* 26(3):331, 2017.

Denaro V, Di Martino A: Current concepts in cervical spine surgery. Editorial comment, *Clin Orthop Relat Res* 469:631, 2011.

DePasse JM, Palumbo MA, Ahmed AK, et al.: Halo-vest immobilization in elderly odontoid fracture patients: evolution in treatment modality and in-hospital outcomes, *Clin Spine Surg* 30(9):E1206, 2017.

Derger T, Place H, Piper C, et al.: Analysis of cervical angiograms in cervical spine trauma patients, does it make a difference? *Clinical Spine Surg* 30:232, 2017.

Dhall SS, Hadley MN, Aarabi B, et al.: Deep venous thrombosis and thromboembolism in patients with cervical spinal cord injuries, *Neurosurgery* 72(Suppl 2):244, 2013.

Dorward IG, Buchowski JM, Stoker GE, Zebala LP: Posterior cervical fusion with recombinant human bone morphogenetic protein 2: complications and fusrion rate at minimum 2-year follow-up, *Clin Spine Surg* 29(6):E319, 2016.

Dunn CJ, Mease S, Issa K, et al.: Low energy chronic traumatic spondylolisthesis of the axis, *Eur Spine J* 28(8):1829, 2017.

Erwood AM, Abel TJ, Grossbach AJ, et al.: Acutely unstable cervical spine injury with normal CT scan findings: MRI detects ligamentous injury, *J Clin Neurosci* 24:165, 2016.

Etter C: Combined anterior screw fixation of an odontoid fracture and the atlanto-axial joints (C1/C2) in a geriatric patient, *Eur Spine J* 2:280, 2016.

Fehlings MG, Vaccaro A, Wilson JR, et al.: Early versus delayed decompression for traumatic cervical spinal cord injury: results of the Surgical Timing in Acute Spinal Cord Injury Study (STASCIS), *PLoS ONE* 7:e32037, 2012.

Feng R, Loewenstern J, Caridi J: Cervical burst fracture in a patient with contiguous 2-level cervical stand-along cages, *World Neurosurg* 105:1041, 2017.

Fredø HL, Rizvi SA, Rezai M, et al.: Complications and long-term outcomes after open surgery for traumatic subaxial cervical spine fractures: a consecutive series of 303 patients, *BMC Surg* 16(1):56, 2016.

Gabriel JP, Muzumdar AM, Khalil S, Ingalhalikar A: A novel crossed rod configuration incorporating translaminar screws for occipitocervical internal fixation: an in vitro biomechanical study, *Spine J* 11:30, 2011.

Gebauer G, Osterman M, Harrop J, Vaccaro A: Spinal cord injury results from injury missed on CT scan: the danger of relying on CT alone for collar removal, *Clin Orthop Relat Res* 470:1652, 2012.

Gelb DE, Aarabi B, Dhall SS, et al.: Treatment of subaxial cervical spinal injuries, *Neurosurgery* 72(Suppl 2):187, 2013.

Gelb DE, Hadley MN, Bizhan A, et al.: Initial closed reduction of cervical spinal fracture-dislocation injuries, *Neurosurgery* 72(Suppl 2):73, 2013.

Glassman DM, Magnusson E, Agel J, et al.: The impact of stenosis and translation on spinal cord injuries in traumatic cervical facet dislocations, *Spine J* 19(4):687, 2019.

Goel A: Expert's comment concerning Grand Rounds case entitled "Low energy chronic traumatic spondylolisthesis of the axis" by C. J. Dunn, S. Mease, K. Issa, K. Sinha, A. Emami (*Eur Spine J*: 2017: DOI 10.007/s00586-01705206-4), *Eur Spine J* 28(8):1833, 2018.

Goode T, Young A, Wilson SP, et al.: Evaluation of cervical spine fracture in the elderly: can we trust our physical examination? *Am Surg* 80:182, 2014.

Grabel ZJ, Armanghani SJ, et al.: Variations in treatment of C2 fractures by time, age, and geographic region in the United States: an analysis of 4818 patients, *World Neurosurg* 113:e535, 2018.

Graffeo CS, Perry A, Puffer RC, et al.: Deadly falls: operative versus nonoperative management of type II odontoid process fracture in octogenarians, *J Neurosurg Spine 26*(1):4, 2017.

Griffith B, Kelly M, Vallee M, et al.: Screening cervical spine CT in the emergency department, phase 2: a prospective assessment of use, *AJNR Am J Neuroradiol* 34:809, 2013.

Gu J, Lei W, Xin A, et al.: Occiput-axis crossing translaminar screw fixation technique using offset connectors: an in vitro biomechanical study, *Clin Neurol Neurosurg 169*:49, 2018.

Guan J, Chen Z, Wu H, et al.: Is anterior release and cervical traction necessary for the treatment of irreducible atlantoaxial dislocation? A systematic review and meta-analysis, *Eur Spine J* 27(60):1234, 2018.

Guo Q, Deng Y, Wang J, et al.: Comparison of clinical outcomes of posterior C1-C2 temporary fixation without fusion and C1-C2 fusion for fresh odontoid fractures, *Neurosurgery* 78(1):77, 2016.

Guo Q, Zhang M, Wang L, et al.: Comparison of atlantoaxial rotation and functional outcomes of two nonfusion techniques in the treatment of Anderson-D'Alonzo type II odontoid fractures, *Spine* 41(12):E751, 2016.

Hadley MN, Walters BC, Bizhan A, et al.: Clinical assessment following acute cervical spinal cord injury, *Neurosurgery* 72(Suppl 2):40, 2013.

Halfpap JP, Cho AA, Rosenthal MD: Cervical spine fracture with vertebral artery dissection, *J Orthop Sports Phys Ther* 46(10):929, 2016.

Hamilton K, Josiah DT, Tierney M, Brooks N: Surgical practice in traumatic spinal fracture treatment with regard to the subaxial cervical injury classification and severity and the thoracolumbar injury classification and severity systems: a review of 58 patients at the University of Wisconsin, *World Neurosurg 127*:e101, 2019.

Harrigan MR, Hadley MN, Dhall SS, et al.: Management of vertebral artery injuries following non-penetrating cervical trauma, *Neurosurgery* 72(Suppl 2):234, 2013.

Harshavardhana NS, Dabke HV: Risk factors for vertebral artery injuries in cervical spine trauma, *Orthop Rev (Pavia)* 6:5429, 2014.

Healy CD, Spilman SK, King BD, et al.: Asymptomatic cervical spine fractures: current guidelines can fail older patients, *J Trauma Acute Care Surg* 83(1):119, 2017.

Helgeson MD, Lehman RA, Sasso RC, et al.: Biomechanical analysis of occipitocervical stability afforded by three fixation techniques, *Spine J* 11:245, 2011.

Hlubeck RJ, Nakaji P: Nonoperative management of odontoid fractures; is halo vest immobilization warranted? *World Neurosurg* 98:839, 2017.

Hohl JB, Lee JY, Horton JA, Rihn JA: A novel classification system for traumatic central cord syndrome: the central cord injury scale (CCIS), *Spine* 35:E238, 2010.

Holla M, Hannink G, Eggen TGE, et al.: Restriction of cervical intervertebral movement with different types of external immobilizers: a cadaveric 3D analysis study, *Spine* 42(20):E1182, 2017.

Holla M, Huisman JM, Verdonschot N, et al.: The ability of external immobilizers to restrict movement of the cervical spine: a systematic review, *Eur Spine J* 25(7):2023, 2016.

Horodyski M, DiPaola CP, Conrad BP, Rechtine 2nd GR: Cervical collars are insufficient for immobilizing an unstable cervical spine injury, *J Emerg Med* 41:513, 2011.

Huang DG, Zhang XL, Hao DJ, et al.: The healing rate of type II odontoid fractures treated with posterior atlantoaxial screw-rod fixation: a retrospective review of 77 patients, *J Am Acad Orthop Surg* 27(5):e242, 2019.

Humphry S, Clarke A, Hutton M, Chan D: Erect radiographs to assess clinical instability in patients with blunt cervical spine trauma, *J Bone Joint Surg* 94A:e174, 2012.

Inagaki T, Kimura A, Makishi G, et al.: Development of a new clinical decision rule for cervical CT to detect cervical spine injury in patients with head or neck trauma, *Emerg Med J* 35(10):614, 2018.

Ishak B, Gnanadev R, Dupont G, et al.: Gerber's ligament - a forgotten structure of the craniocervical junction, *World Neurosurg* 30074(19):S1878–S8750, 2019.

Ishak B, Schneider T, Gimmy V, et al.: A modified posterior C1/C2 fusion technique for the management of traumatic odontoid type II fractures by using intraoperative spinal navigation: midterm results, *J Orthop Trauma* 32(9):e366, 2018.

Ishida W, Ramhmdani S, Xia Y, et al.: Use of recombinant human bone morphogenetic protein-2 at the C1-C2 lateral articulation without posterior structural bone graft in posterior atlantoaxial fusion in adult patients, *World Neurosurg* 123:e69, 2019.

Jiang X, Yao Y, Yu M, et al.: Surgical treatment for subaxial cervical facet dislocations with incomplete or without neurological deficit: a prospective study of 52 cases, *Med Sci Monit* 23:732, 2017.

Joaquim AF, Ghizoni E, Tedeschi H, et al.: Upper cervical injuries—a rational approach to guide surgical management, *J Spinal Cord Med* 37:139, 2014.

Joestl J, Lang N, Bukaty A, Platzer P: A comparison of anterior screw fixation and halo immobilization of type II odontoid fractures in elderly patients at increases risk from anaesthesia, *Bone Joint J* 98-B(9):1222, 2016.

Josten C, Jarvers JS, Glasmacher S, et al.: Anterior transarticular atlantoaxial screw fixation in combination with dens screw fixation for type II odontoid fractures with associated atlanto-odontoid osteoarthritis, *Eur Spine J* 25(7):2210, 2016.

Josten C, Jarvers JS, Glasmacher S, Spiegl UJ: Odontoid fractures in combination with C1 fractures in the elderly treated by combined anterior odontoid and trasarticular C1/2 screw fixation, *Arch Orthop Trauma Surg* 138(11):1525, 2018.

Kakarla UK, Chang SW, Theodore N, Sonntag VKH: Atlas fractures, *Neurosurgery* 66:A60, 2010.

Kalantar BS, Hipp JA, Reitman CA, et al.: Diagnosis of unstable cervical spine injuries: laboratory support for the use of axial traction to diagnose cervical spine instability, *J Trauma* 69:889, 2010.

Kandziora F, Chapman JR, Vaccaro AR, et al.: Atlas fractures and atlas osteosynthesis: a comprehensive narrative review, *J Orthop Trauma* 31(Suppl 4):S81, 2017.

Kanna RM, Shetty AP, Rajasekaran S: Modified anterior-only reduction and fixation for traumatic cervical facet dislocation (AO type C injuries), *Eur Spine J* 27(6):1447, 2018.

Kantelhardt SR, Keric N, Conrad J, et al.: Minimally invasive instrumentation of uncomplicated cervical fractures, *Eur Spine J* 25(1):127, 2016.

Karimi MT, kamali M, Fatoye F: Evaluation of the efficiency of cervical orthoses on cervical fracture: a review of literature, *J Craniovertebr Junction Spine* 7:13, 2016.

Kasliwal MK, Fontes RB, Traynelis VC: Occipitocervical dissociation-incidence, evaluation, and treatment, *Curr Rev Musculoskelet Med* 9(3):247, 2016.

Kepler CK, Vaccaro AR, Chen E, et al.: Treatment of isolated cervical facet fractures; a systematic review, *J Neurosurg Spine* 24(2):347, 2016.

Kepler CK, Vaccaro AR, Fleischman AN, et al.: Treatment of axis body fractures: a systematic review, *Clin Spine Surg* 30(10):442, 2017.

Khan SN, Erickson G, Sena MJ, Gupta MC: use of flexion and extension radiographs of the cervical spine to rule out acute instability in patients with negative computed tomography scans, *J Orthop Trauma* 25:51, 2011.

Khanna P, Chau C, Dublin A, et al.: The value of cervical magnetic resonance imaging in the evaluation of the obtunded or comatose patient with cervical trauma, no other abnormal neurologic findings, and a normal cervical computed tomography, *J Trauma* 72:699, 2012.

Khattab MF, Nageeb Mahmoud A, Saeed Younis A, El-Hawary Y: A simple technique for easier anterior odontoid screw fixation, *Br J Neurosurg* 33(2):135, 2019.

Khelifi A, Saadaoui F: Traumatic spondylolisthesis of the axis, *N Engl J Med* 376(18):1782, 2017.

Kim HS, Cloney MB, Koski TR, et al.: Management of isolated atlas fractures: a retrospective study of 65 patients, *World Neurosurg* 111:e316, 2018.

Kim MS, Kim JY, Kim IS, et al.: The effect of C1 bursting fracture on comparative anatomical relationship between the internal carotid artery and the atlas, *Eur Spine J* 25(1):103, 2016.

Kumar A, Varshney G, Singh PK, et al.: Traumatic atlantoaxial spondyloptosis associated with displaced odontoid fracture: complete reduction via posterior approach using "joint remodeling" technique, *World Neurosurg* 110:609, 2018.

Kurucan E, Bernstein DN, Mesfin A: Surgical management of spinal fractures in ankylosing spondylitis, *J Spine Surg* 4(3):501, 2018.

Lebl DR, Bono CM, Velmahos G, et al.: Vertebral artery injury associated with blunt cervical spine trauma: a multivariate regression analysis, *Spine* 38:1352, 2013.

Lee D, Adeoye AL, Dahdaleh NS: Indications and complications of crown halo vest placement: a review, *J Clin Neurosci* 40:27, 2017.

Leonard R, Belafsky P: Dysphagia following C-spine surgery with anterior instrumentation: evidence from fluoroscopic swallow studies, *Spine* 36:2217, 2011.

Lewkonia P, Dipaola C, Schouten R, et al.: An evidence-based medicine process to determine outcomes after cervical spine trauma: what surgeons should be telling their patients, *Spine* 37:E1140, 2012.

Li C, Duan J, Li L: Anterior submandibular retropharyngeal odontoid osteotomy and posterior atlantoaxial fusion for irreducible atlantoaxial disclocation associated with odontoid fracture malunion, *Eur Spine J* 27(Suppl 3):292, 2018.

Li Z, Li F, Hou S, et al.: Anterior discectomy/corpectomy and fusion with internal fixation for the treatment of unstable hangman's fractures: a retrospective study of 38 cases, *J Neurosurg Spine* 22:387, 2015.

Liu K, Zhang Z: A novel anterior-only surgical approach for reduction and fixation of cervical facet dislocation, *World Neurosurg* 128:e362, 2019.

Liu P, Zhu J, Wang Z, et al.: "Rule of Spence" and Dickman's classification of transverse atlantal ligament injury revisted: discrepancy of prediction on atlantoaxial stability based on clinical outcome of nonoperative treatment for atlas fractures, *Spine* 44(5):E306, 2019.

Lockwood MM, Smith GA, Tanenbaum J, et al.: Screening via CT angiogram after traumatic cervical spine fractures: narrowing imaging to improve cost effectiveness. Experience of a Level 1 trauma center, *J Neurosurg Spine* 24:490, 2016.

Lofrese G, De Bonis P: In response: is conservative treatment really beneficial in elderly patients with unstable odontoid fractures? *Spine* 44(15):E927, 2019.

Longo UG, Denaro L, Campi S, et al.: Upper cervical spine injuries: indications and limits of the conservative management in halo vest. A systematic review of efficacy and safety, *Injury* 41:1127, 2010.

Lopes A, Andrade A, Silva I, et al.: Brain abscess after halo fixation for the cervical spine, *World Neurosurg* 104:1047, 2017.

Lu Y, Lee YP, Bhatia NN, Lee TQ: Biomechanical comparison of C1 lateral mass-C2 short pedicle screw-C3 lateral mass screw-rod construct versus Goel-Harms fixation for atlantoaxial instability, *Spine* 44(7):E393, 2019.

Lukasiewicz AM, Bohl DD, Varthi AG, et al.: Spinal fracture in patients with ankylosing spondylitis: cohort definition, distribution of injuries, and hospital outcomes, *Spine* 41(3):191, 2016.

Lvov I, Grin A, Kordonskiy A, et al.: Minimally invasive posterior transarticular stand-alone screw instrumentation of C1-C2 using a transmuscular approach: a technique description an dresults comparing with posterior midline exposure, *World Neurosurg* 128:e796, 2019.

Machino M, Yukawa Y, Ito K, et al.: Can magnetic resonance imaging reflect the prognosis in patients of cervical spinal cord injury without radiographic abnormality? *Spine* 36:E1568, 2011.

Manoso MW, Moore TA, Agel J, et al.: Floating lateral mass fractures of the cervical spine, *Spine* 41(18):1421, 2016.

Martinez-Del-Campo E, Kalb S, Soriano Barron H, et al.: Computed tomography parameters for atlantooccipital dislocation in adult patients: the occipital condyle-C1 interval, *J Nerosurg Spine* 24(4):535, 2016.

Martinez-Pérez R, Paredes I, Cepeda S, et al.: Spinal cord injury after blunt cervical spine trauma: correlation of soft-tissue damage and extension of lesion, *AJNR Am J Neuroradiol* 35:1029, 2014.

Maung AA, Johnson DC, Barre K, et al.: Cervical spine MRI in patients with negative CT: a prospective, multicenter study of the Research Consortium of New England Centers for Trauma (ReCONECT), *J Trauma Acute Care Surg* 82(2):263, 2017.

Mead II LB, Millhouse PW, Krystal J, Vaccaro AR: C1 fractures: a review of diagnoses, management options, and outcomes, *Curr Rev Musculoskelet Med* 9(3):255, 2016.

Miao DC, Qi C, Wang F, Lu K, Shen Y: Management of severe lower cervical facet dislocation without vertebral body fracture using skull traction and an anterior approach, *Med Sci Monit* 3:24, 2018.

Miller CP, Brubacher JW, Biswas D, et al.: The incidence of non-contiguous spinal fractures and other traumatic injuries associated with cervical spine fractures, *Spine* 36:1532, 2011.

Mueller CA, Peters I, Podlogar M, et al.: Vertebral artery injuries following cervical spine trauma: a prospective observational study, *Eur Spine J* 20:2202, 2011.

Murphy H, Schroeder GD, Shi WJ: Management of hangman's fractures: a systematic review, 31(Suppl 4):S90, 2017.

Musbahi O, Khan AHA, Anwar MO, et al.: Immobilsation in occipital condyle fractures: a systematic review, *Clin Neurol Neurosurg* 173:130, 2018.

Nadeau M, MclLchlin SD, Bailey SI, et al.: A biomechanical assessment of soft-tissue damage in the cervical spine following a unilateral facet injury, *J Bone Joint Surg* 94A:e156, 2012.

Ni B, Guo Q, Lu X, et al.: Posterior reduction and temporary fixation for odontoid fracture. A salvage maneuver to anterior screw fixation, *Spine* 40:E168, 2015.

Ni B, Zhao W, Guo Q, et al.: Comparison of outcomes between C1-C2 screw-hook fixation and C1-C2 screw-rod fixation for treating reducible atlantoaxial dislocation, *Spine* 42(20):1587, 2017.

Niemeier TE, Manoharan SR, Mukherjee A, Theiss SM: Conservative treatment of hangman variant fractures, *Clin Spine Surg* 31(5):E286, 2018.

Nowell M, Nelson R: Traumatic posterior atlantoaxial disclocation with associated C1 Jefferson fracture and bilateral vertebral artery occlusion without odontoid process fracture or neurological deficit, *Eur Spine J*, 2018, https://doi.org/10.1007/s00586-017-5167-7, [Epub ahead of print].

Park J, Scheer JK, Lim TJ, et al.: Biomechanical analysis of Goel technique for C1-2 fusion: laboratory investigation, *J Neurosurg Spine* 14:639, 2011.

Park JH, Kang DH, Lee MK, et al.: Advantages of direct insertion of a straight probe without a guide tube during anterior odontoid screw fixation of odontoid fractures, *Spine* 41(9):E541, 2016.

Passias PG, Poorman GW, Segreto FA, et al.: Traumatic fractures of the cervical spine: analysis of changes in incidence, cause, concurrent injuries, and complications among 488,262 patients from 2005 to 2013, *World Neurosurg* 110:e427, 2018.

Patterson JT, Theologis AA, Sing D, Tay B: Anterior versus posterior approaches fro odontoid fracture stabilization in patients older than 65 years: 30-day morbidity and mortality in a national database, *Clin Spine Surg* 30(8):E1033, 2017.

Peev NA: Understanding the statics and dynamics of the subaxial cervical segments, following C1-C2 fusion, *World Neurosurg* 87:621, 2016.

Pehler S, Jones R, Staggers JR, et al.: Clinical outcomes of cervical facet fractures treated nonoperatively with hard collar or halo immobilization, *Global Spine J* 9(1):48, 2019.

Pimentel L, Diegelmann L: Evaluation and management of acute cervical spine trauma, *Emerg Med Clin North Am* 28:719, 2010.

Pourtaheri S, Emami A, Sinha K, et al.: The role of magnetic resonance imaging in acute cervical spine fractures, *Spine J* 14:2546, 2014.

Prasarn ML, Horodyski MB, Behrend C, et al.: Is it safe to use a kinetic therapy bed for care of patients with cervical spine injuries? *Injury* 46:388, 2015.

Prost S, Barrey C, Blondel B, et al.: Hangman's fracture: management strategy and healing rate in a prospective multi-centre observational study of 34 patient, *Orthop Traumatol Surg Res* 105(4):703, 2019.

Quarrington RD, Jones CF, Tcherveniakov P, et al.: Traumatic subaxial cervical facet subluxation and dislocation: epidemiology, radiographic analyses, and risk factors for spinal cord injury, *Spine J* 18(3):387, 2018.

Radovanovic I, Urquhart JC, Rasoulinejad P, et al.: Patterns of C-2 fracture in elderly: comparison of etiology, treatment, and mortality among specific fracture types, *J Neurosurg Spine* 27(5):494, 2017.

Rayes M, Mittal M, Rengachary SS, Mittal S: Hangman's fracture: a historical and biomechanical perspective: historical vignette, *J Neurosurg* 14:198, 2011.

Reinhold M, Knop C, Kneitz C, Disch A: Spine fractures in ankylosing diseases: recommendations of the spine section of the German Society for Orthopaedics and Trauma (DGOU), *Global Spine J* 8(2 Suppl):56S, 2018.

Reynolds JA, MacDonald JD: Direct C2 pedicle screw fixation for axis body fracture, *World Neurosurg* 93:279, 2016.

Robinson AL, Olerud C, Robinson Y: Surgical treatment improves survival of elderly with axis fracture – a national population-based multiregistry cohort study, *Spine J* 18(10):1853, 2018.

Rose MK, Rosal LM, Gonzalez RP, et al.: Clinical clearance of the cervical spine in patients with distracting injuries: it is time to dispel the myth, *J Trauma Acute Care Surg* 73:498, 2012.

Rozzell CJ, Aarabi B, Dhall SS, et al.: Os odontoideum, *Neurosurgery* 72(Suppl 2):159, 2013.

Rozzelle CJ, Aarabi B, Dhall SS, et al.: Management of pediatric cervical spine and spinal cord injuries, *Neurosurgery* 72(Suppl 2):205, 2013.

Rustagi T, Drazin D, Oner C, et al.: Fractures in spinal ankylosing disorders: a narrative review of disease and injury types, treatment techniques, and outcomes, *J Orthop Trauma* 31(Suppl 4):S57, 2017.

Ryken TC, Aarabi B, Dhall SS, et al.: Management of isolated fractures of the atlas in adults, *Neurosurgery* 72(Suppl 2):127, 2013.

Ryken TC, Hadley MN, Aarabi B, et al.: Management of acute combination fractures of the atlas and axis in adults, *Neurosurgery* 72(Suppl 2):151, 2013.

Ryken TC, Hadley MN, Aarabi B, et al.: Management of isolated fractures of the axis in adults, *Neurosurgery* 72(Suppl 2):132, 2013.

Ryken TC, Hadley MN, Walters BC, et al.: Radiographic assessment, *Neurosurgery* 72(Suppl 2):54, 2013.

Ryken TC, Hurlbert RJ, Hadley MN, et al.: The acute cardiopulmonary management of patients with cervical spinal cord injuries, *Neurosurgery* 72(Suppl 2):84, 2013.

Schoenfeld AJ, Bono CM, Reichmann WM, et al.: Type II odontoid fractures of the cervical spine: do treatment type and medical comorbidities affect mortality in elderly patients? *Spine* 36:879, 2011.

Sadiqi S, Verlaan JJ, Lehr AM: Surgeon reported outcome measure for spine trauma: an international expert survey identifying parameters relevant for the outcome of subaxial cervical spine injuries, *Spine* 41(24):E1453, 2016.

Salunke P, Karthigeyan M, Sahoo SK, Prasad PK: Multiplanar realignment for unstable Hangman's fracture with posterior C2-3 fusion: a prospective series, *Clin Neurol Neurosurg* 169:133, 2018.

Salunke P, Sahoo SK, Krishnan P, et al.: Are C2 pars-pedicle screws alone for type II Hangman's fracture overrated? *Clin Neurol Neurosurg* 141:7, 2016.

Schleicher P, Kobbe P, Kandziora F, et al.: Treatment of injuries to the subaxial cervical spine: recommendations of the spine section of the German Society of Orthopaedics and Trauma (DGOU), *Global Spine J* 8(2 Suppl):25S, 2018.

Schnake KJ, Schroeder GD, Vaccaro AR, Oner C: AOSpine classification systems (subaxial, thoracolumbar), *J Orthop Trauma* 31(Suppl 4):S14, 2017.

Sharpe JP, Magnotti LJ, Weinberg JA, et al.: The old man and the c-spine fracture: impact of the halo vest stabilization in patients with blunt cervical spine fractures, *J Trauma Acute Care Surg* 80(1):76, 2016.

Shatsky J, Bellabarba C, Nguyen Q, Bransford RJ: A retrospective review of fixation of C1 ring fractures – does the transverse atlantal ligament (TAL) really matter? *Spine J* 16(3):272, 2016.

Shin JJ, Kim SJ, Kim TH, et al.: Optimal use of the halo-vest orthosis for upper cervical spine injuries, *Yonsei Med J* 51:648, 2010.

Shousha M, Alhashash M, Allouch H, Boehm H: Surgical treatment of type II odontoid fractures in elderly patients: a comparison of anterior odontoid screw fixation and posterior atlantoaxial fusion using the Magerl-Gallie technique, *Eur Spine J*, 2019, https://doi.org/10.1007/s00586-019-05946-x, [Epub ahead of print].

Singh PK, Garg K, Sawarkar D, et al.: Computed tomography-guided C2 pedicle screw placement for treatment of unstable hangman fractures, *Spine* 39:E1058, 2014.

Teunissen FR, Verbeek BM, Cha TD, Schwab JH: Spinal cord injury after traumatic spine fracture in patients with ankylosing spinal disorders, *J Neurosurg Spine* 27(6):709, 2017.

Theodore N, Aarabi B, Dhall S, et al.: Occipital condyle fractures, *Neurosurgery* 72(Suppl 2):106, 2013.

Theodore N, Aarabi B, Dhall S, et al.: The diagnosis and management of traumatic atlanto-occipital dislocation injuries, *Neurosurgery* 72(Suppl 2):114, 2013.

Theodore N, Aarabi B, Dhall SS, et al.: Transportation of patients with acute traumatic cervical spine injuries, *Neurosurgery* 72(Suppl 2):35, 2013.

Theodore N, Hadley MN, Bizhan A, et al.: Prehospital cervical spinal immobilization after trauma, *Neurosurgery* 72(Suppl 2):22, 2013.

Tobert DG, Le HV, Blucher JA, et al.: The clinical implications of adding CT angiography in the evaluation of cervical spine fractures: a propensity-matched analysis, *J Bone Joint Surgery Am* 100(17):1490, 2018.

Toregrossa F, Grasso G: Conservative management for odontoid cervical fractures: halo or rigid cervical collar? *World Neurosurg* 97:723, 2017.

Umerani MS, Abbas A, Sharif S: Clinical outcome in patients with early versus delayed decompression in cervical spine trauma, *Asian Spine J* 8:427, 2014.

Urrutia J, Zamora T, Campos M, et al.: A comparative agreement evaluation of two subaxial cervical spine injury classification systems: the AOSpine and the Allen and Ferguson schemes, *Eur Spine J* 25(7):2185, 2016.

Vaccaro AR, Kepler CK, Kopjar B, et al.: Functional and quality-of-life outcomes in geriatric patients with type-II dens fracture, *J Bone Joint Surg* 95A:729, 2013.

Walters BC: Methodology of the guidelines for the management of acute cervical spine and spinal cord injuries, *Neurosurgery* 72(Suppl 2):17, 2013.

Wang G, Jiang D, Wang Q, et al.: A novel technique using a pedicle screw and bucking bar for the treatment of hangman's fracture, *Orthop Traumatol Surg Res* 105(4):709, 2019.

Wang H, Wang Q, Ma L, et al.: Predisposing factors of fracture nonunion after posterior C1 lateral mass screws combined with C2 pedicle/laminar screw fixation for type II odontoid fracture, *World Neurosurg* 109:e425, 2018.

Wang J, Chen H, Cao P, et al.: Combined anterior-posterior fixation and fusion for completely dislocated hangman's fracture: a retrospective analysis of 11 cases, *Clin Spine Surg* 30(8):E1050, 2017.

Wang J, Eltorai AEM, DePasse JM, et al.: Variability in treatment for patients with cervical spine fracture and dislocation: an analysis of 107,152 patients, *World Neurosurg* 114:e151, 2018.

Wang L, Gu Y, Chen L, Yang H: Surgery for chronic traumatic atlantoaxial dislocation associated with myelopathy, *Clin Spine Surg* 30(5):E640, 2017.

Wang S, Tian Y, Diebo BG, et al.: Treatment of atlantoaxial dislocations among patients with cervical osseous or vascular abnormalities utilizing hybrid techniques, *J Neurosurg Spine* 29(2):135, 2018.

Waqar M, Van-Popta D, Barone DG, Sarsam Z: External immobilization of odontoid fractures: a systematic review to compare the halo and hard collar, *World Neurosurg* 97:513, 2017.

Werner BC Samartzis D, Shen FH: Spinal fractures in patients with ankylosing spondylitis: etiology, diagnosis, and management, *J Am Acad Orthop Surg* 24(4):241, 2016.

West JL, Palma AE, Vilella L, et al.: Occipital condyle fractures and concomitant cervical spine fractures: implications for management, *World Neurosurg* 115:e238, 2018.

Woods BI, Hohl JB, Braly B, et al.: Mortality in elderly patients following operative and nonoperative management of odontoid fractures, *J Spinal Disord Tech* 27:321, 2014.

Woods RO, Inceoglu S, Akpolat YT, et al.: C1 lateral mass displacement and transverse atlantal ligament failure in Jefferson's fracture: a biomechanical study of the "Rule of Spence", *Neurosurgery* 82(2):226, 2018.

Wu AM, Wang XY, Chi YL, et al.: Management of acute combination atlas-axis fractures with percutaneous triple anterior screw fixation in elderly patients, *Orthop Traumatol Surg Res* 98:894, 2012.

Xu Y, Xiong W, Han SII, et al.: Posterior bilateral intermuscular approach for upper cervical spine injuries, *World Neurosurg* 104:869, 2017.

Yan L, Luo Z, He B, et al.: Posterior pedicle screw fixation to treat lower cervical fractures associated with ankylosing spondylitis: a retrospective study of 35 cases, *BMC Musculoskelet Disord* 18(1):81, 2017.

Zakrison TL, Williams BH: Cervical spine evaluation in the bluntly injured patient, *Int J Surg* 33(Pt B):246, 2016.

Zehnder SW, Lenarz CJ, Place HM: Teachability and reliability of a new classification system for lower cervical spinal injuries, *Spine* 34:2039, 2009.

Zhang Z: Anterior pedicle spreader reduction for unilateral cervical facet dislocation, *Injury* 48(8):1801, 2017.

Zhang Z, Mu Z, Zheng W: Anterior pedicle screw and plate fixation for cervical facet dislocation: case series and technical note, *Spine J* 16(1):123, 2016.

Zhao L, Xu R, Liu J, et al.: Comparison of two techniques for transarticular screw implantation in the subaxial cervical spine, *J Spinal Disord Tech* 24:125, 2011.

Zhao W, Wu Y, Hu W, et al.: Comparison of two posterior three-point fixation techniques for treating reducible atlantoaxial dislocation, *Spine* 44(1):E60, 2019.

Zou HJ, Wu J, Hu Y, et al.: Unilateral vertebral artery injury in a patient with displaced upper cervical spine fractures: the treatment for one case of vertebral artery embolism, *Eur Spine J* 27(Suppl 3):409, 2018.

THORACIC AND LUMBAR SPINE AND SACRUM

Abbasi Fard S, Skoch J, Avila MJ, et al.: Instability in thoracolumbar trauma: is a new definition warranted? *Clin Spine Surg* 30:E1046, 2017.

Abo-Elsoud M, Eldeeb S, Gobba M, Sadek FZ: Biplanar posterior pelvic fixator for unstable sacral fractures: a new fixation technique, *J Orthop Trauma* 32(5):e185, 2018.

Acklin YP, Zderic I, Richards RG, et al.: Biomechanical investigation of four different fixation techniques in sacrum Denis type II fracture with low bone mineral density, *J Orthop Res* 36(6):1624, 2018.

Aebi M: Classification of thoracolumbar fractures and dislocations, *Eur Spine J* 19:S2, 2010.

Aleem IS, Nassr A: Cochrane in CORR®: surgical versus non-surgical treatment for thoracolumbar burst fractures without neurological deficit, *Clin Orthop Relat Res* 474:619, 2016.

Aono H, Ishii K, Tobimatsu H, et al.: Temporary short-segment pedicle screw fixation for thoracolumbar burst fractures: comparative study with and without vertebroplasty, *Spine J* 17(8):1113, 2017.

Aono H, Tobimatsu H, Ariga K, et al.: Surgical outcomes of temporary short-segment instrumentation without augmentation for thoracolumbar burst fractures, *Injury* 47(6):1337, 2016.

Aras EL, Bunger C, Hansen ES, Søgaard R: Cost-effectiveness of surgical versus conservative treatment for thoracolumbar burst fractures, *Spine* 41(4):337, 2016.

Axelsson P, Strömqvist B: Can implant removal restore mobility after fracture of the thoracolumbar segment? *Acta Orthop* 87(5):511, 2016.

Bae JW, Gwak HS, Kim S, et al.: Percutaneous vertebroplasty for patients with metastatic compression fractures of the thoracolumbar spine: clinical and radiological factors affecting functional outcomes, *Spine J* 16(3):355, 2016.

Bakhsheshian J, Dahdaleh NS, Fakurnejad S, et al.: Evidence-based management of traumatic thoracolumbar burst fractures: a systematic review of nonoperative management, *Neurosurg Focus* 37:E1, 2014.

arcellos ALL, da Rocha VM, Guimarães JAM: Current concepts in spondylopelvic dissociation, *Injury* 48(Suppl 6):S5, 2017.

Bederman SS, Hassan JM, Shah KN, et al.: Fixation techniques for complex traumatic transverse sacral fractures, *Spine* 38:E1028, 2013.

Bellabarba C, Fisher C, Chapman JR, et al.: Does early fracture fixation of thoracolumbar spine fractures decrease morbidity or mortality? *Spine* 35:S138, 2010.

Bono CM, Heggeness M, Mick C, et al.: North American Spine Society newly released vertebroplasty randomized controlled trials: a tale of two trials, *Spine J* 10:238, 2010.

Bourghli A, Obeid I, Boissiere L, et al.: Management of a high thoracic chance fracture, *Eur Spine J* 27(7):318, 2018.

Charles YP, Walter A, Schuller S, Steib J-P: Temporary percutaneous instrumentation and selective anterior fusion for thoracolumbar fractures, *Spine* 42(9):E523, 2017.

Chen F, Kang Y, Li H, et al.: Modified pedicle subtraction osteotomy as a salvage method for failed short-segment pedicle instrumentation in the treatment of thoracolumbar fracture, *Clin Spine Surg* 29(3):E120, 2016.

Chen JX, Xu DL, Sheng Sr, et al.: Risk factors of kyphosis recurrence after implant removal in thoracolumbar burst fractures following posterior short-segment fixation, *Int Orthop* 40(6):1253, 2016.

Chou PH, Ma HL, Liu CL, et al.: Is removal of the implants needed after fixation of burst fractures of the thoracolumbar and lumbar spine without fusion? A retrospective evaluation of radiological and functional outcomes, *Bone Joint J* 98-B(1):109, 2016.

Chou PH, MA HL, Wang ST, et al.: Fusion may not be a necessary procedure for surgically treated burst fractures of the thoracolumbar and lumbar spines. A follow-up of at least ten years, *J Bone Joint Surg* 96A:1724, 2014.

Choy W, Smith ZA, Viljoen SV, et al.: Successful treatment of a three-column thoracic extension injury with recumbancy, *Cureus* 8(5):e614, 2016.

Chung HY, Suk KS, Lee HM, et al.: Growing rod technique for the treatment of the traumatic spinopelvic dissociation: a technical trick, *Spine J* 16(3):e209, 2016.

Dayani F, Chen YR, Johnson E, et al.: Minimally invasive lumbar pedicle screw fixation using cortical bone trajectory – screw accuracy, complications, and learning curve in 100 screw placements, *J Clin Neurosci* 61:106, 2019.

Dekutoski MB, Hayes ML, Utter AP, et al.: Pathologic correlation of posterior ligamentous injury with MRI, *Orthopedics* 33:00, 2010.

Dhall SS, Wadhwa R, Yang MY, et al.: Traumatic thoracolumbar spinal injury: an algorithm for minimally invasive surgical management, *Neurosurg Focus* 37:E9, 2014.

De lure F, Lofrese G, De Bonis P, et al.: Vertebral body spread in thoracolumbar burst fractures can predict posterior construct failure, *Spine J* 18(6):1005, 2018.

Diniz JM, Botelho RV: Is fusion necessary for thoracolumbar burst fracture treated with spinal fixation? A systematic review and meta-analysis, *J Neurosurg Spine* 27(5):584, 2017.

D'Oro A, Spoonamore MJ, Cohen JR, et al.: Effects of fusion and conservative treatment on disc degeneration and rates of subsequent surgery after thoracolumbar fracture, *J Neurosurg Spine* 24:476, 2016.

Du JP, Fan Y, Liu JJ, et al.: Decompression for traumatic thoracic/thoracolumbar incomplete spinal cord injury: application of AO spine injury classification system to identify the timing of operation, *World Neurosurg* 116:3867, 2018.

Futamura K, Baba T, Mogami A, et al.: "Within ring"-based sacroiliac rod fixation may overcome the weakness of spinopelvic fixation for unstable pelvic ring injuries: technical notes and clinical outcomes, *Int Orthop* 42(6):1405, 2018.

Gattozzi DA, Friis LA, Arnold PM: Surgery for traumatic fractures of the upper thoracic spine (T1-T6), *Surg Neurol Int* 9:231, 2018.

Gnanenthiran SR, Adie S, Harris IA: Nonoperative versus operative treatment for thoracolumbar burst fractures without neurologic deficit: a meta-analysis, *Clin Orthop Relat Res* 470:567, 2012.

Grobost P, Boudissa M, Kerschbaumer G, et al.: Early versus delayed corpectomy in thoracic and lumbar spine trauma. A long-term clinical and radiological retrospective study, *Orthop Traumatol Surg Res* S1877-0568(18):30390–30396, 2019.

Groen FRJ, Delawi D, Kruyt MC, Oner FC: Extension type fracture of the ankylotic thoracic spine with gross displacement causing esophageal rupture, *Eur Spine J* 25(Suppl 1):A183, 2016.

Grossbach AJ, Dahdaleh NS, Abel TJ, et al.: Flexion-distraction injuries of the thoracolumbar spine: open fusion versus percutaneous pedicle screw fixation, *Neurosurg Focus* E2, 2013.

Guerado E, Cervan AM, Cano JR, Giannoudis PV: Spinopelvic injuries. Facts and controversies, *Injury* 49(3):449, 2018.

He S, Zhang H, Zhao Q, et al.: Posterior approach in treating sacral fracture combied with lumbopelvic dissociation, *Orthopedics* 37:e1027, 2014.

Heintel TM, Dannigkeit S, Fenwick A, et al.: How safe is minimally invasive pedicle screw placement for treatment of thoracolumbar spine fractures? *Eur Spine J* 26(5):1492, 2017.

Hitchen PW, Abode-Iyamah K, Dahdaleh NS, et al.: Nonoperative management in neurologically intact thoracolumbar burst fractures: clinical and radiographic outcomes, *Spine* 41(6):483, 2016.

Hyun SE, Ko JY, Lee E, Ryu JS: The prognostic significance of pedicle enhancement from contrast-enhanced MRI for the further collapse in osteporic vertebral compression fractures, *Spine* 43(22):1586, 2018.

Ibrahim FM, Abd El-Rady Ael-R: Mono segmental fixation of selected types of thoracic and lumbar fractures: a prospective study, *Int Orthop* 40(60):1083, 2016.

Inaba K, Nosanov L, Menaker J, et al.: Prospective derivation of a clinical decision rule for thoracolumbar spine evaluation after blunt trauma: an American Association for the Surgery of Trauma Multi-Institutional Trials Group study, *J Trauma* 78:459, 2015.

Inoue T, Abe M: Esophageal perforation associated with fracture of the upper thoracic spine from blunt trauma: a case report, *Spinal Cord Ser Cases* 2:15034, 2016.

Ituarte F, Wiegers NW, Ruppar T, et al.: Posterior thoracolumbar instrumented fusion for burst fractures: a meta-analysis, *Clin Spine Surg* 32(2):57, 2019.

Jaffray DC, Eisenstein SM, Balain B, et al.: Early mobilisation of thoracolumbar burst fractures without neurology: a natural history observation, *Bone Joint J* 98B:97, 2016.

Janssen I Ryang YM, Gempt J, et al.: Risk of cement leakage and pulmonary embolism by bone cement-augmented pedicle screw fixation of the thoracolumbar spine, *Spine J* 17(6):837, 2017.

Jazini E, Klocke N, Tannous O, et al.: Does lumbopelvic fixation add stability? A cadaveric biomechanical analysis of an unstable pelvic fracture model, *J Orthop Trauma* 31(1):37, 2017.

Jazini E, Weir T, Nwodim E, et al.: Outcomes of lumbopelvic fixation in the treatment of complex sacral fractures using minimally invasive surgical techniques, *Spine J* 17(9):1238, 2017.

Jiang Y, Wang F, Yu X, et al.: A comparative Study on functional recovery, complications, and changes in inflammatory factors in patients with thoracolumbar spinal fracture complicated with nerve injury treated by anterior and posterior decompression, *Med Sci Monit* 25:1164, 2019.

Joaquim AF, Fernandes YB, Cavalcante RAC, et al.: Evaluation of the thoracolumbar injury classification system in thoracic and lumbar spinal trauma, *Spine* 36:33, 2011.

Joaquim AF, Patel AA, Schroeder GD, Vaccaro AR: A simplified treatment algorithm for treating thoracic and lumbar spine trauma, *J Spinal Cord Med* 42(4):416, 2019.

Joaquim AF, Rodrigues SA, DA Silva FS, et al.: Is there an association with spino-pelvic relationships and clinical outcome of type A thoracic and lumbar fractures treated non-surgically? *Int J Spine Surg* 12(3):371, 2018.

Joaquim AF, Schroeder GD, Patell AA, Vaccaro AR: Clinical and radiological outcome of non-surgical management of thoracic and lumbar spinal fracture-dislocations- a historical analysis in the era of modern spinal surgery, *J Spinal Cord Med* 1-7, 2018.

Kakaria UK, Little AS, Chang SW, et al.: Placement of percutaneous thoracic pedicle screws using NeuroNavigation, *World Neurosurg* 74:606, 2010.

Kato S, Murray JC, Kwon BK, et al.: Does surgical intervention or timing of surgery have an effect on neurological recovery in the setting of a thoracolumbar burst fracture? *J Orthop Trauma* 31(Suppl 4):S38, 2017.

Katsura Y, Osborn JM, Cason GW: The epidemiology of thoracolumbar trauma: A meta-analysis, *J Orthop* 13(4):383, 2016.

Kayaci S, Cakir T, Dolgun M, et al.: Aortic injury by thoracic pedicle screw. When is aortic repair required? Literature review and three new cases, *World Neurosurg* 128:216, 2019.

Kelly M, Zhang J, Humphrey CA, et al.: Surgical management of U/H type sacral fractures: outcomes following iliosacral and lumbopelvic fixation, *J spine Surg* 4(2):361, 2018.

Kempen DHR, Delawi D, Altena MC, et al.: Neurological outcome after traumatic transverse sacral fractures: a systematic review of 521 patients reported in the literature, *JBJS Rev* 6(6):e1, 2018.

Kepler Ck, Schroeder GD, Hollern DA, et al.: Do formal laminectomy and timing of decompression for patients with sacral fracture and neurologic deficit affect outcome? *J Orthop Trauma* 31(Suppl 4):S75, 2017.

Khan JM, Marquez-Lara A, Miller AN: Relationship of sacral fractures to nerve injury: is the Denis classification still accurate? *J Orthop Trauma* 31(4):181, 2017.

Khoury L, Change E, Hill D, et al.: Management of thoracic and lumbar spine fractures; is MRI necessary in patients without neurological deficits? *Am Surg* 85(3):306, 2019.

Khurana B, Prevedello LM, Bono CM, et al.: CT for thoracic and lumbar spine fractures: Can CT findings accurately predict posterior ligament complex injury? *Eur Spine J* 27:3007, 2018.

Kingwell SP, Noonan VK, Fisher CG, et al.: Relationship of neural axis level of injury to motor recovery and health-related quality of life in patients with a thoracolumbar spinal injury, *J Bone Joint Surg* 92A:1591, 2010.

Kitzen J, Schontanus MGM, Plasschaert HSW, et al.: Treatment of thoracic or lumbar burst fractures with balloon assisted endplate reduction using tricalcium phosphate cement: histological and radiological evaluation, *BMC Musculoskelet Disord* 18(1):411, 2017.

Klaus JS, Schroeder GD, Vaccaro AR, Oner C: AOSpine classification systems (subaxial, thoracolumbar), *J Orthop Trauma* 31(9):S14, 2017.

Kocanli O, Komur B, Duymuş TM, et al.: Ten-year follow-up results of posterior instrumentation without fusion for traumatic thoracic and lumbar spine fractures, *J Orthop* 13(4):301, 2016.

Kose KC, Inanmaz ME, Isik C, et al.: Shsort segment pedicle screw instrumentation with an index level screw and cantilevered hyperlordotic reduction in the treatment of type-A fractures of the thoracolumbar spine, *Bone Joint J* 96B:541, 2014.

Koshimune K, Itao Y, Sugimoto Y, Kikuchi T: Minimally invasive spinopelvic fixation for unstable bilateral sacral fractures, *Clin Spine Surg* 29:124, 2016.

Kreinest M, Rillig J, Grutzner PA, et al.: Analysis of complications and perioperative data after open or percutaneous dorsal instrumentation following traumatic spinal fracture of the thoracic and lumbar spine: a retrospective cohort study including 491 patients, *Eur Spine J* 26(5):1515, 2017.

Kwan MK, Chan CY, Saw LB, et al.: The safety and strength of a novel medial, partial nonthreaded pedicle screw: a cadaveric and biomechanical investigation, *Clin Spine Surg* 30(3):E297, 2017.

La Maida GA, Ruosi C, Misaggi B: Indications for the monosegmental stabilization of thoraco-lumbar spine fractures, *Int Orthop* 43(1):169, 2019.

Lee HD, Jeon CH, Chung NS, Seo YW: Cost-utility analysis of pedicle screw removal after successful posterior instrumented fusion in thoracolumbar burst fractures, *Spine* 42(15):E926, 2017.

Lee HD, Jeon CH, Won SH, Chung NS: Global sagital imbalance due to change in pelvic incidence after traumatic after traumatic spinopelvic dissociation, 31(7):e195, 2017.

Lee KY, Kim MW, Seok SY, et al.: The relationship between superior disc-endplate complex injury and correction loss in young adult patients with thoracolumbar stable burst fracture, *Clin Orthop Surg* 9(4):465, 2017.

Li K, Li Z, Ren X, et al.: Effect of the percutaneous pedicle screw fixation at the fractured vertebra on the treatment of thoracolumbar fractures, *Int Orthop* 40(6):1103, 2016.

Li Y, Shen Z, Huang M, Wang X: Stepwise resection of the posterior ligamentous complex for stability of a thoracolumbar compression fracture: an in vitro biomechanical investigation, *Medicine (Baltimore)* 96(35):e7873, 2017.

Lindahl J, Mäkinen TJ, Koskinen SK, Söderlund T: Factors associated with outcome of spinopelvic dissociation treated with lumbopelvic fixation, *Injury* 45:1914, 2014.

Liuzza F, Silluzio N, Florio M, et al.: Comparison between posterior sacral plate stabilization versus minimally invasive transiliac-transsacral lag-screw fixation in fractures of sacrum: a single centre experience, *Int Orthop* 43(1):177, 2019.

Lubeleski D, Tharin S, Como JJ, et al.: Surgical timing for cervical and upper thoracic injuries in patients with polytrauma, *J Neurosurg Spine* 31(12):636, 2017.

Marek AP, Morancy JD, Chipman JG: Long-term functional outcomes after traumatic thoracic and lumbar spine fractures, *Am Surg* 84(1):20, 2018.

Martikos K, Greggi T, Faldini C, et al.: Osteporotic thoracolumbar compression fractures: long-term retrospective comparison between vertebroplasty and conservative treatment, *Eur Spine J* 27(Suppl 2):244, 2018.

Matar HE, Hassan K, Duckett SP: Insufficiency sacral fracture-dislocation mimicking suicidal jumper's fracture, *BMJ Case Rep*, 2016(pii):bcr2016216587, 2016.

McAnany SJ, Overley SC, Kim JS, et al.: Open versus minimally invasive fixation techniques for thoracolumbar trauma: a meta-analysis, *Global Spine J* 6:186, 2016.

Mi J, Sun XJ, Zhang K, Zhao CQ, Zhao J: Prediction of MRI findings including disc injury and posterior ligamentous complex injury in neurologically intact thoracolumbar burst fractures by the parameters of vertebral body damage on CT scan, *Injury* 49(2):272, 2018.

Min KS, Zamorano DP, Wahba GM, et al.: Comparison of two-transsacral-screw fixation versus triangular osteosynthesis for transforaminal sacral fractures, *Orthopedics* 37:e754, 2014.

Sp Mohanty, Bhat Sn, Pai Kanhangad M, Gosal GS: Pedicle screw fixation in thoracolumbar and lumbar spine assisted by lateral fluoroscopic imaging: a study to evaluate the accuracy of screw placement, *Musculosckelet Surg* 102(1):47, 2018.

Morgenstern M, von Rüden C, Callsen H, et al.: The unstable thoracic cage injury: the concomitant sternal fracture indicates a severe thoracic spine fracture, *Injury* 47(11):2465, 2016.

Ntilikina Y, Bahlau D, Garnon J, et al.: Open versus percutaneous instrumentation in thoracolumbar fractures: magnetic resonance imaging comparison of paravertebral muscles after implant removal, *J Neurosurg Spine* 27(2):235, 2017.

Nonne D, Capone A, Sanna F, et al.: Suicidal jumper's fracture – sacral fractures and spoinopelvic instability: a case series, *J Med Case Rep* 12(1):186, 2018.

Park SR, Na HY, Kim JM, et al.: More than 5-year follow-up results of two-level and three-level posterior fixations of thoracolumbar burst fractures with load-sharing scores of seven and eight points, *Clin Orthop Surg* 8(1):71, 2016.

Pascal-Moussellard H, Hirsch C, Bonaccorsi R: Osteosynthesis in sacral fracture and lumbosacral dislocation, *Orthop Trumatol Surg Res* 102(Suppl 1):S45, 2016.

Pearson JM, Niemeier TE, McGwin G, Rajaram Manoharan S: Spinopelvic dissociation: comparison of outcomes of percutaneous versus open fixation strategies, *Adv Orthop* 2018:5023908, 2018.

Piltz S, Rubenbauer B, Böcker W, Trentzsch H: Reduction and fixation of displaced U-shaped sacral fractures using lumbopelvic fixation: technical recommendations, *Eur Spine J* 27(12):3025, 2018.

Pulley BR, Cotman SB, Fowler TT: Surgical fixation of geriatric sacral u-type insufficiency fractures: a retrospective analysis, *J Orthop Trauma* 32(12):617, 2018.

Puvanesarajah V, Lina IA, Liauw JA, et al.: Systematic approach for anterior corpectomy through a transthoracic exposure, *Turk Neurosurg* 26(4):646, 2016.

Rajasekaran S, Maheswaran A, Aiyer SN, et al.: Prediction of posterior ligamentous complex injury in thoracolumbar fractures using non-MRI imaging techniques, *Int Orthop* 40(6):1075, 2016.

Rodriguez-Martinez NG, Savardekar A, Nottmeier EW, et al.: Biomechanics of transvertebral screw fixation in the thoracic spine: an in vitro study, *J Neurosurg Spine* 25:187, 2016.

Ruatti S, Kerschbaumer G, Gay E, et al.: Technique for reduction and percutaneous fixation of U- and H-shaped sacral fractures, *Orthop Traumatol Surg Res* 99:625, 2013.

Ruiz Santiago F, Tomás Muñoz P, Moya Sánchez E, et al.: Classifying thoracolumbar fractures: role of quantitative imaging, *Quant Imaging Med Surg* 6(6):772, 2016.

Sadiqi S, Oner FC, Kim JS, Baird EO: What is the best treatment for a thoracolumbar burst fracture in a neurologically intact patient in the absence of posterior ligamentous disruption: surgical treatment, *Clin Spine Surg* 29(9):359, 2016.

Sanders D, Fox J, Starr A, et al.: Transsacral-transiliac screw stabilization: effective for recalcitrant pain due to sacral insufficiency fracture, *J Orthop Trauma* 30(9):e318, 2016.

Santoro G, Ramieri A, Chiarella V, et al.: Thoraco-lumbar fractures with blunt traumatic aortic injury in adult patients: correlations and management, *Eur Spine J* 27(Suppl 2):S248, 2018.

Scheer JK, Bakhsheshian J, Fakurnejad S, et al.: Evidence-based medicine of traumatic thoracolumbar burst fractures: a systematic review of operative management across 20 years, *Global Spine J* 5:73, 2015.

Schroeder GD, Kurd MF, Kepler CK, et al.: The development of a universally accepted sacral fracture classification: a survey of AOSpine and AOTrauma members, *Global Spine J* 6(7):686, 2016.

Shanmuganathan R, Maheswaran A, Aiyer SN, et al.: Prediction of posterior ligamentous complex injury in thoracolumbar fractures using non-MRI imaging techniques, *Int Orthop* 40:1075, 2016.

Shi J, Yue X, Niu N, et al.: Application of a modified thoracoabdominal approach that avoids cutting open the costal portion of diaghragm during anterior thoracolumbar spine surgery, *Eur Spine J* 26(7):1852, 2017.

Sixta S, Moore FO, Ditillo MF, et al.: Screening for thoracolumbar spinal injuries in blunt trauma: an Eastern Association for the Surgery of Trauma practice management guideline, *J Trauma Acute Care Surg* 73:S326, 2012.

Skaggs DL, Avramis I, Myung K, Weiss J: Sacral facet fractures in elite athletes, *Spine* 37:E514, 2012.

Smith WD, Ghazarian N, Christian G: Acute and hyper-acute thoracolumbar corpectomy for traumatic burst fractures using a mini-open lateral approach, *Spine* 43(2):E118, 2018.

Spiegl UJ, Devitt BM, Kasivskiy I, et al.: Comparison of combined posterior and anterior spondylodesis versus hybrid stabilization in unstable burst fractures at the thoracolumbar spine in patients between 60 and 70 years of age, *Arch Orthop Trauma Surg* 138(10):1407, 2018.

Splendiani A, Bruno F, Patriarca L, et al.: Thoracic spine trauma: advanced imaging modality, *Radiol Med* 121(10):2212, 2016.

Starantzis KA, Mirzashahi B, Behrbalk E, et al.: Open reduction and posterior instrumentation of type 3 high transverse sacral fracture-dislocation, *J Neurosurg Spine* 21:286, 2014.

Tian F, Tu LY, Gu Wf, et al.: Percutaneous versus open pedicle screw instrumentation in treatment of thoracic and lumbar spine fractures: A systematic review and meta-analysis, *Medicine (Baltimore)* 97(41):e12535, 2018.

Tian W, Chen WH, Jia J: Traumatic spino-pelvic dissociation with bilateral triangular fixation, *Orthop Surg* 10(3):205, 2018.

Trungu S, Forcato S, Bruzzaniti P, et al.: Minimally invasive surgery for the treatment of traumatic monosegmental thoracolumbar burst fractures: clinical and radiologic outcomes of 144 patients with a 6-year follow-up comparing two groups with or without intermediate screw, *Clin Spine Surg* 32(4):E171, 2019.

Unoki E, Miyakoshi N, Abe E, et al.: Sacropelvic fixation with S2 alar iliac screws may prevent sacroiliac joint pain after multi-segment spinal fusion, *Spine* 44(17):E1024, 2019.

Urquhart JC, Alrehaili OA, Fisher CG, et al.: Treatment of thoracolumbar burst fractures: extended follow-up of a randomized clinical trial comparing orthosis versus no orthosis, *J Neurosurg Spine* 27:42, 2017.

Urrutia J, Besa P, Piza C: Incidental identification of vertebral compression fractures in patients over 60 years old using computed tomography scans showing the entire thoraco-lumbar spine, *Arch Orthop Trauma Surg* 139(11):1497, 2019.

Vaccaro AR, Schroeder GD, Kepler CK, et al.: The surgical algorithm for the AOSpine thoracolumbar spine injury classification system, *Eur Spine J* 25:1087, 2016.

Vanek P, Bradac O, Konopkova R, et al.: Treatment of thoracolumbar trauma by short-segment percutaneous transpedicular screw instrumentation: prospective comparative study with a minimum 2-year follow-up, *J Neurosurg Spine* 20:150, 2014.

Varma R: Does an intraoperative finding of an intact dural sac help to prognosticate neurological recovery in cauda equinal and epiconal injuries in thoracolumbar fractures? An analysis of 31 patients, *Eur Spine J* 25(4):1117, 2016.

Vorlat P, Leirs G, Tajdar F, et al.: Predictors of recovery after conservative treatment of AO-type A thorocolumbar spine fractures without neurological deficit, *Spine* 43(2):141, 2018.

Walker JB, Mitchell SM, Karr SD, et al.: Percutaneous transiliac-transsacral screw fixation of sacral fragility fractures improves pain ambulation, and rate of disposition to home, *J Orthop Trauma* 32(9):452, 2018.

Walters JW, Kopelman TR, Patel AA, et al.: Closed therapy of thoracic and lumbar vertebral body fractures in trauma patients, *Surg Neurol Int* 8:283, 2017.

Wang W, Duan K, Ma M, et al.: Tranexamic acid decreases visible and hidden blood loss without affecting prethrombotic state molecular markers in transforaminal thoracic interbody fusion for treatment of thoracolumbar fracture-dislocation, *Spine* 43(13):E734, 2018.

Williams SK, Quinnan SM: Percutaneous lumbopelvic fixation for reduction and stabilization of sacral fractures with spinopelvic dissociation patterns, *J Orthop Trauma* 30(9):e318, 2016.

Xu JX, Zhou CW, Wang CG, et al.: Risk factors for dural tears in thoracic and lumbar burst fractures associated with vertical laminar fractures, *Spine* 43(11):774, 2018.

Yano S, Aoki Y, Watanabe A, et al.: Less invasive lumbopelvic fixation technique using a percutaneous pedicle screw system for unstable pelvic ring fracture in a patient with severe multiple traumas, *J Neurosurg Spine* 26(2):203, 2017.

Yoshihiro K, Osborn JM, Cason GW: The epidemiology of thoracolumbar trauma: A meta-analysis, *J Orthop* 13:383, 2016.

Yu YH, Lu ML, Tseng IC, et al.: Effect of the subcutaneous route for iliac screw insertion in lumbopelvic fixation for vertical unstable sacral fractures on the infection rate: a retrospective case series, *Injury* 47(10):2212, 2016.

Zhang C, Ouyang B, Li P, et al.: A retrospective study of thoracolumbar fractures treated with fixation and nonfusion surgery of intravertebral bone graft assisted with balloon kyphoplasty, *World Neurosurg* 108:798, 2017.

Zhang R, Yin Y, Li S, et al.: Sacroiliac screw versus a minimally invasive adjustable plate for zone II sacral fractures: a retrospective study, *Injury* 50(3):690, 2019.

Zhang W, Li H, Zhou Y, et al.: Minimally invasive posterior decompression combined with percutaneous pedicle screw fixation for the treatment of thoracolumbar fractures with neurological deficits: a prospective randomized study versus traditional open posterior surgery, *Spine* 41(Suppl 19):B23, 2016.

Zhao Q, Zhang H, Hao D, et al.: Complications of percutaneous pedicle screw fixation in treating thoracolumbar and lumbar fracture, *Medicine (Baltimore)* 97(29):e11560, 2018.

The complete list of references is available online at Expert Consult.com.

SUPPLEMENTAL REFERENCES

GENERAL

American Spinal Injury Association (ASIA): www.asia-spinalinjury.org/publications/index.html. 2006.

Amling M, Posl M, Wening VJ, et al.: Structural heterogeneity within the axis—the main cause in the etiology of dens fractures: a histomorphometric analysis of 37 normal and osteoporotic autopsy cases, *J Neurosurg* 83:330, 1995.

Anderson PA: Nonsurgical treatment of patients with thoracolumbar fractures, *Instr Course Lect* 44:57, 1995.

Anderson PA, Bohlman HH: Anterior decompression and arthrodesis of the cervical spine: long-term motor improvement (two parts), *J Bone Joint Surg* 74A:671, 1992.

Apple DF, Anson C: Spinal cord injury occurring in patients with ankylosing spondylitis: a multicenter study, *Orthopedics* 18:1005, 1995.

Beard VV, Hochschuler SH: Reflex sympathetic dystrophy following spinal surgery, *Semin Spine Surg* 5:153, 1993.

Beaty JH, editor: *Orthopaedic knowledge update, home study syllabus 6*, Rosemont, IL, 1999, American Academy of Orthopaedic Surgeons.

Bhandari M, Tornetta P: Issues in the design, analysis, and critical appraisal of orthopaedic clinical research, *Clin Orthop Relat Res* 413:9, 2003.

Bohlman HH: Pathology and current treatment concepts of acute spine injuries, *Instr Course Lect* 21:108, 1972.

Bosch A, Stauffer ES, Nickel VL: Incomplete traumatic quadriplegia: a ten-year review, *JAMA* 216:473, 1971.

Botte MJ, Byrne TP, Abrams RA, et al.: Halo skeletal fixation: techniques of application and prevention of complications, *J Am Acad Orthop Surg* 4:44, 1996.

Bracken MB: Methylprednisolone and acute spinal cord injury: an update of the randomized evidence, *Spine* 26(Suppl 24):S47, 2001.

Bracken MB, Holford TR: Effects of timing of methylprednisolone or naloxone administration on recovery of segmented and long-tract neurological function in NACSI II, *J Neurosurg* 79:500, 1993.

Bracken MB, Shepard MJ, Collins WF, et al.: A randomized controlled trial of methylprednisolone or naloxone in the treatment of acute spinal cord injury: results of the second National Acute Spinal Cord Injury Study, *N Engl J Med* 322:1405, 1990.

Brightman RP, Miller CA, Rea GL, et al.: Magnetic resonance imaging of trauma to the thoracic and lumbar spine: the importance of the posterior longitudinal ligament, *Spine* 17:541, 1992.

Brown MD, Eismont FJ, Quencer RM: Symposium: intraoperative ultrasonography in spinal surgery, *Contemp Orthop* 11:47, 1985.

Chow YW, Inman C, Pollintine P, et al.: Ultrasound bone densitometry and dual energy x-ray absorptiometry in patients with spinal cord injury: a cross-sectional study, *Spinal Cord* 34:736, 1996.

Clark WK: Spinal cord decompression in spinal cord injury, *Clin Orthop Relat Res* 154:9, 1981.

Cody DD, Goldstein SA, Flynn MJ, et al.: Correlations between vertebral regional bone mineral density (rBMD) and whole bone fracture load, *Spine* 16:146, 1991.

Coleman WP, Benzel D, Cahill DW, et al.: A critical appraisal of the reporting of the National Acute Spinal Cord Injury Studies (II and III) of methylprednisolone in acute spinal cord injury, *J Spinal Disord* 13:165, 2000.

Colterjohn NR, Bednar DA: Identifiable risk factors for secondary neurologic deterioration in the cervical spine–injured patient, *Spine* 20:2293, 1995.

Connolly P, Yuan HA: Cervical spine fractures. In White AH, editor: *Spine care: diagnosis and conservative treatment*, St. Louis, 1995, Mosby.

Cooper C, Atkinson EJ, Fallon WM, et al.: Incidence of clinically diagnosed vertebral fractures: a population-based study in Rochester, Minnesota, 1985-1989, *J Bone Miner Res* 7:221, 1992.

Cotler JM, Herbison GJ, Nasti JF, et al.: Closed reduction of traumatic cervical spine dislocation using traction weights up to 140 pounds, *Spine* 18:386, 1983.

Coyne TJ, Fehlings MG, Wallace MC, et al.: C1-C2 posterior cervical fusion: long-term evaluation of results and efficacy, *Neurosurgery* 37:688, 1995.

Croce MA, Bee TK, Pritchard E, et al.: Does optimal timing for spine fracture fixation exist? *Ann Surg* 233:851, 2001.

Crowther ER: Missed cervical spine fractures: the importance of reviewing radiographs in chiropractic practice, *J Manipulative Physiol Ther* 18:29, 1995.

Danisa OA, Shaffrey CI, Jane JA, et al.: Surgical approaches for the correction of unstable thoracolumbar burst fractures: a retrospective analysis of treatment outcomes, *J Neurosurg* 83:977, 1995.

Delamarter RB, Sherman J, Carr JB: *Spinal cord injury: the pathophysiology of spinal cord damage and subsequent recovery following immediate or delayed decompression*, New York, 1993, Paper presented at Cervical Spine Research Society meeting.

De La Torre JC: Spinal cord injury: review of basic and applied research, *Spine* 6:315, 1981.

Denis F: Spinal instability as defined by the three-column spine concept in acute spinal trauma, *Clin Orthop Relat Res* 189:65, 1984.

Devilee R, Sanders R, deLange S: Treatment of fractures and dislocations of the thoracic and lumbar spine by fusion and Harrington instrumentation, *Arch Orthop Trauma Surg* 114:100, 1995.

Dickman CA, Zabramski JM, Hadley MN, et al.: Pediatric spinal cord injury without radiographic abnormalities: report of 26 cases and review of the literature, *J Spinal Disord* 4:296, 1991.

Dorr LD, Harvey JP, Nickel VL: Clinical review of the early stability of spine injuries, *Spine* 7:545, 1982.

Ebraheim NA, Rupp RE, Savolaine ER, et al.: Posterior plating of the cervical spine, *J Spinal Disord* 8:111, 1995.

Eismont FJ, Arena M, Green B: Extrusion of an intervertebral disc associated with traumatic subluxation or dislocation of cervical facets, *J Bone Joint Surg* 73A:1555, 1991.

Eismont FJ, Clifford S, Goldberg M, et al.: Cervical sagittal spinal canal size in spine injury, *Spine* 9:663, 1984.

Emery SE, Patheia MN, Wilber RG, et al.: Magnetic resonance imaging of posttraumatic spinal ligament injury, *J Spinal Disord Tech* 2:229, 1989.

Fan RS, Schenk RS, Lee CK: Burst fracture of the fifth lumbar vertebra in combination with a pelvic ring injury, *J Orthop Trauma* 9:345, 1995.

Fisher CG, Noonan VK, Smith DE, et al.: Motor recovery, functional status, and health-related quality of life in patients with complete spinal cord injuries, *Spine* 30:220, 2005.

WPJ Fontijne, DeKlerk LWL, Braakman R, et al.: CT scan prediction of neurological deficit in thoracolumbar burst fractures, *J Bone Joint Surg* 74B:683, 1992.

Fowler BL, Dall BE, Rowe DE: Complications associated with harvesting autogenous iliac bone graft, *Am J Orthop* 24:895, 1995.

Fricker R, Gächter A: Lateral flexion/extension radiographs: still recommended following cervical spinal injury, *Arch Orthop Trauma Surg* 113:115, 1994.

Garfin SR, editor: *Complications of spine surgery*, Baltimore, 1989, Williams & Wilkins.

Geisler FH, Dorsey FC, Coleman WP: Recovery of motor function after spinal cord injury: a randomized, placebo-controlled trial with GM-1 ganglioside, *N Engl J Med* 324:1829, 1991.

Geisler FH, Dorsey FC, Coleman WP: GM-1 ganglioside in human spinal cord injury, *J Neurotrauma* 9(Suppl):517, 1992.

Gertzbein SD, Court-Brown CM, Marks P, et al.: The neurological outcome following surgery for spinal fractures, *Spine* 13:641, 1988.

Gold DT: The clinical impact of vertebral fractures: quality of life in women with osteoporosis, *Bone* 18(Suppl 3):185, 1996.

Grabb PA, Pang D: Magnetic resonance imaging in the evaluation of spinal cord injury without radiographic abnormality in children, *Neurosurgery* 35:406, 1994.

Grauer JN, Vaccaro AR, Beinder JM, et al.: Similarities and differences in the treatment of spine trauma between surgical specialties and location of practice, *Spine* 29:685, 2004.

Green BA, Callahan RA, Klore KJ, et al.: Acute spinal cord injury: current concepts, *Clin Orthop Relat Res* 154:125, 1981.

Harris MB, Sethi RK: The initial assessment and management of the multiple-trauma patient with an associated spine injury, *Spine* 31:59, 2006.

Heller JG, Silcox DH, Sutterlin CE: Complications of posterior cervical plating, *Spine* 20:2442, 1995.

Hildingsson C, Hietala SO, Toolanen G, et al.: Negative scintigraphy despite spinal fractures in the multiply injured, *Injury* 24:467, 1993.

Holdsworth FW: Traumatic paraplegia. In Platt H, editor: *Modern trends in orthopaedics (second series)*, New York, 1956, Paul B Hoeber.

Holdsworth FW: Fractures, dislocations, and fracture-dislocations of the spine, *J Bone Joint Surg* 45B:6, 1963.

Holdsworth FW: Fractures, dislocations, and fracture-dislocations of the spine, *J Bone Joint Surg* 52A:1534, 1970.

Holdsworth SF: Review article: fractures, dislocations, and fracture-dislocations of the spine, *J Bone Joint Surg* 52B:1534, 1970.

Hopkins TJ, White AA: Rehabilitation of athletes following spine injury, *Clin Sports Med* 12:603, 1993.

Huang TJ, Hsu RWW, Fan GF, et al.: Two-level burst fractures: clinical evaluation and treatment options, *J Trauma* 41:77, 1996.

Hurlbert RJ: The role of steroids in acute spinal cord injury: an evidence-based analysis, *Spine* 26(24 Suppl):S39, 2001.

Jelsma RK, Rice JF, Jelsma LF, et al.: The demonstration and significance of neural compression after spinal injury, *Surg Neurol* 18:79, 1982.

Kado DM, Browner WS, Palermo L, et al.: Vertebral fractures and mortality in older women: a prospective study: study of osteoporotic fractures research group, *Arch Intern Med* 159:1215, 1999.

Kahnovitz N, Bullough P, Jacobs RR: The effect of internal fixation without arthrodesis on human facet joint cartilage, *Clin Orthop Relat Res* 189:204, 1984.

Kallmes DF, Comstock BA, Heagerty PJ, et al.: A randomized trial of vertebroplasty for osteoporotic spinal fractures, *N Engl J Med* 361:569, 2009.

Karasick D, Huettl EA, Cotler JM: Value of polydirectional tomography in the assessment of the postoperative spine after anterior decompression and vertebral body autografting, *Skeletal Radiol* 21:359, 1992.

Kerwin AJ, Riffen MM, Tepas JJ, et al.: Best practice determination of timing of spinal fracture fixation as defined by analysis of the National Trauma Data Bank, *J Trauma* 65:824, 2008.

Kirkpatrick JS, Wilber RG, Likavec M, et al.: Anterior stabilization of thoracolumbar burst fractures using the Kaneda device: a preliminary report, *Orthopedics* 18:673, 1995.

Kraus JF, Franti CE, Riggins RS, et al.: Incidence of traumatic spinal cord lesions, *J Chronic Dis* 28:471, 1975.

Kreitz BG, Cote P, Cassidy JD: L5 vertebral compression fracture: a series of five cases, *J Manipulative Physiol Ther* 18:91, 1995.

Laborde JM, Bahniuk E, Bohlman HH, et al.: Comparison of fixation of spinal fractures, *Clin Orthop Relat Res* 152:303, 1980.

Leroux JL, Denat B, Thomas E, et al.: Sacral insufficiency fractures presenting as acute low-back pain: biomechanical aspects, *Spine* 18:2502, 1993.

Levi AD, Hurlbert J, Anderson P, et al.: Neurologic deterioration secondary to unrecognized spinal instability following trauma—a multicenter study, *Spine* 31:451, 2006.

Levine AM, McAfee PC, Anderson PA: Evaluation and emergent treatment of patients with thoracolumbar trauma, *Instr Course Lect* 44:33, 1995.

Lyles KW, Gold DT, Shipp KM, et al.: Association of osteoporotic vertebral compression fractures with impaired functional status, *Am J Med* 94:595, 1993.

Mann DC, Dodds JA: Spinal injuries in 57 patients 17 years or younger, *Orthopedics* 16:159, 1993.

Markel DC, Graziano G: A comparison study of treatment of thoracolumbar fractures using the ACE Posterior Segmental Fixator and Cotrel-Dubousset instrumentation, *Orthopedics* 18:679, 1995.

Markel DC, Raskas DS, Graziano GP: A case of traumatic spino-pelvic dissociation, *J Orthop Trauma* 7:562, 1993.

Matsumoto T, Tamaki T, Kawakami M, et al.: Early complications of high-dose methylprednisolone sodium succinate treatment in the follow-up of acute cervical spinal cord injury, *Spine* 26:426, 2001.

McCormack T, Karaikovic E, Gaines RW: The load sharing classification of spine fractures, *Spine* 19:1741, 1994.

McCutcheon EP, Selassie AW, Gu JK, Pickelsimer EE: Acute traumatic spinal cord injury, 1993-2000: a population-based assessment of methylprednisolone administration and hospitalization, *J Trauma* 56:1076, 2004.

McDonnell MF, Glassman SD, Dimar JR, et al.: Perioperative complications of anterior procedures on the spine, *J Bone Joint Surg* 78A:839, 1996.

McLain RF, Benson DR: Urgent surgical stabilization of spinal fractures in polytrauma patients, *Spine* 24:1646, 1999.

McPhee IB: Spinal fractures and dislocations in children and adolescents, *Spine* 6:533, 1981.

Merola A, O'Brien MF, Castro BA, et al.: Histologic characterization of acute spinal cord injury treated with intravenous methylprednisolone, *J Orthop Trauma* 16:155, 2002.

Meyer Jr PR: Emergency room assessment: management of spinal cord and associated injuries. In Meyer Jr PR, editor: *Surgery of spine trauma*, New York, 1989, Churchill Livingstone.

Modic MT, Masaryk T, Paushter D: Magnetic resonance imaging of the spine, *Radiol Clin North Am* 24:229, 1986.

Molina DK, Nichols JJ, Dimalo VJ: The sensitivity of computed tomography (CT) scans in detecting trauma: are CT scans reliable enough for courtroom testimony? *J Trauma* 63:625, 2007.

Montgomery TJ, McGuire Jr RA: Traumatic neuropathic arthropathy of the spine, *Orthop Rev* 22:1153, 1993.

Nagel DA, Edwards WT, Schneider E: Biomechanics of spinal fixation and fusion, *Spine* 16(Suppl):151, 1991.

Oleson CV, Burns AS, Ditunno JF, et al.: Prognostic value of pinprick preservation in motor complete, sensory incomplete spinal cord injury, *Arch Phys Med Rehabil* 86:988, 2005.

Pang D, Pollack IF: Spinal cord injury without radiographic abnormality in children—the SCIWORA syndrome, *J Trauma* 29:654, 1989.

Panjabi MM, Oxland T, Takata K, et al.: Articular facets of the human spine: quantitative three-dimensional anatomy, *Spine* 18:1298, 1993.

Pascal-Moussellard H, Klein JR, Schwab FJ, et al.: Simultaneous anterior and posterior approaches to the spine for revision surgery: current indications and techniques, *J Spinal Disord* 12:206, 1999.

Ploumis A, Ponnappan RK, Bessey JT, et al.: Thromboprophylaxis in spinal trauma surgery: consensus among spine trauma surgeons, *Spine J* 9:530, 2009.

Pollard ME, Apple DF: Factors associated with improved neurologic outcomes in patients with incomplete tetraplegia, *Spine* 28:33, 2003.

Potter PJ, Hayes KC, Hsieh JT, et al.: Sustained improvements in neurological function in spinal cord injured patients treated with oral 4-aminopyridine: three cases, *Spinal Cord* 36:147, 1998.

Poynton AR, O'Farrell DA, Shannon F, et al.: An evaluation of the factors affecting neurological recovery following spinal cord injury, *Injury* 28:545, 1997.

Quencer RM: Intraoperative ultrasound of the spine, *Surg Rounds* 10:17, 1987.

Rechtine GR: Nonoperative management and treatment of spinal injuries, *Spine* 31:S22, 2006.

Riggs BL, Melton III LJ: The worldwide problem of osteoporosis: insights afforded by epidemiology, *Bone* 17:505S, 1995.

Rosenberg N, Lenger R, Weisz I, et al.: Neurological deficit in a consecutive series of vertebral fracture patients with bony fragments within spinal canal, *Spinal Cord* 35:92, 1997.

Rupp RE, Ebraheim NA, Coombs RJ: Magnetic resonance imaging differentiating of compression spine fractures or vertebral lesions caused by osteoporosis or tumor, *Spine* 20:2499, 1995.

Saboe LA, Reid DC, Davic LA, et al.: Spine trauma and associated injuries, *J Trauma* 31:43, 1991.

Sapkas G, Korres D, Babis GC, et al.: Correlation of spinal canal post-traumatic encroachment and neurological deficit in burst fractures of the lower cervical spine (C3-7), *Eur Spine J* 4:39, 1995.

Savolaine ER, Ebraheim NA, Rusin JJ, et al.: Limitations of radiography and computed tomography in the diagnosis of transverse sacral fracture from a high fall, *Clin Orthop Relat Res* 272:122, 1991.

Schlaich C, Minne HW, Bruckner T, et al.: Reduced pulmonary function in patients with spinal osteoporotic fractures, *Osteoporos Int* 8:261, 1998.

Schlegel J, Bayley J, Yuan H, et al.: Timing of surgical decompression and fixation of acute spinal fractures, *J Orthop Trauma* 10:323, 1996.

Schneider RC, Kahn EA: Chronic neurologic sequelae of acute trauma to the spine and spinal cord, part II: the syndrome of chronic anterior spinal cord injury or compression, *J Bone Joint Surg* 41A:449, 1959.

Slucky AV, Eismont FJ: Treatment of acute injury of the cervical spine, *J Bone Joint Surg* 76A:1994, 1882.

Smith MD, Johnson LJ, Perra JH, et al.: A biomechanical study of torque and accuracy of halo pin insertional devices, *J Bone Joint Surg* 78A:231, 1996.

Sobel JW, Bohlman HH, Freehafer AA: Charcot's arthropathy of the spine following spinal cord injury: a report of five cases, *J Bone Joint Surg* 67A:771, 1985.

Southwick WO: Management of fractures of the dens (odontoid process), *J Bone Joint Surg* 62A:482, 1980.

Stambough JL, Lazio BE: Unusual L5 fracture with neurologic involvement, *Orthopedics* 18:1034, 1995.

Stauffer ES, Wood RW, Kelly EG: Gunshot wounds of the spine: the effects of laminectomy, *J Bone Joint Surg* 61A:389, 1979.

Tator CH, Fehlings MG, Thorpe K, et al.: Current use and timing of spinal surgery for management of acute spinal cord injury in North America: results of a retrospective multi-center study, *J Neurosurg* 91:12, 1999.

Tewari MK, Gifti DS, Singh P, et al.: Diagnosis and prognostication of adult spinal cord injury without radiographic abnormality using magnetic resonance imaging: analysis of 40 patients, *Surg Neurol* 63:204, 2005.

Torg JS, Currier B, Douglas R, et al.: Symposium: spinal cord resuscitation, *Contemp Orthop* 30:495, 1995.

Turgut M, Akpinar G, Akalan N, et al.: Spinal injuries in the pediatric age group: a review of 82 cases of spinal cord and vertebral column injuries, *Eur Spine J* 5:148, 1996.

Vaccaro AR, Falatyn SP, Flanders AE, et al.: Magnetic resonance evaluation of the intervertebral disc, spinal ligaments, and spinal cord before and after closed traction reduction of cervical spine dislocations, *Spine* 24:1210, 1999.

Vornanen MJ, Bostman OM, Myllynen PJ: Reduction of bone retropulsed into the spinal canal in thoracolumbar vertebral body compression burst fractures: a prospective randomized comparative study between Harrington rods and two transpedicular devices, *Spine* 20:1699, 1995.

Wilmink JT: MR imaging of the spine: trauma and degenerative disease, *Eur Radiol* 9:1259, 1999.

Wright JG, Swiontkowski MF, Heckman JD: Introducing levels of evidence to the journal, *J Bone Joint Surg* 85A:1, 2003.

Wupperman R, Davis R, Obremskey WT: Level of evidence in spine compared to other orthopedic journals, *Spine* 32:388, 2007.

Xu R, Haman SP, Ebraheim NA, et al.: The anatomic relation of lateral mass screws to the spinal nerves: a comparison of the Magerl, Anderson, and an techniques, *Spine* 24:2057, 1999.

Zdeblick TA: Complications of anterior spinal instrumentation, *Semin Spine Surg* 5:101, 1993.

CERVICAL SPINE

Aarabi B, Koltz M, Ibrahimi D: Hyperextension cervical spine injuries and traumatic central cord syndrome, *Neurosurg Focus* 25:E9, 2008.

Abumi K, Ito M, Taneichi H, Kaneda K: Transpedicular screw fixation for traumatic lesions of the middle and lower cervical spine: description of the techniques and preliminary report, *J Spinal Disord* 7:19, 1994.

Abumi K, Kaneda K: Pedicle screw fixation for nontraumatic lesions of the cervical spine, *Spine* 22:1853, 1997.

Aebi M, Zuber K, Marchesi D: Treatment of cervical spine injuries with anterior plating: indications, techniques, and results, *Spine* 16(Suppl 3):38, 1991.

Allen Jr BL, Ferguson RL, Lehmann R, et al.: Mechanistic classification of closed indirect fractures and dislocations of the lower cervical spine, *Spine* 7:1, 1982.

Amies CP, Acosta F, Nottmeier E: Novel treatment of basilar invagination resulting from an untreated C-1 fracture associated with transverse ligament avulsion: case report and description of surgical technique, *J Neurosurg Spine* 2:83, 2005.

An HS: Internal fixation of the cervical spine: current indications and techniques, *J Am Acad Orthop Surg* 3:194, 1995.

An HS, Gordin R, Renner K: Anatomic considerations for plate-screw fixation of the cervical spine, *Spine* 16:S538, 1991.

Anderson LD, D'Alonzo RT: Fractures of the odontoid process of the axis, *J Bone Joint Surg* 56A:1663, 1974.

Anderson PA, Bohlman HH: Anterior decompression and arthrodesis of the cervical spine: long-term motor improvement, *J Bone Joint Surg* 74A:683, 1992.

Anderson PA, Budorick TE, Easton KB, et al.: Failure of halo vest to prevent in vivo motion in patients with injured cervical spines, *Spine* 16(Suppl 10):S501, 1991.

Anderson PA, Grady MS: Posterior stabilization of the lower cervical spine with lateral mass plates and screws, *Op Tech Orthop* 6:58, 1996.

Anderson PA, Henley MB, Grady MS, et al.: Posterior cervical arthrodesis with AO reconstruction plates and bone grafts, *Spine* 16(Suppl 3):S72, 1991.

Anderson PA, Montesano PX: Morphology and treatment of occipital condyle fractures, *Spine* 13:731, 1988.

Anderson PA, Moore TA, Davis KW, et al.: Cervical spine injury severity score, *J Bone Joint Surg* 89A:1057, 2007.

Aprin H, Harf R: Stabilization of atlantoaxial instability, *Orthopedics* 11:1687, 1988.

Arena MJ, Eismont FJ, Green BA: Intervertebral disc extrusion associated with cervical facet subluxation and dislocation. Paper presented at the Fifteenth Annual Meeting of the Cervical Spine Research Society, Washington, DC, December 2-5, 1987.

Arnold PM, Bryniarski M, McMahon JK: Posterior stabilization of subaxial cervical spine trauma: indications and techniques, *Injury* 36:S-B36, 2005.

Aryan HE, Newman B, Nottmeier EW, et al.: Stabilization of the atlantoaxial complex via C-1 lateral mass and C-2 pedicle screw fixation in a multicenter clinical experience of 102 patients: modification of the Harms and Goel techniques, *J Neurosurg Spine* 8:222, 2008.

Aulino JM, Tutt LK, Kaye JJ, et al.: Occipital condyle fractures: clinical presentation and imaging findings in 76 patients, *Emerg Radiol* 11:342, 2005.

Bailitz J, Starr F, Beecroft M, et al.: CT should replace three-view radiographs as the initial screening test in patients at high, moderate, and low risk for blunt cervical spine injury: a prospective comparison, *J Trauma* 66:1605, 2009.

Ballock RT, Botte MJ, Garfin SR: Complications of halo immobilization. In Garfin SR, editor: *Complications of spine surgery*, Baltimore, 1989, Williams & Wilkins.

Beatson TR: Fractures and dislocations of the cervical spine, *J Bone Joint Surg* 45B:21, 1963.

Bellabarba C, Mirza SK, West A, et al.: Diagnosis and treatment of craniocervical dislocation in a series of 17 consecutive survivors during an 8-year period, *J Neurosurg Spine* 4:429, 2006.

Benzel EC, Hart BL, Ball PA, et al.: Magnetic resonance imaging for the evaluation of patients with occult cervical spine injury, *J Neurosurg* 85:824, 1996.

Beyer CA, Cabanela ME: Unilateral facet dislocations and fracture-dislocations of the cervical spine: a review, *Orthopedics* 15:311, 1992.

Beyer CA, Cabanela ME, Berquist TH: Unilateral facet dislocations and fracture-dislocations of the cervical spine, *J Bone Joint Surg* 73B:977, 1991.

Biffl WL, Ray Jr CE, Moore EE, et al.: Noninvasive diagnosis of blunt cerebrovascular injuries: a preliminary report, *J Trauma* 53:850, 2002.

Blackmore CC, Mann FA, Wilson AJ: Helical CT in the primary trauma evaluation of the cervical spine: an evidence-based approach, *Skeletal Radiol* 29:632, 2000.

Blacksin MF, Lee HJ: Frequency and significance of fractures of the upper cervical spine detected by CT in patients with severe neck trauma, *AJR Am J Roentgenol* 165:1201, 1995.

Bliuc D, Nguyen ND, Milch VE, et al.: Mortality risk associated with low-trauma osteoporotic fracture and subsequent fracture in men and women, *JAMA* 301:513, 2009.

Bloom AI, Neeman Z, Slasky BS, et al.: Fracture of the occipital condyles and associated craniocervical ligament injury: incidence, CT imaging and implications, *Clin Radiol* 52:198, 1997.

Bohlman HH: Pathology and current treatment concepts of cervical spine injuries, *Instr Course Lect* 21:108, 1972.

Bohlman HH: The pathology and current treatment concepts of cervical spine injuries: a critical review of 300 cases, *J Bone Joint Surg* 54A:1353, 1972.

Bohlman HH: Complications of treatment of fractures and dislocations of the cervical spine. In Epps CH, editor: *Complications in orthopaedic surgery*, Philadelphia, 1978, Lippincott.

Bohlman HH: Acute fractures and dislocations of the cervical spine, *J Bone Joint Surg* 61A:1119, 1979.

Bohlman HH: Complications and pitfalls in the treatment of acute cervical spinal cord injuries. In Tator CH, editor: *Early management of acute spinal cord injury*, New York, 1982, Raven.

Bohlman HH: Indications for late anterior decompression and fusion for cervical spinal cord injuries. In Tator CH, editor: *Early management of acute spinal cord injury*, New York, 1982, Raven.

Bohlman HH: Surgical management of cervical spine fractures and dislocations, *Instr Course Lect* 34:163, 1985.

Bohlman HH, Anderson PA: Anterior decompression and arthrodesis of the cervical spine: long-term motor improvement, *J Bone Joint Surg* 74A:671, 1992.

Bohlman HH, Bahniuk E, Gield G, et al.: Spinal cord monitoring of experimental incomplete cervical spinal cord injury, *Spine* 6:428, 1981.

Bohlman HH, Bahniuk E, Raskulinecz G, et al.: Mechanical factors affecting recovery from incomplete cervical spine injury: a preliminary report, *Johns Hopkins Med J* 145:115, 1979.

Bohlman HH, Eismont FJ: Surgical techniques of anterior decompression and fusion for spinal cord injuries, *Clin Orthop Relat Res* 154:57, 1981.

Bono CM, Vaccaro AR, Fehlings M, et al.: Measurement techniques for lower cervical spine injuries. Consensus statement of the Spine Trauma Study Group, *Spine* 31:603, 2006.

Bono CM, Vaccaro AR, Fehlings M, et al.: Measurement techniques for upper cervical spine injuries, *Spine* 32:593, 2007.

Borne GM, Bedou GL, Pinaudeau M: Treatment of pedicular fractures of the axis: a clinical study and screw fixation technique, *J Neurosurg* 60:88, 1984.

Bosch A, Stauffer ES, Nickel VL: Incomplete traumatic quadriplegia: a ten-year review, *JAMA* 216:473, 1967.

Bozbuga M, Ozturk A, Ari Z, et al.: Morphometric evaluation of subaxial cervical vertebrae for surgical application of transpedicular screw fixation, *Spine* 29:1876, 2004.

Bozkus H, Ames CP, Chamberlain RH, et al.: Biomechanical analysis of rigid stabilization techniques for three-column injury in the lower cervical spine, *Spine* 30:915, 2005.

Bransford R, Falicov A, Nguyen Q, Chapman J: Unilateral C-1 lateral mass sagittal split fracture: an unstable Jefferson fracture variant, *J Neurosurg Spine* 10:466, 2009.

Bransford RJ, Stevens DW, Uyeji S, et al.: Halo vest treatment of cervical spine injuries: a success and survivorship analysis, *Spine* 34:1561, 2009.

Bridwell KH, DeWald RL: *Textbook of spinal surgery* (vol 2), New York, 1991, Lippincott-Raven1991.

Brooke DS, Anderson PA, Newell DW, et al.: Compression of anterior and posterior approaches in cervical spinal cord injuries, *J Spinal Disord Tech* 16:229, 2003.

Brooks AL, Jenkins EB: Atlanto-axial arthrodesis by the wedge compression method, *J Bone Joint Surg* 60A:279, 1978.

Brown CV, Antevil J, Sise MJ, et al.: Spiral computed tomography for the diagnosis of cervical, thoracic, and lumbar spine fractures: its time has come, *J Trauma* 58:890, 2005.

Budorick TE, Anderson PA, Rivara FP, et al.: Flexion-distraction fracture of the cervical spine, *J Bone Joint Surg* 73A:1097, 1991.

Campanelli M, Kattner KA, Stroink A, et al.: Posterior C1-C2 transarticular screw fixation in the treatment of displaced type II odontoid fractures in the geriatric population—review of seven cases, *Surg Neurol* 51:596, 1999.

Capen D, Zigler J, Garland D: Surgical stabilization in cervical spine trauma, *Contemp Orthop* 14:25, 1987.

Capen DA, Nelson RW, Zigler JE, et al.: Decompressive laminectomy in cervical spine trauma: a review of early and late complications, *Contemp Orthop* 17:21, 1988.

Carroll C, McAfee PC, Riley Jr LH: Objective findings for diagnosis of "whiplash", *J Musculoskel Med* 3:57, 1986.

Carter DR, Frankel VH: Biomechanics of hyperextension injuries to the cervical spine in football, *Am J Sports Med* 8:302, 1982.

Caspar W: Advances in cervical spine surgery: first experiences with trapezial osteosynthetic plate and new surgical instrumentation for anterior interbody stabilization, *Orthop News* 4:1, 1982.

Castillo M, Mukherji SK: Vertical fractures of the dens, *AJNR Am J Neuroradiol* 17:1627, 1996.

Chen IH, Yang RS, Chen PQ: Plate fixation for anterior cervical interbody fusion, *J Formosa Med Assoc* 90:172, 1991.

Chen JY, Chen WJ, Huang TJ, et al.: Spinal epidural abscess complicating cervical spine fracture with hypopharyngeal perforation, *Spine* 17:971, 1992.

Chin KR, Auerbach JD, Adams SB, et al.: Mastication causing segmental spinal motion in common cervical orthoses, *Spine* 31:430, 2006.

Ching RP, Watson NA, Carter JW, et al.: The effect of post-injury spinal position on canal occlusion in a cervical spine burst fracture model, *Spine* 22:1710, 1997.

Chittiboina P, Wylen E, Ogden A, et al.: Traumatic spondylolisthesis of the axis: a biomechanical comparison of clinically relevant anterior and posterior fusion techniques, *J Neurosurg Spine* 11:379, 2009.

Chiu CW, Haan JM, Cushing BM, et al.: Ligamentous injuries of the cervical spine in unreliable blunt trauma patients: incidence, evaluation, and outcome, *J Trauma* 50:457, 2001.

Choi WG, Vishteh AG, Baskin JJ, et al.: Completely dislocated hangman's fracture with a locked C2-3 facet: case report, *J Neurosurg* 87:757, 1997.

Choueka J, Spivak JM, Kummer FJ, et al.: Flexion failure of posterior cervical lateral mass screws: influence of insertion technique and position, *Spine* 21:462, 1996.

Citron SJ, Wallace RC, Lewis CA, et al.: Quality improvement guidelines for adult diagnostic neuroangiography: cooperative study between ASITN, ASNR, and SIR, *J Vasc Interv Radiol* 14:S257, 2003.

Clark CR: Dens fractures, *Semin Spine Surg* 3:39, 1991.

Clark CR, White AA: Fractures of the dens: a multicenter study, *J Bone Joint Surg* 67A:1340, 1985.

Clark CR, Whitehill R: Two views of the use of methylmethacrylate for stabilization of the cervical spine, *Orthopedics* 12:589, 1989.

Clausen JD, Ryken TC, Traynelis VC, et al.: Biomechanical evaluation of Caspar and cervical spine locking plate systems in a cadaver model, *J Neurosurg* 84:1039, 1996.

Como JJ, Diaz JJ, Dunham M, et al.: Practice management guidelines for identification of cervical spine injuries following trauma: update from the Eastern Association for Surgery of Trauma Practice management Guidelines Committee, *J Trauma* 67:651, 2009.

Cooper PR, Cohen A, Rosiello A, et al.: Posterior stabilization of cervical spine fractures and subluxation using plates and screws, *Neurosurgery* 23:300, 1988.

Coric D, Branch Jr CL, Wilson JA, et al.: Arteriovenous fistula as a complication of C1-2 transarticular screw fixation: case report and review of the literature, *J Neurosurg* 85:340, 1996.

Coric D, Wilson JA, Kelly Jr DL: Treatment of traumatic spondylolisthesis of the axis with nonrigid immobilization: a review of 64 cases, *J Neurosurg* 85:550, 1996.

Cothren CC, Moore EE, Biffl WL, et al.: Cervical spine fracture patterns predictive of blunt vertebral artery injury, *J Trauma* 55:811, 2003.

Coyne TJ, Fehlings MG, Wallace MC, et al.: C1-C2 posterior cervical fusion: long-term evaluation of results and efficacy, *Neurosurgery* 37:688, 1995.

Crenshaw Jr AH, Wood GW, Wood Jr MW, et al.: Fracture and dislocation of the fourth and fifth cervical vertebral bodies with transection of the spinal cord, *Clin Orthop Relat Res* 248:158, 1989.

Crisco JJ, Panjabi MM, Oda T, et al.: Bone graft translation of four upper cervical spine fixation techniques in a cadaver model, *J Orthop Res* 9:835, 1991.

Cusick JF, Yoganandan N, Pintar F, et al.: Cervical spine injuries from high-velocity forces: a pathoanatomic and radiologic study, *J Spinal Disord* 9(1), 1996.

Daentzer D, Flörkemeier T: Conservative treatment of upper cervical spine injuries with the halo vest: an appropriate option for all patients independent of their age? *J Neurosurg Spine* 10:543, 2009.

Daffner RH, Hackney DB, Dalinka MK, et al.: *Suspected spine trauma*, Reston, VA, 2007, American College of Radiology.

Daniels AH, Arthur M, Hart RA: Variability in rates of arthrodesis procedures for patients with cervical spine injuries with and without associated spinal cord injury, *J Bone Joint Surg* 89A:317, 2007.

Davis D, Bohlman H, Walker E, et al.: The pathological findings in fatal craniospinal injuries, *J Neurol* 34:603, 1971.

Davis J: Injuries to the subaxial cervical spine: posterior approach options, *Orthopedics* 20:929, 1997.

Davis JW, Kaups KL, Cunningham MA, et al.: Routine evaluation of the cervical spine in head-injured patients with dynamic fluoroscopy: a reappraisal, *J Trauma* 50:1044, 2001.

Davis JW, Parks SN, Detlefs CL, et al.: Clearing the cervical spine in obtunded patients: the use of dynamic fluoroscopy, *J Trauma* 39:435, 1995.

Deen HG, McGirr SJ: Vertebral artery injury associated with cervical spine fracture, *Spine* 17:230, 1992.

De Iure F, Donthineni R, Boriani S: Outcomes of C1 and C2 posterior screw fixation for upper cervical spine fusion, *Eur Spin J* 18:S2, 2009.

Delamarter RB: *The cervical spine, part III: management of cervical spine injuries*, New Orleans, 1990, Instructional course lecture presented at the Fifty-seventh Annual Meeting of the American Academy of Orthopaedic Surgeons.

Demisch S, Lindner A, Beck R, et al.: The forgotten condyle: delayed hypoglossal nerve palsy caused by fracture of the occipital condyle, *Clin Neurol Neurosurg* 100:44, 1998.

Dickman CA, Crawford NR, Paramore CG: Biomechanical characteristics of C1-2 cable fixations, *J Neurosurg* 85:316, 1996.

Dickman CA, Greene KA, Sonntag VK: Injuries involving the transverse atlantal ligament: classification and treatment guidelines based upon experience with 39 injuries, *Neurosurgery* 38:44, 1996.

Dickman CA, Sonntag VK: Posterior C1-C2 transarticular screw fixation for atlantoaxial arthrodesis, *Neurosurgery* 43:275, 1998.

DiPaola CP, Conrad BP, Horodyski M, et al.: Cervical spin motion generated with manual versus Jackson table turning methods in a cadaveric C1-C2 global instability model, *Spine* 34:2912, 2009.

Donaldson III WF, Heil BV, Donaldson VP, et al.: The effect of airway maneuvers on the unstable C1-C2 segment: a cadaver study, *Spine* 22:1215, 1997.

Donaldson III WF, Lauerman WC, Heil B, et al.: Helmet and shoulder pad removal from a player with suspected cervical spine injury: a cadaver model, *Spine* 23:1729, 1998.

Duane TM, Dechert T, Wolfe LG, et al.: Clinical examination and its reliability in identifying cervical spine fractures, *J Trauma* 62:1405, 2007.

Ducker TB, Bellegarrigue R, Salcman M, et al.: Timing of operative care in cervical spinal cord injury, *Spine* 9:525, 1984.

Duggal N, Chamberlain RH, Park SC, et al.: Unilateral cervical facet dislocation: biomechanics of fixation, *Spine* 30:E164, 2005.

Duggal N, Chamberlain RH, Perez-Garza LE, et al.: Hangman's fracture: a biomechanical comparison of stabilization techniques, *Spine* 32:182, 2007.

Dull ST, Toselli RM: Preoperative oblique axial computed tomographic imaging for C1-C2 transarticular screw fixation: technical note, *Neurosurgery* 37:150, 1995.

Duncan RW, Esses SI: Dens fractures: specifications and management, *Semin Spine Surg* 8:19, 1996.

Dunham CM, Brocker BP, Collier BD, Gemmel DJ: Risks associated with magnetic resonance imaging and cervical collar in comatose, blunt trauma patients with negative comprehensive cervical spine computed tomography and no apparent spinal deficit, *Crit Care* 12:R89, 2008.

Dvorak MF, Fisher CG, Aarabi B, et al.: Clinical outcomes of 90 isolated unilateral facet fractures, subluxations and dislocations treated surgically and nonoperatively, *Spine* 32:3007, 2007.

Dvorak MF, Fisher CG, Fehlings MG, et al.: The surgical approach to subaxial cervical spine injuries: an evidence based algorithm based on the SLIC classification system, *Spine* 32:2620, 2007.

Dvorak MF, Johnson MG, Boyd M, et al.: Long-term health-related quality of life outcomes following Jefferson-type burst fractures of the atlas, *J Neurosurg Spine* 2:411, 2005.

Ebraheim NA, DeTroye RJ, Rupp RE, et al.: Osteosynthesis of the cervical spine with an anterior plate, *Orthopedics* 18:141, 1995.

Ebraheim NA, Hoeflinger MJ, Salpietro B, et al.: Anatomic considerations in posterior plating of the cervical spine, *J Orthop Trauma* 5:196, 1991.

Ebraheim NA, Lu J, Yang H: The effect of translation of the C1-C2 on the spinal canal, *Clin Orthop Relat Res* 351:222, 1998.

Ebraheim NA, Tremains MR, Xu R, et al.: Lateral radiologic evaluation of lateral mass screw placement in the cervical spine, *Spine* 23:458, 1998.

Edwards CC, Matz SO, Levine AM: Oblique wiring technique for rotational injury of cervical spine [abstract], *Orthop Trans* 9:142, 1985.

Eismont FJ, Bohlman HH: Posterior atlanto-occipital dislocation with fractures of the atlas and odontoid process, *J Bone Joint Surg* 60A:397, 1978.

Eismont FJ, Bohlman HH: Posterior methylmethacrylate fixation for cervical trauma, *Spine* 6:347, 1981.

Eismont FJ, Bora F, Bohlman HH: Complete dislocations at two adjacent levels of the cervical spine, *Spine* 9:319, 1984.

Effendi B, Ray D, Cornish B, et al.: Fractures of the ring of the axis. A classification based on the analysis of 131 cases, *J Bone Joint Surg* 63B:319, 1981.

El-Khoury GY, Kathol MH: Radiographic evaluation of cervical spine trauma, *Semin Spine Surg* 3:3, 1991.

Etter C, Coscia M, Jaberg H, et al.: Direct anterior fixation of dens fracture with a cannulated screw system, *Spine* 16:S25, 1991.

Fabris D, Nena U, Gentilucci G, et al.: Surgical treatment of traumatic lesions of the middle and lower cervical spine with Roy-Camille plates, *Ital J Orthop Traumatol* 18:43, 1992.

Fassett DR, Dailey AT, Vaccaro AR: Vertebral artery injuries associated with cervical spine injuries: a review of the literature, *J Spinal Disord Tech* 21:252, 2008.

Fielding JW: Selected observations on the cervical spine in the child. In Ahstrom Jr JP, editor: *Current practice in orthopaedic surgery*, vol 5. St. Louis, 1973, Mosby.

Fielding JW, Cochran GVB, Lawsing III JF, et al.: Tears of the transverse ligament of the atlas: a clinical and biomechanical study, *J Bone Joint Surg* 56A:1683, 1974.

Fielding JW, Francis WR, Hawkins RJ, et al.: Atlantoaxial rotary deformity, *Semin Spine Surg* 3:33, 1991.

Fielding JW, Hawkins RJ: Atlanto-axial rotatory fixation: fixed rotatory subluxation of the atlanto-axial joint, *J Bone Joint Surg* 59A:37, 1977.

Fielding JW, Hawkins RJ, Ratzan SA: Spine fusion for atlanto-axial instability, *J Bone Joint Surg* 58A:400, 1976.

Fielding JW, Hensinger RN: Cervical spine surgery: past, present, and future potential, *Orthopedics* 10:1701, 1987.

Fisher CG, Dvorak MFS, Leith J, Wing PC: Comparison of outcomes for unstable lower cervical flexion teardrop fractures managed with halo thoracic vest versus anterior corpectomy and plating, *Spine* 27:160, 2002.

Foley KT, DiAngelo DJ, Rampersaud YR, et al.: The in vitro effects of instrumentation on multilevel cervical strut-graft mechanics, *Spine* 15:2366, 1999.

Fong S, DuPlessis SJ: Minimally invasive anterior approach to upper cervical spine: surgical technique, *J Spinal Disord Techn* 18:321, 2005.

Francis WR, Fielding JW, Hawkins RJ, et al.: Traumatic spondylolisthesis of the axis, *J Bone Joint Surg* 63B:313, 1981.

Fujimura Y, Nishi Y, Chiba K, et al.: Prognosis of neurological deficits associated with upper cervical spine injuries, *Paraplegia* 33:195, 1995.

Gallie WE: Fractures and dislocations of the cervical spine, *Am J Surg* 46:495, 1939.

Garvey TA, Eismont FJ, Roberti LJ: Anterior decompression, structural bone grafting, and Caspar plate stabilization for unstable cervical spine fractures and/or dislocations, *Spine* 17(Suppl):431, 1992.

Giacobetti FB, Vaccaro AR, Bos-Giacobetti MA, et al.: Vertebral artery occlusion associated with cervical spine trauma: a prospective analysis, *Spine* 22:188, 1997.

Goel A: Treatment of basilar invagination by atlantoaxial joint distraction and direct lateral mass fixation, *J Neurosurg* 1:281, 2004.

Goel A, Laheri V: Plate and screw fixation for atlanto-axial subluxation, *Acta Neurochir* 129:47, 1994.

Goldstein R, Deen Jr HG, Zimmerman RS, et al.: "Preplacement" of the back of the halo vest in patients undergoing cervical traction for cervical spine injuries: a technical note, *Surg Neurol* 44:476, 1995.

Gonzales RP, Fried PO, Bukhalo M, et al.: Role of clinical examination in screening for blunt cervical spine injury, *J Am Coll Surg* 189:152, 1999.

Graber MA, Kathol M: Cervical spine radiographs in the trauma patient, *Am Fam Physician* 59:331, 1999.

Grauer JN, Shafi B, Hilibrand AS, et al.: Proposal of a modified, treatment-oriented classification of odontoid fractures, *Spine J* 5:123, 2005.

Grauer JN, Vaccaro AR, Lee JY, et al.: The timing and influence of MRI on the management of patients with cervical facet dislocations remains highly variable, *J Spinal Disord Tech* 22:96, 2009.

Greene KA, Dickman CA, Marciano F, et al.: Acute axis fractures: analysis of management and outcome in 340 consecutive cases, *Spine* 22:1843, 1997.

Griffen MM, Frykberg ER, Kerwin AJ: Radiographic clearance of blunt cervical spine injury: plain radiograph or computed tomography scan? *J Trauma* 55:222, 2003.

Grob D, Crisco III JJ, Panjabi MM, et al.: Biomechanical evaluation of four different posterior atlantoaxial fixation techniques, *Spine* 17:480, 1992.

Gruenbert MF, Rechtine GR, Chrin AM, et al.: Overdistraction of cervical spine injuries with the use of skull traction: a report of two cases, *J Trauma* 42:1152, 1997.

Guiot B, Fessler RG: Complex atlantoaxial fractures, *J Neurosurg* 91:139, 1999.

Hadley MN: Initial closed reduction of cervical spine fracture-dislocation injuries, *Neurosurgery* 50:S44, 2002.

Hadley MN, Dickman CA, Browner CM, et al.: Acute traumatic atlas fractures: management and long-term outcome, *Adv Orthop Surg* 12:234, 1989.

Hadley MN, Fitzpatrick BC, Volker KH, et al.: Experimental and clinical studies, *Neurosurgery* 30:661, 1992.

Hadley M, Walters B, Grabb P: Occipital condyle fractures, *Neurosurgery* 50:S114, 2002.

Haid RW, Foley KT, Rodts GE, et al.: The Cervical Spine Study Group anterior cervical plate nomenclature, *Neurosurg Focus* 12:1, 2002.

Hamilton A, Webb JK: The role of anterior surgery for vertebral fractures with and without cord compression, *Clin Orthop Relat Res* 300:79, 1994.

Hanssen AD, Cabanela ME, Cass JR: Fractures of the dens (odontoid process), *Adv Orthop Surg* 10:170, 1987.

Harms J, Melcher RP: Posterior C1-C2 fusion with polyaxial screw and rod fixation, *Spine* 26:2467, 2001.

Harris Jr J, Carson GC, Wagner WK: Radiologic diagnosis of traumatic occipitovertebral dislocation: 1. Normal occiptovertebral relations on the lateral radiographs of supine subjects, *AJNR Am J Neuroradiol* 162:881, 1994.

Harris MB, Waguespack AM, Kronlage S: "Clearing" cervical spine injuries in polytrauma patients: is it really safe to remove the collar? *Orthopedics* 20:903, 1997.

Harris TJ, Blackmore CC, Mirza SK, et al.: Clearing the cervical spine in obtunded patients, *Spine* 33:1547, 2008.

Hart R, Saterbak A, Rapp T, Clark C: Nonoperative management of dens fracture non-union in elderly patients without myelopathy, *Spine* 25:1339, 2000.

Haus BM, Harris MB: Case report. Nonoperative treatment of an unstable Jefferson fracture using a cervical collar, *Clin Orthop Relat Res* 466:1257, 2008.

Hayes VM, Silber JS, Siddiqi FN, et al.: Complications of halo fixation of the cervical spine, *Am J Orthop* 34:271, 2005.

Heller JG: Complications of posterior cervical plating, *Semin Spine Surg* 5:128, 1993.

Herkowitz HN, Rothman RH: Subacute instability of the cervical spine, *Spine* 9:348, 1984.

Herr CH, Ball PA, Sargent SK, et al.: Sensitivity of the prevertebral soft tissue measurement of C3 for detection of cervical spine fractures and dislocations, *Am J Emerg Med* 16:346, 1998.

Hoffmann JR, Mower WR, Wolfson AB, et al.: Validation of a set of clinical criteria to rule out injury to the cervical spine in patients with blunt trauma, *N Engl J Med* 343:94, 2000.

Holmes JF, Akkinepalli R: Computed tomography versus plain radiography to screen for cervical spine injury: a meta-analysis, *J Trauma* 58:902, 2005.

Holmes JF, Mirvis SE, Panacek EA, et al.: Variability in computed tomography and magnetic resonance imaging in patients with cervical spine injuries, *J Trauma* 53:524, 2002.

Holness RO, Huestis WS, Howes WJ, et al.: Posterior stabilization with an interlaminar clamp in cervical injuries: technical note and review of the long-term experience with the method, *Neurosurgery* 14:318, 1984.

Hong JT, Sung JH, Son BC, et al.: Significance of laminar screw fixation in the subaxial cervical spine, *Spine* 33:1739, 2008.

Huang CI, Chen IH: Atlantoaxial arthrodesis using Halifax interlaminar clamps reinforced by halo vest immobilization: a long-term follow-up experience, *Neurosurgery* 38:1153, 1996.

Illgner A, Haas N, Tscherne H: A review of the therapeutic concept and results of operative treatment in acute and chronic lesions of the cervical spine: the Hanover experience, *J Orthop Trauma* 5:100, 1991.

Irwin ZN, Arthur M, Mullins RJ, Hart RA: Variations in injury patterns, treatment, and outcome for spinal fracture and paralysis in adult versus geriatric patients, *Spine* 29:769, 2004.

Ivancic PC, Beauchman NN, Tweardy L: Effect of halo-vest components on stabilizing the injured cervical spine, *Spine* 34:167, 2009.

Jacobs B: Cervical fractures and dislocations (C3-7), *Clin Orthop Relat Res* 109:18, 1975.

Jauregui N, Lincoln T, Mubarak S, et al.: Surgically related upper cervical spine canal anatomy in children, *Spine* 18:1939, 1993.

Jeanneret B, Gebhard JS, Margerl F: Transpedicular screw fixation of articular mass fracture-separation: results of an anatomical study and operative technique, *J Spinal Disord* 7:222, 1994.

Jeanneret B, Magerl F, Halter WE, et al.: Posterior stabilization of the cervical spine with hook plates, *Spine* 16:556, 1991.

Jeanneret B, Magerl F, Ward JC: Overdistraction: a hazard of skull traction in the management of acute injuries of the cervical spine, *Arch Orthop Trauma Surg* 110:242, 1991.

Jefferson G: Fracture of the atlas vertebra: report of four cases and a review of those previously recorded, *Br J Surg* 7:407, 1920.

Johnson MG, Fisher CG, Boyd M, et al.: The radiographic failure of single segment anterior cervical plate fixation in traumatic cervical flexion distraction injuries, *Spine* 29:2815, 2004.

Johnson RM, Owen JR, Hart DL, et al.: Cervical orthoses: a guide to their selection and use, *Clin Orthop Relat Res* 154:34, 1981.

Jones ET, Haid Jr R: Injuries to the pediatric subaxial cervical spine, *Semin Spine Surg* 3:61, 1991.

Jónsson Jr H, Bring G, Rauschning W, et al.: Hidden cervical spine injuries in traffic accident victims with skull fractures, *J Spinal Disord* 4:251, 1991.

Jónsson Jr H, Cesarini K, Petrén-Mallmin M, et al.: Locking screw-plate fixation of cervical spine fractures with and without ancillary posterior plating, *Arch Orthop Trauma Surg* 111:1, 1991.

Jónsson Jr H, Rauschning W: Postoperative cervical spine specimens studied with the cryoplaning technique, *J Orthop Trauma* 6:1, 1992.

Julien TD, Frankel B, Traynelis VC, Ryken TC: Evidence-based analysis of odontoid fracture management, *Neurosurg Focus* 8:e1, 2000.

BY Jun: Anatomic study for ideal and safe posterior C1-C2 transarticular screw fixation, *Spine* 23:1703, 1998.

Kadwar E, Uribe JS, Padhya TA, et al.: Management of delayed esophageal perforations after anterior cervical spinal surgery, *J Neurosurg* 11:320, 2009.

Kang JD, Figgie MP, Bohlman HH: Sagittal measurements of the cervical spine in subaxial fractures and dislocations, *J Bone Joint Surg* 76A:1617, 1994.

Kasimatis GB, Panagiotopoulos E, Gliatis J, et al.: Complications of anterior surgery in cervical spine trauma: an overview, *Clin Neurol Neurosurg* 111:18, 2009.

Kast E, Mohr K, Richter HP, et al.: Complications of transpedicular screw fixation in the cervical spine, *Eur Spine J* 15:327, 2006.

Kathol M, El-Khoury GY: Diagnostic imaging of cervical spine injuries, *Semin Spine Surg* 8:2, 1996.

Kaufman WA, Lunsford TR, Lunsford BR, et al.: Comparison of three prefabricated cervical collars, *Orthot Prosthet* 39:21, 1986.

Kerwin GA, Chou KL, White DB, et al.: Investigation of how different halos influence pin forces, *Spine* 19:1078, 1994.

Klein GR, Vaccaro AR, Albert TJ, et al.: Efficacy of magnetic resonance imaging in the evaluation of posterior cervical spine fractures, *Spine* 24:771, 1999.

Koech F, Ackland HM, Varma DK, et al.: Nonoperative management of type II odontoid fractures in the elderly, *Spine* 33:2881, 2008.

Koivikko MP, Kiuru MJ, Koskinen SK, et al.: Factors associated with nonunion in conservatively-treated type-II fractures of the odontoid process, *J Bone Joint Surg* 86B:1146, 2004.

Kontautas E, Ambrozaitis KV, Kalesinskas R, Spakauskas B: Management of acute traumatic atlas fractures, *J Spinal Disord Tech* 18:402, 2005.

Kostuik JP: Indications of the use of halo immobilization, *Clin Orthop Relat Res* 154:46, 1981.

Kraus DR, Stauffer ES: Spinal cord injury as a complication of elective anterior cervical fusion, *Clin Orthop Relat Res* 112:130, 1975.

Landells CD, Van Peteghem PK: Fractures of the atlas: classification, treatment and morbidity, *Spine* 13:450, 1988.

Lander P, Gardner D, Hadjipavlou A: Pseudonotch of the atlas vertebra simulating fracture with computed tomographic diagnosis, *Orthop Rev* 20:614, 1991.

Laxer EB, Aebi M: Management of subaxial cervical spine injuries with internal fixation: the anterior approach, *Semin Spine Surg* 8:27, 1996.

Lee SL, Sena M, Greenholz SK, et al.: A multidisciplinary approach to the development of a cervical spine clearance protocol: process, rationale and initial results, *J Pediatr Surg* 38:358, 2003.

Lee SW, Draper ER, Hughes SP: Instantaneous center of rotation and instability of the cervical spine: a clinical study, *Spine* 22:641, 1997.

Lesoin F, Pellerin P, Villette L, et al.: Anterior approach and osteosynthesis for recent fractures of the pedicles of the axis, *Adv Orthop Surg* 10:130, 1987.

Leventhal MR: Management of lower cervical spine injuries (C4-C7). In Torg JS, editor: *Athletic injuries to the head, neck, and face*, ed 2, St. Louis, 1991, Mosby.

Leventhal MR: Operative management of cervical spine problems in athletes, *Op Tech Sports Med* 1:199, 1993.

Levi AD, Hurlbert RJ, Anderson P, et al.: Neurologic deterioration secondary to unrecognized spinal instability following trauma—a multicenter study, *Spine* 31:451, 2006.

Levine AM, Edwards CC: Treatment of injuries in the C1-C2 complex, *Orthop Clin North Am* 17:31, 1986.

Levine AM, Edwards CC: Fractures of the atlas, *J Bone Joint Surg* 73A:680, 1991.

Levine AM, Mazel C, Roy-Camille R: Management of fracture separations of the articular mass using posterior cervical plating, *Spine* 17:447, 1992.

Levine AM, Rhyne AL: Traumatic spondylolisthesis of the axis, *Semin Spine Surg* 3:47, 1991.

Li F, Chen Q, Xu K: The treatment of concomitant odontoid fracture and lower cervical spine injuries, *Spine* 33:E693, 2008.

Louis R: *Surgery of the spine: surgical anatomy and operative approaches*, New York, 1983, Springer-Verlag.

Lowery GL: *ORION anterior cervical plate system surgical technique manual*, Memphis, 1995, Sofamor Danek.

Lowery GL, McDonough RF: The significance of hardware failure in anterior cervical plate fixation: patients with 2- to 7-year follow-up, *Spine* 23:181, 1998.

Ludwig SC, Kramer DL, Vaccaro AR, Albert TJ: Transpedicle screw fixation of the cervical spine, *Clin Orthop Relat Res* 359:77, 1999.

Lundy DW, Murray HH: Neurological deterioration after posterior wiring of the cervical spine, *J Bone Joint Surg* 79B:948, 1997.

Magerl F, Grob D, Seeman P: Stable dorsal fusion of the cervical spine (C2-T1) using hook plates. In Kehr P, Weidner A, editors: *Cervical spine*, New York, 1987, Springer-Verlag.

Magerl F, Seemann PS: Stable posterior fusion of the atlas and axis by transarticular screw fixation. In Kehr P, Weidner A, editors: *Cervical spine*, New York, 1987, Springer-Verlag.

Majd ME, Vadhva M, Holt RT: Anterior cervical reconstruction using titanium cages with anterior plating, *Spine* 24:1604, 1999.

Majercik S, Tashjian RZ, Biffl WL, et al.: Halo vest immobilization in the elderly: a death sentence? *J Trauma* 59:350, 2005.

Malham GM, Ackland HM, Jones R, et al.: Occipital condyle fractures: incidence and clinical follow-up at a level 1 trauma centre, *Emerg Radiol* 16:291, 2009.

Malik SA, Murphy M, Connolly P, et al.: Evaluation of morbidity, mortality and outcome following cervical spine injuires in elderly patients, *Eur Spine J* 17:585, 2008.

Maroon JC, Bailes JE: Athletes with cervical spine injury, *Spine* 21:2294, 1996.

Maserati MB, Stephens B, Zohny Z, et al.: Occipital condyle fractures: clinical decision rule and surgical management, *J Neurosurg Spine* 11:388, 2009.

Mazur JM, Stauffer ES: Unrecognized spinal instability associated with seemingly "simple" cervical compression fractures, *Spine* 8:687, 1983.

McAfee PC, Bohlman HH, Wilson WL: The triple wire fixation technique for stabilization of acute cervical fracture-dislocations: a biomechanical analysis [abstract], *Orthop Trans* 9:142, 1985.

McAfee PC, Bohlman HH, Ducker TB, et al.: One-stage anterior cervical decompression and posterior stabilization: a study of one hundred patients with a minimum of two years of follow-up, *J Bone Joint Surg* 77A:1791, 1995.

McClelland SH, James RL, Jarenwattananon A, et al.: Traumatic spondylolisthesis of the axis in a patient presenting with torticollis, *Clin Orthop Relat Res* 218:195, 1987.

McCulloch PT, Franc J, Jones DL, et al.: Helical computed tomography alone compared with plain radiographs with adjunct computed tomography to evaluate the cervical spine after high-energy trauma, *J Bone Joint Surg* 87A:2388, 2005.

McGraw RW, Rusch RM: Atlanto-axial arthrodesis, *J Bone Joint Surg* 55B:482, 1973.

McGrory BJ, Klassen RA, Chao EYS, et al.: Acute fractures and dislocations of the cervical spine in children and adolescents, *J Bone Joint Surg* 75A:988, 1993.

McGuire Jr RA, Harkey HL: Modification of technique and results of atlanto-axial transfacet stabilization, *Orthopedics* 18:1029, 1995.

McLain RF, Aretakis A, Moseley TA, et al.: Subaxial cervical dissociation: anatomic and biomechanical principles of stabilization, *Spine* 19:653, 1994.

Meyer Jr PR: Emergency room assessment: management of spinal cord and associated injuries. In Meyer Jr PR, editor: *Surgery of spine trauma*, New York, 1989, Churchill Livingstone.

Miller PR, Fabian TC, Croce MA, et al.: Prospective screening for blunt cerebrovascular injuries: analysis of diagnostic modalities and outcomes, *Ann Surg* 236:386, 2002.

Mirza SK, Krengel III WF, Chapman JR, et al.: Early versus delayed surgery for acute cervical spinal cord injury, *Clin Orthop Relat Res* 359:104, 1999.

Mitchell TC, Sadasivan KK, Ogden AL, et al.: Biomechanical study of atlantoaxial arthrodesis: transarticular screw fixation versus modified Brooks posterior wiring, *J Orthop Trauma* 3:483, 1999.

Moore TA, Vaccaro AR, Anderson PA: Classification of lower cervical spinal injuries, *Spine* 31:S37, 2006.

Morscher E, Sutter F, Jenny H, et al.: Die vordere Verplattung der Halswirbelsaule mit dem Hohlschrauben-Plattensystem aus Titanium, *Chirurg* 57:702, 1986.

Mummaneni PV, Haid RW: Atlantoaxial fixation: overview of all techniques, *Neurol India* 53:408, 2005.

Nguyen GK, Clark R: Adequacy of plain radiography in the diagnosis of cervical spine injuries, *Emerg Radiol* 11:158, 2005.

Noble ER, Smoker WR: The forgotten condyle: the appearance, morphology, and classification of occipital condyle fractures, *AJNR Am J Neuroradiol* 17:507, 1996.

O'Brien PJ, Schweigel JF, Thompson WJ: Dislocation of the lower cervical spine, *J Trauma* 22:710, 1982.

Oda T, Panjabi MM, Crisco 3rd JJ, et al.: Experimental study of atlas injuries, part II: relevance to clinical diagnosis and treatment, *Spine* 16:S466, 1991.

Ohiorenoya D, Hilton M, Oakland CD, et al.: Cervical spine imaging in trauma patients: a simple scheme of rationalising arm traction using zonal divisions of the vertebral bodies, *J Accid Emerg Med* 13:175, 1996.

Olerud C, Jónsson Jr H: Compression of the cervical spine cord after reduction of fracture dislocations, *Acta Orthop Scand* 62:599, 1991.

Osti OL, Fraser RD, Griffiths ER: Reduction and stabilization of cervical dislocations, *J Bone Joint Surg* 71B:275, 1989.

Otis JC, Burstein AH, Torg JS: Mechanisms and pathomechanics of athletic injuries to the cervical spine. In Torg JS, editor: *Athletic injuries to the head, neck, and face*, ed 2, St. Louis, 1991, Mosby.

Padua L, Padua R, LoMonaco M, et al.: Radiculomedullary complications of cervical spinal manipulation, *Spinal Cord* 34:488, 1996.

Pal GP, Routal RV: The role of the vertebral laminae in the stability of the cervical spine, *J Anat* 188:485, 1996.

Pang D, Nemzek WR, Zovickian J: Atlanto-occipital dislocation, part 1: normal occipital condyle-C1 interval in 89 children, *Neurosurgery* 61:514, 2007.

Pang D, Nemzek WR, Zovickian J: Atlanto-occipital dislocation, part 2: the clinical use of (occipital) condyle-C1 interval, comparison with other diagnostic methods, and the manifestation, management, and outcome of atlanto-occipital dislocation in children, *Neurosurgery* 61:995, 2007.

Panjabi MM, Isomi T, Wang JL: Loosening at the screw-vertebra junction in multilevel anterior cervical plate constructs, *Spine* 15:2383, 1999.

Panjabi MM, Oda T, Crisco 3rd JJ, et al.: Experimental study of atlas injuries, part I: biomechanical analysis of their mechanisms and fracture patterns, *Spine* 16(Suppl 10):S460, 1991.

Papadopoulos SM: C6-7 bilateral facet dislocation and herniated disc, *Spinal Frontiers* 1:8, 1994.

Park SH, Sung JK, Lee SH, et al.: High anterior cervical approach to the upper cervical spine, *Surg Neurol* 68:519, 2007.

Pasquale M, Fabian TC: Practice management guidelines for trauma from the Eastern Association for the Surgery of Trauma, *J Trauma* 44:941, 1998.

Paxinos O, Ghanayem AJ, Zindrick MR, et al.: Anterior cervical discectomy and fusion with a locked pate and wedged graft effectively stabilizes flexion-distraction stage 3 injury in the lower cervical spine: a biomechanical study, *Spine* 34:E9, 2008.

Perry J, Nickels VL: Total cervical-spine fusion for neck paralysis, *J Bone Joint Surg* 41A:37, 1959.

Phillips WA, Hensinger RN: The management of rotatory atlanto-axial subluxation in children, *J Bone Joint Surg* 71A:664, 1989.

Pizzutillo PD: Pediatric occipitoatlantal injuries, *Semin Spine Surg* 3:24, 1991.

Pollack Jr CV, Hendey GW, Martin DR, et al.: Use of flexion-extension radiographs of the cervical spine in blunt trauma, *Ann Emerg Med* 38:8, 2001.

Poonnoose PM, Ravichandran G, McClelland MR: Missed and mismanaged injuries of the spinal cord, *J Trauma* 53:314, 2002.

Ralston ME, Chung K, Barnes PD, et al.: Role of flexion-extension radiographs in blunt pediatric cervical spine injury, *Acad Emerg Med* 8:237, 2001.

Reid DC, Leung P: A study of the odontoid process, *Adv Orthop Surg* 12:147, 1989.

Reinhold M, Magerl F, Rieger M, et al.: Cervical pedicle screw placement: feasibility and accuracy of two new insertion techniques based on morphometric data, *Eur Spine J* 16:47, 2007.

Ricciardi JE, Whitecloud III TS: Complications of cervical spine fixation, *Semin Spine Surg* 8:57, 1996.

Richman J: Biomechanics of cervical spine fixation, *Semin Spine Surg* 8:49, 1996.

Richter D, Latta LL, Milne EA, et al.: The stabilizing effects of different orthoses in the intact and unstable upper cervical spine: a cadaver study, *J Trauma* 50:848, 2001.

Ripa DR, Kowell MG, Meyer Jr PR, et al.: Series of ninety-two traumatic cervical spine injuries stabilized with anterior ASIF plate fusion technique, *Spine* 16(Suppl 3):46, 1991.

Rizzolo SJ, Vaccaro AR, Cotler JM: Cervical spine trauma, *Spine* 19:2288, 1994.

Robinson RA, Southwick WO: Indications and techniques for early stabilization of the neck in some fracture dislocations of the cervical spine, *South Med J* 53:565, 1960.

Robinson RA, Southwick WO: Surgical approaches to the cervical spine, *Instr Course Lect* 17:299, 1960.

Rogers WA: Treatment of fracture dislocation of the cervical spine, *J Bone Joint Surg* 24:245, 1942.

Romanelli DA, Dickman CA, Porter RW, et al.: Comparison of initial injury features in cervical spine trauma of C3-C7: predictive outcome with halo-vest management, *J Spinal Disord* 9:146, 1996.

Rommel O, Niedeggen A, Tegenthoff M, et al.: Carotid and vertebral artery injury following severe head or cervical spine trauma, *Cerebrovasc Dis* 9:202, 1999.

Rorabeck CH, Rock MG, Hawkins AJ, et al.: Unilateral facet dislocation of the cervical spine: an analysis of the results of treatment in 26 patients, *Spine* 12:23, 1987.

Roy-Camille R, Saillant G, Laville C, et al.: Treatment of lower cervical spinal injuries C3 to C7, *Spine* 17(Suppl):442, 1992.

Roy-Camille R, Saillant G, Mazel C: Internal fixation of the unstable cervical spine by a posterior-osteosynthesis with plate and screws. In Cervical Spine Research Society, editors: *The cervical spine*, ed 2, Philadelphia, 1989, Lippincott.

Ruf M, Melcher R, Harms J: Transoral reduction and osteosynthesis C1 as a function-reserving option in the treatment of unstable Jefferson fractures, *Spine* 29:823, 2004.

Rumana CS, Baskin DS: Brown-Séquard syndrome produced by cervical disc herniation: case report and literature review, *Surg Neurol* 45:359, 1996.

Rushton SA, Vaccaro AR, Levine MJ, et al.: Bivector traction for unstable cervical spine fractures: a description of its application and preliminary results, *J Spinal Disord* 10:436, 1997.

Ryan MD, Henderson JJ: The epidemiology of fractures and fracture-dislocations of the cervical spine, *Injury* 23:38, 1992.

Sakamoto T, Neo M, Nakamura T: Transpedicular screw placement evaluated by axial computed tomography of cervical pedicle, *Spine* 29:2510, 2004.

Sapkas G, Korres D, Babis GC, et al.: Correlation of spinal canal post-traumatic encroachment and neurological deficit in burst fractures of the lower cervical spine (C3-7), *Eur Spine J* 4:39, 1995.

Sarani B, Waring S, Sonnad S, et al.: Magnetic resonance imaging is a useful adjunct in the evaluation of the cervical spine of injured patients, *J Trauma* 63:637, 2007.

Schatzker J, Rorabeck CH, Waddell JP: Fractures of the dens (odontoid process): an analysis of thirty-seven cases, *J Bone Joint Surg* 53B:392, 1971.

Schlicke LH, Callahan RA: A rational approach to burst fractures of the atlas, *Clin Orthop Relat Res* 154:18, 1981.

Schneider RC, Kahn EA: Chronic neurological sequelae of acute trauma to the spine and spinal cord, part I: the significance of the acute-flexion or "tear-drop" fracture-dislocation of the cervical spine, *J Bone Joint Surg* 38A:985, 1956.

Schneider RC, Kahn EA: Chronic neurological sequelae of acute trauma to the spine and spinal cord, part II: the syndrome of chronic anterior spinal cord injury or compression: herniated intervertebral discs, *J Bone Joint Surg* 41A:449, 1959.

Schulte K, Clark CR, Goel VK: Kinematics of the cervical spine following discectomy and stabilization, *Spine* 14:1116, 1989.

Sciubba DM, McLoughlin GS, Gokaslan ZL, et al.: Are computed tomography scans adequate in assessing cervical spine pain following blunt trauma? *Emerg Med J* 24:803, 2007.

Sciubba DM, Petteys RJ: Evaluation of blunt cervical spine injury, *South Med J* 102:823, 2009.

Seybold EA, Baker JA, Criscitiello AA, et al.: Characteristics of unicortical and bicortical lateral mass screws in the cervical spine, *Spine* 24:2397, 1999.

Shacked I, Ram Z, Hadani M: The anterior cervical approach for traumatic injuries to the cervical spine in children, *Clin Orthop Relat Res* 292:144, 1993.

Shaneyfelt TM, Centor RM: Reassessment of clinical practice guidelines: go gently into that good night, *JAMA* 301:868, 2009.

Shapiro S, Snyder W, Kaufman K, et al.: Outcome of 51 cases of unilateral locked cervical facets: interspinous braided cable for lateral mass plate fusion compared with interspinous wire and facet wiring with iliac crest, *J Neurosurg* 91:19, 1999.

Sherk HH, Schut L, Lane JM: Fractures and dislocations of the cervical spine in children, *Orthop Clin North Am* 7:593, 1976.

Sliker CW, Mirvis SE, Shanmuganathan K: Assessing cervical spine stability in obtunded blunt trauma patients: review of medical literature, *Radiology* 234:733, 2005.

Slone RM, MacMillan M, Montgomery WJ: Spinal fixation, part I: principles, basic hardware, and fixation techniques for cervical spine, *Radiographics* 13:341, 1993.

Smith HE, Vaccaro AR, Maltenfort M, et al.: Trends in surgical management for type II odontoid fracture: 20 years of experience at a regional spinal cord injury center, *Orthopedics* 31:650, 2008.

Smith MD: Cervical spine surgery: fusion of the upper portion of the cervical spine, *Op Tech Orthop* 6:46, 1996.

Sokolowski MJ, Jackson AP, Haak MH, et al.: Acute outcomes of cervical spine injuries in the elderly: atlantoaxial vs subaxial injuries, *J Spinal Cord Med* 30:238, 2007.

Song KJ, Kim GH, Lee KB: The efficacy of the modified classification system of soft-tissue injury in extension injury of the lower cervical spine, *Spine* 33:E488, 2008.

Southwick WO, Robinson RA: Surgical approaches to the vertebral bodies in the cervical and lumbar regions, *J Bone Joint Surg* 631A:39, 1957.

Spector LR, Kim DH, Affonso J, et al.: Use of computed tomography to predict failure of nonoperative treatment of unilateral facet fractures of the cervical spine, *Spine* 31:2827, 2006.

Spence Jr KF, Decker S, Sell KW: Bursting atlantal fracture associated with rupture of the transverse ligament, *J Bone Joint Surg* 52A:543, 1970.

Spivak JM, Chen D, Kummer FJ: The effect of locking fixation screws on the stability of anterior cervical plating, *Spine* 24:334, 1999.

Starr JK, Eismont FJ: Atypical hangman's fractures, *Spine* 18:1954, 1993.

Stauffer ES: Diagnosis and prognosis of acute cervical spinal cord injury, *Clin Orthop Relat Res* 112:9, 1975.

Stauffer ES: Surgical management of cervical spine injuries. In Evarts CM, editor: *Surgery of the musculoskeletal system*, New York, 1983, Churchill Livingstone.

Stauffer ES: Wiring techniques of the posterior cervical spine for the treatment of trauma, *Orthopedics* 11:1543, 1988.

Stauffer ES, Kelly EG: Fracture-dislocations of the cervical spine: instability and recurrent deformity following treatment by anterior interbody fusion, *J Bone Joint Surg* 59A:45, 1977.

Steinmann JC, Anderson PA: Subaxial cervical spine fractures with internal fixation: the posterior approach, *Semin Spine Surg* 8:35, 1996.

Stiell IG, Clement CM, McKnight RD: The Canadian C-spine rule versus the NEXUS low-risk criteria in patients with trauma, *N Engl J Med* 349:2510, 2003.

Stiell IG, Wells GA, Vandemheen KL, et al.: The Canadian C-spine rule for radiography in alert and stable trauma patients, *JAMA* 286:1841, 2001.

Stelfox HT, Velmahos GC, Gettings E, et al.: Computed tomography for early and safe discontinuation of cervical spine immobilization in obtunded multiply injured patients, *J Trauma* 63:630, 2007.

Suh PB, Kostuik JP, Esses SI: Anterior cervical plate fixation with the titanium hollow screw plate system, *Spine* 15:1079, 1990.

Sutterlin CE, McAfee PC, Warden KE, et al.: A biomechanical evaluation of cervical spinal stabilization methods in a bovine model: static and cyclical loading, *Spine* 13:795, 1988.

Sutton DC, Vaccaro AR, Cotler JM: Halo orthosis: indications and application technique, *Op Tech Orthop* 6:2, 1996.

Swank ML, Sutterlin III CE, Bossons CR, et al.: Rigid internal fixation with lateral mass plates in multilevel anterior and posterior reconstruction of the cervical spine, *Spine* 22:274, 1997.

Tan J, Sun G, Qian L, et al.: C1 lateral mass-C2 pedicle screws and crosslink compression fixation for unstable atlas fracture, *Spine* 34:2505, 2009.

Templeton PA, Young JW, Mirvis SE, et al.: The value of retropharyngeal soft tissue measurements in trauma of the adult cervical spine: cervical spine soft tissue measurements, *Skeletal Radiol* 16:98, 1987.

Tessitore E, Momjian A, Payer M: Posterior reduction and fixation of an unstable Jefferson fracture with C1 lateral mass screws, C2 isthmus screws, and crosslink fixation: technical case report, *Op Neurosurg* 63:ONSE100, 2008.

Thalgott JS, Fritts K, Guiffre JM, et al.: Anterior interbody fusion of the cervical spine with coralline hydroxyapatite, *Spine* 24:1295, 1999.

Torg JS: Cervical spinal stenosis with cord neurapraxia and transient quadriplegia, *Sports Med* 20:429, 1995.

Torg JS, Naranja Jr RJ, Pavlov H, et al.: The relationship of developmental narrowing of the cervical spinal canal to reversible and irreversible injury of the cervical spinal cord in football players, *J Bone Joint Surg* 78A:1308, 1996.

Torg JS, Pavlov H, O'Neill MJ, et al.: The axial load teardrop fracture: a biomechanical, clinical, and roentgenographic analysis, *Am J Sports Med* 19:355, 1991.

Torg JS, Sennett B, Pavlov H, et al.: Spear tackler's spine: definition of an entity precluding participation in contact activities, *Am J Sports Med* 21:640, 1993.

Torg JS, Sennett B, Vegso JJ, et al.: Axial loading injuries to the middle cervical spine segment: an analysis and classification of twenty-five cases, *Am J Sports Med* 19:6, 1991.

Torg JS, Vegso JJ, O'Neill MJ, et al.: The epidemiologic, pathologic, biomechanical, and cinematographic analysis of football-induced cervical spine trauma, *Am J Sports Med* 18:50, 1990.

Torre PD, Rinonapoli E: Halo-cast treatment of fractures and dislocations of the cervical spine, *Int Orthop* 16:227, 1992.

Traynelis VC, Donaher PA, Roach RM, et al.: Biomechanical comparison of anterior Caspar plate and three-level posterior fixation techniques in a human cadaver model, *J Neurosurg* 79:96, 1993.

Tribus CB, Corteen DP, Zdeblick TA: The efficacy of anterior cervical plating in the management of symptomatic pseudoarthrosis of the cervical spine, *Spine* 24:860, 1999.

Tsutsumi S, Ueta T, Shiba K, et al.: Effects of the second national acute spinal cord injury study of high-dose methylprednisolone therapy on acute cervical spinal cord injury—results in spinal injuries center, *Spine* 31:2992, 2006.

Tuli S, Tator CH, Fehlings MG, et al.: Occipital condyle fractures, *Neurosurgery* 41:368, 1997.

Vaccaro AR, Albert TJ, Cotler JM: Anterior instrumentation in the treatment of lower cervical spine injuries, *Op Tech Orthop* 6:52, 1996.

Vaccaro AR, Falatyn SP, Flanders AE, et al.: Magnetic resonance evaluation of the intervertebral disc, spinal ligaments, and spinal cord before and after closed traction reduction of cervical spine dislocations, *Spine* 24:1210, 1999.

Vaccaro AR, Hulbert RJ, Patel AA, et al.: The subaxial cervical spine injury classification system. A novel approach to recognize the importance of morphology, neurology, and integrity of the disco-ligamentous complex, *Spine* 32:2365, 2007.

Verheggen R, Jansen J: Hangman's fracture: arguments in favor of surgical therapy for type II and III according to Edwards and Levine, *Surg Neurol* 49:253, 1998.

Vieweg U, Schultheiss R: A review of halo vest treatment of upper cervical spine injuries, *Arch Orthop Trauma Surg* 121:50, 2001.

Walsh GS, Cusimano MD: Vertebral artery injury associated with a Jefferson fracture, *Can J Neurol Sci* 22:308, 1995.

Wang JC, McDonough PW, Endow K, et al.: The effect of cervical plating on single-level anterior cervical discectomy and fusion, *J Spinal Disord* 12:467, 1999.

Waters RL, Adkins RH, Nelson R, et al.: Cervical spinal cord trauma: evaluation and nonoperative treatment with halo-vest immobilization, *Contemp Orthop* 14:35, 1987.

Weiland DJ, McAfee PC: *Enhanced immediate postoperative stability: posterior cervical fusion with triple wire strut technique*, New Orleans, 1989, Paper presented at the Seventeenth Annual Meeting of the Cervical Spine Research Society.

Weir DC: Roentgenographic signs of cervical injury, *Clin Orthop Relat Res* 109:9, 1975.

Weller SJ, Malek AM, Rossitch Jr E: Cervical spine fractures in the elderly, *Surg Neurol* 47:274, 1997.

Wellman BJ, Follett KA, Traynelis VC: Complications of posterior articular mass plate fixation of the subaxial cervical spine in 43 consecutive patients, *Spine* 23:193, 1998.

Wertheim SB, Bohlman HH: Occipitocervical fusion: indications, technique, and long-term results in 13 patients, *J Bone Joint Surg* 69A:833, 1987.

White III AA, Johnson RM, Panjabi MM, et al.: Biomechanical analysis of clinical stability in the cervical spine, *Clin Orthop Relat Res* 109:85, 1975.

White III AA, Panjabi MM: The role of stabilization in the treatment of cervical spine injuries, *Spine* 9:512, 1984.

White III AA, Panjabi MM, Posner I, et al.: Spine stability: evaluation and treatment, *Instr Course Lect* 30:457, 1981.

White III AA, Southwick WO, Panjabi MM: Clinical instability in the lower cervical spine: a review of past and current concepts, *Spine* 1:15, 1976.

Whitehill R: Fractures of the lower cervical spine: subaxial fractures in the adult, *Semin Spine Surg* 3:71, 1991.

Wilson AJ, Marshall RW, Ewart M: Transoral fusion with internal fixation in a displaced hangman's fracture, *Spine* 24:295, 1999.

Wright NM, Lauryssen C: Vertebral artery injury in C1-2 transarticular screw fixation: results of a survey of the AANS/CNS section on disorders of the spine and peripheral nerves. American Association of Neurological Surgeons/Congress of Neurological Surgeons, *J Neurosurg* 88:634, 1998.

Wu JC, Huang WC, Chen YC, et al.: Stabilization of subaxial cervical spines by lateral mass screw fixation with modified Magerl's technique, *Surg Neurol* 70(S1):25, 2008.

Xiao ZM, Zhan XL, Gong DF, et al.: C2 pedicle screw and plate combined with C1 titanium cable fixation for the treatment of atlantoaxial instability not suitable for placement of C1 screw, *J Spinal Disord Tech* 21:514, 2008.

Young R, Thomasson EH: Step-by-step procedure for applying halo ring, *Orthop Rev* 3:62, 1974.

THORACIC AND LUMBAR SPINE AND SACRUM

Abe E, Sato K, Shimada Y, et al.: Thoracolumbar burst fracture with horizontal fracture of the posterior column, *Spine* 22:83, 1997.

Aebi M, Etter C, Kehl T, et al.: Stabilization of the lower thoracic and lumbar spine with internal spinal skeletal fixation system: indications, techniques, and the first results of treatment, *Spine* 12:544, 1987.

Ahlgren BD, Herkowitz HN: A modified posterolateral approach to the thoracic spine, *J Spinal Disord* 8:69, 1995.

Aihara T, Takahashi K, Yamagata M, et al.: Fracture-dislocation of the fifth lumbar vertebra: a new classification, *J Bone Joint Surg* 80B:840, 1998.

Akbarnia BA, Crandall DG, Burkus K, et al.: Use of long rods and a short arthrodesis for burst fractures of the thoracolumbar spine, *J Bone Joint Surg* 76A:1629, 1994.

Akbarnia BA, Fogarth JP, Tayob AA: Contoured Harrington instrumentation in the treatment of unstable spinal fractures (the effect of supplementary sublaminar wires), *Clin Orthop Relat Res* 189:186, 1984.

Akbarnia BA, Gaines Jr R, Keppler L, et al.: *Surgical treatment of fractures and fracture-dislocations of thoracolumbar and lumbar spine using pedicular screw and plate fixation*, Baltimore, 1988, Paper presented at the Twenty-third Annual Meeting of the Scoliosis Research Society.

Allen BL, Ferguson RL: A pictorial guide to the Galveston LRI pelvic fixation technique, *Contemp Orthop* 7:51, 1983.

Allen Jr BL, Ferguson RL: The Galveston technique of pelvic fixation with L-rod instrumentation of the spine, *Spine* 9:388, 1984.

An HS, Simpson JM, Ebraheim NA: Low lumbar burst fractures: comparison between conservative and surgical treatments, *Orthopedics* 15:367, 1992.

Anden U, Lake A, Norwall A: The role of the anterior longitudinal ligament and Harrington rod fixation of unstable thoracolumbar spinal fractures, *Spine* 5:23, 1980.

Anderson PA: Nonsurgical treatment of patients with thoracolumbar fractures, *Instr Course Lect* 44:57, 1995.

Anderson PA, Henley MB, Rivara FP, et al.: Flexion distraction and chance injuries to the thoracolumbar spine, *J Orthop Trauma* 5:153, 1991.

Andreychik DA, Alander DH, Senica KM, et al.: Burst fractures of the second through fifth lumbar vertebrae: clinical and radiographic results, *J Bone Joint Surg* 78A:1156, 1996.

Angtuaco EJC, Binet EF: Radiology of thoracic and lumbar fractures, *Clin Orthop Relat Res* 189:43, 1984.

Aydin E, Solak AS, Tuzuner MM, et al.: Z-plate instrumentation in thoracolumbar spinal fractures, *Bull Hosp Jt Dis* 58:92, 1999.

Baba H, Uchida K, Furusawa N, et al.: Posterior limbus vertebral lesions causing lumbosacral radiculopathy and the cauda equina syndrome, *Spinal Cord* 34:427, 1996.

Barr JD, Barr MS, Lemley TJ, et al.: Percutaneous vertebroplasty for pain relief and spinal stabilization, *Spine* 25:923, 2000.

Bedbrook GM: Treatment of thoracolumbar dislocation and fractures with paraplegia, *Clin Orthop Relat Res* 112:27, 1975.

Been HD: Anterior decompression and stabilization of thoracolumbar burst fractures by the use of the Slot-Zielke device, *Spine* 16:70, 1991.

Bellabarba C, Schildhauer TA, Vaccaro AR, et al.: Complications associated with surgical stabilization of high-grade sacral fracture dislocations with spino-pelvic instability, *Spine* 31:S80, 2006.

Benli IT, Tandogan NR, Kis M, et al.: Cotrel-Dubousset instrumentation in the treatment of unstable thoracic and lumbar spine fractures, *Arch Orthop Trauma Surg* 113:86, 1994.

Benzel EC: Short-segment compression instrumentation for selected thoracic and lumbar spine fractures: the short-rod/two-claw technique, *J Neurosurg* 79:335, 1993.

Berg EE: The sternal-rib complex: a possible fourth column in thoracic spine fractures, *Spine* 18:1916, 1993.

Berlanda P, Bassi G: Surgical treatment of traumatic spinal injuries with cord damage: clinical review of 12 years of experience with the Roy-Camille technique, *Ital J Orthop Traumatol* 17:491, 1991.

Bernstein MP, Mirvis SE, Shanmuganathan K: Chance-type fractures of the thoracolumbar spine: imaging analysis in 53 patients, *Am J Radiol* 187:859, 2006.

Berry GE, Adams S, Harris MB, et al.: Are plain radiographs of the spine necessary during evaluation after blunt trauma? Accuracy of screening torso computed tomography in thoracic/lumbar spine fracture diagnosis, *J Trauma* 59:1410, 2005.

Berry JL, Moran JM, Berg WS, et al.: A morphometric study of human lumbar and selected thoracic vertebrae, *Spine* 12:362, 1987.

Blauth M, Tscherne H, Haas N: Therapeutic concept and results of operative treatment in acute trauma of the thoracic and lumbar spine: the Hanover experience, *J Orthop Trauma* 1:240, 1987.

Böhler L: *Die Technik de Knochenbruchbehandlung Imgrieden und im Kriege*, Verlag non Wilhelm Maudrich, 1929(in German).

Bohlman HH: Current concepts review: treatment of fractures and dislocations of the thoracic and lumbar spine, *J Bone Joint Surg* 67A:165, 1985.

Bohlman HH, Freehafer A, Dejak J: The results of acute injuries of the upper thoracic spine with paralysis, *J Bone Joint Surg* 67A:360, 1985.

Bohlman HH, Kirkpatrick JS, Delamarter RB, et al.: Anterior decompression for late pain and paralysis after fractures of the thoracolumbar spine, *Clin Orthop Relat Res* 300:24, 1994.

Bolesta MJ, Bohlman HH: Mediastinal widening associated with fractures of the upper thoracic spine, *J Bone Joint Surg* 73A:447, 1991.

Bonnin JG: Sacral fractures and injuries to the cauda equina, *J Bone Joint Surg* 27:113, 1945.

Bono CM, Vaccaro AR, Hurlbert RJ, et al.: Validating a newly proposed classification system for thoracolumbar spine trauma: looking to the future of the thoracolumbar injury classification and severity score, *J Orthop Trauma* 20:567, 2006.

Bordurant FJ, Cotler HB, Kulkarni MV, et al.: Acute spinal cord injury: a study using physical examination and magnetic resonance imaging, *Spine* 15:161, 1990.

Borrelli J, Koval KJ, Helfet DL: The crescent fracture: a posterior fracture dislocation of the sacroiliac joint, *J Orthop Trauma* 10:165, 1996.

Bostman OM, Myllynen PJ, Riska EB: Unstable fracture of the thoracic and lumbar spine: the audit of an 8-year series with early reduction using Harrington instrumentation, *Injury* 18:190, 1987.

Bracken MB, Shepard MJ, Collins WF, et al.: A randomized, controlled trial of methylprednisolone or naloxone in the treatment of acute spinal cord injury, *N Engl J Med* 322:1405, 1990.

Bradford DS, Akbarnia BA, Winter RD, et al.: Surgical stabilization of fractures and fracture-dislocations of the thoracic spine, *Spine* 2:185, 1977.

Bradford DS, McBride GG: Surgical management of thoracolumbar spine fractures with incomplete neurologic deficits, *Clin Orthop Relat Res* 218:201, 1987.

Bransford R, Bellabarba C, Thompson JH, et al.: The safety of fluoroscopically-assisted thoracic pedicle screw instrumentation for spine trauma, *J Trauma* 60:1047, 2006.

Broom MJ, Jacobs RR: Update 1988: current status of internal fixation of thoracolumbar fractures, *J Orthop Trauma* 3:148, 1989.

Bryant CE, Sullivan JA: Management of thoracic and lumbar spine fractures with Harrington distraction rods supplemented with segmental wiring, *Spine* 8:532, 1983.

Calenoff L, Chessare JW, Rogers LF, et al.: Multiple level spinal injuries: importance of early recognition, *AJR Am J Roentgenol* 130:665, 1978.

Campbell SE, Phillips CD, Dubovsky E, et al.: The value of CT in determining potential instability of simple wedge-compression fractures of the lumbar spine, *AJNR Am J Neuroradiol* 16:1385, 1995.

Capen DA: Classification of thoracolumbar fractures and posterior instrumentation for treatment of thoracolumbar fractures, *Instr Course Lect* 48:437, 1999.

Carl AL: Sacral spine fractures. In Errico TJ, Bauer RD, Waugh T, editors: *Spinal trauma*, Philadelphia, 1990, Lippincott.

Carl AL, Tranmer BI, Sachs BL: Anterolateral dynamized instrumentation and fusion for unstable thoracolumbar and lumbar burst fractures, *Spine* 22:686, 1997.

Carl AL, Tromanhauser SG, Roger DJ: Pedicle screw instrumentation for thoracolumbar burst fractures and fracture-dislocations, *Spine* 17:S317, 1992.

Carlson GD, Warden KE, Barbeau JM, et al.: Viscoelastic relaxation and regional blood flow response to spinal cord compression and decompression, *Spine* 22:1285, 1997.

Cauley JA, Hochberg MC, Lui LY, et al.: Long-term risk of incident vertebral fractures, *JAMA* 298:2761, 2007.

Chan DPK, Seng NK, Kaan KT: Nonoperative treatment in burst fractures of the lumbar spine (L2-L5) without neurologic deficits, *Spine* 18:320, 1993.

Chang KW: A reduction-fixation system for unstable thoracolumbar burst fractures, *Spine* 17:879, 1992.

Chen WJ, Niu CC, Chen LH, et al.: Back pain after thoracolumbar fracture treated with long instrumentation and short fusion, *J Spinal Disord* 8:474, 1995.

Chipman JG, Deuser WE, Beilman GJ: Early surgery for thoracolumbar spine injuries decreases complications, *J Trauma* 56:52, 2004.

Chiras J, Depriester C, Weill A, et al.: Percutaneous vertebral surgery: techniques and indications, *J Neuroradiol* 24:45, 1997.

Choe DH, Marom EM, Ahrar K, et al.: Pulmonary embolism of polymethyl methacrylate during percutaneous vertebroplasty and kyphoplasty, *AJR Am J Roentgenol* 183:1097, 2004.

Chow GH, Nelson BJ, Gebhard JS, et al.: Functional outcome of thoracolumbar burst fractures managed with hyperextension casting or bracing and early mobilization, *Spine* 21:2170, 1996.

Clark JE: Apophyseal fracture of the lumbar spine in adolescence, *Orthop Rev* 20:512, 1991.

Clohisy JC, Akbarnia BA, Bucholz RD, et al.: Neurologic recovery associated with anterior decompression of spine fractures at the thoracolumbar junction (T12-L1), *Spine* 17(Suppl):325, 1992.

Concato J, Shah N, Horwitz RI: Randomized, controlled trials, observational studies, and hierarchy of research designs, *N Engl J Med* 342:1887, 2000.

Cotrel Y, Dubousset J: *Universal instrumentation (CD) for spinal surgery (technique manual)*, PA, 1985, Greensburg, Stuart.

Cotrel Y, Dubousset J, Guillaumat M: New universal instrumentation for spinal surgery, *Clin Orthop Relat Res* 227:10, 1988.

Court-Brown CM, Gertzbein SD: The management of burst fractures of the fifth lumbar vertebra, *Spine* 12:308, 1987.

Cresswell TR, Marshall PD, Smith RB: Mechanical stability of the AO internal spinal fixation system compared with that of the Hartshill rectangle and sublaminar wiring in the management of unstable burst fractures of the thoracic and lumbar spine, *Spine* 23:111, 1998.

Dai LY, Jiang LS, Jiang SD: Conservative treatment of thoracolumbar burst fractures: a long-term follow-up results with special reference to the load sharing classification, *Spine* 33:2536, 2008.

Dai LY, Jin WJ: Interobserver and intraobserver reliability in the load sharing classification assessment of thoracolumbar burst fractures, *Spine* 30:354, 2005.

Daniaux H, Seykora P, Genelin A, et al.: Application of posterior plating and modifications in thoracolumbar spine injuries, *Spine* 16(Suppl):126, 1991.

Daniels AH, Arthur M, Hart RA: Variability in rates of arthrodesis for patients with thoracolumbar spine fractures with and without associated neurologic injury, *Spine* 32:2334, 2007.

Danisa OA, Shaffrey CI, Jane JA, et al.: Surgical approaches for the correction of unstable thoracolumbar burst fractures: a retrospective analysis of treatment outcomes, *J Neurosurg* 83:977, 1995.

Davies WE, Morris JH, Hill V: An analysis of conservative (nonsurgical) management of thoracolumbar fractures and fracture dislocations with neural damage, *J Bone Joint Surg* 62A:1324, 1980.

Davis LA, Warren SA, Reid DC, et al.: Incomplete neural deficits in thoracolumbar and lumbar spine fractures: reliability of Frankel and Sunnybrook scales, *Spine* 18:257, 1993.

De Klerk LW, Fontijne WP, Stijnen T, et al.: Spontaneous remodeling of the spinal canal after conservative management of the thoracolumbar burst fractures, *Spine* 23:1057, 1998.

Delamarter RB, Bohlman HH, Dodge LD, et al.: Experimental lumbar spinal stenosis: analysis of the cortical evoked potentials, microvasculature, and histopathology, *J Bone Joint Surg* 72A:110, 1990.

Del Bigio MR, Johnson GE: Clinical presentation of spinal cord concussion, *Spine* 14:37, 1989.

Denis F: The three-column spine and its significance in the classification of acute thoracolumbar spinal injuries, *Spine* 8:817, 1983.

Denis F, Armstrong GWD, Searls K, et al.: Acute thoracolumbar burst fractures in the absence of neurologic deficit (a comparison between operative and nonoperative treatment), *Clin Orthop Relat Res* 189:142, 1984.

Denis F, Burkus JK: Diagnosis and treatment of cauda equina entrapment in the vertical lamina fracture of lumbar burst fractures, *Spine* 16:S433, 1991.

Denis F, Burkus JK: Shear fracture-dislocations of the thoracic and lumbar spine associated with forceful hyperextension (lumberjack paraplegia), *Spine* 17:156, 1992.

Denis F, Davis S, Comfort T: Sacral fractures: an important problem, though frequently undiagnosed and untreated: retrospective analysis of two hundred and three consecutive cases, *Orthop Trans* 11:118, 1987.

Denis F, Fuiz H, Searls K: Comparison between square-ended distraction rods and standard round-ended distraction rods in the treatment of thoracolumbar spinal injuries: a statistical analysis, *Clin Orthop Relat Res* 189:162, 1984.

Deramond H, Mathis JM: Vertebroplasty in osteoporosis, *Semin Musculoskelet Radiol* 6:263, 2002.

Devilee R, Sanders R, de Lange S: Treatment of fractures and dislocations of the thoracic and lumbar spine by fusion and Harrington instrumentation, *Arch Orthop Trauma Surg* 114:100, 1995.

DeWald RL: Burst fractures of the thoracic and lumbar spine, *Clin Orthop Relat Res* 189:150, 1984.

Deyo RA, Cherkin DC, Loeser JD, et al.: Morbidity and mortality in association with operations on the lumbar spine, *J Bone Joint Surg* 74A:536, 1992.

Dick W: The "fixateur interne" as a versatile implant for spine surgery, *Spine* 12:882, 1987.

Dickman CA, Yahiro MA, Lu HTC, et al.: Surgical treatment alternatives for fixation of unstable fractures of the thoracic and lumbar spine: a meta-analysis, *Spine* 19(Suppl):2266, 1994.

Dickson JH, Harrington PR, Erwin WD: Harrington instrumentation in the fractured, unstable thoracic and lumbar spine, *Texas Med* 69:91, 1973.

Dickson JH, Harrington PR, Erwin WD: Results of reduction and stabilization of the severely fractured thoracic and lumbar spine, *J Bone Joint Surg* 60A:799, 1978.

Dietemann JL, Runge M, Dosh JC, et al.: Radiology of posterior lumbar apophyseal ring fractures: report of 13 cases, *Neuroradiology* 30:337, 1988.

Dimar II JR, Wilde PH, Glassman SD, et al.: Thoracolumbar burst fractures treated with combined anterior and posterior surgery, *Am J Orthop* 25:159, 1996.

Doerr TE, Montesano PX, Burkus JK, et al.: Spinal canal decompression in traumatic thoracolumbar burst fractures: posterior distraction rods versus transpedicular screw fixation, *J Orthop Trauma* 5:403, 1991.

Donovan DJ, Polly Jr DW, Ondra SL: The removal of a transdural pedicle screw placed for thoracolumbar spine fracture, *Spine* 21:2495, 1996.

Drummond D, Gaudagni J, Keene JS, et al.: Interspinous process segmental spinal instrumentation, *J Pediatr Orthop* 4:397, 1984.

Drummond D, Keene J: A technique of segmental spinal instrumentation without the passing of sublaminar wires, *Mediguide Orthop* 6:1, 1985.

Drummond D, Keene JS, Breed A: The Wisconsin system: a technique of interspinous segmental spinal instrumentation, *Contemp Orthop* 8:29, 1984.

Ebelke DK, Asher MA, Neff JR, et al.: Survivorship analysis of VSP spine instrumentation in the treatment of thoracolumbar and lumbar burst fractures, *Spine* 16:S432, 1991.

Ebraheim NA, Biyani A, Salpietro B: Zone III fractures of the sacrum: a case report, *Spine* 21:2390, 1996.

Edwards CC, Levine AM: Early rod-sleeve stabilization of the injured thoracic and lumbar spine, *Orthop Clin North Am* 17:327, 1986.

Edwards CC, Levine AM: Complications associated with posterior instrumentation for thoracolumbar injuries and their prevention, *Semin Spine Surg* 5:108, 1993.

Eismont FJ, Green BA, Berkowitz BM, et al.: The role of intraoperative ultrasonography in the treatment of thoracic and lumbar spine fractures, *Spine* 9:782, 1984.

Elattrache N, Fadale PD, Fu F: Thoracic spine fracture in a football player, *Am J Sports Med* 21:157, 1993.

Elgafy H, Bellabarba C: Three-column ligamentous extension injury of the thoracic spine: a case report and review of the literature, *Spine* 32:E785, 2007.

Erickson DL, Leider Jr LC, Brown WE: One-stage decompression-stabilization for thoraco-lumbar fractures, *Spine* 2:53, 1977.

Esses SI: The placement and treatment of thoracolumbar spine fractures: an algorithmic approach, *Orthop Rev* 17:571, 1988.

Esses SI: The AO spinal internal fixator, *Spine* 14:373, 1989.

Esses SI, Botsford DJ, Kostuik JP: Evaluation of surgical treatment for burst fractures, *Spine* 15:667, 1990.

Faden AI, Jacobs TP, Patrick DH, et al.: Megadose corticosteroid therapy following experimental traumatic spinal injury, *J Neurosurg* 60:712, 1984.

Farooq N, Pack JC, Pollintine P, et al.: Can vertebroplasty restore normal load-bearing to fractured vertebrae? *Spine* 30:1723, 2005.

Ferguson RL, Allen Jr BL: A mechanistic classification of thoracolumbar spine fractures, *Clin Orthop Relat Res* 189:77, 1984.

Finkelstein JA, Chapman JR, Mirza S: Anterior cortical allograft in thoracolumbar fractures, *J Spinal Disord* 12:424, 1999.

Flesch JR, Leider LL, Erickson D, et al.: Harrington instrumentation and spine fusion for unstable fractures and fracture dislocations of the thoracic and lumbar spine, *J Bone Joint Surg* 59A:143, 1977.

Folman Y, Gepstein R: Late outcome of nonoperative management of thoracolumbar vertebral wedge fractures, *J Orthop Trauma* 17:190, 2003.

Fountain SS, Hamilton RD, Jameson RM: Transverse fractures of the sacrum: a report of six cases, *J Bone Joint Surg 59A* 486, 1977.

Francaviglia N, Bragazzi R, Maiello M, et al.: Surgical treatment of fractures of the thoracic and lumbar spine via the transpedicular route, *Br J Neurosurg* 9:511, 1995.

Fredrickson BE, Yuan HA, Miller H: Burst fractures of the fifth lumbar vertebra, *J Bone Joint Surg* 64A:1088, 1982.

Fribourg D, Tang C, Sra P, et al.: Incidence of subsequent vertebral fracture after kyphoplasty, *Spine* 29:2270, 2004.

Gaebler C, Maier R, Kukla C, et al.: Long-term results of pedicle-stabilized thoracolumbar fractures in relation to the neurological deficit, *Injury* 28:661, 1997.

Gaines RW, Breedlove RF, Munson G: Stabilization of thoracic and thoracolumbar fracture-dislocations with Harrington rods and sublaminar wires, *Clin Orthop Relat Res* 189:195, 1984.

Gaines RW, Humphreys WG: A plea for judgment in management of thoracolumbar fractures and fracture-dislocations: a reassessment of surgical indications, *Clin Orthop Relat Res* 189:36, 1984.

Garcia F, Florez MT, Conejero JA: A butterfly vertebra or a wedge fracture? *Int Orthop* 17:7, 1993.

Garfin S: What the experts say: treatment options for VCF, including balloon kyphoplasty, http://kyphon.com.

Garfin SD, Jacobs RR, Stoll J, et al.: Results of a locking-hook spinal rod for fractures of the thoracic and lumbar spine, *Spine* 15:275, 1990.

Garfin SR, Mowery CA, Guerra Jr J, et al.: Confirmation of the posterolateral technique to decompress and fuse thoracolumbar spine burst fractures, *Spine* 10:218, 1985.

Gertzbein SD, Scoliosis Research Society: Multicenter spine fracture study, *Spine* 17:528, 1992.

Gertzbein SD: Classification of thoracic and lumbar fractures, *Spine* 19:626, 1994.

Gertzbein SD: Neurologic deterioration in patients with thoracic and lumbar fractures after admission to the hospital, *Spine* 19:1723, 1994.

Gertzbein SD: Spine update: classification of thoracic and lumbar fractures, *Spine* 19:626, 1994.

Gertzbein SD, Jacobs RR, Stoll J, et al.: Results of a locking-hook spinal rod for fractures of the thoracic and lumbar spine, *Spine* 15:275, 1990.

Ghanayem AJ, Zdeblick TA: Anterior instrumentation in the management of thoracolumbar burst fractures, *Clin Orthop Relat Res* 335:89, 1997.

Gorczyca JT, Varga E, Woodside T, et al.: The strength of iliosacral lag screws and transiliac bars in the fixation of vertically unstable pelvic injuries with sacral fractures, *Injury* 27:561, 1996.

Grasland A, Pouchot J, Mathieu A, et al.: Sacral insufficiency fractures: an easily overlooked cause of back pain in elderly women, *Arch Intern Med* 56:668, 1996.

Greenfield RT, Grant RE, Bryant D: Pedicle screw fixation in the management of unstable thoracolumbar spine injuries, *Orthop Rev* 21:701, 1992.

Grob D, Scheier HJG, Dvorak J, et al.: Circumferential fusion of the lumbar and lumbosacral spine, *Arch Orthop Trauma Surg* 111:20, 1991.

Grootboom MJ, Govender S: Acute injuries of the upper dorsal spine, *Injury* 24:389, 1993.

Gurr KR, McAfee PC, Shih C: *Biomechanical analysis of posterior instrumentation systems following decompressive laminectomy (an unstable calf spine model)*, NIH grant, Johns Hopkins University School of Medicine, 1987.

Gurwitz GS, Dawson JM, McNamara MJ, et al.: Biomechanical analysis of three surgical approaches for lumbar burst fractures using short-segment instrumentation, *Spine* 18:977, 1993.

Guttmann L: The treatment and rehabilitation of patients with injuries of the spinal cord. In Cope Z, editor: *Medical history of the Second World War: surgery*, London, 1953, His Majesty's Stationery Office.

Guttmann L: A new turning-tilting bed, *Paraplegia* 3:193, 1965.

Guttmann L: Spinal deformities in traumatic paraplegics and tetraplegics following surgical procedures, *Paraplegia* 7:38, 1969.

Ha KI, Han SH, Chung M, et al.: A clinical study of the natural remodeling of burst fractures of the lumbar spine, *Clin Orthop Relat Res* 323:210, 1996.

Hack HP, Zielke K, Harms J: *Spinal instrumentation and monitoring (technique manual)*, PA, 1985, Greensburg, Stuart.

Hak DJ, Baran S, Stahel P: Sacral fractures: current strategies in diagnosis and management, *Orthopedics* 32:752, 2009.

Hanley Jr EN, Eskay ML: Thoracic spine fractures, *Orthopedics* 12:689, 1989.

Hardaker WT, Cook WA, Friedman AH, et al.: Bilateral transpedicular decompression and Harrington rod stabilization in the management of severe thoracolumbar burst fractures, *Spine* 17:162, 1992.

Harkonen M, Kataja M, Keski-Nisula L, et al.: Fractures of the lumbar spine: clinical and radiological results in 94 patients, *Orthop Trauma Surg* 94:43, 1979.

Harrington PR: The history and development of Harrington instrumentation (1973 Nicholas Andry Award Contribution), *Clin Orthop Relat Res* 93:110, 1973.

Harris MB: The role of anterior stabilization with instrumentation in the treatment of thoracolumbar burst fractures, *Orthopedics* 15:347, 1992.

Harris MB, Shi LL, Vacarro AR, et al.: Nonsurgical treatment of thoracolumbar spinal fractures, *Instr Course Lect* 58:629, 2009.

Harrop JS, Vaccaro AR, Hurlbert RJ, et al.: Intrarater and interrater reliability and validity in the assessment of the mechanism of injury and integrity of the posterior ligamentous complex: a novel injury severity scoring system for thoracolumbar injuries, *J Neurosurg Spine* 4:118, 2006.

Hartman MB, Chrin AM, Rechtine GR: Nonoperative treatment of thoracolumbar fractures, *Paraplegia* 33:73, 1995.

Harvey J, Tanner S: Low back pain in young athletes: a practical approach, *Sports Med* 12:394, 1991.

Hatem SF, West OC: Vertical fracture of the central sacral canal: plane and simple, *J Trauma* 40:138, 1996.

Hauser CJ, Visvikis G, Hinrichs C, et al.: Prospective validation of computed tomographic screening of the thoracolumbar spine in trauma, *J Trauma* 55:228, 2003.

Heggeness MH, Doherty BJ: The trabecular anatomy of thoracolumbar vertebrae: implications for burst fractures, *J Anat* 191:309, 1997.

Heinig CF, Chapman TM, Chewning SJ Jr, et al.: Preliminary report on VSP spine fixation system. Unpublished data, 1988.

Herring JA, Wenger DR: Segmental spine instrumentation, *Spine* 7:285, 1982.

Hitchon PW, Torner JC: Recumbency in thoracolumbar fractures, *Neurosurg Clin North Am* 8:509, 1997.

Holdsworth FW, Hardy A: Early treatment of paraplegia from fractures of the thoraco-lumbar spine, *J Bone Joint Surg* 35B:540, 1953.

Horwitz RI, Viscoli CM, Clemens JD, Sadock RT: Developing improved observational methods for evaluating therapeutic effectiveness, *Am J Med* 89:630, 1990.

Hu R, Mustard CA, Burns C: Epidemiology of incident spinal fracture in complete population, *Spine* 21:492, 1996.

Hu SS, Capen DA, Rimoldi RL, et al.: The effect of surgical decompression on neurologic outcome after lumbar fractures, *Clin Orthop Relat Res* 288:166, 1993.

Huang TJ, Chen JY, Shih HN, et al.: Surgical indications in low lumbar burst fractures: experiences with anterior locking plate system and reduction fixation system, *J Trauma* 39:910, 1995.

Hulme PA, Krebs J, Ferguson SJ, et al.: Vertebroplasty and kyphoplasty: a systematic review of 69 clinical studies, *Spine* 31:1983, 2006.

Inaba K, Munera F, McKennely M, et al.: Visceral torso computed tomography for clearance of the thoracolumbar spine in trauma: a review of the literature, *J Trauma* 60:915, 2006.

Isler B: Lumbosacral lesions associated with pelvic ring injuries, *J Orthop Trauma* 4:1, 1990.

Isomi T, Panjabi MM, Kato Y, et al.: Radiographic parameters for evaluating the neurological spaces in experimental thoracolumbar burst fractures, *J Spinal Disord* 13:404, 2000.

Jacobs RR, Asher MA, Snider RK: Thoracolumbar spinal injuries: a comparative study of recumbent and operative treatment in 100 patients, *Spine* 5:463, 1980.

Jacobs RR, Casey MP: Surgical management of thoracolumbar spinal injuries (general principles and controversial considerations), *Clin Orthop Relat Res* 189:22, 1984.

Jacobs RR, Nordwall A, Nachemson A: Reduction, stability and strength provided by internal fixation systems for thoracolumbar spinal injuries, *Clin Orthop Relat Res* 171:300, 1982.

Jacobs RR, Schlaepfer F, Mathys Jr R, et al.: A locking-hook spinal rod system for stabilization of fracture-dislocations and correction of deformities of the dorsolumbar spine: a biomechanical evaluation, *Clin Orthop Relat Res* 189:168, 1984.

James KS, Wenger KH, Schlegel JD, et al.: Biomechanical evaluation of the stability of thoracolumbar burst fractures, *Spine* 19:1731, 1994.

Jane MJ, Freehafer AA, Hazel C, et al.: Autonomic dysreflexia: a cause of morbidity and mortality in orthopedic patients with spinal cord injury, *Clin Orthop Relat Res* 169:151, 1982.

Jelsma RK, Kirsch PT, Jelsma LF, et al.: Surgical treatment of thoracolumbar fractures, *Surg Neurol* 3:156, 1982.

Johnson JR, Leatherman KD, Holt RT: Anterior decompression of the spinal cord for neurologic deficit, *Spine* 8:396, 1983.

Johnson KD, Dadambis A, Seibert GB: Incidence of adult respiratory distress syndrome in patients with multiple musculoskeletal injuries: effect of early operative stabilization of fractures, *J Trauma* 25:375, 1985.

Johnson LP, Nasca RJ, Bonnin JM: Pathoanatomy of a burst fracture, *Surg Rounds Orthop* 2:43, 1988.

Johnston II CE, Ashman RB, Sherman MC, et al.: Mechanical consequences of rod contouring and residual scoliosis in sublaminar segmental instrumentation, *J Orthop Res* 5:206, 1987.

Kahanovitz N, Bullough P, Jacobs RR: The effect of internal fixation without arthrodesis on human facet joint cartilage, *Clin Orthop Relat Res* 189:204, 1984.

Kaneda K, Abumi K, Fujiya M: Burst fractures with neurologic deficits of the thoracolumbar-lumbar spine: results of anterior decompression and stabilization with anterior instrumentation, *Spine* 9:788, 1984.

Kaneda K, Gaines RW: *Kaneda anterior spinal instrumentation for the thoracolumbar spine*, ed 2, Cleveland, 1990, Acromed.

Kaneda K, Taneichi H, Abumi K, et al.: Anterior decompression and stabilization with the Kaneda device for thoracolumbar burst fractures associated with neurological deficits, *J Bone Joint Surg* 79A:69, 1997.

Kaplan SS, Wright NM, Yundt KD, et al.: Adjacent fracture-dislocations of the lumbosacral spine: case report, *Neurosurgery* 44:1134, 1999.

Karjalainen M, Aho AJ, Katevuo K: Operative treatment of unstable thoracolumbar fractures by the posterior approach with the use of Williams plates or Harrington rods, *Int Orthop* 16:219, 1992.

Katonis PG, Kontakis GM, Loupasis GA, et al.: Treatment of unstable thoracolumbar and lumbar spine injuries using Cotrel-Dubousset instrumentation, *Spine* 24:2352, 1999.

Kelly RP, Whitesides Jr TE: Treatment of lumbodorsal fracture-dislocations, *Ann Surg* 167:705, 1968.

Kennedy JG, Soffe KE, McGrath A, et al.: Predictors of outcome in cauda equina syndrome, *Eur Spine J* 8:317, 1999.

Keynan O, Fisher CG, Vaccaro A, et al.: Radiographic measurement parameters in thoracolumbar fractures: a systematic review and consensus statement of the spine trauma study group, *Spine* 31:E156, 2006.

Kim NH, Lee HM, Chun IM: Neurologic injury and recovery in patients with burst fracture of the thoracolumbar spine, *Spine* 24:290, 1999.

King AG: Burst compression fractures of the thoracolumbar spine: pathologic anatomy and surgical management, *Orthopedics* 10:1711, 1987.

Kirkpatrick JS, Wilber RG, Likavec M, et al.: Anterior stabilization of thoracolumbar burst fractures using the Kaneda device: a preliminary report, *Orthopedics* 18:673, 1995.

Korovessis PG, Baikousis A, Stamatakis M: Use of the Texas Scottish Rite Hospital instrumentation in the treatment of thoracolumbar injuries, *Spine* 22:882, 1997.

Korovessis P, Hadjipavlou A, Repantis T: Minimally invasive short posterior instrumentation plus balloon kyphoplasty with calcium phosphate for burst and severe compression lumbar fractures, *Spine* 33:658, 2008.

Korovessis P, Repantis T, Petsinis G, et al.: Direct reduction of thoracolumbar burst fractures by means of balloon kyphoplasty with calcium phosphate and stabilization with pedicle-screw instrumentation and fusion, *Spine* 33:E100, 2008.

Korovessis P, Sidiropoulos P, Dimas A: Complete fracture-dislocation of the thoracic spine without neurologic deficit: case report, *J Trauma* 36:122, 1994.

Kostuik JP: Anterior spinal cord decompression for lesions of the thoracic and lumbar spine: techniques: new methods of internal fixation, results, *Spine* 8:512, 1983.

Kraemer WJ, Schemitsch EH, Lever J, et al.: Functional outcome of thoracolumbar burst fractures without neurological deficit, *J Orthop Trauma* 10:541, 1996.

Krag MH, Weaver DL, Beynnon BD, et al.: Morphometry of the thoracic and lumbar spine related to transpedicular screw placement for surgical spinal fixation, *Spine* 13:27, 1988.

Kramer DL, Rodgers WB, Mansfield FL: Transpedicular instrumentation and short-segment fusion of thoracolumbar fractures: a prospective study using a single instrumentation system, *J Orthop Trauma* 9:499, 1995.

Krompinger WJ, Frederickson BE, Mino DE, et al.: Conservative treatment of fractures of the thoracic and lumbar spine, *Orthop Clin North Am* 17:161, 1986.

Krueger MA, Green DA, Hoyt D, et al.: Overlooked spine injuries associated with lumbar transverse process fractures, *Clin Orthop Relat Res* 327:191, 1996.

Kulkarni MB, McArdle CB, Kopaniky D, et al.: Acute spinal cord injury: MR imaging at 115 T1, *Neuroradiology* 164:837, 1987.

Kupferschmid JP, Weaver ML, Raves JJ, et al.: Thoracic spine injuries in victims of motorcycle accidents, *J Trauma* 29:593, 1989.

Laborde JM, Bahniuk E, Bohlman HH, et al.: Comparison of fixation of spinal fractures, *Clin Orthop Relat Res* 152:305, 1980.

Lafollete BF, Levine MI, McNiesh LM: Bilateral fracture-dislocation of the sacrum, *J Bone Joint Surg* 68A:1099, 1986.

Lee HM, Kim HS, Kim DJ, et al.: Reliability of magnetic resonance imaging in detecting posterior ligament complex injury in thoracolumbar spinal fractures, *Spine* 25:2079, 2000.

Lee JY, Vaccaro AR, Lim MR, et al.: Thoracolumbar injury classification and severity score: a new paradigm for the treatment of thoracolumbar spine trauma, *J Orthop Sci* 10:671, 2005.

Lee JY, Vaccaro AR, Schweitzer KM, et al.: Assessment of injury to the thoracolumbar posterior ligamentous complex in the setting of normal-appearing plain radiography, *Spine J* 7:422, 2007.

Lenarz CJ, Place H, Lenke LG, et al.: Comparative reliability of 3 thoracolumbar fracture classification systems, *J Spinal Disord Tech* 22:422, 2009.

Levine AM, Bosse M, Edwards CC: Bilateral facet dislocations in the thoracolumbar spine, *Spine* 13:630, 1988.

Levine AM, Edwards CC: Low lumbar burst fractures: reduction and stabilization using the modular spine fixation system, *Orthopedics* 1:9, 1988.

Limb D, Shaw DL, Dickson RA: Neurological injury in thoracolumbar burst fractures, *J Bone Joint Surg* 77B:774, 1995.

Lindahl S, Willen J, Nordwall A, et al.: The crush-cleavage fracture: a "new" thoracolumbar unstable fracture, *Spine* 8:559, 1983.

Lindsey RW, Dick W: The fixateur interne in the reduction and stabilization of thoracolumbar spine fractures in patients with neurologic deficit, *Spine* 16(Suppl):140, 1991.

Lindsey RW, Dick W, Nunchuck S, et al.: Residual intersegmental spinal mobility following limited pedicle fixation of thoracolumbar spine fractures with the fixateur interne, *Spine* 18:474, 1993.

Louis R: Fusion of the lumbar and sacral spine by internal fixation with screw plates, *Clin Orthop Relat Res* 203:18, 1986.

Luque ER, Cassis N, Ramirez-Wiella G: Segmental spinal instrumentation in the treatment of fractures of the thoracolumbar spine, *Spine* 7:312, 1982.

Macmillan M, Stauffer ES: Transient neurologic deficits associated with thoracic and lumbar spine trauma without fracture or dislocation, *Spine* 15:466, 1990.

Magerl FP: Stabilization of the lower thoracic and lumbar spine with external skeletal fixation, *Clin Orthop Relat Res* 189:125, 1984.

Magerl F, Aebi M, Gertzbein SD, et al.: A comprehensive classification of thoracic and lumbar injuries, *Eur Spine J* 3:184, 1994.

Maiman DJ, Pintar F, Yoganandan N, et al.: Effects of anterior vertebral grafting on the traumatized lumbar spine after pedicle screw-plate fixation, *Spine* 18:2423, 1993.

Mann KA, McGowan DP, Fredrickson BE, et al.: A biomechanical investigation of short segment spinal fixation for burst fractures with varying degrees of posterior disruption, *Spine* 15:407, 1990.

Markel DC, Graziano GP: A comparison study of treatment of thoracolumbar fractures using the ACE Posterior Segmental Fixator and Cotrel-Dubousset instrumentation, *Orthopedics* 18:679, 1995.

McAfee PC: Biomechanical approach to instrumentation of the thoracolumbar spine: a review article, *Adv Orthop Surg* 8:313, 1985.

McAfee PC, Bohlman HH: Anterior decompression of traumatic thoracolumbar fractures with incomplete paralysis through the retroperitoneal approach, *Orthop Trans* 8:392, 1984.

McAfee PC, Bohlman HH: Complications following Harrington instrumentation for fractures of the thoracolumbar spine, *J Bone Joint Surg* 67A:672, 1985.

McAfee PC, Bohlman HH, Yuan HA: Anterior decompression of traumatic thoracolumbar fractures with incomplete neurological deficit using a retroperitoneal approach, *J Bone Joint Surg* 67A:89, 1985.

McAfee PC, Levine AM, Anderson PA: Surgical management of thoracolumbar fractures, *Instr Course Lect* 44:47, 1995.

McAfee PC, Werner FW, Glisson RR: A biomechanical analysis of spinal instrumentation systems in thoracolumbar fractures: comparison of traditional Harrington side traction instrumentation with segmental spinal instrumentation, *Spine* 10:204, 1985.

McAfee PC, Yuan HA, Fredrickson BE, et al.: The value of computed tomography in thoracolumbar fractures, *J Bone Joint Surg* 64A:461, 1983.

McAfee PC, Yuan HA, Lasda NA: The unstable burst fracture, *Spine* 7:365, 1982.

McBride GG: Surgical stabilization of thoracolumbar fractures using Cotrel-Dubousset rods, *Semin Spine Surg* 2:24, 1990.

McCrory BJ, VanderWilde RS, Currier BL: Diagnosis of subtle thoracolumbar burst fractures: a new radiographic sign, *Spine* 18:2282, 1993.

McDonough PW, Davis R, Tribus C, et al.: The management of acute thoracolumbar burst fractures with anterior corpectomy and Z-plate fixation, *Spine* 29:1901, 2004.

McFarland EG, Giangarra C: Sacral stress fractures in athletes, *Clin Orthop Relat Res* 329:240, 1996.

McGuire Jr RA: The role of anterior surgery in the treatment of thoracolumbar fractures, *Orthopedics* 20:959, 1997.

McGuire RA, Freeland AE: Flexion-distraction injury of the thoracolumbar spine, *Orthopedics* 15:379, 1992.

McHenry TP, Mirza SK, Wang JJ, et al.: Risk factors for respiratory failure following operative stabilization of thoracic and lumbar spine fractures, *J Bone Joint Surg* 88A:997, 2006.

Mehta S, Auerbach JD, Born CT, et al.: Sacral fractures, *J Am Acad Orthop Surg* 14:656, 2006.

Mehta JS, Reed MR, McVie JL, et al.: Weight-bearing radiographs in thoracolumbar fractures: do they influence management? *Spine* 29:564, 2004.

Meldon SW, Moettus LN: Thoracolumbar spine fractures: clinical presentation and the effect of altered sensorium and major injury, *J Trauma* 39:1110, 1995.

Mermelstein LE, McLain RF, Yerby SA: Reinforcement of the thoracolumbar burst fractures with calcium phosphate cement: a biomechanical study, *Spine* 23:664, 1998.

Meves R, Avanzi O: Correlation between neurological deficit and spinal canal compromise in 198 patients with thoracolumbar and lumbar fractures, *Spine* 30:787, 2005.

Meves R, Avanzi O: Correlation among canal compromise, neurologic deficit, and injury severity in thoracolumbar burst fractures, *Spine* 31:2137, 2006.

Meyer PR: Complications of treatment of fractures and dislocations of the dorsolumbar spine. In Epps CH, editor: *Complications in orthopaedic surgery*, Philadelphia, 1978, Lippincott.

Mirza SK, Mirza AJ, Chapman JR, Anderson PA: Classifications of thoracic and lumbar fractures: rationale and supporting data, *J Am Acad Orthop Surg* 10:364, 2002.

Miyakoshi N, Abe E, Shimada Y, et al.: Anterior decompression with single segmental spinal interbody fusion for lumbar burst fracture, *Spine* 24:67, 1999.

Moorman CT, Richardson WJ, Fitch RD, et al.: Flexion-distraction injuries to the lumbar spine in children, *J South Orthop Assoc* 1:296, 1992.

Morgan FH, Wharton W, Austin GN: The results of laminectomy in patients with incomplete spinal cord injuries, *Paraplegia* 9:14, 1971.

Mozes GC, Kollender Y, Sasson AA: Transpedicular screw-rod fixation in the treatment of unstable lower thoracic and lumbar fractures, *Bull Hosp Jt Dis* 53:37, 1993.

Mumford J, Weinstein JN, Spratt KF, et al.: Thoracolumbar burst fractures: the clinical efficacy and outcome of nonoperative management, *Spine* 18:955, 1993.

Munro AHG, Irwin CG: Interlocked articular processes complicating fracture-dislocation of the spine, *Br J Surg* 25:621, 1938.

Myllynen P, Bostman O, Riska E: Recurrence of deformity after removal of Harrington's fixation of spine fractures (seventy-six cases followed for 2 years), *Acta Orthop Scand* 59:497, 1988.

Nagai H, Shimizu K, Shikata J: Chylous leakage after circumferential thoracolumbar fusion for correction of kyphosis resulting from fracture: report of three cases, *Spine* 22:2766, 1997.

Nagel DA, Koogle TA, Piziali RL, et al.: Stability of the upper lumbar spine following progressive disruptions in the application of individual internal and external fixation devices, *J Bone Joint Surg* 63A:62, 1981.

Nicoll EA: Fractures of the dorso-lumbar spine, *J Bone Joint Surg* 31B:376, 1949.

Noojin FK, Malkani AL, Haikal L, et al.: Cross-sectional geometry of the sacral ala for safe insertion of iliosacral lag screws: a computed tomography model, *J Orthop Trauma* 14:31, 2000.

Nork SE, Jones CD, Harding SP, et al.: Percutaneous stabilization of U-shaped sacral fractures using iliosacral screws: technique and early results, *J Orthop Trauma* 15:238, 2001.

Oda T, Panjabi MM: Pedicle screw adjustments affect stability of thoracolumbar burst fracture, *Spine* 26:2328, 2001.

Oda T, Panjabi MM, Kato Y: The effects of pedicle screw adjustments on the anatomical reduction of thoracolumbar burst fractures, *Eur Spine J* 10:505, 2001.

Okuyama K, Abe E, Chiba M, et al.: Outcome of anterior decompression and stabilization for thoracolumbar unstable burst fractures in the absence of neurologic deficits, *Spine* 21:620, 1996.

Olerud C, Sjöström L, Jónsson H, et al.: Posterior reduction of a pathologic spinal fracture: a case of indirect anterior dual decompression, *Acta Orthop Scand* 63:345, 1992.

Oner FC, van-Gils AP, Dhert WJ, et al.: MRI findings of thoracolumbar spine fractures: a categorisation based on MRI examinations of 100 fractures, *Skeletal Radiol* 28:433, 1999.

Oner FC, van-der-Rijt RR, Ramos LM, et al.: Changes in the disc space after fractures of the thoracolumbar spine, *J Bone Joint Surg* 80B:833, 1998.

Osebold WR, Weinstein SL, Sprague BL: Thoracolumbar spine fractures: results of treatment, *Spine* 6:13, 1981.

Osti OL, Fraser RD, Cornish BL: Fractures and fractures-dislocations of the lumbar spine: a retrospective study of 70 patients, *Int Orthop* 11:323, 1987.

Ozturk C, Ersozlu S, Aydinli U: Importance of greenstick lamina fractures in low lumbar burst fractures, *Int Orthop* 30:295, 2006.

Panjabi MM, Kifune M, Wen L, et al.: Dynamic canal encroachment during thoracolumbar burst fractures, *J Spinal Disord* 8:39, 1995.

Panjabi MM, Oxland TR, Kifune M, et al.: Validity of the three-column theory of thoracolumbar fractures: a biomechanic investigation, *Spine* 20:1122, 1995.

Panjabi MM, Oxland TR, Lin RM, et al.: Thoracolumbar burst fracture: a biomechanical investigation of its multidirectional flexibility, *Spine* 19:578, 1994.

Parfenchuck TA, Chambers J, Goodrich JA, et al.: Lumbar spine arthrodesis: a comparison of hospital costs between 1986 and 1993, *Am J Orthop* 24:854, 1995.

Patel AA, Dailey A, Brodke DS, et al.: Thoracolumbar spine trauma classification: the Thorcolumbar Injury Classification and Severity Score system and case examples, *J Neurosurg Spine* 10:201, 2009.

Patel AA, Vaccaro AR, Albert TJ, et al.: The adoption of a new classification system: time-dependent variation in interobserver reliability of the thoracolumbar injury severity score classification system, *Spine* 32:E105, 2007.

Pattee GA, Bohlman HH, McAfee PC: Compression of a sacral nerve as a complication of screw fixation of the sacro-iliac joint, *J Bone Joint Surg* 68A:769, 1986.

Pearch M, Protek I, Shepherd J: Three-dimensional x-ray analysis of normal movement in the lumbar spine, *Spine* 9:294, 1984.

Peh WC, Ooi GC: Vacuum phenomena in the sacroiliac joints and in association with sacral insufficiency fractures: incidence and significance, *Spine* 22:1997, 2005.

Pflugmacher R, Agarwal A, Kandziora F, et al.: Balloon kyphoplasty combined with posterior instrumentation for the treatment of burst fractures of the spine—1-year results, *J Orthop Trauma* 23:126, 2009.

Pinzur MS, Meyer Jr PR, Lautenschlager EP, et al.: Measurement of internal fixation device: a report in experimentally produced fractures of the dorsolumbar spine, *Orthopedics* 2:28, 1979.

Post MJD, Green BA, Stokes NA, et al.: Value of computed tomography in spinal trauma, *Spine* 7:417, 1982.

Pringle RG: The conservative management of spinal injured patients, *Semin Orthop* 4:34, 1989.

Purcell GA, Markolf KL, Dawson EG: Twelfth thoracic-first lumbar vertebral mechanical stability of fractures after Harrington rod instrumentation, *J Bone Joint Surg* 63A:71, 1981.

Rao S, Patel A, Schildhauer T: Osteogenesis imperfecta as a differential diagnosis of pathologic burst fractures of the spine, *Clin Orthop Relat Res* 289:113, 1993.

Rea GL, Zerick WR: The treatment of thoracolumbar fractures: one point of view, *J Spinal Disord* 8:368, 1995.

Rechtine GR: Nonsurgical treatment of thoracic and lumbar fractures, *Instr Course Lect* 48:413, 1999.

Rechtine GR, Bono PL, Cahill D, et al.: Postoperative wound infection after instrumentation of thoracic and lumbar fractures, *J Orthop Trauma* 15:566, 2001.

Rhea JT, Sheridan RL, Mullins ME, Novelline RA: Can chest and abdominal trauma CT eliminate the need for plain films of the spine? Experience with 329 multiple trauma patients, *Emerg Radiol* 8:99, 2001.

Rhyne III A, Banit D, Laxer E, et al.: Kyphoplasty: report of eighty-two thoracolumbar osteoporotic vertebral fractures, *J Orthop Trauma* 18:294, 2004.

Rihn JA, Anderson DT, Sasso RC, et al.: Emergency evaluation, imaging, and classification of thoracolumbar injuries, *Instr Course Lect* 58:619, 2009.

Riska EB: Antero-lateral decompression as a treatment of paraplegia following vertebral fracture in the thoraco-lumbar spine, *Int Orthop* 1:22, 1977.

Robertson PA, Sherwood MJ, Hadlow AT: Lumbosacral dislocation injuries: management and outcomes, *J Spinal Disord Tech* 18:232, 2005.

Rodger RM, Missiuna P, Ein S: Entrapment of bowel within a spinal fracture, *J Pediatr Orthop* 11:783, 1991.

Roy-Camille R, Saillant G, Gagna G, et al.: Transverse fracture of the upper sacrum: suicidal jumpers' fracture, *Spine* 10:838, 1985.

Roy-Camille R, Saillant G, Mazel C: Plating of thoracic, thoracolumbar, and lumbar injuries with pedicle screw plates, *Orthop Clin North Am* 17:147, 1986.

Roy-Camille R, Saillant G, Mazel C, et al.: *Posterior spinal fixation with transpedicular screws and plates*, Paris, 1961, Groupe Hopitalier, La Pitié Salpétriere.

Rumball K, Jarvis J: Seat-belt injuries of the spine in young children, *J Bone Joint Surg* 74B:572, 1992.

Rupp RE, Ebraheim NA, Chrissos MG, et al.: Thoracic and lumbar fractures associated with femoral shaft fractures in the multiple trauma patient: occult presentations and implications for femoral fracture stabilization, *Spine* 19:556, 1994.

Sachs BL, Makley JT, Carter JR, et al.: Primary osseous neoplasms of the thoracic and lumbar spine, *Orthop Trans* 8:422, 1984.

Sagi HC, Militano U, Caron T, et al.: A comprehensive analysis with minimum 1-year follow-up of vertically unstable transforaminal sacral fractures treated with triangular osteosynthesis, *J Orthop Trauma* 23:313, 2009.

Saiki K, Hirabayashi S, Sakai H, et al.: Traumatic anterior lumbosacral dislocation caused by hyperextension mechanism in preexisting L5 spondylolysis: a case report and review of literature, *J Spinal Disord Tech* 19:455, 2006.

Samberg LC: Fracture-dislocation of the lumbosacral spine, *J Bone Joint Surg* 57A:1107, 1975.

Sapkas G, Efstathiou P, Makris A, et al.: Thoracolumbar burst fractures: correlation between post-traumatic spinal canal stenosis and initial neurological deficit, *Bull Hosp Jt Dis* 55:36, 1996.

Saraste H: The etiology of spondylolysis: a retrospective radiographic study, *Acta Orthop Scand* 56:253, 1985.

Sasani M, Özer F: Single-stage posterior corpectomy and expandable cage placement for treatment of thoracic or lumbar burst fractures, *Spine* 34:E33, 2008.

Sasso RC, Best NM, Reilly TM, McGuire RA: Anterior-only stabilization of three-column thoracolumbar injuries, *J Spinal Disord Tech* 18:S7, 2005.

Sasso RC, Cotler HB: Posterior instrumentation and fusion for unstable fractures and fracture-dislocations of the thoracic and lumbar spine: a comparative study of three fixation devices in 70 patients, *Spine* 18:450, 1993.

Sasso RC, Cotler HB, Reuben JD: Posterior fixation of thoracic and lumbar spine fractures using DC plates and pedicle screws, *Spine* 16:S134, 1991.

Savolaine ER, Ebraheim NA, Stitgen S, et al.: Aortic rupture complicating a fracture of an ankylosed thoracic spine, *Clin Orthop Relat Res* 272:137, 1991.

Scapinelli R, Candiotto S: Spontaneous remodeling of the spinal canal after burst fractures of the low thoracic and lumbar region, *J Spinal Disord* 8:486, 1995.

Schildhauer TA, Bellabarba C, Nork SE, et al.: Decompression and lumbopelvic fixation for sacral fracture-dislocations with spino-pelvic dissociation, *J Orthop Trauma* 20:447, 2006.

Schildhauer TA, Josten C, Muhr G: Triangular osteosynthesis of vertically unstable sacrum fractures: a new concept allowing early weight bearing, *J Orthop Trauma* 12:307, 1998.

Schildhauer TA, Ledoux WR, Chapman JR, et al.: Triangular osteosynthesis and iliosacral screw fixation for unstable sacral fractures: a cadaver and biomechanical evaluation under cyclic loads, *J Orthop Trauma* 17:22, 2003.

Schmidek HH, Smith DA, Kristiansen TK: Sacral fractures, *Neurosurgery* 15:735, 1984.

Schnaid E, Eisenstein SM, Drummond-Webb J: Delayed post-traumatic cauda equina compression syndrome, *J Trauma* 25:1099, 1985.

Schnee CL, Ansell LV: Selection criteria and outcome of operative approaches for thoracolumbar burst fractures with and without neurological deficit, *J Neurosurg* 86:48, 1997.

Schweitzer KM, Vaccaro AR, Lee JY, et al.: Confusion regarding mechanisms of injury in the setting of thoracolumbar spinal trauma: a survey of the Spine Trauma Study Group (STSG), *J Spinal Disord Tech* 19:528, 2006.

Seibel R, La Duca J, Hassett JM, et al.: Blunt multiple trauma (ISS36), femur traction, and the pulmonary failure-septic state, *Ann Surg* 202:283, 1985.

Sethi MK, Schoenfeld AJ, Bono CM, et al.: The evolution of thoracolumbar injury classification systems, *Spine J* 9:780, 2009.

Seybold EA, Sweeney CA, Fredrickson BE: Functional outcome of low lumbar burst fractures: a multicenter review of operative and nonoperative treatment, *Spine* 24:2154, 1999.

Shaffrey CI, Shaffrey ME, Whitehill R, et al.: Surgical treatment of thoracolumbar fractures, *Neurosurg Clin North Am* 8:519, 1997.

Shen WJ, Shen YS: Nonsurgical treatment of three-column thoracolumbar junction burst fractures without neurologic deficit, *Spine* 24:412, 1999.

Shirado O, Kaneda K: Lumbosacral fracture-subluxation associated with bilateral fractures of the first sacral pedicles: a case report and review of the literature, *J Orthop Trauma* 9:354, 1995.

Shirado O, Kaneda K, Tadano S, et al.: Influence of disc degeneration on mechanism of thoracolumbar burst fractures, *Spine* 17:286, 1992.

Shono Y, McAfee PC, Cunningham BW: Experimental study of thoracolumbar burst fractures: a radiographic and biomechanical analysis of anterior and posterior instrumentation systems, *Spine* 19:1711, 1994.

Siebenga J, Leferink VJ, Segers MJ, et al.: Treatment of traumatic thoracolumbar spine fractures: a multicenter prospective randomized study of operative versus nonsurgical treatment, *Spine* 31:2881, 2006.

Silverman SL: The clinical consequences of vertebral compression fracture, *Bone* 13(Suppl):27, 1992.

Singer BR: The functional prognosis of thoracolumbar vertebrae fractures without neurological deficit: a long-term follow-up study of British Army personnel, *Injury* 26:519, 1995.

SLACK Incorporated: Kyphoplasty. www.slackinc.com.

Slosar Jr PJ, Patwardhan AG, Lorenz M, et al.: Instability of the lumbar burst fracture and limitations of transpedicular instrumentation, *Spine* 20:1452, 1995.

Soref J, Axdorph G, Bylund P, et al.: Treatment of patients with unstable fractures of the thoracic and lumbar spine: a follow-up of surgical and conservative treatment, *Acta Orthop Scand* 53:369, 1982.

Soumalainen O, Pääkkönen M: Fracture-dislocation of the lumbar spine without paraplegia: a case report, *Acta Orthop Scand* 55:466, 1984.

Spivak JM, Vaccaro AR, Cotler JM: Thoracolumbar spine trauma, part I: evaluation and classification, *J Am Acad Orthop Surg* 3:345, 1995.

Spivak JM, Vaccaro AR, Cotler JM: Thoracolumbar spine trauma, part II: principles of management, *J Am Acad Orthop Surg* 3:353, 1995.

Stadhouder A, Buskens E, de Klerk LW, et al.: Traumatic thoracic and lumbar spinal fractures: operative or nonoperative treatment. Comparison of two treatment strategies by means of surgeon equipoise, *Spine* 33:1006, 2008.

Stadhouder A, Öner FC, Wilson KW, et al.: Surgeon equipoise as an inclusion criterion for the evaluation of nonoperative versus operative treatment of thoracolumbar spinal injuries, *Spine J* 8:975, 2008.

Stahlman GC, Wyrsch RB, McNamara MJ: Late-onset sternomanubrial dislocation with progressive kyphotic deformity after a thoracic burst fracture, *J Orthop Trauma* 9:350, 1995.

Stanislas MJ, Latham JM, Porter KM, et al.: A high-risk group for thoracolumbar fractures, *Injury* 29:15, 1998.

Stauffer ES: Spinal cord injury syndromes, *Semin Spine Surg* 3:87, 1991.

Stauffer ES, Neil JL: Biomechanical analysis of structural stability of internal fixation in fractures of the thoracolumbar spine, *Clin Orthop Relat Res* 112:159, 1975.

Steffee AD, Sitkowski DJ: Posterior lumbar interbody fusion and plates, *Clin Orthop Relat Res* 227:99, 1988.

Stovall Jr DO, Goodrich A, MacDonald A, et al.: Pedicle screw instrumentation for unstable thoracolumbar fractures, *J South Orthop Assoc* 5:165, 1996.

Strange-Vognsen HH, Lebech A: An unusual type of fracture in the upper sacrum, *J Orthop Trauma* 5:299, 1991.

Sullivan JA: Sublaminar wiring of Harrington distraction rods for unstable thoracolumbar spine fractures, *Clin Orthop Relat Res* 189:178, 1984.

Taguchi T, Kawai S, Kaneko K, et al.: Operative management of displaced fractures of the sacrum, *J Orthop Sci* 4:347, 1999.

Taylor RS, Fritzell P, Taylor RJ: Balloon kyphoplasty in the management of vertebral compression fractures: an updated systematic review and meta-analysis, *Eur Spine J* 16:1085, 2007.

Taylor RS, Taylor RJ, Fritzell P: Balloon kyphoplasty and vertebroplasty for vertebral compression fractures: a comparative systematic review of efficacy and safety, *Spine* 31:2747, 2006.

Templeman D, Goulet J, Duwelius PJ, et al.: Internal fixation of displaced fractures of the sacrum, *Clin Orthop Relat Res* 329:180, 1996.

Tewes DP, Fisher DA, Quick DC, et al.: Lumbar transverse process fractures in professional football players, *Am J Sports Med* 23:507, 1995.

Thomas JC Jr: The Wiltse system of pedicle screw fixation. Unpublished data.

Todiere A: Severe displaced fracture of the thoracic spine without neurologic lesion: a case report, *Ital J Orthop Traumatol* 18:411, 1992.

Tötterman A, Glott T, Madsen JE, et al.: Unstable sacral fractures: associated injuries and morbidity at 1 year, *Spine* 31:E628, 2006.

Trafton PG, Boyd CA: Computed tomography of thoracic and lumbar spine injuries, *J Trauma* 24:506, 1984.

Trammell TR, Rapp G, Maxwell KM, et al.: Luque interpeduncular segmental fixation of the lumbosacral spine, *Orthop Rev* 57:20, 1991.

Transfeldt EE, White D, Bradford DS, et al.: Delayed anterior decompression in patients with spinal cord and cauda equina injuries of the thoracolumbar spine, *Spine* 15:953, 1990.

Tsou PM, Wang J, Khoo L, et al.: A thoracic and lumbar spine injury severity classification based on neurologic function grade, spinal canal deformity, and spinal biomechanical stability, *Spine J* 6:636, 2006.

Vaccaro AR: Combined anterior and posterior surgery for fractures of the thoracolumbar spine, *Instr Course Lect* 48:443, 1999.

Vaccaro AR, Lee JY, Schweitzer KM, et al.: Assessment of injury to the posterior ligamentous complex in thoracolumbar spine trauma, *Spine J* 6:524, 2006.

Vaccaro AR, Lim MR, Hurlbert J, et al.: Surgical decision making for unstable thoracolumbar spine injuries: results of a consensus panel review by the spine trauma study group, *J Spinal Disord Tech* 19:1, 2006.

Vaccaro AR, Rihn JA, Saravanja D, et al.: Injury of the posterior ligamentous complex of the thoracolumbar spine: a prospective evaluation of the diagnostic accuracy of magnetic resonance imaging, *Spine* 34:E841, 2009.

Vaccaro AR, Zeiller SC, Hulbert RJ, et al.: The thoracolumbar injury severity score: a proposed treatment algorithm, *J Spinal Disord Tech* 18:209, 2005.

Vanichkachorn JS, Vaccaro AR: Nonoperative treatment of thoracolumbar fractures, *Orthopedics* 20:948, 1997.

van Loon JL, Slot GH, Pavlov PW: Anterior instrumentation of the spine in thoracic and thoracolumbar fractures: the single rod versus the double rod Slot-Zielke device, *Spine* 21:734, 1996.

Verlaan JJ, Diekerhof CH, Buskens E, et al.: Surgical treatment of traumatic fractures of the thoracic and lumbar spine: a systematic review of the literature on techniques, complications, and outcome, *Spine* 29:803, 2004.

Villarraga ML, Bellezza AJ, Harrigan TP, et al.: The biomechanical effects of kyphoplasty on treated and adjacent nontreated vertebral bodies, *J Spinal Disord Tech* 18:84, 2005.

Vincent KA, Benson DR, McGahan JP: Intraoperative ultrasonography for reduction of thoracolumbar burst fractures, *Spine* 14:387, 1989.

Vollmer DG, Gegg C: Classification and acute management of thoracolumbar fractures, *Neurosurg Clin North Am* 8:499, 1997.

Vornanen MJ, Bostman OM, Myllynen PJ: Reduction of bone retropulsed into the spinal canal in thoracolumbar vertebral body compression burst fractures: a prospective randomized comparative study between Harrington rods and two transpedicular devices, *Spine* 20:1699, 1995.

Vornanen M, Bostman O, Keto P, et al.: The integrity of intervertebral disks after operative treatment of thoracolumbar fractures, *Clin Orthop Relat Res* 297:150, 1993.

Wang XY, Dai LY, Xu HZ, et al.: The load-sharing classification of thoracolumbar fractures: an in vitro biomechanical validation, *Spine* 32:1214, 2007.

Weinstein JN, Collalto P, Lehmann TR: Long-term follow-up of nonoperatively treated thoracolumbar spine fractures, *J Orthop Trauma* 1:152, 1987.

Wenger DR, Carollo JJ: The mechanics of thoracolumbar fractures stabilized by segmental fixation, *Clin Orthop Relat Res* 189:89, 1984.

Wenger DR, Carollo JJ, Wilkerson JA, et al.: Laboratory testing of segmental spinal instrumentation vs traditional Harrington instrumentation for scoliosis treatment, *Spine* 7:265, 1982.

Wenger DR, Miller S, Wilkerson J: *Evaluation of fixation sites for segmental instrumentation of human vertebrae*, Montreal, 1981, Paper presented at the Sixteenth Annual Meeting of the Scoliosis Research Society.

Whang PG, Vaccaro AR, Poelstra KA, et al.: The influence of fracture mechanism and morphology on the reliability and validity of two novel thoracolumbar injury classification systems, *Spine* 32:791, 2007.

White RR, Newberg A, Seligson D: Computerized tomographic assessment of the traumatized dorsolumbar spine before and after Harrington instrumentation, *Clin Orthop Relat Res* 146:149, 1980.

Whitesides Jr TE, Shah SGA: On the management of unstable fractures of the thoracolumbar spine: rationale for use of anterior decompression and fusion and posterior stabilization, *Spine* 1:99, 1976.

Wilber RG, Thompson GH, Shaffer JW, et al.: Postoperative neurological deficits in segmental spinal instrumentation, *J Bone Joint Surg* 66A:1178, 1984.

Wilcox RK, Boerger TO, Allen DJ, et al.: A dynamic study of thoracolumbar burst fractures, *J Bone Joint Surg* 85A:2184, 2003.

Wilcox RK, Boerger TO, Hall RM: Measurement of canal occlusion during the thoracolumbar burst fracture process, *J Biomech* 35:381, 2002.

Willin J, Anderson J, Toomoka K, et al.: The natural history of burst fracture at the thoracolumbar junction, *J Spinal Disord* 3:39, 1990.

Willen J, Dahiiof AG, Nordwall A: Paraplegia in unstable thoracolumbar injuries: a study of conservative and operative treatment regarding neurological improvement and rehabilitation, *J Rehab Med* 9:195, 1983.

Wood K, Butterman G, Mehbod A, et al.: Operative compared with nonoperative treatment of a thoracolumbar burst fracture without neurological deficit: a prospective randomized study, *J Bone Joint Surg* 85A:773, 2003.

Wood KB, Garvey TA, Gundry C, et al.: Magnetic resonance imaging of the thoracic spine: evaluation of asymptomatic individuals, *J Bone Joint Surg* 77A:1631, 1995.

Wood KB, Khanna G, Vaccaro AR, et al.: Assessment of two thoracolumbar fracture classification systems as used by multiple surgeons, *J Bone Joint Surg* 87A:1423, 2005.

Yazici M, Atilla B, Tepe S, et al.: Spinal canal remodeling in burst fractures of the thoracolumbar spine: a computerized tomographic comparison between operative and nonoperative treatment, *J Spinal Disord* 9:409, 1996.

Yazici M, Gulman B, Sen S, et al.: Sagittal contour restoration and canal clearance in burst fractures of the thoracolumbar junction (T12-L1): the efficacy of timing of the surgery, *J Orthop Trauma* 9:491, 1995.

Yi L, Jingping B, Gele J, et al.: Operative versus non-operative treatment for thoracolumbar burst fractures without neurological deficit (review), *Cochrane Database Syst Rev* 8(4):CD005079, 2006.

York DH, Watts C, Raffensberger M, et al.: Utilization of somatosensory evoked cortical potentials in spinal cord injury, *Spine* 8:832, 1983.

Zdeblick TA: *Z-plate anterior thoracolumbar instrumentation: surgical technique, Memphis*, TN, 2006, Danek Medical.

Zdeblick TA, Shirado O, McAfee PC, et al.: Anterior spinal fixation after lumbar corpectomy: a study in dogs, *J Bone Joint Surg* 73A:527, 1991.

Zelle BA, Gruen GS, Hunt T, Speth SR: Sacral fractures with neurological injury: is early decompression beneficial? *Int Orthop* 28:244, 2004.

Zindrick MR: The role of transpedicular fixation systems for stabilization of the lumbar spine, *Orthop Clin North Am* 22:333, 1991.

Zindrick MR, Wiltse LL, Doornik A, et al.: Analysis of the morphometric characteristics of the thoracic and lumbar pedicles, *Spine* 12:160, 1987.

Zoltan JD, Gilula LA, Murphy WA: Unilateral facet dislocation between the fifth lumbar and first sacral vertebrae: case report, *J Bone Joint Surg* 61A:767, 1979.

Zou D, Yoo JU, Edwards WT, et al.: Mechanics of anatomic reduction of thoracolumbar burst fractures, *Spine* 18:195, 1993.

CHAPTER 6

INFECTIONS AND TUMORS OF THE SPINE

Keith D. Williams

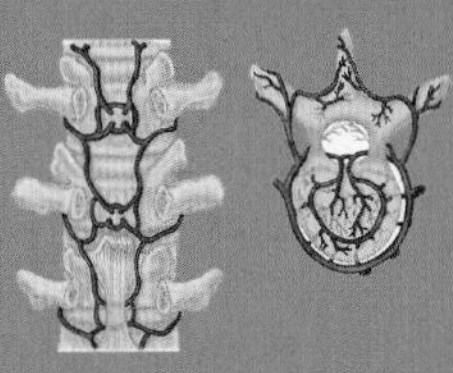

INFECTIONS OF THE SPINE

Spinal infections are relatively uncommon but serious conditions, accounting for 3% to 5% of all osteomyelitis cases. Unfortunately, delays in diagnosis and treatment are common due to the manner in which these infections present. Symptoms may be vague, and there are no pathognomonic clinical signs or definitive laboratory tests to make the diagnosis. Spinal infections can be categorized into different groups based on location of infection, mode of transmission, and infecting pathogen. The location can be in the vertebral body, disc space, paraspinal region, or epidural space. Transmission of the infection can occur by hematogenous seeding, contiguous spread, or direct inoculation. Pathogens can be gram positive, with *Staphylococcus aureus* being the most common, gram negative, fungal, or acid-fast.

SPINAL ANATOMY

Knowledge of the structure and composition of the spinal elements is essential to understanding spinal infections. The nucleus pulposus is avascular in adults, receiving nutrients through perforations in the cartilaginous end plates of the intervertebral discs. Coventry et al. in 1945, in a microscopic study, found that in adults older than 30 years of age there is no direct vascular supply to the disc. They noted multiple openings in the end plates of the vertebral bodies. These allow for the transport of nutrients through the end plates into the central portion of the adult disc.

The microvasculature of the vertebral bony end plates contains vessels oriented obliquely. These were found to originate from the circumferential vessels fed from the arterial plexus outside the perichondrium and from nearby metaphyseal marrow vessels. The bony end plate, which is vascular, seems to be the anatomic area in which the arterial supply ends. The perforations in the cartilaginous end plates of the disc may allow the ingress of bacterial or fungal pathogens into the disc. Hematogenous spread of infection is more commonly arterial than venous.

PYOGENIC VERTEBRAL OSTEOMYELITIS AND DISCITIS

Pyogenic vertebral osteomyelitis and discitis represent 3% to 5% of all cases of pyogenic osteomyelitis. There is a bimodal age distribution with a small peak in childhood and then a larger spike in adulthood around the age of 50. Males are affected more frequently than females. Pyogenic osteomyelitis and discitis are most common in the lumbar spine (50% to 60%), followed by thoracic (30% to 40%) and cervical spine (10%). Seventeen percent of infected patients present with neurologic deficits. Infections higher in the spine are more likely to present with neurologic deficit. Infections in the cervical and thoracic regions are also more likely to be multifocal with noncontiguous foci of infection. The reported incidence of distant foci of infection ranges from 10% to 35% and requires imaging of the entire spine. The most common organism reported is *S. aureus* (65%). Drug abusers have been noted to more likely have *Pseudomonas aeruginosa* infections. Infections caused by *Enterococci* and *Streptococci* species are associated with endocarditis as the primary source of infection.

Pyogenic vertebral osteomyelitis and discitis usually result from the hematogenous spread of pyogenic bacteria. The bacteria may originate from an infection in the urinary tract, respiratory tract, soft tissue, or elsewhere. The arterial spread of infection originates in the endplate of the vertebra. The highly vascular end plate is an area with high volume and slow blood flow—an environment that provides conditions conducive for microorganism seeding and growth. Blood borne organisms sludging in these low-flow anastomoses can lead to a local suppurative infection. This infection can cause tissue necrosis, bony collapse, and spread of the infection into the adjacent intervertebral disc spaces, the epidural space, or into paravertebral structures. In addition, the insertion of fibers of the anterior longitudinal ligament described by Coventry appears to serve as conduits for infection of the intervertebral disc, particularly tuberculosis. The course of the infection varies with the infecting organism and the patient's immune status. The infection itself may create a malnourished condition that compromises the immune system.

Neurologic deficit from spinal infection may occur early or late. Early-onset deficits frequently suggest epidural extension of an abscess. Late-onset deficits may be caused by the development of significant kyphosis, vertebral collapse with retropulsion of bone and debris, late abscess formation in more indolent infections, or delay in diagnosis. A recent longitudinal hospital database study by Issa et al. found that the incidence of vertebral osteomyelitis was 4.8/100,000 admissions and has been increasing over recent decades. Mortality was found to be 2.1% and was higher for males, older patients, and those with a higher comorbidity score. In particular, congestive heart failure, cerebrovascular disease, liver disease, hepatitis C, and renal disease were associated with higher mortality risks.

CLINICAL PRESENTATION

The most common presenting symptom of spinal infection is back pain or neck pain. No pathognomonic features of the pain occur with vertebral osteomyelitis or discitis, which can lead to a delay in diagnosis. Pain often is worse at night and can occur with changes in position, ambulation, and other forms of activity. The intensity of the pain varies from mild to extreme. Constitutional symptoms include anorexia, malaise, night sweats, intermittent fever, and weight loss. Spinal deformity may be a late presentation of the disease. Neurologic deficits are a serious complication but rarely are the presenting complaint. A history of an immune-suppressing disease or a recent infection, or both, is common.

Temperature elevation, if present, usually is minimal. Localized tenderness over the involved area is the most common physical sign. Sustained paraspinal spasm also is indicative of the acute process. Limitation of motion of the involved spinal segments because of pain is frequent. Torticollis may result from infection in the cervical spine, and bizarre posturing and physical positions that could be considered psychogenic in origin are possible. Other possible findings include the Kernig sign (severe tightness of the hamstring) and generalized weakness. Clinical findings in elderly and immunosuppressed individuals may be minimal.

Because of the depth of the spine, abscess formation is difficult to identify unless it points superficially. Frequently, these areas of abscess pointing are some distance from the primary process. A paraspinal abscess commonly presents as a swelling in the groin below the Poupart ligament (inguinal ligament) because of extension along the psoas muscle.

The development of neurologic signs should suggest the possibility of neural compression from abscess formation, bone collapse, or direct neural infection. Neurologic findings rarely are radicular and more frequently involve multiple myotomes and dermatomes. As might be expected, neurologic symptoms become more frequent at higher spinal levels; they are most frequent with infections in the cervical and thoracic areas and are least common with infections in the lumbar region. When neurologic symptoms appear, they can progress rapidly unless active decompression or drainage is undertaken.

LABORATORY STUDIES

The erythrocyte sedimentation rate (ESR) is used to help identify and clinically monitor spinal infections. The ESR is not diagnostic and indicates only an inflammatory process. The ESR is elevated in 71% to 97% of children with vertebral osteomyelitis. In 37% of adults with osteomyelitis, the rate is greater than 100 mm/h, and in 67%, rates greater than 50 mm/h are noted. The ESR normally is elevated after surgery (approximately 25 mm/h), peaking at 5 days but may stay elevated for 4 weeks. Persistent elevation of the ESR 4 weeks after surgery, with associated clinical findings, indicates the presence of infection.

C-reactive protein (CRP) has proven to be a more sensitive marker for early detection of postoperative spine infections when compared with ESR. CRP levels tend to peak within the first 2 postoperative days and then decline rapidly. A continued elevation of the CRP in the immediate postoperative period (4 to 7 days) or a second rise is a strong indicator of an infection. Thelander and Larsson compared the CRP with the ESR as an indicator of infection after surgery on the spine, including microscopic and conventional disc excision and anterior and posterior spinal fusion. They noted in all patients that results of both tests were elevated initially after the surgery, but in all the patients the CRP value had returned to normal by 14 days whereas the ESR took much longer to return to normal. The CRP also can be used to monitor the antibiotic treatment of an infection because of its rapid return to normal with resolution of the infection. The ESR may be elevated for weeks in a treated infection.

More recently, procalcitonin (PCT) has been found to be a useful marker for infection generally. Aljabi et al. found PCT to be a more sensitive and specific infection marker than CRP in 200 postoperative patients. In addition, the biokinetics of PCT were not affected by the surgical procedure. Other biomarkers such as presepsin are also being evaluated to help identify infection.

Leukocytosis is not especially helpful in diagnosing spinal infection. White blood cell counts may decrease in infants and debilitated patients. High white blood cell counts may indicate areas of infection other than the spine. Blood cultures are helpful if positive, which usually occurs in times of active sepsis with a febrile illness, and may be adequate for the diagnosis and treatment of osteomyelitis, but this occurrence is rare.

IMAGING TECHNIQUES

The purpose of diagnostic techniques is confirmation of the clinical impression. Because clinical findings are nonspecific, imaging findings play a key role in the diagnosis of spinal infection. In spinal infection, no single diagnostic technique is 100% effective as a confirmatory test. Culture of the organism from the infected tissue is the most definitive test, but

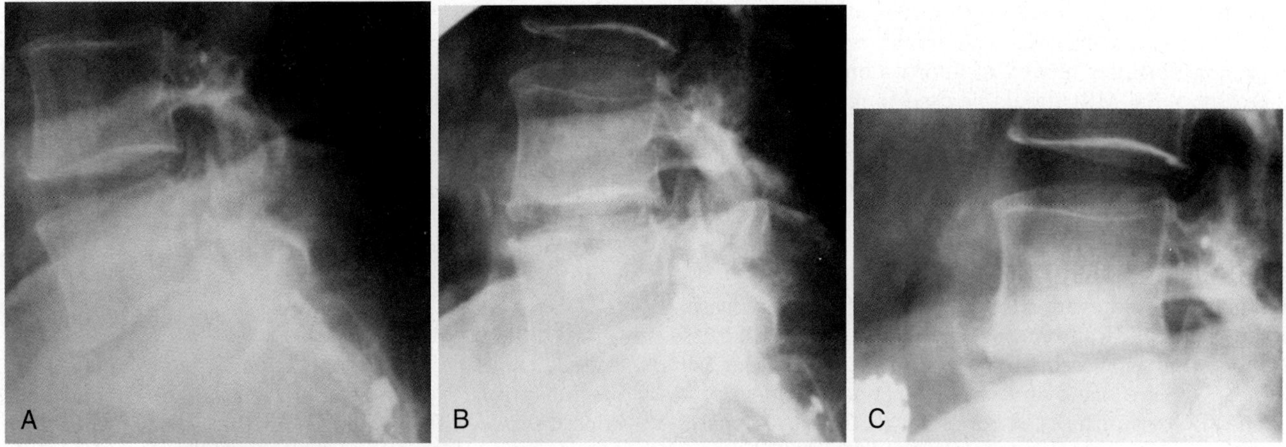

FIGURE 6.1 Radiographic appearance of spinal osteomyelitis. **A,** Minimal disc space narrowing but normal end plate and subchondral region. **B,** Reduction of disc height associated with destruction of endplate and development of subchondral lytic defects. **C,** After successful treatment, note sclerotic vertebra and large osteophyte. (From Acker JD, Wood GW II, Moinuddin M, et al: Radiologic manifestations of spinal infection, *State Art Rev Spine* 3:403, 1989.)

results may be falsely negative even under the most optimal conditions. Likewise, all imaging and laboratory studies may be inconclusive, depending on the time at which they are done relative to the onset of infection.

RADIOGRAPHY

Plain radiographs of the involved area are the most common initial study in patients with spinal infection. Radiographic findings, which appear 2 weeks to 3 months after the onset of the infection, include disc space narrowing, vertebral end plate irregularity or loss of the normal contour of the end plate, defects in the subchondral portion of the end plate, and hypertrophic (sclerotic) bone formation (Fig. 6.1). Occasionally, paravertebral soft-tissue masses may be noted with involvement of nearby areas of the spine. Late radiographic findings may include vertebral collapse, segmental kyphosis, and bony ankylosis. The sequence of events may range from 2 to 8 weeks for early findings to more than 2 years for later findings. The only definable abnormality on plain radiographs and CT scans related specifically to tuberculosis is fine calcification in the paravertebral soft-tissue space.

COMPUTED TOMOGRAPHY

CT adds another dimension to the plain radiographs. CT identifies paravertebral soft-tissue swelling and abscesses much more readily and can monitor changes in the size of the spinal canal. Some clinicians prefer CT to radiography for determining clinical progress. Findings with CT are similar to findings with plain radiographs, including lytic defects in the subchondral bone, destruction of the end plate with irregularity or multiple holes visible in the cross-sectional views, sclerosis near the lytic irregularities, hypodensity of the disc, flattening of the disc itself, disruption of the circumferential bone near the periphery of the disc, and soft-tissue density in the epidural and paraspinal regions. Postmyelogram CT more clearly defines compression of the neural elements by abscess or bone impingement and helps determine whether the infection extends to the neural structures themselves, but there is a risk of seeding the subarachnoid space.

MAGNETIC RESONANCE IMAGING

MRI with and without contrast is the imaging modality of choice for identifying spinal infection. MRI has a reported sensitivity of 96% and specificity of 93% for spinal infections. The entire spine should be imaged because of the frequency of noncontiguous infection. MRI (T1 hypointense and T2 hyperintense) identifies infected and normal tissues and best determines the full extent of the infection. MRI does not differentiate between pyogenic and non-pyogenic infections and cannot eliminate the need for diagnostic biopsy. To detect infection, T1- and T2-weighted views in the sagittal plane should be obtained. T1-weighted images have a decreased signal intensity in the vertebral bodies and disc spaces in patients with vertebral osteomyelitis. The margin between the disc and the adjacent vertebral body cannot be differentiated. In T2-weighted images, the signal intensity is increased in the vertebral disc and is markedly increased in the vertebral body. Abscesses in the paravertebral soft tissue around the thecal sac can be readily identified as areas of increased signal intensity on T2-weighted sequences. Fat-suppression techniques improve the sensitivity of T2 and postgadolinium T1 sequences. In recent years, the addition of diffusion-weighted imaging (DWI) has been used to characterize fluid collections to differentiate spondylodiscitis from benign reactive marrow changes. MRI also is useful to identify primary spinal cord infections (myelitis) without epidural or bone involvement. The addition of gadolinium enhances the delineation of epidural abscesses and to delineate further the extent of spinal infection.

Using serial MRI to follow the response to treatment of spine infections may not be clinically useful depending on what is being evaluated. Follow-up MRI has shown that bony findings of vertebral body enhancement, marrow edema, and compression fractures often appeared unchanged or worse in the setting of clinical improvement. Soft-tissue findings of paraspinal abscesses, epidural abscesses, and T2 disc space abnormalities tended to improve on follow-up MRI. Therefore, serial MRI should be used to monitor soft-tissue findings not bony findings. Furthermore, the clinical findings, such as decreased pain and improved neurologic function, seem to be better indicators than an improvement seen on MRI.

RADIONUCLIDE SCANNING

Radionuclide studies are relatively effective in identifying spinal infection and can be used as an adjunct to MRI. These techniques include technetium-99m (^{99m}Tc) bone scan, gallium-67 (^{67}Ga) scan, and indium-111–labeled leukocyte (^{111}In WBC) scan. The ^{99m}Tc bone scan has three basic phases: angiogram, blood pool images, and delayed static images. In infection, diffuse increased activity is seen on the blood pool images; the diffuse activity becomes focally increased on delayed views. This marked reactivity may persist for months. Bone scans are generally positive in patients with infection, but they are not specifically diagnostic of infection and false-negatives do occur. The ^{67}Ga scan is a good adjunct to ^{99m}Tc scanning for the detection of osteomyelitis, especially the soft-tissue infection that accompanies spondylodiscitis. A sensitivity of 90%, specificity of 100%, and accuracy of 94% in patients having combined ^{99m}Tc and ^{67}Ga scanning for infection have been reported. ^{67}Ga scans alone are not as accurate as the combination of ^{99m}Tc scan and a ^{67}Ga scan for identifying infection. They also do not identify the type of organism involved. Because the ^{67}Ga scan changes rapidly with the resolution of the acute active infection, it may be useful to document clinical improvement.

The ^{111}In WBC scan is useful in detecting abscesses but it is not reliable in acute infections. False-negative ^{111}In WBC scans have been reported in chronic infections also. Neoplastic noninfectious inflammatory lesions may lead to similar false-positive results with all scanning techniques. One major advantage of ^{111}In WBC scanning is that it differentiates between noninfectious lesions, such as hematomas or seromas and true infection, all which may appear as a mass or an abscess-like cavity on MRI or CT. Differentiation is important in the postoperative evaluation of potential infections.

DIAGNOSTIC BIOPSY

Biopsy of the suspected lesion is the best method of determining infection and identifying the causative agent so that appropriate antibiotics can be administered. Current guidelines from the Infectious Disease Society of America recommend direct tissue biopsy with image guidance when clinical and imaging findings suggest spinal infection and blood cultures are negative. These same guidelines recommend withholding antibiotics in hemodynamically stable patients without neurologic deficits until after biopsy is done. Biopsy may be obtained percutaneously through a CT-guided needle procedure or by an open procedure. Biopsy, however, may not yield a pathogen. Administration of antibiotics before biopsy, inadequate biopsy, or the elapse of a long period between the onset of the disease and the biopsy may result in a negative biopsy. A systematic review by McNamara et al. found an average yield of 48% for the diagnosis of spondylodiscitis using CT-guided biopsy. Open surgical biopsy results are reported positive in 76% of patients. Obtaining core biopsies of subchondral bone may improve diagnostic yield. Often abscess fluid is sterile and should not be sought for biopsy.

Negative results from percutaneous biopsy should not preclude open biopsy if there is good clinical evidence of infection. Razak, Kamari, and Roohi reported only 22% positive results with percutaneous biopsy and 93% positive results with open biopsy. Marschall et al. likewise demonstrated that open biopsy had a higher microbiologic yield than needle biopsies.

DIFFERENTIAL DIAGNOSIS

The differential diagnosis of spinal osteomyelitis should include primary and metastatic malignancies, metabolic bone diseases with pathologic fractures, and infections in contiguous and related structures, including the psoas muscle, hip joint, abdominal cavity, and genitourinary system. Rheumatoid arthritis and ankylosing spondylitis and Charcot spinal arthropathy may also cause findings resembling osteomyelitis of the spine. Acquired immunodeficiency syndrome may be another underlying factor in these infections. Myelitis from bacterial infection also has similar findings and distinctive MRI findings.

NONOPERATIVE TREATMENT

Antibiotic treatment for vertebral osteomyelitis and discitis infections in adults is the primary therapy. Surgery is reserved for disease progression despite appropriate antimicrobial therapy, spinal instability with spinal cord or cauda equina compression or impending significant neural compression, and drainage of an epidural abscess. The antibiotic is chosen according to the positive stains, cultures, and sensitivities of the organism. Response to treatment is evaluated by observing clinical symptoms and serially following CRP levels and PCT levels. Failure of antibiotic therapy suggests the presence of a multiorganism infection, and repeat biopsy, including open biopsy, should be considered. Consideration should also be given to surgical debridement of sequestered bone and abscess drainage if there is no clinical improvement with antibiotic therapy.

The time for discontinuing antibiotic therapy also varies. Collert suggested that antibiotic therapy should be continued until the ESR returns to normal. Unfortunately the ESR can stay elevated for a prolonged period even in a treated infection. CRP values decline more rapidly and may be a better gauge to base discontinuance of antibiotics, but currently this factor is still being studied. Intravenous antibiotics usually are continued for about 6 weeks and are followed by oral antibiotics as indicated by the CRP, ESR, and clinical response.

With an adequate biopsy and a reliable patient who responds rapidly to antibiotics, hospitalization and bed rest usually are required only for the primary symptoms. Home-administered intravenous antibiotics allow the patient to complete treatment out of the hospital. A major risk with this technique is late pathologic fracture of the infected bone. In patients who are at risk for fracture or are in pain, a brace is used. If ambulatory therapy is chosen, thorough education and close monitoring of the patient are mandatory.

PROGNOSIS

Even if an absolute diagnosis is not made, most spinal infections resolve symptomatically and radiographically within 9 to 24 months of onset. Recurrence of infection and periods of decreased immune response are always possible, as are delayed complications of kyphosis, paralysis, and myelopathy. These risks are greatest during the period when the infection is controlled but the bone is still soft, when the healing process has not advanced to the point where solid bone has formed around the infected tissue. Bracing is strongly recommended in these patients.

OPERATIVE TREATMENT

Surgical intervention is indicated when medical management has failed, when there is a neurologic deficit from either an abscess, or instability with deformity, or when a diagnosis is not otherwise possible. The location of the infection, extent of bony destruction, and presence of neurologic involvement dictate the surgical approach and the surgical objectives. Several recent studies have reported endoscopic procedures to obtain biopsy material for culture and abscess drainage with results similar to open biopsy. Posterior-only surgery is generally not indicated in patients with spondylodiscitis, although some with a significant epidural abscess component may be appropriate for posterior decompression only. Because vertebral osteomyelitis and discitis typically affect the vertebral bodies and discs, an approach that allows thorough debridement of this area and reconstruction is usually necessary. Surgical planning is nuanced, and the need for posterior stabilization is determined primarily by the stability and length of the anterior construct. In the cervical spine, an anterior-only approach often is adequate; however, supplemental posterior instrumentation may also be required, as shown by Ackshota et al. in a study of 56 patients with multilevel cervical corpectomy. The vertebral body can be accessed from an anterior or posterior approach in the thoracic or lumbar spine. Whether an anterior, posterior, or combined approach is used, the objective of surgery is to perform a thorough debridement with decompression of the neural elements and stabilization of the spine with correction of the deformity. Often this requires a corpectomy and the need for anterior reconstruction with an interbody graft or cage. The interbody graft can be an allograft or autograft bone strut, and a mesh or expandable cage can be packed with allograft or autograft. Various studies have shown that all these interbody devices are acceptable. Often supplementation with anterior and/or posterior instrumentation is needed for added stability and to correct deformity.

SPECIFIC INFECTIONS

INFECTIONS IN CHILDREN

Primary pyogenic spinal infections are uncommon in children. These infections have been divided into three clinical presentations based on the age of the child. Neonatal spondylodiscitis is rare, but the most serious form occurs between birth and 6 months and usually is due to *S. aureus.* This infection often is multifocal and associated with septicemia, causing some to consider it differently from spondylodiscitis in older children. The second group is infantile spondylodiscitis, which occurs from 6 months to 4 years of age. About 50% to 60% of all cases occur in this age group. Dayer et al. found that these infections are more often caused by *Kingella kingae.* The juvenile/adolescent group of children are those between 4 and 16 years of age. In this group *S. aureus* again is the most common pathogen. In children who are old enough, the syndrome frequently is associated with difficulty in walking, irritability, and sudden inability to stand or walk comfortably. Most reports indicate that the cause is hematogenous spread of a bacterial infection, although trauma also has been implicated, and males are more commonly afflicted. When positive, most blood culture reports are positive for *S. aureus.* Unfortunately, blood cultures are positive in only about 10% of cases. Even needle aspirations provide negative cultures in over 50% of patients, making it difficult to recommend due to the associated risks.

The average age at onset is 4 to 5 years, although the age group most commonly affected are 6 months to 4 years of age. Symptoms usually are present for 4 weeks before hospitalization, and the lumbar spine is most commonly affected. Physical findings are limited. The child may refuse to walk or may cry when walking, and spinal flexion may be limited and so painful that the child holds himself or herself erect. Physical findings directly related to the spine are rare. Neurologic findings are uncommon but are ominous when present. In older children, abdominal pain may be a presenting symptom. Other, less frequent symptoms include hamstring tightness and spinal tenderness.

Diagnosing disc space infection (vertebral osteomyelitis) in children is difficult early, and plain radiographs usually are negative. There may be a mild febrile reaction, but patients do not appear systemically ill. Laboratory investigation often reveals only a mildly elevated CRP and ESR in most patients, and patients usually are afebrile. The ESR has been found to be elevated more often than the CRP, and elevated platelet counts also are common. Polymerase chain reaction tests have become a very useful tool in the past decade, especially in diagnosing *K. kingae* using a throat swab. Older children are more likely to present with fever and laboratory findings of acute illness. The best test to identify the infection is MRI with and without gadolinium, or a combination of bone scanning and ^{67}Ga scanning, although there is a significant radiation dose with nuclear medicine studies. These scans are not always diagnostic, and other possibilities, including inflammatory processes and tumors, may give false-positive results. Spondylodiscitis represents a continuum of disease. Most commonly the disc and the vertebrae on both sides of the disc space are affected; however, in a small portion of patients, discitis affects only the disc, and in others only vertebral osteomyelitis occurs. The treatment of discitis in children is organism-specific intravenous antibiotics and bed rest without immobilization until the child can walk and move around comfortably and then oral antibiotics for an additional period of time. Most patients are symptom free within several months. Spontaneous fusion occurs in about 25% of patients. Surgical procedures rarely are required, and persistent back pain rarely is a problem in children. Cast or brace immobilization has been recommended if pain or difficulty in walking persists; most frequently this is necessary in older children. Surgical treatment rarely is needed in children except in tuberculosis and other caseating diseases that have not responded well to antibiotics alone.

Special situations involving patients with immune suppression, suspected drug use, tumorous conditions, or poor response to conservative treatment require more vigorous evaluation by needle aspiration biopsy for culture and sensitivity. CT-guided percutaneous biopsy, with the patient under sedation, makes this a relatively safe procedure, but rates of positive culture are disappointingly low. Definitive diagnosis and organism-specific antibiotic treatment constitute the most efficient method of dealing with these infections.

SPINAL EPIDURAL ABSCESS (SEA)

Epidural infections have a low reported incidence of 2 to 10 cases per 10,000 hospital admissions per year and have increased with an aging population. The incidence of this infection is increased in immunosuppressed patients and intravenous drug users. Morbidity and mortality can be high with epidural infections when significant neurologic deficits are present and when the diagnosis is delayed. The neurologic risk is highest in the cervical spine and lowest in the lumbar spine below the conus. Fortunately, most SEAs occur in the lower lumbar region. The causes of infection are the same as those for osteomyelitis and discitis: direct extension from infected adjacent structures, which is by far the most common; hematogenous spread; and iatrogenic inoculation. Epidural abscess usually spans three to five vertebral segments. Longitudinal and circumferential extension of epidural infections is believed to be limited by the spinal canal anatomy. Using cryomicrotome sectioning, Hogan showed that the epidural space is discontinuous circumferentially and longitudinally. A SEA caused by direct extension from a vertebral osteomyelitis usually is on the ventral side of the canal anterior to the thecal sac, and extension from an infected facet joint often presents with an abscess posterior to the thecal sac.

The clinical findings are similar to those of osteomyelitis but with several distinct differences: (1) a more rapid development of neurologic symptoms (days instead of weeks), (2) a more acute febrile illness, and (3) signs of meningeal irritation, including radicular pain with a positive straight-leg raising test and neck rigidity. The classic progression of the disease is generalized spinal ache, nerve root pain, weakness, and finally paralysis, which can occur within 7 to 10 days. The diagnosis of SEA is based primarily on MRI with gadolinium. This study can determine the presence of contiguous spondylodiscitis or facet infection, whether the SEA is anterior or posterior to the thecal sac, and the spinal levels of involvement. Diagnosing a SEA quickly after presentation of the patient may allow medical management if there is no neurologic involvement. SEA without neurologic involvement and a known organism usually can be managed with antibiotic therapy alone, which in recent years has led to a trend away from surgical management. Medical management does require close clinical follow-up, as cases that progress to neurologic deficit have a worse prognosis. The clinical course is more important than follow-up imaging in determining a change to operative management.

There is controversy over the etiology of neurologic impairment. Some authors believe that it is the result of mechanical compression, whereas others implicate vascular changes. At least the initial neurologic deficits appear to be mechanical and usually can be reversed with decompression within 36 hours. Although progression of the process is usually slow enough to allow evaluation and preparation without endangering the patient, failure to provide prompt drainage in the cervical and thoracic spine can result in serious neurologic deficit and possibly death. Purported independent predictors of failure of nonoperative management of SEAs include age over 65 years, diabetes, methicillin-resistant *S. aureus*, elevated CRP, and WBC counts; however, to date these have not been validated. Nonoperative medical management demands close observation and more active intervention if necessary. Medical management should be avoided in patients with cervical SEA. Alton et al. reported a 75% failure rate and unacceptably poor motor score outcomes with medical management of cervical SEA when compared with surgical management. They recommended that all patients with cervical SEA have early decompression to optimize motor function. In addition management of contiguous infection is important. SEA resulting from spondylodiscitis with spinal instability and collapse with neurologic compromise is more likely than SEA caused by spinal instability from posterior element infection.

The primary methods of treatment are appropriate antibiotic therapy and surgical drainage. Antibiotic treatment should be based on culture results whenever possible. Blood cultures and CT-guided biopsy of the infected adjacent structures and aspiration of paraspinal abscesses are appropriate. While there are reports of SEA decompression by CT-guided aspiration, this is not our recommendation and has significant technical limitations. Antibiotics should be held until cultures are obtained in patients who are hemodynamically and neurologically stable. Most cases of SEA are caused by gram-positive bacteria, *S. aureus*, *Staphylococcus* sp., enterococci, coagulase-negative staphylococci, and streptococci. Empiric therapy should provide coverage for these organisms.

The method of surgical treatment requires an accurate assessment of the location of the abscess and the presence of an associated osteomyelitis. Acute or chronic isolated dorsal (posterior), lateral, and some ventral (anterior) infections are best treated with total laminectomy for drainage, with closure over drains or secondary closure at a later date. Epidural infections associated with osteomyelitis are best exposed by anterior or posterolateral exposures that allow treatment of the osteomyelitis and the epidural infection. Laminectomy in patients with ventral (anterior) osteomyelitis results in late deformity and collapse, so posterior instrumentation should be used.

Other intraspinal infections include subdural spinal abscess and spinal cord abscess. These infections are rare. Subdural spinal abscesses progress at a slower pace than epidural abscesses and can be confused with tumors. Treatment requires durotomy without opening the arachnoid mater, thorough debridement, and dural closure if possible. Spinal cord abscesses cause pronounced incontinence and long tract signs. They frequently are confused with intramedullary tumors and transverse myelitis. In both of these conditions, the bone scan is normal, but the ^{67}Ga scan should be positive. MRI, preferably with gadolinium contrast, is extremely helpful in defining the extent of the abscess. Some spinal cord abscesses can be treated successfully with antibiotics alone. Tung et al. noted that weakness at follow-up was associated with 50% or more narrowing of the central canal, peripheral contrast enhancement, and abnormal spinal cord signal intensity. Incomplete recovery was associated with abscess size and the severity of canal narrowing.

SURGICAL SITE INFECTIONS

Postoperative infections are usually pyogenic and occur shortly after an operation. Preventive measures should be taken to decrease the risk of infection. The most common source for surgical site infection (SSI) is contamination of the surgical wound by the patient's endogenous skin flora, most often *S. aureus*. A consistent and systematic approach is necessary to minimize the risk of SSI. Patient selection

TABLE 6.1

Recommendations for Minimizing Spinal Wound Infections

PREOPERATIVE RECOMMENDATIONS

- Whenever possible, identify and treat all infections remote to the surgical site before the elective procedure.
- Postpone elective operations on patients with remote site infections until the infection has resolved.
- Have patient use 2% chlorhexidine gluconate disposable cloth wipes the night before surgery and again in the holding area before the procedure.
- Do not remove hair preoperatively unless it will interfere with the operation.
- If hair is removed, remove immediately before the operation, preferably with electric clippers.
- Control serum blood glucose such that preoperative hemoglobin A1c is 7% or lower in in all diabetic patients. Avoid hyperglycemia perioperatively.
- Encourage tobacco cessation; at a minimum, instruct patients to abstain from smoking cigarettes, cigars, or pipes or from any other form of tobacco consumption (e.g., chewing/dipping) for at least 30 days before elective operation.

OPERATING ROOM

- Prophylactic antibiotics should be given 30 min prior to the incision and redose after 3-4 h or 1500 mL blood loss.
- Do not use flash sterilization for instruments or equipment.
- Reduce traffic in and out of the operating room.
- Release soft-tissue retraction regularly.
- Irrigate regularly.
- Irrigate wound with dilute povidone-iodine solution (35 mL aqueous Betadine 10% solution/1000 mL saline) before wound closure.
- Consider adding 1 g of vancomycin powder to bone graft before implantation and placing 1 g of vancomycin powder in the wound after fascial closure.
- Maintain strict aseptic techniques.
- Close and seal wounds.
- Maintain sterile dressings in the immediate postoperative period unless the wound is chemically sealed.

POSTOPERATIVE MANAGEMENT

- Concomitant infections (e.g., urinary tract infections, pneumonia) should be aggressively evaluated and treated.
- Sterile dressings should be maintained for 48 h.
- Nutritional status of the patient should be carefully maintained, particularly during the postoperative period.

Modified from Singh K, Heller JG: Postoperative spinal infections, *Contemp Spine Surg* 6:61, 2005.

criteria and medical optimization including glycemic control (hemoglobin A1c <7%), cessation of nicotine at least 4 weeks preoperatively, decreased preoperative skin bacterial burden, appropriate antibiotic prophylaxis, antiseptic skin preparation, aseptic surgical techniques, and perioperative management are among other important measures (Table 6.1). Patients with instrumentation have been found to have significantly higher ESR and CRP values than patients without instrumentation, but these parameters normally decrease after surgery unless infection is present. Patients with postoperative infection usually have a renewed elevation of these parameters. Wound drainage occurs commonly at an average of 3 to 5 days after surgery; however, fever is less common. There usually is back pain and tenderness to palpation with wound erythema. Deep wound infections can occur up to 90 days postoperatively.

The Spine Patient Outcome Research Trial study of lumbar degenerative conditions showed the overall incidence of infection to be 2% after procedures for disc herniation, 2.5% after spinal stenosis surgery, and 4% after surgery for degenerative spondylolisthesis. Other studies have put the rate of infection after all spinal infections at 1.9% to 4.4%. Although this number is small, postoperative spinal infections are costly and, more important, can have a significant effect on a patient's clinical outcome. There are conflicting data on the association of preoperative lumbar epidural steroid administration and SSI. A retrospective study by Hartveldt et al. of 5311 patients did not find an increased risk of SSI in their cohorts after lumbar epidural steroid injection (LESI). In a Medicare database review, however, Yang et al. did find an increased risk of SSI if LESI occurred within 90 days of surgery.

Procedure-related risk factors associated with postoperative infection include duration of the surgical procedure, patient hypothermia, number of people in the operating room, dural tear, blood loss, transfusion of packed red blood cells, retained wound drain, and instrumentation.

Use of topical intrawound vancomycin powder has been shown in most studies to decrease the risk of SSI. A recent meta-analysis showed that vancomycin powder is protective against SSI. Edin et al. reported no signs of tissue toxicity with vancomycin use and that it had little or no effect on osteoblasts at doses used in the surgical wound, which is usually 1 g. A systematic review by Lemans et al. found that intrawound povidone iodine irrigation led to a similar reduction in SSI and intrawound antibiotics.

Surgical treatment of wound infection involves obtaining cultures followed by initial debridement and wound irrigation, with primary closure done in layers over a drain if the wound is deemed "clean" after the procedure. The patient is started on broad-spectrum intravenous antibiotics until cultures yield a pathogen. Once the organism is obtained with sensitivities, the antibiotic may be changed. The patient stays

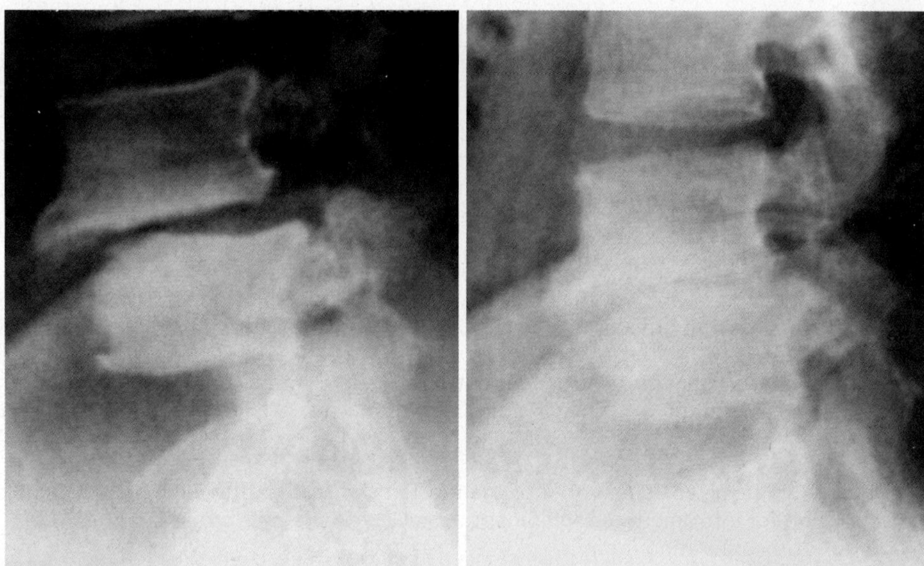

FIGURE 6.2 Brucellosis of lumbar spine. Note vertebral sclerosis, spondylolisthesis, steplike irregularity in anterior vertebral body, and anterior osteophytes. (From Lifeso RM, Harder E, McCorkell SJ: Spinal brucellosis, *J Bone Joint Surg* 67B:345, 1985.)

on intravenous antibiotics usually for 6 weeks, and if there is clinical improvement and normalization of the ESR and CRP, intravenous antibiotics will be switched to oral antibiotics for roughly another 4 weeks. It is important to consult an infectious disease specialist for these patients.

Repeat irrigation and debridement of the wound with cultures and layered closure over drains is done at 48-hour intervals until the wound is without drainage and the patient is improving. Instrumentation should be assessed at the time of debridement in patients with early SSI. Well-fixed implants should be left in place. If repeat debridement is required, MRI is used to evaluate for osteomyelitis or intradiscal abscess formation. Kanayama et al. suggested that, if MRI evidence of vertebral osteomyelitis or spondylodiscitis was present, the implants should be removed. They found that with implant removal in this circumstance the infection could be better treated. Implant retention led to frequent implant failure, which made salvage more difficult because of increased bone loss and deformity from persistent infection.

Numerous authors have shown that most infections can be treated without removal of the instrumentation. Instrumentation can be removed when the fusion is solid to avoid chronic suppressive antibiotics. Bone graft pieces that are not attached to soft tissue should be removed at the time of the initial debridement. This is also our method of treatment of acute postoperative infections. Recalcitrant wounds may require negative pressure wound therapy, V-Y flaps, or free flaps when bone or implants are exposed. Recent literature has shown negative pressure wound therapy to be useful in treating postoperative spinal infections. The technique involves packing a debrided wound with gauze or foam dressing. A drain is placed over the dressing, and then the wound is sealed with a drape. The end of the drain is attached to a vacuum to produce negative pressure. The dressing is changed sterilely every 2 to 3 days until the wound can be closed.

BRUCELLOSIS

Brucellosis results in a noncaseating, acid-fast–negative granuloma caused by a gram-negative capnophilic coccobacillus. This infection occurs most frequently in individuals involved in animal husbandry and meat processing (workers in abattoirs). Pasteurization of milk and antibiotic treatment of animals have led to a significant decrease in the incidence of this disease. Symptoms include polyarthralgia, fever, malaise, afternoon or night sweats, anorexia, and headache. Psoas abscesses are found in 12% of patients. Bone involvement, most frequently of the spine, occurs in 2% to 30% of patients. The lumbar spine is the most frequently involved spinal region.

Radiographic changes of steplike erosions of the margin of the vertebral body require 2 months or more to develop. Disc space thinning and vertebral segment ankylosis by bridging are similar to changes in other forms of osteomyelitis (Fig. 6.2). CT and MRI may show soft-tissue involvement. Moehring noted that ^{67}Ga scanning is not helpful in sacroiliac infections. MRI may be helpful in the early identification of the disease but has not been reported for this specific infection. The diagnosis usually is indicated by *Brucella* titers of 1 : 80 or greater; confirmatory cultures also should be done, if possible, using special techniques. Treatment usually consists of antibiotic therapy for 4 months and close monitoring of the *Brucella* titers. Persistence of a titer of 1 : 160 or greater after 4 months of treatment may indicate recurrence or resistance of the infection. Indications for surgical treatment are the same as for tubercular spinal infections. Because of the indolent nature of this disease, it can be mistaken for a degenerative process. Nas et al. recommended 6 months of antibiotic therapy (rifampicin and doxycycline) with surgery for spinal cord compression, instability, or radiculopathy.

FUNGAL INFECTIONS

Fungal infections generally are noncaseating, acid-fast–negative infections. They usually occur as opportunistic infections in immunocompromised patients. Difficulty in diagnosis often leads to delayed treatment. Symptoms usually develop slowly. Pain is less prominent as a physical symptom than in other forms of spinal osteomyelitis. Laboratory and radiographic findings are similar to those of pyogenic infections. Tubercular infection and tumors are the primary differential diagnoses. Direct culture by biopsy is the only method of absolute determination of the infecting organism.

Aspergillus and *Candida* infections were the most common fungal pathogens in a review by Ganesh et al. *Aspergillus* is an opportunistic infection and the most common fungus affecting the spine. Pain, tenderness, and an elevated ESR and CRP are the most common symptoms, but white blood cell elevations are rare. Ganesh et al. found that half of patients with spinal aspergillosis had undergone a recent surgery and 71% had lung infection with *Aspergillus*. In addition, 75% of patients with candidiasis had undergone recent surgery and almost a quarter had a malignancy. The lumbar spine is the area most commonly involved with fungal infection. Mortality is quite high with these opportunistic infections. With aspergillosis, there was 26% mortality with surgical and medical management, while mortality was 60% with medical management alone. With *Candida* infections they reported no mortality with combined treatment and 29% mortality with medical management alone. About 37% of patients presented with neurologic deficits; half of these recovered completely and most of the remaining patients had a residual deficit. Some of the case reports did not specify neurologic recovery status. Medical management is complex in these patients and infectious disease consultation is needed. The operative indications are significant neurologic deficit, spinal instability, and failure to respond to medical management. Imaging with MRI is crucial, and CT is helpful to best characterize bone destruction.

■ TUBERCULOSIS

Despite spinal tuberculosis being one of the oldest diseases known, dating back to 3400 BCE and being described by Pott in 1779, it remains a relevant problem throughout the world. The worldwide incidence is over 10 million cases/year. Before the advent of effective chemotherapy, time and surgery for paralysis were the only treatment options. Laminectomy initially was performed for paralysis, but the results were disappointing until Ménard accidentally opened an abscess and the patient improved. Many patients treated in this manner died as a result of a secondary bacterial infection, and the practice was abandoned. Posterior spinal fusion, as described by Hibbs and Albee, was the preferred operation to prevent deformity and promote healing by internal immobilization. The first radical debridement and bone grafting procedure for abscess formation was reported in 1934. After the development of satisfactory chemotherapeutic agents, more aggressive surgery was attempted, including costotransversectomy with bone grafting and radical debridement as popularized by Hodgson.

Tubercular bone and joint infections currently account for 2% to 3% of all reported cases of *Mycobacterium tuberculosis*. Spinal tubercular infections account for one third to one half of the bone and joint infections. The thoracolumbar spine is the most commonly infected area. The incidence of infection seems to increase with age, but males and females are almost equally infected. With current medical management, surgical treatment is not commonly needed, outcomes are generally good, and neurologic deficits often improve.

Pathologically, the infection is characterized by acid-fast–positive, caseating granulomas with or without purulence. Tubercles composed of monocytes and epithelioid cells, forming minute masses with central caseation in the presence of Langerhans-type giant cells, are typical on microscopic examination. Abscesses expand, following the path of least resistance, and contain necrotic debris. Skin sinuses form, drain, and heal spontaneously. Bone reaction to the infection varies from intense reaction to no reaction. In the spine the infection spares the intervertebral discs and spreads beneath the anterior and posterior longitudinal ligaments. Epidural infection is more likely to result in permanent neurologic damage. Spinal tuberculosis involves the anterior vertebral body initially. Progressive bone destruction leads to the characteristic gibbus deformity. Spread occurs under the anterior longitudinal ligament, initially sparing the discs of adults but not of children because of disc vascularity in young children.

Slowly progressive constitutional symptoms are predominant in the early stages of the disease, including weakness, malaise, night sweats, fever, and weight loss. Back pain is present in 70% at presentation. Progressive pain is a late symptom associated with bone collapse and paralysis. About 30% of patients present with neurologic deficits in less developed countries but less commonly in the United States and other developed countries. Cervical involvement can cause hoarseness because of recurrent laryngeal nerve paralysis, dysphagia, and respiratory stridor (known as *Millar asthma*). These symptoms may result from anterior abscess formation in the neck. Sudden death has been reported with cervical disease after erosion into the great vessels. Neurologic signs usually occur late and may wax and wane. Motor function and rectal tone are good prognostic predictors.

Laboratory studies suggest chronic disease. Findings include anemia, hypoproteinemia, and mild elevation of ESR and CRP. ESR has been found to be normal in over 50% of patients. Skin testing may be helpful but is not diagnostic. The test is contraindicated in patients with prior tuberculous infection because of the risk of skin slough from an intense reaction and is not useful in patients with suspected reactivation of the disease. Early radiographic findings include a subtle decrease in one or more disc spaces and localized osteopenia. Later findings include vertebral collapse, called "concertina collapse" by Seddon because of its resemblance to an accordion. CT and MRI show bone involvement and paraspinal abscess formation. MRI is preferred because it can demonstrate epidural abscess formation.

Definitive diagnosis depends on culture of the organism and requires biopsy of the lesion. Percutaneous techniques with radiographic or CT control usually are adequate. Percutaneous thoracoscopic, laparoscopic, or endoscopic biopsy are other reported options. Open biopsy may be required if needle biopsy is dangerous or nonproductive or if other open procedures are required.

Delayed diagnosis and missed diagnosis are common. Differential diagnoses include pyogenic and fungal infections, secondary metastatic disease, primary tumors of bone (e.g., osteosarcoma, chondrosarcoma, myeloma, eosinophilic granuloma, and aneurysmal bone cyst [ABC]), sarcoidosis, giant cell tumors (GCTs) of bone, and bone deformities such as Scheuermann disease.

TREATMENT OF THORACIC AND LUMBAR TUBERCULAR SPINAL INFECTION

With early diagnosis and medical treatment, the prognosis is generally good, and fusion of the involved level occurs 80% of the time. Definitive diagnosis by culture of a biopsy specimen is important because of the toxicity of the chemotherapeutic agents and the length of treatment required. Multidrug therapy is the primary treatment, using a combination of isoniazid, rifampicin, pyrazinamide, ethambutol, and streptomycin. Patients with normal immune system function may require only 6 months of therapy, whereas others may require 18 to 24 months of therapy. Reasons for extended treatment include HIV infection or other cause of immune compromise and infection by drug-resistant organisms. The most common surgical indications cited in the literature include neurologic deficit, severe kyphosis, pain due to spinal instability, failure of medical therapy, large paraspinal or epidural abscess, and more than four levels of vertebral involvement.

If surgical treatment is planned, multidrug therapy should be instituted at least 3 to 6 weeks before surgery to suppress the infection in most patients. During this time of medical treatment, nutritional support should be initiated to correct hypoproteinemia and manage other comorbidities such as hypertension or diabetes. MRI and upright plain radiographs should be obtained to determine all involved levels because skip lesions are common. In addition, the location and extent of abscesses and neurologic compression should be determined. Plain radiographs are important to determine the severity of spinal deformity and instability.

The surgical approach and technique have continued to evolve, and medical management has improved. The optimal approach and technique depend on a number of patient-specific factors. The development of posterior spondylectomy techniques, expandable titanium cages, and pedicle screw instrumentation systems are some of the most impactful surgical changes over recent decades. Wang et al. retrospectively reviewed a series of 184 patients who were treated with posterior-only, anterior-only, or combined anterior and posterior debridement and reconstruction. Their findings are consistent with those from a number of other authors and demonstrated that posterior-only patients had fewer perioperative complications and slightly better outcomes at long-term follow-up. It is important to note that most authors with similar studies have included an anterior debridement through a costotransversectomy or transpedicular approach. In addition, the use of longer constructs extending two levels above and below the affected levels in the thoracic and lumbar spine allows better kyphosis correction and maintenance of correction. Correction of kyphosis is achieved by using temporary rods during debridement and progressively using rod contouring, altering table position, and applying compression along the rods. These same techniques can be used with shorter constructs to achieve satisfactory results, especially when the initial kyphosis is less severe and involves fewer infected vertebrae, as shown recently by Liu et al. in a series of 66 patients with a minimum 5-year follow-up. Some authors have described placement of anterior load-sharing constructs of allograft or structural autograft in addition to titanium cages of various designs, whereas others add only posterior morsellized autograft or allograft all from a posterior approach. Neurologic improvement also is equivalent regardless of the approach that is used as demonstrated by Wang et al. Anterior surgery is most helpful when more direct visualization is needed for neural decompression or when a large abscess is more anteriorly located around the great vessel or other vital structures.

TREATMENT OF CERVICAL TUBERCULAR SPINAL INFECTIONS

Cervical tuberculosis is a rare disease with a high complication rate. Hsu and Leong reported a 42.5% spinal cord compression rate in 40 patients. Children younger than 10 years old were more likely to develop abscesses, whereas older children were more likely to develop tetraparesis. Drainage and chemotherapy were adequate for the younger children. For older patients, these researchers recommended radical anterior debridement and strut grafting followed by chemotherapy. Cervical laminectomy resulted in increased kyphosis, subluxation, and neurologic deficits. A more recent retrospective study by Yin et al. showed that cervical tuberculosis infections could be treated with anterior-only, posterior-only and combined anterior and posterior approaches. In the subaxial spine, one- or two-level involvement was treated with anterior debridement and anterior grafting and instrumentation. Patients with more than two levels of involvement had anterior debridement and grafting followed by posterior stabilization. Posterior stabilization was reserved for upper cervical infections where anterior reconstruction was not feasible and posterior occipital cervical fusion was used. In a small case series, Xing et al. had good results with combined anterior decompression and posterior occipitocervical fixation. Preoperative traction has been reported to improve kyphosis prior to surgery.

ATYPICAL TUBERCULAR INFECTIONS

Reports of atypical tubercular infections are limited to isolated case reports, usually in individuals who are elderly or immunocompromised by disease or medication. These atypical infections require more aggressive surgical intervention because of the lack of antibiotic sensitivity and the risk of progression with standard tubercular therapy. The clinical manifestations and aggressive surgical treatment of atypical tubercular spinal infections and mycobacterial infections are similar.

ABSCESS DRAINAGE BY ANATOMIC LEVEL

Any abscess cavity around the spine and pelvis can be drained as summarized in the following techniques. Reconstructive techniques are covered in other sections.

CERVICAL SPINE

If the cervical spine is involved, the abscess may be present retropharyngeally, in the posterior triangle of the neck, or supraclavicular area. The tuberculous detritus may also gravitate downward under the prevertebral fascia to form a mediastinal abscess.

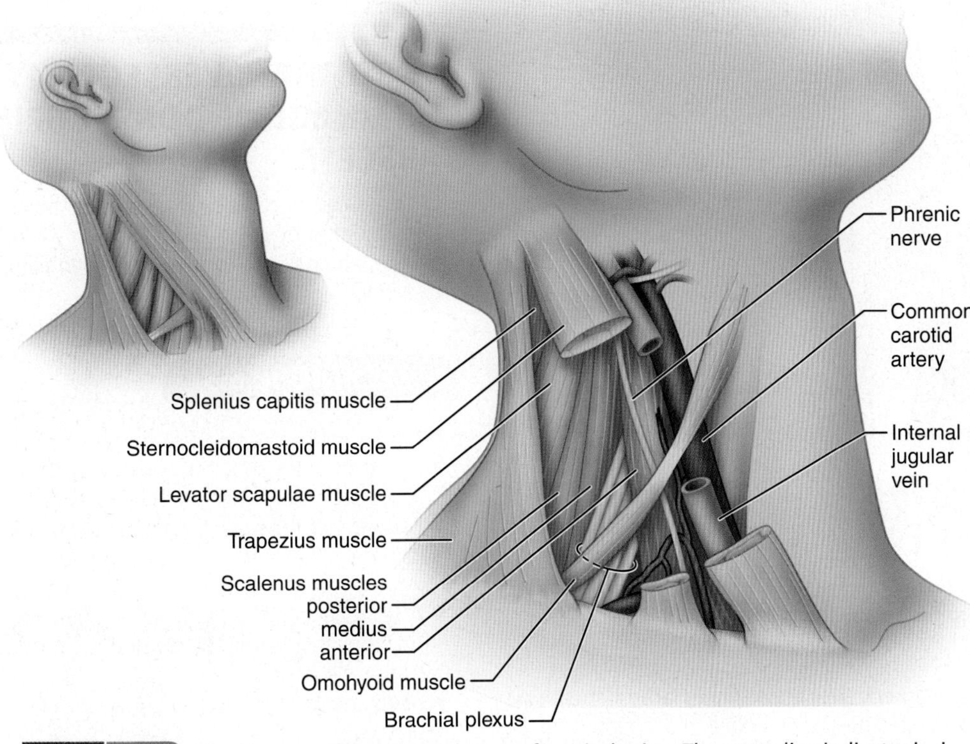

FIGURE 6.3 Drainage of tuberculous abscess of cervical spine. The green line indicates incision for extraoral approach (inset). **SEE TECHNIQUE 6.1.**

DRAINAGE OF RETROPHARYNGEAL ABSCESS THROUGH POSTERIOR TRIANGLE OF THE NECK

Drainage of a retropharyngeal abscess through an incision in the posterior wall of the pharynx is warranted only in an emergency, as indicated by cyanosis and respiratory difficulty. This approach can be used if only abscess drainage is planned, without spinal reconstruction. Usually drainage should be through an extraoral approach (Fig. 6.3).

TECHNIQUE 6.1

- Make a 5- to 6-cm incision along the posterior border of the sternocleidomastoid muscle, centered at the junction of its middle and upper thirds.
- Incise the superficial layer of cervical fascia and protect the spinal accessory nerve that pierces the sternocleidomastoid muscle and runs obliquely across the posterior triangle deep to the sternocleidomastoid.
- Retract the sternocleidomastoid muscle anteriorly.
- Using blunt dissection, expose the levator scapulae and scalenus muscles.
- Staying anterior to the levator scapulae and anterior scalene, displace the carotid sheath containing the carotid artery, internal jugular vein, and vagus nerve anteriorly. The brachial plexus exits between the scalenus anterior and the scalenus medius. Palpate the abscess in front of the transverse processes and bodies of the vertebrae. Be aware that the sympathetic chain is superficial to the longus capitis.
- Puncture the abscess wall with a hemostat, enlarge the opening, and gently but thoroughly evacuate the abscess.
- If the abscess is unusually large and symptoms are severe, do not close the wound; if the abscess is not large and symptoms are not severe, close the wound in layers.
- A tracheostomy set should be available postoperatively at the bedside in case the patient develops respiratory difficulty from edema of the larynx.

ANTERIOR CERVICAL APPROACH TO DRAINAGE OF RETROPHARYNGEAL ABSCESS

The anterior aspect of the cervical vertebrae is exposed as for standard anterior disc excision. This technique allows exposure from C2 to C7. A transverse incision is possible if only two or three vertebrae are involved. A longitudinal incision is made along the medial border of the sternocleidomastoid muscle if longer exposure is necessary. This approach allows bony reconstruction to be done at the time of abscess drainage.

TECHNIQUE 6.2

- Place the patient supine on the operating table with endotracheal anesthesia administered through a noncollapsible tube. The insertion of a small nasogastric tube may facilitate the positive identification of the esophagus.
- Place a small roll between the scapulas; the shoulders can be pulled downward with tape to allow easy radiography.

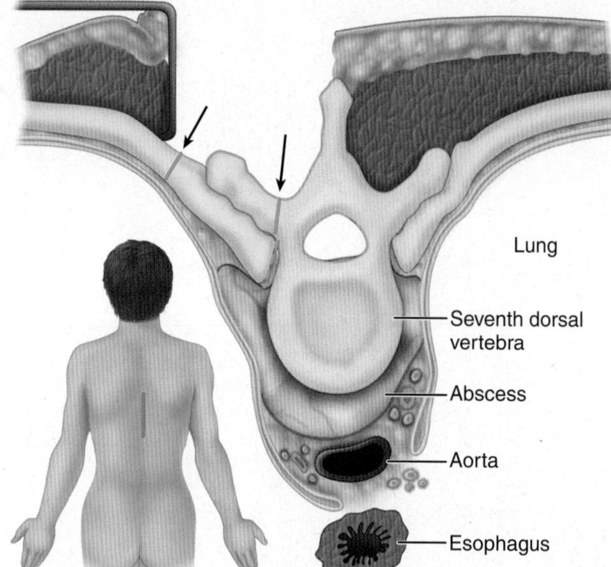

FIGURE 6.4 Costotransversectomy to drain tuberculous abscess of dorsal spine. **SEE TECHNIQUE 6.3.**

- Slightly extend the neck over a small roll placed beneath it. Place a head halter on the mandible and occiput and apply several pounds of traction if bony reconstruction is planned.
- Prepare and drape the area from the mandible to the upper chest.
- Place the incision at the appropriate level based on surface anatomy; the cricoid is usually at C5-C6 level.
- Undermine the subcutaneous tissue superficial to the platysma fascia cephalad and caudally to allow expansion of the exposure. Divide the platysma muscle longitudinally in the direction of its fibers.
- Open the cervical fascia along the medial border of the sternocleidomastoid muscle.
- Develop a plane between the sternocleidomastoid laterally and the omohyoid and sternohyoid medially.
- Palpate the carotid artery in this plane and gently retract it laterally with a finger.
- With combined blunt and sharp dissection divide the pretracheal fascia attachment to the carotid sheath, develop a relatively avascular plane between the carotid sheath laterally and the thyroid, trachea, and esophagus medially.
- Insert handheld retractors initially.
- Dissect free the filmy connective tissue on the posterolateral aspect of the esophagus along the entire exposed wound to prevent ballooning of the esophagus above and below the retractor.
- Expose the prevertebral fascia and open the abscess cavity. Thoroughly debride and irrigate the abscess cavity.
- Insert a hypodermic needle into this material and obtain a lateral radiograph to confirm the proper level. Proceed with reconstruction if planned.
- Drain the wound in a standard fashion.
- Do not close the neck fascia, but let it fall together. The skin can be loosely closed or left open for delayed closure.

DORSAL SPINE

COSTOTRANSVERSECTOMY FOR DRAINAGE OF DORSAL SPINE ABSCESS

Most abscesses caused by disease of the dorsal spine can be evacuated by costotransversectomy (Fig. 6.4). This procedure, originally performed by Haidenhaim, was described by Ménard in 1894.

TECHNIQUE 6.3

- Make a midline incision over three spinous processes. Reflect the periosteum and soft tissues laterally from the spinous processes and laminae on the side containing the abscess.
- Expose fully the middle transverse process and resect it at its base. Hemilaminectomy or laminectomy can be added if there is an epidural component to drain.
- After reflecting the periosteum from the contiguous rib, resect its medial end by division 5 cm from the tip of the transverse process.
- Bevel and smooth the end of the rib; avoid puncturing the pleura.
- After resecting the rib(s), doubly ligate and divide the neurovascular bundle.
- Open the abscess by blunt dissection close to the vertebral body. An elevator can be used to detach the rib head from vertebral body. Usually pus will pour into the wound when the rib head is removed. The opening should be large enough to permit thorough exploration and evacuation of the cavity and removal of all debris. If resection of more than one rib is necessary, enlarge the initial incision accordingly.
- Close the wound in layers. The wound can be dusted with streptomycin powder before closure if desired.

LUMBAR SPINE

DRAINAGE OF PARAVERTEBRAL ABSCESS

TECHNIQUE 6.4

- Make a 7.5- to 10-cm longitudinal incision 3-5 cm lateral to the midline parallel to the spinous processes.
- Divide the lumbodorsal fascia in line with the incision and pass a hemostat bluntly around the lateral and anterior borders of the erector spinae muscles to the transverse processes (Fig. 6.5).
- Usually the abscess is encountered immediately; if it is not, puncture the layer of lumbodorsal fascia that separates the quadratus lumborum muscle from the erector spinae group and force the hemostat along the anterior border of the transverse processes.
- After thorough evacuation of the abscess, close the incision in layers.

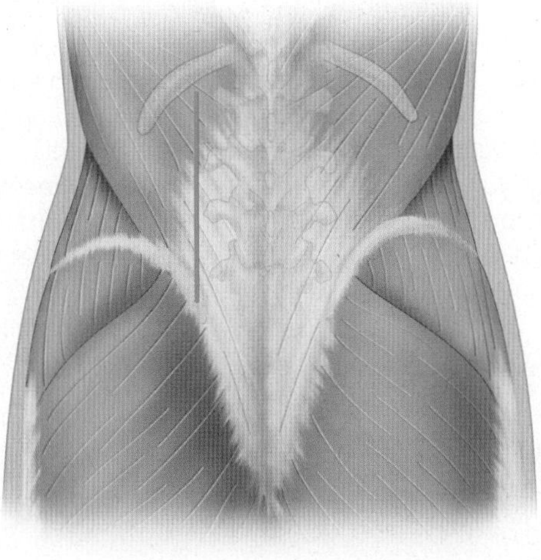

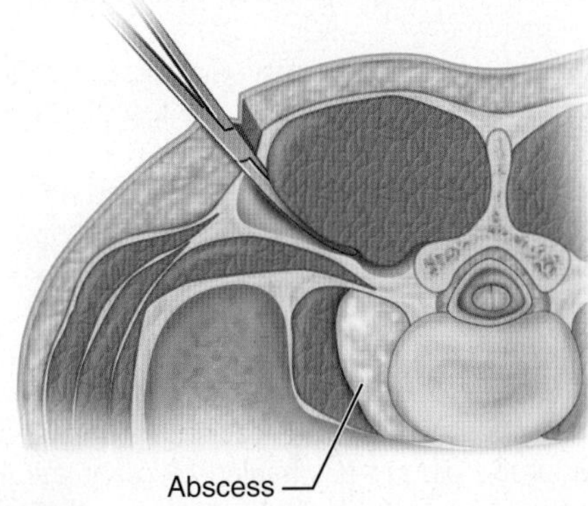

FIGURE 6.5 Drainage of paravertebral abscess. **SEE TECHNIQUE 6.4.**

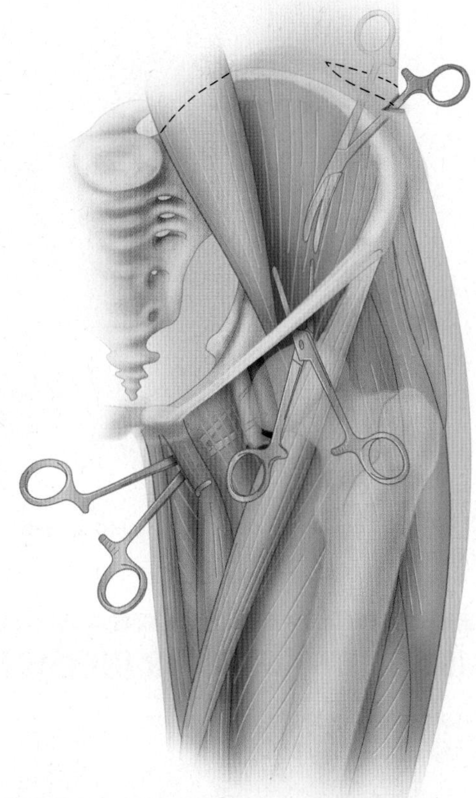

FIGURE 6.6 Drainage of psoas abscess. Hemostat in adductor region is pointed toward inferior edge of acetabulum; abscess usually is located near junction of femoral head and neck.

PELVIS

PSOAS ABSCESS

Psoas abscesses are entirely extraperitoneal and follow the course of the iliopsoas muscle. Drainage can be done posteriorly through the Petit triangle, by a lateral incision along the crest of the ilium, or anteriorly under the Poupart ligament, depending on the size of the abscess and the area in which it appears. Occasionally, an abscess burrows beneath the Poupart ligament and is seen subcutaneously in the proximal third of the thigh in the adductor region (Fig. 6.6).

DRAINAGE THROUGH THE PETIT TRIANGLE

The sides of the Petit triangle are formed by the lateral margin of the latissimus dorsi muscle and the medial border of the obliquus externus abdominis muscle and its base by the crest of the ilium. The floor of the triangle is the obliquus internus abdominis muscle.

TECHNIQUE 6.5

- Make a 7.5-cm incision 2.5 cm proximal to and parallel with the posterior crest of the ilium, beginning lateral to the erector spinae group of muscles (Fig. 6.7).
- After exposure of the Petit triangle, bluntly dissect through the obliquus internus abdominis muscle directly into the abscess.
- After thorough evacuation of the abscess, close the incision in layers.

POSTOPERATIVE CARE Because flexion contracture of the hip usually accompanies a psoas abscess, Buck traction should be used to correct the deformity and relax the spastic muscles until the hip is fully extended.

DRAINAGE BY LATERAL INCISION

TECHNIQUE 6.6

- Make a 10-cm incision along the middle third of the crest of the ilium and free the attachments of the internal and external obliquus abdominis muscles.
- With a hemostat, puncture the abscess, which can be palpated as a fluctuant extraperitoneal mass on the inner surface of the wing of the ilium.
- Avoid rupture of the peritoneum.

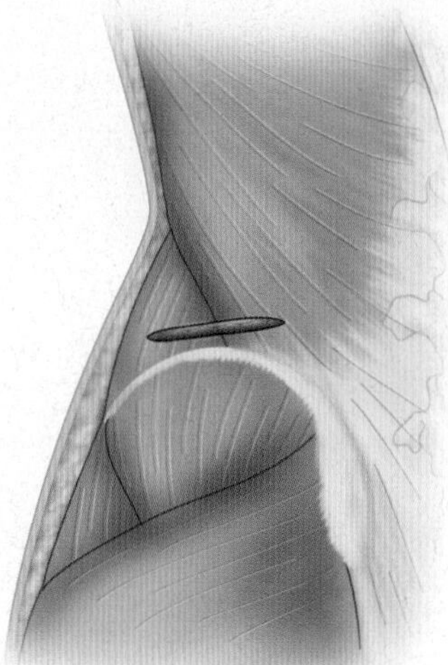

FIGURE 6.7 Drainage of pelvic abscess through Petit triangle. SEE TECHNIQUE 6.5.

DRAINAGE BY ANTERIOR INCISION

TECHNIQUE 6.7

- Begin a longitudinal skin incision at the anterior superior spine and continue it distally for 5-7.5 cm on the anterior aspect of the thigh.
- Identify the sartorius muscle and carry the dissection deep to its medial border to the level of the anterior inferior spine. Protect the femoral nerve, which lies just medial to this area.
- Insert a long hemostat along the medial surface of the wing of the ilium under the Poupart ligament and puncture the abscess.
- Separate the blades of the hemostat to enlarge the opening and permit complete evacuation.
- Close the incision in layers.

Drainage by Ludloff Incision. When a psoas abscess points subcutaneously in the adductor region of the thigh, drainage is accomplished by a Ludloff incision, as described in other chapter. Weinberg described a method of excising a psoas abscess when simpler treatment has failed or is likely to fail because of the size of the abscess, its chronicity, or involvement with mixed bacterial infection. He removed the abscess and any bony or cartilaginous sequestra lodged in the tract or in the diseased vertebrae.

COCCYGECTOMY FOR DRAINAGE OF A PELVIC ABSCESS

Lougheed and White noted that when tuberculosis involves the lower lumbar and lumbosacral areas, soft-tissue abscesses may gravitate into the pelvis, forming a large abscess anterior to the sacrum. These soft-tissue abscesses may point to the skin on the anterior surface of the thigh or above the iliac crest, but drainage at these sites alone is insufficient, resulting only in a chronically draining sinus despite antibacterial therapy. The pelvic abscess usually can be seen radiographically by retrograde injection of an opaque contrast medium. Lougheed and White devised a method of establishing dependent drainage posteriorly by coccygectomy. Their results in treatment of 10 patients by this method were uniformly good. The wound usually healed within 6 to 8 weeks, and the spinal lesions all became inactive.

TECHNIQUE 6.8

(LOUGHEED AND WHITE)

- Make a 15-cm elliptical incision over the coccyx, removing a strip of skin.
- After freeing the coccyx from soft tissues, disarticulate it from the sacrum.
- With careful hemostasis, carry the dissection upward, staying close to the sacrum until the resulting pyramidal tunnel communicates with the abscess cavity.
- After evacuating the purulent matter, insert an irrigating catheter to the top of the cavity and pack the wound with iodoform gauze.

POSTOPERATIVE CARE For 2-3 weeks, the wound is irrigated through the catheter several times daily with a solution of streptomycin. The packing is changed at intervals until the wound has healed by granulation tissue from within.

RADICAL DEBRIDEMENT AND ARTHRODESIS–DORSOLATERAL APPROACH

TECHNIQUE 6.9

(ROAF ET AL.)

- Expose the dorsal spine through a dorsolateral approach. Maintain careful hemostasis throughout.
- Select the side with the larger abscess shadow, or, in the absence of an abscess, use the left side; make a curved incision. Begin posteriorly 3.8 cm from the midline and 7.5 cm proximal to the center of the lesion and curve distally and laterally to a point 12.5 cm from the midline at the center of the lesion; continue medially and distally, ending 3.8 cm from the midline and 7.5 cm distal to the center of the lesion (Fig. 6.8).
- Divide the superficial and deep fascia and the underlying muscles down to the ribs in the line of the incision. Retract the flap of the skin and muscle medially. Now locate the rib opposite the center of the focus and remove 7.5-10 cm of this rib and the one proximal and distal in the following manner.

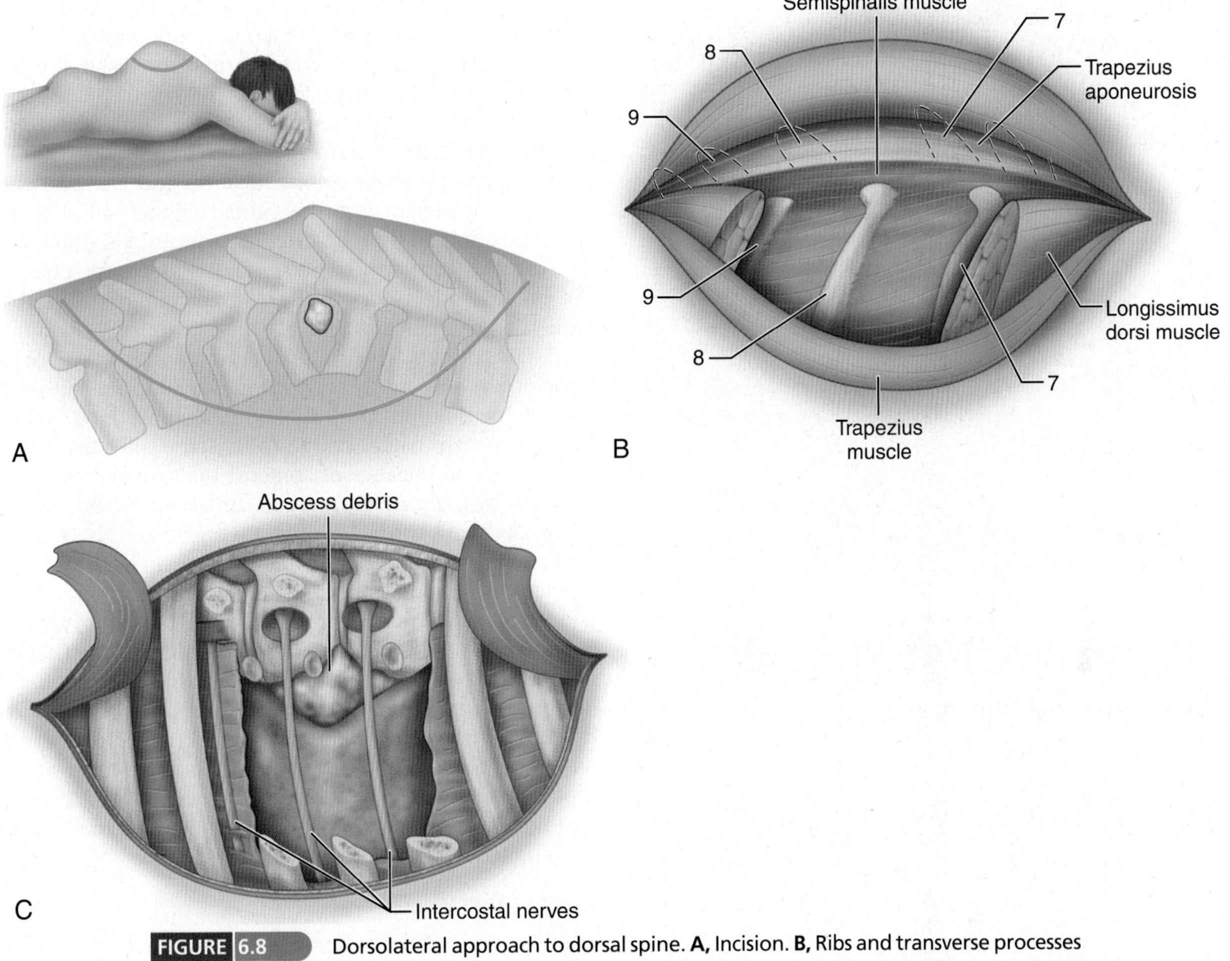

FIGURE 6.8 Dorsolateral approach to dorsal spine. **A,** Incision. **B,** Ribs and transverse processes exposed. **C,** Ribs and transverse processes resected, and abscess and vertebral bodies exposed. **SEE TECHNIQUE 6.9.**

- Free the ribs with a periosteal elevator and divide them with rib shears 7.5-10 cm from the tips of the transverse processes.
- Resect each at the tip of the transverse process.
- Divide under direct vision the ligaments and muscles attached to the rib heads and transverse processes and resect these bony parts.
- Identify two and preferably three intercostal nerves and trace them medially to the intervertebral foramina. These nerves, as they pass into the foramina, indicate the level of the cord in the spinal canal.
- Expose the intercostal vessels near the spinal column and cut them between clamps.
- Divide the intercostal muscles near the vertebral column.
- Separate the pleura from the spinal column by blunt dissection, exposing the lateral and anterolateral aspects of the vertebral bodies. Avoid perforating the pleura because it is often adherent and thickened; if a perforation occurs, suture it at once.
- Locate the center of the lesion by passing a finger into the wound anterior to the vertebral bodies. Remove all pus, granulation tissue, and necrotic matter.
- Occasionally, one or more vertebral bodies may be sequestrated and lying free in the abscess cavity. Usually two or three small bony sequestra and pieces of necrotic disc material are found. If the paravertebral shadow, thought to be an abscess, is found to be mainly fibrous tissue, it is more difficult to find the lesion. Under these circumstances, using radiographic control, explore the bone with a fine gouge, burr, and rongeur.
- After thorough debridement, decide whether bone grafts are advisable. The simplest method of grafting is to pack the cavity with bone chips.
- A more extensive procedure may be undertaken. With a chisel or gouge, roughen the lateral and anterolateral aspects of the diseased vertebral bodies and, if possible, of one healthy vertebra above and below and cut a groove in them, passing from healthy bone above to healthy bone below.
- Wedge a full-thickness rib graft into the groove and sink it deeply within the vertebral bodies.
- Place cancellous bone chips obtained from the remaining portion of the resected ribs into the groove and laterally along the roughened surface of the vertebral bodies.
- If the pleura has been accidentally opened, drain the pleural cavity with a chest tube inserted through a small stab incision in the eighth intercostal space in the midaxillary line and connected to an underwater seal for 48 hours after surgery.

BOX 6.1

Radiographic Diagnosis of Spine Tumors According to Age and Location

Diagnosis According to Age

10 to 30 Years Old

Aneurysmal bone cyst
Ewing sarcoma
Giant cell carcinoma
Histiocytosis X
Osteoblastoma
Osteoid osteoma
Osteochondroma
Osteosarcoma

30 to 50 Years Old

Chondrosarcoma
Chordoma
Hodgkin disease
Hemangioma

Older Than 50 Years

Metastatic
Myeloma

Diagnosis According to Location

Vertebral Body

Chordoma
Giant cell carcinoma
Hemangioma
Histiocytosis X
Metastatic disease
Multiple myeloma

Posterior Elements

Aneurysmal bone cyst
Osteoblastoma
Osteoid osteoma
Osteochondroma

Adjacent Vertebrae

Aneurysmal bone cyst
Chondrosarcoma
Chordoma

Multiple Vertebrae

Histiocytosis X
Metastatic
Myeloma

From Chabot M, Herkowitz HN: Spine tumors: patient evaluation, *Semin Spine Surg* 7:260, 1995.

TUMORS OF THE SPINE

BENIGN TUMORS

Of all primary benign bone tumors, 8% occur in the spine or sacrum. Benign lesions have a predilection for younger patients, usually occurring in the first three decades of life, with 60% of benign lesions identified in the second and third decades (Box 6.1). The location of the lesion along the spinal column and its topographic location on the vertebra itself can provide information regarding diagnosis (Figs. 6.9 and 6.10). Typically, benign lesions are in the posterior elements, anteriorly located lesions tend to be malignant (76%).

During operative treatment of tumors, certain fundamentals must be followed to maintain function and anatomy and to minimize the risk of recurrence or instability. These principles are most important in the region of the spinal cord. For cervical and thoracic lesions, the spinal cord must of course be preserved. However, nerve roots vary in importance depending on anatomic location and can be resected if long-term benefit is to be gained. Some paired vascular structures, including the vertebral arteries, also can be singly resected. In the thoracic spine, laminectomy alone does not provide safe access to the anterior column. The risk of paralysis is significant, and alternative approaches must be used. For patients who are unable to tolerate a thoracotomy, a costotransversectomy is a reasonable and safe approach to the anterior column. With aggressive lesions, the spinal canal may be contaminated. Nerve roots serve only the intercostal muscles, so sacrifice of some of the thoracic nerve roots does not severely affect function, unless numerous roots are taken. As more thoracic roots are sacrificed, there is some effect on chest cage function and respiration because of interference with intercostal innervation. Sacral tumors requiring wide excision are rare. Combined approaches often are necessary for wide excision and require complex reconstruction to stabilize the ilia to the distal lumbar spine. Resection of the sacrum and its associated nerve roots also affects continence. If both S1 nerve roots and a single S2 nerve root are preserved, 50% of patients retain continence. If only a single S3 root is taken, with S1 and S2 undisturbed, bowel and bladder function are retained. The nature of the tumor to be resected often dictates the anatomic level of resection.

■ STABILITY

Stability considerations after resection are different in adult and pediatric patients. In the cervical and thoracic regions, laminectomy creates instability in an immature spine, so arthrodesis should be done. The adult spine seems to tolerate laminectomy better, and some biomechanical considerations are useful when choosing instrumentation and fusion procedures. Instability created by anterior resection increases as more vertebral body is resected. As a rule of thumb, fusion should be done when any significant amount of vertebral body is resected. The exception to this is curettage; if adequate bone graft is placed after curettage, fusion usually is unnecessary. After anterior fusion, with or without instrumentation, immobilization with a thoracic lumbar sacral orthosis (TLSO) generally is recommended. When incorporation of fusion bone is identified, usually 3 to 6 months postoperatively, the orthosis is discontinued.

Determination of instability after posterior spinal resections is not as straightforward as after anterior procedures. Important bony and ligamentous structures posteriorly contribute individually to overall stability in the intact spine. Soft-tissue restraints include the supraspinous, interspinous, and posterior longitudinal ligaments, the ligamentum flavum, and the facet capsules. The spinous processes, laminae, pars interarticularis, facet joints individually on the left and right, and posterior vertebral wall provide bony stability. Point systems have been created to assist in the determination of stability. Bridwell assigned 25% of posterior vertebral stability for each stabilizing structure, including the midline osteoligamentous complex (laminae, spinous processes, and intervening ligaments); each of the two facet joint complexes (left and right); and the posterior vertebral wall, disc, and

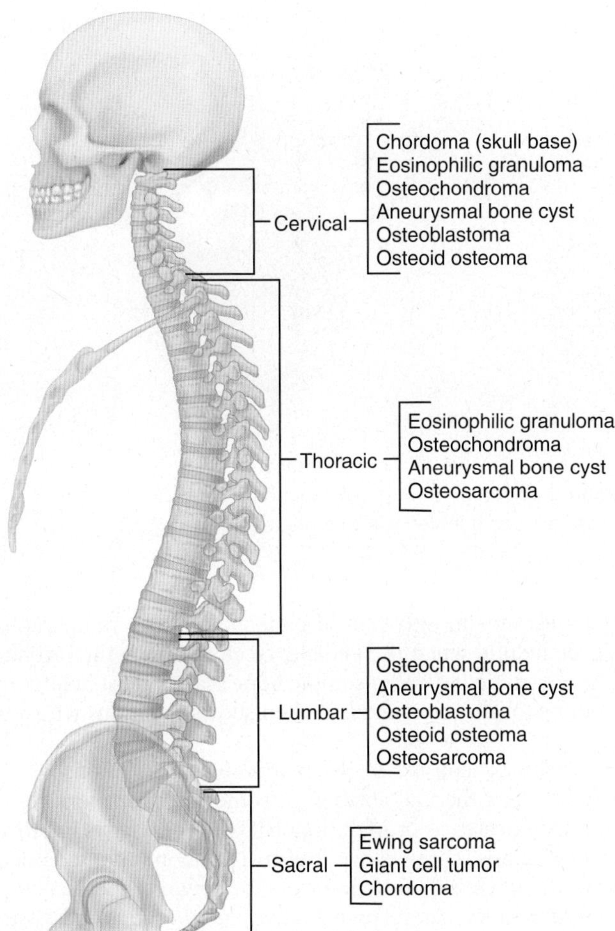

FIGURE 6.9 Distribution of the most common locations for primary osseous lesions in the pediatric spinal column. (From Ravindra VM, Eli IM, Schmidt MH, et al: Primary osseous tumors of the pediatric spinal column: review of pathology and surgical decision making, *Neurosurg Focus* 41:E3, 2016.)

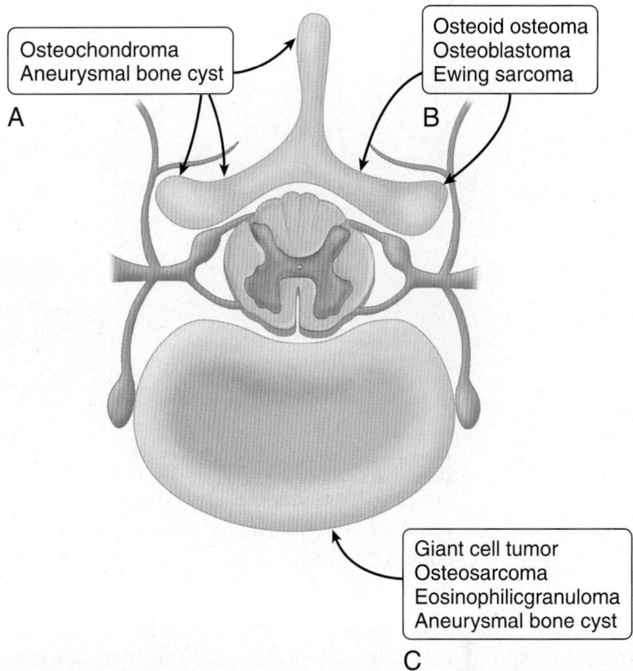

FIGURE 6.10 Most common topographical locations for the occurrence of each of the possible primary osseous lesions in the pediatric spinal column. *A,* Lesions that occur along the facet joint, laminar arch, and spinous process. *B,* Lesions that can occur at the facet joint or pedicle or along the laminar arches or pars interarticularis. C, Lesions that occur along the vertebral body. (From Ravindra VM, Eli IM, Schmidt MH, et al: Primary osseous tumors of the pediatric spinal column: review of pathology and surgical decision making, *Neurosurg Focus* 41:E3, 2016.)

annulus. Violation of two of the four complexes, or disruption of 50% of the stabilizing structures, is an indication for instrumentation and fusion. Bony involvement by tumors also contributes to impending pathologic fracture and instability. Considerations for impending instability or for determining stability after fracture include more than 50% collapse of the vertebral body, translation, segmental kyphosis of more than 20 degrees above normal, and involvement of anterior and posterior columns.

CLASSIFICATION AND ADJUVANT TREATMENTS

As with tumors in other locations, the Enneking classification is useful in determining treatment of spinal tumors (Fig. 6.11). Stage 1 tumors (e.g., osteoid osteoma, eosinophilic granuloma, osteochondroma, and hemangioma) are latent and typically require no treatment. If surgery is necessary, often intralesional excision is all that is required, with or without adjuvants such as liquid nitrogen, phenol, or polymethylmethacrylate (PMMA). Stage 2 lesions are active, become symptomatic, and usually require en bloc excision (i.e., removal of the tumor as a whole, as opposed to piecemeal). Examples of stage 2 lesions include osteoid osteoma, osteoblastoma, eosinophilic granuloma, more aggressive hemangiomas, osteochondroma, and ABCs. Aggressive lesions are characterized as stage 3. Despite being classified as benign tumors, lesions such as GCTs and osteoblastomas are locally aggressive and have a tendency to recur. Wide excision is indicated for these lesions and consists of removal of the tumor with a cuff of normal tissue if possible. A marginal excision would result in a biopsy specimen that includes the reactive zone around the tumor. The exact type of excisional biopsy often is dictated by the anatomy of the spine and the location of the tumor.

A number of adjuvant treatments have been developed in recent years to help manage benign spine tumors of various types. These include denosumab, bisphosphonates, doxycycline, selective arterial embolization, and thermal ablation. Denosumab is a monoclonal antibody that targets the receptor of activator nuclear factor kappa-B ligand (RANKL). This receptor is important for the mediation of osteolysis by the multinucleated giant cells of GCT. Targeting RANKL with denosumab has shown efficacy in myeloma and metastatic disease and more recently by Branstetter et al. in GCT. Because of concerns about disease progression with discontinuation and reports of sarcomatous change during denosumab therapy, the indications remain unclear. Selective arterial embolization is recommended in the treatment of GCT and ABC of the spine. Care must be taken, especially in the lower thoracic spine, to identify the anterior spinal artery of Adamkiewicz; paralysis has been reported due to selective arterial embolization. Doxycycline is an antibiotic that has been shown to have certain antitumor properties, including inhibition of

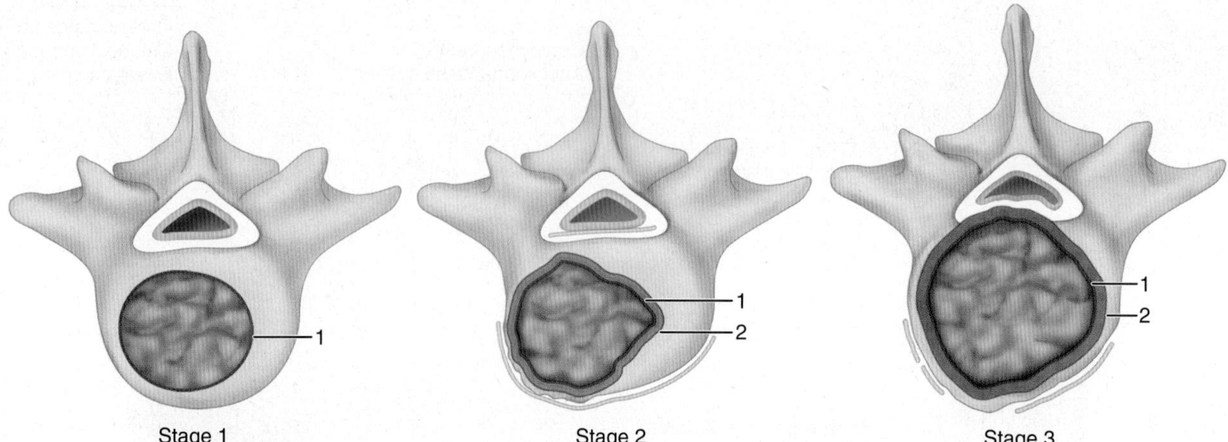

FIGURE 6.11 Enneking staging of benign spinal tumors. Capsule of tumor is indicated by *1*, and reactive pseudocapsule is indicated by *2*. Stage 3 aggressive benign tumors can expand through posterior vertebral wall and compress cord. Pseudocapsule is vascularized reactive tissue and can adhere to dura.

osteoblastic cell function and possibly osteoclast apoptosis and inhibition of matrix metalloproteinase. Thermal ablation has been used primarily in treating osteoid osteoma.

POSTERIOR ELEMENT TUMORS

OSTEOID OSTEOMA

Osteoid osteoma is a lesion of bony origin that was first described by Jaffe in 1935. These lesions are most common in the spine (42%), affect men more often than women, and occur most often in the second decade of life. The lumbar spine is the most common location, the cervical next, and the thoracic last, and the lesion is almost invariably located in the posterior elements. A few cases of osteoid osteomas of vertebral bodies have been reported. This lesion is not locally aggressive and is defined by a size of less than 2 cm; larger lesions are classified as osteoblastomas.

Pain is the primary complaint in 83% of patients, is worse at night with awakening in nearly 30%, and is relieved by aspirin in 27%. Because of the location in the posterior elements, radiculopathy occurs in 28% of patients. A painful scoliosis may result, with the lesion usually present at the apex of the curve in the concavity. Although various curve types may result, the usual structural features of vertebral rotation normally present in idiopathic scoliosis are absent. The resultant scoliosis is rigid and rapidly progressive. Saifuddin et al., in a meta-analysis of spinal osteoid osteoma and osteoblastoma, determined that (1) 63% of patients had scoliosis, (2) scoliosis was significantly more common with osteoid osteomas than with osteoblastomas, (3) lesions were more common in the thoracic and lumbar regions than in the cervical region and more common in the lower cervical region than in the upper cervical region, and (4) lesions were more commonly located to one side of the midline. They concluded that these findings support the concept that in patients with spinal osteoid osteoma or osteoblastoma, scoliosis is secondary to asymmetric muscle spasm.

Diagnosis can be difficult because early radiographs may appear normal. Frequently, a sclerotic lesion of the posterior elements is all that is apparent, and even this may be a subtle asymmetry. Later, the usual configuration of a central nidus with surrounding sclerosis may be found, but it is typical in appearance in only half of patients. Oblique radiographs can be helpful when the pedicle, facet, and pars interarticularis are studied. A radioisotopic bone scan is most helpful in accurate localization, and CT often shows the nidus which is less than 1.5 cm in size.

Treatment consists of observation for small lesions which may involute, thermal ablation in some cases, or more commonly surgical excision of the lesion if symptoms fail to improve or the scoliosis is progressive. Thermal ablation is not indicated if the lesion is less than 10 mm from the neural elements. Nidus excision requires careful preoperative planning and can be confirmed by specimen CT. Several studies have shown benefit from intraoperative CT and three-dimensional (3D) navigation to accurately locate the lesion and excise it. If the spine is considered unstable because of facet or pedicle removal, a single-level fusion is done simultaneously. Complete excision should result in improvement in the angular degree of the scoliosis, although resolution is less likely in patients 9 to 13.5 years old. Scoliosis persists in 20% to 30% of patients after successful resection. Curves that persist for more than 18 months after resection may require treatment. Brace management may be necessary in immature patients, and regular follow-up is advised. Surgery for spinal deformity usually is deferred until after treatment and resection of the osteoid osteoma and follows the same principles as for idiopathic scoliosis. Prompt relief of pain is the best postoperative indicator of successful removal of the tumor.

OSTEOBLASTOMA

Osteoblastoma accounts for 10% of all spinal tumors, and 32% appear in the spine. Similar to osteoid osteoma, osteoblastoma occurs most commonly in the second and third decades, with a male-to-female ratio of 2 : 1. These lesions almost always involve the pedicle or posterior elements or both, although contiguous levels may be affected. The predominant spinal region affected is the cervical region (40%), followed by the lumbar (23%), thoracic (21%), and sacral regions (17%). Osteoblastoma may be misdiagnosed as an osteosarcoma, Ewing sarcoma, lymphoma, or ABC, which all are high on the list of differential diagnoses. Differentiation from osteoid osteoma is based on size—these lesions exceed 2 cm. Neurologic deficits are relatively common because of the large size of osteoblastomas.

Radiographic evaluation reveals a destructive, expansile lesion with a thin rim of cortical bone. Lytic features are predominant and occur in 50%, with purely blastic changes in 20%. Bone scanning always is positive and is helpful in identification. Although MRI is useful in identifying a soft-tissue mass, it may confuse the picture. A "flare" reaction may occur, suggesting extracompartmental extension and confusing the diagnosis of a benign lesion. As with other bony lesions, CT is best for definition of the extent of the tumor and for identification of the nidus.

Wide excision, if possible, is the treatment of choice. The tumor recurs 9 years after resection in 10% to 20% of patients with intralesional excision. The best indication of successful removal is relief of preoperative pain. Because of the possibility of recurrence and malignant transformation, however, long-term CT follow-up is mandatory. Operative treatment is necessary for recurrences because these lesions are not radiosensitive. A case report by Reynolds et al. found that a preoperative course of denosumab caused tumor regression and simplified surgical management.

OSTEOCHONDROMA

Although rarely symptomatic, osteochondroma is the most common benign primary bone tumor. Half of patients with symptomatic tumors are younger than 20 years old, which is consistent with the growing cartilaginous cap. Males are affected three times more often than females, with most lesions protruding eccentrically from the neural arch. Because the spinal canal is occupied by spinal cord in the thoracic and cervical spine, lesions here are more frequently symptomatic. Ninety-one percent of spinal osteochondromas occur in the cervical and upper thoracic spine, although the lumbar spine and sacrum also are affected. The lack of symptoms may result in underdiagnosis of lesions in the lumbar and sacral regions.

Radiographic evaluation often is diagnostic, with the lesions found most often in the posterior elements. Because of the radiolucent cartilaginous cap, however, MRI or myelography may be necessary to determine if impingement of the neural structures is present. These lesions are slow growing and require excision only if symptomatic. Malignant transformation occurs in less than 1% of tumors and is suspected when symptoms are rapid in onset with growth of a previously stable osteochondroma. A cartilaginous cap larger than 1 cm also is suspect. En bloc excision including all of the cartilaginous cap is done, with neurologic recovery the rule and recurrence the exception. If there is recurrence, however, reoperation is recommended because malignant transformation has occurred in 10% of patients.

ANEURYSMAL BONE CYST

ABCs are relatively uncommon, accounting for only 1% to 2% of benign bone tumors. Although predominantly a posterior element lesion, an ABC may expand to include the pedicle and vertebral body. Of all ABCs, 11% to 30% occur in the spine and are most frequent in patients younger than 20 years old. There does not seem to be a gender preference. Back pain is the predominant symptom in 95% of patients, although muscle spasms causing spinal rigidity or scoliosis also may be present. The differential diagnosis includes GCTs, tuberculosis, fibrous dysplasia, eosinophilic granuloma, Ewing sarcoma, and osteoblastoma.

The characteristic radiographic finding with ABCs is an expansile lesion with a reactive rim of cortical bone outlining the lesion as it expands from the cortex, although this may be absent in 30%. Another characteristic feature is that these lesions may affect contiguous levels. Arteriography may show a lesion with multiple septa and blood-filled spaces. MRI with gadolinium enhancement also shows the fluid levels within the septations.

Selective arterial embolization may be successful, although some may require repeated embolizations. Low-dose irradiation has had limited success, with few side effects when dosages are less than 30 Gy. Radiation alone is successful, however, in only approximately 50%. Surgery has remained the standard of care for ABCs. After embolization to decrease intraoperative blood loss, en bloc excision is preferred when possible because recurrence rates are low with this technique. Embolization must be undertaken with caution, especially in the lower thoracic spine to avoid paraplegia. Intralesional resection by curettage and bone grafting is done if en bloc resection is not possible. With intralesional curettage, the recurrence ranges from 13% to 60%. Any instability created must be treated at the time of surgery and often requires a single-level fusion in skeletally immature patients. Shiels et al. reported a series of ABCs treated with intralesional doxycycline with radiographic improvement in 18 of 21. Only five patients had spinal ABCs.

VERTEBRAL BODY TUMORS

Typical benign lesions found in the vertebral bodies include hemangiomas, eosinophilic granulomas, and GCTs. Historically, lesions such as these were considered surgically inaccessible when in the vertebrae. The older literature recommended irradiation or chemotherapy. Although this still may be appropriate in special circumstances, such as in highly radiosensitive malignant tumors, angular deformity with potential paraplegia may result because of subsequent spinal instability. Benign tumors are best treated without irradiation to avoid secondary sarcomatous change. Optimal treatment of aggressive benign or solitary malignant tumors usually is anterior resection of the tumor for cure or for tumor debulking.

HEMANGIOMA

Hemangioma is a common hamartomatous lesion, present in 10% to 12% of autopsy specimens. Most of these lesions are clinically silent and are detected only incidentally during evaluation for other problems. Occurrence may be single or multiple with contiguous levels affected, but the vertebral body is the most common location, especially in the lumbar and lower thoracic regions. The posterior elements are involved in 10% to 15% of patients; however, this is atypical and indicative of an aggressive lesion. Patients with symptomatic hemangiomas most commonly have pain (60%), neurologic compromise (30%), or symptomatic fracture (10%). Epidural cavernous hemangiomas are rare. Several case reports can be found in the recent literature. Differentiation from metastatic lesions can be clinically difficult, but dynamic contrast MRI can be helpful.

Radiographs detect larger lesions, which have vertical striations and coarse, thick trabeculae, described as a "corduroy" vertebra. Expansion may be noted in aggressive hemangiomas, with expansion of the vertebral body. Axial CT shows a classic "polka dot" appearance. Bone scanning is not particularly helpful because lesions may be either hot or cold. MRI has become the standard for diagnosing these lesions. Typical hemangiomas are identified by increased intensity on T1- and T2-weighted sequences and can be differentiated from Paget disease because pagetic bone has more cortical thickening and affects the entire vertebral body. Aggressive hemangiomas can involve the entire vertebral body, may be expansile, and may have a soft-tissue component, which is differentiated from typical hemangioma by hypointensity on T1-weighted images and hyperintensity on T2-weighted images.

Most hemangiomas do not require treatment, and other causes of pain must be excluded. For rare symptomatic lesions, radiation is successful in 50% to 80%. Embolization also is useful, especially in patients with progressive neurologic deficits, and may provide temporary relief of pain. Vertebroplasty has been used successfully for treatment of aggressive hemangiomas by stabilizing pathologic bone with an injection of bone cement into the vertebral body. Use of inflatable bone tamps has had similarly good short-term results. Direct intralesional injection of ethanol has been reported to be effective in obliterating symptomatic vertebral hemangiomas. CT angiography is required before injection to identify functional vascular spaces of the hemangioma and to direct needle placement. Less than 15 mL of ethanol should be used because pathologic fractures of the involved vertebrae have been reported in two patients who received 42 mL and 50 mL. For progressive neurologic deficit, radiation alone may be successful in arresting progression. With neurologic deficit and fracture, however, surgery with en bloc resection is necessary to remove an aggressive hemangioma, and embolization should be done preoperatively to minimize bleeding intraoperatively.

EOSINOPHILIC GRANULOMA

Eosinophilic granuloma is most common in patients younger than 10 years old, but it can occur well into adulthood, with reported cases in the eighth decade. It typically is a solitary lesion of bone, with 7% to 15% occurring in the spine, and has a predilection for the cervical or thoracic region. Symptoms usually include pain, muscular rigidity, and neurologic deficits; systemic symptoms may occur. The classic radiographic finding is vertebra plana seen as a complete collapse of the vertebral body on the lateral view. Bone scans are cold, and MRI often reveals a flare reaction on T2-weighted images, which can be mistaken for a malignant lesion. Differential diagnoses include Ewing sarcoma, ABC, infection, tuberculosis, leukemia, and neuroblastoma. Because radiographic findings are not pathognomonic, biopsy is necessary.

When the diagnosis is made, immobilization and observation alone often are sufficient treatment unless there is significant neurologic deficit. These lesions typically regress spontaneously over time with some, although incomplete, restoration of vertebral deformity. Follow-up is important to detect instability. Operative intervention, including curettage and grafting, may speed healing. There presently is no role for radiation in the treatment of eosinophilic granuloma. Recurrence is unusual, and resolution of neurologic deficits usually occurs as the tumor regresses.

GIANT CELL TUMOR

GCT is the most prevalent benign tumor of the sacrum, rarely affecting other spinal sites, and is second only to hemangioma as the most common benign spinal neoplasm. These benign tumors can be locally aggressive. GCTs account for 4% to 5% of all primary bone tumors, occurring most often between the third and fifth decades. Females are affected twice as frequently as males, and 1% to 18% of GCTs occur in the spine. Because of its lytic appearance, differential diagnoses include ABCs, osteoblastoma, and metastasis.

Pain is the most common complaint and often has been present a long time before diagnosis. Neurologic deficits occur in 20% to 80% of patients with GCTs of the spine. Radiographs show the lesions as lytic, septated, and expansile, often with cortical breakthrough and an associated soft-tissue mass. More than 50% of these lesions involve the vertebral body only. When present in the sacrum, the lesion is in the proximal aspect and eccentrically located. The cervical spine is the second most common location in the spine behind the sacrum.

Because of the aggressive nature of these lesions, en bloc resection with wide margins is necessary. The addition of denosumab has been beneficial in treating unresectable GCT. Despite aggressive operative treatment, a 10% to 80% recurrence rate has been reported. Preoperative embolization is recommended. Embolization, denosumab, and radiation are reserved for lesions that cannot be resected or excised completely or in which surgery would result in significant functional morbidity. Doses ranging from 3500 to 4500 cGy are safe and effective in controlling GCT. If intralesional excision is done, adjuvant cryotherapy should be considered. Metastases occur in 1% to 11% of patients, with a 10% incidence of sarcomatous change.

PRIMARY MALIGNANT TUMORS

Almost all patients with malignancies of the spine have pain. More than 95% seek medical care for pain, with radiculopathy occurring in about 20% of these patients.

CLASSIFICATION

The Enneking classification of malignant tumors also is useful for spinal tumors: stage I, low grade; stage II, high grade; and stage III, regional or distant metastases (Fig. 6.12). The site of the tumor is indicated by A, intracompartmental, or B, extracompartmental. This classification scheme is useful in determining if marginal or wide excision is best. Radical excision is impossible in the spine.

OSTEOSARCOMA

Primary osteosarcoma of the spine is rare, accounting for only 3% of all osteosarcomas, and frequently is fatal. Pain is the most common presenting complaint, but neurologic symptoms also are present in 70% of patients. These tumors are anterior column tumors, and 95% affect the vertebral body. Men and women are equally affected. Secondary osteosarcomas, which occur most commonly after irradiation or develop in patients with Paget disease, affect patients in their 60s. Soft-tissue extension, or extracompartmental disease, is the rule at the time of diagnosis, which is evident on MRI or at surgery.

Radiographs may show a lytic, blastic, or mixed picture affecting the vertebral body. Bone scanning is useful in identifying multicentric or metastatic disease, and axial CT scans are useful in delineating the bony anatomy. Intensive radiation therapy and chemotherapy are the primary treatments.

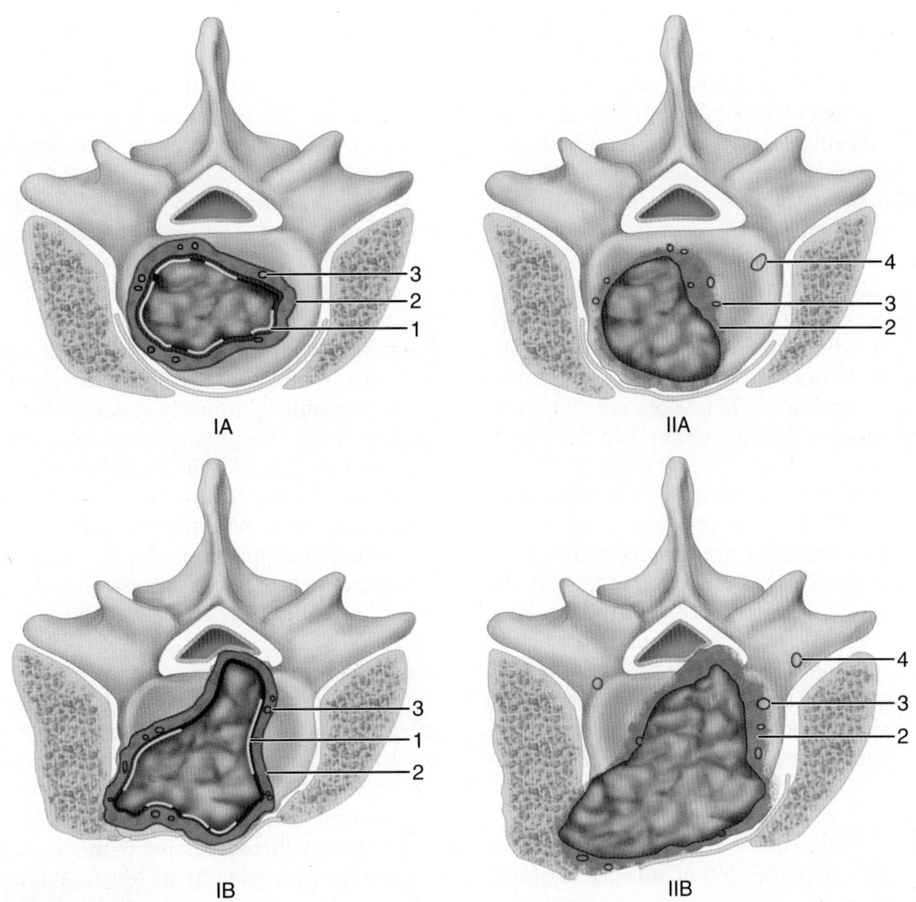

FIGURE 6.12 Enneking staging of malignant spinal tumors. Capsule of tumor is indicated by *1*, pseudocapsule is indicated by *2*, island of tumor within pseudocapsule (satellites) is indicated by *3* and at distance (skip metastases) is indicated by *4*. Types IB and IIB tumors can compress cord if expanding posteriorly. Pseudocapsule is more or less infiltrated by neoplastic tissue, which can have direct contact with dural sac.

Surgery is recommended when wide resection is possible with adjuvant radiation therapy. The risk of local recurrence has been shown to be five times greater in patients with positive resection margins than in patients with tumor-free resection margins. Wide or marginal excision of the tumors improves survival; therefore, chemotherapy and at least marginal excision should be done if possible. Patients with metastases, large tumors, and sacral tumors have a poor prognosis. No association, however, has been found between the affected spinal region and outcome. Total sacrectomy and reconstruction with PMMA, plate-and-screw devices, and custom-made prostheses have been reported to be successful in the treatment of sacral osteosarcoma. Pombo et al. in a systematic review that included 108 cases confirmed that patients with Enneking-appropriate resections (wide or marginal) had longer survival and fewer recurrences or metastases than those with intralesional or contaminated margins.

EWING SARCOMA

Another anterior column primary bone tumor, Ewing sarcoma, is a permeative lesion that affects the spine only 3.5% to 8% of the time, with half of these tumors found in the sacrum. Neurologic deficits are present in many patients because of soft-tissue extension, and constitutional symptoms are common. Radiographic findings are confusing, with vertebra plana apparent in some patients, which may be confused with eosinophilic granuloma. Generally, these tumors are lytic, with a soft-tissue mass identified on MRI. Surgical resection and reconstruction and decompression may be indicated for tumors causing neurologic compromise and for potential instability to preserve neurologic function. Long-term survival is possible with this tumor. Systematic review by Berger et al. identified 28 cases of spinal Ewing sarcoma treated surgically. The 1-, 2-, and 5-year survival rates were 82%, 75%, and 57%, respectively. Patients younger than 14 and older than 20 years had substantially better prognoses than those aged 14 to 20 years; however, other studies have shown that multiagent chemotherapy without surgery may have similar results. There is a predilection for Ewing sarcoma to involve the sacrum and pelvis more so than other areas of the spine, often with large soft-tissue components. Radiation therapy is often also recommended for sacral lesions. The AO Spine Knowledge Forum Tumor has recommended surgery for spinal Ewing sarcoma when a wide or marginal excision is possible, along with neoadjuvant and postoperative chemotherapy.

CHORDOMA

Primarily a tumor of adults, chordoma is an uncommon tumor that can occur at all spine levels but most often affects the sacrum and coccyx followed by the cervical spine. It originates embryologically from the notochord remnants and, as such, usually is a midline tumor. It is relatively slow growing but relentless in progression with high recurrence rates when a wide excision is not obtained. Symptoms usually are indolent with a palpable mass in the sacrum anteriorly on rectal examination. Men are affected twice as often as women, and the tumor affects an older population, with peak incidences during the fifth and seventh decades.

Radiographs reveal a lytic lesion in the midline of the sacrum with variable calcification. Bone scans often are negative because of the indolent biologic behavior of these tumors. MRI provides excellent delineation of the anterior soft-tissue extension that typically occurs with these tumors. Treatment involves a wide en bloc excision where feasible, which may be impossible in the craniocervical junction and in the proximal sacrum without sacrifice of the S2 nerve roots. Radiation therapy may be the primary treatment modality in these areas. The 5-year survival for chordomas is reported to be 45% to 67%. Bowel and bladder continence are retained only if both the S2 roots and one of the S3 roots are preserved. If for any reason the tumor is incised during excision, recurrence may be as high as 64%. As a result, great care is needed in resection of these tumors and radiation should be used for tumors with incisional margins. Long-term survival may approach 50% to 75% if marginal resection or better is achieved. A large database study of 1598 patients by Lee et al. found the disease-specific survival to be 71% at 5 years and 57% at 10 years.

■ MULTIPLE MYELOMA

Plasmacytoma is the single-lesion variety of multiple myeloma and is rare, accounting for only 3% of plasma cell dyscrasias. This diagnosis carries a 60% 5-year survival rate. Thereafter, gradual progression to multiple myeloma occurs, although extended survival has been reported. Multiple myeloma, in contrast, accounts for 1% of newly diagnosed malignancies and is uniformly fatal within 4 years of diagnosis in all patients when spinal disease is diagnosed. Men and women are equally affected during the sixth to eighth decades. These tumors result from unregulated proliferation of plasma cells, causing systemic manifestations. Diagnosis is confirmed by the presence of at least 10% abnormal plasma cells, lytic bone lesions, and monoclonal gammopathy diagnosed on serum protein electrophoresis or urine protein electrophoresis. Anemia and elevation of sedimentation rate also are characteristic on laboratory studies. Protein electrophoresis may be negative in 3% of patients with myeloma, which requires a low threshold for bone marrow aspiration in patients at risk. Treatment of plasmacytoma and multiple myeloma is irradiation, with operative intervention reserved for patients with neurologic deficits or progression despite maximal chemotherapy and irradiation. A Cochrane review in 2017 found that some bisphosphonates reduced vertebral but not other fractures and did not improve overall survival or disease progression-free survival. In addition, the risk of osteonecrosis of the jaw was 1/1000 patients.

METASTATIC TUMORS

Metastatic tumors are the most common malignant lesions found in bone, present 40 times more often than all primary malignant bone tumors combined. Metastatic disease involves the spine in 50% to 85% of patients. The spine is the most common site of skeletal metastasis. Metastatic spread to the spine favors the thoracic region (70%), followed by the lumbar spine (20%), the cervical spine, and the sacrum. The vertebral body is the most common site of metastasis, followed by the pedicle and then the posterior elements. Ninety percent of tumors are extradural, 5% are intradural, and 1% are intramedullary. Breast, lung, and prostate are the most frequent tumors to metastasize to the spine, followed by thyroid, renal, and gastrointestinal cancer. Lymphoma is another tumor that commonly affects the spine and must be considered. Advances in chemotherapy, radiation therapy, and other cancer therapies have resulted in a significant improvement in survival for many of these types of cancer. With the improved survival, previously silent spinal metastases are becoming clinically apparent and significantly impair quality of life. The management of metastatic spinal lesions has been significantly impacted by stereotactic body radiotherapy and other advanced radiation delivery methods. This technique can allow durable local tumor control with many different tumor histologic types. Surgery is most useful for significant neurologic compression and deficit and significant spinal instability. The goals of decompression and restoration of stability can be accomplished with less radical surgery in some cases.

The chief complaint in most patients is pain, although 36% of spinal metastases do not cause symptoms. Pain usually is progressive and unremitting, and often no relief occurs even with rest or at night. A previous history of cancer, regardless of how remote, must prompt a search for metastatic disease in patients with progressive pain. Neurologic symptoms or signs may be present but are less frequent, occurring in 5% to 20% of patients with spinal metastases. For patients with thoracic metastasis, however, the rate of neurologic symptoms increases to 37%, probably because less space is available for the spinal cord available at this level compared with compression of the nerve roots in the lumbar spine. In patients who develop neurologic deterioration and paraparesis, only 25% to 35% regain lost motor function. According to a systematic review by Kumar et al., patients who present with significant neurologic deficits or incontinence benefit from a loading dose of IV dexamethasone 10 mg and 16 mg/day orally, with a rapid taper. Patients who are paraplegic or have complete bowel or bladder dysfunction are not likely to regain function regardless of treatment, especially if the deficit has persisted more than 12 hours. Rapid onset of symptoms over less than 24 hours also indicates a poor prognosis for neurologic recovery, in contrast to a lesion with a slower onset of symptoms. With aggressive treatment, 60% of patients who retain the ability to walk before treatment of spinal metastasis maintain this function after treatment. In a study comparing radiation with surgery for patients with metastatic cord compression and neurologic symptoms, those who received surgery had greater benefits in terms of ambulation ability than those who had radiation. Imaging often is inconclusive and nondiagnostic in these patients. Plain radiographs of the spine are inconclusive in many with metastatic disease. The most useful skeletal screening study is bone scanning, which identifies most lesions larger than 2 mm, although false-negative studies occur in 5%. Multiple myeloma, breast, nasopharyngeal, lung, and renal tumors are the most likely neoplasms to appear falsely negative on bone scans. Use of CT is helpful in delineating soft-tissue extension from the bone or into the bone from extrinsic sources. Also, certain features of the CT

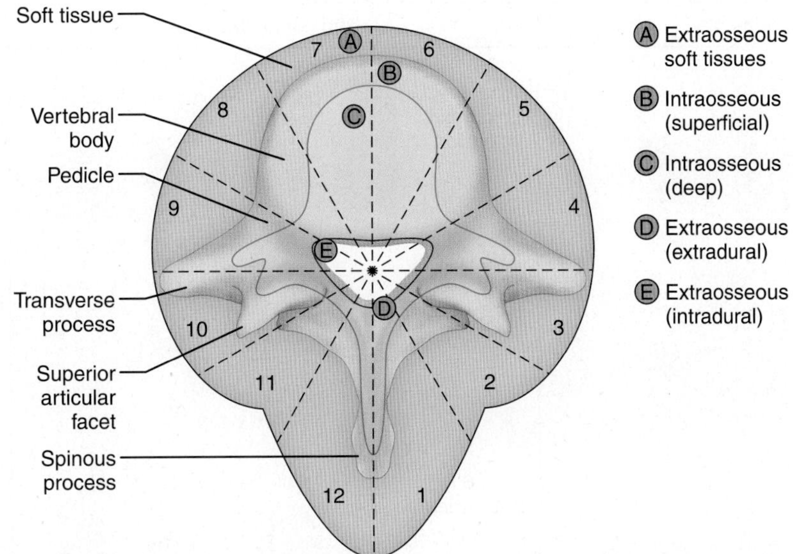

FIGURE 6.13 Weinstein-Boriani-Biagini surgical staging system. In this classification, the spine is divided radially into 12 equal segments (clock face) in the axial plane and examined in five layers from superficial to deep plane. (From Ciftdemir M, Kaya M, Selcuk E, et al: Tumors of the spine, *World J Orthop* 7:109, 2016.)

scan are useful in determining whether a compression fracture is a result of osteoporosis or metastasis. Osteoporotic compression fractures reveal no evidence of cortical destruction, homogeneous involvement of the vertebral body, localized pathology, and the absence of a soft-tissue mass. MRI is the imaging modality of choice and is more useful in evaluating soft-tissue masses, neural elements, and vertebral body lesions. Characteristic features of metastatic lesions are hypointensity on T1-weighted images, with enhancement on T2-weighted images and gadolinium-enhanced T1-weighted images. The STIR sequences are the most sensitive, demonstrating hyperintense tumor and suppressed marrow fat signal.

Myelography occasionally is necessary for tumors not well defined by other, less invasive, procedures but should be used cautiously because it can precipitate neurologic deterioration in 16% to 24% of patients, necessitating immediate decompression.

CLASSIFICATION

Dewald et al. developed a classification of spinal metastases that incorporates the extent of bony involvement, the presence of deformity, and the immune status of the patient. These factors were used to recommend surgical treatment for metastatic spinal disease. Other researchers have contributed newer classification schemes, including the Weinstein-Boriani-Biagini surgical staging system (Fig. 6.13). This system incorporates a radially oriented division of the vertebra into 12 equal sections, like the face of a clock. The center is in the spinal canal. It also includes five layers extending from extraosseous to intradural. Tomita et al. developed a prognostic scoring system incorporating tumor characteristics and presence and type of visceral and bony metastases. The prognostic score can be used to determine treatment goals and surgical strategy (Fig. 6.14 and Table 6.2).

The newest framework is the Neurologic, Oncologic, Mechanical stability, and Systemic (NOMS) (Table 6.3), which was developed to provide a comprehensive assessment of spinal metastatic disease. This system allows complex decision-making and improves communication among all members of the treating team. The neurologic considerations assess the presence of radiculopathy/myelopathy and the degree of neural compression passed on the Epidural Spinal Cord Compression scale (Fig. 6.15). The oncologic assessment evaluates the predicted local tumor control from radiation, chemotherapy, or surgery. The mechanical stability assesses spinal instability caused by pathologic fracture and serves as an independent indication for procedure-based interventions such as percutaneous cement augmentation. The systemic assessment is to evaluate the disease status and comorbidities of the patient, which help predict the ability of the patient to tolerate any proposed intervention and the overall survival.

OPERATIVE TREATMENT

Indications for surgical decompression can include the requirement of tissue for diagnosis; treatment of an isolated lesion; treatment of a fracture causing instability, pain, or spinal canal compromise; radioresistant tumors, which usually include gastrointestinal and kidney metastases; recurrent tumor in a previously irradiated field; neurologic symptoms that are progressive despite adjuvant measures; and potential instability. The development of stereotactic body radiotherapy has impacted these indications, but this modality is not universally available. Operative procedures can be extensive and involve significant blood loss; the patient must be in a physical state that allows for survival of the proposed procedure. Expected survival of more than 6 weeks is a relative indication for surgery in the presence of unremitting or progressive symptoms, although general physical condition also is important in operative decision-making (see Table 6.3). In patients with a reasonable long-term survival, bone grafting is recommended rather than PMMA because of the likely failure of such materials. Adjunctive radiation therapy must

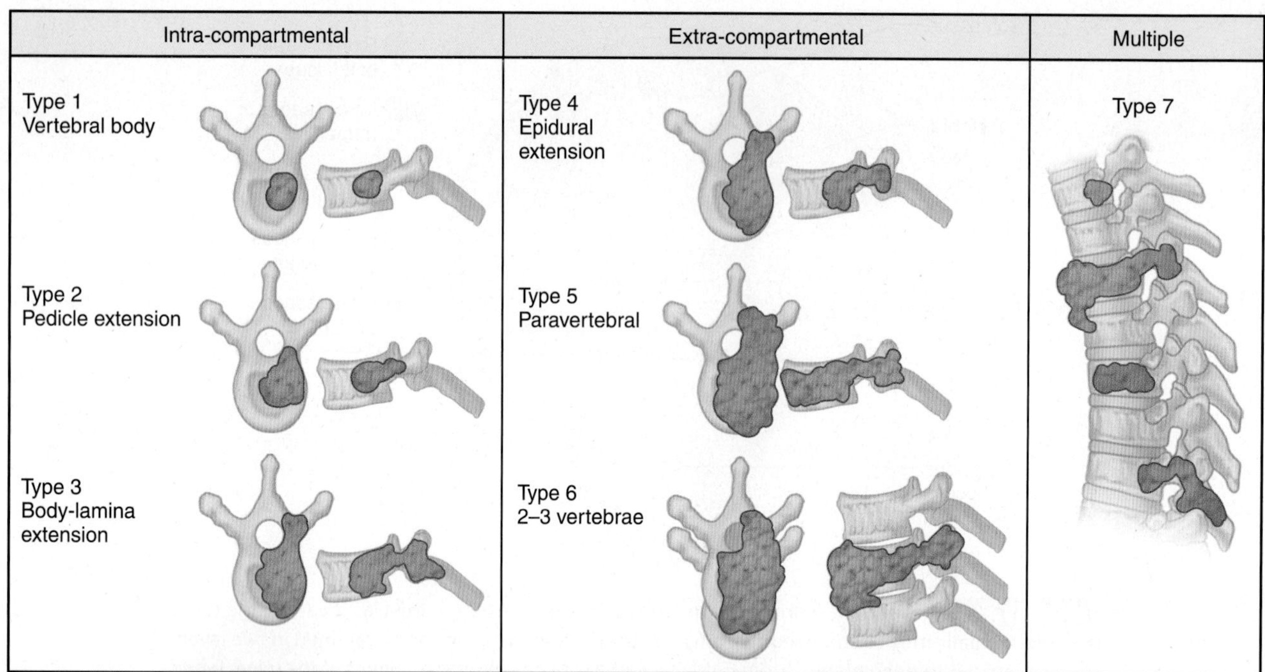

FIGURE 6.14 Tomita et al. surgical classification of spinal tumors. (From Ciftdemir M, Kaya M, Selcuk E, et al: Tumors of the spine, *World J Orthop* 7:109, 2016.)

TABLE 6.2

Surgical Strategy for Spinal Metastases

POINT	SCORING SYSTEM			PROGNOSTIC SCORE	TREATMENT GOAL	SURGICAL STRATEGY
	PROGNOSTIC FACTORS					
	PRIMARY TUMOR	VISCERAL METASTASES	BONE METASTASES*			
1	Slow growth (breast, thyroid, etc.)		Solitary or isolated	2	Long-term local control	Wide or marginal excision
				3		
2	Moderate growth (kidney, uterus, etc.)	Treatable	Multiple	4	Middle-term local control	Marginal or intra-lesional excision
				5		
4	Rapid growth (lung, stomach, etc.)	Untreatable		6	Short-term palliation	Palliative surgery
				7		
				8	Terminal care	Supportive care
				9		
				10		

No visceral metastases = 0 points.
*Bone metastases: including spinal metastases.
From Ciftdemir M, Kaya M, Selcuk E, et al: Tumors of the spine, *World J Orthop* 7:109, 2016.

be planned carefully, however, to allow for incorporation of grafts when used. This is best accomplished by performing the irradiation preoperatively or delaying it until at least 3 weeks postoperatively if possible to improve fusion rates. Because of the hypercoagulable state of malignancy, especially in patients with paraplegia, the use of a preoperative inferior vena cava filter also should be considered as should anticoagulation therapy perioperatively.

Laminectomy has been shown to be of little value in the treatment of progressive paralysis caused by malignant spinal tumors in the anterior column. Successful results using this approach have been reported in only 30% to 40% of patients and are inferior to the results obtained with radiation alone. Radical laminectomy for tumor resection is of value, however, and should be considered when compression is caused by lesions in the posterior elements compressing the

TABLE 6.3

Current Neurologic, Oncologic, Mechanical, and Systemic (NOMS) Decision Framework

NEUROLOGIC	ONCOLOGIC	MECHANICAL	SYSTEMIC	DECISION
Low-grade ESCC + no myelopathy	Radiosensitive	Stable		cEBRT
	Radiosensitive	Unstable		Stabilization followed by cEBRT
	Radiosensitive	Stable		SRS
	Radiosensitive	Unstable		Stabilization followed by SRS
High-grade ESCC ± no myelopathy	Radiosensitive	Stable		cEBRT
	Radiosensitive	Unstable		Stabilization followed by cEBRT
	Radiosensitive	Stable	Able to tolerate surgery	Decompression/stabilization followed by SRS
	Radiosensitive	Stable	Able to tolerate surgery	cEBRT
	Radiosensitive	Unstable	Able to tolerate surgery	Decompression/stabilization followed by SRS
	Radiosensitive	Unstable	Able to tolerate surgery	Stabilization followed by cEBRT

cEBRT, Conventional external beam radiation; *ESCC,* epidural spinal cord compression; *SRS,* stereotactic radiosurgery.
Low-grade ESCC is defined as grade 0 or 1 on Spine Oncology Study Group scoring system. High-grade ESCC is defined as grade 2 or 3 on the ESCC scale.
From Barzilai O, Fisher CG, Bilsky MH: State of the art treatment of spinal metastatic disease, *Neurosurgery* 82:757, 2018.

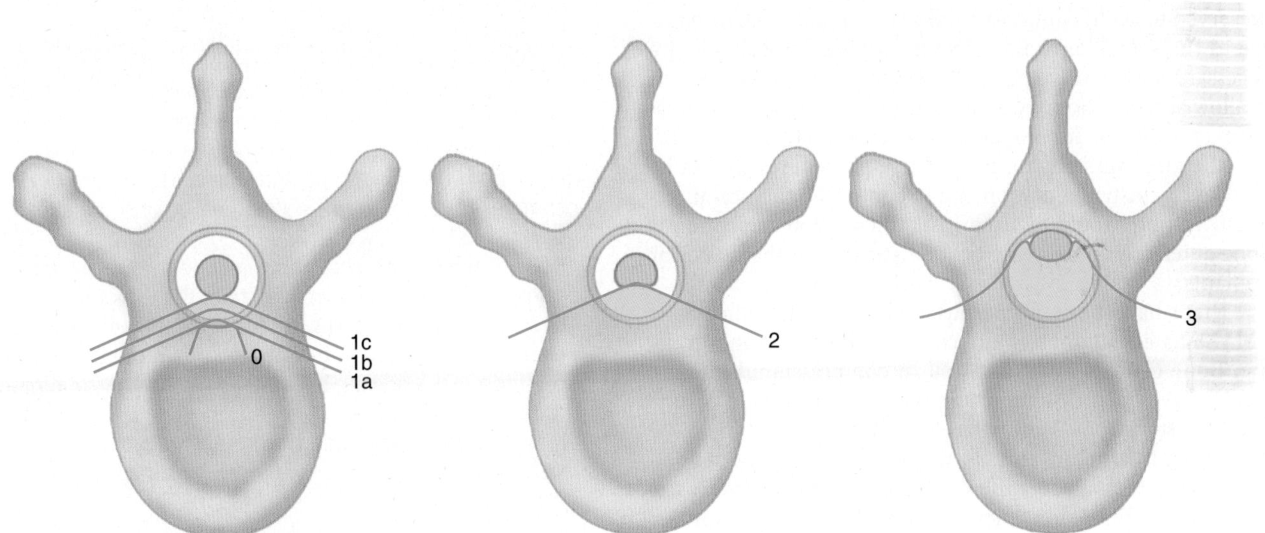

FIGURE 6.15 Schematic representation of the six-point epidural spinal cord compression scale (ESCC) grading scale. A grade of *0* indicates bone-only disease; *1a,* epidural impingement, without deformation of the thecal sac; *1b,* deformation of the thecal sac, with spinal cord abutment; *1c,* deformation of the thecal sac with spinal cord abutment, but without cord compression. *2,* Spinal cord compression, but with CSF visible around the cord. *3,* Spinal cord compression, with cerebral spinal fluid (CSF) visible around the cord. (From Bilsky MH, Laufer I, Fourney DR, et al: Reliability analysis of the epidural spinal cord compression scale, *J Neurosurg Spine* 13:324, 2010.)

dura. Careful evaluation of diagnostic images is necessary for appropriate preoperative planning of the operative approach and subsequent procedures.

Because of the predominant vertebral body location of malignant tumors, anterior decompression is most often necessary to remove the pathologic process responsible for neurologic deterioration and pain. Other indications for anterior surgery include pathologic kyphosis with an intact posterior osteoligamentous complex. Improvement in pain is possible in 80% to 95% of patients, with restoration of neurologic function in 75%. Decompression often creates instability that requires reconstruction with instrumentation, allografts, and occasionally structural bone cement. Although circumferential instrumentation is definitely superior in stabilization, anterior instrumentation alone often suffices if the posterior osteoligamentous complex is intact and resection is less than a complete spondylectomy. Additional posterior decompression and stabilization in a combined approach often are necessary if the spinal canal is compressed anteriorly and posteriorly or if the posterior column is attenuated. If exposure of anterior and posterior columns is necessary, a two-stage approach combined under one anesthesia or a simultaneous approach can be used. High-grade instability, contiguous vertebral involvement, destruction of anterior and posterior columns, and need for en bloc resection are indications for these approaches. Stable fixation is possible with structural grafting anteriorly and anterior instrumentation. Segmental instrumentation can be applied posteriorly if necessary to provide the most rigid surgical constructs.

For patients with anterior column involvement who are unable to tolerate a thoracotomy or for patients with circumferential spinal cord or neural constriction, a costotransversectomy is useful in the thoracic spine and a posterior approach is useful in the lumbar spine. Excision is often intralesional, but decompression often is acceptable with the ability to restore stability using structural grafts or devices anteriorly with segmental instrumentation posteriorly. Techniques are available that allow en bloc resection or total spondylectomy from posterior approaches. The morbidity of a thoracotomy is avoided, which is a necessity in some patients, especially patients with symptomatic metastasis from lung cancer. By excising the rib head, intercostal neurovascular bundle, and transverse process on the side of the lesion, the anterior and middle columns are accessible to about the midline using special curets. If the pedicle is uninvolved, this medial wall is preserved to avoid contamination of the spinal canal or damage to the spinal cord. Bilateral approaches occasionally are necessary for extensive posterior vertebral body involvement to allow access to both sides of the middle column. Care must be taken with soft-tissue extension to avoid inadvertent entry into the great vessels anteriorly. These procedures should be followed by instrumentation and fusion, and structural interbody grafting should be used if significant bony resection is done anteriorly to decrease tension stresses on the posterior implants.

There have been numerous reports on the efficacy of PMMA as an adjunct to internal fixation and bone grafting. Bone cement functions well in compression; however, results have been disappointing on the tension side of spinal reconstructions. Failure has been noted at a mean of 200 days after treatment, and its use has been recommended for patients with a short life expectancy or in salvage cases. Generally, if life expectancy is more than 3 to 6 months, bone graft incorporation is possible. Fear of neural injury from the use of PMMA has been a frequent concern. Wang et al. showed that, although the temperature of the curing cement may reach 176°F to 194°F, the temperature measured beneath an intact lamina and under Gelfoam covering the dura at a laminar defect was significantly less (45°C). Later examination of the spinal cord in test animals did not show evidence of neural injury. Injury from the use of the material near the spinal cord has not been reported. PMMA can be used to augment existing internal fixation devices; however, loosening is to be expected. If long-term survival is expected, provision for bone grafting and graft incorporation must be made.

Percutaneous vertebroplasty has been reported to be effective treatment for osteolytic spinal metastases and multiple myelomas. Cortet et al. reported decreased pain within 48 hours of vertebroplasty in 97% of patients with beneficial effects maintained in 89% at 3 months and 75% at 6 months. Although leakage of the cement outside the vertebral body occurred in 29, only two patients developed severe nerve root pain, owing to leakage into a neural foramen. Vertebroplasty should be done only in centers with experienced neurosurgeons or orthopaedic surgeons because of the possibility of severe complications. It important to determine if the pain is caused by pathologic fracture, which will respond to cement augmentation, or by pathologic destruction by tumor, which may not respond to augmentation.

ANTERIOR EXCISION OF SPINAL TUMOR

TECHNIQUE 6.10

- Approach the diseased spine using the standard anterior approach for that spinal segment from the side of the most prominent tumor mass, but choose an approach that allows for more radical or extensive exposure if necessary.
- Identify normal bone and disc cranially and caudally.
- Ligate segmental vessels first to allow discectomy, which is carried to the posterior longitudinal ligament. Ligation of the segmental vessel at the level of vertebral body involvement may be difficult because of encasement by soft-tissue extension.
- En bloc resection of tumor is possible if lesions are anteriorly situated. If intralesional decompression is planned, create an access portal within the vertebral body anterior to the tumor and use curets to pull tumor tissue anteriorly away from the spinal canal into the void. This allows decompression without forcing material against the already compressed dura.
- Piecemeal resection commonly is done for metastatic lesions; however, for en bloc resection, the tumor must not be violated. In these cases, osteotomize the pedicles after discectomy to allow en bloc resection. Be prepared for a cerebrospinal fluid leak because adherence of the tumor to the dura is possible.
- If any extension of tumor is present into the posterior elements, a staged posterior procedure for completion of vertebrectomy is done.
- When resection of tumor is complete, prepare for fixation. For patients with expected long-term survival of more than 6 months, place allograft or autograft for structural support. These grafts include allograft femur, humerus, fibula, and iliac crest. Autograft fibula and iliac crest are the best autograft options unless a structural spacer, such as a mesh cage, is applied.
- Bone cement is a consideration in patients with a poor expected survival and allows for irradiation and immediate compressive strength when combined with anterior instrumentation. Cover the exposed dura or posterior longitudinal ligament or both with Gelfoam and use small brain spatulas to isolate the spinal cord from PMMA.
- Insert PMMA in a semiliquid or doughy state. Use of a reinforcement device is recommended before placing PMMA; this may include Harrington or other hook-rod implants used as a distraction device, Steinmann pins, or a mesh titanium cage that engages the vertebral bodies and will be covered with PMMA to provide a smooth external surface.

- Remove excess cement prior to polymerization, which is especially important in the cervical spine where a large mass of cement can cause dysphagia. Avoid allowing the cement to contact the dura. As soon as the cement has been trimmed, begin continuous irrigation of the wound with normal saline. This theoretically keeps perineural temperatures at a minimum; although owing to cerebrospinal fluid convection, this may be unnecessary.
- Anterior instrumentation is added to provide maximal fixation. Numerous implants that are of low profile and provide at least four fixation points are available. For optimal fixation, place vertebral body screws in a bicortical fashion. If a later posterior instrumentation construct is planned, slight modification of screw placement is necessary to allow for placement of pedicle screws if these are to be used. Under these circumstances, identify the pedicle, and simply keep the vertebral body screws just inferior to these structures.
- When fixation is complete and compression of the interbody construct is maintained, test the construct for stability before closing. Remove and replace the cement and metal fixation if it is loose.
- Close the wound in the standard fashion.
- If corpectomy of more than a single level is done or if posterior column involvement is present, a combined approach with posterior instrumentation is preferred.

POSTOPERATIVE CARE Rigid immobilization is preferable after these procedures, especially when the bone quality is in question because of osteoporosis or other metabolic causes. A TLSO is typically worn when getting out of bed and while up; however, it is unnecessary for the patient to wear this during sleep. When the graft incorporates over the next 3-6 months, the TLSO is discontinued. Radiation is deferred for 3 weeks if possible if grafting is used. Great attention is paid to nutrition during the perioperative period, and parenteral or enteral supplementation may be required.

COSTOTRANSVERSECTOMY FOR INTRALESIONAL EXCISION OF SPINAL TUMOR

TECHNIQUE 6.11

- Using a standard posterior incision or a paramedian incision, expose the spinous processes and transverse processes bilaterally over the levels of anticipated instrumentation (see chapter 1).
- When radiographic localization is complete, identify and expose the rib at the level and side of the pathologic process.
- To perform corpectomy, usually it is necessary to expose three ribs subperiosteally and disarticulate them at the costotransverse articulation and to excise the medial 8-10 cm of the ribs. Removal of the transverse processes aids in vertebral body exposure.
- When the ribs are removed, use peanut dissectors to elevate the pleura bluntly from the vertebral bodies.
- Create working portals between the intercostal neurovascular bundles for placement of retractors and instruments. During this step of the procedure, headlight illumination or microscope is mandatory to see into the retropleural space.
- Laminectomy or facetectomy can be done if necessary for posterior decompression. Ligation of the segmental vessels is possible, if necessary, under direct observation.
- Retention of the intercostal nerves is preferable; however, these can be sacrificed if they interfere with proper decompression. The tradeoff is chest wall anesthesia, intercostal paralysis, and potentially upper abdominal muscle paralysis below T7.
- Perform discectomy above and below the affected vertebral body in the standard fashion.
- For intralesional resection, remove the tumor with curets and rongeurs to the level of the posterior longitudinal ligament or dura as necessary. Brisk bleeding as the tumor is curetted is to be expected but is minimized by preoperative embolization. Intermittent packing of the tumor also helps to control bleeding, with continuation of the procedure after bleeding subsides. When the tumor is excised, hemostasis usually occurs without much difficulty.
- This approach can be useful in patients unable to tolerate thoracotomy when an anterior pathologic process is predominant and stabilization is necessary. Instrumentation is necessary for stabilization and can be used posteriorly at any time during the procedure. Early placement of implants also can be helpful to distract the ligamentous structures and disc during the decompression and allow provisional rod placement if substantial anterior bone will be removed.
- Before closure, maintain positive-pressure ventilation momentarily while irrigation is allowed to cover the pleura. This is done to inspect the pleura for leaks that usually would necessitate placement of a chest tube.
- After bone grafting, standard closure is done over drains.

TRANSPEDICULAR INTRALESIONAL EXCISION FOR TUMOR OF THE SPINE

Posterolateral excision is indicated for patients with tumors that involve the anterior, middle, and posterior columns simultaneously. This is done without the risks or the extensive exposure required for a simultaneous approach.

TECHNIQUE 6.12

- If a transpedicular approach is to be used, make a midline incision to expose the pathologic level.
- When identification of the correct level is confirmed, decompression can be done or posterior instrumentation can be placed. Because of the destabilization that occurs with laminectomy and pedicle resection, place posterior instrumentation before completion of the procedure. By placing instrumentation initially, a temporary rod can be placed if aggressive vertebral body removal is planned to provide stability during vertebral body removal.

- Begin decompression as the pedicle that leads into the tumor is sounded and use sequentially larger curets to remove bone through this access site. Leave the medial pedicle wall as a barrier for tumor to the spinal canal if the pedicle itself is not involved with tumor.
- Hemilaminectomy is helpful to expose the medial border of the pedicle to avoid medial penetration, unless adequate decompression requires laminectomy, in which case this is done before the transpedicular decompression.
- Resect the lateral wall of the pedicle with a Leksell rongeur, which allows medialization of the curets.
- If the posterior vertebral body wall is retropulsed, resect the medial pedicle border as well.
- If compression is bilateral, a bilateral transpedicular approach is necessary.
- When the pedicle is resected, a reverse-angle curet or even a posterior lumbar interbody fusion (PLIF) tamp can be placed ventral to the dura, against the tumor or retropulsed posterior vertebral wall so that it is tamped or pushed back into the vertebral body. Decancellation of the middle column often is necessary before this maneuver to create a space for the bone that is reduced.
- When the retropulsed material is pushed anteriorly, resect it with curets and pituitary rongeurs.
- Anterior column grafting depends on the procedure performed.
- Take care that morcellized graft is not retropulsed into the spinal canal after placement, creating the same problem the procedure was intended to correct.
- Perform appropriate bone grafting and instrumentation. If a large anterior vertebral body was resected, a structural device should be placed in addition to posterior segmental spinal instrumentation.

POSTOPERATIVE CARE Patients are fitted for a TLSO, and immobilization is continued after the procedure for 3-6 months. Mobilization is started on the first postoperative day. Anticoagulants are not used in partial vertebrectomy patients immediately postoperatively because of the inherent risk of epidural hematoma, so lower extremity antiembolism stockings and compression foot devices are used until the patient is ambulatory. A vena cava filter should be considered for high-risk patients. Radiation is deferred, if possible, for at least 3 weeks when autogenous or allograft bone is used.

REFERENCES

INFECTION

BIOLOGY, DIAGNOSIS, AND TREATMENT OF SPINAL INFECTION

Ackshota N, Nash A, Bussey I, et al.: Outcomes of multilevel vertebrectomy for spondylodiscitis, *Spine J* 19:285, 2019.

Adogwa O, Elsamidicy AA, Sergesketter A, et al.: Prophylactic use of intraoperative vancomycin powder and postoperative infection: an analysis of microbiological patterns in 1200 consecutive surgical cases, *J Neurosurg Spine* 27(3):328, 2017.

Adsul N, Kalra KL, Jain N, et al.: Thoracic cryptococcal osteomyelitis mimicking tuberculosis: a case report, *Surg Neurol Int* 10:81, 2019.

Alduraibi AK, Naddaf S, Alzayed MF: FDG PET/CT of spinal brucellosis, *Clin Nucl Med* 44(6):465, 2019.

Aljabi Y, Manca A, Ryan J, Elshawary A: Value of procalcitonin as a marker of surgical site infection following spinal surgery, *Surgeon* 17:97, 2019.

Alshafai NS, Gunness VRN: The high cervical anterolateral retropharyngeal approach, *Acta Neurochir Suppl* 125:147, 2019.

Anderson PA, Savage JW, Vaccaro AR, et al.: Prevention of surgical site infection in spine surgery, *Neurosurgery* 80:S114, 2017.

Balcescu C, Odeh K, Rosinski A, et al.: High prevalence of multifocal spine infections involving the cervical and thoracic regions: a case for imaging the entire spine, *Neurospine* 2019, (E-pub ahead of print).

Bhavan KP, Marschall J, Olsen MA, et al.: The epidemiology of hematogenous vertebral osteomyelitis: a cohort study in a tertiary care hospital, *BMC Infect Dis* 10:158, 2010.

Brinjikji W, Everist BM, Wald JT, et al.: Association between imaging findings and microbiological findings for image-guided biopsies for spine infections, *J Neurosurg Sci* 61(6):589, 2017.

Caroom C, Tullar JM, Benton Jr G, et al.: Intrawound vancomycin powder reduces surgical site infections in posterior cervical fusion, *Spine* 38:1183, 2013.

Chaichana KL, Bydon M, Santiago-Dieppa DR, et al.: Risk of infection following posterior instrumented lumbar fusion for degenerative spine disease in 817 consecutive cases, *J Neurosurg Spine* 20:45, 2014.

Chen SH, Chen WJ, Wu MH, et al.: Postoperative infection in patients undergoing posterior lumbosacral spinal surgery: a pictorial guide for diagnosis and early treatment, *Clin Spine Surg* 31(6):225, 2018.

Cho C, Gotto M: Spinal brucellosis, *N Engl J Med* 379:e28, 2018.

Choi EJ, Kim SY, Kim HG, et al.: Percutaneous endoscopic debridement and drainage with four different approach methods for the treatment of spinal infection, *Pain Physician* 20(6):E933, 2017.

Cox M, Curtis B, Patel M, et al.: Utility of sagittal MR imaging of the whole spine in cases of known or suspected single-level spinal infection: overkill or good clinical practice? *Clin Imaging* 51:98, 2018.

Dayer R, Alahrani MM, Saran N, et al.: Spinal infections in children: a multicentre retrospective study, *Bone Joint Lett J* 100-B(4):542, 2018.

Dietz N, Sharma M, Alhourani A, et al.: Outcomes of decompression and fusion for treatment of spinal infection, *Neurosurg Focus* 46(1):E7, 2019.

Dunn RN, Castelein S, Held M: Impact of HIV on spontaneous spondylodiscitis, *Bone Joint Lett J* 101-B:617, 2019.

Elgafy H, Raberding CJ, Mooney ML, et al.: Analysis of a ten step protocol to decrease postoperative spinal wound infection, *World J Orthop* 9(11):271, 2018.

Emamian S, Fox MG, Boatman D, et al.: *Spinal blastomycosis, unusual musculoskeletal presentation with literature review, Skeletal Radiol* 2019, (Epub ahead of print).

Elsamadicy AA, Wang TY, Back AG, et al.: Impact of intraoperative steroids on postoperative infection rates and length of hospital stay: a study of 1200 spine surgery patients, *World Neurosurg* 96:429, 2016.

Esmaeilnejad-Ganji SM, Esmaeilnejad-Ganji SMR: Osteoarticular manifestations of human brucellosis: a review, *World J Orthop* 10(2):54, 2019.

Ghobrial GM, Thakkar V, Andrews E, et al.: Intraoperative vancomycin use in spinal surgery, *Spine* 39:550, 2014.

Hartveldt S, Janssen SJ, Wood KB, et al.: Is there an association of epidural corticosteroid injection with postoperative surgical site infection after surgery for lumbar degenerative spine disease? *Spine* 41(19):1542, 2016.

Issa K, Diebo B, Faloon M, et al.: The epidemiology of vertebral osteomyelitis in the United States from 1998 to 2013, *Clin Spine Surg* 31(2):E102, 2018.

Iwata E, Scarborough M, Bowden G, et al.: The role of histology in the diagnosis of spondylodiscitis: correlation with clinical and microbiological findings, *Bone Joint Lett J* 101-B(3):246, 2019.

Joo HS, Ha JK, Hwang CJ, et al.: Lumbar cryptococcal osteomyelitis mimicking metastatic tumor, *Asian Spine J* 9(5):798, 2015.

Kanayama M, Hashimoto T, Shigenobu K, et al.: MRI-based decision making of implant removal in deep wound infection after instrumented lumbar fusion, *Clin Spine Surg* 30(2):E99, 2017.

Khalil JG, Gandhi SD, Park DK, Fischgrund JS: Cutibacterium acnes in spine pathology: pathophysiology, diagnosis, and management, *J Am Acad Orthop Surg* 27:E633, 2019.

Khan NR, Thompson CJ, DeCuypere M, et al.: A meta-analysis of spinal surgical site infection and vancomycin powder, *J Neurosurg Spine* 21:974, 2014.

Kimura H, Shikata J, Odate S, Soeda T: Pedicle screw fluid sign: an indication on magnetic resonance imaging of a deep infection after posterior spinal instrumentation, *Clin Spine Surg* 30(4):169, 2017.

Koakutsu T, Sato T, Aizawa IE, Kushimoto S: Postoperative changes in presepsin level and values predictive of surgical site infection after spinal surgery. A single-center, prospective observational study, *Spine* 43:578, 2018.

Koutsoumbelis S, Hughes AP, Girardi FP, et al.: Risk factors for postoperative infection following posterior lumbar instrumented arthrodesis, *J Bone Joint Surg* 93A:1627, 2011.

Lavi ES, Pal A, Bleicher D, et al.: MR imaging of the spine: urgent and emergent indications, *Semin Ultrasound CT MRI* 39:551, 2018.

Lemans JVC, Wijdicks SPJ, Boot W, et al.: Intrawound treatment for prevention of surgical site infections in instrumented spinal surgery: a systematic comparative effectiveness review and meta-analysis, *Global Spine J* 9(2):219, 2019.

Liang C, Wei W, Liang X, et al.: Spinal brucellosis in huylunbuir, China, 2011-2016, *Infect Drug Resist* 12:1565, 2019.

Lim S, Edelstein AI, Patel AA, et al.: Risk factors for postoperative infections following single-level lumbar fusion surgery, *Spine* 43:215, 2018.

Lin CY, Chang CC, Chen YJ: New strategy for minimally invasive endoscopic surgery to treat infectious spondylodiscitis in the thoracolumbar spine, *Pain Physician* 22(3):281, 2019.

Mao Y, Li Y, Cui X: Percutaneous endoscopic debridement and drainage for spinal infection: systemic review and meta-analysis, *Pain Physician* 22(4):323, 2019.

McNamara AL, Dickerson EC, Gomez-Hassan DM, Cinti SK, Srinivasan A: Yield of image-guided needle biopsy for infectious discitis: a systematic review and meta-analysis, *AJNR Am J Neuroradiol* 38(10):2021, 2017.

Raghavan M, Lazzeri E, Palestro CJ: Imaging of spondylodiscitis, *Semin Nucl Med* 48(2):131, 2018.

Nota SPFT, Braun Y, Ring D, Schwab JH: Incidence of surgical site infection after spine surgery: what is the impact of the definition of infection? *Clin Orthop Relat Res* 473:1612, 2015.

Pahys JM, Pahys JR, Cho SK, et al.: Methods to decrease postoperative infections following posterior cervical spine surgery, *J Bone Joint Surg* 95A:549, 2013.

Radcliff KE, Neusner AD, Millhouse PW, et al.: What is new in the diagnosis and prevention of spine surgical site infections, *Spine J* 15:336, 2015.

Rao SB, Vasquez G, Harrop J, et al.: Risk factors for surgical site infections following spinal fusion procedures: a case-control study, *Clin Infect Dis* 53:686, 2011.

Rustemi O, Raneri F, Alvaro L, et al.: Single-approach vertebral osteosynthesis in the treatment of spinal osteolysis by spondylodiscitis, *Neurosurg Focus* 46(1):E9, 2019.

Sagreto FA, Beyer GA, Grieco P: Vertebral osteomyelitis: a comparison of associated outcomes in early versus delayed surgical treatment, *Int J Spine Surg* 12(6):703, 2018.

Sertic M, Parkes, Mattiassi S, et al.: The efficacy of computed tomography-guided percutaneous spine biopsies in determining a causative organism in cases of suspected infection: a systematic review, *Can Assoc Radiol J* 70:96, 2019.

Shillingford JN, Laratta JL, Reddy H, et al.: Postoperative surgical site infection after spine surgery: an update from the Scoliosis Research Society (SRS) morbidity and mortality database, *Spine Deformity* 6:634, 2018.

Strom RG, Pacione D, Kalhorn SP, Frempong-Boadu AK: Decreased risk of wound infection after posterior cervical fusion with routine local application of vancomycin powder, *Spine* 38:991, 2013.

Talbott JF, Shah VN, Uzelac A, et al.: Imaging-based approach to extradural infections of the spine, *Semin Ultrasound CT MRI* 39(6):570, 2018.

Thakkar V, Ghobrial GM, Maulucci CM, et al.: Nasal MRSA colonization: impact on surgical site infection following spine surgery, *Clin Neurol Neurosurg* 125:94, 2014.

Theologis AA, Demirkiran G, Callahan M, et al.: Local intrawound vancomycin powder decreases the risk of surgical site infections in complex adult deformity reconstruction, *Spine* 39:1875, 2014.

Theologis AA, Lansdown D, McClellan RT, et al.: Multilevel corpectomy with anterior column reconstruction and plating for subaxial cervical osteomyelitis, *Spine* 41:E1088, 2016.

Torres C, Zakhari N: Imaging of spine infection, *Semin Roentgenol* 52(1):17, 2017.

Tu L, Liu X, Gu W, et al.: Imaging-assisted diagnosis and characteristics of suspected spinal brucellosis: a retrospective study of 72 cases, *Med Sci Monit* 24:2647, 2018.

Waheed G, Soliman MAR, Ali AM, Aly MH: Spontaneous spondylodiscitis: review, incidence, management, and clinical outcome in 44 patients, *Neurosurg Focus* 46(1):E10, 2019.

Wang B, Fintelmann FJ, Kamath RS, et al.: Limited magnetic resonance imaging of the lumbar spine has high sensitivity for detection of acute fractures, infection, and malignancy, *Skeletal Radiol* 45(12):1687, 2016.

Wang AJ, Huang KT, Smith TR, et al.: Cervical spine osteomyelitis: a systematic review of instrumented fusion in the modern era, *World Neurosurg* 120:35632, 2018.

Weinstein JN, Tosteson TD, Lurie JD, et al.: Surgical versus nonoperative treatment for lumbar spinal stenosis four-year results of the spine patient outcomes research trial, *Spine* 35:1329, 2010.

Xiong L, Pan Q, Jin G, et al.: Topical intrawound application of vancomycin powder in addition to intravenous administration of antibiotics: a meta-analysis on the deep infection after spinal surgeries, *Orthop Traumatol Surg Res* 100:785, 2014.

Yang S, Werner BC, Cancienne JM, et al.: Preoperative epidural injections are associated with increased risk of infection after single-level lumbar decompression, *Spine J* 16:191, 2016.

PYOGENIC INFECTIONS

Canoui E, Zarrouk V, Canoui-Poitrine F, et al.: Surgery is safe and effective when indicated in the acute phase of hematogenous pyogenic vertebral osteomyelitis, *Infect Dis* 51(4):268, 2019.

Courjon J, Lamaignen A, Ghout I, et al.: Pyogenic vertebral osteomyelitis of the elderly: characteristics and outcomes, *PloS One* 12(12): e0188470, 2017.

Davis WT, April MD, Mehta S, et al.: High risk clinical characteristics for pyogenic spinal infection in acute neck or back pain: prospective cohort study, *Am J Emerg Med* 2019, pii:S0735-6757(19)30336-5.

Griffith-Jones W, Nasto LA, Pola E, et al.: Percutaneous suction and irrigation for the treatment of recalcitrant pyogenic spondylodiscitis, *J Orthop Traumatol* 19(1):10, 2018.

Kim UJ, Bae JY, Kim SE, et al.: Comparison of pyogenic postoperative and native vertebral osteomyelitis, *Spine J* 19(5):880, 2019.

Kim J, Jang SB, Sim SW, et al.: Clinical effect of early bisphosphonate treatment for pyogenic vertebral osteomyelitis with osteoporosis: an analysis by the Cox proportional hazard model, *Spin J* 19(3):418, 2019.

Kim J, Lee SY, Jung JH, et al.: The outcome following spinal instrumentation in haemodialyzed patients with pyogenic spondylodiscitis, *Bone Joint Lett J* 101-B:75, 2019.

Korovessis P, Repantis T, Hadjipavlou AG: Hematogenous pyogenic spinal infection: current perceptions, *Orthopedics* 35:885, 2012.

Lemaignen A, Ghout I, Dinh A, et al.: Characteristics of risk factors for severe neurological deficit in patients with pyogenic vertebral osteomyelitis: a case-control study, *Medicine* 96(21):e6387, 2017.

Lin CP, Ma HL, Wang ST, et al.: Surgical results of long posterior fixation with short fusion in the treatment of pyogenic spondylodiscitis of the thoracic and lumbar spine: a retrospective study, *Spine* 37:E1572, 2012.

Marschall J, Bhavan KP, Olsen MS, et al.: The impact of prebiopsy antibiotics on pathogen recovery in hematogenous vertebral osteomyelitis, *Clin Infect Dis* 52(7):867, 2011.

Von der Hoeh NH, Voelker A, Hofmann A, et al.: Pyogenic spondylodiscitis of the thoracic spine: outcome of 1-stage posterior versus 2-stage posterior and anterior spinal reconstruction in adults, *World Neurosurg* 120:e297, 2018.

INFECTIONS IN CHILDREN

Dayer R, Alzahrani MM, Saran N, et al.: Spinal infections in children. A multicentre retrospective study, *Bone Joint Lett J* 100-B:542, 2018.

Fucs PM, Meves R, Yamada HH: Spinal infections in children: a review, *Int Orthop* 36:387, 2012.

Ho AK, Shrader MW, Falk MN, Segal LS: Diagnosis and initial management of musculoskeletal coccidioidmomycosis in children, *J Pediatr Orthop* 34:571, 2014.

Ryan SL, Sen A, Staggers K, et al.: Texas Children's Hospital Spine Study Group: a standardized protocol to reduce pediatric spine surgery infection: a quality improvement initiative, *J Neurosurg Pediatr* 14:259, 2014.

Sandler AL, Thompson D, Goodrich JT, et al.: Infections of the spinal subdural space in children: a series of 11 contemporary cases and review of all published reports. A multinational collaborative effort, *Childs Nerv Syst* 29:105, 2013.

Scheuerman O, Landau D, Schwarz M, et al.: Cervical disciitis in children, *Pediatr Infect Dis J* 34(7):794, 2015.

Sponseller PD, Jain A, Shah SA, et al.: Deep wound infections after spinal fusion in children with cerebral palsy: a prospective cohort study, *Spine* 38:2023, 2013.

EPIDURAL SPACE INFECTION

Alton TB, Patel AR, Bransford RJ, et al.: Is there a difference in neurologic outcome in medical versus early operative management of cervical epidural abscesses? *Spine J* 15:10, 2015.

Babic M, Simpfendorfer CS, Berbari EF: Update on spinal epidural abscess, *Curr Opin Infect Dis* 32:265, 2019.

Du JY, Schell AJ, Kim C, et al.: 30-day mortality following surgery for spinal epidural abscess, *Spine* 44:E500, 2018.

Howie BA, Davidson IU, Tanenbaum JE, et al.: Thoracic epidural abscesses: a systematic review, *Global Spine J* 8(4S):68S, 2018.

Kim SD, Melikian R, Ju KL, et al.: Independent predictors of failure of nonoperative management of spinal epidural abscesses, *Spine J* 14:1673, 2014.

Patel AR, Alton TB, Bransford RJ, et al.: Spinal epidural abscesses: risk factors, medical versus surgical management, a retrospective review of 128 cases, *Spine J* 14:326, 2014.

Ran B, Chen X, Zhong Q, et al.: CT-guided minimally invasive treatment for extensive spinal epidural abscess: a case report and literature review, *Eur Spin J* 27(Suppl 3):380, 2017.

Shah A, Yang H, Ogink PT, Schwab JH: Independent predictors of spinal epidural abscess recurrence, *Spine J* 18:1837, 2018.

Stratton A, Gustafson K, Thomas K, James MT: Incidence and risk factors for failed medical management of spinal epidural abscess: a systematic review and meta-analysis, *J Neurosurg Spine* 26:81, 2017.

Vakili M, Crum-Cianflone NF: Spinal epidural abscess: a series of 101 cases, *Am J Med* 130:1458, 2017.

FUNGAL INFECTIONS

Ganesh D, Gottlieb J, Chan S, et al.: Fungal infections of the spine, *Spine* 40:E719, 2015.

Iwata A, Ito M, Abumi K, et al.: Fungal spinal infection treated with percutaneous posterolateral endoscopic surgery, *J Neurol Surg Cent Eur Neurosurg* 75:170, 2014.

Shweikeh F, Zyck S, Sweiss F, et al.: Aspergillus spinal epidural abscess: case presentation and review of the literature, *Spinal Cord Series and Cases* 20184:19, 2018.

Sohn YJ, Yun JH, Yun KW, et al.: Aspergillus terreus spondylodiscitis in an immunocompromised child, *Pediatr Infect Dis J* 38(2):161, 2019.

TUBERCULOSIS

Agarwal A, Kant KS, Kumar A, Shaharyar A: One-year multidrug treatment for tuberculosis of the cervical spine in children, *J Orthop Surg (Hong Kong)* 23(2):168, 2015.

Ali A, Musbahi O, White VLC, Montgomery AS: Spinal tuberculosis. A literature review, *JBJS Reviews* 7(1):e9, 2019.

Assaghir YM, Refae HH, Alam-Eddin M: Anterior versus posterior debridement fusion for single-level dorsal tuberculosis: the role of graft-type and level of fixation on determining the outcome, *Eur Spine J* 25:3884, 2016.

Boachie-Adjei O, Papadopoulos EC, Pellisé F, et al.: Late treatment of tuberculosis-associated kyphosis: literature review and experience from a SRS-GOP site, *Eur Spine J* 22(Suppl 4):641, 2013.

Boody BS, Tarazona DA, Vaccaro AR: Evaluation and management of pyogenic and tubercular spine infections, *Cur Rev Musculoskel Med* 11:643, 2018.

Cao G, Rao J, Cai Y, et al.: Analysis of treatment and prognosis of 863 patients with spinal tuberculosis in Guizhou Province, *BioMed Res Int* 2018:3265735, 2018.

Chandra SP, Singh A, Goyal N, et al.: Analysis of changing paradigms of management in 179 patients with spinal tuberculosis over a 12-year period and proposal of a new management algorithm, *World Neurosurg* 80:190, 2013.

Dean A, Zyck S, Toshkezi G, et al.: Challenges in the diagnosis and management of spinal tuberculosis: case series, *Cureus* 11(1):e3855, 2019.

De la Garza Ramos R, Goodwin CR, Abu-Bonsrah N, et al.: The epidemiology of spinal tuberculosis in the United States: an analysis of 2002-2011 data, *J Neurosurg Spine* 26:507, 2017.

D'souza AR, Mohapatra B, Bansal ML, Das K: Role of posterior stabilization and transpedicular decompression in the treatment of thoracic and thoracolumbar TB. A retrospective evaluation, *Clin Spine Surg* 30(10):E1426, 2017.

Dumont RA, Keen NN, Bloomer CW, et al.: Clinical utility of diffusion-weighted imaging in spinal infections, *Clin Neuroradiol* 29(3):515, 2019.

Dunn RN, Husien MB: Spinal tuberculosis. Review of current management, *Bone Joint Lett J* 100-B:425, 2018.

Gao M, Sun J, Jiang Z, et al.: Comparison of tuberculous and brucellar spondylitis on magnetic resonance images, *Spine* 42(2):113, 2017.

Hogan JI, Hurtado RM, Nelson SB: Mycobacterial musculoskeletal infections, *Infect Dis Clin N Am* 31:369, 2017.

Huang Z, Liu J, Ma K: Posterior versus anterior approach surgery for thoracolumbar spinal tuberculosis, *J Coll Physicians Surg Pak* 29(2):187, 2019.

Kaloostian PE, Gokaslan ZL: Current management of spinal tuberculosis: a multimodal approach, *World Neurosurg* 80:64, 2013.

Kanna RM, Babu N, Kannan M, et al.: Diagnostic accuracy of whole spine magnetic resonance imaging in spinal tuberculosis validated through tissue studies, *Eur Spine J* 2019, (Epub ahead of print).

Khanna K, Sabharwal S: Spinal tuberculosis: a comprehensive review for the modern spine surgeon, *Spine J* 000:1, 2019.

Li Z, Lei F, Xiu P, et al.: Surgical management for middle or lower thoracic spinal tuberculosis (T5-T12) in elderly patients: posterior versus anterior approach, *J Orthop Sci* 24:68, 2019.

Liao JC, Lai PL, Chen LH, Niu CC: Surgical outcomes of infectious spondylitis after vertebroplasty, and comparisons between pyogenic and tuberculosis, *BMC Infect Dis* 18(1):555, 2018.

Liu C, Lin L, Wang W, et al.: Long-term outcomes of vertebral column resection for kyphosis in patients with cured spinal tuberculosis: average 8-year follow-up, *J Neurosurg Spine* 24:777, 2016.

Liu Z, Zhang P, Zeng H, et al.: A comparative study of single-stage transpedicular debridement, fusion, and posterior long-segment versus short-segment fixation for the treatment of thoracolumbar spinal tuberculosis in adults: minimum five year follow-up outcomes, *Int Orthop* 42:1883, 2018.

Luo C, Wang X, Wu P, Ge L, et al.: Single-stage transpedicular decompression, debridement, posterior instrumentation, and fusion for thoracic tuberculosis with kyphosis and spinal cord compression in aged individuals, *Spine J* 16:154, 2016.

Marais S, Ros I, Mitha A, et al.: Spinal tuberculosis: clinicoradiological findings in 274 patients, *Clin Infec Dis* 67(1):89, 2018.

Mohan K, Rawall S, Pawar UM, et al.: Drug resistance patterns in 111 cases of drug-resistant tuberculosis spine, *Eur Spine J* 22(Suppl 4):647, 2013.

Pan Z, Luo J, Yu L, et al.: Debridement and reconstruction improve postoperative sagittal alignment in kyphotic cervical spinal tuberculosis, *Clin Orthop Relat Res* 475:2084, 2017.

Pang X, Shen X, Wu P, et al.: Thoracolumbar spinal tuberculosis with psoas abscesses treated by one-stage posterior transforaminal lumbar debridement, interbody fusion, posterior instrumentation, and postural drainage, *Arch Orthop Trauma Surg* 133:765, 2013.

Rachdi I, Fekih Y, Daoud F, et al: Cervical Pott's disease revealed by retropharyngeal abscess, *Presse Med* 47(10):918, 2018.

Rajasekaran S, Khandelwal G: Drug therapy in spinal tuberculosis, *Eur Spine J* 22(Suppl 4):587, 2013.

Shi J, Yue X, Niu N, et al.: Application of a modified thoracoabdominal approach that avoids cutting open the costal portion of diaphragm during anterior thoracolumbar spine surgery, *Eur Spine J* 26(7):1852, 2017.

Soares Do Brito J, Tirado A, Fernandes P: Surgical treatment of spinal tuberculosis complicated with extensive abscess, *Iowa Orthop J* 34:129, 2014.

Stratton A, Gustafson K, Thomas K, James MT: Incidence and risk factors for failed medical management of spinal epidural abscess: a systematic review and meta-analysis, *J Neurosurg Spine* 26(1):81, 2017.

Ukunda UNF, Lukhele MM: The posterior-only surgical approach in the treatment of tuberculosis of the spine, *Bone Joint Lett J* 100-B:1208, 2018.

Vaishnav B, Suthar N, Shaikh S, Tambile R: Clinical study of spinal tuberculosis presenting with neuro-deficits in Western India, *Indian J Tuberc* 66(1):81, 2019.

Wang L-J, Zhang H-Q, Tang M-X, et al.: Comparison of three surgical approaches for thoracic spinal tuberculosis in adults, *Spine* 42:808, 2017.

Wang S-T, Ma H-L, Lin C-P, et al.: Anterior debridement may not be necessary in the treatment of tuberculous spondylitis of the thoracic and lumbar spine in adults, *Bone Joint Lett J* 98-B:834, 2016.

Wang Y-X, Zhang H-Q, Liao W, et al.: One-stage posterior focus debridement, interbody graft using titanium mesh cages, posterior instrumentation and fusion in the surgical treatment of lumbo-sacral spinal tuberculosis in the aged, *Int Orthop* 40:1117, 2016.

Wu W, Li Z, Lin R, et al.: Anterior debridement, decompression, fusion, and instrumentation for lower cervical spine tuberculosis, *J Orthop Sci* 2019, (Epub ahead of print).

Xing S, Gao Y, Gao K, et al.: Anterior cervical retropharyngeal debridement combined with occipital cervical fusion to upper cervical tuberculosis, *Spine* 41:104, 2016.

Yao Y, Zhang H, Liu M, et al.: Prognostic factors for recovery of patients after surgery for thoracic spinal tuberculosis, *World Neurosurg* 105:327, 2017.

Yin XH, He BR, Liu ZK, Hao DJ: The clinical outcomes and surgical strategy for cervical spine tuberculosis. A retrospective study in 78 cases, *Medicine* 97(27):e11401, 2018.

Yin XH, Yan L, Yang M, et al.: Posterolateral decompression, bone graft fusion, posterior instrumentation, and local continuous chemotherapy in the surgical treatment of thoracic spinal tuberculosis, *Medicine* 97(51):e13822, 2018.

Zhang N, Zeng X, He L, et al.: The value of MR imaging in comparative analysis of spinal infection in adults: pyogenic versus tuberculous, *World Neurosurg* 2019, (Epub ahead of print).

Zhu G, Jiang LY, Yi Z, et al.: Sacroiliac joint tuberculosis: surgical management by posterior open-window focal debridement and joint effusion, *BMC Musculoskelet Disord* 18(1):504, 2017.

Zhu Z, Hao D, Wang B, et al.: Selection of surgical treatment approaches for cervicothoracic spinal tuberculosis: a 10-year case review, *PloS One* 13(2):e0192581, 2018.

Zou DX, Zhou JL, Zhou XX, Jiang XB: Clinical efficacy of CT-guided percutaneous huge ilio-psoas abscesses drainage combined with posterior approach surgery for the management of dorsal and lumbar spinal tuberculosis in adults, *Orthop Traumatol* 103:1251, 2017.

TUMORS

Ahmed AT, Abdel-Rahman O, Morsy M, et al.: Management of sacrococcygeal chordoma. A systematic review and meta-analysis of observational studies, *Spine* 43:E1157, 2018.

Ailon T, Torabi R, Fisher CG, et al.: Management of locally recurrent chordoma of the mobile spine and sacrum: a systematic review, *Spine* 41(Suppl 20):S193, 2016.

Alhumaid I, Abu-Zaid A: Denosumab therapy in the management of aneurysmal bone cysts: a comprehensive literature review, *Cureus* 11(1):e3989, 2019.

Alshafai NS, Gunness VRN: The high cervical anterolateral retropharyngeal approach, *Acta Neurochir Suppl* 125:147, 2019.

Amelot A, Moles A, Cristini J, et al.: Predictors of survival in patients with surgical spine multiple myeloma metastases, *Surgical Oncol* 25:178, 2016.

Amendola L, Cappuccio M, De Iure F, et al.: En bloc resections for primary spinal tumors in 20 years of experience: effectiveness and safety, *Spine J* 14:2608, 2014.

Anderson K, Ismaila N, Flynn PJ, et al.: Role of bone-modifying agents in multiple myeloma: American Society of clinical oncology clinical practice guideline update, *J Clin Oncol* 36(8):812, 2018.

Bakar D, Tanenbaum JE, Phan K, et al.: Decompression surgery for spinal metastases: a systematic review, *Neurosurg Focus* 41(2):E2, 2016.

Bakker SH, Jacobs WCH, Pondaag W, et al.: Chordoma: a systematic review of the epidemiology and clinical prognostic factors predicting progression-free and overall survival, *Eur Spine J* 27(12):3043, 2018.

Barakat S, Alsingaby H, Shousha M, et al.: Early recurrence of a solid variant of aneurysmal bone cyst in a young child after resection: technique and literature review and two-year follow-up after corpectomy, *J Am Acad Orthop Surg* 26(10):369, 2018.

Barzilai O, Boriani S, Fisher CG, et al.: Essential concepts for the management of metastatic spine disease: what the surgeon should know and practice, *Global Spine J* 9(1):98S, 2019.

Barzilai O, Fisher CG, Bilsky MH: State of the art treatment of spinal metastatic disease, *Neurosurgery* 82(6):757, 2018.

Barzilai O, McLaughlin L, Lis E, et al.: Outcome analysis of surgery for symptomatic spinal metastases in long-term cancer survivors, *J Neurosurg Spine* 31:285, 2019.

Barzilai O, McLaughlin L, Amato M-K, et al.: Predictors of quality of life improvement after surgery for metastatic tumors of the spine: prospective cohort study, *Spine J* 18:1109, 2018.

Berger GK, Nisson PL, James WS, et al.: Outcomes in different age groups with primary Ewing sarcoma of the spine: a systematic review of the literature, *J Neurosurg Spine* 30:664, 2019.

Branstetter D, Rohrbach K, Huang LY, et al.: RANK and RANK ligand expression in primary human osteosarcoma, *J Bone Oncol* 4(3):59, 2015.

Buchowski JM, Sharan AD, Gokasaln ZL, Yamada J: *Modern techniques in the treatment of patients with metastatic spine disease, Instructional Course Lecture #308*, San Francisco, 2012, American Academy of Orthopaedic Surgeons, Annual meeting.

Cai W, Yan W, Huang Q, et al.: Surgery for plasma cell neoplasia patients with spinal instablity or neurological impairment caused by spinal lesions as the first clinical manifestation, *Eur Spine J* 24(8):1761, 2015.

Cazzato RL, Auloge P, Dalili D, et al.: Percutaneous image-guided cryoablation of osteoblastoma, *AJR Am J Roentgenol* 16:1, 2019.

Chandra SP, Singh P, Kumar R, et al.: Long-term outcome of treatment of vertebral body hemangiomas with direct ethanol injection short-segment stabilization, *Spine J* 19(1):131, 2019.

Charest-Morin R, Boriani S, Fisher C, et al.: Benign tumors of the spine, *Spine* 41(20S):S178, 2016.

Charest-Morin R, Dea N, Fisher CG: Health-related quality of life after spine surgery for primary bone tumor, *Curr Treat Options Oncol* 17(2): 9, 2016.

Charest-Morin R, Dirks MS, Patel S, et al.: Ewing sarcoma of the spine. Prognostic variables for survival and local control in surgically treated patients, *Spine* 9:622, 2018.

Chaudhry SR, Tsetse C, Chennan SE: Early recognition and diagnosis of Ewing sarcoma of the cervical spine, *Radiol Case Rep* 14(2):160, 2018.

Chemelik JR, Walek P, et al.: Deep convolutional neural network-based segmentation and classification of difficult to define metastatic spinal lesions in 3D CT data, *Med Imag Anal* 49:76, 2018.

Choi D, Bilsky M, Fehlings M, et al.: Spine oncology-metastatic spine tumors, *Neurosurgery* 80(3S):S131, 2017.

Ciftdemir M, Kaya M, Selcuk E, Yalniz E: Tumors of the spine, *World J Orthop* 7(2):109, 2016.

Cossu G, Terrier LM, Benboubker L: Spinal metastases in multiple myeloma: a high-risk subgroup for ISS III patients, *Surg Oncol* 27(2):321, 2018.

D'Amore T, Boyce B, Mesfin A: Chordoma of the mobile spine and sacrum: clinical management and prognosis, *J Spine Surg* 4(3):546, 2018.

De la Garza Ramos R, Longo M, Gelfand Y, et al.: Timing of prophylactic anticoagulation and its effect on thromboembolic events after surgery for metastatic tumors of the spine, *Spine* 44(11):e650, 2019.

Denaro L, Berton A, Ciuffreda M, et al.: Surgical management of chordoma: a systematic review, *J Spinal Cord Med* 2018, (Epub ahead of print).

Elsamadicy AA, Adogwa O, Sergesketter A, et al.: Posterolateral thoracic decompression with anterior column cage reconstruction versus decompression alone for spinal metastases with cord compression: analysis of perioperative complications and outcomes, *J Spine Surg* 3(4):609, 2017.

Esteban Cuesta H, Martel Villagran J, Bueno Horcajadas A, et al.: Percutaneous radiofrequency ablation in osteoid osteoma: tips and tricks in special scenarios, *Eur J Radiol* 102:169, 2018.

Faddoul J, Faddoul Y, Kobaiter-Maarrawi S, et al.: Radiofrequency ablation of spinal osteoid osteoma: a prospective study, *J Neurosurg Spine* 26:313, 2017.

Frassanito P, D'Onofrio GF, Pennisi G, et al.: Multimodal management of aggressive recurrent aneurysmal bone cyst of spine: case report and review of literature, *World Neurosurg* 126:423, 2019.

Gibbs WN, Nael K, Doshi AH, Tanenbaum LN: Spine oncology imaging and intervention, *Radiol Clin N Am* 47:377, 2019.

Gokaslan ZL, Yamada J, Buchowski JM, Sharan AD: *Modern techniques in the treatment of patients with metastatic spine disease, Instructional Course Lecture #308*, San Diego, CA, 2011, American Academy of Orthopaedic Surgeons, annual meeting.

Gokaslan ZL, Zadnik PL, Sciubba DM, et al.: Mobile spine chordoma: results of 166 patients from the AO Spine Knowledge Form Tumor database, *J Neurosurg Spine* 24(4):644, 2016.

Goldschlager T, Dea N, Boyd M, et al.: Giant cell tumors of the spine: has denosumab changed the treatment paradigm? *J Neurosurg Spine* 22:526, 2015.

Groot OQ, Ogink PT, Paulino Pereira NR, et al.: High risk of symptomatic venous thromboembolism after surgery for spine metastatic bone lesions: a retrospective study, *Clin Orthop Relat Res* 477(7):1674, 2019.

Hao DJ, Sun HH, He BR, et al.: Accuracy of CT-guided biopsies in 158 patients with thoracic spinal lesions, *Acta Radiol* 52:1015, 2011.

Hauschild O, Lüdemann M, Engelhardt M, et al.: Aneurysmal bone cyst (ABC): treatment options and proposal of a follow-up regime, *Acta Orthop Belg* 82(3):474, 2016.

Henrichs MP, Beck L, Gosheger G, et al.: Selective arterial embolization of aneurysmal bone cysts of the sacrum: a promising alternative to surgery, *Fortschr Röntgenstr* 188:53, 2016.

Hesla C, Tsagozis P, Jebsen N, et al.: Improved prognosis for patients with Ewing sarcoma in the sacrum compared with the innominate bones. The Scandinavian Sarcoma Group experience, *J Bone Joint Surg Am* 98:199, 2016.

Hillin TJ, Anchala P, Friedman MV, Jennings JW: Treatment of metastatic posterior vertebral body osseous tumors by using a targeted bipolar radiofrequency ablation device: technical note, *Radiology* 273:261, 2014.

Honstad A, Polly DW, Hunt MA: A novel, minimally invasive resection of a pediatric cervical spine osteoblastoma, *JBJS Case Connect* 5:e108, 2015.

Huh A, Villeli N, Martinez D, et al.: Denosumab treatment for a residual giant cell tumor of the clivus: a case report and review of the literature, *World Neurosurg* 118:98, 2018.

Hussain AK, Vig KS, Cheung ZB: The impact of metastatic spinal tumor location on 30-day perioperative mortality and morbidity after surgical decompression, *Spine* 43(11):E648, 2018.

Itshayek E, Candanedo C, Fraifeld S, et al.: Ambulation and survival following surgery in elderly patients with metastatic epidural spinal cord compression, *Spine J* 18(7):1211, 2018.

Ji X, Wang S, Oner FC, et al.: Surgical management of Enneking stage 3 aggressive vertebral hemangiomas with neurological deficit by one stage posterior total en bloc spondylectomy: a review of 23 cases, *Spine* 2019, (Epub ahead of print).

Jia Q, Chen G, Cao J: Clinical features and prognostic factors of pediatric spine giant cell tumors: report of 31 clinical cases in a single center, *Spine J* 19:1232, 2019.

Kadhim M, Binitie O, O'Toole P, et al.: Surgical resection of osteoid osteoma and osteoblastoma of the spine, *J Pediatr Orthop B* 26:362, 2017.

Kieser DC, Mazas S, Cawley DT, et al.: Bisphosphonate therapy for spinal aneurysmal bone cysts, *Dur Spine J* 27(4):851, 2018.

Kim JM, Losina E, Bono CM, et al.: Clinical outcome of metastatic spinal cord compression treated with surgical excision + radiation versus radiation therapy alone: a systematic review of literature, *Spine* 37:78, 2012.

Kumar A, Weber WH, Gokaslan Z, et al.: Metastatic spinal cord compression and steroid treatment. A systematic review, *Clin Spine Surg* 30:156, 2017.

Kumar N, Malhotra R, Zaw AS, et al.: Evolution in treatment strategy for metastatic spine disease: presently evolving modalities, *Eur J Surg Oncol* 43(9):1784, 2017.

Kumar N, Patel R, Wadhwa AC, et al.: Basic concepts in metal work failure after metastatic spine tumour surgery, *Eur Spine J* 27(4):806, 2018.

Kumar R, Meis JM, Amini B, et al.: Giant cell tumor of cervical spine presenting as acute asphyxia: successful surgical resection after down-staging with denosumab, *Spine* 42(10):E629, 2017.

Lange T, Stehling C, Fröhlich B, et al.: Denosumab: a potential new and innovative treatment option for aneurysmal bone cysts, *Eur Spine J* 22:1417, 2013.

Lau D, Chou D: Posterior thoracic corpectomy with cage reconstruction for metastatic spinal tumors: comparing the mini-open approach to the open approach, *J Neurosurg Spine* 23:217, 2015.

Laufer I, Bilsky MH: Advances in the treatment of metastatic spine tumors: the future is not what it used to be, *J Neurosurg Spine* 30:299, 2019.

Lawton AJ, Lee KA, Cheville AL, et al.: Assessment and management of patients with metastatic spinal cord compression: a multidisciplinary review, *J Clin Oncol* 37(1):61, 2019.

Le R, Tran JD, Lizaso M, et al.: Surgical intervention vs. radiation therapy: the shifting paradigm in treating metastatic spinal disease, *Cureus* 10(10):e3406, 2018.

Lee IJ, Lee RJ, Fahim DK: Prognostic factors and survival outcome in patients with chordoma in the United States: a population-based analysis, *World Neurosurg* 104:346, 2017.

Lei M, Li J, Liu Y, et al.: Who are the best candidates for decompressive surgery and spine stabilization in patients with metastatic spinal cord compression? A new scoring system, *Spine* 41(18):1469, 2016.

Li B, Li J, Miao W, et al.: Prognostic analysis of clinical and immunohistochemical factors for patients with spinal schwannoma, *World Neurosurg* 120:e617, 2018.

Li B, Zhang H, Zhou P, et al.: Prognostic significance of pretreatment plasma D-dimer levels in patients with spinal chordoma: a retrospective cohort study, *Eur Spine J* 28:1480, 2019.

Liu JK, Laufer I, Bilsky MH: Update on management of vertebral column tumors, *CNS Oncol* 3:137, 2014.

Liu X, Han SB, Yang SM, et al.: Percutaneous albumin/doxycycline injection versus open surgery for aneurysmal bone cysts in the mobile spine, *Eur Spine J* 28:1529, 2019.

Louie PK, Khan JM, Miller I, Colman MW: All-posterior total en bloc spondylectomy for thoracic spinal tumors, *Ann Transl Med* 7(1):227, 2019.

Luksanapruksa P, Buchowski JM, Singhatanadgige W, Bumpass DB: Systematic review and meta-analysis of en bloc vertebrectomy compared with intralesional resection for giant cell tumors of the mobile spine, *Global Spine J* 6:798, 2016.

Luksanapruksa P, Buchowski JM, Singhatanadgige W, et al.: Management of spinal giant cell tumors, *Spine J* 16:259, 2016.

Ma Y, Xu W, Yin H, et al.: Therapeutic radiotherapy for giant cell tumor of the spine: a systematic review, *Eur Spine J* 2015, [Epub ahead of print].

Madaelil TP, Long JR, Wallace AN, et al.: Preoperative fiducial marker placement in the thoracic spine: a technical report, *Spine* 42(10):E624, 2017.

Matsumoto Y, Harimaya K, Kawaguchi K, et al.: Dumbbell scoring system: a new method for the differential diagnosis of malignant and benign spinal dumbbell tumors, *Spine* 41(20):E1230, 2016.

Mazonakis M, Tzedakis A, Lyraraki E, Damilakis J: Symptomatic vertebral hemangiomas, *Med Phys* 43(4):1841, 2016.

Meng T, Jin J, Jiang C, et al.: Molecular targeted therapy in the treatment of chordoma: a systematic review, *Frontiers in Oncology* 9:1, 2019.

Mesfin A, Sciubba DM Dea N, et al.: Changing the adverse event profile in metastatic spine surgery: an evidence-based approach to target wound complications and instrumentation failure, *Spine* 41(Suppl 20):S262, 2016.

Mhaskar R, Kumar A, Miladinovic B, Djulbegovic B: Bisphosphonates in multiple myeloma: an updated network meta-analysis (review), *Cochrane Database Syst Rev* 12, 2017, Art. No.: CD03188.

Miller JA, Bowen A, Morisada MV, et al.: Radiologic and clinical characteristics of vertebral fractures in multiple myeloma, *Spine J* 15(10):2149, 2015.

Mirzaei L, Daal SEJ, Schreuder HWB, Bartels RHMA: The neurological compromised spine due to Ewing sarcoma. What first: surgery or chemotherapy? Therapy, survival, and neurological outcome of 15 cases with primary Ewing sarcoma of the vertebral column, *Neurosurgery* 77:718, 2015.

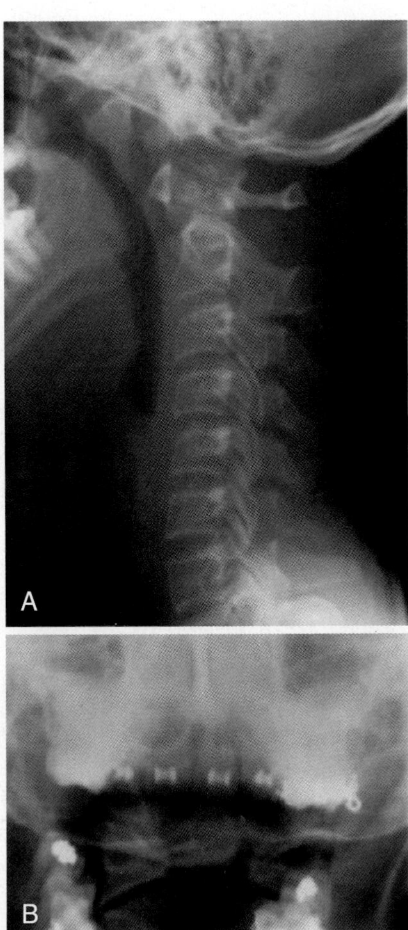

FIGURE 7.4 Lateral radiograph **(A)** and open-mouth odontoid radiograph **(B)** showing os odontoideum.

distance from the posterior aspect of the odontoid or axis to the nearest posterior structure. Fielding reported that most symptomatic patients in his study had an average of 1 cm of movement. Cineradiography can also be helpful in determining motion around the C1-2 articulation.

Watanabe, Toyama, and Fujimura described two radiographic measurements that correlate with neurologic signs and symptoms. They found that if there is a sagittal plane rotation angle of more than 20 degrees or an instability index of more than 40%, a patient is likely to have neurologic signs and symptoms. The instability index is measured from lateral flexion and extension radiographs. Minimal and maximal distances are measured from the posterior border of the C2 body to the posterior arc of the atlas. The instability index is calculated by the following equation:

Instability index = **maximal** distance − **minimal** distance +
minimal distance +
maximal distance × 100 (%)

The sagittal plane rotation angle is measured by the change in the atlantoaxial angle between flexion and extension (Fig. 7.5). MRI can be useful in identifying reactive retrodental lesions that can occur with chronic instability. This reactive tissue is not seen on routine radiographs but can be responsible for a decrease in the space available for the spinal cord and compressive myelopathy. The prognosis of os odontoideum depends on the clinical presentation. The prognosis is good if only mechanical symptoms (torticollis or neck pain) or transient neurologic symptoms exist. It is poor if neurologic deficits slowly progress.

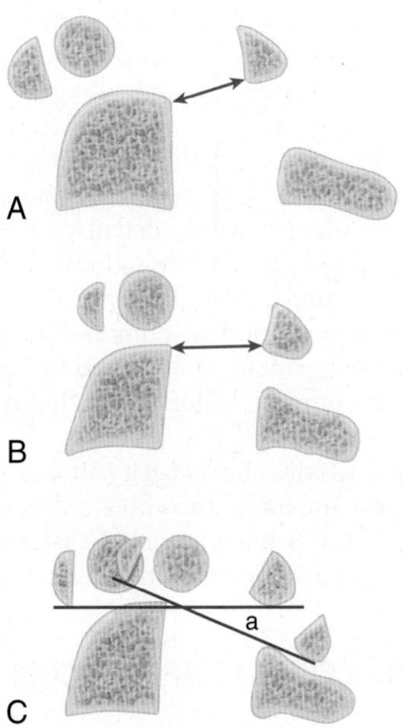

FIGURE 7.5 Radiographic parameters. Minimal **(A)** and maximal **(B)** distance from posterior border of body of C2 to posterior atlantal arch. **C,** Change of atlantoaxial angle between flexion and extension position. *a,* sagittal plane rotation.

BOX 7.1

Indications for Operative Stabilization of Os Odontoideum

- Neurologic involvement (even transient)
- Instability of greater than 5 mm posteriorly or anteriorly
- Progressive instability
- Persistent neck complaints

TREATMENT

The primary concern in congenital anomalies of the odontoid is that an already abnormal atlantoaxial joint can subluxate or dislocate with minor trauma and cause permanent neurologic damage or even death. Patients with local symptoms usually improve with conservative treatment and immobilization. The indications for operative stabilization are: (1) neurologic involvement (even if this is transient), (2) instability of more than 5 mm anteriorly or posteriorly, (3) progressive instability, and (4) persistent neck complaints associated with atlantoaxial instability and not relieved by conservative treatment (Box 7.1).

Prophylactic operative stabilization of odontoid instability of less than 5 mm in asymptomatic patients is controversial. Because it may be difficult or impossible to restrict a child's activities, the safety of stability without restriction of activity must be weighed against the possible complications of surgery.

The decision concerning prophylactic arthrodesis must be made after discussion with the patient and family concerning potential risks of operative and nonoperative treatment. Delayed neurologic injury has been reported in three patients who initially received conservative treatment. We, therefore, recommend prophylactic stabilization of os odontoideum.

In patients with neurologic deficits, skull traction can be used before surgery to achieve reduction. Achieving and maintaining reduction are probably the most important aspects in the treatment of this anomaly. Dlouhy et al. found that the transverse ligament anterior and inferior to the ossicle was the most common factor preventing reduction of an os odontoideum.

Before C1-2 fusion, the integrity of the posterior arch of C1 must be documented. Incomplete development of the posterior ring of C1 is uncommon (3 cases in 1000) but is reported to occur with increased frequency in patients with os odontoideum.

POSTERIOR CERVICAL APPROACHES

ATLANTOAXIAL FUSION

Many variations of two basic techniques of atlantoaxial fusion exist (Box 7.2). The Gallie and the Brooks and Jenkins techniques have been the most frequently used for posterior atlantoaxial fusion (Figs. 7.6 to 7.8). The Gallie technique has the advantage of using only one wire passed beneath the lamina of C1, but tightening the wire can cause the unstable C1 vertebra to displace posteriorly and fuse in a dislocated position (Fig. 7.6). The Brooks and Jenkins technique has the disadvantage of requiring sublaminar wires at C1 and C2 but gives greater resistance to rotational movement, lateral bending, and extension. The wire varies in size from 22 gauge to 18 gauge, depending on the age of the patient and the size of the spinal canal. Songer cables may also be used instead of wires for the Brooks and Jenkins fusion. In a very young child, wire fixation may be unnecessary; instead, the graft is placed along the decorticated fusion site, and a halo or Minerva cast is used for postoperative immobilization. With the use of fluoroscopy and image-guided systems, C1-2 transarticular screws or C1-2 screw and rod fixation can be used for stabilization in appropriately sized children and is often the preferred fixation method.

POSTERIOR ATLANTOAXIAL FUSION

TECHNIQUE 7.1

(GALLIE)

- Carefully intubate the patient in the supine position while the patient is on a stretcher. Place the patient prone on the operating table with the head supported by traction, maintaining the head-thorax relationship at all times during turning. Obtain a lateral cervical spine radiograph to ensure proper alignment before surgery.

BOX 7.2

Posterior Fusion Techniques

Atlantoaxial Fusion

Gallie

Advantage: One wire passed beneath lamina of C1.

Disadvantage: Wire may cause unstable C1 vertebra to displace posteriorly and fuse in dislocated position; need for postoperative halo immobilization.

Brooks and Jenkins

Advantage: Greater resistance to rotational movement, lateral bending, and extension.

Disadvantage: Requires sublaminar wires at C1 and C2.

Harms and Melcher

Advantage: Individual placement of polyaxial screws simplifies technique and involves less risk to C1-C2 facet joint and vertebral artery.

Disadvantages: Possible irritation of the C2 ganglion from instrumentation. Technique is not possible in patients with aberrant course of the vertebral artery (20%).

Magerl and Seeman

Advantage: Significant improvement in fusion rates over traditional posterior wire stabilization and bone grafting techniques.

Disadvantage: Technically demanding and must be combined with Gallie or Brooks fusion for maximum stability.

Occipitocervical Fusion

Occipital Rod and Screw Fusion

Cone and Turner; Willard and Nicholson; Rogers

Required when other bony anomalies occur at occipitocervical junction.

Wertheim and Bohlman

Wires passed through outer table of skull at occipital protuberance instead of through inner and outer tables near foramen magnum.

Lessens risk of danger to superior sagittal and transverse sinuses (which are cephalad to occipital protuberance).

Koop, Winter, Lonstein

No internal fixation used.

Autogenous corticocancellous iliac bone graft.

Dormans et al.

Stable fixation is achieved by exact fit of autogenous iliac crest bone graft and fixation of the spinous process with button wire and fixation of the occiput with wires through burr holes.

Can be used in high-risk patients (Down syndrome) with increased stabilization and shorter immobilization time.

Contoured Rod, Screw, or Contoured Plate Fixation

Has the advantage of achieving immediate stability of the occipitocervical junction.

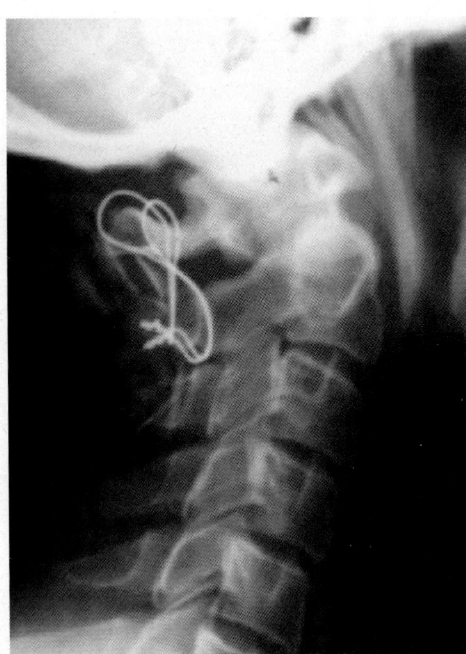

FIGURE 7.6 Posterior translation of atlas after C1-2 posterior Gallie fusion.

- Prepare and drape the skin in a sterile fashion and inject a solution of epinephrine (1:500,000) intradermally to aid hemostasis.
- Make a midline incision from the lower occiput to the level of the lower end of the fusion, extending it deeply within the relatively avascular midline structures, the intermuscular septum, or ligamentum nuchae. Do not expose any more than the area to be fused to decrease the chance of spontaneous extension of the fusion.
- By subperiosteal dissection, expose the posterior arch of the atlas and the laminae of C2.
- Remove the muscular and ligamentous attachments from C2 with a curet or periosteal elevator; dissect laterally along the atlas to prevent injury to the vertebral arteries and vertebral venous plexus that lie on the superior aspect of the ring of C1, less than 2 cm lateral to the midline.
- Expose the upper surface of C1 no farther laterally than 1.5 cm from the midline in adults and 1 cm in children. Decortication of C1 and C2 is generally unnecessary.
- From below, pass a wire loop of appropriate size upward under the arch of the atlas directly or with the aid of a nonabsorbable suture, which can be passed with an aneurysm needle.
- Pass the free ends of the wire through the loop, grasping the arch of C1 in the loop.
- Take a corticocancellous graft from the iliac crest and place it against the laminae of C2 and the arch of C1 beneath the wire.
- Pass one end of the wire through the spinous process of C2 and twist the wire on itself to secure the graft in place.
- Irrigate the wound and close it in layers with suction drainage tubes.

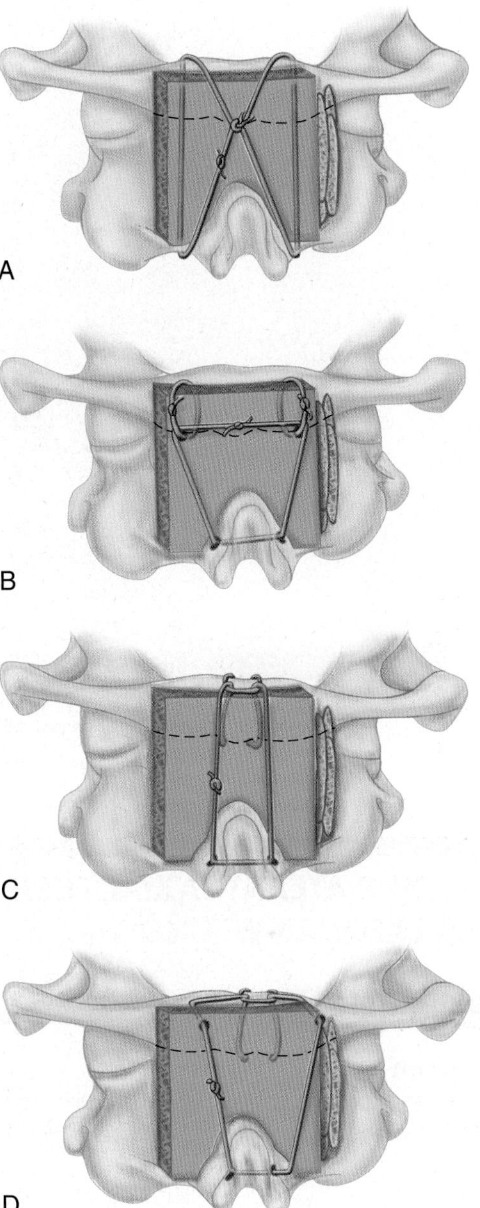

FIGURE 7.7 Fielding's modifications of wire techniques for holding graft in place. **A,** Wire passes under laminae of atlas and axis and is tied over graft. **B,** Wire passes through holes drilled in laminae of atlas and through spine of axis; holes are drilled through graft. **C,** Wire passes under laminae of atlas and through spine of axis and is tied over graft. This method is used most frequently. **D,** Wire passes under laminae of atlas and through spine of axis; holes are drilled through graft. **SEE TECHNIQUE 7.1.**

Fielding described several modifications of the Gallie fusion, as shown in Figure 7.7.

POSTOPERATIVE CARE The patient is immobilized in a Minerva cast, halo cast or halo vest, or a cervicothoracic orthosis. Immobilization usually is continued for 12 weeks.

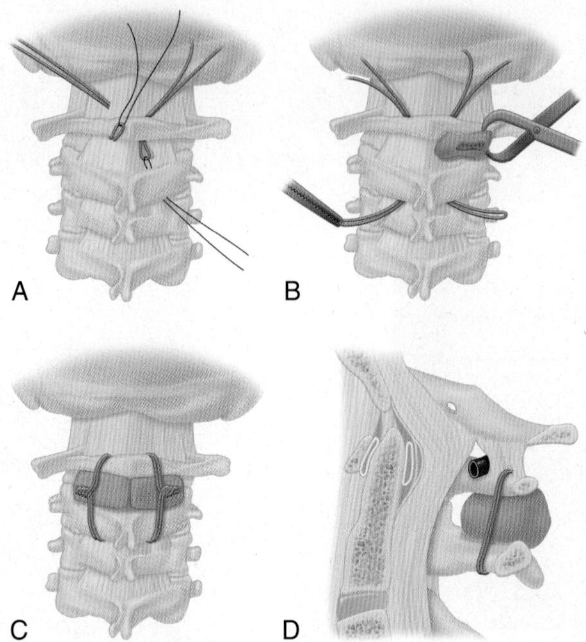

FIGURE 7.8 Brooks-Jenkins technique of atlantoaxial fusion. **A,** Insertion of wires under atlas and axis. **B,** Wires in place with graft being inserted. **C** and **D,** Bone grafts secured by wires (anteroposterior and lateral views). **SEE TECHNIQUE 7.2.**

POSTERIOR ATLANTOAXIAL FUSION USING LAMINAR WIRING

TECHNIQUE 7.2

(BROOKS AND JENKINS)

- Intubate and turn the patient onto the operating table as for the Gallie technique (Technique 7.1). Prepare and drape the operative site as described.
- Expose C1 and C2 through a midline incision.
- Using an aneurysm needle, pass a Mersilene suture from cephalad to caudad on each side of the midline under the arch of the atlas and then beneath the laminae of C2 (Fig. 7.8A). These sutures serve as guides to introduce two doubled 20-gauge wires. The size of the wire used varies depending on the size and age of the patient.
- Obtain two full-thickness bone grafts 1.25 to 3.5 cm from the iliac crest and bevel them so that the apex of the graft fits in the interval between the arch of the atlas and the lamina of the axis (Fig. 7.8B).
- Fashion notches in the upper and lower cortical surfaces to hold the circumferential wires and prevent them from slipping.
- Tighten the doubled wires over the graft and twist them on each side (Fig. 7.8C and D).
- Irrigate and close the wound in layers over suction drains.

POSTOPERATIVE CARE The postoperative care is the same as that for the Gallie technique.

C1-2 FIXATION WITH TRANSARTICULAR SCREWS AND WITH SCREW AND RODS (HARMS TECHNIQUE)

Adult instrumentation and fusion techniques may be used in the pediatric cervical spine. The use of this instrumentation is dependent on the preoperative anatomy that would allow appropriate size screws to be placed safely. Adult instrumentation of the cervical spine usually can be used in adolescents and preteens. For smaller children, the use of these adult instrumentation techniques becomes more difficult but can be used safely in certain patients. Wang et al. reported good results in the management of pediatric atlantoaxial instability with C1-2 transarticular screw fixation and fusion, using a 3.5-mm screw in children of 4 years of age. Originally described for adult patients, it is technically demanding and requires fluoroscopic or stereotactic assistance for the proper placement of the transarticular screw (Fig. 7.9). Harms and Melcher reported posterior C1-C2 fusion using polyaxial screw and rod fixation in adults and children with good results. They cited the following advantages: individual placement of polyaxial screws in C1 and C2 allows direct manipulation of C1 and C2, simplifying reduction and fixation; superior and medial placement of the C2 screw carries less risk to the vertebral artery; the integrity of the posterior arch of C1 is not necessary for stable fixation (Fig. 7.10). Please refer to Chapter 5 for transarticular screw fixation technique in adults.

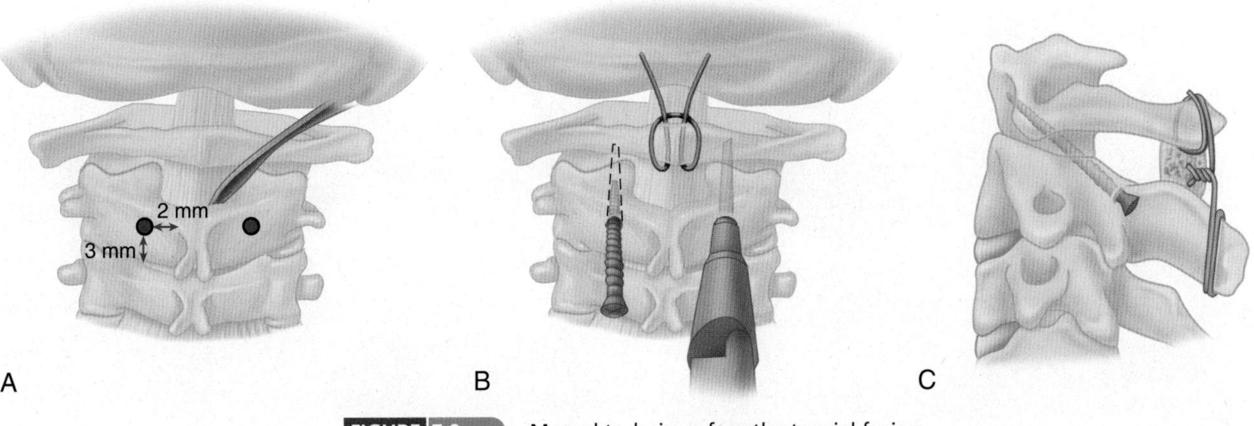

FIGURE 7.9 Magerl technique for atlantoaxial fusion.

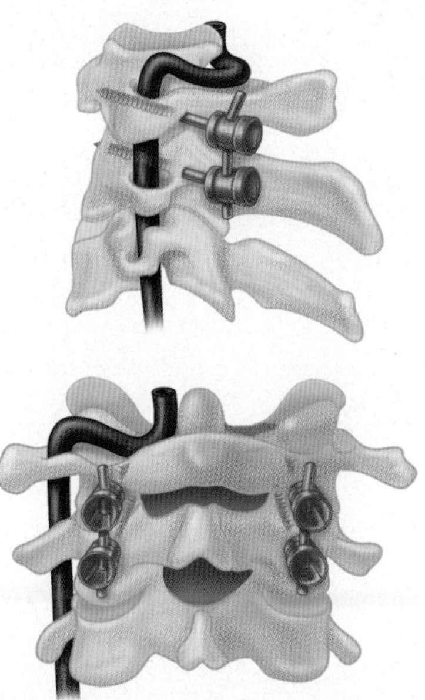

FIGURE 7.10 Harms and Melcher technique. Upper cervical spine after C1-C2 fixation by polyaxial screw and rod fixation.

TRANSLAMINAR SCREW FIXATION OF C2

Translaminar screw fixation can be used as an alternative to polyaxial screw and rod fixation when the C2 isthmus or pedicle cannot be instrumented. Approximately 20% of patients have an abnormal path of the vertebral artery that will prevent placement of the C2 screw in Harms and Melcher's technique. Translaminar screw fixation may also be used in the lower cervical spine if needed.

TECHNIQUE 7.3

- Place the patient prone with the head in a neutral position in a Mayfield head holder.
- Expose the posterior arch of C1 and the spinous process, laminae, and medial and lateral masses of C2.
- Create a small cortical window at the junction of the C2 spinous process and the lamina on the left, close to the rostral margin of the C2 lamina (Fig. 7.11A).
- Using a hand drill, carefully drill along the length of the contralateral (right) lamina, with the drill visually aligned along the angle of the exposed contralateral laminar surface.
- Palpate the length of the drill hole with a small ball probe to verify that no cortical breakthrough into the spinal canal has occurred.
- Insert a 4-mm diameter polyaxial screw along the same trajectory. In the final position, the screw head is at the junction of the spinous process and lamina on the left, with the length of the screw within the right lamina.
- Create a small cortical window at the junction of the spinous process and lamina of C2 on the right, close to the caudal aspect of the lamina.
- Using the same technique as above, insert a 4-mm diameter screw into the left lamina, with the screw head remaining on the right side of the spinous process.
- Place appropriate rods into the screw heads and attach to C1 screws or lateral mass screws below C2 (Fig. 7.11B).

POSTOPERATIVE CARE The patient is immobilized in a cervical or cervicothoracic orthosis for 8 to 12 weeks.

OCCIPITOCERVICAL FUSION

When other bony anomalies occur at the occipitocervical junction, such as absence of the posterior arch of C1, the fusion can extend up to the occiput. The following technique for occipitocervical fusion includes features of techniques described by Cone and Turner, Rogers, Willard and Nicholson, and Robinson and Southwick.

TECHNIQUE 7.4

- Approach the base of the occiput and the spinous processes of the upper cervical vertebrae through a longitudinal

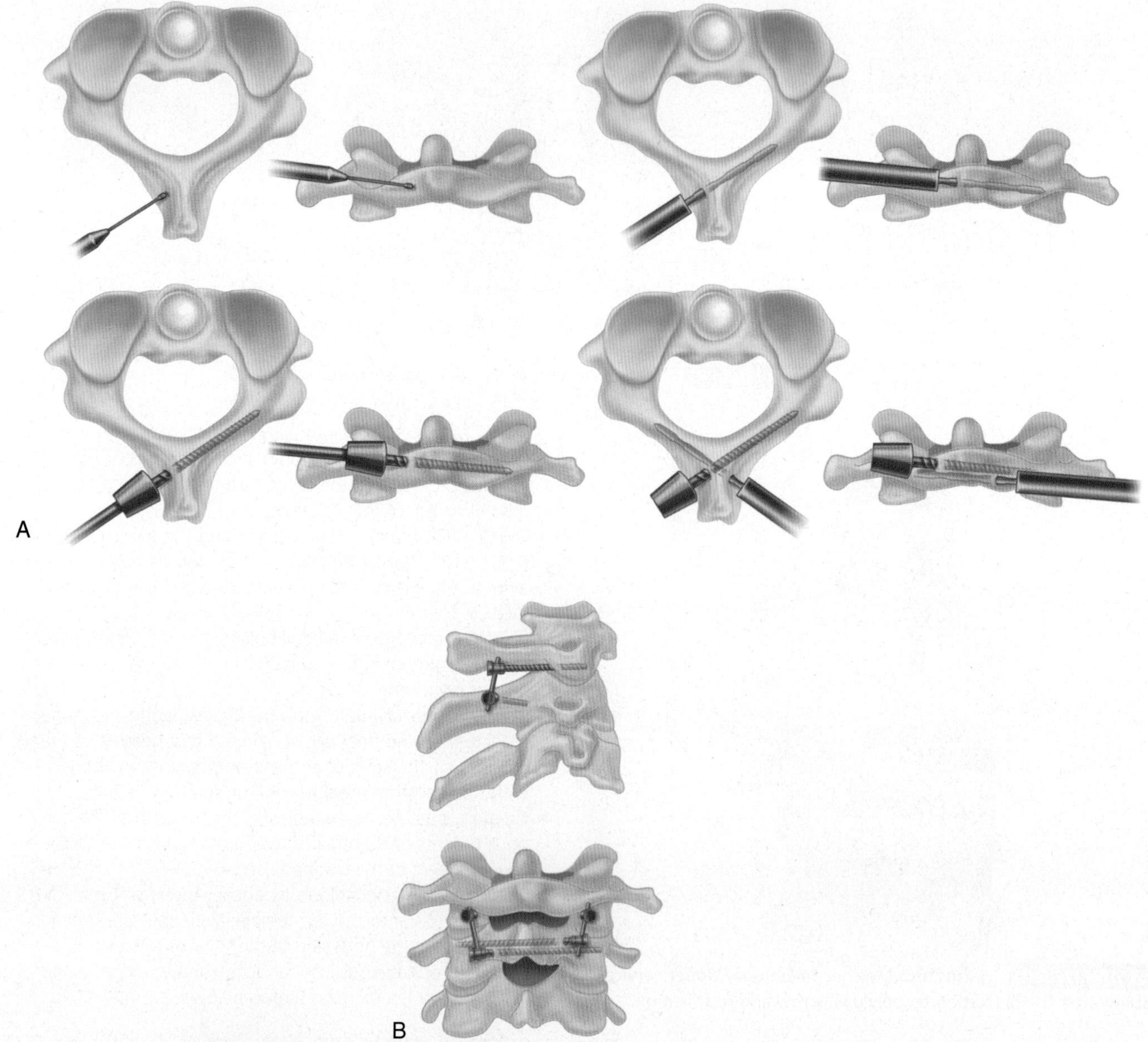

FIGURE 7.11 **A,** C2 translaminar screw placement. **B,** Lateral and anteroposterior views of completed C1-C2 fixation with C1 lateral mass screws connected to C2 laminar screws. **SEE TECHNIQUE 7.3.**

midline incision, extending it deeply within the relatively avascular intermuscular septum.

- Expose the entire field subperiosteally.
- Dissect the posterior occiput laterally to the level of the external occipital protuberance.
- Make two burr holes in the posterior occiput about 7 mm from the foramen magnum and 10 mm lateral to the midline (Fig. 7.12).
- Separate the dura from the inner table of the skull by blunt dissection with a right-angle dissector.
- Pass short lengths of wire through the holes in the occiput and through the foramen magnum.
- Pass wires beneath the posterior arch of C1 on either side if the arch is intact.
- Drill holes in the outer table of the spinous processes of C2 and C3, completing them with a towel clip or Lewin clamp, and pass short lengths of wire through the holes.
- Obtain a corticocancellous graft from the iliac crest and make holes at appropriate intervals to accept the ends of the wires.
- Pass the wires through the holes in the graft and lay the graft against the occiput and the laminae of C2 and C3.
- Tighten the wires to hold the graft firmly in place (Fig. 7.12, *inset*).
- Lay thin strips of cancellous bone around the cortical grafts to aid in fusion.

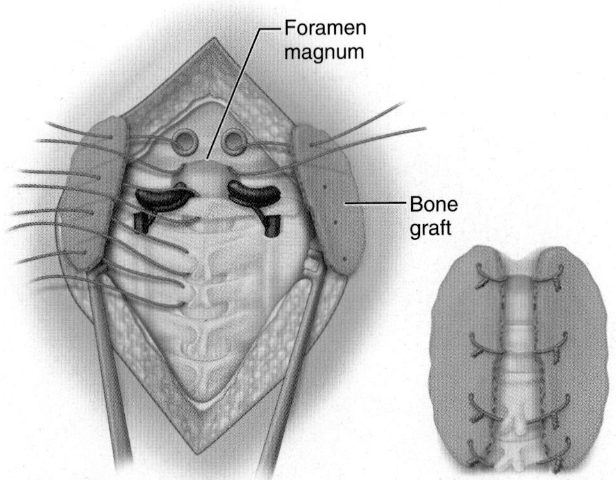

FIGURE 7.12 Robinson and Southwick method of occipitocervical fusion. **SEE TECHNIQUE 7.4.**

- Inspect the graft and wires to ensure that they do not impinge on the dura or vertebral arteries. Irrigate and close the wound in layers over suction drains.

  Robinson and Southwick passed individual wires beneath the laminae of C2 and C3 instead of through the spinous processes (Fig. 7.12).

POSTOPERATIVE CARE Some form of external support is recommended. This support may vary from a Minerva cast or halo vest or halo cast to a cervicothoracic brace, depending on the degree of preoperative instability and the stability of fixation.

OCCIPITOCERVICAL FUSION PASSING WIRES THROUGH TABLE OF SKULL

Wertheim and Bohlman described a technique of occipitocervical fusion similar to that described by Grantham et al. in which wires are passed through the outer table of the skull at the occipital protuberance instead of through the inner and outer tables of the skull near the foramen magnum. Superior to the foramen magnum the occipital bone is very thin, but at the external occipital protuberance, it is thick and allows passage of wires without passing through both tables. The transverse and superior sagittal sinuses are cephalad to the protuberance and are out of danger.

TECHNIQUE 7.5

(WERTHEIM AND BOHLMAN)

- Stabilize the spine preoperatively with cranial skeletal traction with the patient on a turning frame or cerebellar headrest.
- Place the patient prone and obtain a lateral radiograph to document proper alignment.
- Prepare the skin and inject the subcutaneous tissue with a solution of epinephrine (1:500,000).
- Make a midline incision extending from the external occipital protuberance to the spine of the third cervical vertebra.
- Sharply dissect the paraspinous muscles subperiosteally with a scalpel and a periosteal elevator to expose the occiput and cervical laminae, taking care to stay in the midline to avoid the paramedian venous plexus.
- At a point 2 cm above the rim of the foramen magnum, use a high-speed diamond burr to create a trough on either side of the protuberance, making a ridge in the center (Fig. 7.13A). With a towel clip, make a hole in this ridge through only the outer table of bone.
- Loop a 20-gauge wire through the hole and around the ridge and loop another 20-gauge wire around the arch of the atlas.
- Pass a third wire through a drill hole in the base of the spinous process of the axis and around this structure; three separate wires are used to secure the bone grafts on each side of the spine (Fig. 7.13B).
- Expose the posterior iliac crest and obtain a thick, slightly curved graft of corticocancellous bone of premeasured length and width.
- Divide this horizontally into two pieces and place three drill holes in each graft (Fig. 7.13C).
- Decorticate the occiput and anchor the grafts in place with the wires on both sides of the spine (Fig. 7.13D). Pack additional cancellous bone around and between the two grafts.
- Close the wound in layers over suction drains.

POSTOPERATIVE CARE A rigid cervical orthosis or a halo cast is worn for 6 to 16 weeks, followed by a soft collar that is worn for an additional 6 weeks.

OCCIPITOCERVICAL FUSION WITHOUT INTERNAL FIXATION

Koop, Winter, and Lonstein described a technique of occipitocervical fusion without internal fixation for use in children. The spine is decorticated, and autogenous corticocancellous iliac bone is placed over the area to be fused. In children with vertebral arch defects, an occipital periosteal flap is reflected over the bone defect to provide an osteogenic tissue layer for the bone grafts. A halo cast is used for postoperative stability.

TECHNIQUE 7.6

(KOOP ET AL.)

- After the administration of endotracheal anesthesia, apply a halo frame with the child supine.
- Turn the child prone and secure the head with the neck in slight extension by securing the halo frame to a traction frame.

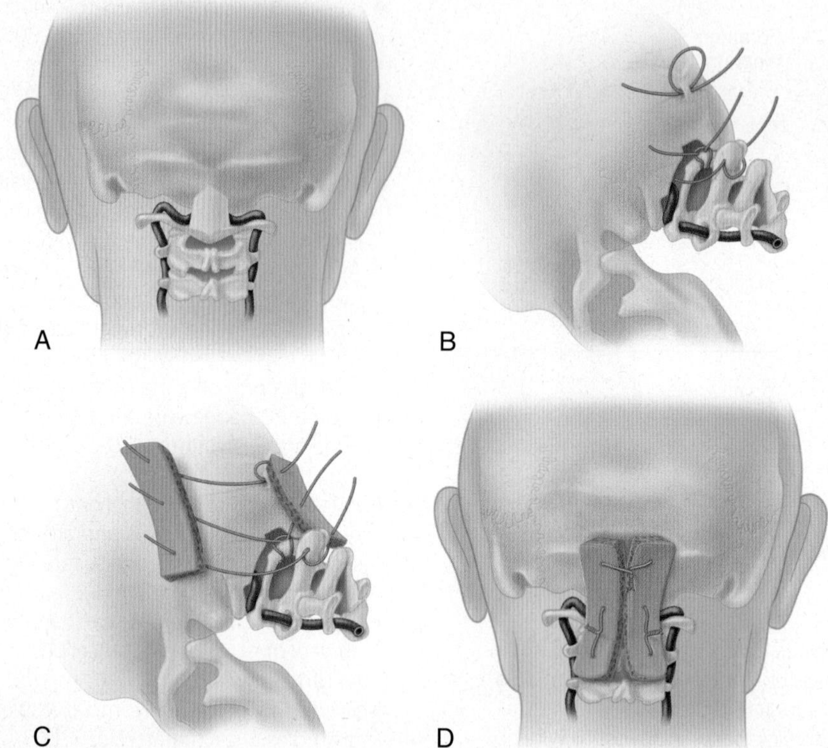

FIGURE 7.13 Wertheim and Bohlman method of occipitocervical fusion. **A,** Burr is used to create a ridge in external occipital protuberance; hole is made in the ridge. **B,** Wires are passed through outer table of occiput, under arch of atlas, and through spinous process of axis. **C,** Grafts are placed on wires. **D,** Wires are tightened to secure grafts in place. **SEE TECHNIQUE 7.5.**

- Make a midline incision. In patients with intact posterior elements, expose the vertebrae by sharp dissection.
- Decorticate the exposed vertebral elements and lay strips of autogenous cancellous iliac bone over the decorticated bone. Expose only the vertebrae to be included in the fusion. In patients with defects in the posterior elements, do not expose the dura, if possible.
- At the level of the occiput, dissect the nuchal tissue from the periosteum and retract it laterally (Fig. 7.14A).
- Elevate the occipital periosteum in a triangular-based flap attached near the margin of the foramen magnum.
- Reflect this flap caudally to cover the defects in the posterior vertebral elements and suture it in place (Fig. 7.14B).
- Decorticate the occiput and the remaining exposed vertebral elements with an air drill (Fig. 7.14C).
- Lay strips of autogenous cancellous bone in place over the entire area (Fig. 7.14D).
- Close the wound in layers over a suction drain.
- Turn the child supine and apply a halo cast.

POSTOPERATIVE CARE The halo cast is worn until union is radiographically evident, usually at about 5 months. When union is documented by lateral flexion and extension radiographs, the halo cast is removed, and a soft collar is worn for 1 month.

OCCIPITOCERVICAL FUSION USING CROSSED WIRING

Dormans et al. described occipitocervical fusion using a different wiring technique in 16 children with an average age of 9.6 years (range 2.5 to 19.3 years). Fusion was achieved in 15 patients. Complications included pin track infection (four patients), pneumonia (one patient), additional level of fusion (one patient), and graft fracture and nonunion (one patient). The use of wire fixation, combined with inherent stability of the bone-graft construct, allowed for removal of the halo device relatively early (6 to 12 weeks).

TECHNIQUE 7.7

(DORMANS ET AL.)

- After halo ring application, place the patient prone and secure the halo frame to the operating table. Confirm alignment of the occiput and cervical spine with lateral radiographs.
- Expose the midline from the occiput to the second or third cervical vertebra. Limit the lateral dissection to avoid damaging the vertebral arteries.

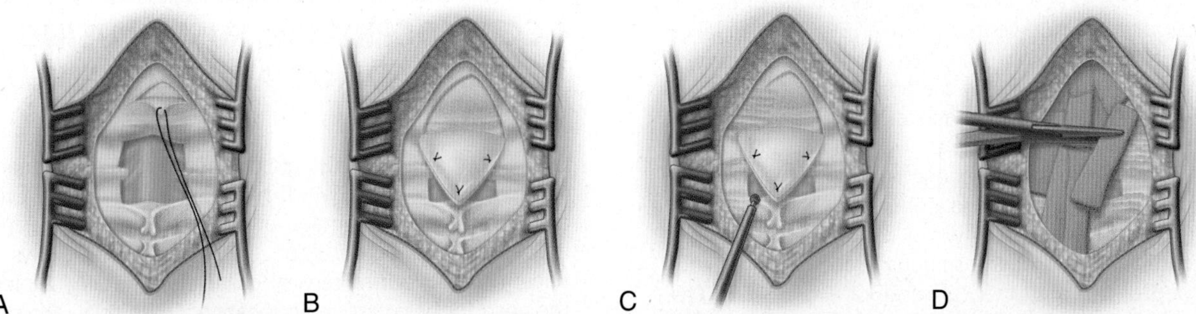

FIGURE 7.14 Koop, Winter, and Lonstein method of occipitocervical fusion used when posterior arch of C1 is absent. **A,** Exposure of occiput, atlas, and axis. **B,** Reflection of periosteal flap to cover defect in atlas. **C,** Decortication of exposed vertebral elements. **D,** Placement of autogenous cancellous iliac bone grafts. **SEE TECHNIQUE 7.6.**

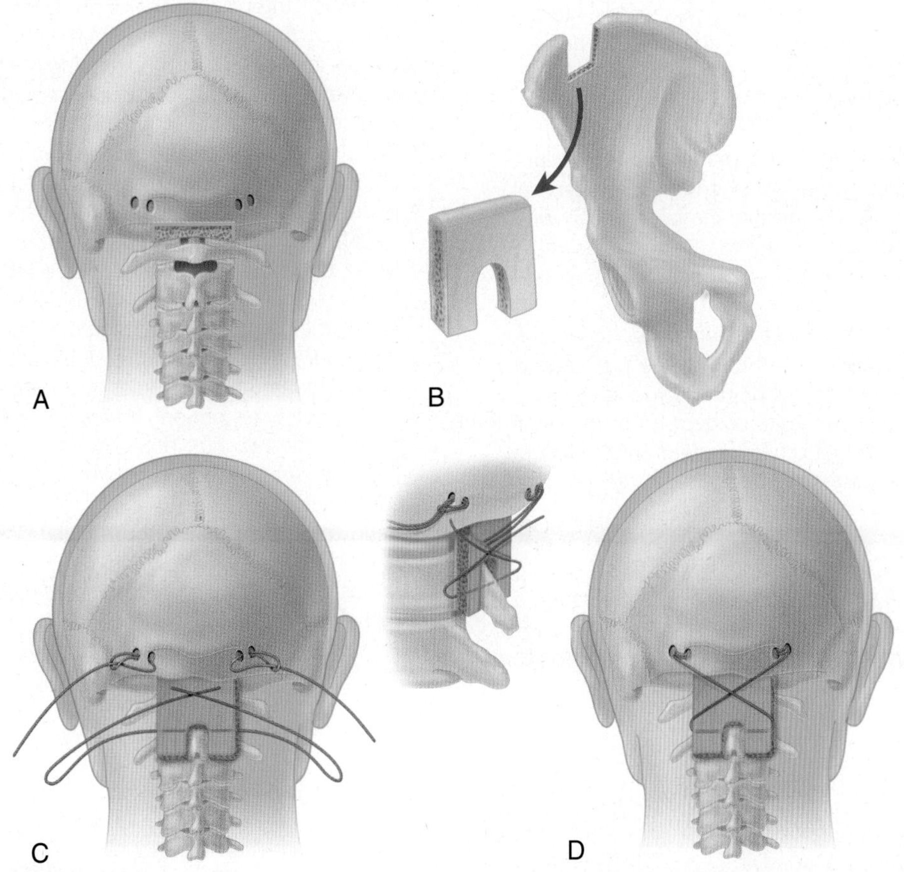

FIGURE 7.15 Occipitocervical fusion as described by Dormans et al. **A,** Placement of burr holes. **B,** Corticocancellous graft obtained from iliac crest. **C,** Looped 16- or 18-gauge wires passed through burr holes and looped on themselves. Graft positioned into occipital trough and around spinous process of cervical vertebra at caudal extent of fusion and locked into place by precise contouring of bone. **D,** Wires crossed, twisted, and cut. **SEE TECHNIQUE 7.7.**

- In patients who require decompression because of cervical stenosis or for removal of a tumor, remove the arch of the first or second cervical vertebra, or both, with or without removal of a portion of occipital bone to enlarge the foramen magnum.
- Use a high-speed drill to make four holes through both cortices of the occiput, aligning them transversely with two on each side of the midline and leaving a 1-cm osseous bridge between the two holes of each pair. Place the holes caudad to the transverse sinuses (Fig. 7.15A).
- Fashion a trough into the base of the occiput to accept the cephalad end of the bone graft.
- Obtain a corticocancellous graft from the iliac crest and shape it into a rectangle, with a notch created in the

inferior base to fit around the spinous process of the second or third cervical vertebra (Fig. 7.15B). The caudal extent of the intended fusion (the second or third cervical vertebra) is determined by the presence or absence of a previous laminectomy, congenital anomalies, or level of instability.

- Pass a looped 16- or 18-gauge Luque wire through the burr holes on each side and loop it onto itself.
- Pass Wisconsin button wires (Zimmer, Warsaw, IN) through the base of the spinous process of either the second or the third cervical vertebra (Fig. 7.15C). Pass the wire that is going into the left arm of the graft through the spinous process from right to left. Place the graft into the occipital trough superiorly and around the spinous process of the vertebra that is to be at the caudal level of the arthrodesis (the second or third cervical vertebra).
- Contour the graft precisely so that it fits securely into the occipital trough and around the inferior spinous process before the wires are tightened.
- Cross the wires, twist, and cut (Fig. 7.15D).
- Obtain a radiograph at this point to assess the position of the graft and wires and the alignment of the occiput and cephalad cervical vertebrae. Extension of the cervical spine can be controlled by positioning of the head with the halo frame, by adjustment of the size and shape of the graft, and, to a lesser extent, by appropriate tightening of the wires.
- For patients who have not had a decompression, pass the sublaminar wire caudally to the ring of the first cervical vertebra to secure additional fixation. In young children, this may be difficult or undesirable because of the small size of the ring of the first cervical vertebra or the failure of formation of the posterior arch of the first cervical vertebra.

POSTOPERATIVE CARE A custom halo orthosis or halo cast is worn until a solid fusion is obtained; thereafter, a cervical collar is worn for 1 month.

OCCIPITOCERVICAL FUSION USING CONTOURED ROD AND SEGMENTAL ROD FIXATION

Occipitocervical fusion using a contoured rod and segmental wire or cable fixation, which has been described by several authors, has the advantage of achieving immediate stability of the occipitocervical junction. This stability allows the patient to move in a cervical collar after surgery, avoiding the need for halo cast immobilization. Smith et al. described occipitocervical arthrodesis using a contoured plate instead of a rod for fixation.

TECHNIQUE 7.8

Figure 7.16

- Approach the base of the occiput and the spinous processes of the upper cervical vertebrae through a longitudinal midline incision, extending it deeply within the relatively avascular intermuscular septum.
- Expose the entire field subperiosteally.
- Carry the dissection proximally above the inion and laterally to the level of the external occipital protuberance.
- Make a template of the intended shape of the stainless-steel rod with the appropriate length of Luque wire.
- Make two burr holes on each side, about 2 cm lateral to the midline and 2.5 cm above the foramen magnum. Avoid the transverse and sigmoid sinus when making these burr holes. Leave at least 10 mm of intact cortical bone between the burr holes to ensure solid fixation.
- Pass Luque wires or Songer cables in an extradural plane through the two burr holes on each side of the midline. Pass the wires or cables sublaminar in the upper cervical spine.
- Bend the rod to match the template; this usually has a head-neck angle of about 135 degrees and slight cervical lordosis. A Bend Meister (Sofamor/Danek, Memphis) may be helpful in bending the rod.

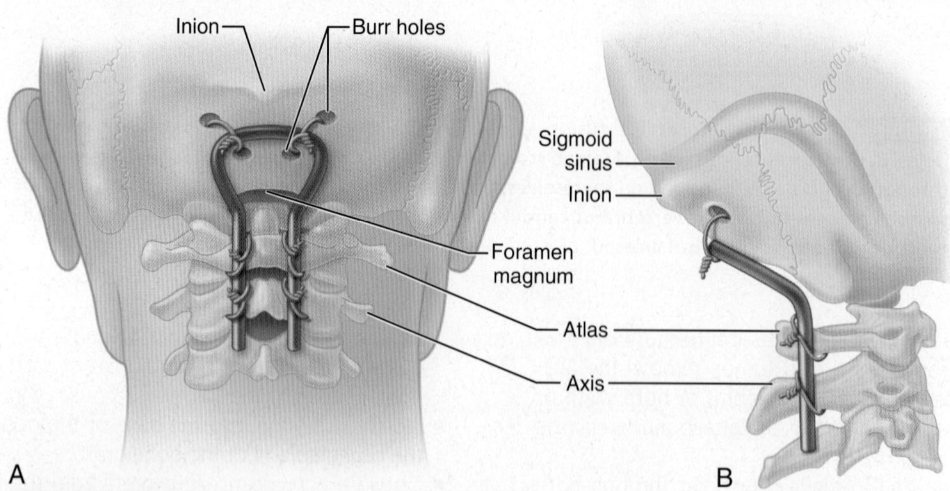

FIGURE 7.16 **A** and **B**, Occipitocervical fusion using contoured rod and segmental wire or cable fixation. **SEE TECHNIQUE 7.8.**

- Secure the wires or cables to the rod.
- Decorticate the spine and occiput and perform autogenous cancellous bone grafting.

POSTOPERATIVE CARE A Philadelphia collar or an occipitocervical orthosis is worn until the fusion is stable.

OCCIPITOCERVICAL FUSION USING A CONTOURED OCCIPITAL PLATE, SCREW, AND ROD FIXATION

This technique uses an adjustable-angle rod and a contoured occipital plate (Vertex Select, Medtronic, Memphis, TN) for fixation.

TECHNIQUE 7.9

Figure 7.17

- Expose the spine posteriorly as described in Technique 7.8.
- Adjust the angle of each rod for the most preferable alignment; tighten the internal set screws to lock the angle. Further bend the rods to best fit the patient's anatomy. Cut both ends of the rods to the required lengths.
- Position the rods in the previously placed cervical implants to determine the proper occipital plate size and make adjustments, if necessary, to align the rod.
- Position the occipital plate in the midline (occipital keel) between the external occipital protuberance and the posterior border of the foramen magnum. Contour the plate for an anatomic fit against the occiput. Avoid repeated bending of the plate because this may compromise its integrity. It may be necessary to contour the bone of the occiput.
- With an appropriate-size drill bit and guide that match the screw diameter, drill a hole in the occiput to the desired predetermined depth. Drilling must be done through the occipital plate to ensure proper drilling depth.
- Tap the hole, using a gauge to verify the depth. The occipital bone is very dense, and each hole should be completely tapped.
- Insert the appropriate size occipital screw and provisionally tighten it. Insert the rest of the screws as above and hand-tighten each.
- Place the rods into the implants and stabilize them by tightening the set screws. Perform final tightening of the occipital plate set screws and recheck all connections of the final construct before wound closure.

POSTOPERATIVE CARE Immobilize the cervical spine in an orthosis for 8 to 12 weeks.

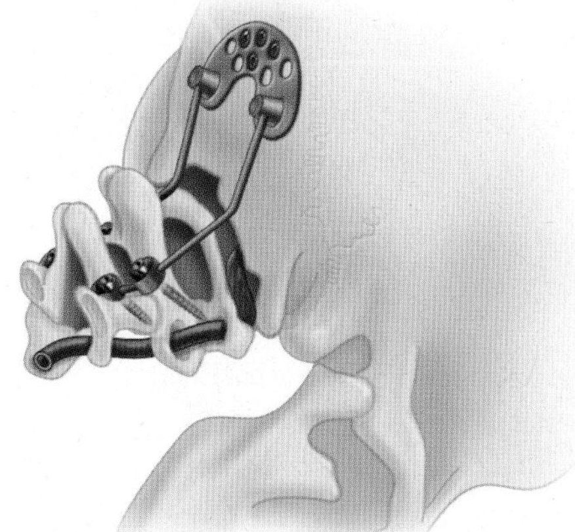

FIGURE 7.17 Occipitocervical fusion using contoured occipital plate, screw, and rod fixation (Vertex Select, Medtronic, Memphis). **SEE TECHNIQUE 7.9.**

ANTERIOR CERVICAL APPROACHES

C1-2 subluxation or dislocation sometimes cannot be reduced with traction. If a patient has no neurologic deficits, a simple in situ posterior fusion can be done with little increase in risk. Posterior decompression by laminectomy has been associated with increased morbidity and mortality. Posterior decompression increases C1-2 instability unless accompanied by fusion from the occiput to C2 or C3. If posterior stabilization cannot be performed because of the clinical situation or anterior subluxation associated with cord compression is present, then an anterior approach should be considered. A subtotal maxillectomy, lateral retropharyngeal approach, or transoral approach can be used. The retropharyngeal approach usually is preferred because of the increased incidence of wound complications and infection associated with the transoral and maxillectomy approaches (Box 7.3).

TRANSORAL APPROACH

Fang and Ong achieved fusion by placing rectangular grafts into similarly shaped graft beds extending from the lateral mass of the atlas to the lateral mass and body of the axis. If only an anterior decompression is performed, a posterior fusion and stabilization should also be done. Most authors recommend posterior fusion for stabilization before decompression, but it can be done after decompression depending on stability.

TECHNIQUE 7.10

(FANG AND ONG)

- Parenteral prophylactic antibiotics are given based on preoperative nasopharyngeal cultures. Endotracheal intubation is achieved using a noncollapsible tube and cuff. If extensive dissection is anticipated, a tracheostomy should be performed.
- Place the patient in the Trendelenburg position and insert a mouth gag to provide retraction. Identify the vertebral bodies by palpation.
- The ring of the first vertebra has a midline anterior tubercle, and the disc between the second and third vertebrae is prominent, providing another localizing landmark. Make a longitudinal incision in the midline of the posterior pharynx (Fig. 7.18A). The soft palate can be divided

in the midline, making paresis after retraction less likely, or it can be folded back on itself.

- Continue the midline dissection down to bone and reflect the tissue laterally to the outer margin of the lateral masses of the axis (Fig. 7.18B). Beyond these margins are the vertebral arteries, and care should be taken not to harm them. The soft-tissue flap can be retracted using long stay sutures.
- After the procedure is complete, irrigate and close the wound loosely with interrupted absorbable sutures. Continue antibiotics for at least 3 days after surgery.

BOX 7.3

Anterior Cervical Approaches

Transoral (Fang et al.)
High incidence of wound complications and infection

Transoral Mandible-Splitting and Tongue-Splitting (Hall, Denis, and Murray)
More extensive exposure of upper cervical spine

Subtotal Maxillectomy (Cocke et al.)
Extended maxillotomy and subtotal maxillectomy are used when exposure of base of skull is necessary and cannot be obtained by other approaches

Lateral Retropharyngeal (Whitesides and Kelly)
Extension of classic Henry approach to vertebral artery
Sternocleidomastoid muscle everted and retracted posteriorly
Dissection in plane posterior to carotid sheath
Potential for postoperative edema and airway obstruction

Modifications of Robinson and Southwick Approach (Deandrade and Macnab)
Anterior to sternocleidomastoid muscle
Dissection anterior to carotid sheath
Risk of injury to superior laryngeal nerve

Mcafee et al.
Exposure from atlas to body of C3
No posterior dissection of carotid sheath
No entrance into oral cavity
Adequate for insertion of iliac or fibular strut grafts

TRANSORAL MANDIBLE-SPLITTING AND TONGUE-SPLITTING APPROACH

Hall, Denis, and Murray described a mandible-splitting and tongue-splitting transoral approach to the cervical spine that gives more extensive exposure of the upper cervical spine than the approach of Fang and Ong.

TECHNIQUE 7.11

(HALL, DENIS, AND MURRAY)

- Apply a halo cast preoperatively and perform a tracheostomy through the fourth tracheal ring.
- With the patient under general anesthesia, prepare the operative field with povidone-iodine (Betadine) and drape it to exclude the halo cast and tracheostomy tube.
- Make an incision from the anterior gum margin through both surfaces of the lower lip and down over the middle of the mandible to the hyoid cartilage (Fig. 7.19A).
- Divide the tongue in the midline with electrocautery.
- Place traction sutures to allow better exposure of the midline raphe.
- Remove the lower incisor and make a step-cut with an oscillating saw in the mandible.
- Split the tongue longitudinally to the epiglottis through its central raphe (Fig. 7.19B).
- Fold the uvula on itself and suture it to the roof of the soft palate; retract the mandible and tongue down on each side to improve exposure.
- Open the mucosa over the posterior wall of the oral pharynx to expose the anterior cervical spine from the first cervical vertebra to the upper portion of the fifth cervical vertebra (Fig. 7.19C).
- Divide the anterior longitudinal ligament in the midline and reflect it laterally to allow enough exposure for removal of the anterior portion of the cervical spine and placement of bone grafts for fusion.
- Fix the posterior pharyngeal flap with 3-0 chromic suture.
- Thread a suction drain through the nose and insert it deep into the pharyngeal flap.

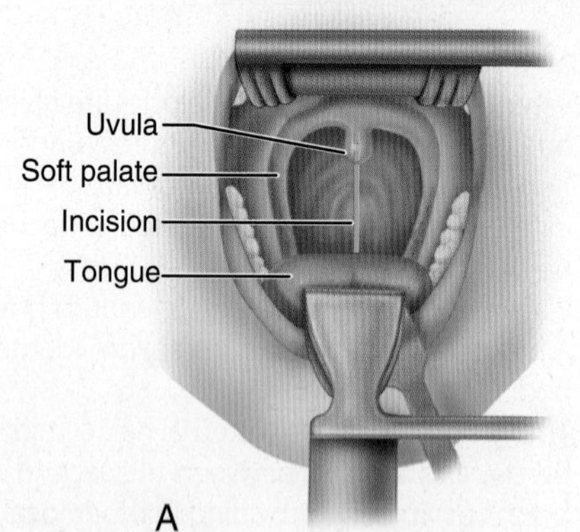

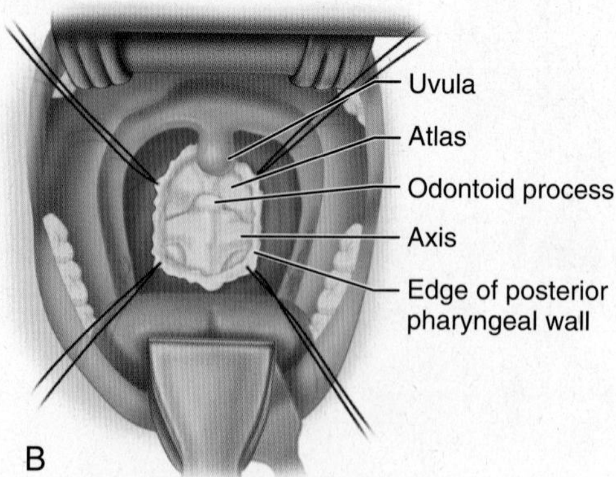

FIGURE 7.18 **A and B,** Transoral approach to upper cervical spine for exposure of anterior aspect of atlas and axis. **SEE TECHNIQUE 7.10.**

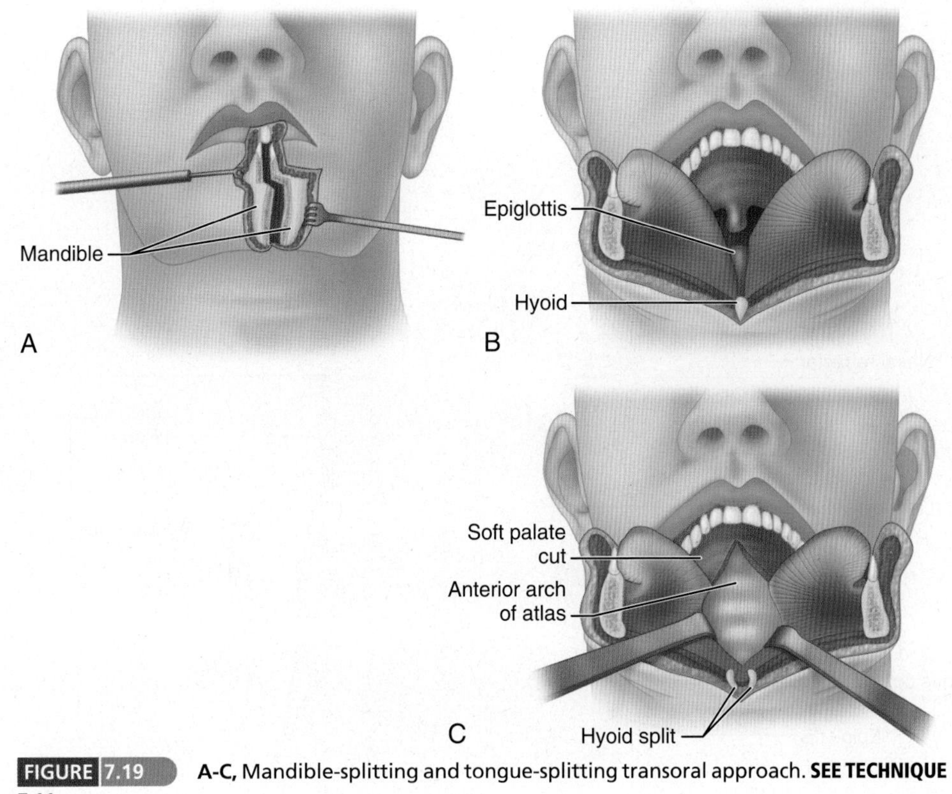

FIGURE 7.19 A-C, Mandible-splitting and tongue-splitting transoral approach. **SEE TECHNIQUE 7.11.**

- Repair the tongue with 2-0 and 3-0 chromic sutures and fix the mandible with wires inserted through drill holes on each side of the osteotomy.
- Close the infralingual mucosa with 3-0 chromic sutures and close the subcutaneous tissue and skin.
- Preoperative and postoperative antibiotics are recommended.

POSTOPERATIVE CARE A halo cast is worn until fusion is evident on radiographs. The halo cast is removed, and a soft collar is worn for 1 month.

SUBTOTAL MAXILLECTOMY

Cocke et al. described an extended maxillotomy with subtotal maxillectomy to be used when exposure of the base of the skull is needed and cannot be obtained by other approaches. This approach is technically demanding and requires a thorough knowledge of head and neck anatomy. A team of surgeons, including an otolaryngologist, a neurosurgeon, and an orthopaedist, should perform this surgery. Please refer to older editions of *Campbell's Operative Orthopaedics* for the complete description.

Endoscopic approaches have also been described for anterior resection of the odontoid. The endoscopic approaches to the odontoid and anterior ring of C1 may be sublabial, transoral, or transcervical (Fig. 7.20).

LATERAL RETROPHARYNGEAL APPROACH

The lateral retropharyngeal approach described by Whitesides and Kelly is an extension of the classic approach of Henry to the vertebral artery. In this approach, the sternocleidomastoid muscle is everted and retracted posteriorly. The remainder of the dissection follows a plane posterior to the carotid sheath.

TECHNIQUE 7.12

(WHITESIDES AND KELLY)

- Make a longitudinal incision along the anterior margin of the sternocleidomastoid muscle. At the superior end of the muscle, carry the incision posteriorly across the base of the temporal bone.
- Divide the muscle at its mastoid origin.
- Partially divide the splenius capitis muscle at its insertion in the same area.
- At the superior pole of the incision is the external jugular vein, which crosses the anterior margin of the sternocleidomastoid; ligate and divide this vein. Branches of the auricular nerve also may be encountered and may require division.
- Evert the sternocleidomastoid muscle and identify the spinal accessory nerve as it approaches and passes into the muscle.
- Divide and ligate the vascular structures that accompany the nerve.

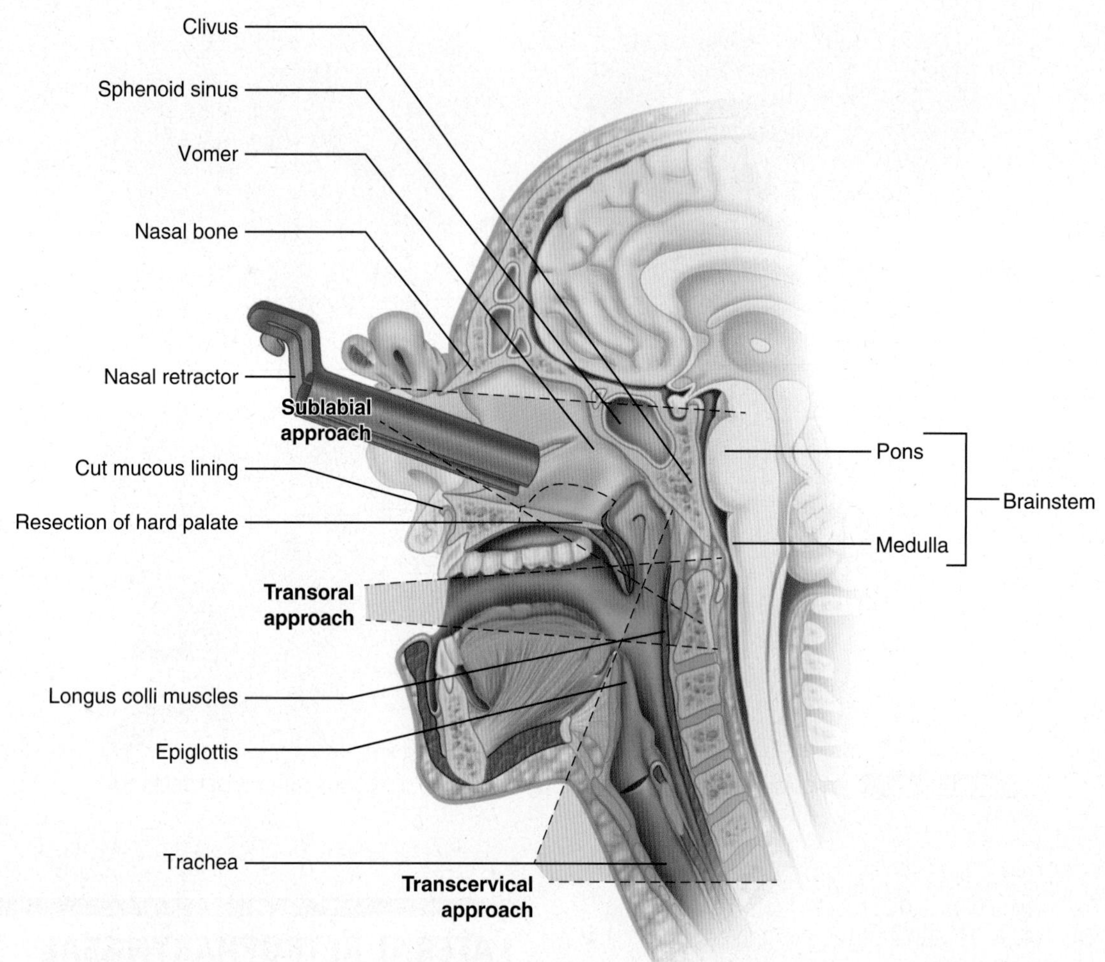

FIGURE 7.20 **Endoscopic approaches to the cervical spine: relevant anatomy and operative angles for sublabial, transoral, and transcervical approaches to the cervical spine.** (From Bettegowda C, Shajari M, Suk I, et al: Sublabial approach for the treatment of symptomatic basilar impression in a patient with Klippel-Feil syndrome, *Neurosurgery* 69[ONS Suppl 1]:ons77, 2011.)

- Develop the approach posterior to the carotid sheath and anterior to the sternocleidomastoid muscle (Fig. 7.21A). The transverse processes of all the exposed cervical vertebrae are palpable in this interval.
- Using sharp and blunt dissection, develop the plane between the alar and prevertebral fascia along the anterior aspect of the transverse processes of the vertebral bodies. The dissection plane is anterior to the longus colli and capitis muscles and the overlying sympathetic trunk and superior cervical ganglion. (An alternative approach is to elevate the longus colli and capitis muscles from their bony insertion on the transverse processes and retract the muscles anteriorly, but this approach can disrupt the sympathetic rami communicantes and cause Horner syndrome.)
- When the vertebral level is identified, make a longitudinal incision to bone through the anterior longitudinal ligament.
- Dissect the ligament and soft tissues subperiosteally to expose the vertebral bodies.
- For fusion, place corticocancellous strips in a longitudinal trough made in the vertebral bodies.
- Irrigate and close the wound in layers over a suction drain in the retropharyngeal space.

POSTOPERATIVE CARE Because of the potential for postoperative edema and airway obstruction, the patient should be monitored closely. Traction may be required for 1 to 2 days after surgery. When the traction is removed, the patient is immobilized in a cervicothoracic brace or halo vest or halo cast.

deAndrade and Macnab described an approach to the upper cervical spine that is an extension of the approach described by Robinson and Southwick and Bailey and Badgley. This approach is anterior to the sternocleidomastoid muscle (Fig. 7.21B), but the dissection is anterior to the carotid sheath rather than posterior. This approach carries an increased risk of injury to the superior laryngeal nerve.

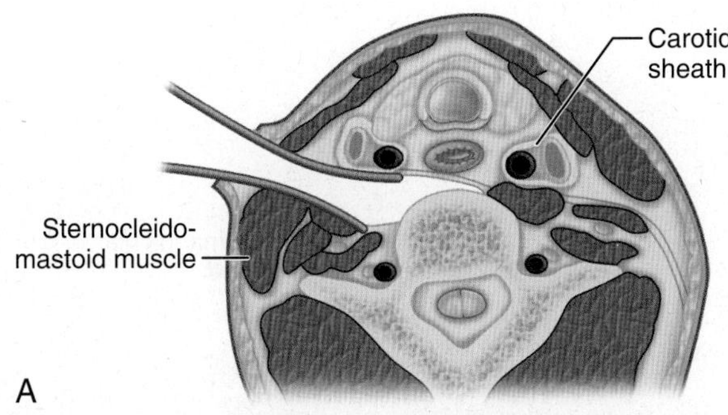

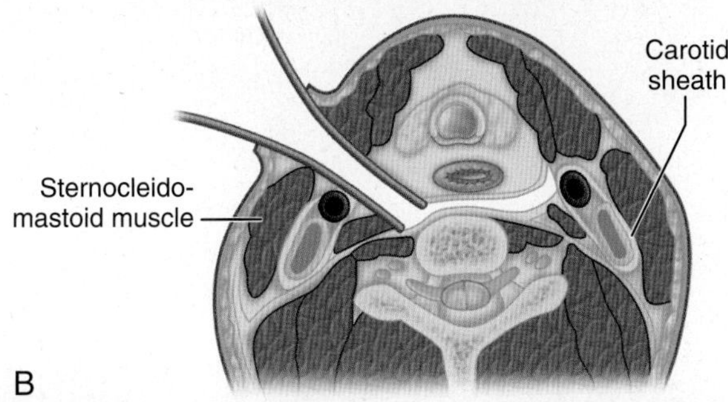

FIGURE 7.21 Lateral retropharyngeal approach to cervical spine. **A,** Whitesides and Kelly approach anterior to sternocleidomastoid muscle and posterior to carotid sheath. **B,** DeAndrade and Macnab approach anterior to sternocleidomastoid muscle and anteromedial to carotid sheath. **SEE TECHNIQUE 7.12.**

ANTERIOR RETROPHARYNGEAL APPROACH

McAfee et al. used a superior extension of the anterior approach of Robinson and Smith to the cervical spine. This approach provides exposure from the atlas to the body of the third cervical vertebra without the need for posterior dissection of the carotid sheath or entrance into the oral cavity and gives adequate exposure for insertion of iliac or fibular strut grafts.

TECHNIQUE 7.13

(MCAFEE ET AL.)

- Place the patient supine on an operative wedge turning frame and perform a neurologic examination. Monitor the spinal cord during the operation using cortically recorded somatosensory-evoked potentials.
- Apply Gardner-Wells tongs with 4.5 kg of traction, if not already in place. Carefully extend the neck with the patient awake. Mark the maximal point of safe extension and do not exceed this at any time during the operative procedure.
- Perform fiberoptic nasotracheal intubation with the patient under local anesthesia. When the airway has been secured, place the patient under general anesthesia. Keep the patient's mouth free of all tubes to prevent any depression of the mandible inferiorly that may compromise the operative exposure.
- Make a modified transverse submandibular incision (the incision can be made on the right or left side depending on the surgeon's preference) (Fig. 7.22A). Provided the dissection does not extend caudally to the fifth cervical vertebra, this exposure is sufficiently superior to the right recurrent laryngeal nerve to prevent damage to this structure.
- Carry the incision through the platysma muscle and mobilize the skin and superficial fascia in the subplatysmal plane of the superficial fascia.
- Locate the marginal mandibular branch of the facial nerve with the aid of a nerve stimulator and by ligating and dissecting the retromandibular veins superiorly. Branches of the mandibular nerves usually cross the retromandibular vein superficially and superiorly. By ligating this vein as it joins the internal jugular vein and by keeping the dissection deep and inferior to the vein as the exposure is extended superiorly, the superficial branches of the facial nerve are protected.
- Free the anterior border of the sternocleidomastoid muscle by longitudinally transecting the superficial layer of deep cervical fascia.
- Locate the carotid sheath by palpation.
- Resect the submandibular salivary gland and suture its duct to prevent a salivary fistula. Identify the posterior belly of the digastric muscle and the stylohyoid muscle.
- Divide and tag the digastric tendon for later repair. Division of the digastric and stylohyoid muscles allows mobilization of the hyoid bone and the hypopharynx medially (Fig. 7.22B).
- Free the hypoglossal nerve from the base of the skull to the anterior border of the hypoglossal muscle and retract it superiorly throughout the remainder of the procedure (Fig. 7.22C).
- Continue the dissection between the carotid sheath laterally and the larynx and pharynx anteromedially.
- Beginning inferiorly and progressing superiorly, the following arteries and veins may need to be ligated for exposure: the superior thyroid artery and vein, the lingual artery and vein, and the facial artery and vein (Fig. 7.22C).
- Free the superior laryngeal nerve from its origin near the nodose ganglion to its entrance into the larynx (Fig. 7.22D).
- Transect the alar and prevertebral fascia longitudinally to expose the longus colli muscles (Fig. 7.22E).
- Ensure orientation to the midline by noting the attachment of the right and left longus colli muscles as they converge toward the anterior tubercle of the atlas. Detach the longus colli muscles from the anterior surface of the atlas and axis.
- Divide the anterior longitudinal ligament and expose the anterior surface of the atlas and axis. Do not carry the dissection too far laterally and damage the vertebral artery.
- McAfee et al. used a fibular or bicortical iliac strut graft contoured into the shape of a clothespin. The anterior body of C2 and the discs of C2 and C3 can be removed. Place the two prongs of the clothespin superiorly to straddle the anterior arch of the atlas. Tamp the inferior edge of the graft into the superior aspect of the body of C3, which is undercut to receive the graft. If the anterior aspect of the atlas must be removed, the superior aspect of the graft can be secured to the clivus.
- Begin closure by approximation of the digastric tendon.

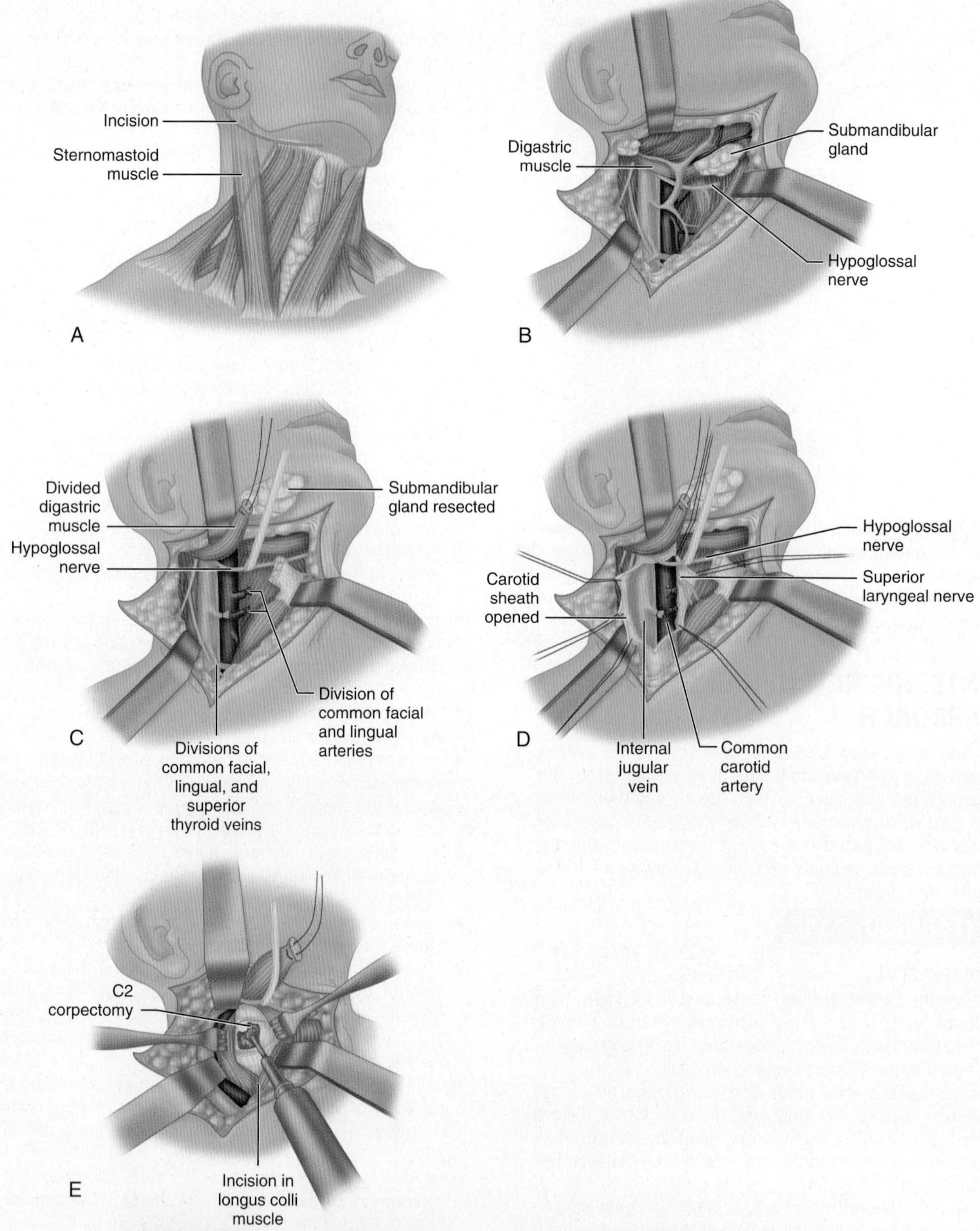

FIGURE 7.22 Anterior retropharyngeal approach to upper cervical spine described by McAfee et al. **A,** Submandibular incision. Lower limb of incision is used only if midcervical vertebrae must be exposed. **B** and **C,** Submandibular gland is resected, and digastric tendon is divided. Superior thyroid artery and vein also are divided. **D,** Hypoglossal nerve and superior laryngeal nerve are mobilized. Contents of carotid sheath are mobilized laterally, and hypopharynx is mobilized medially. **E,** Longus colli muscle is dissected laterally to expose anterior aspect of atlas and axis. **SEE TECHNIQUE 7.13.**

- Place suction drains in the retropharyngeal space and the subcutaneous space.
- Suture the platysma and skin in the standard fashion.
- If the spine has been made unstable by the anterior decompression, perform a posterior cervical or occipitocervical fusion.
- If the hypopharynx has been inadvertently entered, have the anesthesiologist insert a nasogastric tube intraoperatively.
- Close the hole in two layers with absorbable sutures.

POSTOPERATIVE CARE Parenteral antibiotics effective against anaerobic organisms should be added to the routine postoperative prophylactic antibiotics. The nasogastric tube is left in place for 7 to 10 days. Skull traction is maintained with the head elevated 30 degrees to reduce hypopharyngeal edema. Nasal intubation is maintained for 48 hours. If extubation is not possible in 48 to 72 hours, a tracheostomy can be performed. The Gardner-Wells tongs are removed 2 to 4 days after surgery, and a halo vest is applied and is worn for about 3 months. When the halo vest is removed, a cervical collar is worn for an additional month.

HALO VEST IMMOBILIZATION

The halo device, introduced by Perry and Nickel in 1959, provides immobilization for an unstable cervical spine and can be used for preoperative traction in certain situations. Successful use of the halo has been shown in infants and children with instabilities caused by injuries or by cervical malformations, although complications are more frequent in children than adults.

Most authors agree that the halo device provides the best immobilization of the cervical spine of all external immobilization methods, but reports have shown increased spinal motion (up to 70% of normal) and loss of reduction while in the halo. The halo vest has been well accepted by adult patients, and the vest can usually be easily fitted; in children, however, proper fit is rarely achieved with a prefabricated halo vest, and the use of a halo cast or custom-molded halo vest is a better choice.

Mubarak et al. recommended the following steps in the fabrication of a custom halo for a child: (1) the size and configuration of the head are obtained with the use of a flexible lead wire placed around the head; (2) the halo ring is fabricated by constructing a ring 2 cm larger in diameter than the wire model; (3) a plaster mold of the trunk is obtained for the manufacture of a custom bivalved polypropylene vest; and (4) linear measurements are made to ensure appropriate length of the superstructure. CT helps determine bone structure to plan pin sites to avoid suture lines or congenital malformations.

Skull thickness in children varies greatly up to age 6 years; it increases between ages 10 and 16 years, after which it is similar to that in adults. One study found that a 2-mm skull could be completely penetrated with a 160-lb load, which is below the recommended torque pressure for adult skulls.

Mubarak et al. described a technique for the application of a halo device in children younger than 2 years old. This multiple-pin technique differs from previously accepted recommendations in older children regarding pin number, pin placement, and torque. With multiple pins, significantly less torque can be used, allowing a greater range of pin placement sites in areas where the skull might otherwise be considered too thin. Perpendicular halo pin insertion has been recommended in an immature skull because this configuration results in increased load at the pin-bone interface and increases stability. Skull development is important to consider in halo device application in patients younger than 2 years old. Cranial suture interdigitation may be incomplete, and fontanels may be open anteriorly in patients younger than 18 months old and posteriorly in patients younger than 6 months. Because of this, the halo device probably should not be used in children younger than 18 months old.

APPLICATION OF HALO DEVICE

Halo device applications for children in this age group require a custom-made halo ring and plastic jacket. Ten to twelve standard halo skull pins can be used. When constructed, the halo ring is applied with the patient under general anesthesia. In older children and adolescents, local anesthesia can be used.

TECHNIQUE 7.14

(MUBARAK ET AL.)

- Place the patient supine, with the head supported by an assistant or a cupped metal extension that cradles the head. If a metal extension is used, do not place the neck in flexion; a child's head is relatively large in proportion to the body.
- Shave the immediate areas of pin insertion and prepare the skin with antiseptic solution.
- Infiltrate the skin and the periosteum in the selected areas with local anesthetic.
- Support the halo ring around the patient's head with the application device or the help of an assistant. Hold it below the area of greatest diameter of the skull, just above the eyebrows, and about 1 cm above the tips of the ears.
- Select the pin sites carefully so that the pins enter the skull as nearly perpendicular as possible. The best position for the anterior pins is in the anterolateral aspect of the skull, above the lateral two thirds of the orbit, and below the greatest circumference of the skull; this area is a relatively safe zone. Avoid the temporalis muscle because penetration of this muscle by the halo pin can be painful and may impede mandibular motion during mastication or talking; the bone in this area also is very thin, and pin loosening is likely.
- Place the posterior pins directly diagonal from the anterior pins, if possible, and inferior to the equator of the skull. Introduce the pins through the halo frame and tighten two diagonally opposed pins simultaneously.
- Ensure that the patient's eyes are closed while the pins are tightened to ensure that the forehead skin is not anchored in such a way as to prevent the eyelids from closing after application of the halo ring.
- In an infant or young child, insert 10 pins to finger tightness or 2 in-lb anterolaterally and posteriorly (Fig. 7.23A). If the skull thickness is of great concern, use finger tightness only to prevent penetrating the skull.

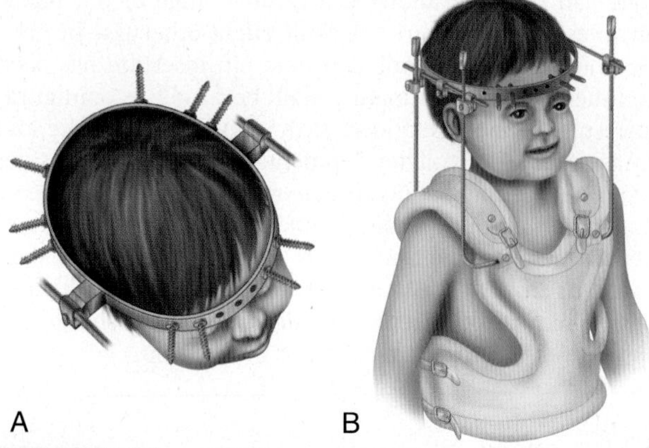

FIGURE 7.23 **A,** Ten pin placement sites for infant halo ring attachment using multiple-pin, low-torque technique. Usually, four pins are placed anteriorly, avoiding temporal area, and remaining six pins are placed in occipital area. **B,** Custom halo vest and light superstructure. **SEE TECHNIQUE 7.14.**

- In slightly older children, use 2 in-lb of torque (for halo device application in adults, see chapter 5).
- In adolescents near skeletal maturity whose skull thickness is nearly that of an adult (as determined by CT), torque pressure can be increased to 6 to 8 in-lb.
- Secure the pins to the halo device with the appropriate lock nuts or set screws.
- Apply the polypropylene vest and superstructure after the halo ring and pins are in place (Fig. 7.23B).

POSTOPERATIVE CARE The pins are cleansed daily at the skin interface with hydrogen peroxide or a small amount of povidone-iodine solution. The pins are retightened once at 48 hours after application.

COMPLICATIONS

Complications include pin loosening, infection, pin site bleeding, and dural puncture. If a pin becomes loose, it can be retightened, provided the resistance is met. If no resistance is met, the pin should be removed, and another pin inserted in an alternative site. If drainage develops around a pin, oral antibiotics and local skin care are begun. If the drainage does not respond to these measures or if cellulitis or an abscess develops, the pin should be removed, and another pin should be inserted at an alternative site. If dural puncture occurs, the pin should be removed, and another pin inserted at an alternative site; the patient should receive prophylactic antibiotic therapy. The dural tear usually heals in 4 or 5 days, at which time antibiotics can be discontinued.

BASILAR IMPRESSION

Basilar impression (basilar invagination) is a rare deformity in which there is an indention of the skull floor by the upper cervical spine. The tip of the odontoid is more cephalad than normal. The odontoid may protrude into the foramen magnum and encroach on the brainstem, causing neurologic symptoms because of the limited space available for the brainstem and spinal cord. Neurologic damage can be caused by direct pressure from the odontoid or from other constricting structures around the foramen magnum, circulatory compromise of the vertebral arteries, or impairment of cerebrospinal fluid flow. It is important that the orthopaedist be familiar with basilar impression and its presentation because this spinal deformity often goes unrecognized or is misdiagnosed as a posterior fossa tumor, bulbar palsy of polio, syringomyelia, amyotrophic lateral sclerosis, spinal cord tumor, or multiple sclerosis.

Basilar impression can be primary (congenital) or secondary (acquired). Primary basilar impression is a congenital structural abnormality of the craniocervical junction that often is associated with other vertebral defects (atlantooccipital fusion, Klippel-Feil syndrome, Arnold-Chiari malformation, syringomyelia, odontoid anomalies, hypoplasia of the atlas, and bifid posterior arch of the atlas); these associated conditions can cause the predominant symptoms. The incidence of primary basilar impression in the general population is 1%. Secondary basilar impression is an acquired deformity of the skull resulting from systemic disease that causes softening of the osseous structures at the base of the skull, such as Paget disease, osteomalacia, rickets, osteogenesis imperfecta, rheumatoid arthritis, neurofibromatosis, and ankylosing spondylitis. Secondary basilar impression occurs more commonly in types III and IV than in type I osteogenesis imperfecta.

Basilar impression causes neurologic symptoms because of crowding of the neural structures as they pass through the foramen magnum. Clinical presentation varies, and patients with severe basilar impression may be totally asymptomatic. Symptoms usually appear during the second and third decades of life, probably because of increased ligamentous laxity and instability with age and decreased tolerance to compression of the spinal cord and vertebral arteries.

Most patients with basilar impression have short necks, asymmetry of the face or skull, and torticollis, but these findings are not specific for basilar impression and can be seen in patients with other congenital vertebral anomalies. Headache in the distribution of the greater occipital nerve is a frequent complaint. DeBarros et al. divided the signs and symptoms into two categories: those caused by pure basilar impression and those caused by the Arnold-Chiari malformation. They found that symptoms caused by pure basilar impression were primarily motor and sensory disturbances, such as weakness and paresthesia in the limbs, whereas patients with Arnold-Chiari malformation had symptoms of cerebellar and vestibular disturbances, such as ataxia, dizziness, and nystagmus. Involvement of the lower cranial nerves also occurs in basilar impression. The trigeminal, vagus, glossopharyngeal, and hypoglossal nerves may be compressed as they emerge from the medulla oblongata. DeBarros et al. also noted sexual disturbances, such as impotence and reduced libido in 27% of their patients.

Compression of the vertebral arteries as they pass through the foramen magnum is another source of symptoms. Bernini et al. found a significantly higher incidence of vertebral artery anomalies in patients with basilar impression and atlantooccipital fusion. Symptoms caused by vertebral artery insufficiency, such as dizziness, seizures, mental deterioration, and syncope, can occur alone or in combination with other symptoms of basilar impression. Children with occipitocervical

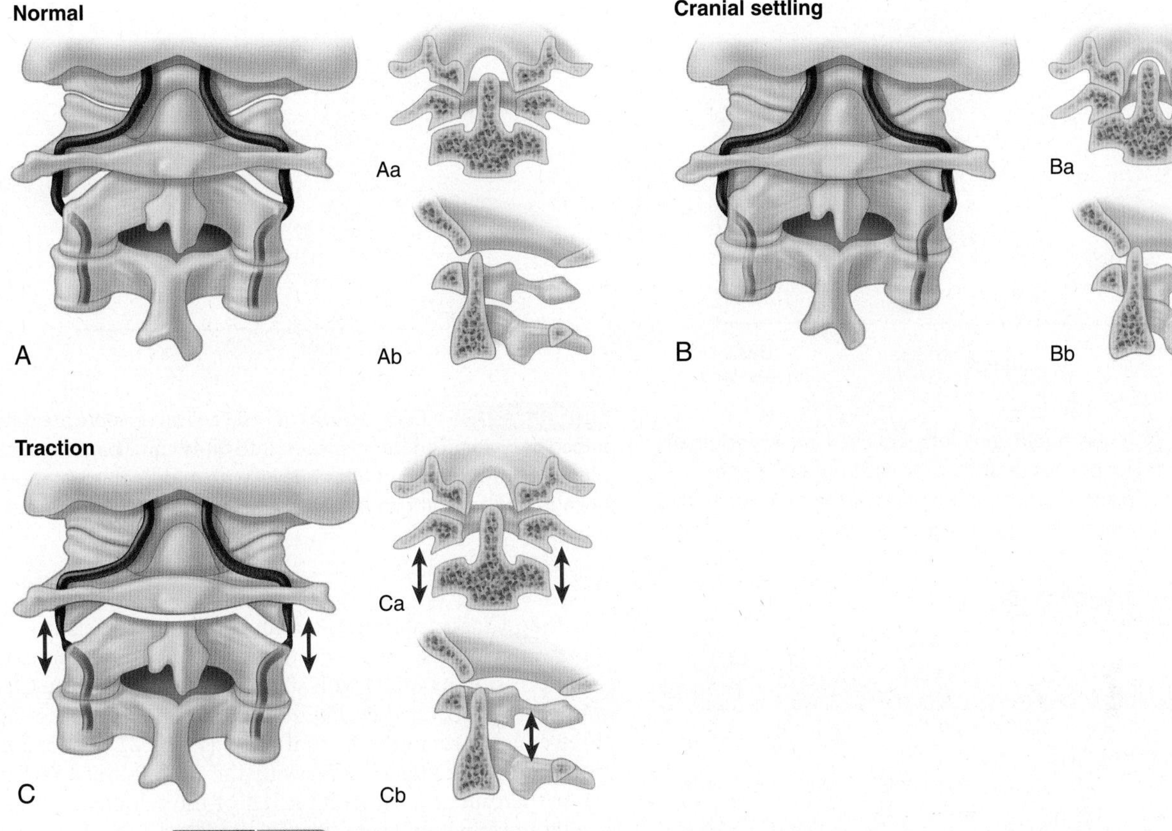

FIGURE 7.24 Schematic diagram showing cranial settling and possible vertebral artery injuries resulting from traction. **A,** Normal position of vertebral artery. *Aa* and *Ab,* Normal vertebral alignment. **B,** Position of vertebral artery after cranial settling. *Ba* and *Bb,* Vertebral alignment in cranial settling. **C,** Effect of traction on vertebral arteries. *Ca* and *Cb,* Effect of vertebral alignment.

anomalies may be more susceptible to vertebral artery injury and brainstem ischemia if skull traction is applied (Fig. 7.24).

RADIOGRAPHIC FINDINGS

Numerous measurements have been suggested for diagnosing basilar impression (Box 7.4), reflecting the difficulty of evaluating this area of the spine radiographically, and several methods of evaluation (plain radiography, CT, and MRI) may be needed to confirm the diagnosis. The most commonly used measurements are the lines of Chamberlain, McGregor, McRae, and Fischgold and Metzger. The Chamberlain, McGregor, and McRae lines are made on lateral radiographs of the skull (Fig. 7.25); the Fischgold and Metzger lines are made on an anteroposterior view (Fig. 7.26).

The Chamberlain line is drawn from the posterior edge of the hard palate to the posterior border of the foramen magnum. Symptomatic basilar impression can occur when the odontoid tip extends above this line. There are two disadvantages to the Chamberlain line: the posterior tip of the foramen magnum is difficult to define on the standard lateral view, and the posterior tip of the foramen magnum is often invaginated. McGregor modified the Chamberlain line by drawing a line from the upper surface of the posterior edge of the hard palate to the most caudal point of the occipital curve, which is much easier to identify on a standard lateral radiograph. The position of the tip of the odontoid is measured in relation to the McGregor line, and a point 4.5 mm above this line is considered the upper limit of normal. The McRae line determines the anteroposterior dimension of the foramen magnum and is formed by drawing a line from the anterior tip of the foramen magnum to the posterior tip. McRae observed that if the tip of the odontoid is below this line, then the patient usually is asymptomatic.

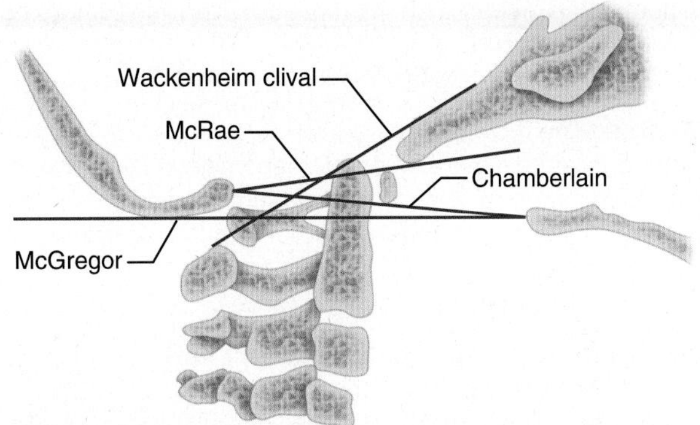

FIGURE 7.25 Base of skull and upper cervical spine showing location of McRae, McGregor, Chamberlain, and Wackenheim lines.

The lateral lines of McGregor and Chamberlain have been criticized because the anterior reference point (the hard palate) is not part of the skull, and measurements can be distorted by an abnormal facial configuration or a

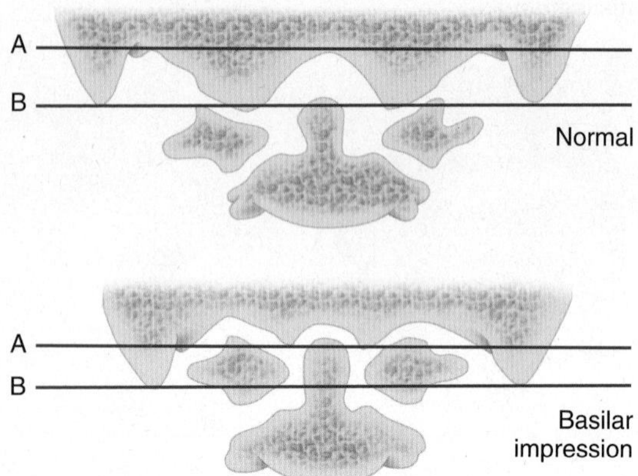

FIGURE 7.26 Fischgold and Metzger lines. Line was originally drawn from lower pole of mastoid process *B*, but because of variability in size of mastoid processes, these researchers recommended drawing the line between digastric grooves *A*.

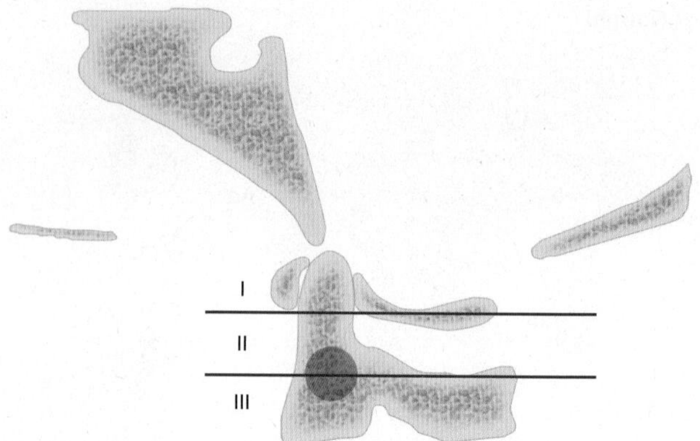

FIGURE 7.27 Clark stations of first cervical vertebra are determined by dividing odontoid process into three equal parts in sagittal plane. If anterior ring of atlas is level with middle third (station *II*) or caudal third (station *III*) of odontoid process, basilar impression is present.

BOX 7.4

Measurements for Diagnosing Basilar Impression: Lateral Radiograph

Chamberlain Line

Extends from posterior edge of hard palate to posterior border of foramen magnum

Symptomatic basilar impression may occur if tip of odontoid is above this line

McGregor Line

Extends from upper surface of posterior edge of hard palate to most caudal point of occipital curve

Easier to identify on standard lateral view

Odontoid tip greater than 4.5 mm above this line considered an abnormal finding

Routine screening test; landmarks easily identified

McRae Line

Anteroposterior dimension of foramen magnum; line extends from anterior tip of foramen magnum to posterior tip

Patient usually asymptomatic if tip of odontoid is below this line

Helpful to determine clinical significance

Fischgold and Metzger (Digastric) Line

Extends between two digastric grooves (junction of medial aspect of mastoid process at base of skull)

Line normally passes 10.7 mm above odontoid tip and 11.6 mm above atlantooccipital joint

Confirms diagnosis

high-arched palate. To resolve these problems, Fischgold and Metzger described a method of assessing basilar impression that uses an anteroposterior tomogram or CT with anteroposterior reconstruction views (Fig. 7.26). This assessment is based on a line drawn between the two digastric grooves (the junction of the medial aspect of the mastoid process at the base of the skull). Normally, the digastric line passes above the odontoid tip (10.7 mm) and the atlantooccipital joint (11.6 mm).

The Clark station, Redlund-Johnell criterion, and Ranawat criterion have been found useful to measure basilar impression in adults with rheumatoid arthritis. The Clark station is determined by dividing the odontoid process into three equal parts in the sagittal plane (Fig. 7.27). If the anterior ring of the atlas is level with the middle third (station II) or the caudal third (station III) of the odontoid process, basilar invagination is present. The Redlund-Johnell criterion is the distance between the McGregor line and the midpoint of the caudal margin of the second cervical vertebral body. Basilar invagination is present if the measurement is less than 34 mm in men and less than 29 mm in women. The Ranawat criterion is the distance between the center of the second cervical pedicle and the transverse axis of the atlas. Basilar invagination is present if this distance is less than 15 mm in men and less than 13 mm in women. The Redlund-Johnell and Ranawat criteria may not be applicable in small children.

The McGregor line is used as a routine screening test because the landmarks for this line can be defined easily on a standard lateral radiograph. If more information is needed, an MRI of the craniovertebral junction is used to confirm the diagnosis of basilar impression. CT and MRI are recommended; CT provides better osseous detail and MRI provides superior soft-tissue resolution. "Functional" MRI obtained with the cervical spine in flexion and then extension shows the dynamics of spinal cord compression caused by vertebral instability or anomaly.

TREATMENT

Conservative treatment of symptomatic patients with a collar or cervical orthosis has not been successful. Many patients with basilar impression have no neurologic symptoms, and some have minimal symptoms with no sign of progressive neurologic damage. These patients can be observed and examined periodically; surgery is indicated if the clinical picture becomes worse. The indications for surgery are based on the clinical symptoms and not on the degree of basilar impression. When a patient becomes symptomatic, progression of the disease and symptoms is likely.

If symptoms are caused by anterior impingement from the odontoid, stabilization in extension by an occipital C1-2 fusion is indicated. If symptoms and impingement persist, anterior excision of the odontoid can be done after posterior stabilization. Posterior impingement requires suboccipital craniectomy and laminectomy of C1 and possibly C2 to decompress the brainstem and spinal cord. The dura may need to be opened during this procedure to check for a tight posterior dural band that may be causing the symptoms instead of the bony abnormalities. Posterior fusion is recommended in addition to decompression if stability is in question.

ATLANTOOCCIPITAL FUSION

Atlantooccipital fusion (occipitalization) is a partial or complete congenital fusion between the atlas and the base of the occiput ranging from a complete bony fusion to a bony bridge or even a fibrous band uniting one small area of the atlas and occiput. Occipitalization is a failure of segmentation between the fourth occipital sclerotome and the first spinal sclerotome. This condition can lead to chronic atlantoaxial instability or basilar invagination and can produce a wide range of symptoms because of spinal cord impingement and vascular compromise of the vertebral arteries. The incidence of atlantooccipital fusion has been reported to be 1.4 to 2.5 per 1000 children, affecting males and females equally. Symptoms usually appear in the third and fourth decades of life. Atlantooccipital fusion frequently is associated with congenital fusion between C2 and C3 (reportedly in 70% of patients). Kyphosis and scoliosis are also frequently associated with this deformity. Other associated congenital anomalies, such as anomalies of the jaw, incomplete cleft of the nasal cartilage, cleft palate, external ear deformities, cervical ribs, and urinary tract anomalies, occur in 20% of patients with atlantooccipital fusion.

Patients with atlantooccipital fusion commonly have low hairlines, torticollis, short necks, and restricted neck movement. Many patients complain of a dull, aching pain in the posterior occiput and the neck, with episodic neck stiffness, but symptoms vary depending on the area of spinal cord impingement. If the impingement is anterior, pyramidal tract signs and symptoms predominate; if the impingement is posterior, posterior column signs and symptoms predominate.

The shape and position of the odontoid are the keys to neurologic symptoms. When the odontoid lies above the foramen magnum, a relative or actual basilar impression is present. If the odontoid lies below the foramen magnum, the patient usually is asymptomatic. In this condition, the odontoid may be excessively long and angulated posteriorly, decreasing the anteroposterior diameter of the spinal canal. Autopsy findings have shown the brainstem indented by the abnormal odontoid. Anterior spinal cord compression with pyramidal tract irritation causes muscle weakness and wasting, ataxia, spasticity, pathologic reflexes (Babinski and Hoffman), and hyperreflexia. Posterior compression causes loss of deep pain, light touch, proprioception, and vibratory sensation. Nystagmus is a common finding. Cranial nerve involvement can cause diplopia, dysphagia, and auditory disturbances. Disturbances of the vertebral artery result in syncope, seizures, vertigo, and an unsteady gait.

Neurologic symptoms generally begin in the third and fourth decades of life, possibly because the older patient's spinal cord and vertebral arteries become less resistant to compression. Symptoms may be initiated by trauma or infection in the pharynx or nasopharynx.

RADIOGRAPHIC FINDINGS

Because this anomaly ranges from complete incorporation of the atlas into the occiput to a small fibrous band connecting part of the atlas to the occiput, routine radiographs usually are difficult to interpret, and CT or MRI may be needed to show the occipitocervical fusion (Fig. 7.28). Most commonly, the anterior arch of the atlas is assimilated into the occiput and displaced posteriorly relative to the occiput. About half of patients have a relative basilar impression caused by loss of height of the atlas. Posterior fusion usually is a small bony fringe or a fibrous band that frequently is not evident on a radiograph. This fringe is directed downward and into the spinal canal and can cause neurologic symptoms. Gholve et al. classified fusion of C1 to the occiput into four zones. Zone 1 is a fused anterior arch, zone 2 a fusion of the lateral masses, zone 3 a fused posterior arch, and zone 4 a combination of the zones (Fig. 7.29). In their 30 patients, zone 4 (a combination of zones) was the most common, and patients with zone 2 fusion had the highest prevalence

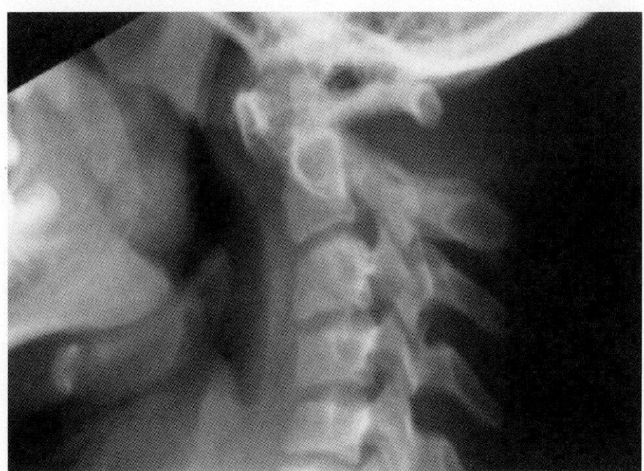

FIGURE 7.28 Lateral radiograph of patient with occipital cervical synostosis.

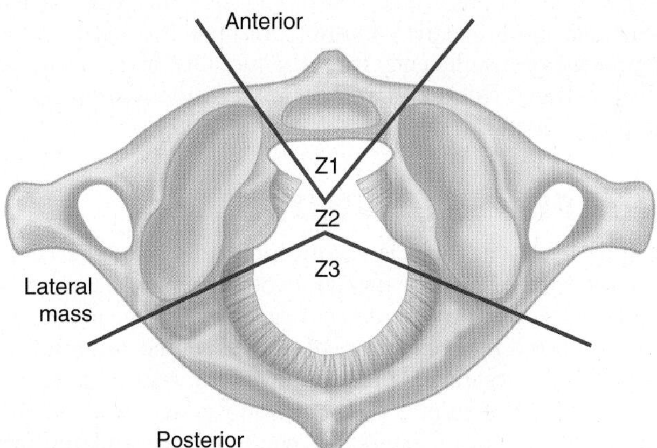

FIGURE 7.29 Morphologic classification of fusion of C1 to the occiput according to the anatomic site of occipitalization: *Z1,* a fused anterior arch; *Z2,* fused lateral masses; *Z3,* a fused posterior arch; and *Z4,* a combination of fused zones. (Redrawn from Gholve PA, Hosalkar HS, Ricchetti ET, et al: Occipitalization of the atlas in children. Morphologic classification, associations, and clinical relevance, J Bone Joint Surg Am 89:571, 2007.)

of spinal canal encroachment. Flexion and extension lateral cervical spine views should be part of the initial evaluation because of the frequency of atlantoaxial instability. McRae and Barnum measured the distance from the posterior aspect of the odontoid to the posterior arch of the atlas or the posterior lip of the foramen magnum, whichever was closer. When the distance was 19 mm or less, a neurologic deficit usually was present in their series. A sagittal diameter of 13 mm has been associated with neurologic symptoms. This measurement should be made on a flexion view because maximal narrowing of the canal usually occurs in flexion. Myelography or MRI can detect areas of encroachment on the spinal cord or medulla and is especially useful when a constricting fibrous band occurs posteriorly. Flexion and extension MRI often is needed to identify the pathology.

TREATMENT

Patients who have minor symptoms or become symptomatic after minor trauma or infection can be treated nonoperatively with immobilization in cervical orthosis. When neurologic symptoms occur, cervical spine fusion or decompression is indicated. Anterior symptoms usually are caused by a hypermobile odontoid; preliminary reduction of the odontoid with traction, followed by fusion from the occiput to C2, usually relieves the symptoms. If the odontoid is irreducible, the appropriateness of either in situ fusion without reduction or fusion with excision of the odontoid, with its associated risks and complications, must be determined. Posterior signs and symptoms usually are caused by bony compression or compression from a dural band. When this is documented by MRI or myelography, suboccipital craniectomy, excision of the posterior arch of the atlas, and removal of the dural band are indicated. This may need to be combined with a posterior fusion to prevent instability. Surgical results have been variable.

IDIOPATHIC ATLANTOOCCIPITAL INSTABILITY

Idiopathic atlantooccipital instability has been reported in five patients in one study. Neurologic signs included vertigo, syncope, and projectile vomiting, presumably caused by vertebral artery insufficiency from the mobility at the occipital-C1 junction. Posterior atlantooccipital fusion was successful in these patients.

KLIPPEL-FEIL SYNDROME

Klippel-Feil syndrome is a congenital fusion of the cervical vertebrae that may involve two segments, a congenital block vertebra, or the entire cervical spine. Congenital cervical fusion is a result of failure of normal segmentation of the cervical somites during the third to eighth week of gestation. The skeletal system may not be the only system affected during this time; cardiorespiratory, genitourinary, and auditory systems frequently are involved. In most patients, the exact cause is unknown. One proposed cause is a primary vascular disruption during embryonic development that results in fusion of the cervical vertebrae and other associated anomalies. Studies have suggested that this may be an inherited condition in some patients and have found autosomal dominant inheritance in those with C2-3 fusion. Evidence of a familial Klippel-Feil syndrome gene locus has been identified on the long arm of chromosome 8. Maternal alcoholism has also been suggested as a causative factor; a 50% incidence of cervical vertebral fusions has been found on radiographs of infants with fetal alcohol syndrome.

Occipitalization of the atlas, hemivertebrae, and basilar impression occur frequently in patients with Klippel-Feil syndrome, but their isolated occurrence is not considered part of this syndrome. The classic features of Klippel-Feil syndrome are a short neck, low posterior hairline, and limited range of neck motion. Patients may consult an orthopaedist because of neurologic problems, because of signs of instability of the cervical spine, or for cosmetic reasons. Because many patients are asymptomatic, the actual incidence of this condition is unknown, but estimates in the literature range from 1 in 42,400 births to 3 in 700. There is a slight male predominance (1.5:1). Feil classified the syndrome into three types: type I, block fusion of all cervical and upper thoracic vertebrae; type II, fusion of one or two pairs of cervical vertebrae; and type III, cervical fusion in combination with lower thoracic or lumbar fusion. Minimally involved patients with Klippel-Feil syndrome lead normal, active lives with no significant restrictions or symptoms. More severely involved patients have a good prognosis if genitourinary, cardiopulmonary, and auditory problems are treated early. Samartzis et al. developed the following radiographic classification: type I, a single congenitally fused cervical segment; type II multiple noncontiguous, congenitally fused segments; and type III multiple contiguous, congenitally fused cervical segments. Patients with type I have more long-term axial neck pain, and those with type II and III are more likely to have radiculopathy and myelopathy.

In patients with Klippel-Feil syndrome, neurologic compromise, ranging from radiculopathy to quadriplegia to death, can occur. The neurologic symptoms are caused by occipitocervical anomalies, instability, or degenerative joint and disc disease. Instability and degenerative joint disease are common when two fused areas are separated by a single open interspace. Patients with multiple short areas of fusion (three or more vertebrae) separated by more than one open interspace do not develop instability or degenerative joint disease as frequently, possibly because of a more equal distribution of stress in the cervical spine. Three patterns of cervical spine fusion with a potentially poor prognosis because of late instability or degenerative joint disease have been identified. Pattern 1 is fusion of C1-2 with occipitalization of the atlas. This pattern concentrates the motion of flexion and extension at the atlantoaxial joint; the odontoid becomes hypermobile and may dislocate posteriorly, narrowing the spinal canal and causing neurologic compromise. Pattern 2 is a long fusion with an abnormal occipitocervical junction, concentrating the forces of flexion, extension, and rotation through an abnormal odontoid or poorly developed C1 ring; with time, this abnormal articulation becomes unstable. This pattern should be differentiated from a long fusion with a normal C1-2 articulation and occipitocervical junction. Patients with pattern 2 are at high risk for instability and neurologic problems and have a normal life expectancy. Pattern 3 is a single open interspace between two fused segments with cervical spine motion concentrated at the single open interspace, which becomes hypermobile and causes instability and degenerative joint disease. On a lateral radiograph, the cervical spine with this pattern appears to hinge at an open segment.

BOX 7.5

Conditions Commonly Associated With Klippel-Feil Syndrome

Scoliosis
Most frequent orthopaedic complication (60%)
Obtain radiographs of entire spine

Renal Abnormalities
Occur in approximately 30%
Usually asymptomatic
Obtain ultrasound or intravenous pyelogram

Cardiovascular Anomalies
Found in 4%–14%
Ventricular septal defects most common

Deafness
Occurs in approximately 30%
Obtain audiometric testing

Synkinesis (Mirror Movements)
Occurs in approximately 20%
May restrict bimanual activities
Usually decreases with age

Respiratory Anomalies
Failure of lobe formation
Ectopic lungs
Restriction of lung function by shortened trunk, scoliosis, rib fusion, or deformed costovertebral joints

Sprengel Deformity
Occurs in approximately 20%
Unilateral or bilateral
Increases unsightly appearance
May affect shoulder motion

ASSOCIATED CONDITIONS

Several congenital problems have been associated with congenital fusion of the cervical vertebrae, most commonly scoliosis, renal abnormalities, Sprengel deformity, deafness, synkinesis, and congenital heart defects (Box 7.5).

SCOLIOSIS

The most common orthopaedic anomaly is scoliosis. Studies have shown that 60% to 70% of patients with Klippel-Feil syndrome have scoliosis (curves >15 degrees), kyphosis, or both. Xue found that patients with congenital scoliosis have a 5.4% incidence of Klippel-Feil syndrome. These patients may require treatment and should be followed closely until growth is complete. Two types of scoliosis have been identified. The first is congenital scoliosis caused by vertebral anomalies. The second occurs in a normal-appearing spine below an area of congenital scoliosis or cervical fusion; this type of curve tends to be progressive. Progression may be controlled with a brace. Surgery may be required to prevent progression in both types of scoliosis associated with Klippel-Feil syndrome. Radiographs of the entire spine should be obtained because a progressive curve may not be appreciated until significant deformity has occurred if attention is focused just on the congenital scoliosis or cervical fusion.

RENAL ANOMALIES

About one third of patients with Klippel-Feil syndrome have urogenital anomalies. Because the cervical vertebrae and genitourinary tract differentiate at the same time in the embryo, fetal maldevelopment between 4 and 8 weeks of development may produce genitourinary anomalies and Klippel-Feil syndrome. These renal anomalies usually are asymptomatic, and children with Klippel-Feil syndrome should be evaluated with an ultrasound, intravenous pyelogram, or MRI because the renal problems can be life threatening. The most common renal anomaly is unilateral absence of the kidney. Other anomalies include malrotation of kidneys, ectopic kidney, horseshoe kidney, and hydronephrosis from ureteropelvic obstruction.

CARDIOVASCULAR ANOMALIES

The reported incidence of cardiovascular anomalies in children with Klippel-Feil syndrome ranges from 4.2% to 29%. Ventricular septal defects, alone or in combination, are the most common anomaly. Patients may have significant dyspnea and cyanosis. Other reported cardiovascular anomalies include mitral valve insufficiency, coarctation of the aorta, right-sided aorta, patent ductus arteriosus, pulmonic stenosis, dextrocardia, atrial septal defect, aplasia of the pericardium, patent foramen ovale, single atrium, single ventricle, and bicuspid pulmonic valve.

DEAFNESS

Approximately 30% of children with Klippel-Feil syndrome have some degree of hearing loss. McGaughran, Kuna, and Das reported that 80% of the 44 patients they studied had some type of audiologic abnormalities. Several reports document conduction defects with ankylosis of the ossicles, footplate fixation, or absence of the external auditory canal. Other reports suggest a sensorineural defect. There is no common anatomic lesion, and the hearing loss may be conductive, sensorineural, or mixed. All patients with Klippel-Feil syndrome should have audiometric testing. Early detection of hearing defects in a young child may improve speech and language development by permitting early initiation of speech and language training.

SYNKINESIS

Synkinesis (mirror movements) is involuntary paired movements of the hands and occasionally of the arms. One hand is unable to move without a similar reciprocal motion of the opposite hand. Synkinesis can be observed in normal children younger than 5 years old and is present in 20% of patients with Klippel-Feil syndrome. Synkinesis may be so severe as to restrict bimanual activities. The mirror movements become less obvious with increasing age and usually are not clinically obvious after the second decade of life.

In autopsy studies, incomplete decussation of the pyramidal tract in the upper cervical spinal cord has been observed, suggesting that an alternative extrapyramidal path is required to control motion in the upper extremity. Clinically normal patients with Klippel-Feil syndrome have been shown to have electrically detectable paired motion in the opposite extremity. These patients may be clumsier in two-handed activities. Occupational therapy can help the child disassociate the mirror movements and improve bimanual dexterity.

RESPIRATORY ANOMALIES

Pulmonary complications involving failure of lobe formation, ectopic lungs, or restrictive lung disease resulting from a shortened trunk, scoliosis, rib fusion, and deformed costovertebral joints have been reported.

■ SPRENGEL DEFORMITY

Sprengel deformity occurs in about 20% of patients with Klippel-Feil syndrome and can be unilateral or bilateral. Descent of the scapula coincides with the period of development of Klippel-Feil anomalies, and maldevelopment during this time (3 to 8 weeks of gestation) can cause both anomalies. Sprengel deformity increases the unsightly appearance of an already short neck and can affect the range of shoulder motion.

■ CERVICAL RIBS

Cervical ribs occur in 12% to 15% of patients with Klippel-Feil syndrome. When evaluating a patient with neurologic symptoms, the presence of a cervical rib and associated thoracic outlet syndrome should be investigated.

CLINICAL FINDINGS

The classic clinical presentation of Klippel-Feil syndrome is the triad of a low posterior hairline, a short neck, and limited neck motion (Fig. 7.30). This triad indicates almost complete cervical involvement and may be clinically evident at birth; however, fewer than half of patients with Klippel-Feil syndrome have all parts of the triad. Many patients with Klippel-Feil syndrome have a normal appearance, and the syndrome is diagnosed through incidental radiographs. Shortening of the neck and a low posterior hairline are not constant findings and may be overlooked; webbing of the neck (pterygium colli) is seen in severe involvement. The most constant

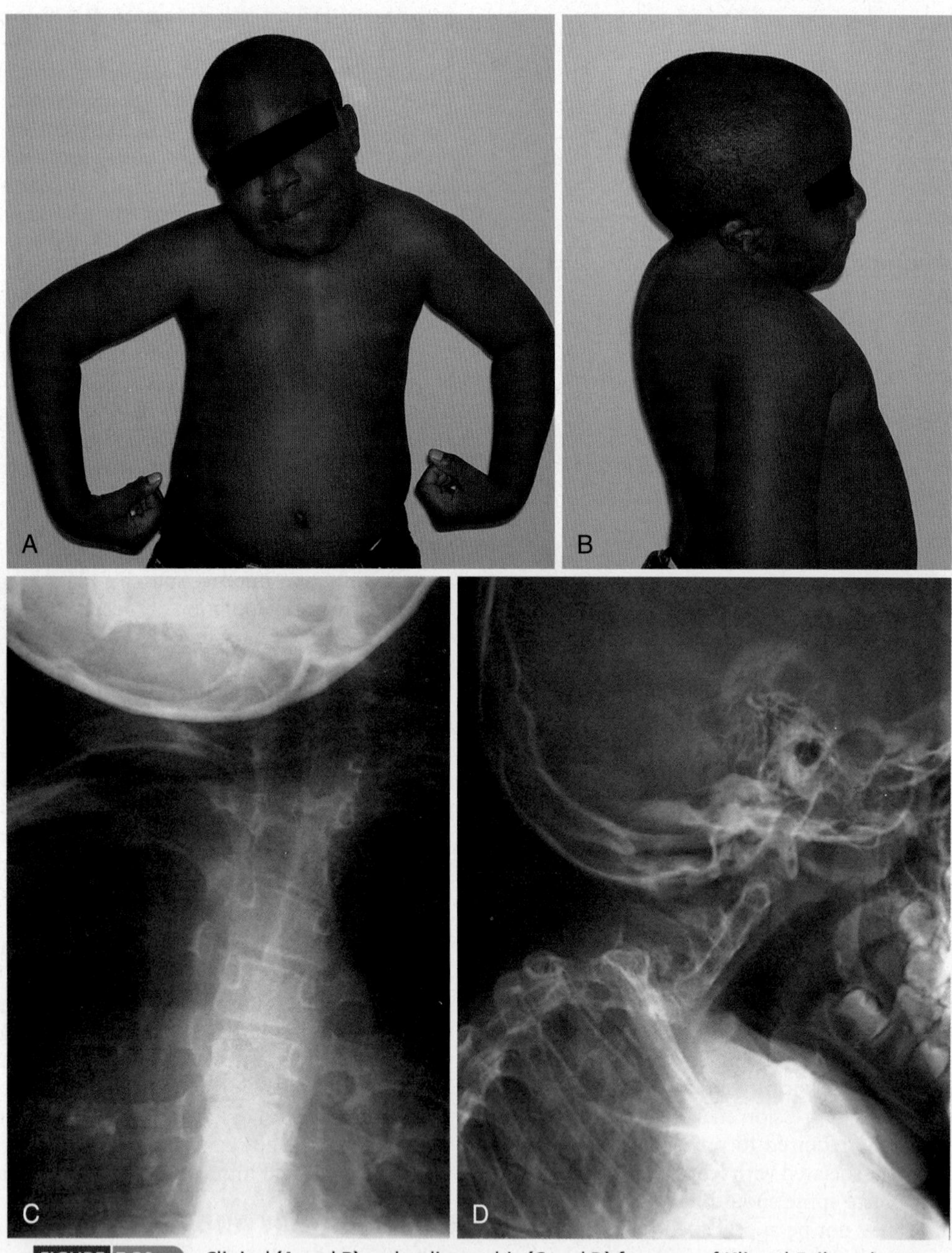

FIGURE 7.30 Clinical **(A and B)** and radiographic **(C and D)** features of Klippel-Feil syndrome in young boy.

clinical finding is limitation of neck motion. Rotation and lateral bending are affected more than flexion and extension. If fewer than three vertebrae are fused or if the lower cervical vertebrae are fused, motion is only slightly limited. Hensinger reported that some of his patients had almost full flexion and extension through only one open (unfused) interspace.

Symptoms usually are not caused by the fused cervical vertebrae but by open segments adjacent to areas of synostosis that become hypermobile in response to increased stress placed on the area. Symptoms can be caused by mechanical or neurologic problems. Mechanical problems are caused by stretching of the capsular and ligamentous structures near the hypermobile segment, resulting in early degenerative arthritis with pain localized to the neck. Neurologic problems result from direct irritation of or impingement on a nerve root or from compression of the spinal cord. Involvement of the nerve root alone causes radicular symptoms; spinal cord compression can cause spasticity, hyperreflexia, muscle weakness, and even complete paralysis.

RADIOGRAPHIC FINDINGS

Routine radiographs, CT scans, and MR images may be useful in the evaluation of Klippel-Feil syndrome. Adequate radiographs can be difficult to obtain in severely involved children, but initial examination should include anteroposterior, odontoid, and lateral flexion and extension views of the cervical spine. Lateral flexion-extension views are the most important to identify atlantoaxial instability or instability near an open segment between two congenitally fused areas (Fig. 7.31). Spinal canal narrowing can occur from degenerative osteophytes or from congenital spinal stenosis. If enlargement of the spinal canal is evident on radiographs, syringomyelia, hydromyelia, or Arnold-Chiari malformation should be suspected. In young patients with Klippel-Feil syndrome, serial lateral flexion-extension views should be obtained to evaluate instability at the atlantoaxial joint or at an open interspace between fused areas. Development of congenital or idiopathic scoliosis should be documented by radiographic examination of the entire spine. Besides vertebral fusion, flattening and widening of involved vertebral bodies and absent disc spaces are common findings. In young children, the spine may appear normal because of the lack of ossification. The posterior elements usually are the first to ossify and fuse, which aids in early diagnosis of Klippel-Feil syndrome. CT and MRI are helpful in diagnosing nerve root and spinal cord impingement by osteophyte formation. To evaluate instability and the risk of neurologic compromise, a flexion and extension MRI may be needed to give the soft-tissue definition necessary to show instability or spinal cord compromise.

TREATMENT

Mechanical symptoms caused by degenerative joint disease usually respond to a cervical collar and analgesics. Neurologic symptoms should be evaluated carefully to locate the exact

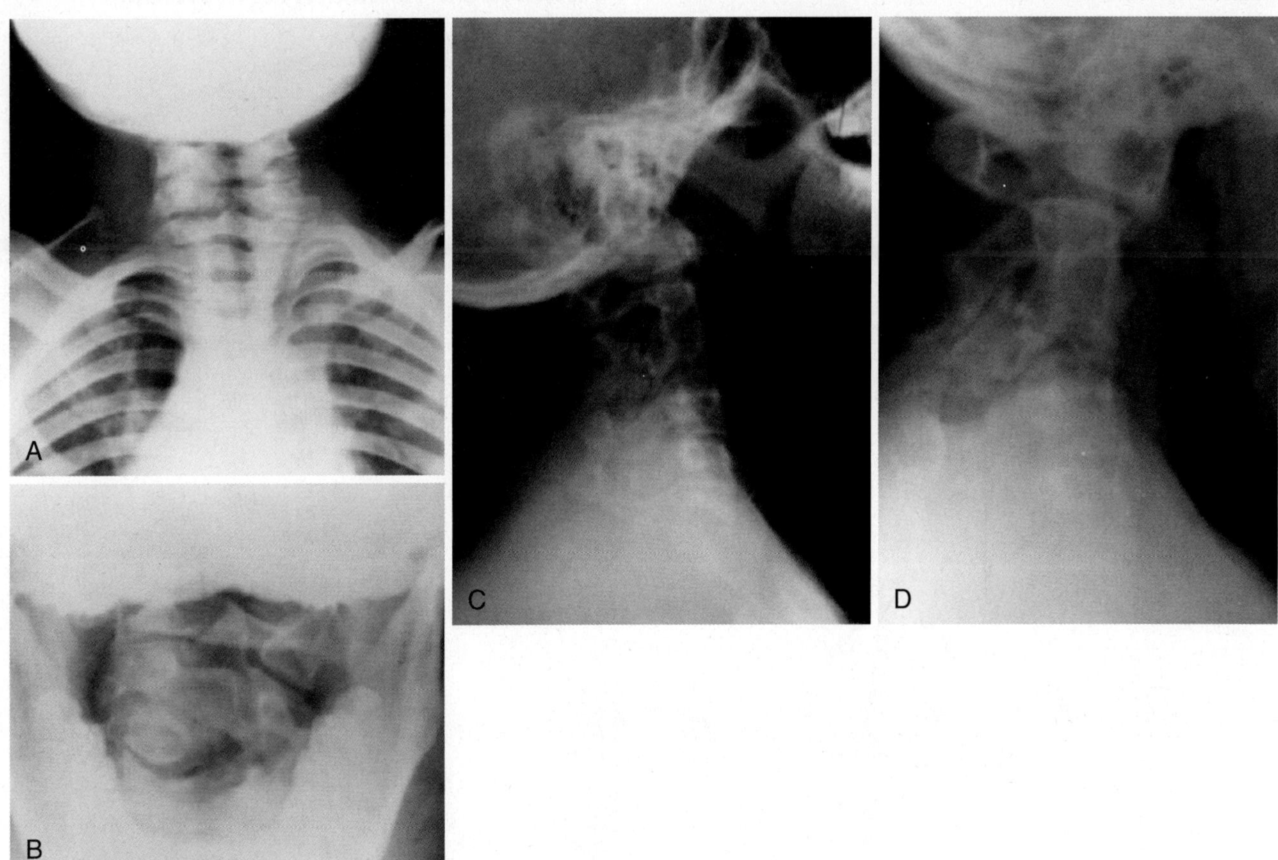

FIGURE 7.31 Radiographic features of Klippel-Feil syndrome in adolescent. **A,** Posteroanterior view shows congenital anomalies of cervical spine and left Sprengel deformity. **B,** Open-mouth odontoid view shows bony anomalies of cervical spine. **C,** Extension view shows odontoid in normal position. **D,** Flexion view shows increased atlantodens interval.

pathologic condition; surgical stabilization with or without decompression may be required. Prophylactic fusion of a hypermobile segment is controversial. The risk of neurologic compromise must be weighed against the further reduction in neck motion, and this decision must be made for each patient individually. Depending on the type of anatomic deformity and location of instability, a posterior fusion, anterior fusion, or a combined anterior and posterior fusion may be needed. If anterior decompression and fusion are needed, this can be done with an anterior approach. Anterior decompression and interbody fusion can be performed with plate and screw fixation similar to adults if the anatomy allows for this (see chapter 5). Cosmetic improvement after surgery has been limited, but surgical correction of Sprengel deformity can significantly improve appearance, and occasionally soft-tissue procedures such as Z-plasty and muscle resection improve cosmesis. Bonola described a method of rib resection to obtain an apparent increase in neck length and motion, but this is an extensive procedure with significant risk. Partial thoracoplasty is performed as a two-stage procedure: removal of the upper four ribs on one side and, after the patient has recovered from the first surgery, removal of the upper four ribs on the other side.

POSTERIOR FUSION OF C3-7

TECHNIQUE 7.15 *Figure 7.32*

- Administer general anesthesia with the patient supine.
- Turn the patient prone on the operating table, maintaining traction and proper alignment of the head and neck. The head can be positioned in a headrest or maintained in skeletal traction.
- Obtain radiographs to confirm adequate alignment of the vertebrae and to localize the vertebrae to be exposed. There is a high incidence of extension of the fusion mass when extra vertebrae or spinous processes are exposed in the cervical spine.
- Make a midline incision over the chosen spinous processes and expose the spinous process and laminae subperiosteally to the facet joints.
- If the spinous process is large enough, make a hole in the base of the spinous process with a towel clip or Lewin clamp.
- Pass an 18-gauge wire through this hole, loop it over the spinous process, and pass it through the hole again.
- Make a similar hole in the base of the spinous process of the inferior vertebra to be fused.
- Pass the wire through this hole, loop it under the inferior aspect of the spinous process, and pass it back through the same hole.
- Tighten the wire and place corticocancellous bone grafts along the exposed lamina and spinous processes.
- Close the wound in layers.
- If the spinous process is too small to pass wires, an in situ fusion can be performed and external immobilization can be used.

POSTOPERATIVE CARE The patient should wear a rigid cervical orthosis until a solid fusion is documented radiographically.

POSTERIOR FUSION OF C3 TO C7 USING 16-GAUGE WIRE AND THREADED KIRSCHNER WIRES

TECHNIQUE 7.16

(HALL)

- Pass the threaded Kirschner wires through the bases of the spinous processes of the vertebrae to be fused, followed by a figure-of-eight wiring with a 16-gauge wire.
- After the 16-gauge wire has been tightened around the threaded Kirschner wires, pack strips of corticocancellous and cancellous bone over the posterior arches of the vertebrae to be fused (Fig. 7.33).
- Exposure and postoperative care are similar to those described for a Rogers posterior fusion and wiring.

Posterior instrumentation techniques (see chapter 5) that are used in the adult spine (plate or rods and lateral

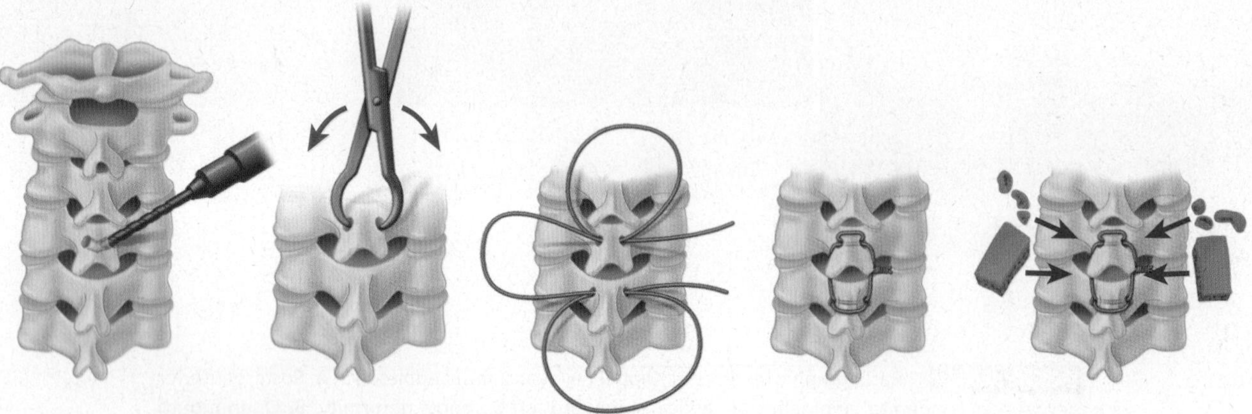

FIGURE 7.32 Modified Rogers wiring of cervical spine for posterior fusion. **SEE TECHNIQUE 7.15.**

mass screws) can be used in the pediatric cervical spine. Before the techniques are used, the size of the lateral masses must be evaluated to ensure there would be adequate room to place these screws.

POSTERIOR FUSION WITH LATERAL MASS SCREW FIXATION

Lateral mass screw fixation of the lower cervical spine can be used in older children or adolescents. The instrumentation should be matched to the size of the child. Techniques described differ primarily in the entry points and screw trajectories.

TECHNIQUE 7.17

(ROY-CAMILLE)

- Create an entry point for the screw 5 mm medial to the lateral edge and midway between the facet joint or at the center of the rectangular posterior face of the lateral mass (Fig. 7.34A).
- Direct the drill perpendicular to the posterior wall of the vertebral body with a 10-degree lateral angle (Fig. 7.34B). This trajectory takes the exit slightly lateral to the vertebral artery and below the existing nerve root. Use lateral fluoroscopic imaging to avoid penetration of the subadjacent facet.
- Set the depth guide to 10 to 12 mm to avoid penetration beyond the anterior cortex. For men the lateral mass depth from C3 to C6 ranges from 6 to 14 mm (average 8.7 mm) and in women 6 to 11 mm (average 7.9 mm). The depth can be increased if the local anatomy permits. If additional 20% of pullout strength with bicortical fixation is desired, place the screw to exit at the junction of the lateral mass and transverse process (Fig. 7.34C).

POSTERIOR FUSION WITH LATERAL MASS SCREW AND ROD FIXATION

TECHNIQUE 7.18

- Select an entry portal 1 mm medial to the center of the lateral mass.
- Drill the lateral mass 25 to 35 degrees laterally and 15 degrees cephalad (parallel to the plane of the facet joint) for C3 to C6 (Fig. 7.35). The drilling should be 10 to 25 degrees medially and 25 degrees superiorly at C2 to avoid injuring the vertebral artery. Use a hand drill with a stop

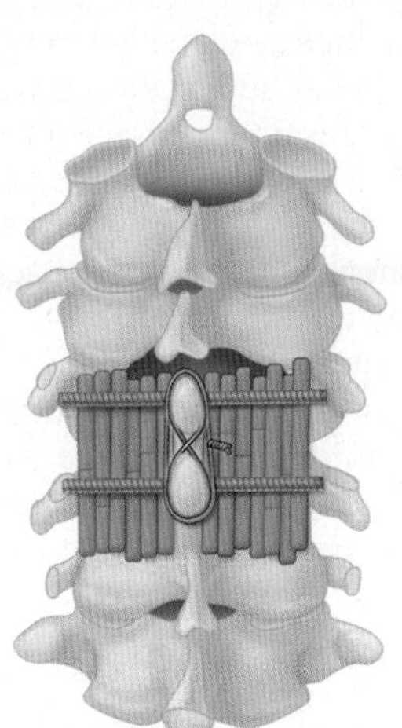

FIGURE 7.33 Hall technique of fixation for posterior arthrodesis of cervical spine. **SEE TECHNIQUE 7.16.**

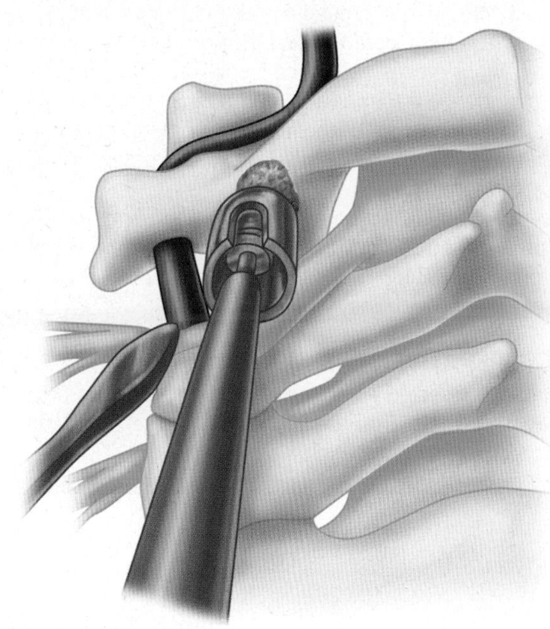

FIGURE 7.35 Posterior lateral mass screw and rod fixation. Drilling lateral mass for screw insertion. **SEE TECHNIQUE 7.18.**

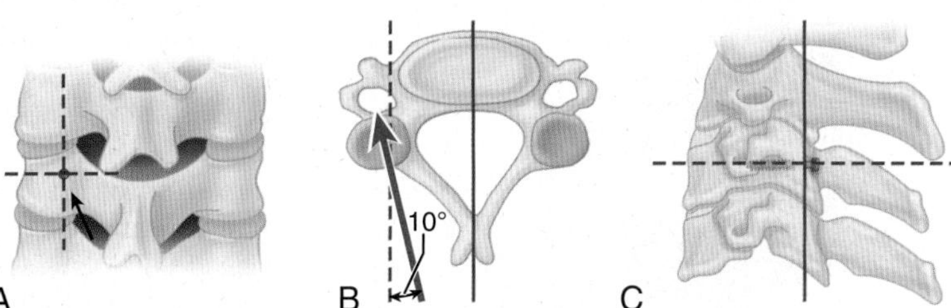

FIGURE 7.34 Roy-Camille technique of lateral mass screw insertion. **A,** Screw entry point. **B,** Drill directed perpendicular to posterior wall of vertebral body at 10-degree angle. **C,** Final screw position. **SEE TECHNIQUE 7.17.**

guide to prevent drilling of the opposite cortex. Tap the drill hole if necessary.

- Insert the proper length polyaxial screw into each lateral mass to be instrumented and check the position of the screws with posteroanterior and lateral C-arm images. Make adjustments as necessary.
- Insert the prebent rods into the screw head fixtures. Tighten the rods to the screws.

POSTOPERATIVE CARE A cervical orthosis (cervical collar) is applied and worn for 6 to 8 weeks. Halo device immobilization may be considered if there is suboptimal fixation.

RIB RESECTION

TECHNIQUE 7.19

(BONOLA)

- Bonola described partial thoracoplasty with the use of local anesthesia, but general anesthesia can be used.
- Through a right paravertebral incision midway between the spinous processes and the medial margin of the scapula, divide the trapezius and rhomboid muscles to expose the posterior aspect of the first four ribs (Fig. 7.36A).
- Cut these ribs with a rib cutter a few centimeters from the costovertebral joint.
- Continue the dissection anteriorly along the ribs, dividing and removing the ribs as far anteriorly as the dissection allows (Fig. 7.36B).
- Close the wound in layers.

POSTOPERATIVE CARE A cervical collar is fitted to help mold the resected area. The second stage of the procedure is performed on the opposite side after the patient has recovered from the initial surgery.

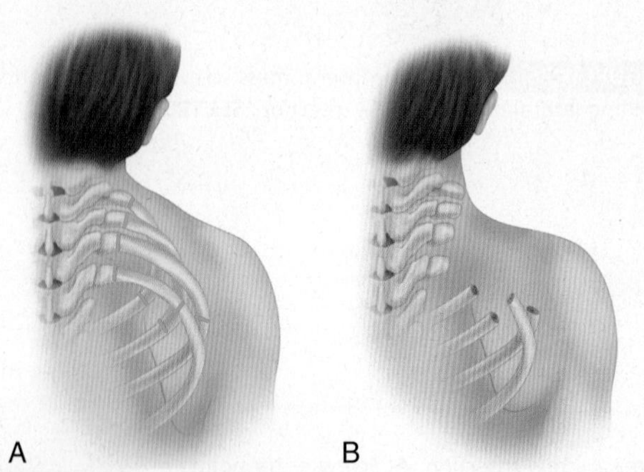

FIGURE 7.36 **A** and **B**, Bonola partial thoracoplasty for treatment of short neck in Klippel-Feil syndrome. **SEE TECHNIQUE 7.19.**

ATLANTOAXIAL ROTATORY SUBLUXATION

Atlantoaxial rotatory subluxation is a common cause of childhood torticollis, but the subluxation and torticollis usually are temporary. Rarely do they persist and become what is best described as atlantoaxial rotatory "fixation." Atlantoaxial rotatory subluxation occurs when normal motion between the atlas and axis becomes limited or fixed, and it can occur spontaneously, can be associated with minor trauma, or can follow an upper respiratory tract infection. The cause of this subluxation is not completely understood. Various causes that have been proposed include hyperemic decalcification of the arch of the atlas, causing inadequate attachment of the transverse ligaments; inflammation of the synovial fringes that act as an obstruction to reduction of subluxation; and disruption of one or both of the alar ligaments with an intact transverse ligament. A meniscus-like synovial fold in the C1-2 facet joints, which is primarily noted in children, caused subluxation in one study. Most authors now agree that the subluxation is related to increased laxity of ligaments and capsular structures caused by inflammation or trauma.

Fielding and Hawkins classified atlantoaxial rotatory subluxation into four types (Fig. 7.37): type I, simple rotatory displacement without anterior shift of C1; type II, rotatory displacement with an anterior shift of C1 on C2 of 5 mm or less; type III, rotatory displacement with an anterior shift of C1 on C2 greater than 5 mm; and type IV, rotatory displacement with a posterior shift. Type I displacement is the most common and occurs primarily in children. Type II is less common but has greater potential for neurologic damage. Types III and IV are rare but have high potential for neurologic damage.

Atlantoaxial rotatory subluxation usually occurs in children after an upper respiratory tract infection or minor or major trauma. The head is tilted to one side and rotated to the opposite side with the neck slightly flexed (the "cock robin" position). The sternocleidomastoid muscle on the long side is often in spasm in an attempt to correct this deformity. When the subluxation is acute, attempts to move the head cause pain. Patients can increase the deformity but cannot correct the deformity past the midline. With time, muscle spasms subside and the torticollis becomes less painful but the deformity persists. A careful neurologic examination should determine any neurologic compression or vertebral artery compromise.

RADIOGRAPHIC FINDINGS

Adequate radiographs of the cervical spine can be difficult to obtain in children with torticollis. Initial examination should include anteroposterior and odontoid views of the cervical spine. On the open-mouth odontoid view, the lateral mass that is rotated forward appears wider and closer to the midline and the opposite lateral mass appears narrower and farther away from the midline (Fig. 7.38). Apparent overlapping may obscure one of the facet joints of the atlas and axis. On the lateral view, the anteriorly rotated lateral mass appears wedge-shaped in front of the odontoid. The posterior arch of the atlas may appear to be assimilated into the occiput because of the head tilt. A lateral radiograph of the skull may show the relative position of C1 and C2 more clearly than a lateral radiograph of the cervical spine. Lateral flexion and extension views should be obtained to document any atlantoaxial instability. Cineradiography confirms the diagnosis by

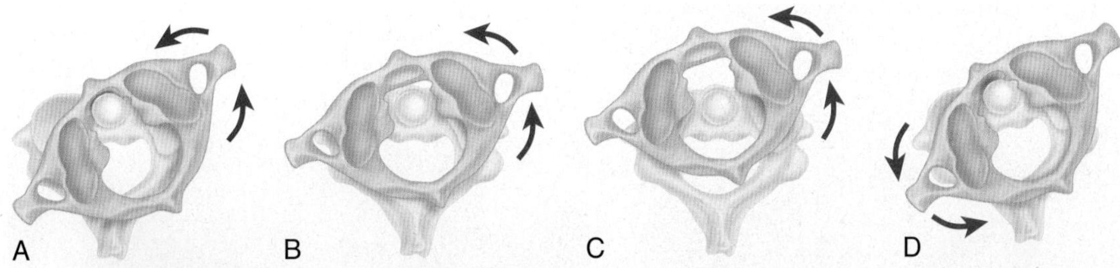

FIGURE 7.37 Fielding and Hawkins classification of rotatory displacement. **A,** Type I, simple rotatory displacement without anterior shift; odontoid acts as pivot. **B,** Type II, rotatory displacement with anterior displacement of 3-5 mm; lateral articular process acts as pivot. **C,** Type III, rotatory displacement with anterior displacement of more than 5 mm. **D,** Type IV, rotatory displacement with posterior displacement.

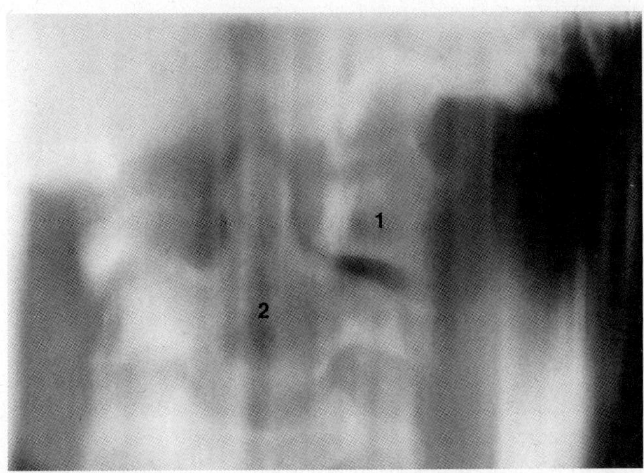

FIGURE 7.38 Atlantoaxial rotatory subluxation. Note lateral masses (1 and 2).

BOX 7.6

Treatment Plan for Rotatory Subluxation

Nonoperative Treatment

Present less than 1 week: immobilization in soft collar, analgesics, bed rest for 1 week; if no spontaneous reduction: hospitalization, halo traction

Present more than 1 week but less than 1 month: hospitalization, head halter, cervical collar 4-6 weeks

Present more than 1 month: hospitalization, halo traction, cervical collar 4-6 weeks

Indications for Operative Treatment

Neurologic involvement

Anterior displacement

Failure to achieve and maintain correction of deformity that exists longer than 3 months

Recurrence of deformity after an adequate trial of conservative management consisting of at least 6 weeks of immobilization

showing the movement of atlas and axis as a single unit but is difficult to perform during the acute stage because movement of the neck is painful. Cineradiography is not routinely used because of the increased radiation exposure. CT with the head rotated as far to the left and right as possible during scanning to confirm the loss of normal rotation at the atlantoaxial joint confirms the diagnosis of rotatory subluxation. McGuire et al. classified the findings on dynamic CT scans (DCTS) into three stages: stage 0, torticollis but normal DCTS; stage 1, limitation of motion (<15 degrees difference between C1 and C2, but C1 crosses the midline of C2); and stage 2, fixed (C1 does not cross midline of C2). They found a significant trend between increasing intensity of treatment and stage of DCTS findings. The usefulness of DCTS, however, for the diagnosis of atlantoaxial rotatory subluxation has been questioned. MRI may be beneficial for the evaluation of ligamentous pathology or spinal cord compression.

TREATMENT

The treatment plan should be based on the duration of the subluxation (Box 7.6). If rotatory subluxation has existed less than 1 week, immobilization in a soft collar, analgesics, and bed rest for 1 week are recommended. If reduction does not occur spontaneously, hospitalization and traction are indicated. If rotatory subluxation is present for longer than 1 week, but less than 1 month, hospitalization and cervical traction are indicated. Head-halter traction generally is used, but when torticollis persists longer than 1 month, halo traction may be required. Traction is maintained until the deformity corrects, then a cervical collar is worn for 4 to 6 weeks. Nonoperative treatment should be used only if no significant anterior displacement or instability is seen on radiographic evaluation.

Fielding listed the following as indications for operative treatment: (1) neurologic involvement, (2) anterior displacement, (3) failure to achieve and maintain correction if the deformity exists for longer than 3 months, and (4) recurrence of the deformity after an adequate trial of conservative management consisting of at least 6 weeks of immobilization. If operative treatment is indicated, a C1-2 posterior fusion is performed (Fig. 7.39). Fielding and Hawkins recommended preoperative traction for 2 to 3 weeks to correct the deformity as much as possible. Fusion is performed with the head in a neutral position. Halo immobilization is continued for 6 weeks after surgery to maintain correction while the fusion becomes solid. This can be accomplished with a halo cast or halo vest. Immobilization is continued until there is radiographic evidence of fusion. C1-C2 fusion with the Harms technique may assist in reduction and can avoid the use of a halo immobilization (Fig. 7.40).

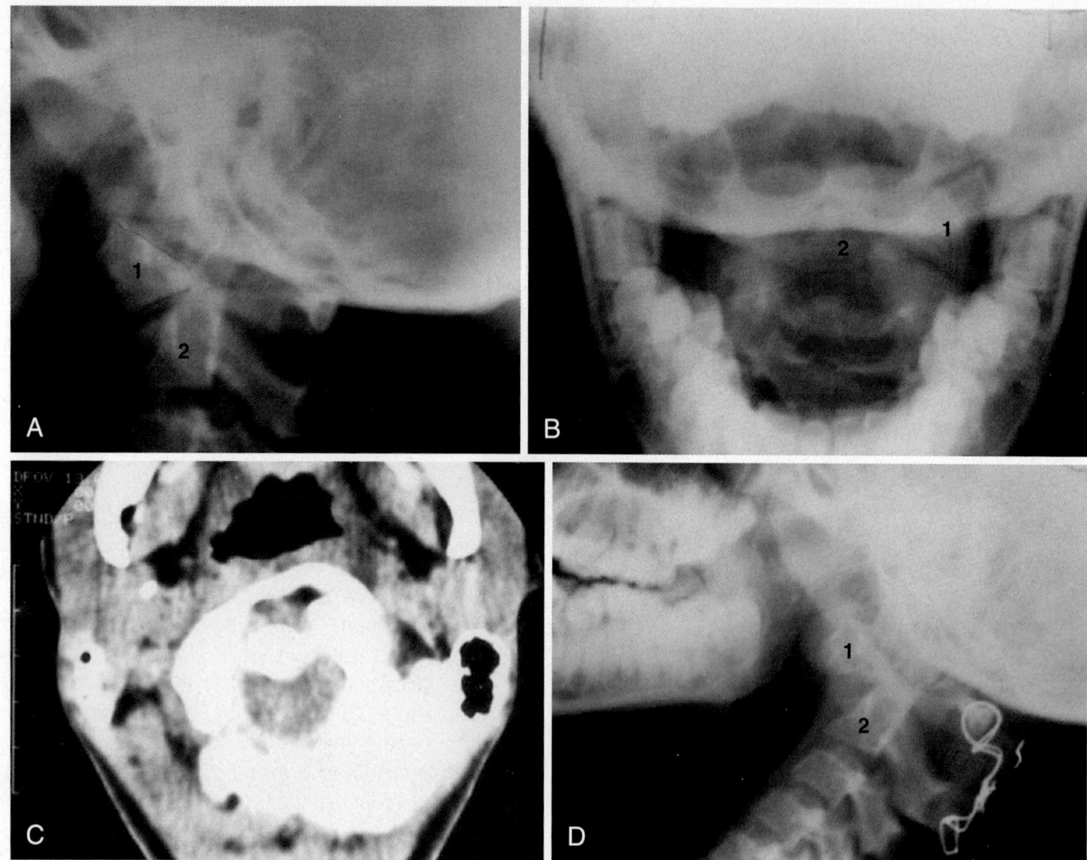

FIGURE 7.39 Atlantoaxial rotatory fixation. **A,** Lateral radiograph shows wedge-shaped mass anterior to odontoid. **B,** Open-mouth odontoid view. **C,** CT scan. **D,** After C1-2 in situ fusion.

CERVICAL INSTABILITY IN DOWN SYNDROME

In children with Down syndrome, generalized ligamentous laxity caused by the underlying collagen defect can result in atlantoaxial and atlantooccipital instability. Pizzutillo and Herman made a distinction between cervical instability and hypermobility in patients with Down syndrome. Instability implies pathologic intersegmental motion that jeopardizes neurologic integrity. Hypermobility refers to increased excursions that occur in the cervical spine of patients with Down syndrome compared with normal controls but do not result in loss of structural integrity of the anatomic restraints that protect neural tissues. Atlantoaxial instability, first described by Spitzer, Rabinowitch, and Wybar in 1961, occurs in 10% to 20% of children with Down syndrome. Instability can occur at more than one level and in more than one plane. Atlantooccipital instability also can occur in patients with Down syndrome; the incidence has been reported to be 60%. Despite these reports of atlantoaxial and atlantooccipital instability in patients with Down syndrome, the exact natural history related to this instability is unknown. In patients with Down syndrome, differentiating those with hypermobility and those with clinically significant instability may be difficult.

The cervical spine in children with Down syndrome may be associated with congenital anomalies of the upper cervical spine, but whether the cervical anomalies are the cause or the result of ligamentous laxity is still controversial.

NEUROLOGIC FINDINGS

Neurologic symptoms are present in 1% to 2.6% of patients with cervical instability. Instability is usually discovered on routine screening examinations or on cervical radiographs obtained for other reasons. Progressive instability leading to neurologic symptoms is most common in boys older than 10.5 years of age. Involvement of the pyramidal tract usually results in gait abnormalities, hyperreflexia, and motor weakness. Other neurologic symptoms include neck pain, occipital headaches, and torticollis. Detailed neurologic examination is often difficult in patients with Down syndrome, and somatosensory-evoked potentials may be beneficial in documenting neurologic involvement.

RADIOGRAPHIC FINDINGS

Radiographic screening for atlantoaxial instability in Down syndrome patients is controversial. Routine screening in preschool patients and re-screening every decade had been recommended in the past but the present AAP guidelines stress the inability for screening radiographs to predict any future risk of developing atlantoaxial instability. The emphasis now for screening is based on symptoms or positive physical exam findings during annual well-child checks to obtain screening radiographs.

Radiographic examination should include anteroposterior, flexion and extension lateral, and odontoid views. CT scans in flexion and extension or cineradiography in flexion and extension also may be needed to evaluate the

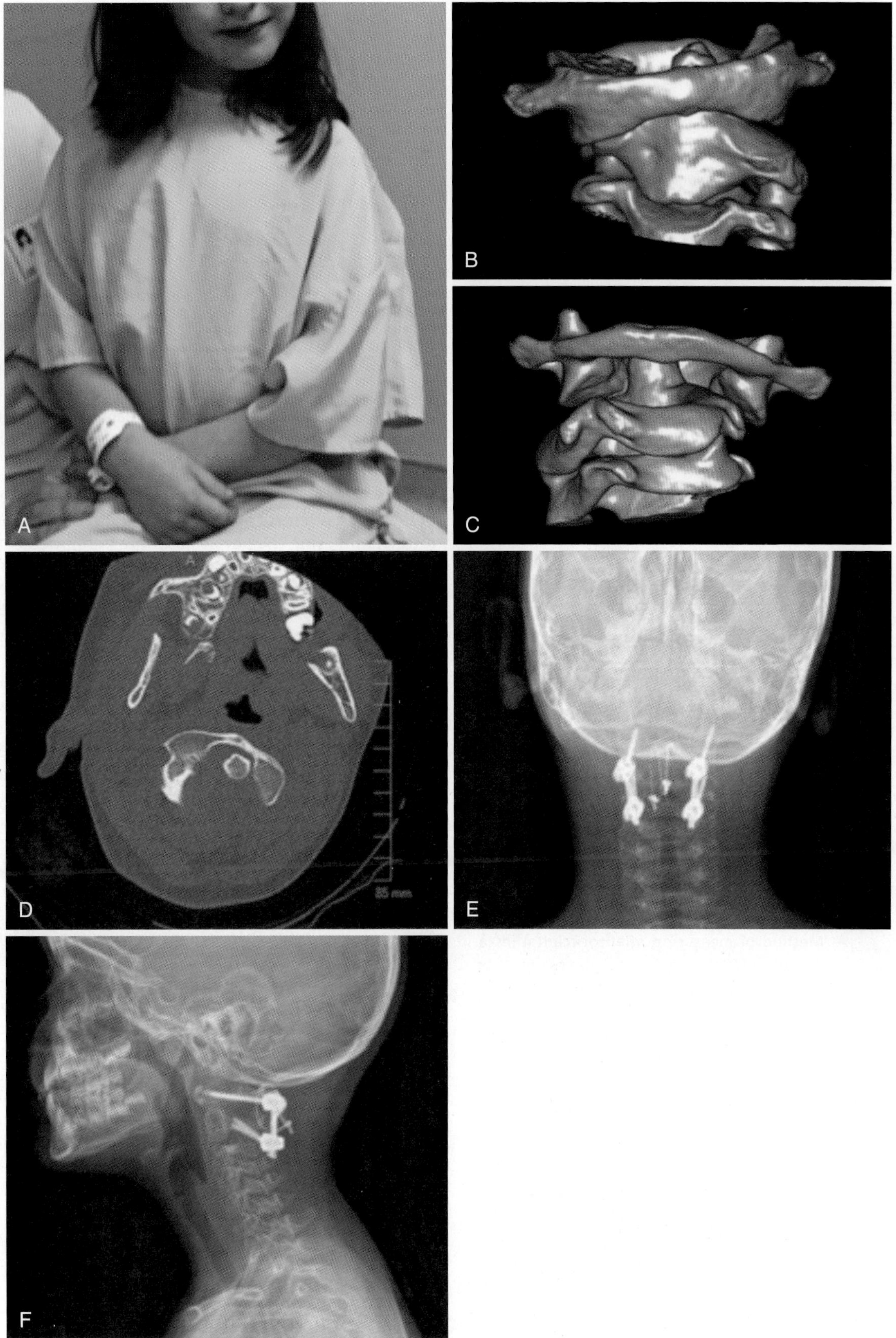

FIGURE 7.40 **A,** Child with rotary subluxation of C1 on C2. Note the direction of head tilt and rotation of the neck. **B** and **C,** CT posteroanterior and anteroposterior reconstructions documenting rotary subluxation. **D,** CT showing subluxation. **E** and **F,** After posterior C1-C2 fusion. (From Warner WC, Hedequist DJ: Cervical spine injuries in children. In Waters PM, Skaggs DL, Flynn JM, editors: *Rockwood and Wilkins' fractures in children*, ed 9, Philadelphia, Wolters Kluwer, 2020, p 800.)

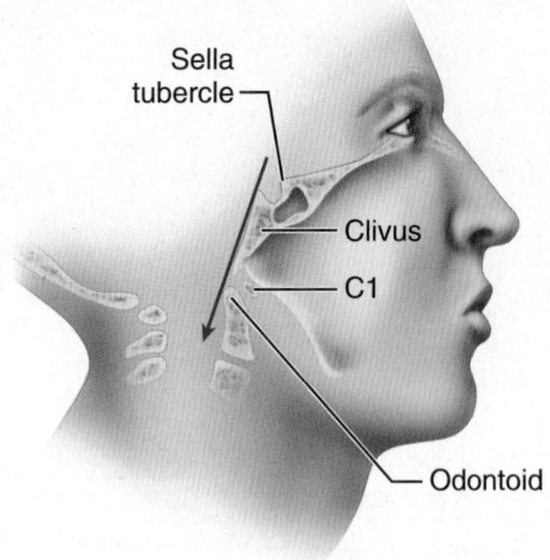

FIGURE 7.41 Drawing of Wackenheim clivus-canal line. This line is drawn along the clivus into the cervical spinal canal and should pass just posterior to the tip of the odontoid.

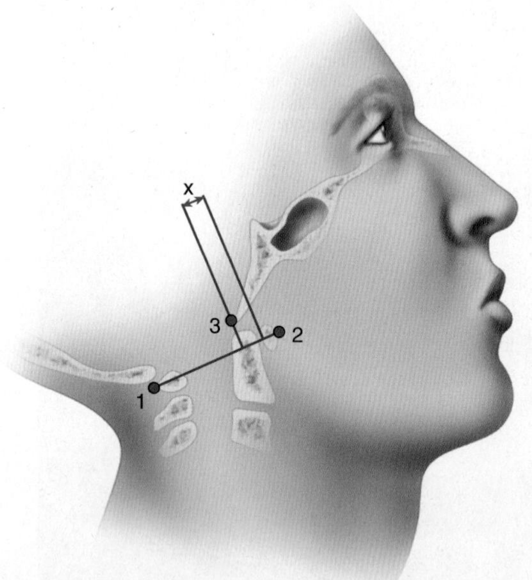

FIGURE 7.42 Method of measuring atlantooccipital instability according to Wiesel and Rothman. These lines are drawn on flexion and extension lateral radiographs, and translation should be no more than 1 mm. Atlantal line joins points *1* and *2*. Line drawn perpendicular to atlantal line at posterior margin of anterior arch of atlas. Point *3* is basion. *x* is distance from point *3* to perpendicular line measured in flexion and extension. Difference represents anteroposterior translation.

occipitoatlantal joint and the atlantoaxial joint for instability. MRI is useful in detecting any spinal cord signal changes in suspected instability and neurologic compromise in these patients in whom it is often difficult to obtain a detailed neurologic examination. Radiographic evidence of atlantooccipital instability is not as well defined as that for atlantoaxial instability, but the measurements described by Wackenheim (Fig. 7.41), Wiesel and Rothman (Fig. 7.42), Powers (Fig. 7.43), and Tredwell et al. are helpful. A Powers ratio of more than 1.0 is indicative of abnormal anterior translation of the occiput, and, according to Parfenchuck et al., a ratio of less than 0.55 indicates posterior translation. However, some

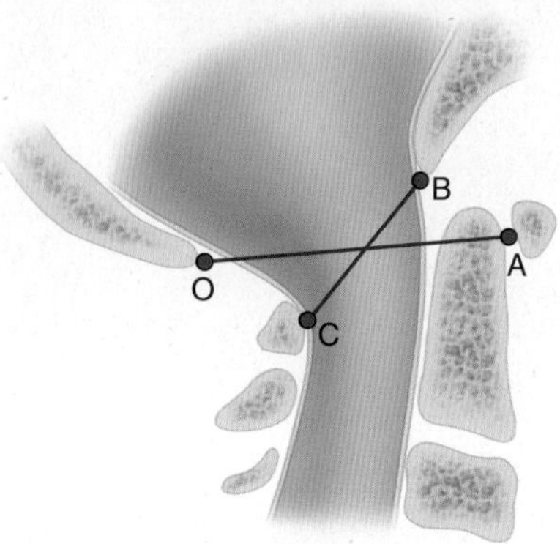

FIGURE 7.43 Powers ratio is determined by drawing a line from the basion *(B)* to the posterior arch of the atlas *(C)* and a second line from the opisthion *(O)* to the anterior arch of the atlas *(A)*. The length of line *BC* is divided by the length of line *OA*. A ratio greater than 1 is diagnostic of anterior atlantooccipital translation, and a ratio less than 0.55 is diagnostic of posterior translation.

studies have reported the poor reproducibility and reliability of these measurement techniques in children with Down syndrome, hindering the physician in providing well-supported treatment recommendations. CT scans in flexion and extension or cineradiography may be needed to give better detail and information about possible atlantooccipital instability.

An atlantodens interval (ADI) of 4.5 to 5 mm indicates instability in normal pediatric patients. Increased ADI in patients with Down syndrome has not been directly correlated with an increase in neurologic compromise. This suggests that radiographs of the cervical spine in Down syndrome must be evaluated by standards specific to that population and not by traditional standards for general pediatric patients because this may result in overdiagnosis of a pathologic process. Neurologic compromise occurs with a similar incidence in individuals with Down syndrome who have a normal ADI and those with an ADI from 4 to 10 mm. In Down syndrome, an ADI of less than 4.5 mm is normal; an ADI of 4.5 to 10 mm is considered hypermobile but not unstable unless neurologic findings are present; and an ADI of more than 10 mm is considered unstable, and the patient is at risk for neurologic compromise because of the decrease in the space available for the spinal cord.

Nakamura et al. described two diagnostic radiographic measurements for atlantoaxial instability in Down syndrome patients: the C1/4 space available for cord (SAC) ratio and the C1 inclination angle. The C1/4 SAC ratio was defined as the ratio of the anteroposterior diameter of the spinal canal at the C1 level to the anteroposterior diameter of the spinal canal at the C4 level. A normal ratio is 1.2; a ratio of <0.86 was at risk of symptomatic instability. The C1 inclination angle is defined as the angle formed between a line perpendicular to the tangent at the posterior surface of the body of C2 and the line connecting the centers of the anterior and posterior arches of C1. A normal value is 15 degrees; values less than 10 degrees were likely to have symptomatic instability.

TREATMENT

Hypermobility of the occipitoatlantal junction has been observed in more than 60% of patients with Down syndrome, but this usually is not associated with neurologic risk. If hypermobility of this joint is documented and the patient is neurologically normal, then restriction of high-risk activities is recommended. If there is hypermobility and a neurologic deficit or an abnormal signal change in the spinal cord on MRI, then an occiput to C2 or 3 fusion is recommended.

When the ADI is less than 4.5 mm, no restriction of activities is necessary. In those who have an ADI of 4.5 to 10 mm with no neurologic symptoms, high-risk activities are limited. If there is a neurologic deficit or spinal cord changes on MRI, a C1-2 fusion is indicated. If the ADI is 10 mm or more, posterior fusion and instrumentation are recommended. Before fusion and instrumentation, the unstable C1-2 joint should be reduced by traction. If reduction cannot be obtained, an in situ fusion reduces the risk of neurologic compromise.

Complications are relatively common after cervical fusions in children with Down syndrome. Segal et al. reported frequent graft resorption after 10 posterior fusions and suggested as causes inadequate inflammatory response and collagen defects. Msall et al. reported the frequent development of instability above and below C1-2 fusion in patients with Down syndrome. Postoperative immobilization in a halo cast or halo vest should be continued for as long as possible because graft resorption 6 months after fusion has been reported. More stable fixation may decrease this complication.

C1-C2 transarticular screw fixation (Figs. 7.9 and 7.10) or occiput to C2 instrumentation with plates or rods (Techniques 7.8 and 7.9) can be used successfully and give greater stability than wire fixation.

FAMILIAL CERVICAL DYSPLASIA

Saltzman et al. described a familial cervical dysplasia that affects the first cervical vertebra. Nine of 12 family members from three generations were affected by this inherited form of cervical vertebral dysplasia. The mode of transmission of this disorder is autosomal dominant, with apparently complete penetrance and variable expressivity. Most patients are asymptomatic, and clinical presentation varies from an incidental finding on radiographic examination to a passively correctable head tilt. Symptoms such as suboccipital headaches or decreased cervical motion may be present. CT scan and three-dimensional reconstructions best delineate the anatomic pathology. MRI is useful in identifying the potential for neurologic compromise and the need for surgical stabilization. If surgery is required for stabilization, an occiput-to-C2 fusion is usually needed.

CONGENITAL ANOMALIES OF THE ATLAS

Dubousset and Winter et al. described congenital hemiatlas or hypoplasia of the atlas that can cause marked torticollis if left untreated. Dubousset reported 17 patients with absence of the facet of C1 that led to severe, progressive, fixed torticollis. Initially, the deformity or torticollis was flexible, but with time it became fixed.

In most patients, the deformity is noted at birth as a lateral translation of the head on the trunk, with some degree of lateral tilt and rotation. The sternocleidomastoid muscle is not tight and there is often aplasia of the muscles in the nuchal concavity of the tilted side. Neurologic signs such as headaches, vertigo, or myelopathy occur in about 25% of patients. Plain radiographs are often difficult to interpret, and the diagnosis usually is made by CT. Other spinal cord anomalies may be detected by MRI, such as Arnold-Chiari malformations and stenosis of the foramen magnum. Angiography should be obtained preoperatively because vertebral arterial anomalies may occur on the aplastic side. This disorder has been classified into three types: type I is an isolated hemiatlas, type II is a partial or complete aplasia of one hemiatlas with other associated anomalies of the cervical spine, and type III is a partial or complete atlantooccipital fusion and symmetric or asymmetric hemiatlas aplasia, with or without anomalies of the odontoid and lower cervical spine. Initially, the patient should be observed for progression of the deformity. Bracing will not stop progression of the deformity. Dubousset recommended using a halo cast to gradually correct the torticollis and obtain an acceptable position of the head and neck, followed by posterior fusion from occiput to C2. Seven of his 17 patients required surgical correction. Although the age at which the torticollis could be corrected was not specified, Dubousset obtained good results in patients 13 and 15 years of age.

LARSEN SYNDROME

Larsen syndrome is a rare disorder that may have vertebral anomalies such as spina bifida, hypoplastic vertebrae, cervical kyphosis, and anteroposterior dissociation. Patients with cervical kyphosis that may eventually lead to anteroposterior dissociation are difficult to treat. This is potentially the most serious manifestation of Larsen syndrome because of the risk of paralysis. The natural history of cervical kyphosis is variable. Both static and dynamic flexion and extension radiographs should be obtained to document the degree of deformity and any instability. Treatment is also variable and is based on the age of the patient, amount and flexibility of the kyphosis, and the presence of any neurologic deficits. Johnston et al. advocated early posterior fusion in patients with Larsen syndrome and cervical kyphosis. They found gradual improvement of the cervical kyphosis from continued anterior vertebral body growth when a solid posterior fusion was obtained. In one patient, excessive lordosis occurred after posterior-only fusion. Sakaura et al. recommended posterior spinal fusion for patients with mild and flexible cervical kyphosis and anterior decompression and circumferential arthrodesis for those with severe kyphotic deformity or in patients with neurologic deficits. The potential for dural ectasia should be considered in patients with Larsen syndrome. Jain et al. listed CT or MRI findings of enlargement of the dural sac, vertebral body scalloping, narrowing of the pedicles, and an enlarged spinal canal as highly indicative of dural ectasia.

POSTERIOR SPINAL FUSION FOR CERVICAL KYPHOSIS THROUGH A LATERAL APPROACH

TECHNIQUE 7.20

(SAKAURA ET AL.)

- Place the patient in the right decubitus position.
- Make an incision along the posterior margin of the sternocleidomastoid muscle (Fig. 7.44A) and bluntly dissect

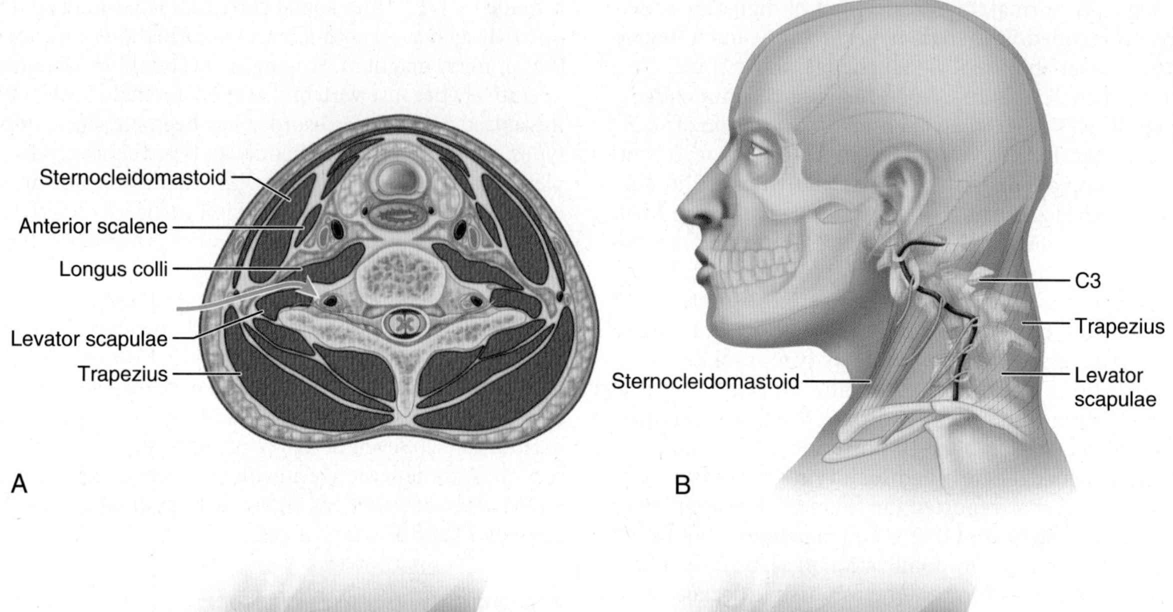

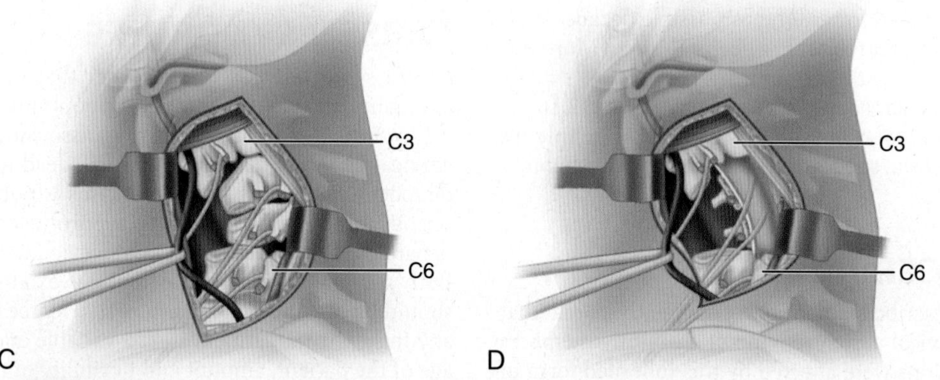

FIGURE 7.44 Sakaura et al. anterior decompression and arthrodesis through a lateral approach. **A,** Axial image of lateral approach to cervical spine. **B,** Vertebral artery and C4-C6 nerve roots posterior to the vertebral artery. **C,** Vertebral artery anteriorly dislocated by resecting transverse processes from C3 to C6. **D,** Subtotal removal of C4 and C5 bodies and cutting of posterior longitudinal ligament. (A from Sakaura H, Matsuoka T, Iwasaki M, et al: Surgical treatment of cervical kyphosis in Larsen syndrome, *Spine* 32:E39-44, 2007.) **SEE TECHNIQUE 7.20.**

fascia of the posterior triangle of the neck to identify the levator scapulae muscle.

- Retract the carotid sheath and sternocleidomastoid muscle ventrally and the levator scapulae muscle dorsally to expose the scalene muscles.
- Identify the phrenic nerve and carefully dissect the insertions of the anterior scalene muscles from the anterior tubercles of the transverse processes from the C3 to C6 vertebrae. Also, dissect the longus colli and capitis muscles from the anterior tubercles to identify the anterior aspect of the cervical spine.
- Identify the vertebral artery and C4 to C6 nerve roots lying posterior to the vertebral artery (Fig. 7.44A and B). Retract the vertebral artery anteriorly and resect the transverse process from C3 to C6 (Fig. 7.44C).
- Release and cut the tight cartilaginous tissue and anterior longitudinal ligaments attaching to the cervical vertebrae ventrally.
- Using a surgical microscope, expose the lateral aspect of the dura from C4 to C5 by removing the left lateral masses and pedicles of the C4 and C5 vertebrae with a rongeur and a diamond-headed airtome. This allows removal of the vertebral bodies of the C4 and C5 vertebrae including the discs between C3 and C4 and C5 and C6 with clear exposure of the nerve roots and dura.
- Remove the vertebral bodies and discs starting at the middle of the bodies and discs. Using a diamond burr, thin the dorsal cortices of the bodies to the width of the spinal canal.
- If the kyphosis cannot be manually corrected, then insert a thin spatula between the posterior longitudinal ligament and dura to avoid dural injury and cut the posterior longitudinal ligament at the middle of the exposed area (Fig. 7.44D). The vertebrae become slightly mobile, and the dura shifts ventrally. Under manual correction, insert an appropriate size strut from the tibia.
- Immobilize the patient in a halo device.

POSTOPERATIVE CARE The patient is immobilized in a halo cast or vest or a cervicothoracic orthosis for 12 weeks.

STERNAL-SPLITTING APPROACH TO THE CERVICOTHORACIC JUNCTION

Mulpuri et al. described a sternal splitting approach to the cervicothoracic junction in children that is useful for complex spinal deformities around the cervicothoracic junction. The approach requires the assistance of a cardiothoracic surgeon.

TECHNIQUE 7.21

(MULPURI ET AL.)

- Make a standard extensile anterior cervical spine approach, incorporating an anterior sternal extension (Fig. 7.45A).
- Complete the neck dissection in a standard fashion.
- Make an incision along the medial border of the sternomastoid muscle, extending down to the sternal notch.

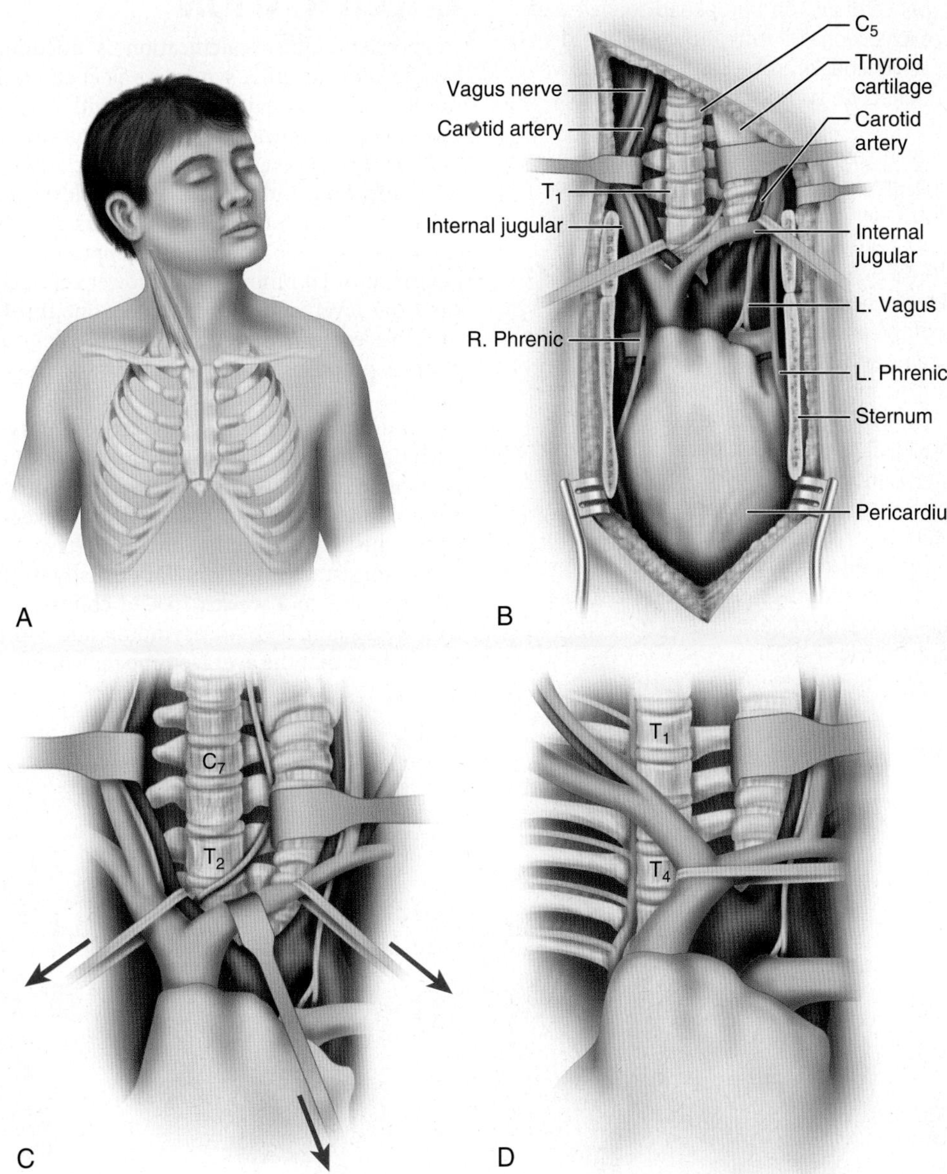

FIGURE 7.45 Mulpuri et al. sternal-split approach to cervicothoracic junction. **A,** Incision for right-sided approach. **B,** Sternum is opened, thymus gland is resected, and brachiocephalic trunk is mobilized to allow contiguous access to anterior cervical spine and upper thoracic spine. **C,** Retraction of trachea, esophagus, and innominate artery provides access to lower cervical spine and upper thoracic spine. **D,** Medial displacement of brachiocephalic trunk allows more distal access to thoracic spine. **SEE TECHNIQUE 7.21.**

- Retract the sternomastoid muscle laterally with the neurovascular sheath, including the carotid artery, the jugular vein, and the vagus nerve. Division of the omohyoid, sternohyoid, and sternothyroid muscles facilitates extensile exposure.
- Extend the incision as a midline sternotomy approach.
- Use blunt digital dissection to mobilize the retrosternal soft tissues.
- Split the sternum using a sternal saw in a standard fashion.
- After opening the sternum, resect the thymus gland to provide exposure as well as mobilize and control the brachiocephalic trunk with a vessel loop.
- At this point, the anterior cervical spine and upper thoracic spine can be accessed contiguously (Fig. 7.45B).
- If necessary, the pericardium can be opened to increase mobility of the brachiocephalic trunk; however, the dissection of the brachiocephalic trunk can be done down to the pericardial reflection without opening the pericardium.
- Retract the trachea and esophagus slightly away from the midline with a right-angle retractor.
- Place a deep right-angle retractor under the innominate artery and pull it forward and downward as necessary to provide access to the lower cervical and upper thoracic spine (Fig. 7.45C).
- The distal extent of the exposure at this point depends on the patient's anatomy and deformity; in most patients, T4 can now be accessed and disc removal and instrumentation can be done safely. Aggressive distal exposure places the recurrent laryngeal nerve under traction and must be done carefully. Although left-sided anterior cervical approaches typically are preferred because of the distal course of the recurrent laryngeal nerve on that side, Mulpuri et al. used a right-sided approach with mobilization of the brachiocephalic trunk because medial displacement of the trunk exposes more segments of the thoracic spine on the right side (Fig. 7.45D).
- After completion of the orthopaedic procedure, obtain hemostasis and approximate the sternum with wires or sutures depending on the age of the child.
- Reattach the sternothyroid and omohyoid muscles.
- Close the neck incision in usual fashion. A small Silastic drain may be required under the sternothyroid muscle if hemostasis is a problem in the cervical portion of the approach.
- Place a mediastinal tube as in cardiac surgical procedures.

INTERVERTEBRAL DISC CALCIFICATION

Intervertebral disc calcification is uncommon in children but does occur. This syndrome is characterized by an acute onset of cervical pain associated with torticollis and limited motion of the cervical spine. Although no definite cause has been identified, suggested causes include metabolic disease, local infection, and trauma. Most children with vertebral disc calcification are 5 months to 11 years old, and boys are more frequently affected than girls. Symptomatic disc calcification occurs most commonly in the lower cervical spine, usually at the C6-7 level, and approximately one third of patients have multiple levels involved. In children, calcification involves the nucleus pulposus, in contrast to the process in adults, which involves the annulus fibrosus (Fig. 7.46).

The most common symptoms of intervertebral disc calcification are neck pain, limitation of motion, and torticollis. Radicular pain or signs of nerve root compression are rare. Approximately 25% of patients have fever, 30% of patients have a history of trauma, and 15% have a history of upper respiratory tract infection. Pain usually begins suddenly and persists for 2 to 3 weeks; 75% of children are asymptomatic by 3 weeks, and 95% are asymptomatic within 6 months. Dai et al. found that the average time for symptoms to resolve was

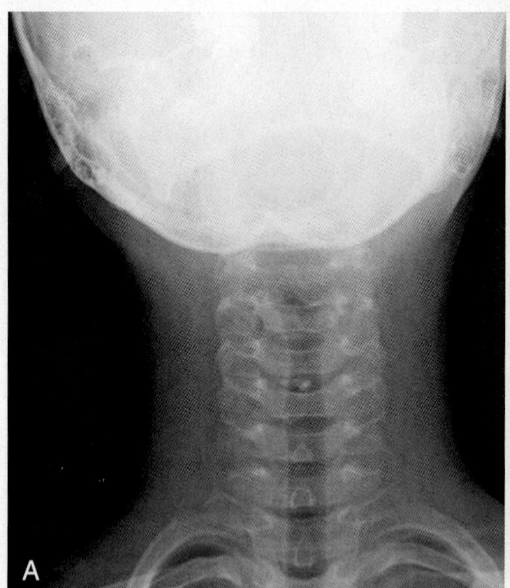

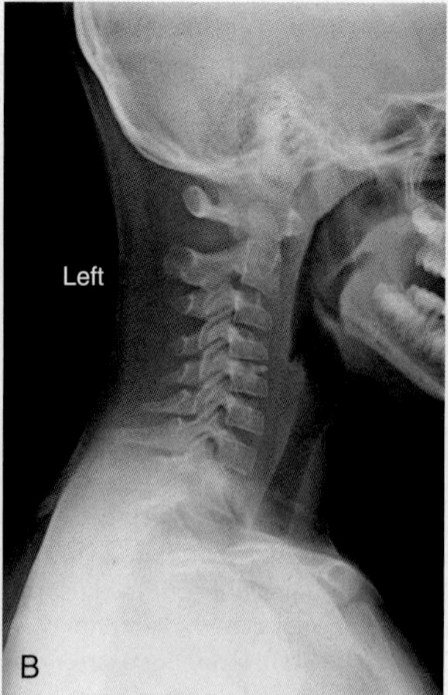

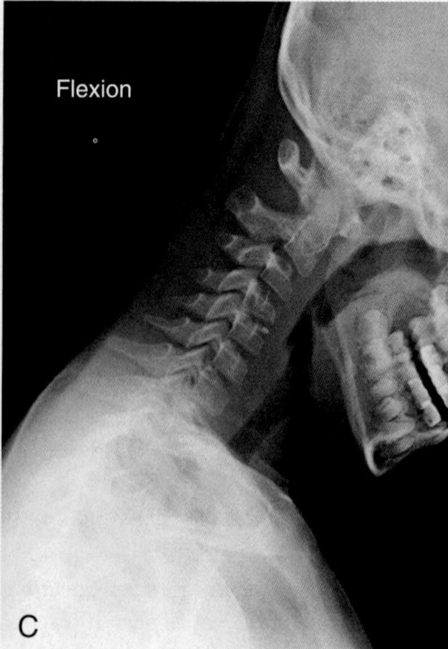

FIGURE 7.46 Intervertebral disc calcification in an 8-year-old boy.

34 days, and resolution of the calcifications was seen on radiographs by 15 months. Neurologic deficits, if present, improve in 90% of patients. Disc herniation is rare, but posterior herniations can cause spinal cord compression, and anterior herniations may result in dysphagia.

Appropriate treatment consists of rest, cervical immobilization, and analgesics. Rarely, symptomatic nerve root or spinal cord impingement requires anterior discectomy and fusion. The long-term effects of intervertebral disc calcification are unknown, but permanent changes around the adjacent vertebral bodies that may be associated with early degenerative changes have been reported in young adults.

REFERENCES

EMBRYOLOGY AND GROWTH AND DEVELOPMENT

Bapuraj JR, Bruzek AK, Tarpeh JK, et al.: Morphometric changes at the craniocervical junction during childhood, *J Neurosurg Pediatr*1–9, 2019, [Epub ahead of print].

Hita-Contreras F, Roda O, Martinez-Amat A, et al.: Embryonic and early fetal period development and morphogenesis of human craniovertebral junction, *Clin Anat* 27:337, 2014.

Kim HJ: Cervical spine anomalies in children and adolescents, *Curr Opin Pediatr* 25:72, 2013.

McKay SD, Al-Omari A, Tomlinson LA, Dormans JP: Review of cervical spine anomalies in genetic syndromes, *Spine (Phila Pa 1976)* 37:E269, 2012.

O'Brien Sr WT, Shen P, Lee P: The dens: normal development, developmental variants and anomalies, and traumatic injuries, *J Clin Imaging Sci* 5:38, 2015.

Pesenti S, Lafage R, Lafage V, et al.: Cervical facet orientation varies with age in children: an MRI study, *J Bone Joint Surg Am* 100:e57, 2018.

SURGICAL APPROACHES

Dalbayrak S, Yaman O, Yilmaz M, et al.: Results of the transsternal approach to cervicothoracic junction lesions, *Turk Neurosurg* 24:720, 2014.

Farah K, Pech-Gourg G, Graillon T, et al.: A new minimally invasive technique for primary unstable C2 spondylolysis in an 8-year-old child: a case report and review of the literature, *World Neurosurg* 115:79, 2018.

Harel R, Nulman M, Cohen ZR, et al.: Anterior cervical approach for the treatment of axial or high thoracic levels, *Br J Neurosurg*, 2018 May 10, [Epub ahead of print].

Yu M, Diao Y, Sun Y, et al.: Evaluation of a combined approach to the correction of congenital cervical or cervicothoracic scoliosis, *Spine J* 19:803, 2019.

ANOMALIES OF THE ODONTOID

Arvin B, Fournier-Gosselin MP, Fehlings MG: Os odontoideum: etiology and surgical management, *Neurosurgery* 66:A22, 2010.

Dlouhy BJ, Policeni BA, Menezes AH: Reduction of atlantoaxial dislocation prevented by pathological position of the transverse ligament in fixed, irreducible os odontoideum: operative illustrations and radiographic correlates in 41 patients, *J Neurosurg Spine* 27:20, 2017.

Kim IS, Hong JT, Jang WY, et al.: Surgical treatment of os odontoideum, *J Clin Neurosci* 18:481, 2011.

Klimo Jr P, Coon V, Brockmeyer D: Incidental os odontoideum: current management strategies, *Neurosurg Focus* 31:E10, 2011.

Koppula R, Singh A, Roberti F: Endoscopic transnasal resection of an Os odontoideum with preservation of the atlas: a short anatomic report, *Minim Invasive Neurosurg* 54:276, 2011.

Mazzatenta D, Zoli M, Mascari C, et al.: Endoscopic endonasal odontoidectomy: clinical series, *Spine (Phila Pa 1976)* 39:846, 2014.

Park JS, Cho DC, Sung JK: Feasibility of C2 translaminar screw as an alternative or salvage of C2 pedicle screws in atlantoaxial instability, *J Spinal Disord Tech* 25:254, 2012.

Perdikakis E, Skoulikaris N: The odontoid process: various configuration types in MR examinations, *Eur Spine J* 23:1077, 2014.

Weng C, Tian W, Li ZY, et al.: Surgical management of symptomatic os odontoideum with posterior screw fixation performed using the Magerl and Harms techniques with intraoperative 3-dimensional fluoroscopy-based navigation, *Spine (Phila Pa 1976)* 37:1839, 2012.

White D, Al-Mahfoudh R: The role of conservative management in incidental os odontoideum, *World Neurosurg* 88:695, 2016.

Yen YS, Chang PY, Huang WC, et al.: Endoscopic transnasal odontoidectomy without resection of nasal turbinates: clinical outcomes of 13 patients, *J Neurosurg Spine* 21:929, 2014.

Zwagerman NT, Tormenti MJ, Tempel ZJ, et al.: Endoscopic endonasal resection of the odontoid process: clinical outcomes in 34 adults, *J Neurosurg* 128:923, 2018.

Zygourakis CC, Cahill KS, Proctor MR: Delayed development of os odontoideum after traumatic cervical injury: support for a vascular etiology, *J Neurosurg Pediatr* 7:201, 2011.

BASILAR IMPRESSION

Cobanoglu M, Bauer JM, Campbell JW, et al.: Basilar impression in osteogenesis imperfecta treated with staged halo traction and posterior decompression with short-segment fusion, *J Craniovertebr Junction Spine* 9:212, 2018.

Dasenbrock HH, Clarke MJ, Bydon A, et al.: Endoscopic image-guided transcervical odontoidectomy: outcomes of 15 patients, *Neurosurgery* 70:359, 2012.

Hedequist D, Bekelis K, Emans J, Proctor MR: Single stage reduction and stabilization of basilar invagination after failed prior fusion surgery in children with Down's syndrome, *Spine* 35:E128, 2010.

Pinter NK, McVige J, Mechtler L: Basilar invagination, basilar impression, and platybasia: clinical and imaging aspects, *Curr Pain Heacache Rep* 20:49, 2016.

Smith JS, Shaffrey CI, Abel MF, Menezes AH: Basilar invagination, *Neurosurgery* 66:39, 2010.

Yu Y, Hu F, Zhang X, et al.: Endoscopic transnasal odontoidectomy combined with posterior reduction to treat basilar invagination: technical note, *J Neurosurg Spine* 19:637, 2013.

ATLANTOOCCIPITAL FUSION

Iyer RR, Tuite GF, Meoded A, et al.: A modified technique for occipitocervical fusion using compressed iliac crest allograft results in a high rate of fusion in the pediatric population, *World Neurosurg* 107:342, 2017.

Jeszenszky D, Fekete TF, Lattig F, et al.: Intraarticular atlantooccipital fusion for the treatment of traumatic occipitocervical dislocation in a child: a new technique for selective stabilization with nine years follow-up, *Spine (Phila Pa 1976)* 35:E421, 2010.

Kennedy BC, D'Amico RS, Youngerman BE, et al.: Long-term growth and alignment after occipitocervical and atlantoaxial fusion with rigid internal fixation in young children, *J Neurosurg Pediatr* 17:94, 2016.

Sharma DK, Sharma D, Sharma V: Atlantooccipital fusion: prevalence and its development and clinical correlation, *J Clin Diagn Res* 11:AC01, 2017.

Vedantam A, Hansen D, Briceno V, et al.: Patient-reported outcomes of occipitocervical and atlantoaxila fusions in children, *J Neurosurg Pediatr* 19:85, 2017.

KLIPPEL-FEIL SYNDROME

Bettegowda C, Sharjari M, Suk I, et al.: Sublabial approach for the treatment of symptomatic basilar impression in a patient with Klippel-Feil syndrome, *Neurosurgery* 69(ONS Suppl 1):ons77, 2011.

Gruber J, Saleh A, Bakhsh W, et al.: The prevalence of Klippel-Feil syndrome: a computed tomography-based analysis of 2,917 patients, *Spine Deform* 6:448, 2018.

Moses JT, Williams DM, Rubert PT, et al.: The prevalence of Klippel-Feil syndrome in pediatric patients: analysis of 831 CT scans, *J Spine Surg* 5:66, 2019.

Ogihara N, Takahashi J, Hirabayashi H, et al.: Surgical treatment of Klippel-Feil syndrome with basilar invagination, *Eur Spine J* 22(Suppl 3):S380, 2013.

Samartzis D, Kalluri P, Herman J, et al.: Cervical scoliosis in the Klippel-Feil patients, *Spine* 36:E1501, 2011.

Xue X, Shen J, Zhang J, et al.: Klippel-Feil syndrome in congenital scoliosis, *Spine (Phila Pa 1976)* 39:E1343, 2014.

ATLANTOAXIAL ROTATORY SUBLUXATION

Beier AD, Vachhrajani S, Bayerl SH, et al.: Rotatory subluxation: experience from the Hospital for Sick Children, *J Neurosurg Pediatr* 9:144, 2012.

Hannonen J, Perhomaa M, Salokorpi N, et al.: Interventional magnetic resonance imaging as a diagnostic and therapeutic method in treating acute pediatric atlantoaxial rotatory subluxation, *Exp ther Med* 18:18, 2019.

Iaccarino C, Franceca O, Piero S, et al.: Grisel's syndrome: non-traumatic atlantoaxial rotatory subluxation—report of five cases and review of the literature, *Acta Neurochir Suppl* 125:279, 2019.

Mifsud M, Abela M, Wilson NI: The delayed presentation of atlantoaxial rotatory fixation in children: a review of the management, *Bone Joint J* 98-B:715, 2016.

Neal KM, Mohamed AS: Atlantoaxial rotatory subluxation in children, *J Am Acad Orthop Surg* 23:382, 2015.

Ozalp H, Hamzaogl V, Avci E, et al.: Early diagnosis of Grisel's syndrome in children with favorable outcome, *Child's Nerv Syst* 35:113, 2019.

Spiegel D, Shrestha S, Sitoula P, et al.: Atlantoaxial rotatory displacement in children, *World J Orthop* 8:836, 2017.

Wang S, Yan M, Passias PG, et al.: Atlantoaxial rotatory fixed dislocation: report on a series of 32 pediatric cases, *Spine (Phila Pa 1976)* 41:E725, 2016.

Wu X, Li Y, Tan M, et al.: Long-term clinical and radiologic postoperative outcomes after C1-C2 pedicle screw techniques for pediatric atlantoaxial rotatory dislocation, *World Neurosurg* 115:e404, 2018.

CERVICAL INSTABILITY IN DOWN SYNDROME

Ando K, Kobayashi K, Ito K, et al.: Occipitocervical or C1-C2 fusion using allograft bone in pediatric patients with Down syndrome 8 years of age or younger, *J Pediatr Orthop B* 28:405, 2019.

Bull MJ, Committee on Genetics: Health supervision for children with Down syndrome, *Pediatrics* 128:393, 2011.

Dedlow ER, Siddiqi S, Fillipps DJ, et al. Symptomatic atlantoaxial instability in an adolescent with trisomy 21 (Down's syndrome), *Clin Pediatr (Phila)* 52:633–638, 2013.

Hankinson TC, Anderson RC: Craniovertebral junction abnormalities in Down syndrome, *Neurosurgery* 66(Suppl 3):32, 2010.

Hofler RC, Pecoraro N, Jones GA: Outcomes of surgical correction of atlantoaxial instability in patients with Down syndrome: systematic review and meta-analysis, *World Neurosurg*, 2018 Feb 18, [Epub ahead of print].

Ito K, Imagama S, Ito Z, et al.: Screw fixation for atlantoaxial dislocation related to Down syndrome in children younger than 5 years, *J Pediatr Orthop B* 26:86, 2017.

Nakamura N, Inaba Y, Aota Y, et al.: New radiological parameters for the assessment of atlantoaxial instability in children with Down syndrome: the normal values and the risk of spinal cord injury, *Bone Joint J* 98-B:1704–1710, 2016.

Nakamura N, Inaba Y, Oba M, et al.: Novel 2 radiographical measurements for atlantoaxial instability in children with Down syndrome, *Spine (Phila Pa 1976)* 39:E1566, 2014.

Scollan JP, Alhammoud A, Tretiakov M, et al.: The outcomes of posterior arthrodesis for atlantoaxial subluxation in Down syndrome patients: a meta-analysis, *Clin Spine Surg* 31:300, 2018.

Tomlinson C, Campbell A, Hurley A, et al.: Sport preparticpation screening for asymptomatic atlantoaxial instability in patients with Down syndrome, *Clin J Sport Med*, 2018 Aug 15, [Epub ahead of print].

Warner WC, Hedequist DJ: Cervical spine injuries in children. In Waters PM, Skaggs DL, Flynn JM, editors: *Rockwood and Wilkins' fractures in children*, ed 9, Philadelphia, Wolters Kluwer, 2020, p 800.

LARSEN SYNDROME

Jain VV, Anadio JM, Chang G, et al.: Dural ectasia in a child with Larsen syndrome, *J Pediatr Orthop* 34:e44, 2014.

McKay SD, Al-Omari A, Tomilson LA, et al.: Review of cervical spine anomalies in genetic syndromes, *Spine (Phila Pa 1976)* 37:E269, 2012.

Mohindra S, Savardekar A: Management of upper cervical kyphosis in an adolescent with Larsen's syndrome, *Neurol India* 60:262, 2012.

Yonekura T, Kamiyama M, Kimura K, et al.: Anterior mediastinal tracheostomy with a median mandibular splitting approach in a Larsen syndrome patient with posterior cervical arthrodesis, *Pediatr Surg Int* 31:1001, 2015.

INTERVERTEBRAL DISC CALCIFICATION

Bajard X, Renault F, Benharrats T, et al.: Intervertebral disc calcification with neurological symptoms in children: report of conservative treatment in two cases, *Childs Nerv Syst* 26:973, 2010.

Chu J, Wang T, Pei S, Yin Z: Surgical treatment for idiopathic intervertebral disc calcification in a child: case report and review of the literature, *Childs Nerv Syst* 31:123, 2015.

Ho C, Chang S, Fulkerson D, et al.: Children presenting with calcified disc herniation: a self-limiting process, *J Radiol Case Rep* 6:11, 2012.

Sasagawa T, Hashimoto F, Nakamura T, et al.: A pediatric case of single-level idiopathic cervical intervertebral disk calcification with symptom relapse 1 year after initial onset, *J Pediatr Orthop* 34:282, 2014.

Wu XD, Chen HJ, Yuan W, et al: Giant calcified thoracic disc herniation in a child: a case report and review of the literature, *J Bone Joint Surg Am* 92:1992, 2010.

The complete list of references is available online at Expert Consult.com.

CHAPTER 8

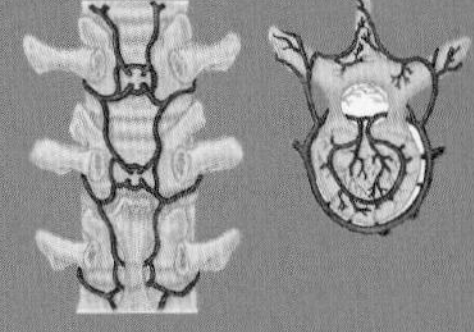

SCOLIOSIS AND KYPHOSIS

William C. Warner Jr., Jeffrey R. Sawyer

SCOLIOSIS

The word *scoliosis* is derived from the Greek word meaning "crooked." Scoliosis is defined as a lateral deviation of the normal vertical line of the spine. The lateral curvature of the spine also is associated with rotation of the vertebrae. This produces a three-dimensional deformity of the spine that occurs in the sagittal, frontal, and coronal planes.

The Scoliosis Research Society (SRS) recommends that idiopathic scoliosis be classified according to the age of the patient when the diagnosis is made. Infantile scoliosis occurs from birth to 3 years of age; juvenile idiopathic scoliosis, between the ages of 4 and 10 years; and adolescent idiopathic scoliosis, between 10 years of age and skeletal maturity. This traditional chronologic definition of scoliosis is important because major differences exist between the subtypes (Table 8.1).

Scoliosis also can be classified based on the cause and associated conditions. Idiopathic scoliosis is the most common type, but the exact cause of this type of scoliosis is not known. Congenital scoliosis is caused by a failure in vertebral formation or segmentation of the involved vertebrae. Scoliosis also can be classified based on associated conditions, such as neuromuscular disorders (cerebral palsy, muscular dystrophy, or other neuromuscular disorders), associated syndromes, or generalized disease (neurofibromatosis, Marfan syndrome, bone dysplasia, tumors, or as a result of irradiation).

A distinction should be made between early-onset and late-onset scoliosis because the deformity may affect cardiopulmonary development. During childhood, not only do the lungs grow in size, but also the alveoli and arteries multiply and the pattern of vascularity changes. The alveoli in the pulmonary tree increase by about 10-fold between infancy and 4 years of age and are not completely developed until 8 years of age. Scoliotic deformity limits the space available for lung growth, and children who develop significant scoliosis before the age of 5 years generally have disabling dyspnea or cardiorespiratory failure. Currently, according to the classification as it relates to treatment, some infantile and early juvenile curves are being identified as early-onset scoliosis.

INFANTILE IDIOPATHIC SCOLIOSIS

Infantile idiopathic scoliosis is a structural, lateral curvature of the spine occurring in patients younger than age 3 years. James, who first used the term *infantile idiopathic scoliosis,* noted that these curves occurred before 3 years of age, were more frequent in boys than in girls, and were primarily thoracic and convex to the left.

Wynne-Davies noted plagiocephaly in 97 children in whom curves developed in the first 6 months of life; the flat side of the head was on the convex side of the curve. Other associated conditions that she found were intellectual impairment in 13%, inguinal hernias in 7.4% of boys with progressive scoliosis, developmental dislocation of the hip in 3.5%, and congenital heart disease in 2.5% of all patients. This led her to believe that the etiologic factors of infantile idiopathic scoliosis are multiple, with a genetic tendency that is either "triggered" or prevented by external factors.

Infantile idiopathic scoliosis is more common in Europe than in North America. In the early 1970s, infantile scoliosis was seen in 41% of patients with idiopathic scoliosis in Great Britain compared with less than 1% in the United States. This difference was believed to be from infant positioning (Fig. 8.1). Supine positioning was recommended in Europe, and prone positioning was recommended in the United States. Since the change to prone positioning, the incidence of infantile idiopathic scoliosis has declined in Great Britain from 41% to 4%.

Most curves in infantile idiopathic scoliosis are self-limiting and spontaneously resolve (70% to 90%); however, some curves may be progressive, usually increasing rapidly, are often difficult to manage, and may result in significant deformity and pulmonary impairment. Unfortunately, when

TABLE 8.1

Classification of Idiopathic Scoliosis by Age

PARAMETER	INFANTILE	JUVENILE	ADOLESCENT
Age at presentation	Birth to 3 yr	4-9 yr	10-20 yr
Male:female	1:1 to 2:1	<6 yr: 1:3 >6 yr: 1:6	1:6
Incidence	United States: 2%-3% Great Britain: 30%	United States: 12%-15% Great Britain: 12%-15%	United States: 85% Great Britain: 55%
Curve types	Left thoracic L:R (2:1) Left thoracic/right lumbar	Right thoracic R:L (6:1)	Right thoracic R:L (8:1)
Associated findings	Mental deficiency, congenital hip dysplasia, plagiocephaly, congenital heart defects	None	None
Risk of cardiopulmonary compromise	High	Intermediate	Low
Risk of curve progression	<6 mo: low >1 yr: high	67%	23%
Rate of curve progression	Gradual progression: 2-3 degrees/yr Malignant progression: 10 degrees/yr	Progression at puberty: 6 degrees/yr Malignant progression: 10 degrees/yr	1-2 degrees/mo during puberty
Curve resolution	<1 yr: 90% >1 yr: 20%	20%	Rare
Curve magnitude and maturity	Gradual progression: 70-90 degrees Malignant progression: >90 degrees	Progression at puberty: 50-90 degrees Malignant progression: >90 degrees	Curves >90 degrees are rare
Orthotic management	Effective at delaying and slowing rate of progression Ultimate progression: 100%	Decreases rate of progression until puberty (failure rate: 30%-80%)	Effectively controls curves <40 degrees (success rate: 75%-80%)
Surgical treatment	Instrumentation without fusion <8 yr After 8 yr: ASF-PSF After 11 yr: PSF	Instrumentation without fusion <8 yr After 8 yr: ASF-PSF After 1 yr: PSF	PSF with instrumentation ASF if younger than 11 yr with open triradiate cartilage
Risk of crankshaft	High	High	Low

ASF, Anterior spinal fusion; *PSF,* posterior spinal fusion.
Modified from Mardjetko SM: Infantile and juvenile scoliosis. In Bridwell KH, DeWald RL, editors: *The textbook of spinal surgery*, ed 2, Philadelphia, 1997, Lippincott-Raven.

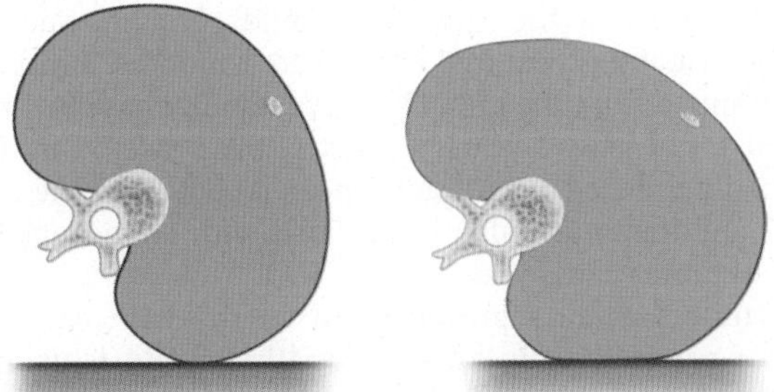

FIGURE 8.1 Diagram illustrates postural molding of thorax when infant is laid supine and partly turned toward the side.

a curve is mild, no absolute criteria are available for differentiating the two types and predicting progression. James et al. found that those with resolving scoliosis generally had a deformity that was noted before 1 year of age; most had smaller curves at presentation, and none had compensatory curves. Lloyd-Roberts and Pilcher found that curves associated with plagiocephaly or other molding abnormalities were more likely to be resolving, indicating an intrauterine positioning cause of this scoliosis. According to James, when compensatory or secondary curves develop or when the curve measures more than 37 degrees by the Cobb method when first seen, the scoliosis probably will be progressive.

Mehta developed a method to differentiate resolving from progressive curves in infantile idiopathic scoliosis based on measurement of the rib-vertebral angle (RVA). She evaluated the relationship of the convex rib head and vertebral body of the apical vertebra by drawing one line perpendicular to the apical vertebral endplate and another from the midneck to the midhead of the corresponding rib; the angle formed by the intersection of these lines is the RVA (Fig. 8.2). The RVA difference (RVAD) is the difference between the values of the RVAs on the concave and convex sides of the curve. Mehta reported that 83% of the curves

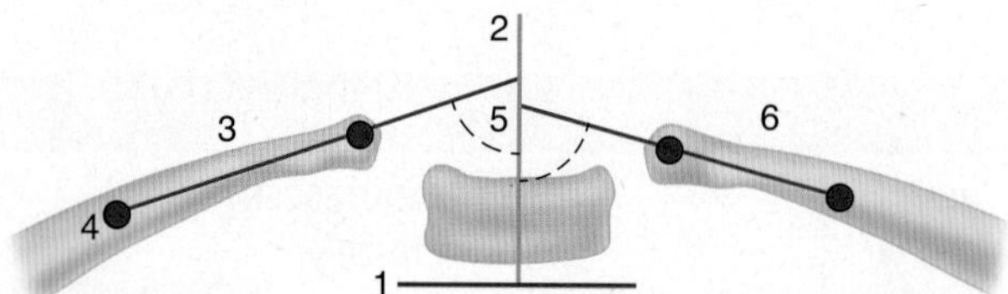

FIGURE 8.2 Construction of rib-vertebral angle (RVA) and rib–vertebral angle difference (RVAD). *(1)* Draw line parallel to bottom of apical vertebra (apical vertebral endplate). *(2)* Draw line perpendicular to line drawn in Step 1. *(3)* Find midpoint of head of rib. Find midpoint of neck of rib. These landmarks are estimated and mental note is taken. *(4)* Draw line from midpoint of head of rib to midpoint of neck of rib to line from Step 2. *(5)* Resulting angle is RVA for one side. *(6)* To calculate RVAD, calculate RVA for other side. Use lines created in Steps 1 and 2, and repeat Steps 3-5 for other side. (From Corna J, Sanders JO, Luhmann SJ, et al: Reliability of radiographic measures for infantile idiopathic scoliosis, *J Bone Joint Surg* 94A:e86, 2012.)

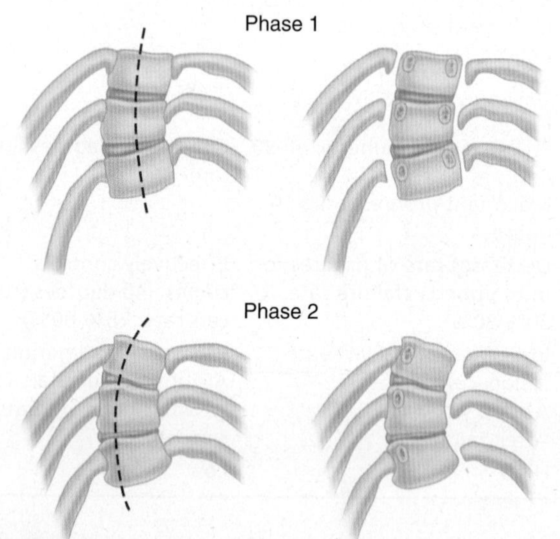

FIGURE 8.3 Two phases in progression of infantile scoliosis as seen on posteroanterior radiographs. *Phase 1*: rib head on convex side does not overlap vertebral body. *Phase 2*: rib head on convex side overlaps vertebral body. (Redrawn from Herring JA, editor: *Tachdjian's pediatric orthopaedics*, ed 4, Philadelphia, 2008, Elsevier, p 337.)

resolved if the RVAD measured less than 20 degrees and that 84% of the curves progressed if the RVAD was greater than 20 degrees. She described a two-phase radiographic appearance based on the relationship of the apical ribs with the apical vertebra. In phase 1, the rib head on each side of the apical vertebra does not overlap the vertebral body. In phase 2, the rib head overlaps the convex side of the vertebral body. Phase 2 curves are progressive, and therefore the measurement of RVAD is unnecessary. These measurements are helpful in predicting curve progression, but the curves must be monitored closely to prevent severe progression with the resultant risk of restricted pulmonary disease. These measurements are helpful in predicting curve progression, but Corona et al. noted that these measurements should be used with care because of some variability of more than 10 degrees in 18% of paired observations. This highlights the necessity of closely monitoring curves both clinically and radiographically to prevent severe progression with the resultant risk of restricted pulmonary disease (Fig. 8.3).

An increased incidence of neural axis abnormalities (Chiari malformation, syrinx, low-lying conus, and brainstem tumor) has been noted on magnetic resonance imaging (MRI) in patients with infantile idiopathic scoliosis (21.7%). MRI evaluation is now recommended for infantile scoliosis for curves measuring more than 20 degrees. These patients usually require sedation for MRI. Pahys found a smaller percentage (13%) of patients with infantile scoliosis and intraspinal anomalies. Because of the need for sedation to obtain the MRI, close observation may be a reasonable alternative.

TREATMENT

Because of the favorable natural history in 70% to 90% of patients with infantile idiopathic scoliosis, active treatment often is not required. If the initial curve is less than 25 degrees and the RVAD is less than 20 degrees, observation with radiographic follow-up every 6 months is recommended. Most resolving curves correct by 3 years of age (Fig. 8.4); however, follow-up should continue even after resolution because scoliosis may recur in adolescence.

CASTING

Treatment options for children with progressive infantile idiopathic scoliosis curves include serial casting, bracing, and later fusion; preoperative traction to correct the curve followed by fusion; and growing rod or vertical expandable prosthetic titanium rib (VEPTR) instrumentation without fusion (Synthes, West Chester, PA). Once the diagnosis of a progressive curve is made based on either a progressive Cobb angle or an RVAD of more than 20 degrees, rib phase 2, or a double curve, treatment is recommended. An orthotist can make a satisfactory thoracolumbosacral orthosis (TLSO) or cervicothoracolumbosacral orthosis (CTLSO) for curves that are not too large. Progression of many infantile curves can be prevented and significant improvement can be obtained with the use of a well-fitting orthosis during the early period of skeletal growth. In a very young child, serial casting with general anesthesia may be required until the child is large enough for a satisfactory orthosis. The interval between cast changes is determined by the rate of the child's growth, but a cast change usually is required every 2 to 3 months. Brace wear is continued full time until the curve stability has been maintained for at least 2 years. At that point, brace wear can be gradually reduced. McMaster reported control of the curves in 22 children with infantile scoliosis with an average brace time of more than 6 years.

Sanders et al. reported good results with early casting for progressive infantile idiopathic scoliosis using the technique of Cotrel and Morel (extension, derotation, flexion) cast correction. Best results were achieved if casting was started before 20 months of age and in curves less than 60 degrees. Cast correction in older patients with curves of more than 60 degrees frequently resulted in curve improvement (Fig. 8.5). Casts were changed every 2 to 4 months based on age and growth of the child. Once curves were corrected to less than 10 degrees, a custom-molded brace was used.

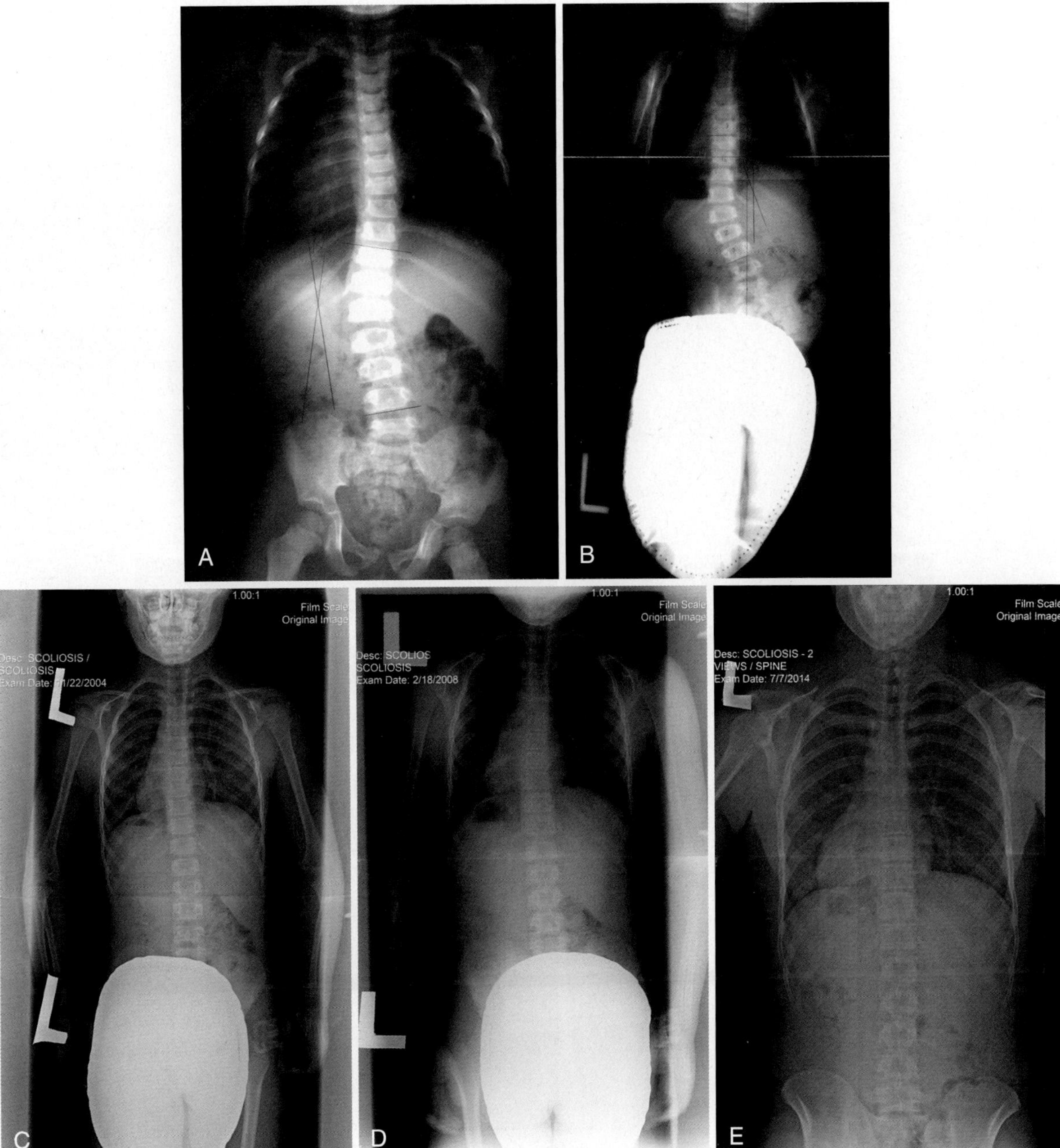

FIGURE 8.4 **A,** Infantile scoliosis in 3-year-old child. **B,** At 4 years of age. **C,** At 6 years of age, curve has greatly improved and by 10 years of age **(D)** has resolved. **E,** At follow-up at age 16, there is no curve progression.

CASTING FOR IDIOPATHIC SCOLIOSIS

A proper casting table is crucial for this procedure. Although a standard Risser frame will suffice, it is quite large for small children. Sanders et al. have designed a table that leaves the head, arms, and legs supported but the body free for cast application.

TECHNIQUE 8.1

- Intubate the patient; thoracic pressure during cast molding can make ventilation temporarily difficult.
- Use a silver-impregnated shirt as the innermost layer. Head halter and pelvic traction also are used to assist in stabilizing the patient and in narrowing the body (Fig. 8.6A).
- A mirror slanted under the table is useful for viewing rib prominence, the posterior cast, and molds.
- Apply a thin layer of Webril with occasional felt on bony prominences.
- If there is a lumbar curve, flex the hips slightly to decrease lumbar lordosis and facilitate curve correction.
- Plaster is usually preferred over fiberglass because it is more moldable. The pelvic portion is the foundation of the cast and should be well molded.

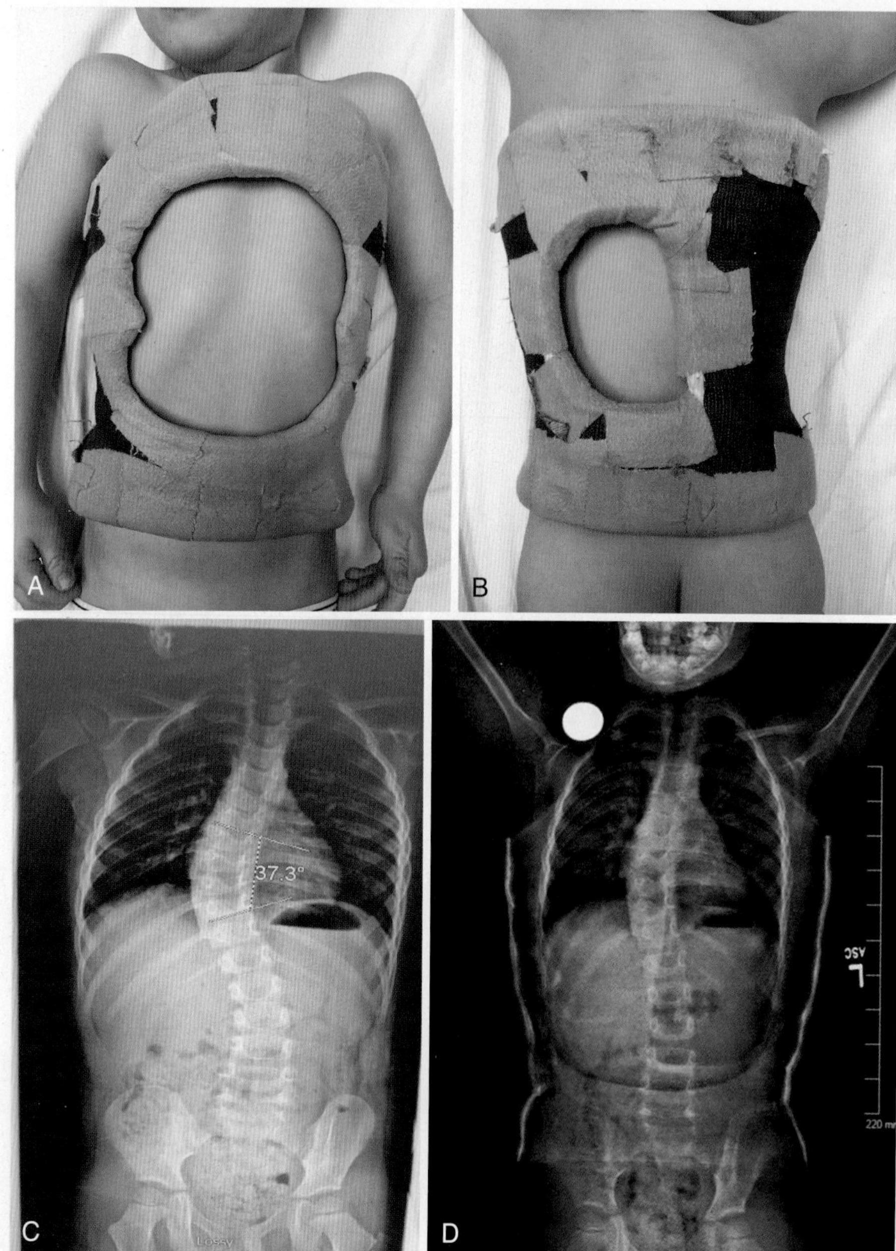

FIGURE 8.5 **A** and **B,** Mehta cast. **C,** Before cast wear. **D,** After 9 months of cast wear.

- Apply pressure to the posteriorly rotated ribs with an attempt to anteriorly rotate these ribs to create a more normal chest configuration with counterrotation applied through the pelvic mold and upper torso. This is a derotation maneuver and should not push the ribs toward the spine in an attempt to correct the curve (Fig. 8.6B).
- If the apex is T9 or below, an underarm cast can be used, but the original technique used an over-the-shoulder cast.
- Create an anterior window to relieve the chest and abdomen while preventing the lower ribs from rotating. Create a posterior window on the concave side to allow the depressed concave ribs and spine to move posteriorly (Fig. 8.6C).

OPERATIVE TREATMENT

If a curve is severe or increases despite the use of an orthosis or casting, surgical stabilization is needed. Ideally, surgery should not only stop progression of the curve but also allow continued growth of the thorax and development of the pulmonary tree. Growing rods can be used to control curve progression and still allow for growth of the spine (Video 8.1). This usually requires surgery every 6 months to lengthen the rods (see Technique 8.2 and Video 8.2). The use of magnetically controlled growing rods (MCGR), such as the MAGEC Spinal Bracing and Distraction System (NuVasive, Aliso Viejo, CA), may help avoid a return for surgical lengthening every 6 months; however, these should be used in carefully selected patients because of the size and stiffness of the magnetic implants. Rib-based instrumentation, such as VEPTR, has been reported as another alternative to correct the curve and allow for continued growth

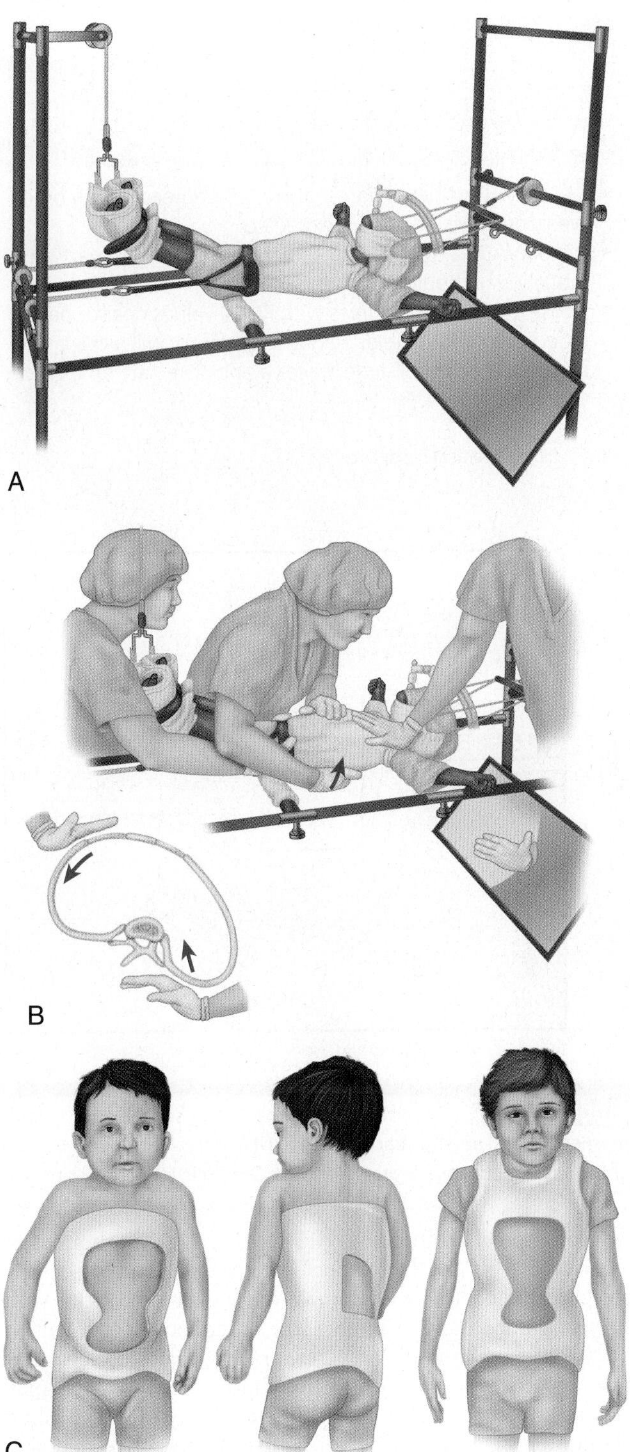

FIGURE 8.6 **A,** Position on table with traction applied to halter and pelvis. **B,** Example of correction maneuver for derotation of left thoracic curve. **C,** Underarm cast with windows. (Redrawn from Sanders JO, D'Astous J, Fitzgerald M, et al: Derotational casting for progressive infantile scoliosis, *J Pediatr Orthop* 29:581, 2009.) **SEE TECHNIQUE 8.1.**

of the spine, potentially decreasing the rate of autofusion seen with standard growing rods (see Technique 8.45). Schulz et al. reported this to be a safe and effective treatment of progressive curves in this patient population. When surgical fusion is necessary, a relatively short anterior and posterior arthrodesis should be considered, including only the structural or primary curve. Combined anterior and posterior arthrodesis is necessary to prevent the "crankshaft" phenomenon. The problem with this approach is that it leaves the child with a straight, shortened spine rather than a deformed spine of near-normal length. Karol reported that, despite early fusion surgery, revision surgery was required in 24% to 39% of patients. Restrictive pulmonary disease, defined as forced vital capacity less than 50% of normal, occurs in 43% to 64% of patients who have early fusion surgery. Thoracic growth after early surgery is an average of 50% of that seen in children with scoliosis who did not have early surgery. Because of the deleterious effect on the developing thoracic cage and lung function, fusionless instrumentation techniques are preferred.

JUVENILE IDIOPATHIC SCOLIOSIS

Juvenile idiopathic scoliosis appears between the ages of 4 and 10 years. Multiple patterns can occur, but the convexity of the thoracic curve usually is to the right. Juvenile idiopathic scoliosis accounts for 12% to 21% of idiopathic scoliosis cases. The female-to-male ratio is 1:1 in children between 3 and 6 years of age. This ratio increases with age, with the ratio of 4:1 from 6 to 10 years of age, and reaches a female-to-male ratio of 8:1 by the time the children are 10 years of age. The natural history of juvenile idiopathic scoliosis is usually slow to moderate progression until the pubertal growth spurt. Lonstein found that 67% of patients younger than age 10 years showed curve progression and that the risk of progression was 100% in patients younger than 10 years who had curves of more than 20 degrees. Robinson and McMaster reported curve progression in 95% of children with juvenile idiopathic scoliosis. Of those patients followed to maturity, 86% required spinal fusion. Most juvenile curves are convex right thoracic curve or double thoracic curve patterns and closely resemble those of adolescent idiopathic scoliosis. Few patients with juvenile idiopathic scoliosis have thoracolumbar or lumbar curves. Dobbs et al. modified the adolescent idiopathic scoliosis classification system of Lenke for juvenile idiopathic scoliosis (see Fig. 8.33). (There are the same six curve types, but instead of using side-bending radiographs to distinguish structural from nonstructural minor curves the authors used the deviation from the midline of the apex of the curve from the C7 plumb line for thoracic curves and the center sacral vertical line (CSVL) for thoracolumbar and lumbar curves. If the apex of the curve is completely off the line, a structural minor curve is present; if the apex is not off the line, a nonstructural minor curve is present.)

As in infantile idiopathic scoliosis, a high incidence of neural axis abnormalities has been found on MRI in children younger than 11 years with scoliosis (26.7%). Some may argue about the need for MRI in a routine preoperative workup, but most would agree that specific factors indicating a need for further MRI evaluation include pain, rapid progression, left thoracic deformity, neurologic abnormalities (alterations in the superficial abdominal reflex), and other neurologic findings, such as loss of bowel or bladder control. If operative intervention is planned, then preoperative MRI evaluation is recommended.

TREATMENT

Although it is likely to progress and often requires surgery, juvenile idiopathic scoliosis is treated according to guidelines similar to those for adolescent idiopathic scoliosis. For curves of less than 20 degrees, observation is indicated, with examination and standing posteroanterior radiographs every 4 to 6 months. Evidence of progression on the radiographs as indicated by a change of at least 5 to 7 degrees warrants brace treatment. If the curve is not progressing, observation is continued until skeletal maturity.

Although much of the earlier literature concerning orthotic treatment of juvenile idiopathic scoliosis had emphasized the Milwaukee brace, a TLSO is used for thoracic curves with the apex at T8 or below. Initially, the brace is worn full time (22 of 24 hours). If the curve improves after at least 1 year of full-time bracing, the hours per day of brace wear can be decreased gradually to a nighttime-only bracing program, which is much more tolerable, especially when the child reaches puberty. However, the patient is carefully observed for any sign of curve progression during this weaning process. If curve progression is noted, a full-time bracing program is resumed.

The success of nonoperative treatment is variable; 27% to 56% require spinal fusion for progressive curves. It often is not possible to predict which curves will increase from the curve pattern, the degree of curvature, or the patient's age at the time of diagnosis. Serial RVAD measurements have been useful to evaluate brace treatment; several guidelines can be formulated for evaluating brace treatment (Box 8.1).

Evidence of progression should be obtained before a brace is applied, unless the curve is greater than 30 degrees when the juvenile patient is first seen. Some curves, even in the range of 20 to 30 degrees, did not progress during a period of several months in one study; Mannherz et al. found progressive RVAD of more than 10 degrees over time to be associated with curve progression, and more frequent curve progression was noted in patients with less than 20 degrees of thoracic kyphosis. Double major curves tended to progress most often. Charles et al. reported that juvenile curves of more than 30 degrees had a 100% risk of progression to a surgical range, underscoring the importance of beginning treatment in curves of more than 30 degrees.

Kahanovitz, Levine, and Lardone found that patients who wore a Milwaukee brace part time (after school and at night) had good outcomes with curves of less than 35 degrees and RVADs of less than 20 degrees. Patients with curvatures of greater than 45 degrees at the onset of bracing and whose RVADs exceeded 20 degrees all eventually underwent spinal fusion. Patients with curvatures from 35 to 45 degrees at the onset of bracing had much less predictable prognoses. The part-time brace program consisted of wearing the brace after school and all night for approximately a year. The patients were then kept in the brace at night only for another 2.5 years. The brace was at that point worn every other night for an average of 1.2 years. Bracing generally was discontinued completely at an average of about 14 years of age. Individually, however, the number of hours spent wearing the brace depended on the amount of improvement and stability of the curvature. Part-time brace treatment may afford these children the social and psychologic benefits not provided by a full-time brace program. Jarvis et al. reported the successful management (prevention of surgery) with part-time bracing in patients with juvenile idiopathic scoliosis. The Milwaukee brace may be preferred because it does not cause chest wall compression in these young patients. A total-contact TLSO often is prescribed, but rib cage distortion is possible because of the lengthy time the child must wear the brace. Robinson and McMaster found that the level of the most rotated vertebra at the apex of the primary curve was the most useful factor in determining the prognosis of patients with juvenile idiopathic scoliosis. Patients who had a curve apex at T8, T9, or T10 had an 80% chance of requiring spinal arthrodesis by 15 years of age. Khoshbin et al. reported that 50% of their patients progressed to surgery despite brace treatment. The operative rate was higher for patients with curves of more than 30 degrees at the start of brace treatment.

BOX 8.1

Evaluation of Brace Treatment of Juvenile Idiopathic Scoliosis by the Rib–Vertebral Angle Difference

- If the RVAD values progress above 10 degrees during brace wear, progression can be expected.
- If the RVAD values decline as treatment continues, part-time brace wear should be adequate.
- Those patients with curves with RVAD values near or below 0 degrees at the time of diagnosis generally will require only a short period of full-time brace wear before part-time brace wear is begun.

RVAD, Rib–vertebral angle difference.

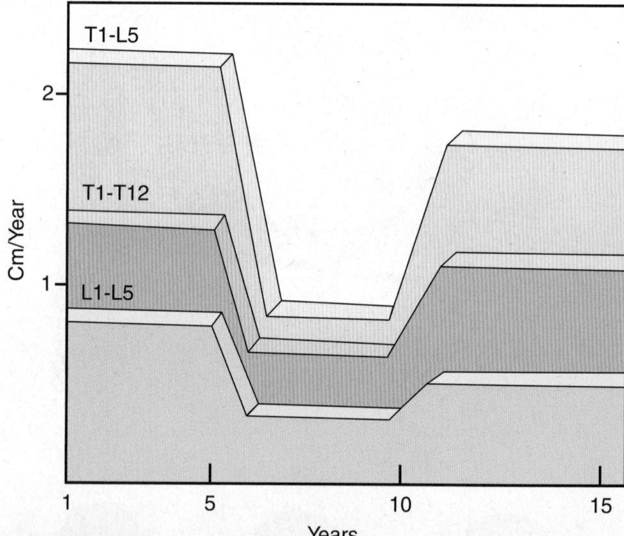

FIGURE 8.7 Growth velocity of T1-L5 segment, thoracic segment T1-12, and lumbar segment L1-L5. (From Dimeglio A: Growth of the spine before age 5 years, *J Pediatr Orthop B* 1:102, 1993.)

Even if the curve progresses, bracing may slow progression and delay surgery until the child is older, which may avoid a short trunk and lessen the possibility of a crankshaft phenomenon. If orthotic treatment fails, operative management of the curve should be considered. Important considerations in the operative treatment of patients with juvenile idiopathic scoliosis are the expected loss of spinal height and the limited chest wall growth and lung development after spinal fusion. Another important consideration is the crankshaft phenomenon. With a solid posterior fusion, continued anterior growth of the vertebral bodies causes the vertebral body and discs to bulge laterally toward the convexity and to pivot on the posterior fusion, causing loss of correction, increase in vertebral rotation, and recurrence of the rib hump. Dimeglio found that during the first 5 years of life the spine from T1 to S1 grows more than 2 cm a year. Between the ages of 5 and 10 years, it grows 0.9 cm per year, and then it grows 1.8 cm per year during puberty (Fig. 8.7). A solid spinal fusion stops the longitudinal growth in the posterior elements, but the vertebral bodies continue to grow anteriorly.

There is no full agreement about the exact parameters for which a child requires anterior and posterior fusions to prevent crankshaft deformity (Figs. 8.8 and 8.9). Shufflebarger and Clark recommended that patients with a Risser sign of grade 0 or 1, a Tanner grade of less than 2, and a significant three-dimensional deformity have a preliminary anterior periapical fusion before posterior instrumentation and fusion. Sanders et al. noted that 10 of 43 patients with triradiate cartilage developed a crankshaft deformity after posterior-only fusion. An open triradiate physis in the pelvis indicates the need for supplementary anterior fusion. With superior correction and rotational control available with pedicle screw instrumentation, perhaps the need for anterior fusions could be lessened.

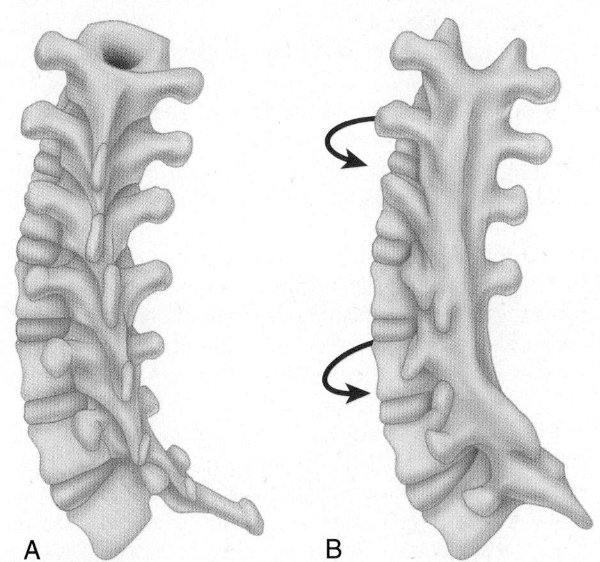

FIGURE 8.8 Crankshaft phenomenon. **A,** Spine with scoliosis. **B,** Despite solid posterior fusion, continued anterior growth causes increase in deformity.

If the child is younger than 8 years, is small, and has a curve that cannot be controlled by nonoperative means, the ideal treatment is a growing rod system without fusion or growth modulation techniques. If the child is 9 or 10 years of age or large, growing rods or growth modulation may still be used but instrumentation and fusion may be appropriate. A combined anterior and posterior spinal fusion to avoid the crankshaft phenomenon may be needed, but with the use of pedicle screws to allow better correction and derotation of the spine, an anterior fusion may not be necessary.

GROWING ROD INSTRUMENTATION

Growing rod instrumentation is a technique of posterior instrumentation that is sequentially lengthened to allow longitudinal growth while still attempting to control progressive spinal deformity.

Currently, growing rod techniques include the use of (1) a single growing rod, (2) dual growing rods, (3) VEPTR rods, (4) Luque trolley, and (5) Shilla technique. MCGR can help decrease the rate of surgical lengthening and can be used in a single- or dual-rod configuration, although a higher rate of rod failure occurs with single-rod instrumentation.

The growing rod techniques should be considered in a patient with significant growth remaining and a reliable family that will follow-up during treatment. This procedure usually is considered for patients younger than 10 years of age who have a curve of 60 degrees or more. Surgery typically is required every 6 months to lengthen the construct. A TLSO often is necessary for at least the first 3 to 6 months to protect the upper and lower levels of the instrumentation. Dual growing rods have been found to be effective in controlling severe spinal deformities and allowing spinal growth. With the use of dual rods, an apical fusion does not appear to be necessary during the course of treatment. Dual-rod techniques have been associated with a lower rate of complications than single-rod techniques, most commonly rod breakage and anchor failure.

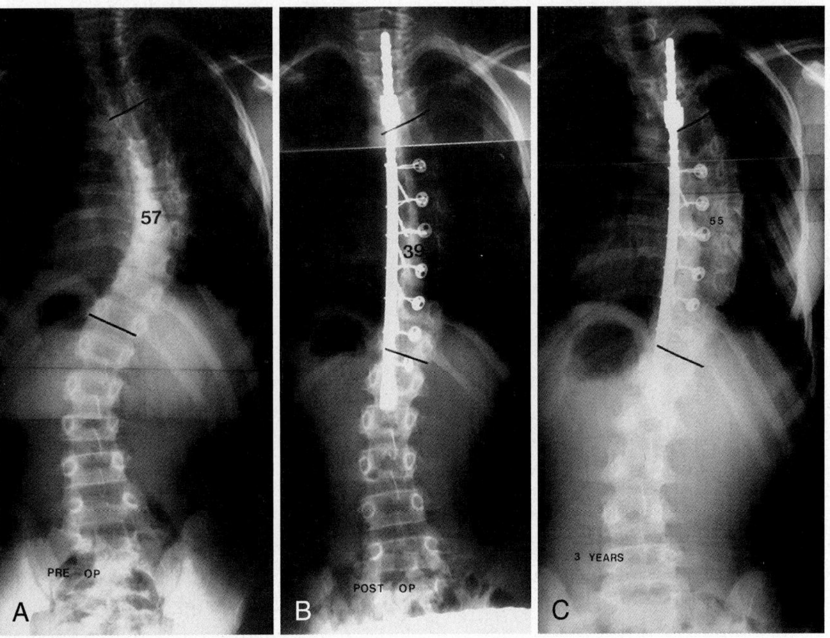

FIGURE 8.9 Fifty-seven-degree curve **(A)** was corrected to 39 degrees with posterior fusion and instrumentation **(B)**. **C,** Three years after surgery, deformity has recurred because of crankshaft phenomenon.

DUAL GROWING ROD INSTRUMENTATION WITHOUT FUSION

A spinal instrumentation system that is appropriate for the child's size is used and should include both pedicle screws and hooks for fixation. If the child weighs less than 30 lb, an infant spinal set may be necessary. If the infant set is used, the rod is quite flexible, and therefore some additional protection in the form of external immobilization is necessary until the system can be converted to a pediatric rod system of a larger diameter.

TECHNIQUE 8.2

- Place the patient prone on the operating table or frame; prepare and drape the back in the routine sterile fashion.
- Take care to select the stable vertebrae at both ends of the curve and make a single, long, straight incision into the subcutaneous tissue from the upper to the lower neutral vertebrae. Alternatively, cranial and caudal incisions can be made over the end vertebrae and the rods can be tunneled between them. Dede et al. described preservation of motion segments by using the "stable-to-be vertebra" on bending or traction films as the lowest instrumented vertebra. The stable-to-be vertebra is the vertebra that is transected by the center sacral line on traction or bending films (Fig. 8.10).
- Confirm appropriate levels with a radiograph.
- Carry the dissection down to the lamina and spinous process of the end vertebrae.
- Strip the periosteum from the concave and convex lamina out to the facet joint of the two vertebrae selected for instrumentation at each end of the curve.
- The upper and lower foundations for the growth rods can be done with either pedicle screws or hooks. If pedicle screws are used, especially in the upper thoracic spine, the use of a sublaminar wire or tape at the same level can be helpful in preventing axial pullout of the screws. If hooks are used to form the upper claw, insert a pedicle hook onto the lower of the two upper vertebrae and another superior transverse process hook on the upper of the two vertebrae on both the concave and convex sides.
- Form the lower claw by placing a supralaminar hook on the upper vertebra and the infralaminar hook on the lower vertebra. If it is anatomically feasible, pedicle screw fixation can be used in both the upper and lower foundations.
- Use two rods on the concave side and two rods on the convex side.
- Contour the rods to the natural contours of thoracic kyphosis and lordosis.
- Insert the rods under direct vision and use the appropriate set screws to hold the rods in the hooks or pedicle screws. Alternatively, tunnel the rods between the two incisions using a chest tube for guidance and to prevent intrathoracic penetration of the rod.
- Join the rods together with a low-profile growth rod connector (Fig. 8.11).
- Use local autograft and allograft bone to pack around the upper and lower foundation sites.
- Do not attempt subperiosteal dissection between the hook sites to minimize the risk of autofusion.

POSTOPERATIVE CARE The child is placed in an orthosis for the first 6 months depending on the quality of the anchor fixation. At that time, the orthosis can be discontinued if the anchor sites are solidly fused. The rods routinely are lengthened every 6 months depending on the growth rate of the child. Lengthening is performed by exposing the connector and loosening the set screws. Distraction is applied, and the set screws are retightened. Lengthenings are stopped when no further distraction can be achieved. Sankar et al. found that with successive lengthenings, there is a law of diminishing returns: repeated lengthenings had decreased gains in length with each subsequent lengthening over time. When no further distraction can be achieved, patients have typically undergone "final arthrodesis." This usually necessitates removal of the rods, and in our experience, if the proximal and distal anchors are still solidly fixed and well fused, they can be used as part of the final construct (Figs. 8.12 and

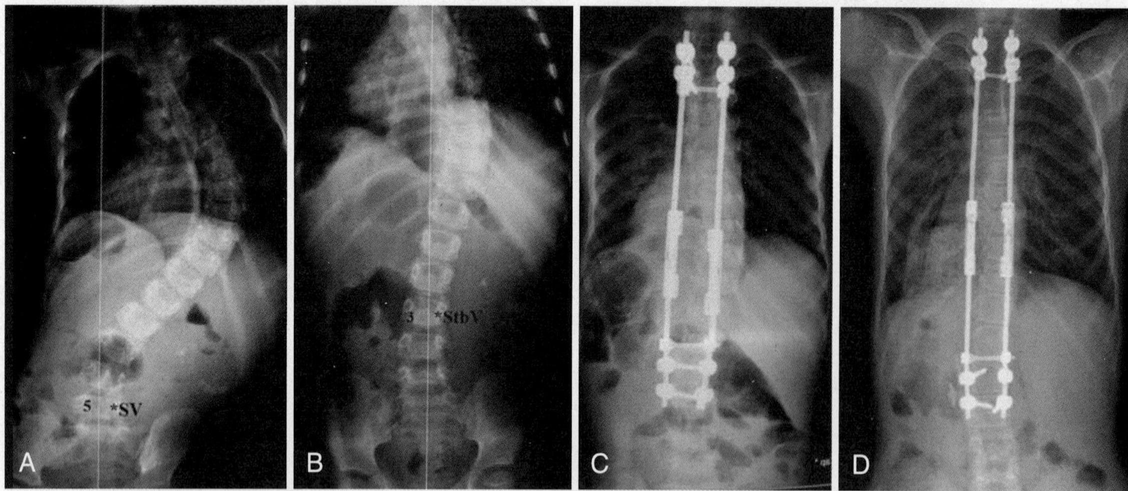

FIGURE 8.10 **The "stable-to-be vertebra" (StbV) is vertebra most closely bisected by central sacral vertical (SV) line. A, In this patient, stable-to-be vertebra is at L5. B, On traction radiograph, it is at L3. C, The patient was treated with growing rod instrumentation extending to L3. D, At 6-year follow-up, correction is well maintained with no evidence of distal adding on.** (From Dede O, Demirkiran G, Bekmez S, et al: Utilizing the "stable-to-be vertebra" saves motion segments in growing rods treatment of early-onset scoliosis, *J Pediatr Orthop* 36:336, 2016.)

8.13). "Final arthrodesis" in this setting has been associated with very little curve correction and a high complication rate. For this reason, patients with good deformity correction, sagittal and coronal balance, and well-fixed implants may be able to be observed with implants in place.

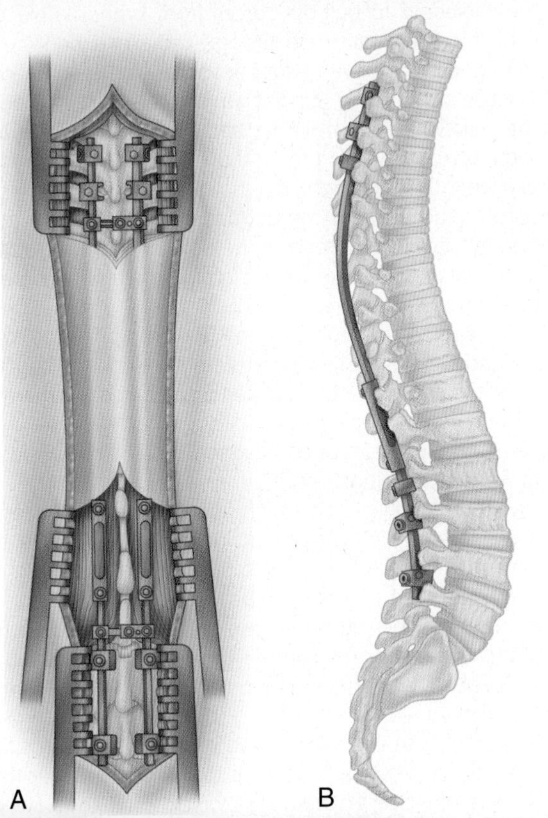

FIGURE 8.11 Technique of dual-rod instrumentation. **A,** Anteroposterior view. **B,** Lateral view showing construct contoured to maintain sagittal alignment. Extended tandem connectors are placed in thoracolumbar spine to minimize profile. **SEE TECHNIQUE 8.2.**

Other growing rod constructs include the Luque trolley and the Shilla technique. These techniques allow apical control while guiding the growth of the spine along the rod system. The Luque trolley consists of sublaminar wires and rods without fusion. The Shilla technique consists of a nonlocking pedicle screw implant. The apex of the deformity is fixed and fused with pedicle screws while the ends of the construct are instrumented with screws that are not locked to the rod. This theoretically allows for apical control of the deformity and continued axial lengthening of the spine with growth. While techniques such as that of Shilla have been shown to decrease the number of surgical episodes for patients, concerns exist about wear debris and implant prominence.

SHILLA GUIDED GROWTH SYSTEM

TECHNIQUE 8.3

(MCCARTHY ET AL.)

- Careful assessment of upright coronal and sagittal films, along with analysis of the flexibility of the curve by bending or traction films, is necessary to determine the location of the apical vertebral segments (Fig. 8.14). The apical three or four vertebral segments that are least corrected through flexibility testing are the apical levels for fusion and maximal correction.
- Place small needle markers in the spinous processes and obtain a radiograph to identify spinal levels.
- Make a single midline incision and perform subperiosteal dissection to only the apical levels.
- Incise the fascia 1 cm off the midline on both sides of the spinous processes from cephalad to caudad, merging with the subperiosteal dissection at the apex.
- Place bilateral fixed-head pedicle screws throughout the apical levels.

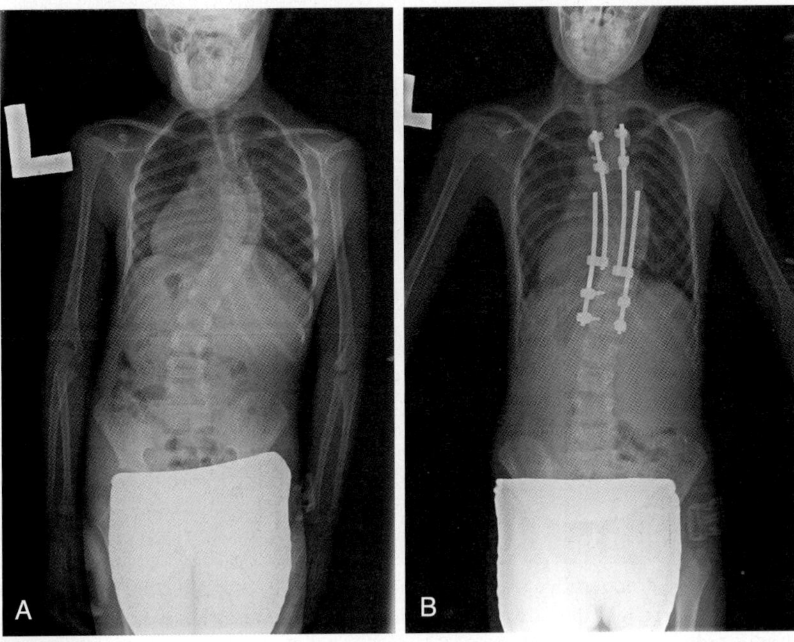

FIGURE 8.12 **A,** Posteroanterior radiograph of child with infantile scoliosis treated with dual growing rods **(B).**

- Perform Ponte osteotomies (see Technique 8.24) between the apical segments if needed to enhance correction in all planes. Apical decortication is necessary for fusion of these levels.
- Place the growth guidance screws through the muscular layer with fluoroscopic visualization of bone. Use a cannulated polyaxial screw of sufficient diameter to fill the pedicle. A Jamshidi trocar system is helpful in placing the screw in the center of the pedicle.
- The location of the guidance screws depends on the curve; the screw should extend far enough into the lumbar spine to maintain the lordosis and coronal correction. Avoid stopping the caudal instrumentation at the thoracolumbar junction because this may lead to prominence with flexion.
- Place the guidance screws at bilateral locations or staggered, making sure that they are separated by enough distance on the rod to allow for easy sliding.
- Because the guidance screws at the top of the construct are subjected to pull-out forces from kyphosis, place a sublaminar or transverse process cable or FiberWire (3 mm) one level above the upper screws to protect them.
- Choose a rod of the appropriate diameter for the size of the child, generally 4.5 mm, and contour it into normal sagittal curves, leaving the rod one vertebral level long at each length for growth.
- Before placement of the permanent rods, place a temporary (provisional) rod on the convex side and attach it loosely at the apex and one growing screw above and below the apex.
- Roll the provisional rod into a neutral position in the coronal and sagittal positions, translate it toward the concavity of the curve with coronal benders, and hold it there by tightening the apical plugs.
- Attach the permanent concave rod to the screws and remove the provisional rod.
- Derotate the apical levels with tube derotation devices or a vertebral column derotation device while holding the rods in place with vise grips to prevent rod rotation.
- The fixed-head screws lock the rods at the apical screws through the locking set screws that fix to the rods. The guidance screw caps capture the rods in the guidance screw head, leaving room for movement of the rod within the screw head.
- If needed to help maintain rod rotation, use a crosslink just below the apical fixation. If the child is younger than 5 years old, use a sliding type of crosslink to allow for growth in the canal diameter.
- Use the torque/countertorque device to snap off the caps at a preset torque pressure.
- Place bone graft at the apex only.
- Close the wound in routine fashion, using a small drain if necessary.

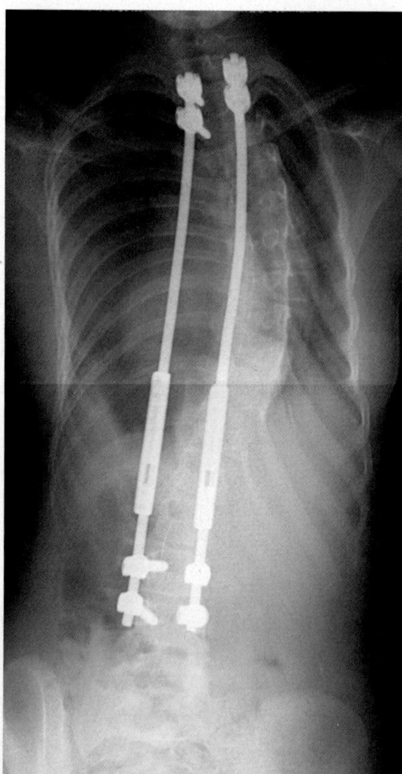

FIGURE 8.13 Growing rods. **SEE TECHNIQUE 8.2.**

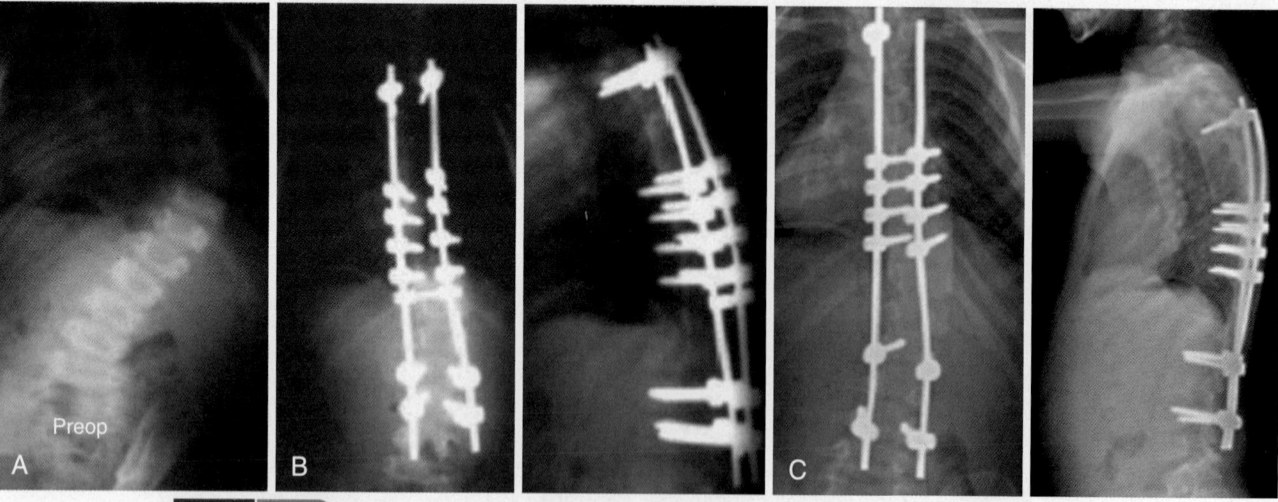

FIGURE 8.14 **A,** Preoperative standing radiograph of a 3-year-old child with infantile idiopathic scoliosis. **B,** Three-month postoperative radiographs after insertion of Shilla rods. **C,** Five-year postoperative radiographs. (From Medtronic: *Shilla Growth Guidance System*, 2012, Memphis, TN.) **SEE TECHNIQUE 8.3.**

POSTOPERATIVE CARE The child is immobilized for 3 months. A bivalved form-fitting turtle-shell brace is used during daytime until the apical fusion is solid. A protective brace is not necessary after this period of immobilization unless excessively vigorous activities are expected.

Growing rods do have potential complications, and complications are common. Bess et al. found at least one complication in 58% of patients with early-onset scoliosis who were treated with growing rods; submuscular placement of the rod resulted in fewer complications than subfascial placement. The most common complications are (1) rod breakage, (2) hook displacement or failure of proximal or distal fixation points, (3) infection, (4) skin breakdown over prominent rods, and (5) autofusion of the spine. Cahill et al. reported autofusion in 89% of children treated with growing rods. Arthrodesis after growing rod treatment has been associated with minimal curve correction in the coronal and sagittal planes, minimal gain in thoracic height, and a complication rate approaching 30% due primarily to spine stiffness, osteopenia from stress shielding, and infection from multiple previous surgical lengthenings. For these reasons, it may be reasonable for patients with well-balanced curves to be observed long term with their implants left in place, avoiding the risks of arthrodesis. A follow-up study of 100 patients treated with growing rods found that at 4-year follow-up, there was a 20% rate of unplanned return to the operating room, primarily for infection, device problems, and curve progression, highlighting the fact that "final arthrodesis" may not be final.

Rib-based instrumentation systems such as VEPTR can be used as a growing rod system (see Technique 8.45). The constructs can be rib-to-rib, rib-to-spine, or rib-to-pelvis. This has the advantage of minimal exposure of the spine and a theoretical decreased risk of spontaneous fusion of the spine. Another technique is to use a claw construct around ribs to act as the proximal attachment for dual growing rods. The advantage to using ribs as anchors instead of the spine is the preservation of motion between vertebrae, thereby preventing or delaying spontaneous fusion. The procedure is contraindicated in patients with kyphosis (upper thoracic kyphosis is poorly controlled with rib anchors) and patients who cannot tolerate repeated surgical procedures. This technique uses traditional spine implants with hooks that fit around the ribs. It is important to place the hook as close as possible to the transverse process to prevent the hook from sliding laterally (Fig. 8.15A,B). The rate of proximal (rib) anchor failure is inversely related to the number of rib anchor points, and ideally six to eight rib anchors (three or four on each side) should be used. Outriggers often can be used to increase the number of anchor points as well (Fig. 8.16).

GROWING ROD ATTACHMENT USING RIB ANCHORS

TECHNIQUE 8.4

(SANKAR AND SKAGGS)

- Position the patient prone, taking care to pad all bony prominences. Neuromonitoring is essential when performing this procedure and should include both the upper and lower extremities because of the proximity of the upper instrumentation to the brachial plexus when the second and third ribs are used. Fixation to the first rib should be avoided.
- Make a midline skin incision or two separate incisions at the top and bottom of the construct, depending on the surgery.
- Dissect through the subcutaneous tissues and elevate a flap superficial to the paraspinal muscles laterally past the transverse processes. Confirm the location fluoroscopically.
- Alternatively, if the patient has multiple fused ribs and an open thoracostomy is planned, place the patient in the lateral decubitus position. Make a curvilinear J-shaped incision, starting halfway between the medial edge of the scapula and the posterior spinous process of T1-T2. Carry the incision distally and laterally across the 10th rib. Transect the muscle layers in line with the skin incision down to the level of the ribs and elevate an anterior flap to the costochondral junction. The paraspinal muscles are elevated from lateral to medial to the tips of the transverse process. In patients with multiple rib fusions and stiff chest walls, an opening wedge thoracostomy is indicated.
- For most patients, a thoracostomy usually is not necessary and has been shown to disrupt pulmonary function. The use of distraction-based rib implants is effective in opening up the rib spaces. Standard spine hooks can be used. Make a 5-mm transverse incision just distal to the neurovascular bundle using cautery (lateral to the transverse process). Make sure that the dissection on the top of the rib is immediately adjacent to the transverse process only (see Fig. 8.15A). If the soft tissues are dissected too far laterally, hooks tend to slide down. Use a Freer elevator to dissect the soft tissue anterior to the rib (see Fig. 8.15B). Preserve the periosteum around the rib to allow the rib to hypertrophy in response to stress.
- If a specialized device cradle is necessary, use a similar insertion technique, except stay subperiosteal with the rib dissection. Use a Freer elevator in both a superior and inferior direction around the rib to create a channel. Insert the rib cradle cap into the superior end of the channel and the rib cradle into the inferior end of the channel. Align the two devices and connect them with the cradle cap lock.
- Place a conventional upgoing spinal hook into the interval between the periosteum and pleura using a standard hook inserter or partial rod. Usually a second upgoing hook is placed around an adjacent rib to share the load.
- After proximal fixation, attention is turned to placement of the distal anchor. Through the same incision, subperiosteally dissect the lamina of the intended vertebrae. Either single-level fixation with a downgoing supralaminar hook or, more commonly, two-level fixation with pedicle screws can be used. If single-level fixation is used, preserve the interspinous ligament to avoid progressive kyphosis of the distal segment with distraction. If pedicle screws are used, place them at two adjacent levels because plowing of the implants could injure nerve roots.
- If two-level distal anchoring is chosen, use a narrow rongeur to destroy the facet joint and place cancellous crushed allograft into the joint. Decorticate the exposed bone and place bone graft before the rod to maximize bony contact.

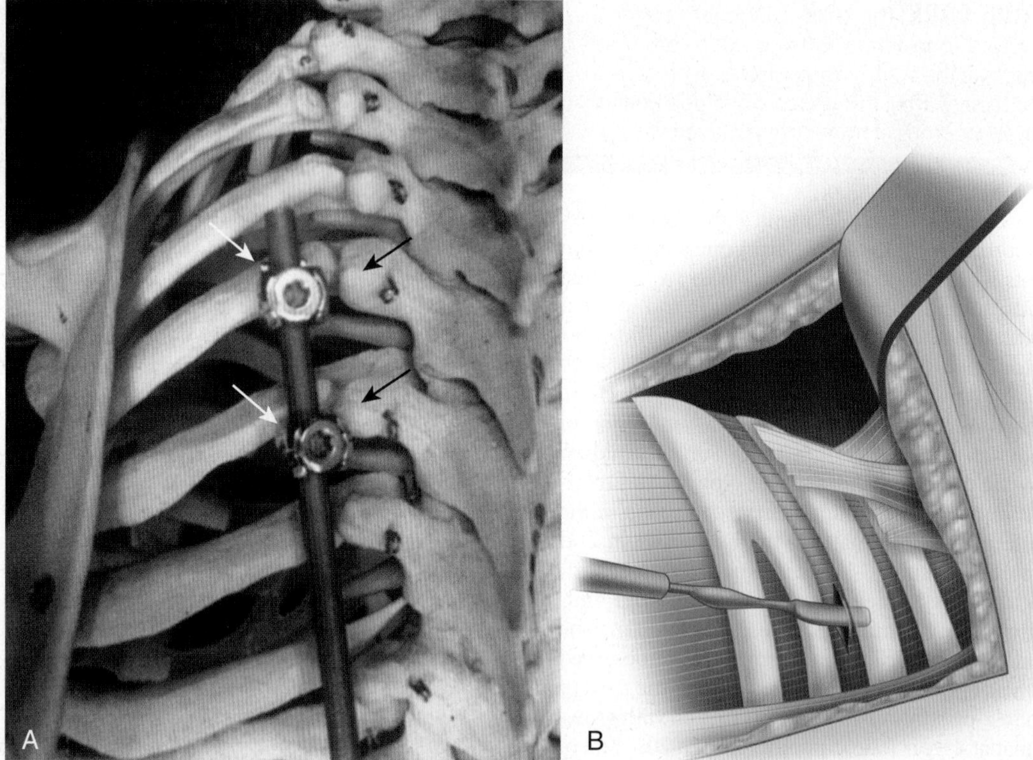

FIGURE 8.15 **A,** Model of thoracic spine with ribs. Correct placement of rib anchors *(white arrows)* lateral to tips of transverse processes *(black arrows).* **B,** Dissection of soft tissue anterior to rib. (From Sankar WN, Skaggs DL: Rib anchors in distraction-based growing spine implants. In Wang JC, editor: *Advanced reconstruction spine*, Rosemont, IL, 2011, American Academy of Orthopaedic Surgeons.) **SEE TECHNIQUE 8.4.**

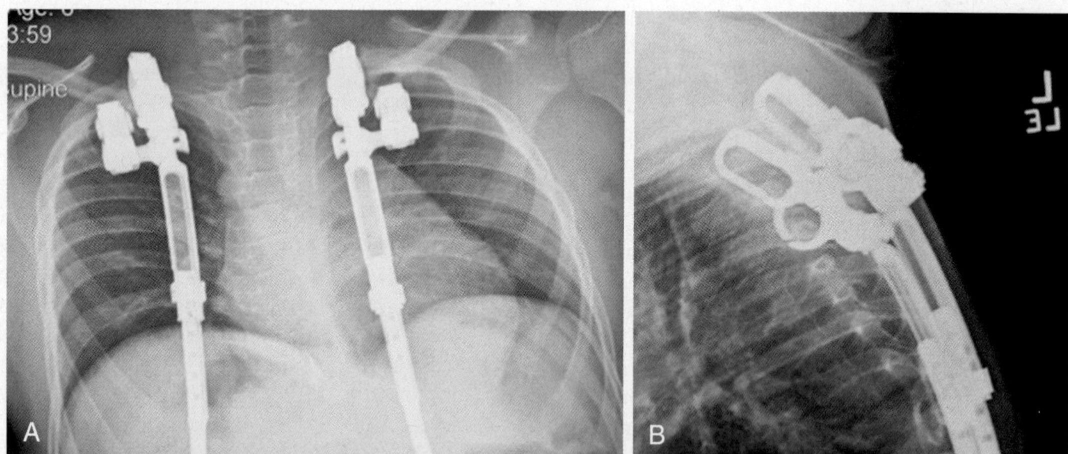

FIGURE 8.16 Anterior-posterior and lateral radiographs of 8-year-old girl with neuromuscular scoliosis and rib-based fixation with outriggers. **A,** Note that outriggers allow increased number of rib anchor points. **B,** Use of specialized rib cradles allows fixation of multiple ribs in same cradle, increasing strength of anchor.

- If one incision was used and if separate upper and lower rods were used, they can be connected with a longitudinal growing rod connector or side-to-side connector with the rods overlapping. It is prudent to use more than one connector. If two separate incisions were used for exposure, a soft-tissue tunnel should be made between the two anchor sites for passage of the rods using a chest tube to facilitate safe passage of the rod.

- Although unilateral rods are less invasive, there are fewer anchor points to share the load, and balancing the curve can be problematic. Dual rods are more stable and less prone to breakage and loss of fixation and make balancing the spine easier. When dual rods are used, a crosslink should be avoided because, although biomechanically more stable, use of a crosslink has been associated with catastrophic spinal cord injury when screw pull-out occurs. Screw pull-out with a crosslink typically occurs posteriorly along the axis of the pedicle, avoiding the spinal cord. The crosslink will not allow the screw to pull out along the trajectory of the pedicle and can pull out directly into the spinal cord.

- If an opening wedge thoracostomy was performed, a second rib-to-rib device can be used laterally to assist in correction and to reduce the load on the medial rib-to-spine device. Place the superior cradle around the same ribs that have the medial hybrid device and place the inferior cradle on a stable rib no lower than the 10th rib.
- Before wound closure, fill the upper anchor site with warm saline and perform a Valsalva maneuver to look for a pleural leak. If bubbles are present, place a Hemovac (Zimmer, Inc., Warsaw, IN) or chest tube into the pleural space for a few days.
- Close the wound in layers using 1-0 braided absorbable suture for the musculocutaneous flap, a 2-0 suture for the dermis, and a running 3-0 monofilament absorbable suture for the final subcuticular layer.

See also Videos 8.1 and 8.2

POSTOPERATIVE CARE Physical therapy is started on the first day after surgery. A TLSO should be used for 3 months if the arthrodesis was at a distal anchor site. Patients may return to sports at 3 months. Lengthenings are planned for every 6 months after the initial surgery.

GUIDED GROWTH AND PHYSEAL STAPLING

Growth modulation is an attempt to apply the principles of guided growth in the lower extremities with physeal stapling. Intervertebral stapling is used to produce a tethering effect on the convex side of the spine. This tether theoretically will allow for continued growth on the concave side of the spine deformity and gradual correction of the deformity with growth. Devices that have been used for this growth modulation are a flexible titanium clip, a nitinol staple, and, more recently, an anterior spinal tether using anterior vertebral body screws and a polypropylene cord.

ANTERIOR VERTEBRAL TETHERING

With the development and FDA approval of anterior vertebral tethering, the use of vertebral body stapling has dropped dramatically. Purported advantages of anterior vertebral tethering over posterior spinal fusion include that it allows the spine to grow and remain flexible, it is one-time surgery, and a later fusion can be done if needed. The indications for this technique have not been well established, but it is most likely beneficial for patients with enough growth remaining to substantially alter the shape of the spine and is most suited for primary thoracic curves with typical hypokyphotic apices (Fig. 8.17). Suggested contraindications include patients with no remaining growth, patients younger than 8 years of age, patients with curves of less than 40 degrees or more than 65 degrees, and patients with left-sided curves, pulmonary disease limiting single-lung ventilation, previous ipsilateral chest surgery, or poor bone quality.

TECHNIQUE 8.5

- With the use of single-lung ventilation and the patient in the lateral decubitus position, make a thoracoscopic approach.
- With fluoroscopy, mark the screw trajectories in the coronal plane, planning for three posterior axillary line 15-mm portals for screw placement. Use an 11-mm anterior axillary line portal for endoscopic placement.
- Open the pleura longitudinally 1 cm anterior to the rib heads.
- Coagulate and divide the segmental vessels and retract them anteriorly with sponges placed between the spine and the great vessels.
- Place bicortical transverse vertebral body screws through pronged washers using fluoroscopy to guide the screw trajectory.
- Introduce the tethering cord through a portal and capture it with a set screw into the proximal vertebral body screw. Adjust the portals to the appropriate interspace used to place the adjacent screws, and remove the long end of the tether from the chest through that portal, allowing a tensioning device to take slack out of the tether as the next set screw is tightened.
- Repeat this sequence for each screw, with more or less compression applied as indicated based on the deformity (generally more compression at the apex and less to none at the ends).
- Cut the tether distally and close the pleura over the device with the endoscopic suturing technique. Place a chest tube and reinflate the lungs.

POSTOPERATIVE CARE The patient recovers in the hospital for 4 to 5 days. A thoracolumbosacral orthosis is recommended for 3 months after surgery. Noncontact activities can be resumed after 3 months.

INSTRUMENTATION WITH FUSION

If a child is older than 9 or 10 years or is unable to cooperate with the demands of growth rods, instrumentation and spinal fusion should be considered. A combined anterior and posterior procedure should be considered if the patient is deemed at risk for the crankshaft phenomenon (see Figs. 8.7 and 8.8). However, with the use of pedicle screw fixation and the ability to get better correction of vertebral body rotation and the Cobb angle, an anterior fusion rarely is used.

Preferably, if an anterior procedure is performed, the anterior release and fusion are done without sacrificing the segmental vessels. Anterior instrumentation is not used if posterior instrumentation is scheduled as a second procedure. Posteriorly, a multiple-hook or pedicle screw segmental system is most commonly used. Many of these systems have a variety of different size hooks, pedicle screws, and rods, depending on the size of the child. Karol et al., however, found that patients with proximal thoracic deformity who required fusion of more than four segments, especially the upper thoracic, were at higher risk for the development of restrictive pulmonary disease. There was a significant correlation between poor pulmonary function and the proximal level of the thoracic fusion and the percentage of thoracic vertebrae fused.

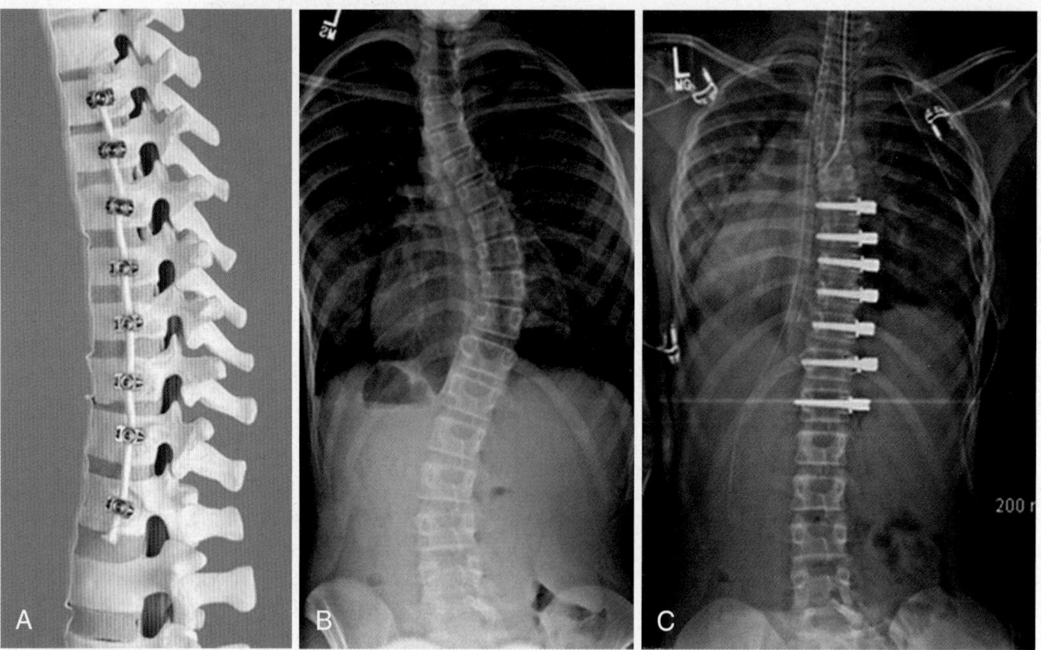

FIGURE 8.17 **A,** Anterior vertebral body tethering. **B,** Before tethering. **C,** After tethering. (From *Shriners Hospital for Children Philadelphia Newsletter*, June 18, 2014.) **SEE TECHNIQUE 8.5.**

ADOLESCENT IDIOPATHIC SCOLIOSIS

Adolescent idiopathic scoliosis is present when the spinal deformity is recognized after the child is 10 years of age but before skeletal maturity. This is the most common type of idiopathic scoliosis. The characteristics of adolescent idiopathic scoliosis include a three-dimensional deformity of the spine with lateral curvature plus rotation of the vertebral bodies. Most idiopathic curves are lordotic or hypokyphotic in the thoracic region, and this may represent an important factor in the etiology of idiopathic scoliosis.

ETIOLOGY

The exact cause of idiopathic scoliosis remains unknown. The consensus is that there is a hereditary predisposition and its actual cause is multifactorial. There are many proposed etiologic factors, but these can be divided into six general categories: (1) genetic factors, (2) neurologic disorders, (3) hormonal and metabolic dysfunctions, (4) skeletal growth, (5) biomechanical factors, and (6) environmental and lifestyle factors. The role of a genetic component in the cause of scoliosis is supported by several studies demonstrating an increased incidence of scoliosis in family members. Riseborough and Wynne-Davies found scoliosis in 11% of first-degree relatives of 207 patients with scoliosis. Genetic studies of families in which multiple members are affected have suggested several sites within the genome that appear to be linked to scoliosis. Currently genetic testing is being evaluated as a prognostic test for the risk of curve progression. Abnormalities in the central nervous system also have been thought to play a role in causing scoliosis. These neurologic factors can be divided into two major groups: neuroanatomic and neurophysiologic dysfunction. Studies have reported anatomic abnormalities in the midbrain, pons, and medulla and the vestibular system in scoliosis patients. Hindbrain abnormalities with cervicothoracic syrinx and low-lying cerebellar tonsils, with or without an abnormal cerebrospinal fluid dynamic, have been reported in patients with adolescent idiopathic scoliosis. Abnormalities of equilibrium and vestibular function have been noted as a possible cause. Differential growth between the right and left sides of the spine and a relative overgrowth of the anterior spinal column compared with the posterior column, resulting in a relative thoracic lordosis, have been postulated to cause scoliosis. Hormone abnormalities that have been proposed as causes are abnormalities in growth hormone, estrogen, melatonin, calmodulin, and leptin. Biomechanical causes are thought to be a result of asymmetric loading of the immature spine, which in turn causes asymmetric growth, resulting in a progressive deformity. Possible environmental or lifestyle factors include nutrition, diet, calcium and vitamin D intake, and exercise level. In summary, the exact cause of scoliosis remains unknown and may be multifactorial. Current research continues to try to better define these proposed causes.

NATURAL HISTORY

A knowledge of the natural history and prevalence of idiopathic scoliosis is essential to determine if treatment is necessary. Three important questions need to be answered:

What is the prevalence of idiopathic scoliosis in the general population?

What is the likelihood of curve progression necessitating treatment in a child with scoliosis?

What problems may occur in adult life if scoliosis is left untreated and the curve progresses?

Idiopathic scoliotic curves of more than 10 degrees are estimated to occur in 2% to 3% of children younger than 16 years of age. Larger curves of more than 30 degrees are estimated to occur in 0.15% to 0.3% of children. Weinstein created a table of calculations that show decreasing prevalence with increasing curve magnitude (Table 8.2). The importance

TABLE 8.2

Adolescent Idiopathic Scoliosis Prevalence

COBB ANGLE (DEGREES)	FEMALE:MALE	PREVALENCE (%)
>10	1.4-2:1	2-3
>20	5.4:1	0.3-0.5
>30	10:1	0.1-0.3
>40		<0.1

From Weinstein SL: Adolescent idiopathic scoliosis: prevalence and natural history. In Weinstein SL, editor: *The pediatric spine: principles and practice*, New York, 2001, Raven.

BOX 8.2

Factors Related to Progression of Adolescent Idiopathic Scoliosis

- Girls > boys
- Premenarchal
- Risser sign of 0
- Double curves > single curves
- Thoracic curves > lumbar curves
- More severe curves

of these prevalence studies is that small degrees of scoliosis are common but larger curves occur much less frequently. Fewer than 10% of children with curves of 10 degrees or more require treatment.

Once scoliosis has been discovered in a child, the curve must be evaluated for the probability of progression, defined as an increase of 5 degrees or more measured by the Cobb measurement over two or more visits. What is unknown is whether this progression will continue and what the final curve will be. Spontaneous improvement is rare, occurring in 3% of adolescents with idiopathic scoliosis, most of whom have curves of less than 11 degrees. Certain factors have been found to be related to curve progression (Box 8.2). Progression is more likely in girls than in boys. The time of curve progression in adolescent idiopathic scoliosis generally is during the rapid adolescent growth known as the peak height velocity (PHV), which usually occurs before menses in females and is about 8 cm per year for girls and 9.5 cm per year for boys. The incidence of progression decreases as the child gets older and approaches skeletal maturity. The incidence of progression also has been found to be related to curve patterns. In general, double curves are more likely to progress than single curves and single thoracic curves tend to be more progressive than single lumbar curves. The incidence of progression also increases with the curve magnitude. Bunnell estimated that the risk of progression for a 20-degree curve is approximately 20% and the risk for a 50-degree curve is 90%, and Sanders developed a chart to predict progression of a curve when a patient is first seen (Fig. 8.18). Historically, the Risser staging based on the ossification of the iliac crest was used to assess skeletal maturity and subsequent risk of curve progression. While simple and readily available on routine spine radiographs, its reliability has been questioned because of the variability of ossification of the iliac crest apophysis and the fact that Risser staging correlates poorly

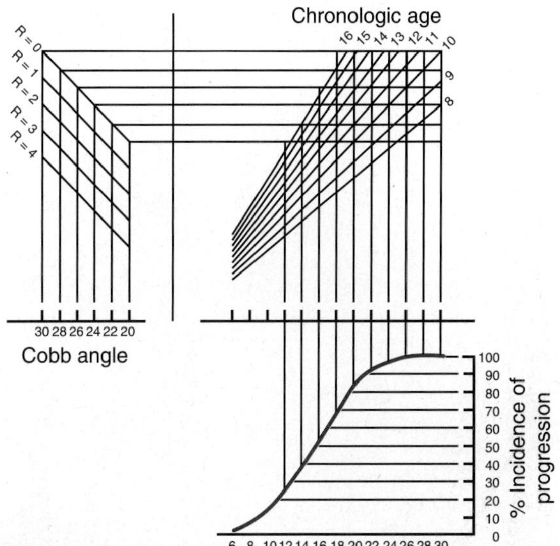

FIGURE 8.18 Logistic projection of probability of Lenke type I and type 3 curves progressing to surgery assuming greater than 50-degree threshold. (From Sanders JO, Khoury JG, Kishan S, et al: Predicting scoliosis progression from skeletal maturity: a simplified classification during adolescence, *J Bone Joint Surg Am* 90:551, 2008.)

to predicting PHV. Sanders et al. developed a simplified classification of skeletal maturity based on hand radiographs that has been shown to correlate highly with curve behavior (Fig. 8.19). The natural history of adolescent idiopathic scoliosis in adulthood is difficult to study because of the challenges in obtaining long-term follow-up data. In general, patients with smaller curves, less than 30 degrees, will do well in adulthood with little or no associated morbidity.

The incidence of back pain in the general population is between 60% and 80%, and the incidence in patients with idiopathic scoliosis is comparable. Patients with lumbar or thoracolumbar curves, especially those with translatory shifts at the lower end of the curves, have a slightly greater incidence of backache than patients with other curve patterns, but this is rarely disabling and is unrelated to the presence of osteoarthritic changes on radiographic examination.

In a 50-year follow-up study, the incidence of back pain in scoliosis patients was 77% compared with 37% in control subjects. Chronic back pain was reported by 61% of the scoliosis group and 35% of the control subjects. However, the ability of scoliosis patients to perform activities of daily living and work was similar to that of the control subjects. The location of pain has been variable in studies and generally unrelated to the location or magnitude of the curve. In contrast, lumbar and thoracolumbar curves may arise in adult life and cause severe pain and discomfort. This degenerative type of scoliosis should not be confused with the natural history of untreated adolescent idiopathic scoliosis. Ultimately, it is important to determine whether the pain is related to scoliosis before treatment determinations are made.

A direct correlation has been noted between decreasing vital capacity and increasing curve severity due to restrictive lung disease and is seen in large thoracic curves, greater than 100 degrees. One study found significant respiratory impairment (pulmonary function <65% predicted) in 19% of their preoperative patients with adolescent idiopathic scoliosis. The decrease in pulmonary function correlated with the severity

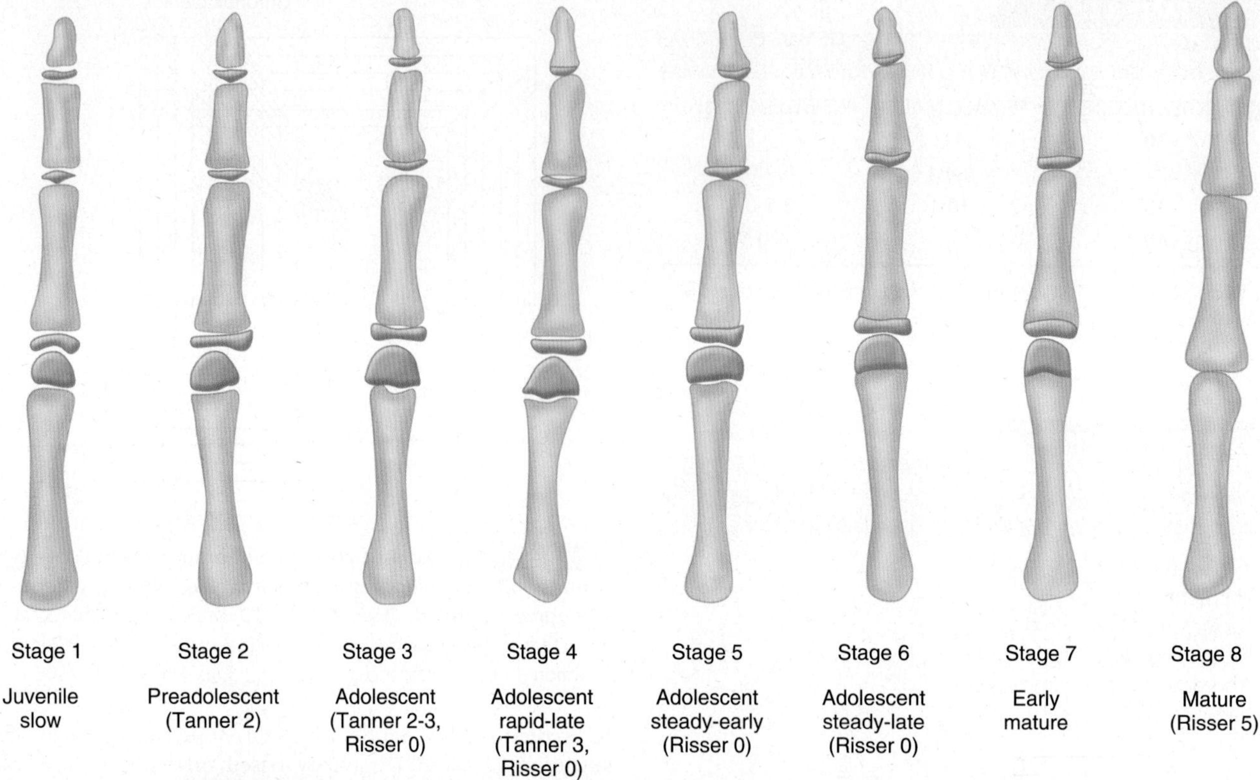

FIGURE 8.19 **Sanders classification of skeletal maturity.** (From Crawford AH, et al: Clinical and radiographic evaluation of the scoliotic patient. In Newton PO, O'Brien MF, Shufflebarger HL, et al, editors: *Idiopathic scoliosis: the Harms Study Group treatment guide*, New York, 2010, Thieme, p 60.)

of the main thoracic curve and sagittal plane hypokyphosis and was seen in patients with curves of 70 to 80 degrees. Death in patients with adult idiopathic scoliosis also seems to be related to thoracic curves greater than 100 degrees, with resultant cor pulmonale. With modern surgical techniques, death from cor pulmonale from adolescent idiopathic scoliosis is extremely rare.

The psychologic effect of scoliosis has been studied by numerous authors. Unhappiness with the appearance often is correlated with the size of the rib prominence. Middle-aged patients tolerate the psychologic effects of scoliosis better than teenagers; however, many adult patients seeking treatment for untreated adolescent idiopathic scoliosis are most concerned with the cosmetic aspects of the disorder.

Curves may continue to progress throughout adult life. Weinstein et al. identified multiple factors that predict the likelihood of curve progression after maturity (Table 8.3). In general, curves in any area of less than 30 degrees at skeletal maturity did not tend to progress in adult life. Larger curves were more likely to progress throughout adult life, especially thoracic curves between 50 and 75 degrees. Lumbar curves also tend to progress in adulthood in curves less than 50 degrees if they are accompanied by a transitory shift between the lower vertebrae.

TABLE 8.3

Progression Factors in Curves More Than 30 Degrees at Skeletal Maturity

THORACIC	LUMBAR	THORACOLUMBAR
Cobb >50 degrees	Cobb >30 degrees	Cobb >30 degrees
Apical vertical rotation >30 degrees	Apical vertical rotation >30 degrees	Apical vertical rotation >30%
Mehta angle >30 degrees	Curve direction Relation L5 to intercrest line Translatory shifts	Translatory shifts

From Weinstein SL: Natural history, *Spine* 24:2592, 1999.

PATIENT EVALUATION

The initial evaluation of the patient should include a thorough history, physical and neurologic examinations, and spine radiographs.

Most patients with scoliosis present for evaluation because of the appearance of their spine deformity. The prevalence of back pain for most adolescent idiopathic scoliosis patients is similar to that in the general population. Further workup may be needed if the patient's back pain is persistent, interferes with daily activities, occurs at night, or is associated with any abnormal neurologic findings. Menarchal status, patient and parental height, and family history of scoliosis should be determined. Scoliosis occurs three times more frequently in children whose parents are affected and seven times more frequently if a sibling is affected. Also, if the parents or siblings have been treated for scoliosis, this may suggest a greater likelihood of curve progression in the patient. Surgical history is important in identifying scoliosis associated with congenital heart disease or with a prior thoracotomy.

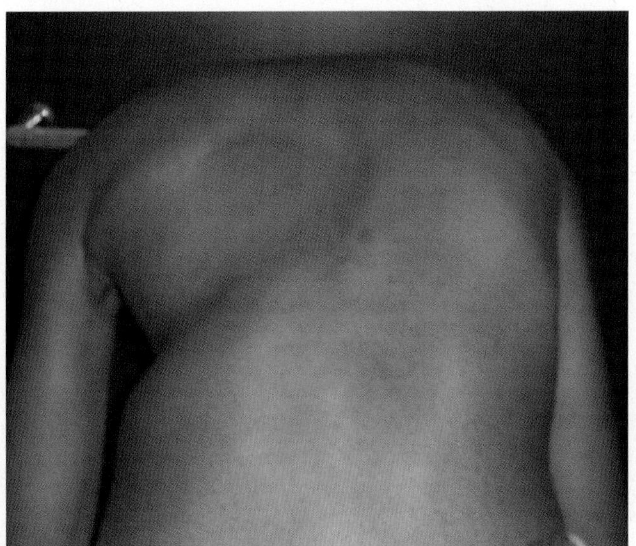

FIGURE 8.20 Adams forward bending test. Note right thoracic rib prominence and left lumbar prominence in patient with thoracolumbar curve.

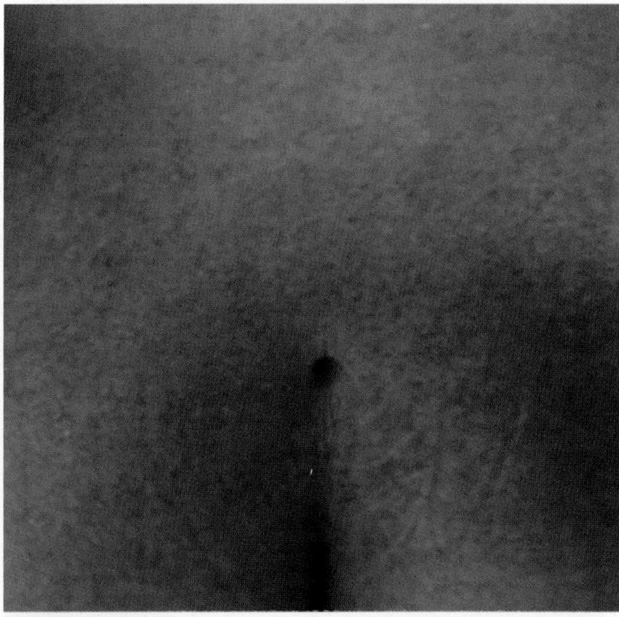

FIGURE 8.21 Sacral dimple may be sign of congenital scoliosis.

On physical examination, the height of the patient should be measured. Serial measurement of height will detect when PHV is occurring associated with an increase in progression of the curve. The best clinical test for evaluating spinal curvature is the Adams forward bending test (Fig. 8.20). As the patient bends forward at the waist until the spine is horizontal, the trunk is observed for rotation from behind (to assess midthoracic and lumbar rotation) and from the front (to assess upper thoracic rotation). The knees should be straight, the feet together, the arms dependent, and the palms in opposition. Because of vertebral rotation, this will produce a rib prominence in the thoracic region or a paraspinal fullness in the lumbar region. An angle of more than 7 degrees is considered abnormal and usually correlates with a curve of 15 to 20 degrees. The sagittal plane should also be examined for excessive kyphosis or lordosis. Limb lengths should be evaluated because a discrepancy may cause a pelvic tilt and a compensatory scoliosis.

On inspection of the spine, the examiner should look for any dimpling (Fig. 8.21), hair patches, or skin abnormalities, such as hemangiomas or café au lait spots. Asymmetry of the shoulder, scapula, ribs, and waistline should be noted. Spinal balance can be determined by the alignment of the head over the pelvis. The head should be positioned directly above the gluteal crease. This can be assessed by dropping a plumb line from the base of the skull or from the spinous process of C7. The plumb line should not deviate from the center of the gluteal crease by more than 1 to 2 cm. In the sagittal plane, the spine is usually hypokyphotic. If hypokyphosis is absent clinically and radiographically, then a syrinx should be ruled out by MRI. A thorough neurologic examination should be done to determine if an intraspinal neoplasm or a neurologic disorder is the cause of scoliosis. Particular attention should be given to the abdominal reflexes because often they are the only neurologic abnormality found with some intraspinal disorders.

RADIOGRAPHIC EVALUATION

Posteroanterior and lateral radiographs of the spine, including the iliac crest distally and most of the cervical spine proximally, should be made with the patient standing. Inclusion of the iliac crest and the cervical spine generally requires 14 × 36-inch cassettes or digital equipment that allows accurate splicing of images. Patients should stand with their knees locked, with feet shoulder width apart, and looking straight ahead. The patient's shoulders are flexed forward, the elbows are fully flexed, and the fists should rest on the clavicles. The organs most at risk from radiation are the maturing breasts, and radiation is decreased by a factor of 5 to 11 by use of the posteroanterior view. Faster radiographic film and rare-earth screens also reduce the patient's exposure to radiation. New low-dose, digital slot-scanning techniques require approximately one eighth the radiation of standard radiographs and allow the creation of three-dimensional models to aid with surgical planning when necessary.

Although no absolutely accurate method is available for determining skeletal maturity as an adolescent progresses through puberty, various radiographic parameters can be used to assess maturity. The most common method is assessment of bone age at the hand and wrist and development of the iliac apophysis (Risser sign), triradiate cartilage, olecranon apophysis ossification, and digital ossification.

The Risser sign is a measurement based on the ossification of the iliac apophysis, which is divided into four quadrants. The Risser sign proceeds from grade 0, no ossification, to grade 4, in which all four quadrants of the apophysis have ossification. Risser grade 5 is when the apophysis has fused completely to the ilium when the patient is skeletally mature. The Risser sign may not be as useful for predicting curve progression because of variations in the normal ossification patterns and because grade 1 has been found to begin after the period of rapid adolescent growth or PHV.

The PHV has been reported by several authors to be a better maturity indicator than the Risser sign, chronologic age, or menarchal age. PHV is calculated from serial height measurements and is expressed as centimeters of growth per year. Average values of PHV are 8 cm per year in girls and 9.5 cm per year in boys. Little et al., in a study of 120 girls with scoliosis, found that PHV reliably predicted cessation of growth (3.6 years after PHV in 90%) and likelihood of curve progression.

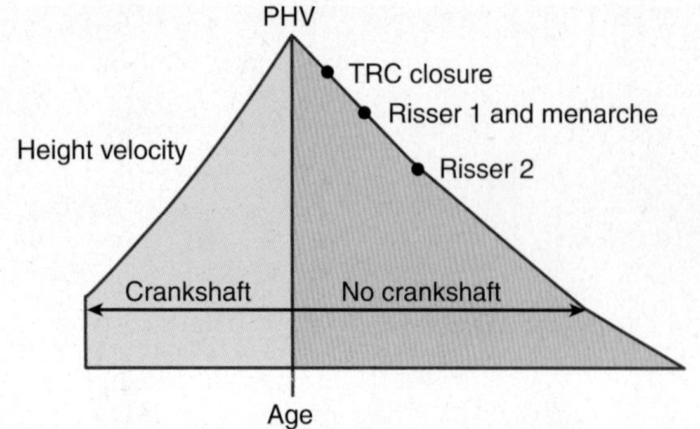

FIGURE 8.22 Height velocity. Triradiate cartilage (TRC) closure occurs after period of peak height velocity (PHV) and before Risser grade 1 and menarche. (Modified from Sanders JO, Little DG, Richards BS: Prediction of the crankshaft phenomenon by peak height velocity, *Spine* 22:1352, 1997.)

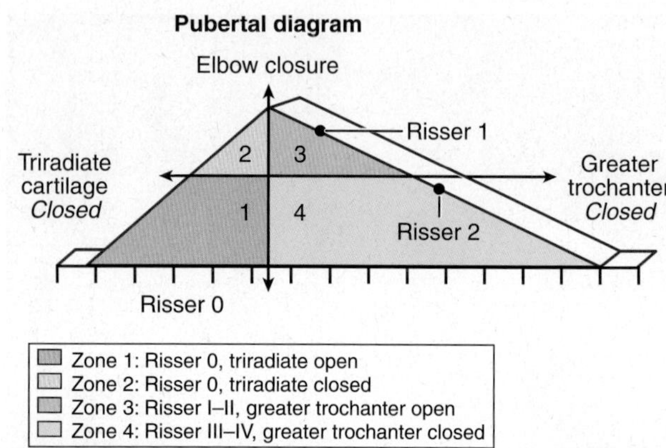

FIGURE 8.23 Pubertal diagram divided into four zones. Zone 1, ascending side, triradiate cartilage open, bone age between 11 and 13 years in girls and boys (Risser 0). Zone 2, ascending side, triradiate cartilage closed, bone age between 11 and 13 years in girls and between 13 and 15 years in boys (Risser 0). Zone 3, descending side, elbow closed but greater trochanter not fused, bone age between 13 and 16 years in girls and between 15 and 18 years in boys (Risser 1 to 2). Zone 4, descending side, elbow closed and greater trochanter fused, bone age between 13 and 16 years in girls and between 15 and 18 years in boys (Risser 3 to 4). (Redrawn from Dimeglio A, Canavese F, Charles P: Growth and adolescent idiopathic scoliosis: when and how much? *J Pediatr Orthop* 31:S28, 2011.)

Of 60 patients with curves of more than 30 degrees at PHV, 50 (83%) had curve progression to 45 degrees or more; of 28 with curves of 30 degrees or less at PHV, only one (4%) progressed to 45 degrees or more. Little et al. found similar results in boys with scoliosis and reported a 91% accuracy rate for predicting progression to 45 degrees or more. In both girls and boys, they found the PHV to be superior to the Risser sign, chronologic age, and menarchal age as a maturity indicator.

The triradiate cartilage begins to ossify in the early stages of puberty. In girls it is completely ossified after the period of PHV and before Risser grade 1 and menarche. In boys it is in the early stages of ossification when puberty begins. Sanders et al. found a higher rate of crankshaft phenomenon after posterior spinal fusion in patients at or before PHV as indicated by an open triradiate cartilage. These findings, however, may not be as common with modern pedicle screw fixation, which is more rigid and provides three-column fixation that may be more resistant to crankshaft than posterior hooks, which control only the posterior column of the spine (Fig. 8.22).

Other methods for evaluating maturity and the risk of curve progression are based on hand and wrist or elbow radiographs. The Sauvegrain method determines skeletal age from anteroposterior and lateral radiographs of the left elbow. It is a 27-point system based on four anatomic structures about the elbow: lateral condyle, trochlea, olecranon apophysis, and the proximal radial epiphysis. Skeletal age is determined from this score. Charles et al. reported a simple but reliable method to assess maturity based on the olecranon apophysis and allowed skeletal age to be determined at regular 6-month intervals from the age of 11 to 13 years in girls and from 13 to 15 years in boys. They found that this information complemented the Risser grade 0 and triradiate cartilage closure information (Figs. 8.23 and 8.24).

Both the Tanner-Whitehouse-III Radius-Ulna-Short Bones (RUS) score, based on the radiographic appearance of the epiphyses of the distal radius, ulna, and small bones of the hands, and the digital skeletal age maturity scoring system, based on the metacarpals and phalanges, highly correlate with PHV and curve progression. However, these systems are cumbersome and not very practical to use in a busy clinical setting. Because of this, Sanders et al. reported a simplified classification based on the epiphyses of the phalanx, metacarpal, and distal radius. They were able to demonstrate that this method reliably predicted maturity and probability of progression to surgery (see Fig. 8.19 and Table 8.4).

Approximately 10% of patients with presumed adolescent idiopathic scoliosis have a neurologic abnormality. An MRI should be used when there is a concern for a neurologic etiology, such as a Chiari malformation, syringomyelia, or intraspinal tumor, for the scoliosis and is most commonly used when curves are left thoracic, rapidly progressing, or painful, or the physical examination is unreliable or concerning. Another valuable sign is lack of thoracic apical lordosis or hyperkyphosis.

■ MEASUREMENT OF CURVES

The Cobb method of measurement recommended by the Terminology Committee of the SRS (Fig. 8.25) consists of three steps: (1) locating the superior end vertebra, (2) locating the inferior end vertebra, and (3) drawing intersecting perpendicular lines from the superior surface of the superior end vertebra and from the inferior surface of the inferior end vertebra. The angle of deviation of these perpendicular lines from a straight line is the angle of the curve. If the endplates are obscured, the pedicles can be used instead. The end vertebra of the curve is the one that tilts the most into the concavity of the curve being measured. In general, on moving away from the apex of the curve, the next intervertebral space below the inferior end vertebra or above the superior end vertebra is wider on the concave side of the curve. Within the curve, the intervertebral spaces usually are wider on the convex side and narrower on the concave side. When significantly wedged, the vertebrae themselves, rather than the intervertebral disc spaces, may be wider on the convex side of the curve and narrower on the concave side. The reported interobserver and intraobserver variations in Cobb measurements average 5 to 7 degrees. The same levels should be measured between visits and variability should be taken into account in determining whether a curve is truly progressing.

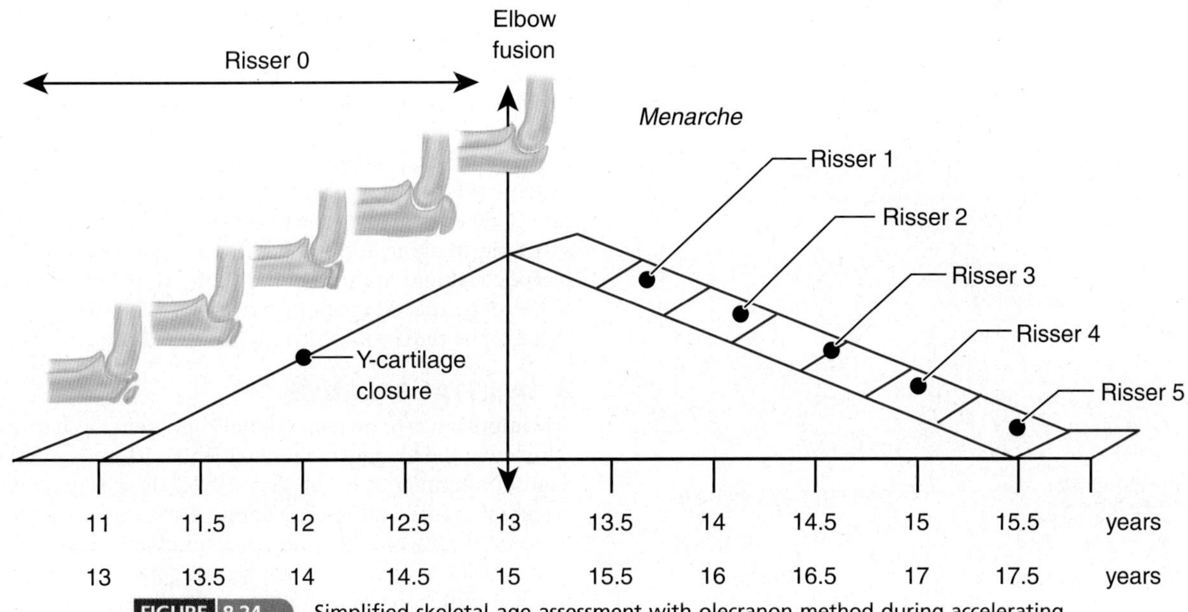

FIGURE 8.24 Simplified skeletal age assessment with olecranon method during accelerating pubertal growth phase of peak height velocity and Risser grade 0 from ages of 11 to 13 years in girls and from 13 to 15 years in boys, with a decelerating growth phase after elbow fusion. Y-cartilage closure = triradiate cartilage closure. (Redrawn from Charles YP, Dimeglio A, Canavese F, Dauers JP: Skeletal age assessment from the olecranon for idiopathic scoliosis at Risser grade 0, *J Bone Joint Surg* 89A:737, 2007.)

TABLE 8.4

Logistic Projection of the Probability of Lenke Type 1 and Type 3 Curves Progressing to Surgery Assuming a Threshold of More Than 50 Degrees*,†

CURVE (DEGREES)	STAGE 1	STAGE 2	STAGE 3	STAGE 4	STAGE 5	STAGE 6	STAGES 7 AND 8
10	2% (0%-40%)	0% (0%-15%)	0% (0%-0%)	0% (0%-0%)	0% (0%-0%)	0% (0%-0%)	0% (0%-1%)
15	23% (4%-69%)	11% (1%-58%)	0% (0%-2%)	0% (0%-0%)	0% (0%-0%)	0% (0%-0%)	0% (0%-7%)
20	84% (40%-98%)	92% (56%-99%)	0% (0%-14%)	0% (0%-1%)	0% (0%-1%)	0% (0%-1%)	0% (0%-26%)
25	99% (68%-100%)	100% (92%-100%)	29% (3%-84%)	0% (0%-5%)	0% (0%-5%)	0% (0%-2%)	0% (0%-64%)
30	100% (83%-100%)	100% (98%-100%)	100% (47%-100%)	0% (0%-27%)	0% (0%-22%)	0% (0%-11%)	0% (0%-91%)
35	100% (91%-100%)	100% (100%-100%)	100% (89%-100%)	0% (0%-79%)	0% (0%-65%)	0% (0%-41%)	0% (0%-98%)
40	100% (95%-100%)	100% (100%-100%)	100% (98%-100%)	15% (0%-99%)	0% (0%-94%)	0% (0%-83%)	0% (0%-100%)
45	100% (98%-100%)	100% (100%-100%)	100% (100%-100%)	88% (2%-100%)	1% (0%-99%)	0% (0%-98%)	0% (0%-100%)

*Unshaded cells correspond with combinations of curve size and maturity stage for which surgery would be a plausible treatment if more than 50 degrees at maturity is accepted as the threshold for surgical treatment. Shaded cells correspond with combinations for which surgery would not be a plausible treatment.
†Cells with wide 95% confidence intervals (shown in parentheses) correspond with groups that had too few patients for accurate estimates (or groups that had no patients) and should be interpreted with caution.
Reproduced from Sanders JO, Khoury JG, Kishan S, et al.: Predicting scoliosis progression from skeletal maturity: a simplified classification during adolescence, *J Bone Joint Surg* 90A:540, 2008.

VERTEBRAL ROTATION

Because of the three-dimensional nature of adolescent idiopathic scoliosis, accurate assessment of vertebral rotation both preoperatively and postoperatively is important. The two most commonly used methods of determining vertebral rotation from plain radiographs are those of Nash and Moe and of Perdriolle and Vidal. In the method of Nash and Moe, if the pedicles are equidistant from the sides of the vertebral bodies, no vertebral rotation is present (0 rotation). The grades progress to grade IV rotation, in which the pedicle is past the center of the vertebral body (Fig. 8.26). It may be difficult to assess postoperative rotation because of the instrumentation

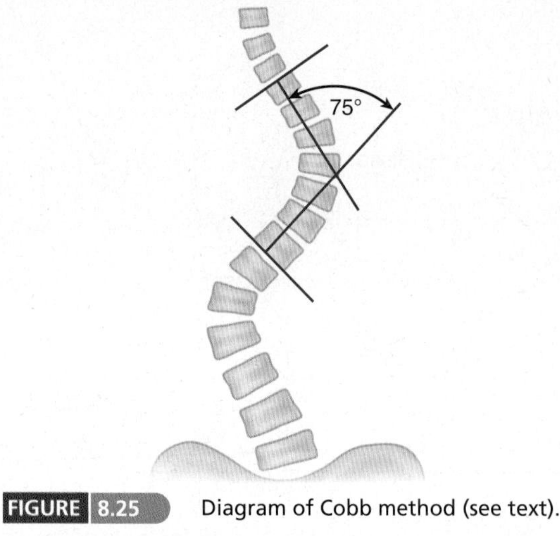

FIGURE 8.25 Diagram of Cobb method (see text).

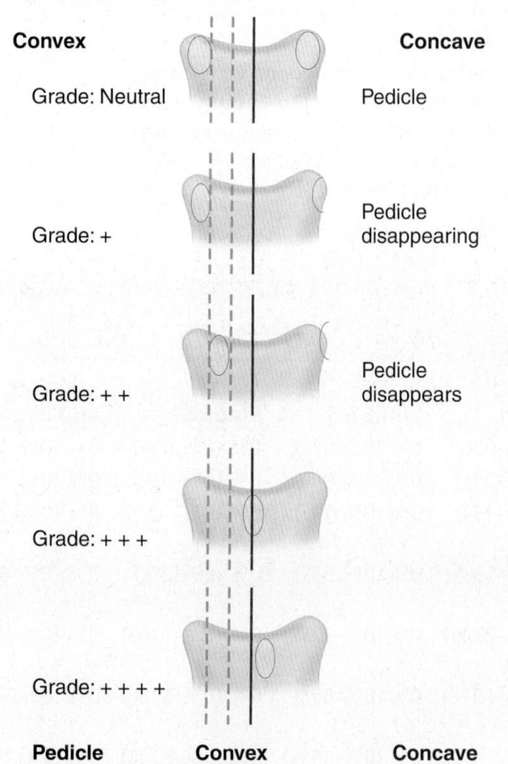

Pedicle	Convex	Concave
Grade: Neutral	No asymmetry	No asymmetry
Grade: +	Migrates within first segment	May start disappearing
	Early distortion	Early distortion
Grade: + +	Migrates to second segment	Gradually disappears
Grade: + + +	Migrates to middle segment	Not visible
Grade: + + + +	Migrates past midline to concave side of vertebral body	Not visible

FIGURE 8.26 Pedicle method of determining vertebral rotation. Vertebral body is divided into six segments and grades 0 to 4+ are assigned, depending on location of pedicle within segments. Because pedicle on concave side disappears early in rotation, pedicle on convex side, easily visible through wide range of rotation, is used as standard.

obscuring the measurement landmarks. Kuklo et al. evaluated the utility of alternative radiographic measures of vertebral rotation. They found that the rib hump as measured on the lateral radiograph (Fig. 8.27A) and the apical vertebral body-rib ratio (Fig. 8.27B) showed a strong correlation with vertebral rotation and can be used when CT is not feasible or when instrumentation obscures the landmarks necessary for rotation to be evaluated by the other techniques. New slot digital scanning imaging techniques (EOS Imaging, Paris, France) provide fast and accurate three-dimensional reconstructions of the spine that can better determine vertebral body rotation without the radiation exposure from a CT scan.

SAGITTAL BALANCE

The importance of normal sagittal alignment has become recognized in the management of patients with spinal deformity. Sagittal alignment can be considered on a segmental (two vertebral bodies and intervening disc), regional (cervical, thoracic, thoracolumbar junction, lumbar, lumbosacral), or global basis. Global spinal alignment generally is considered to be an indication of overall sagittal balance.

Overall spinal sagittal balance is determined by a plumb line dropped from the dens, which should fall anterior to the thoracic spine, posterior to the lumbar spine, and through the posterior superior corner of S1 (Fig. 8.28). Because the dens is difficult to evaluate on long scoliosis films, the plumb line usually is dropped from the middle of the C7 vertebral body. This plumb line is called the sagittal vertebral axis. A positive sagittal vertebral axis is considered present when the plumb line is anterior to the anterior aspect of S1. A negative sagittal vertebral axis occurs when this plumb line passes posterior to the anterior body of S1 (Fig. 8.29). The overall sagittal balance is probably a more important measurement than regional and segmental measurements. In general, for sagittal balance to be maintained, lumbar lordosis should measure 20 to 30 degrees more than the kyphosis. If overall sagittal balance is not considered, correction to the normal range of lordosis without similar correction of the kyphotic thoracic spine can lead to significant sagittal imbalance (Fig. 8.30).

In the thoracic spine, the normal sagittal curvature is kyphotic and typically is 30 to 40 degrees in adolescents. The kyphosis begins at the first thoracic vertebra and reaches its maximal segmental kyphosis at T6 or T7. Ranges of thoracic kyphosis in normal patients, both adults and children, have been reported. Although the kyphosis begins at T1, this vertebra often cannot be seen on standing long-cassette lateral films. The T4 or T5 vertebra is more easily seen and measured. Gelb et al. found that the upper thoracic kyphosis from T1 to T5 in 100 adults averaged 14 ± 8 degrees. Adding this number to the kyphosis measured from T5 to T12 provides a reasonable estimate of overall regional kyphosis.

The normal regional lumbar sagittal alignment is lordotic. The normal apex of this lordosis is at the vertebral body of L3 or L4 or the disc space itself. The segments at L4-L5 and L5-S1 account for 60% of the overall lumbar lordosis. It is important to remember that the lumbar discs account for 47 degrees of the lordosis (78%); the vertebral bodies themselves account for only12 degrees. This emphasizes the importance of preserving disc height during anterior procedures for the treatment of spinal deformities. Because 40% of the total lumbar lordosis is in the L5-S1 segment, it is important to be able to measure to the top of the sacrum, although this can be difficult on standing lateral images. The lumbar lordosis is a dependent variable based on the amount of kyphosis. For

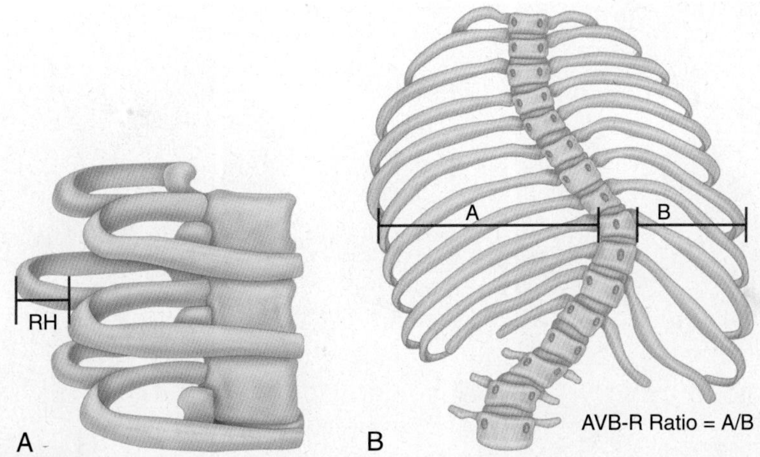

FIGURE 8.27 **A,** Diagram of measurement technique for assessing rib hump (RH) deformity. RH is linear distance between left and right posterior rib prominences at apex of rib deformity on lateral radiograph. **B,** Diagram of measurement technique for apical vertebral body/rib ratio (AVB-R). AVB-R is ratio of linear measurements from lateral borders of apical thoracic vertebrae to chest wall on anteroposterior radiographs. (Redrawn from Kuklo TR, Potter BK, Lenke WG: Vertebral rotation and thoracic torsion in adolescent idiopathic scoliosis: what is the best radiographic correlate? *J Spinal Disord Tech* 18:139, 2005.)

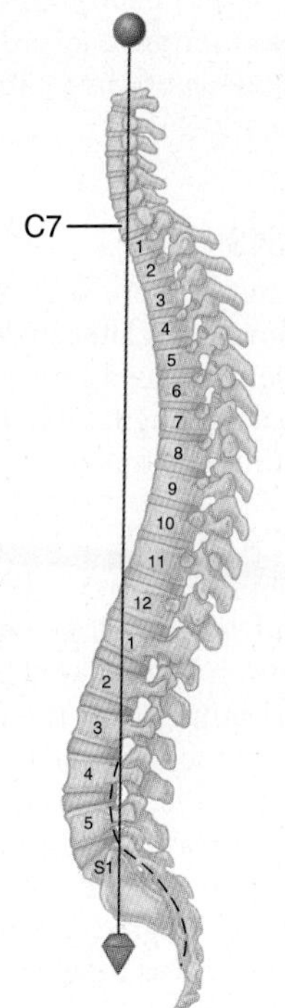

FIGURE 8.28 C7 sagittal plumb line is useful measurement of sagittal balance. Plumb line dropped from middle of C7 vertebral body falls close to posterosuperior corner of S1 vertebral body.

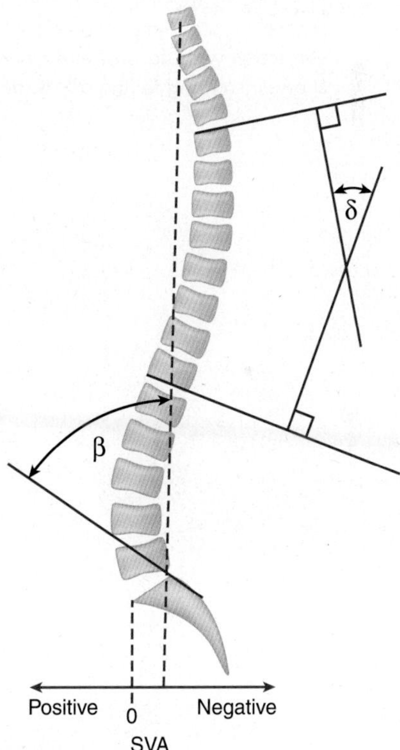

FIGURE 8.29 Method of measurement of various parameters of sagittal spinal alignment. Sagittal vertical axis (SVA) is horizontal distance from C7 plumb line to front corner of sacrum. Positive values indicate position anterior to sacrum; negative values are through or behind sacrum. β, Angle of sacral inclination, is angle subtended by tangent to posterior border of S1 and vertical axis. δ, Cobb angle between two vertebrae.

sagittal balance to be maintained, lordosis generally is 20 to 30 degrees larger than thoracic kyphosis.

The orientation of the sacrum, the sacral slope, and the pelvic incidence are closely associated with the characteristics of lumbar lordosis and location of the apex of lumbar lordosis (Fig. 8.31). A sacral slope of less than 35 degrees and a low pelvic incidence are associated with a relatively flat, short lumbar lordosis. A sacral slope of more than 45 degrees and a high pelvic incidence are associated with a long, curved lumbar lordosis.

The thoracolumbar junction is the transition area from a relatively rigid kyphotic thoracic spine to a relatively mobile lordotic lumbar spine. Bernhardt and Bridwell showed that the thoracolumbar junction is nearly straight. This relationship must be maintained during reconstructive procedures to prevent a junctional kyphosis.

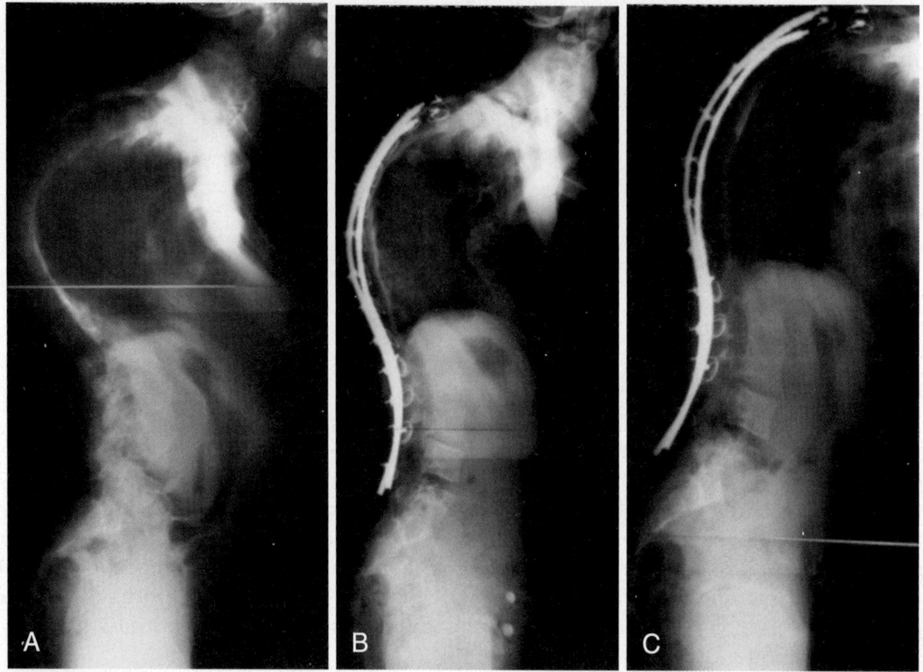

FIGURE 8.30 **A,** Preoperative standing lateral radiograph in patient with neuromuscular scoliosis. **B,** Standing lateral view 1 month later indicates imbalance between kyphosis and lordosis correction with signs of early increasing thoracic kyphosis. **C,** Further follow-up of same patient shows increasing falling off of thoracic kyphosis above instrumentation.

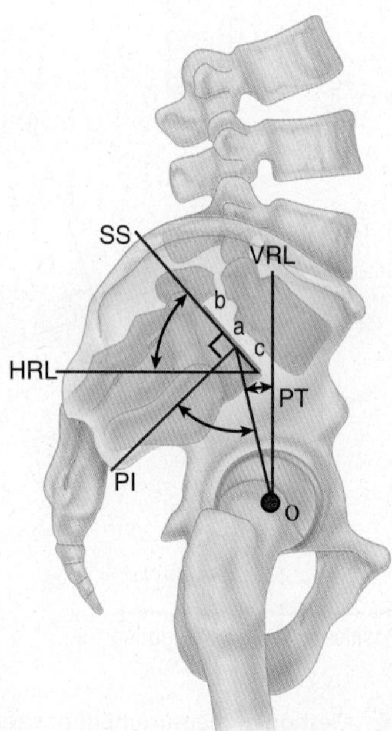

FIGURE 8.31 Sacral slope (SS) is angle subtended by horizontal reference line (HRL) and sacral endplate line (bc). SS shares common reference line (bc) with pelvic incidence (PI) and pelvic tilt (PT). PI is measured from static anatomic structures. PT and SS depend on angular position of sacrum/pelvis in relation to femoral heads, which changes with standing, sitting, and lying down. Relationship of PT and SS is affected by lumbosacropelvic flexion and extension. *VRL,* Vertical reference line. (From Jackson R, Kanemura T, Kawakami N, Hales C: Lumbopelvic lordosis and pelvic balance on repeated standing lateral radiographs of adult volunteers and untreated patients with constant low back pain, *Spine* 25:575–586, 2000.)

CURVE PATTERNS

Idiopathic scoliosis curves were first descriptively classified by Ponseti and Friedman and later by King. These classification systems have been replaced by the Lenke classification, which uses the coronal and sagittal planes to help guide treatment decisions including fusion levels.

LENKE CLASSIFICATION

Measurements are obtained from standard posteroanterior, lateral, and right and left bending radiographs. The three steps in this classification system are (1) identification of the primary curve, (2) assignment of the lumbar modifier, and (3) assignment of the thoracic sagittal modifier. The first step is to identify the primary curve. These curves should be divided by region: proximal thoracic, main thoracic, and thoracolumbar or lumbar. Curves are considered to be structural curves if they are more than 25 degrees on posteroanterior radiographs and do not bend to less than 25 degrees on side-bending radiographs. Based on these measurements the curve can be classified into six types (Fig. 8.32). The second step is to determine the lumbar spine modifier. This is determined by drawing a vertical line upward from the center of the sacrum (CSVL). The lumbar spine modifier is then determined by the relationship of the CSVL to the concave pedicle of the apical lumbar vertebra and can be assigned into A, B, or C. In type A, the CSVL is between the pedicles; in type B, it is between the medial pedicle wall and the lateral vertebra; and in type C, it is medial to the entire vertebra. The third step is to determine the thoracic sagittal modifier. The sagittal modifier is hypokyphotic (<10 degrees), normal (10 to 40 degrees), or hyperkyphotic (>40 degrees). Using this technique, fusion levels can be chosen so that the major and structural minor curves are included in the instrumentation and the nonstructural curves

Curve type

Type	Proximal thoracic	Main thoracic	Thoracolumbar/ lumbar	Curve description
1	Nonstructural	Structural (major)	Nonstructural	Main thoracic (MT)
2	Structural	Structural (major)	Nonstructural	Double thoracic (DT)
3	Nonstructural	Structural (major)	Structural	Double major (DM)
4	Structural	Structural (major)	Structural	Triple major (TM)
5	Nonstructural	Nonstructural	Structural (major)	Thoracolumbar/lumbar (TL/L)
6	Nonstructural	Structural	Structural (major)	Thoracolumbar/lumbar—structural MT (Lumbar curve > thoracic by ≥ 10°)

Structural Criteria

Proximal thoracic: Side-bending Cobb ≥ 25°
T2-T5 kyphosis ≥ 120°

Main thoracic: Side-bending Cobb ≥ 25°

Thoracolumbar/lumbar: Side-bending Cobb ≥ 25°
T10-L2 kyphosis ≥ +20°

Location of Apex
(SRS definition)

Curve	Apex
Thoracic	T2-T11-12 Disc
Thoracolumbar	T12-L1
Lumbar	L1-2 Disc-L4

Modifiers

Lumbar Spine Modifier	Center Sacral Vertical Line (CSVL) to Lumbar Apex
A	CSVL between pedicles
B	CSVL touches apical body(ies)
C	CSVL completely medial

A B C

Thoracic Sagittal Profile T5-T12		
–	(Hypo)	< 10°
N	(Normal)	10°–40°
+	(Hyper)	> 40°

Curve type (1–6) + Lumbar spine modifier (A, B, or C) + Thoracic sagittal modifier (–, N, or +)
Classification (e.g., 1 B +): ___________

FIGURE 8.32 Curve types and criteria for structural curves and location of apex. (From Lenke LG, Betz RR, Harms J, et al: Adolescent idiopathic scoliosis: a new classification to determine extent of spinal arthrodesis, *J Bone Joint Surg* 83A:1169, 2001.)

excluded. In addition, this classification allows better organization of similar curve patterns and provides comparisons of various treatment methods.

NONOPERATIVE TREATMENT

Various methods have been used to treat adolescent idiopathic scoliosis over the years, including physical therapy, manipulation, and electrical stimulation, but there is no scientific evidence supporting their effectiveness. The two most widely accepted nonoperative techniques for idiopathic scoliosis are observation and bracing, often in conjunction with Schroth-based physical therapy.

OBSERVATION

Because mild scoliosis is frequent in the general population and few individuals have curves that require treatment, no method is reliable for accurately predicting at the initial evaluation which curves will progress. For these reasons, observation, except in patients with large curves, should be the initial form of treatment. Attempts have been made to monitor external contours with measurement of the rib hump, measurement of the trunk rotation angle with a "scoliometer," and use of contour devices such as surface topography scanning; however, these techniques have very limited, if any, clinical application. For this reason, radiographic evaluation remains the mainstay of observation. Because of intraobserver and interobserver variability in radiographic measurement, an increase of 5 or more degrees is considered progression. In general, the frequency of radiographic follow-up is driven by where the patient is in their development relative to their PHV (Table 8.5).

TABLE 8.5

Suggested Follow-up Frequency for Adolescent Idiopathic Scoliosis

AGE	PEAK HEIGHT VELOCITY	CURVE MAGNITUDE	FREQUENCY
Young	Before	<20 degrees	6 mo
Young	Before	>20 degrees	4 mo
Mid	In	All	4 mo
Older	After	<20 degrees	None
Older	After	>30 degrees	Annually to maturity*

*Should be followed every 5 years after skeletal maturity.

Curves of 30 to 40 degrees in skeletally mature patients generally do not require treatment, but because studies indicate a potential for progression in adult life, these patients should be observed with yearly standing posteroanterior radiographs for 2 to 3 years after skeletal maturity and then every 5 years.

ORTHOTIC TREATMENT

The goal of brace treatment is to limit further curve progression and avoid surgery. A small amount of correction may occur while in the brace, but the curve will generally settle to its pretreatment degree of curvature once the brace is discontinued. Brace correction of spinal curves is thought to occur through molding of the spine, trunk, and rib cage during growth, specifically through transverse loading of the spine through the use of corrective pads. The efficacy of brace treatment for patients with adolescent idiopathic scoliosis remains controversial. Numerous studies in the literature support the effectiveness of an orthosis in preventing curve progression and the need for surgical intervention. However, there are other studies that suggest bracing may not be effective. A large bracing study showed successful treatment in 72% of braced patients compared with 48% success with observation and concluded that bracing significantly decreased progression of high-risk curves to the threshold of surgery and that the benefit of bracing increased with longer hours of brace wear.

The SRS Committee on Bracing and Nonoperative Management has recommended standardization of criteria for adolescent idiopathic scoliosis brace studies so that valid and reliable comparisons can be made. The optimal inclusion criteria consist of age 10 years or older when a brace is prescribed, Risser grades 0 to 2, primary curve angles of 25 to 40 degrees, no prior treatment, and, if female, either premenarchal or less than 1 year postmenarchal. Bracing is recommended for a flexible curve of 25 degrees or more in a growing child with documented progression. Although surgery usually is indicated for curves in the 40- to 50-degree range in growing children, orthotic treatment may be considered for some curves in an effort to delay surgery to allow further maturation and spinal growth. Orthotic treatment is not used in patients with curves of more than 50 degrees.

Underarm braces (Boston, Wilmington, and Miami) have replaced the Milwaukee brace in most centers. However, these low-profile braces work best in patients whose curve apex is at T7 or lower. The Charleston and Providence nighttime bending braces hold the patient in maximal side-bending correction and are worn only at night for 8 to 10 hours. These braces are best suited for single thoracolumbar or lumbar curves.

The orthoses were originally intended to be worn 23 hours a day, but concern about compliance has led to part-time bracing regimens. Most part-time bracing protocols call for approximately 16 hours or less of brace wear each day. A meta-analysis of the literature found a relationship between the duration of brace wear per day and prevention of curve progression, suggesting that the more time that is spent in a brace, the less likely it will be for the curve to progress. Another study found that the total number of hours of brace wear correlated with the lack of curve progression and inversely correlated with the need for surgical treatment. This effect was most significant in patients who were at Risser grade 0 or 1 or with an open triradiate cartilage at the beginning of treatment. Curves did not progress in 82% of patients who wore the brace more than 12 hours per day compared with only 31% of those who wore the brace less than 7 hours per day.

The SpineCor brace (Biorthex Inc., Boucherville, Quebec, Canada) is an adjustable, flexible, dynamic brace with the cited advantages of simplicity of use, comfort, increased mobility, high patient compliance, and effectiveness. Outcomes of clinical studies indicate that prevention of curve progression is better with the brace than with no treatment, but comparative studies have shown it to be less effective than rigid orthoses in preventing curve progression. It appears to provide the greatest benefit for children between the juvenile and early adolescent stages, generally between the ages of 6 and 11 years, with Cobb angles of less than 30 degrees in whom other forms of bracing have failed.

OPERATIVE TREATMENT

Operative treatment is considered if the curve is likely to reach a magnitude that can be expected to become troublesome in adulthood. Although most authors recommend surgery when the curve reaches 50 degrees, other factors need to be considered. Smaller lumbar and thoracolumbar curves may cause significant trunk shift, coronal decompensation, and cosmetic deformity. Double 50-degree curves are not as cosmetically unacceptable as single curves, and if progression occurs in skeletally mature patients, it is likely to be gradual. In an immature patient, surgery may be considered for curves between 40 and 50 degrees, because of the high likelihood of growth-dependent progression. Surgery is more likely to be required in a patient with a curve that progresses despite brace treatment. Patients with significant back pain should have further evaluation before surgery for neurologic abnormalities. Thoracic lordosis also should be considered because it has a detrimental effect on pulmonary function, and bracing worsens thoracic lordosis. The general indications for operative treatment are summarized in Box 8.3.

PREOPERATIVE PREPARATION

Preoperative preparation is essential for an optimal surgical outcome. Aspirin-containing products or nonsteroidal

BOX 8.3

Indications for Operative Treatment of Idiopathic Scoliosis

- Increasing curve in growing child
- Severe deformity (>50 degrees) with asymmetry of trunk in adolescent
- Pain uncontrolled by nonoperative treatment
- Thoracic lordosis
- Significant cosmetic deformity

antiinflammatory agents should be discontinued before surgery because these medications may increase surgical blood loss and oral contraceptives should be discontinued because of the risk of deep venous thrombosis postoperatively. Preoperative radiographic evaluation with posteroanterior, lateral, and side-bending films of the thoracic and lumbar spine are necessary to determine fusion levels. Advanced imaging, most commonly MRI but also CT and myelography, occasionally are needed to rule out conditions such as syringomyelia, diastematomyelia, and tethered cord.

Patients with adolescent idiopathic scoliosis should have preoperative pulmonary function studies if they have a history of poor exercise tolerance, a curve of more than 60 degrees associated with a history of reactive airway disease, or a curve of more than 80 degrees. Patients with larger thoracic curves, thoracic lordosis, and coronal imbalance may be at higher risk of pulmonary impairment, but some patients with smaller curves may have clinically relevant pulmonary impairment. In fact, in some patients the pulmonary impairment may be out of proportion to the severity of the scoliosis. In rare cases with very large curves, a tracheostomy should be considered with a vital capacity of less than 30% of predicted normal. Ideally this should be done preoperatively to allow healing and pulmonary optimization.

With advances in perioperative anesthetic techniques, such as the use of hypotensive anesthesia during surgical exposure and the use of antifibrinolytic agents, most commonly tranexamic acid, the need for transfusion following surgical treatment for scoliosis has decreased dramatically. The use of tranexamic acid has been shown in large multicenter studies, as well as randomized studies, to correlate with decreased blood loss, decreased cell-saver volume, and need for postoperative transfusion. In rare cases, preoperative autologous blood donations and/or preoperative erythropoietin can be used in patients who qualify to decrease the risk of homologous blood transfusions.

INTRAOPERATIVE CONSIDERATIONS

Because spinal surgery has the potential for significant blood loss, two large-bore intravenous lines are needed, and an arterial line is necessary for continuous blood pressure monitoring. An indwelling urinary catheter is used to monitor urinary output. Electrocardiographic leads, blood pressure cuff, and a pulse oximeter also are necessary.

Spinal cord monitoring using both spinal somatosensory-evoked potentials and motor-evoked potentials has become the standard of care during scoliosis surgery because it facilitates timely diagnosis of neurologic injury, allowing the surgeon time to correct the etiology before permanent neurologic harm occurs. A large series of surgically treated scoliosis patients found that the use of electrophysiology had a sensitivity of 100% and specificity of 87% and all events had an identifiable episode that led to the change.

Cervical and cortical leads to the surgical area can record stimulation of the distal sensory nerves and can alert the surgeon to possible alteration of spinal cord transmission. Preoperative monitoring for a "baseline" is helpful for comparison during the operative procedure. When somatosensory-evoked potentials are used, multiple recording sites must be used, including cortical, subcortical, and peripheral sites, and certain inhalation agents, such as halothane and isoflurane, should be avoided, as should diazepam and droperidol. The somatosensory-evoked potential is a useful adjunct for monitoring spinal cord function, but it is not infallible, and false-positive and false-negative results have been reported. An important limitation of the somatosensory-evoked potential is that it measures only the integrity of the sensory system.

The use of motor-evoked potentials will monitor the spinal cord motor tracts. The combination of motor-evoked potentials and somatosensory-evoked potentials can significantly decrease the chance of unrecognized injury to the spinal cord. Transcranial electrical stimulation of the motor cortex generates an electrical impulse that descends the corticospinal tract and enters the peripheral muscle, where this electrical impulse can be recorded. This allows monitoring of the ventral spinal cord, which is vulnerable to cord ischemia. For this reason, motor-evoked potentials are more sensitive to mean arterial pressure and hypotensive anesthesia, and changes in motor-evoked potentials occur more rapidly than in somatosensory-evoked potentials after a neurologic injury.

Triggered electromyographic monitoring is useful to detect a possible breach in the pedicle wall by a pedicle screw. A threshold of less than 6 mA should alert the surgeon to a possible breach.

The first available spinal cord monitoring technique was the Stagnara wake-up test, described by Vauzelle, Stagnara, and Jouvinroux in 1973. In this test, the anesthesia is decreased or reversed after correction of the spinal deformity. The patient is brought to a conscious level and asked to move both lower extremities. Once voluntary movement is noted, anesthesia is returned to the appropriate level and the surgical procedure is completed. With the widespread use of somatosensory and motor-evoked potentials, this technique is rarely used because of the risk of awaking a prone, intubated patient but is useful if concerns about the quality of the motor and somatosensory-evoked potentials exists or a spinal cord injury is suspected. The ankle clonus test has been reported as an alternative to the wake-up test. Clonus should be present for a brief period on emergence from anesthesia. The absence of clonus during this time is abnormal.

Hypotensive anesthesia, in which mean arterial blood pressure is kept at 65 mm Hg, is an effective way to decrease intraoperative blood loss. An arterial line is essential during this type of anesthesia. Care also must be taken in reducing blood pressure so that it does not lead to ischemia of the spinal cord. Hypotensive anesthesia should not be considered in patients with a heart condition or in patients with spinal cord compression in whom a decrease in arterial blood supply might restrict an already compromised spinal cord blood flow. Antifibrinolytics have been shown to reduce intraoperative blood loss, percent blood loss, and the need for postoperative transfusion, with the most commonly used being tranexamic acid. They are typically used in conjunction with other techniques such as hypotensive anesthesia, judicious use of crystalloids, and a cell saver to decrease surgical blood loss and rate of transfusion.

The cell saver is used in most institutions and has been shown to save approximately 50% of the red cell mass, thereby reducing the need for intraoperative blood transfusions. The cell saver is contraindicated in patients with malignant disease or infection. Care must be taken when using microfibrillar products such as Gelfoam and topical clotting agents such as thrombin to avoid direct aspiration of these, which can lead to microclot embolization. Thorough irrigation of the wound after the use of these products is recommended before resuming cell saver use. Certain substances such as antibiotics including bacitracin, as well as betadine and hydrogen peroxide, can cause red cell lysis. The surgeon should try to estimate preoperatively if enough blood will be salvaged to make the cell saver cost-effective.

SURGICAL GOALS

The goals of surgery for spinal deformity are to correct or improve the deformity, to maintain sagittal balance, to preserve or improve pulmonary function, to minimize morbidity or pain, to maximize postoperative function, and to improve or at least not to harm the function of the lumbar spine. To accomplish these goals in patients with idiopathic scoliosis, surgical techniques may include anterior, posterior, or combined anterior and posterior procedures. The surgical indications, techniques, and procedures are divided into anterior and posterior sections.

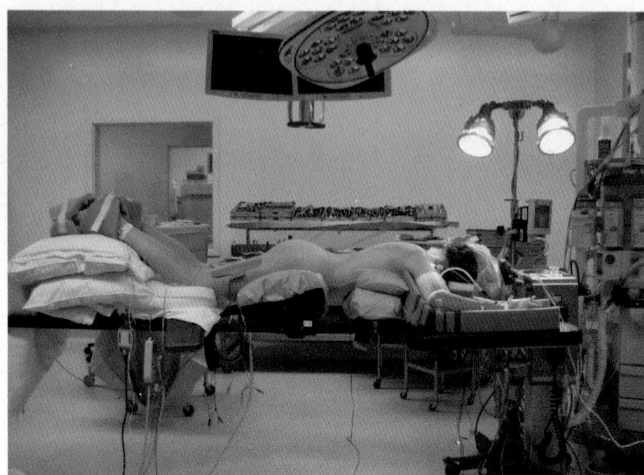

FIGURE 8.33 Patient positioning on Jackson table with hips in extension to maintain lumbar lordosis. **SEE TECHNIQUE 8.6.**

POSTERIOR SURGERIES FOR IDIOPATHIC SCOLIOSIS

The posterior approach to the spinal column is the most commonly used. It is familiar to all orthopaedic surgeons and offers a safe and extensile approach that exposes the entire vertebral column.

TECHNIQUE 8.6

- Position the patient prone on a Jackson table (Mizuho OSI, Union City, CA) with the arms carefully supported and the elbows padded. The Jackson table eliminates intraabdominal pressure and helps reduce blood loss (Fig. 8.33).
- Do not abduct the shoulders more than 90 degrees to prevent pressure or stretch on the brachial plexus.
- The Jackson table maintains the hips in extension, which will maintain the lumbar lordosis, which is extremely important in obtaining proper sagittal alignment of the spine with instrumentation. The knees are well padded and slightly flexed to relieve some pressure from the hamstring muscles.
- Carefully pad the pressure points. The upper pads of the frame should rest on the chest and not in the axilla to avoid pressure on any nerves from the brachial plexus.
- When the patient is positioned on the frame with the hips flexed, lumbar lordosis is partially eliminated. If the fusion is to be extended into the lower lumbar spine, elevate the knees and thighs so that the patient lies with the hip joints extended to maintain normal lumbar lordosis.
- Scrub the patient's back with a surgical soap solution for 5 to 10 minutes and prepare the skin with an antiseptic solution. Drape the area of the operative site and use a plastic Steri-Drape (3M, St. Paul, MN) to seal off the skin.
- Make the skin incision in a straight line from one vertebra superior to the proposed fusion area to one vertebra inferior to it. A straight scar improves the postoperative appearance of the back (Fig. 8.34A). Make the initial incision through the dermal layer only. Infiltrate the intradermal and subcutaneous areas with an epinephrine solution (1:500,000).
- Deepen the incision to the level of the spinous processes and use self-retaining Weitlaner retractors to retract the skin margins. Control bleeding with an electrocautery. Identify the interspinous ligament between the spinous processes; this often appears as a white line. As the incision is deepened, keep the Weitlaner retractors tight to help with exposure and to minimize bleeding. Now incise the cartilaginous cap overlying the spinous processes as close to the midline as possible (Fig. 8.34B). This midline may vary because of rotation of the spinous processes.
- With use of a Cobb elevator and electrocautery, expose the spinous processes subperiosteally after the cartilaginous caps have been moved to either side.

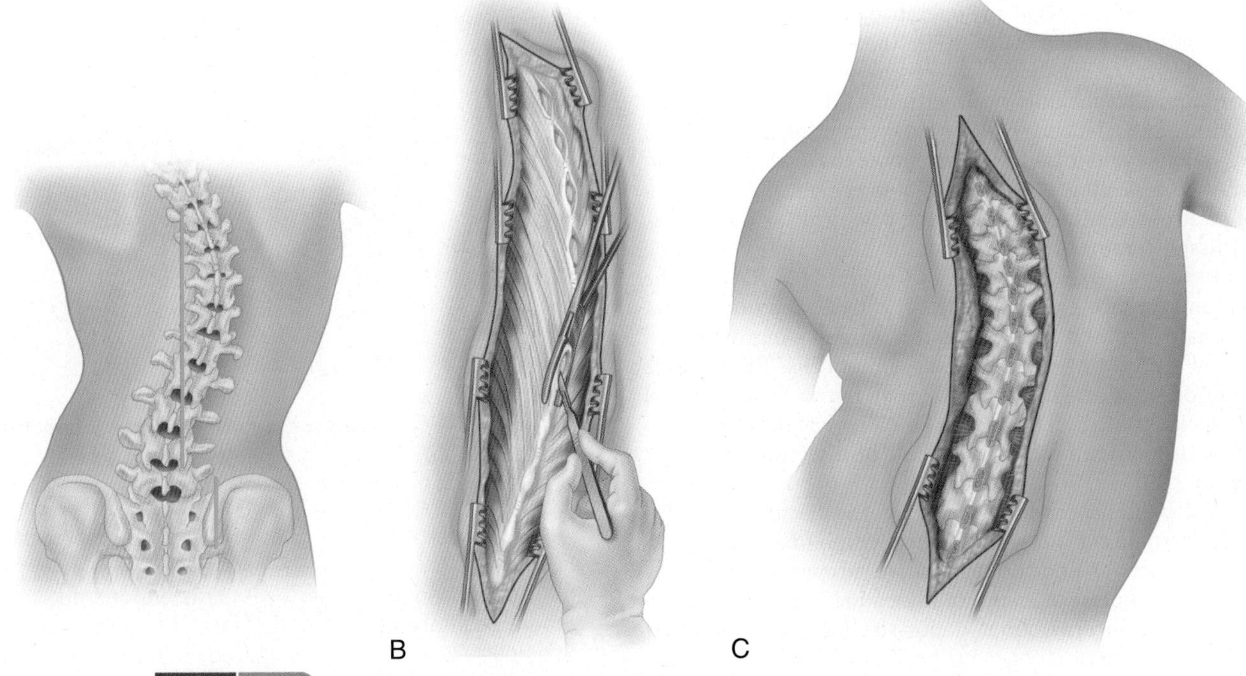

FIGURE 8.34 **A,** Skin incisions for posterior fusion and autogenous bone graft. **B,** Incisions over spinous processes and interspinous ligaments. **C,** Weitlaner retractors used to maintain tension and exposure of spine during dissection. **SEE TECHNIQUE 8.6.**

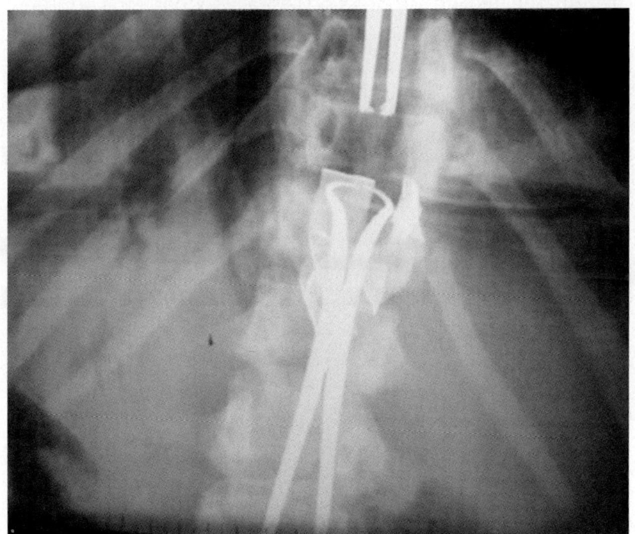

FIGURE 8.35 Intraoperative fluoroscopy showing towel clip in the spinous process of T11, which lies over the body of T12. See text. **SEE TECHNIQUE 8.6.**

- After several of the spinous processes have been exposed, move the Weitlaner retractors to a deeper level and maintain tension for retraction and hemostasis.
- After exposure of all spinous processes, a localizing radiograph can be obtained (Fig. 8.35). Alternatively, the T12 rib and the L1 transverse process can be used to localize the levels. Continue the subperiosteal exposure of the entire area to be fused, keeping the retractors tight at all times (Fig. 8.34C). It is easier to dissect from caudad to cephalad because of the oblique attachments of the short rotator muscles and ligaments of the spine.

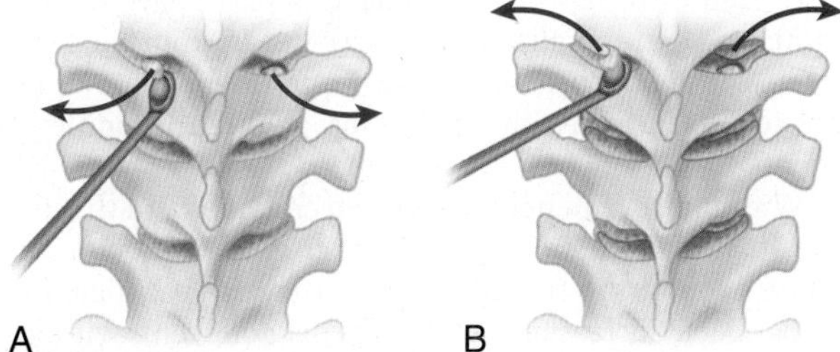

FIGURE 8.36 **A** and **B,** Cobb curets used to clean facets of ligament attachments. **SEE TECHNIQUE 8.6.**

- Extend the subperiosteal dissection first to the facet joints on one side and then the other side, deepening the retractors as necessary. Continue the dissection laterally to the ends of the transverse processes on both sides.
- Coagulate the branch of the segmental vessel just lateral to each facet.
- Place the self-retaining retractors deeper to hold the entire incision open and exposed.
- Sponges soaked in the 1:500,000 epinephrine solution can be used to maintain hemostasis.
- Use a curet and pituitary rongeur to completely clean the interspinous ligaments and the facets of all ligamentous attachments and capsule, proceeding from the midline laterally (Fig. 8.36) to decrease the possibility of the curet's slipping and penetrating the spinal canal.
- The entire spine is now exposed from one transverse process to another, all soft tissue has been removed, and the spine is ready for instrumentation and arthrodesis as indicated by the procedure chosen.

POSTERIOR ARTHRODESIS

The long-term success of any operative procedure for scoliosis depends on a solid arthrodesis. The classic extraarticular Hibbs technique has been replaced by intraarticular fusion techniques that include the facet joints. The success of spinal arthrodesis depends on surgical preparation of the fusion site, systemic and local factors, ability of the graft material to stimulate a healing process, and biomechanical features of the graft positioning. To obtain the best field for the fusion, soft-tissue trauma should be minimal and avascular tissue should be removed from the graft bed. The surface of the bone and the facets should be decorticated to provide a large, maximally exposed surface area for vascular ingrowth and to allow delivery of more osteoprogenitor cells. The patient's condition should be optimized through nutrition and control of associated medical problems. Smoking has been found to inhibit fusion significantly and should be discontinued before surgery.

While autogenous bone graft from the iliac crest remains the "gold standard" for graft material, combining osteogenic, osteoconductive, and osteoinductive properties, it rarely is used in routine adolescent idiopathic scoliosis surgery because of concerns about donor-site morbidity. Another excellent source of autogenous bone is rib obtained from a thoracoplasty. Allografts, which avoid donor site morbidity, are most commonly used, provide osteoconductive properties, and have been shown to produce results equal to those of autogenous iliac crest graft in young patients. Several alternative graft materials include tricalcium phosphate, hydroxyapatite, and demineralized bone matrix. Bone morphogenetic protein can supply osteoinductive properties but has not been routinely used in multilevel fusions required in adolescent patients.

With improvements in surgical techniques and the inclusion of intraarticular fusion, together with meticulous dissection around the transverse processes, the pseudarthrosis rate has been decreased to 2% or less in adolescents with idiopathic scoliosis.

FACET FUSION

TECHNIQUE 8.7

(MOE)

- Expose the spine to the tips of the transverse processes as previously described (see Technique 8.6).
- Begin a cut over the cephalad articular processes at the base of the lamina and carry it along the transverse process almost to its tip. Bend this fragment laterally to lie between the transverse processes, leaving it hinged if possible.
- Thoroughly remove the cartilage from the superior articular process.
- Make another cut in the area of the superior articular facet with the Cobb gouge, beginning medially and working laterally to produce another hinged fragment. Alternatively, an ultrasonic bone scalpel (Misonix, Farmingdale, NY) can be used to decrease blood loss and the risk of spinal cord injury.

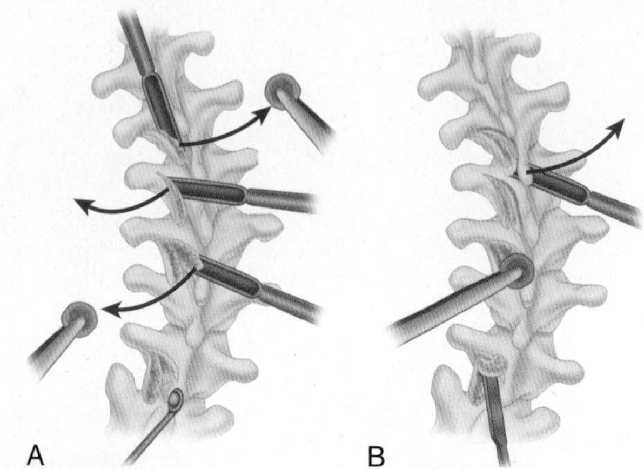

FIGURE 8.37 **A** and **B,** Moe technique of thoracic facet fusion. **SEE TECHNIQUE 8.7.**

- Place cancellous bone graft in the defect created (Fig. 8.37).
- In the lumbar spine, the facet joints are oriented in a more sagittal direction and a facet fusion is best accomplished by removal of the adjoining joint surface with a small osteotome or a needle-nose rongeur. This creates a defect that is packed with cancellous bone (Fig. 8.38).
- Decorticate the entire exposed spine with Cobb gouges from the midline, progressing laterally so that if the gouge were to slip it would be moving away from the spinal canal. Alternatively, a high-speed burr can be used to decorticate the spine, decreasing the risk of spinal cord penetration.

FACET FUSION

TECHNIQUE 8.8

(HALL)

- First, sharply cut the inferior facet with a gouge, remove this bone fragment to expose the superior facet cartilage, and remove this cartilage with a sharp curet. Alternatively, an ultrasonic bone scalpel (Misonix, Farmingdale, NY) can be used to decrease blood loss and the risk of spinal cord injury.
- Create a trough by removing the outer cortex of the superior facet and add cancellous bone grafts (Fig. 8.39).
- Proceed with decortication as described in the Moe technique.

BONE GRAFTING

Autogenous iliac crest bone graft has been considered the gold standard. The harvest of autogenous bone graft from the ilium adds to surgical time and can introduce the potential for intraoperative and postoperative morbidity associated with

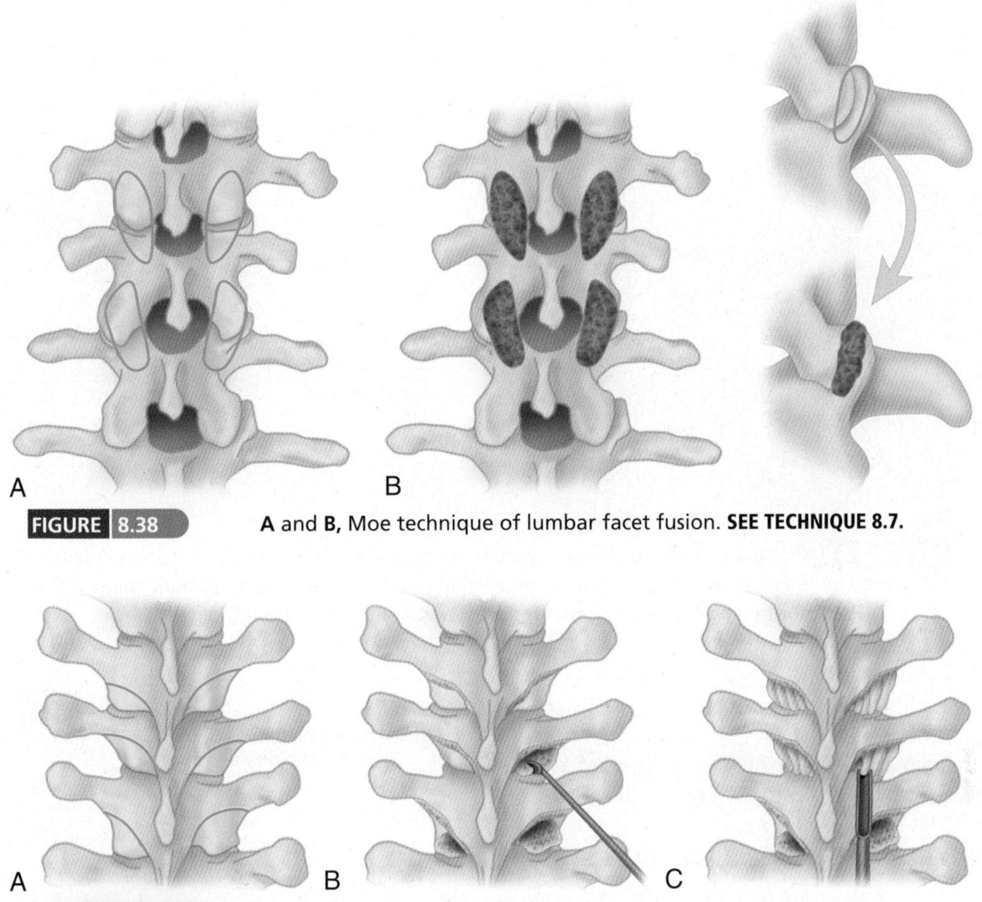

FIGURE 8.38 **A** and **B,** Moe technique of lumbar facet fusion. **SEE TECHNIQUE 8.7.**

FIGURE 8.39 **A-C,** Hall technique of thoracic facet fusion. **SEE TECHNIQUE 8.8.**

the procedure. With the use of modern-day rigid segmental instrumentation, the rate of pseudarthrosis with allograft is extremely low and equal to that with the use of autogenous graft. For these reasons, autogenous iliac crest bone graft is rarely if ever used in routine adolescent idiopathic scoliosis surgery. The time saved by using allograft in many cases offsets the additional cost. In rare revision settings or poor healing environments, the use of iliac crest autogenous graft can be helpful.

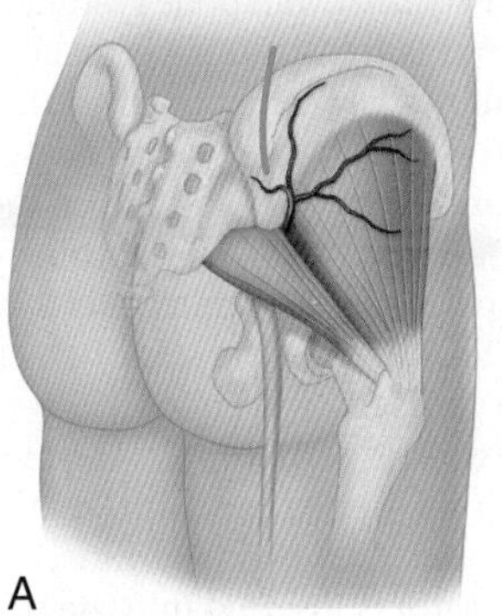

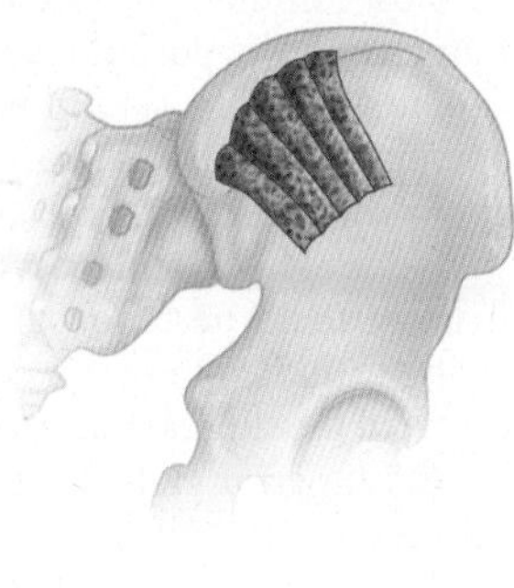

FIGURE 8.40 **A,** Superior gluteal artery as it emerges from area of sciatic notch. **B,** Cortical and cancellous strips removed from outer table of ilium for autogenous bone graft. **SEE TECHNIQUE 8.9.**

AUTOGENOUS ILIAC CREST BONE GRAFT

TECHNIQUE 8.9

- Make an incision over the iliac crest to be used (Fig. 8.40A). If the original incision extends far enough distally into the lumbar spine, the iliac crest can be exposed through the same incision by subcutaneous dissection.
- Infiltrate the intradermal and subcutaneous areas with 1:500,000 epinephrine solution.
- Expose the cartilaginous apophysis overlying the posterior iliac crest and split it in the middle.
- With a Cobb elevator, expose the ilium subperiosteally.
- The superior gluteal artery emerges from the area of the sciatic notch (see Fig. 8.40A) and should be carefully avoided during the bone grafting procedure.
- If bicortical grafts are desired, expose the posterior crest of the ilium on the inner side and obtain two or three strips of bicortical graft with a large gouge. Otherwise, take cortical and cancellous strips from the outer table of the ilium (Fig. 8.40B).
- Place these bone grafts in a kidney basin and cover them with a sponge soaked in saline or blood.
- Control bleeding from the iliac crest with bone wax or Gelfoam.

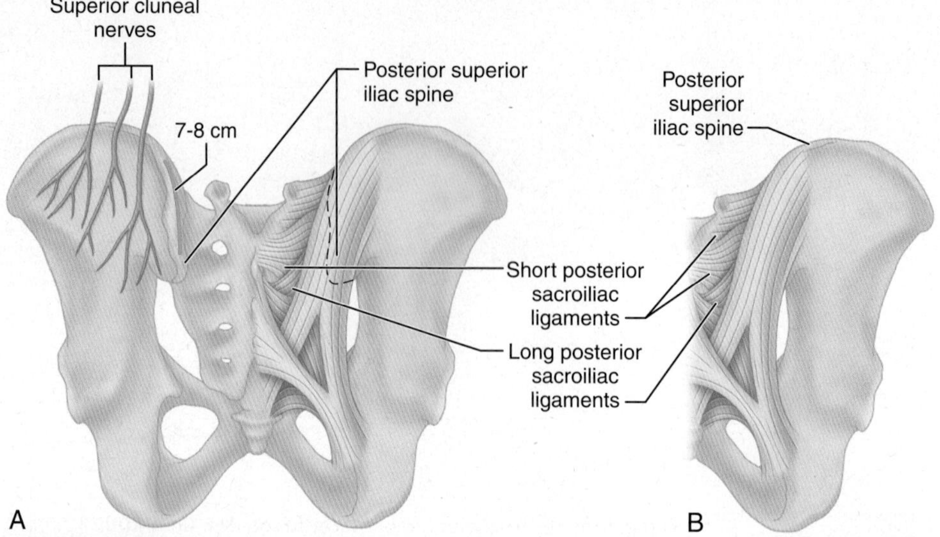

FIGURE 8.41 **A,** Superior cluneal nerve may be injured during harvest of bone graft from iliac crest. Limited incision *(green line)*, staying within 8 cm of posterior superior iliac spine, avoids nerve. **B,** Posterior ligament complex provides most of stability of sacroiliac joint.

- Approximate the cartilaginous cap of the posterior iliac crest with an absorbable stitch.
- Place a suction drain at the donor site and connect it to a separate reservoir to monitor postoperative bleeding here separately from the spinal fusion site.

COMPLICATIONS OF BONE GRAFTING

The most common complication associated with bone graft harvesting from the posterior iliac crest is transient or permanent numbness over the skin of the buttock caused by injury of the superior cluneal nerves (Fig. 8.41A). The superior cluneal nerves supply sensation to a large area of the buttocks and pierce the lumbodorsal fascia and cross the posterior iliac crest beginning 8 cm lateral to the posterior superior iliac spine. A limited incision, staying within 8 cm of the posterior superior iliac spine, which will avoid the superior cluneal nerves, is recommended.

The superior gluteal artery exits the pelvis, enters the gluteal region through the superiormost portion of the sciatic notch, and sends extensive branches to the gluteal muscles. Care should be taken when a retractor is inserted into the sciatic notch. Injury to the superior gluteal artery will cause massive hemorrhage, and the artery generally retracts proximally into the pelvis. Control of the bleeding frequently requires bone removal from the sciatic notch to obtain sufficient exposure. It may be necessary to pack the wound, turn the patient, and have a general surgeon locate and ligate the hypogastric artery. Ureteral injury also can occur in the sciatic notch from the sharp tip of a retractor.

Most of the stability of the sacroiliac joint is provided by the posterior ligamentous complex (Fig. 8.41B). Injury to the sacroiliac joint from removal of these ligaments can range from clinical symptoms of instability to dislocation. Dislocation of the sacroiliac joint as a complication of full-thickness graft removal from the posterior ilium has been reported. If a full-thickness graft is obtained, it should not be obtained too close to the sacroiliac joint (Fig. 8.42).

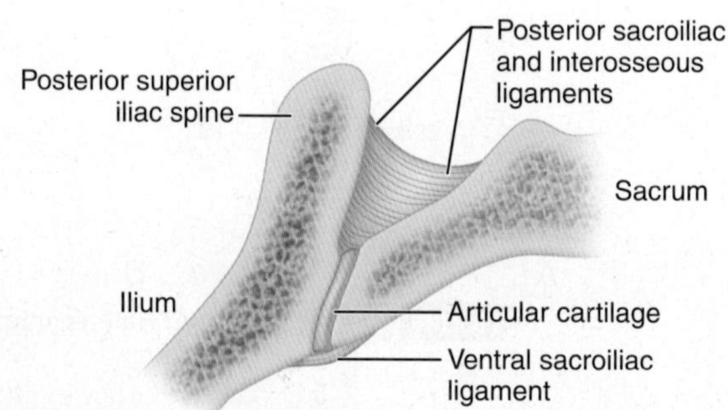

FIGURE 8.42 Axial view of sacroiliac joint. Full-thickness graft should not be obtained too close to sacroiliac joint to avoid damage to posterior ligamentous complex.

POSTERIOR SPINAL INSTRUMENTATION

The goals of instrumentation in scoliosis surgery are to correct the deformity as much as possible and to stabilize the spine in the corrected position while the fusion mass becomes solid. The fusion mass in a well-corrected spine is subjected to much lower bending moments and tensile forces than is the fusion mass in an uncorrected spine.

In 1962, Harrington introduced the first effective instrumentation system for scoliosis. For more than 30 years, use of the Harrington distraction rod, combined with a thorough posterior arthrodesis and immobilization in a cast or brace for 6 to 9 months, was the standard surgical treatment of adolescent idiopathic scoliosis. Despite its success, the Harrington instrumentation system had several disadvantages. Correction with this system is achieved with distraction, leading to loss of normal sagittal balance and creating a flatback deformity (Fig. 8.43). Because this rod was anchored only at the ends of the construct, minimal rotational correction was obtained and anchor failure due to lamina failure was common. While transformative at its time, Harrington instrumentation has been replaced by more modern segmental instrumentation systems using multiple anchors, most commonly pedicle screws and hooks, which allow more

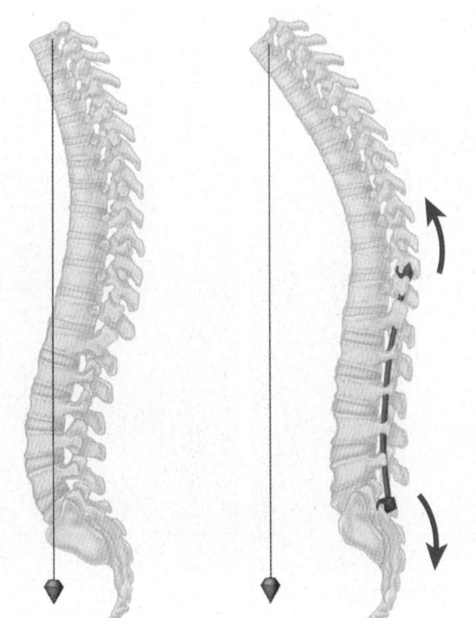

FIGURE 8.43 Effects of distraction rod in lumbar spine. If contouring for lordosis is inadequate, lumbar spine can be flattened by distracting force. Also note kyphotic deformity just superior to distraction rod.

powerful correction, rotational control, and better correction of sagittal plane deformity.

Posterior segmental spinal instrumentation systems provide multiple points of fixation to the spine and apply compression, distraction, and rotation forces through the same rod. These systems generally do not require any postoperative immobilization. They provide better coronal plane correction and better control in the sagittal plane. Hypokyphosis in the thoracic spine can be reduced and lumbar lordosis preserved when the instrumentation extends to the lower lumbar spine. With the use of pedicle screws there appears to be better transverse plane correction (vertebral rotation). These systems generally have implant failure and pseudarthrosis rates lower than those of Harrington instrumentation (Video 8.3).

Three kinds of devices are available for fixation of posterior segmental instrumentation: pedicle screws, sublaminar wires/tapes, and hooks.

CORRECTION MANEUVERS

A variety of techniques and maneuvers can be used to achieve correction of spinal deformity, and the specific technique used should be customized to each patient and his or her curve characteristics, making a thorough knowledge of each of these techniques essential. Correction of a scoliotic curve also can be obtained by translating the apex of the curve into a more normal position. Translation can be achieved by a rod derotation maneuver described by Cotrel and Dubousset; this is accomplished by connecting the precontoured concave rod to each fixation site and then rotating the rod approximately 90 degrees into the sagittal plane. This essentially converts the pre-existing scoliosis to kyphosis. This en bloc derotation maneuver results in a lateral translation of the apical vertebrae or an in situ relocation of the apex of the treated curve.

Pure translation is another method for correcting curves. This can be achieved with sublaminar wires or a reduction screw on the concave side. The rod is contoured into the desired amount of coronal and sagittal plane correction and placed into the proximal and distal fixation sites. The spine is then slowly and sequentially pulled to the precontoured rods using sublaminar wires or reduction screws.

In situ contouring is another correction technique. With the use of appropriate bending tools, in situ contouring in both the coronal and sagittal planes can improve spinal alignment in scoliosis. A cantilever technique can be used to reduce spinal deformity. With this technique the precontoured rod is inserted and fixed either proximally or distally and then sequentially reduced into each fixation site with a cantilever maneuver. This is usually followed by appropriate compression and distraction to finalize the correction. With the use of monoaxial and uniplanar pedicle screws, correction can be obtained by en bloc vertebral derotation over three or four apical vertebral segments or by direct segmental vertebral rotation in which the derotation maneuver is applied to individual vertebral segments.

Finally, distraction on the concave side of a thoracic curve will decrease scoliosis and thoracic kyphosis. Compression applied on the convex side of a lumbar curve will correct scoliosis and allow for restoration or maintenance of lumbar lordosis. Distraction and compression are the primary modes of correction when hooks are used due to their limited ability to rotate or translate the spine.

SEGMENTAL INSTRUMENTATION: PEDICLE SCREWS

PEDICLE FIXATION

Pedicle screw fixation from the posterior approach into the vertebral body has become the most popular form of spinal fixation because of the ability to facilitate greater three-dimensional curve correction (Fig. 8.44). While commonly used, there is still no evidence on the optimal number and placement of screws. Larson observed that early adopters of pedicle screw placement recommended higher screw densities, with two screws at every level. A recent expert consensus panel recommended an intermediate density (1.6 screws/level) with higher densities at the ends of the construct and at the apex. Several studies have shown no significant difference in curve correction between high- and low-density screw constructs. Because screw density correlates with intraoperative blood loss and surgical time, the screw density and the purpose of each screw in the construct should be carefully considered. In addition, implants make up 30% to 50% of the total surgical cost, so small changes in screw density can lead to cost savings that equal or exceed those of accelerated discharge pathways.

In studies comparing hook fixation with thoracic pedicle screw fixation, thoracic posterior-only pedicle screw constructs were found to provide better correction than hook constructs. For each screw used there also is a risk of screw malposition. With a freehand technique, the rate of screw malposition is between 5% and 15%, which is experience dependent. The highest risk for malplacement is in the upper thoracic spine because of the smaller pedicle diameter at these levels. A recent meta-analysis comparing freehand to navigation-assisted pedicle screw techniques found the overall breach rate to be lower using navigation (7.9% vs. 9% to 17%); there were no screw-related complications in the navigation group, but there were 0 to 1.7% in the non-navigation group. The disadvantages of CT-based navigation are the cost,

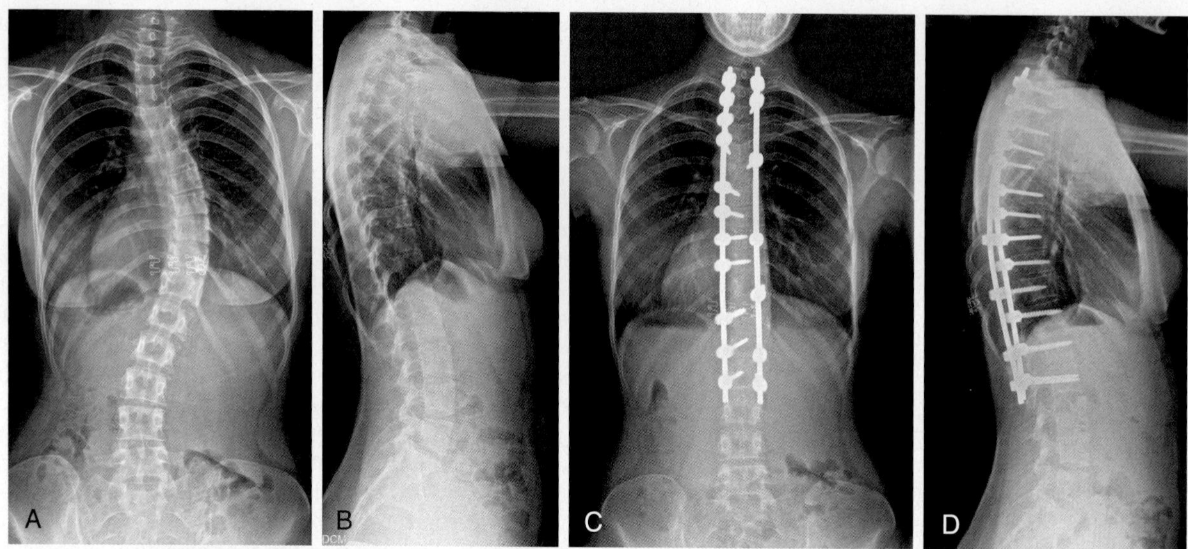

FIGURE 8.44 **A** and **B**, Preoperative anteroposterior and lateral radiographs of patient with idiopathic scoliosis treated with lumbar and thoracic pedicle screws. **C** and **D**, Postoperative posteroanterior and lateral radiographs.

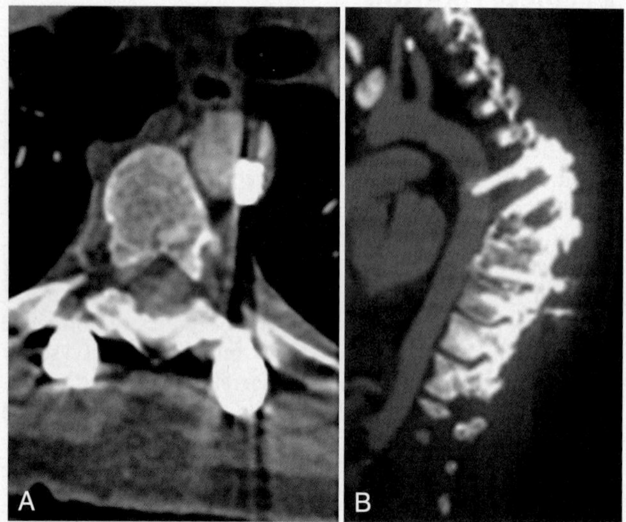

FIGURE 8.45 **A**, Axial CT showing far lateral penetration and aortic impingement of thoracic pedicle screw. **B**, Sagittal reconstruction. Note aortic arch and heart.

time, and radiation exposure. Newer techniques, such as the use of three-dimensional models, robotic-assisted drill hole placement, and patient-specific custom drill jigs, are under investigation. There is no consensus on the optimal treatment of a malplaced screw because most are asymptomatic; however, because of the potential for severe complications including aortic or esophageal erosion (Fig. 8.45) and the relatively low risk of screw removal, a low threshold should exist for removal of malplaced screws.

A thorough knowledge of the pedicle anatomy is necessary for the use of pedicle fixation. The pedicle connects the posterior elements to the vertebral body. Medial to the pedicle are the epidural space, nerve root, and dural sac. The exiting nerve root at the level of the pedicle is close to the medial and caudal cortex of the pedicle (Fig. 8.46). Close to the lateral and superior aspects of the pedicle cortex is the nerve root from the level above. At the L3 and L4 vertebral bodies, the common iliac artery and veins lie directly anterior to the pedicles (Fig. 8.47). In the sacral region, the great vessels and their branches lie laterally along the sacral ala. In the midline of the sacrum, a variable middle sacral artery can lie directly anterior to the S1 vertebral body. Anterior penetration of a vertebral body can occur without being apparent on the radiograph unless a "near-approach" view is obtained (Fig. 8.48).

In a study of the size of pedicles in mature and immature spines, the transverse pedicle width at the L5 and L4 levels reached 8 mm or more in children 6 to 8 years of age, but transverse width at L3 approaching 8 mm was not seen until 9 to 11 years of age (Fig. 8.49). The distance to the anterior cortex increased dramatically from the youngest age group until adulthood at all levels (Fig. 8.50). In patients with spinal deformities, the pedicles, especially the concave pedicles, often are deformed, and care must be taken in insertion of any pedicle fixation.

Four anatomic types of pedicles exist (Fig. 8.51): type A has a large cancellous channel in which the pedicle probe can be smoothly inserted without difficulty; type B has a small cancellous channel in which the probe fits snugly; type C is a cortical channel in which the probe must be tapped with

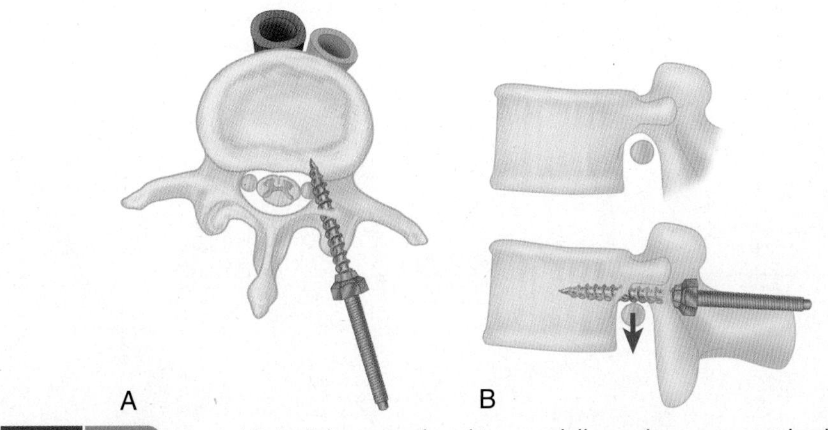

FIGURE 8.46 **A,** and **B,** Pedicle screw placed too caudally causing nerve root impingement.

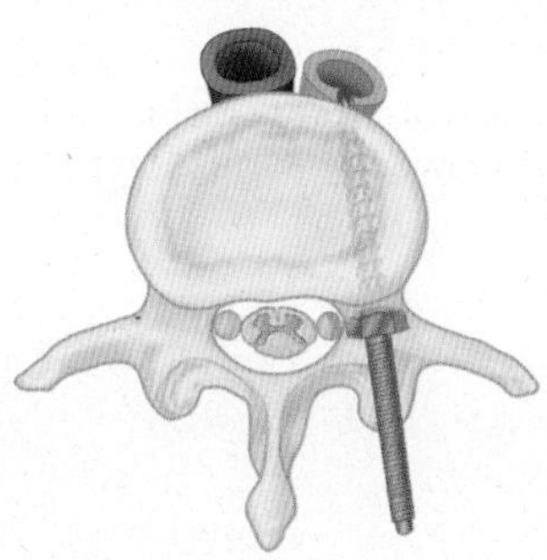

FIGURE 8.47 Vascular damage by insertion of screw beyond anterior cortex.

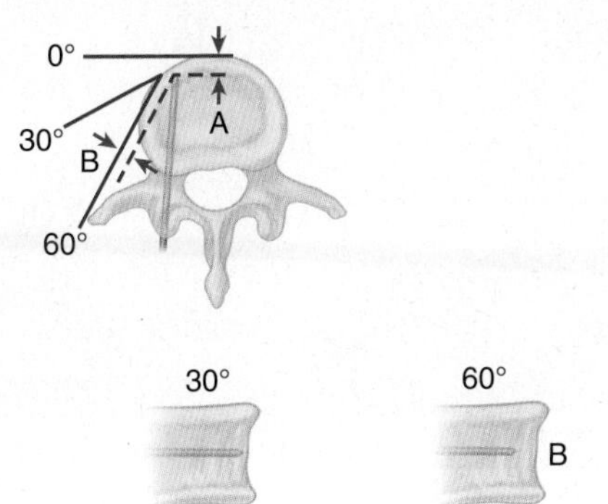

FIGURE 8.48 Near-approach radiographic view to decrease likelihood of anterior screw penetration. When drill (or screw or probe) tip is actually at anterior cortex, lateral view (0 degrees) misleadingly shows tip still to be some distance (*A*) away from cortex. When angle of view is too oblique (60 degrees), tip appears to be some distance (*B*) from cortex. Only when view is tangent to point of penetration (30 degrees in this illustration) does tip appear most nearly to approach actual breakthrough.

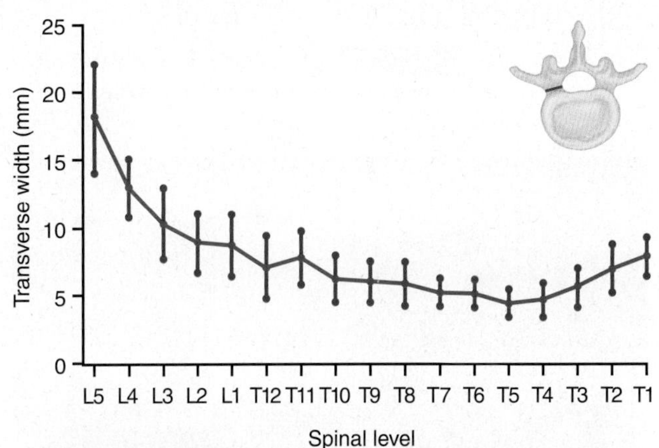

FIGURE 8.49 Transverse pedicle isthmus widths.

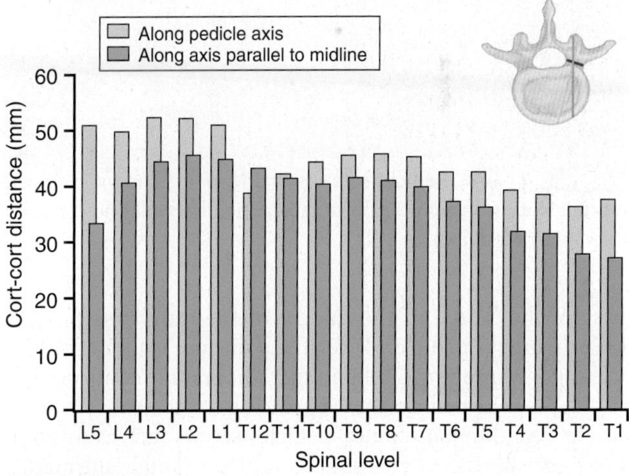

FIGURE 8.50 Distance to anterior cortex through pedicle angle axis versus through line parallel to midline axis of vertebra.

a mallet to enter the body; and type D is an absent pedicle channel that requires a juxtapedicular screw position. Type A and B pedicles do not require special techniques for probe insertion, whereas type C and especially type D pedicles do require special methods. Pedicles located on the concave (compression) side of the curves were found to be significantly smaller than those on the convex side, regardless of whether they were cancellous or cortical. Of 1021 pedicles in which pedicle screws were placed, 61% were type A, 29.2% were type B, 6.8% were type C, and 3% were type D. CT validated the morphologic evaluation and description of the four pedicle types.

Various methods have been described for identifying the pedicle and placing the pedicle screw, but basic steps include (1) clearing the soft tissue, (2) exposing the cancellous bone of the pedicle canal by decortication at the intersection of the

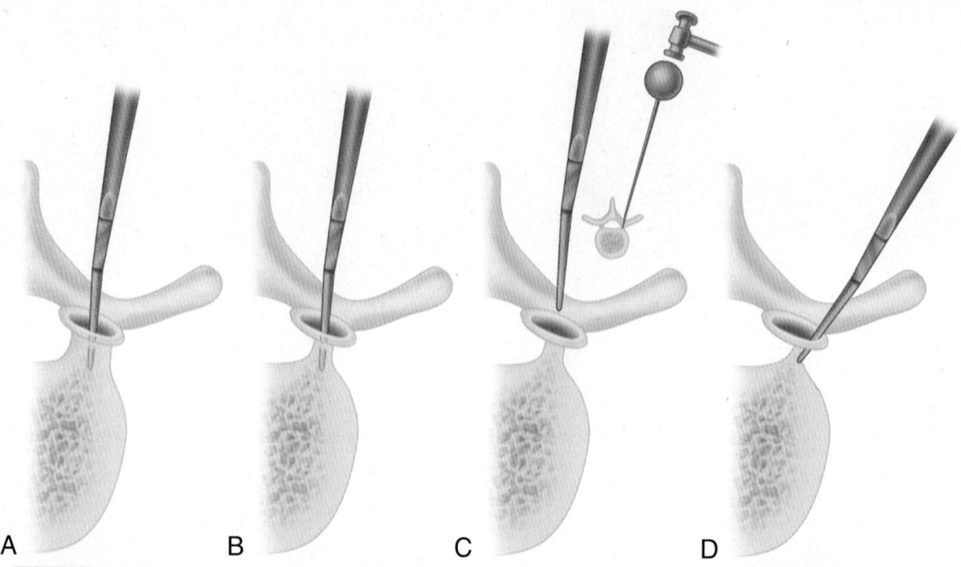

FIGURE 8.51 Pedicle channel classification (see text). (From Watanabe K, Lenke KG, Matsumoto M, et al: A novel pedicle channel classification describing osseous anatomy, *Spine* 35:1836, 2010.)

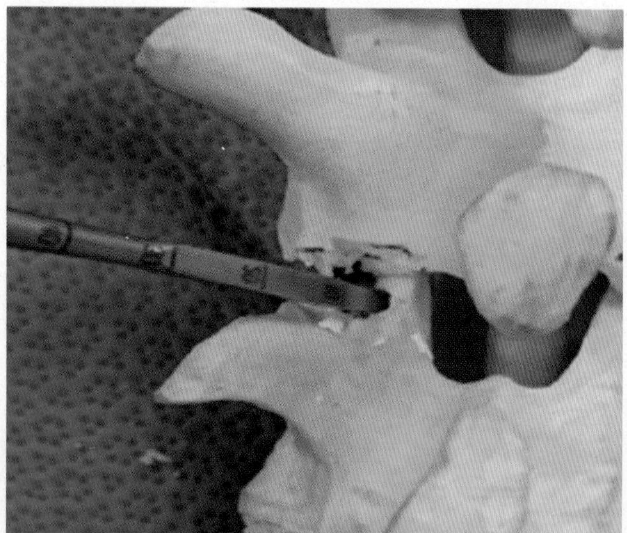

FIGURE 8.52 Pedicle screw starting point shown on bone model. Note starting point is at lateral pedicle wall and centered in cranio-caudal axis.

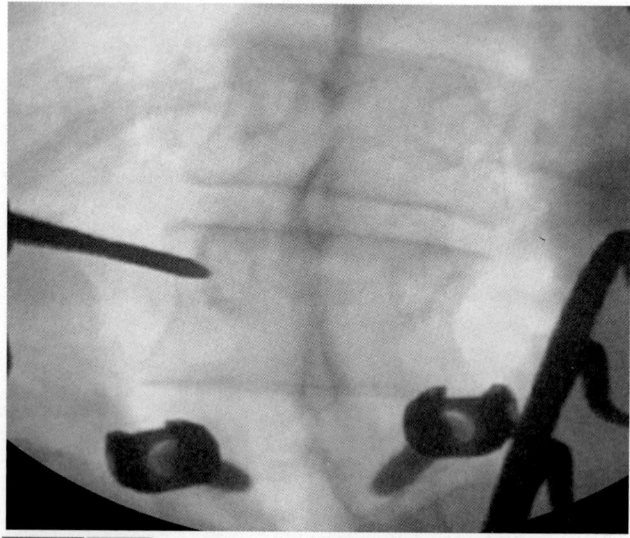

FIGURE 8.53 Pedicle screw starting point using fluoroscopic assistance.

base of the facet and the middle of the transverse process, (3) probing the pedicle, (4) verifying the four walls of the pedicle canal by probing or obtaining radiographic confirmation, (5) tapping the pedicle, and (6) placing the screw.

In the lumbar spine, pedicle screws are commonly inserted with use of anatomic landmarks, and confirmatory radiographs are obtained. Because of the deformed pedicles associated with scoliosis, many surgeons use fluoroscopic guidance. Freehand pedicle screw placement in the thoracic spine, which reduces patient and surgeon radiographic exposure, may be safe in experienced hands and evidence suggests that lower medial breach rates are associated with surgeon experience. The technique significantly reduces exposure of both the surgeon and the patient to radiation. Because of the tight confines of the pedicle in the thoracic spine and the frequently altered normal anatomy, we still use fluoroscopy to identify the entry site into the thoracic pedicle and to confirm screw placement (Figs 8.52 and 8.53). Frameless stereotactic technology allows three-dimensional navigation and is more commonly being used to guide and confirm pedicle screw placement. It has been shown to have a greater accuracy rate than other techniques but is associated with higher radiation exposure. It is important to have knowledge of and proficiency with multiple techniques to optimize the technique used based on the patient's diagnosis and anatomy, as well as resources available.

INSERTION OF LUMBAR PEDICLE SCREWS

Zindrick described a "pedicle approach zone" (Fig. 8.54) that is decorticated before the pedicle is cannulated with either a probe or pedicle awl. The awl is carefully advanced until resistance is felt. An intraoperative radiograph or

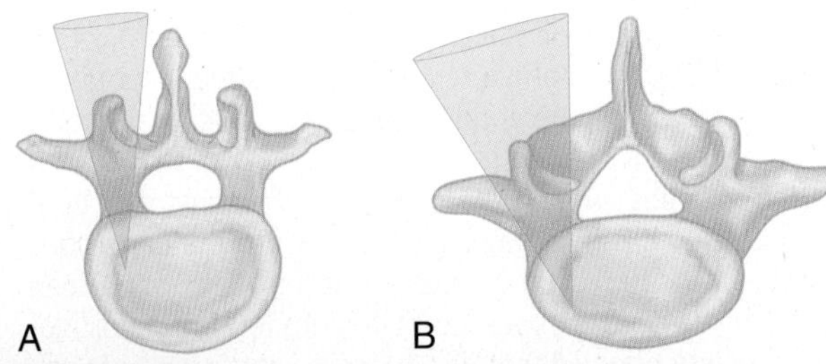

FIGURE 8.54 **A,** Funnel-shaped pedicle approach zone in upper lumbar region (L1). **B,** Funnel-shaped pedicle approach zone in lower lumbar region (L5). With increased pedicle size, pedicle approach zone funnel increases, especially in lower lumbar spine, allowing more latitude in pedicle screw insertion than in smaller upper lumbar and thoracic pedicles. (From Zindrick MR: Clinical pedicle anatomy, *Spine: State of the Art Reviews* 6:11, 1992.)

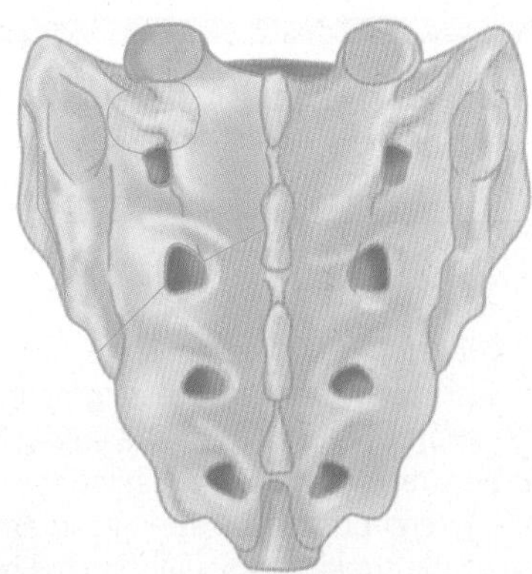

FIGURE 8.56 Coronal posterior view of contribution of sacrum and posterior element to pedicle approach zone.

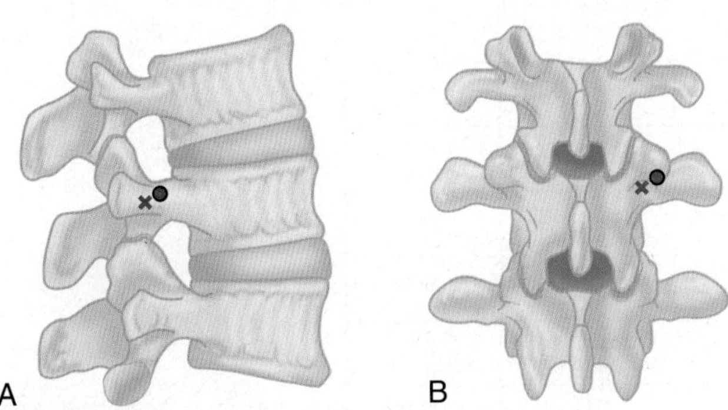

FIGURE 8.55 Entrance points for pedicle screw placement in lumbar spine as described by Roy-Camille (X) and Weinstein (•). **A,** Lateral view. **B,** Posterior view. Weinstein approach reduces interference with upper uninvolved lumbar motion segment.

C-arm image can be used to verify correct position. The pedicle awl should pass relatively easily and should not be forced into the pedicle. In addition to radiographs or image intensification, laminotomy and medial pedicle wall exposure can be done to help confirm the intrapedicular passage of the instrument. Once satisfactory entry into the pedicle has been achieved and palpation from within the pedicle finds solid bone margins along the pedicle wall throughout 360 degrees, the screw can be inserted. If the screws are self-tapping, the screw itself is inserted. If the screws require tapping, the tap is inserted first and then the screw. The common entry points in the lumbar spine are shown in Figure 8.55. The position of the pedicle in the sacrum is shown in Figure 8.56. In the lumbar spine, a medially directed screw allows the use of a longer screw and spares the facet joint, with less chance of injury to the common iliac vessels. Similarly, a medially directed sacral screw reduces the possibility of injury to anterior structures if the screw penetrates the anterior cortex.

When pedicle screws are used in the lumbar spine, screws usually are placed at every level on both the convex and concave sides. Each individual vertebra can be better derotated if it is instrumented on both sides (see deformity correction by direct vertebral rotation in Technique 8.10). In choosing the lowest instrumented vertebra, the standing posteroanterior films and the bending films must be considered. Bending films should be used in choosing the lowest instrumented lumbar vertebra. Instrumentation is stopped at the vertebra just above the first disc space that opens in the concavity of the lumbar curve on the bending film away from the concavity. Unless the curve is very flexible, the lower instrumented vertebra should at least touch the center sacral line on the standing posteroanterior radiograph.

BOX 8.4

Advantages and Disadvantages of Thoracic Pedicle Screws

Advantages
- When they are optimally placed, the screws are completely external to the spinal canal (supralaminar and infralaminar hooks, in contrast, are within the canal itself).
- Stronger fixation is possible than with hook implants.
- The screws are attached to all three columns, providing a rigid triangular crosslinked construct with a posterior-only implant.
- Facet joints, laminae, and transverse processes are free of implants; therefore, theoretically, there is more surface area for decortication.
- There is superior coronal correction and axial derotation.
- Most studies have shown slightly shorter fusion lengths than with hook constructs. With improved correction, there is a decreased need for anterior procedures and thoracoplasties.

Disadvantages
- The implants add significantly to the cost of the procedure.
- The potential complications in insertion of thoracic pedicle screws include injury to the spinal cord, nerve roots, pleural cavity, and aorta.
- Radiation exposure is significant to the surgeon and patient if routine fluoroscopy is used.

INSERTION OF THORACIC PEDICLE SCREWS

The routine use of thoracic pedicle screws in adolescent idiopathic scoliosis has become more common. The advantages and disadvantages of thoracic screws are given in Box 8.4.

THORACIC PEDICLE SCREW INSERTION TECHNIQUES

TECHNIQUE 8.10

- Clean the facet joints of all capsular tissue. Perform a partial inferior articular process facetectomy to enhance fusion and to improve exposure of the entry site for the thoracic pedicle screws (Fig. 8.57A). Seeing the transverse processes, the lateral portion of the pars interarticularis, and the base of the superior articular process helps identify the starting points (Fig. 8.58). In general, start the screw insertion from the neutrally rotated, most distal vertebra to be instrumented. Anatomic landmarks can be used as a guide for starting points and screw trajectory (Fig. 8.57B). Fixed-angle screws provide superior rotation in the thoracic spine and lumbar spine. Multiaxial screws can be used if needed.
- Perform a posterior cortical breach with a high-speed burr. A pedicle "blush" suggests entrance into the cancellous bone at the base of the pedicle, but this may not be seen in smaller pedicles because of the limited intrapedicular cancellous bone. Alternatively, screw starting points can be confirmed fluoroscopically (Fig. 8.59).
- Use a thoracic gearshift probe to find the cancellous soft spot indicating entrance into the pedicle.
- Point the tip first laterally to avoid perforation of the medial cortex (Fig. 8.57C).
- Advance the tip 20 to 25 mm until the tip is anterior to (past) the spinal canal (Fig. 8.57D).

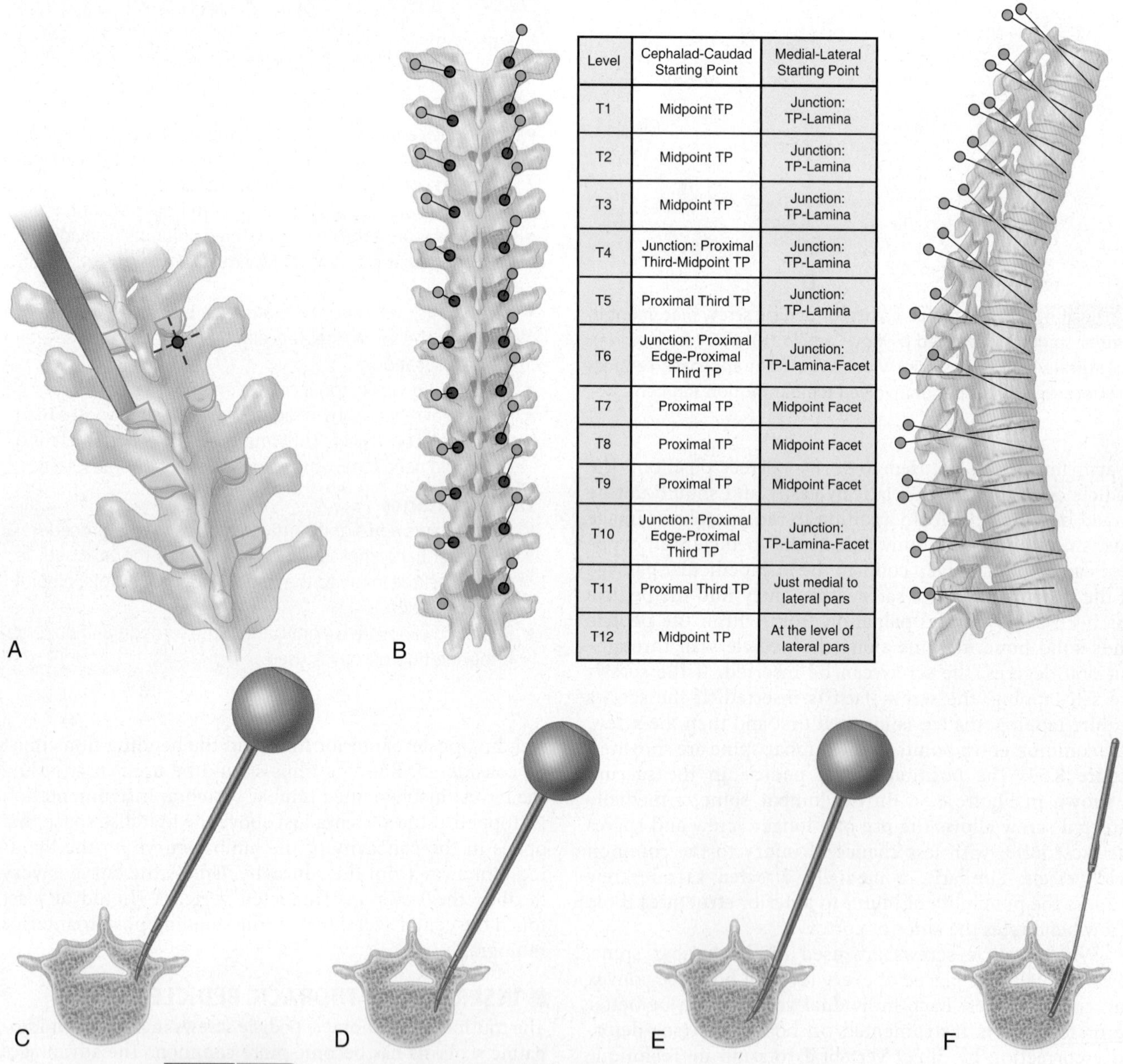

Level	Cephalad-Caudad Starting Point	Medial-Lateral Starting Point
T1	Midpoint TP	Junction: TP-Lamina
T2	Midpoint TP	Junction: TP-Lamina
T3	Midpoint TP	Junction: TP-Lamina
T4	Junction: Proximal Third-Midpoint TP	Junction: TP-Lamina
T5	Proximal Third TP	Junction: TP-Lamina
T6	Junction: Proximal Edge-Proximal Third TP	Junction: TP-Lamina-Facet
T7	Proximal TP	Midpoint Facet
T8	Proximal TP	Midpoint Facet
T9	Proximal TP	Midpoint Facet
T10	Junction: Proximal Edge-Proximal Third TP	Junction: TP-Lamina-Facet
T11	Proximal Third TP	Just medial to lateral pars
T12	Midpoint TP	At the level of lateral pars

FIGURE 8.57 **A-T,** Thoracic pedicle screw insertion technique with use of CD Horizon Legacy spinal deformity system. See text for description. (Medtronic Sofamor Danek.) **SEE TECHNIQUE 8.10.**

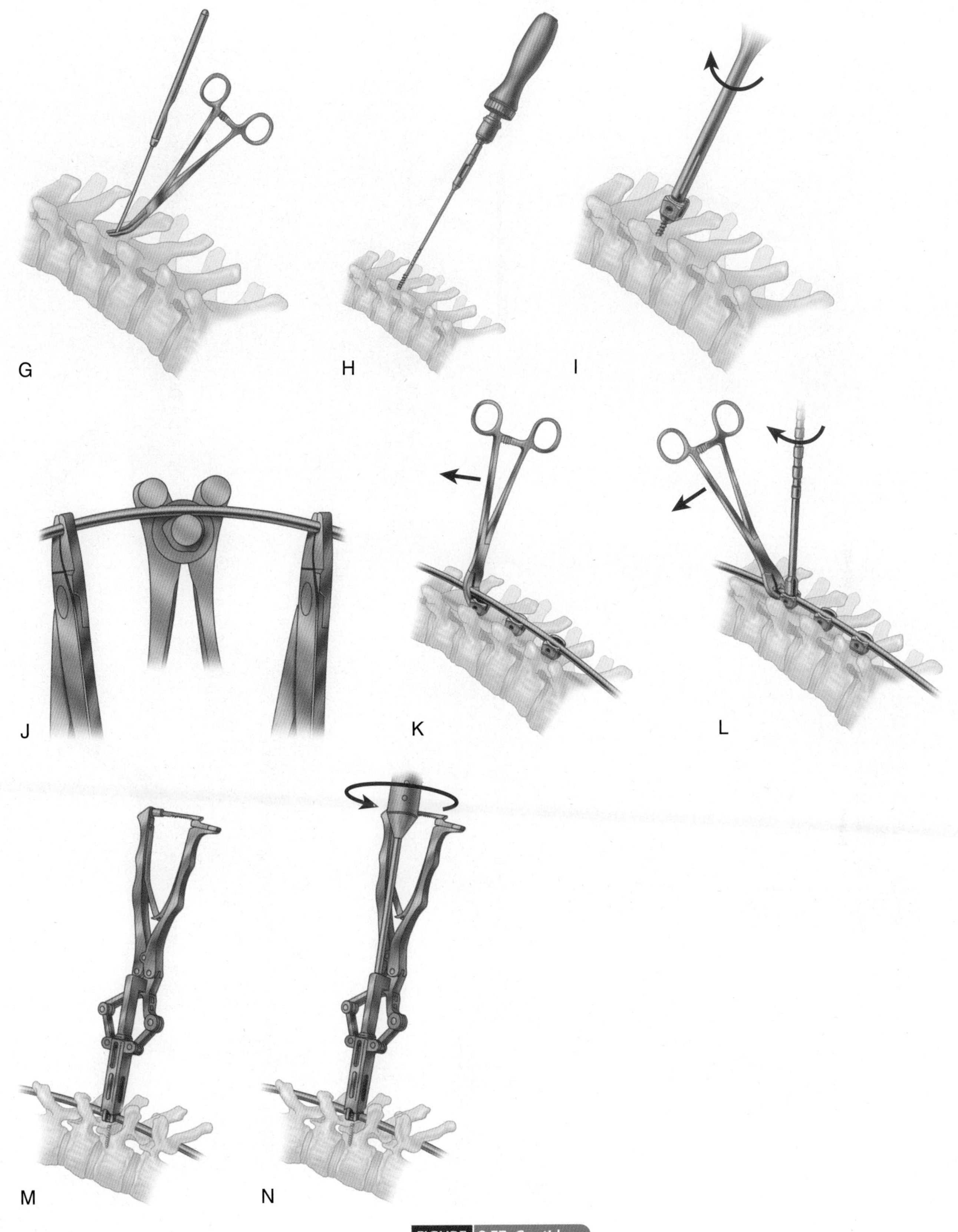

FIGURE 8.57, Cont'd

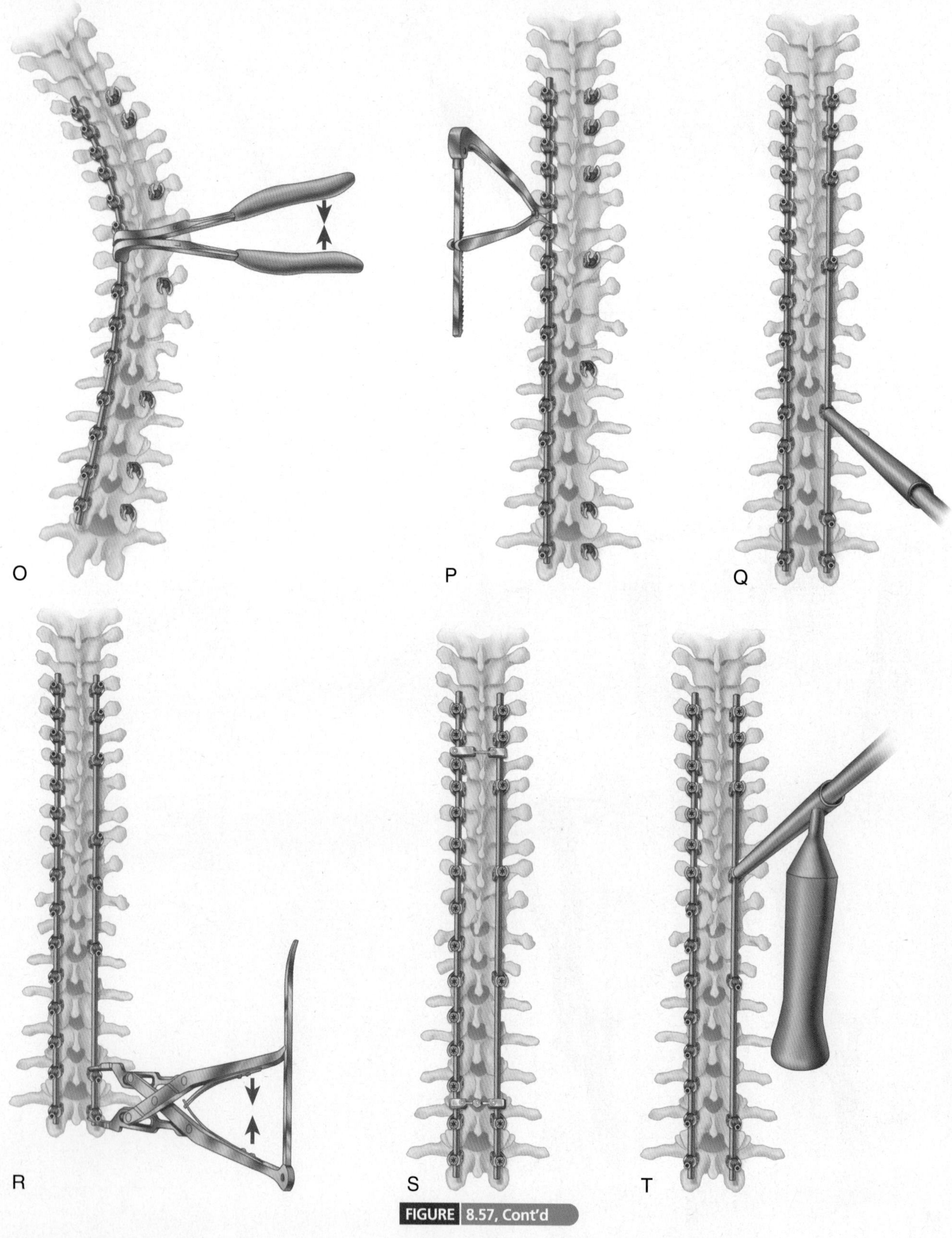

FIGURE 8.57, Cont'd

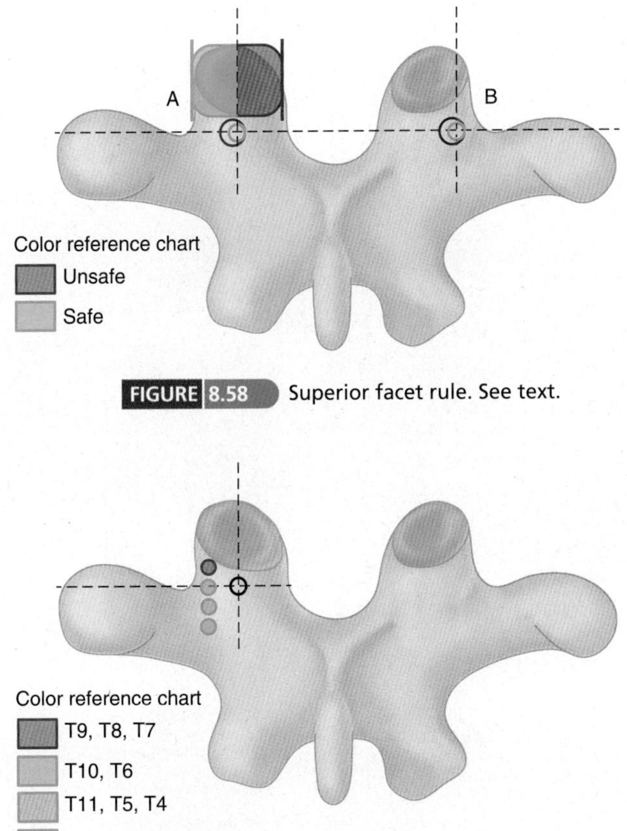

FIGURE 8.58 Superior facet rule. See text.

FIGURE 8.59 Pedicle starting point. See text.

- Remove the gearshift probe to reorient it so that the tip points medially and then place the probe carefully back into the base of the prior hole and advance it to the desired depth (Fig. 8.57E). The average depth is 30 to 40 mm in the lower thoracic region, 20 to 30 mm in the midthoracic region, and 20 to 30 mm in the proximal thoracic region in adolescents.
- Rotate the probe in a 180-degree arc to ensure adequate room for the screw. Probing of the pedicle with the gearshift should proceed in a smooth and consistent manner with a snug feel. Any sudden advancement of the gearshift or loss of resistance suggests penetration into soft tissue and pedicle wall or vertebral body violation.
- Once the gearshift probe is removed, view the track to make sure that only blood is coming out and not cerebrospinal fluid.
- With use of a flexible ball-tipped probe, advance the feeler probe to the base (floor) of the hole to confirm five distinct bony borders: the floor and four walls (medial, lateral, superior, and inferior) (Fig. 8.57F). Take special care in feeling the walls to the first 10 to 15 mm of the track, as breaches here are at the depth of the spinal canal.
- If a soft-tissue breach is palpated, consider leaving the screw out. If it is a critical screw, redirect it. With the feeler probe at the base of the pedicle track, mark the length of the track with a hemostat and measure it (Fig. 8.57G).
- Undertap the pedicle track by 0.5 to 1 mm of the final screw diameter (Fig. 8.57H). After tapping, always palpate the tapped pedicle track again with the flexible feeler probe. This second palpation will allow identification of distinct bony ridges, confirming the intraosseous position of the track.
- Select the appropriate screw diameter and length by the preoperative radiographs, as well as by intraoperative measurement.
- Slowly advance the screw down the pedicle to ensure proper tracking while allowing viscoelastic expansion (Fig. 8.57I-T). This can be done safely using power or manual drivers.
- Confirm intraosseous screw placement.
- On the anteroposterior image intensification, make sure the screws are positioned correctly relative to each other. Screws should not go past the midline on the true anteroposterior image. For any screw that needs to be removed, re-probe the screw hole to ensure that there is no medial breach. Use the lateral image primarily to gauge the length of the screws. No screw should extend past the anterior border of the vertebral body.
- Use electromyographic stimulation with real-time monitoring of the appropriate thoracic nerve root, recording from the intercostal and/or rectus abdominis musculature. Below T12, the lumbar pedicle screws are tested by monitoring the appropriate lumbar nerve root. A triggered electromyographic threshold of less than 6 mA or a significant decrease from the average of all other screws may indicate a pedicle wall breach by the screw. If this is the case, remove the screw and palpate the pedicle wall before deciding whether to replace or to discard the screw.

FUSION LEVELS AND SCREW PLACEMENT

The most widely used classification and guide for fusion levels is the Lenke classification. A review of this classification gave the following recommendations to aid in selecting fusion levels:

1. All Lenke structural curves should be included in the fusion and instrumentation.
2. The upper instrumented vertebra should not end at a kyphotic disc.
3. T2 is selected as the upper instrumented vertebra when the left shoulder is elevated, T1 tilt is more than 5 degrees, and/or significant rotational prominences or trapezial fullness accompanies the proximal thoracic curve.
4. In lumbar modifier A curves, the lower instrumented vertebra is the vertebra touching the center sacral vertebral line; however, the spine is fused one or two levels farther distal when L4 is tilted in the direction of the thoracic curve.

In lumbar modifier B and C curves, the thoracolumbar stable vertebra is selected as the lower instrumented vertebra.

The lower instrumented vertebra in lumbar structural curves is influenced by curve flexibility (proposed by the lower instrumented vertebra translation) and rotation and correction on bending radiographs.

Even with these guidelines and using Lenke's classification, selection of fusion and instrumentation levels must be individualized for each patient.

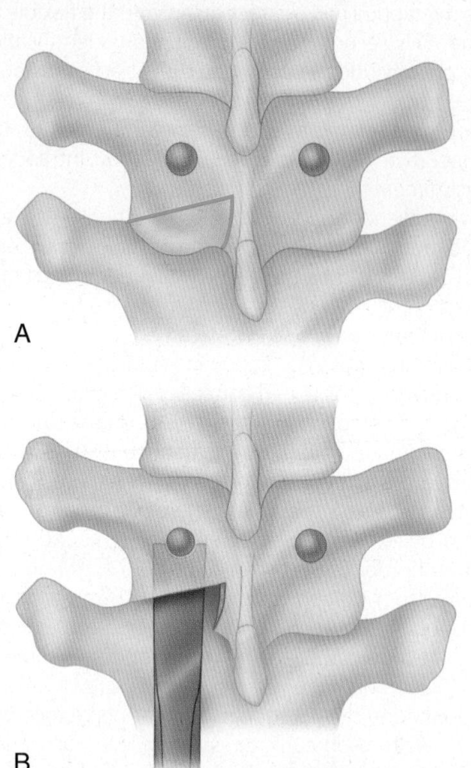

FIGURE 8.60 Pedicle hook implantation. **A** and **B,** Hook site preparation and placement. **SEE TECHNIQUE 8.11.**

HOOK SITE PREPARATION AND PLACEMENT

Before the widespread use of pedicle screw fixation, hook fixation was the most common method of spinal fixation. Hook fixation is still a useful technique in situations where pedicle screw fixation is not safe, possible, or available. There are basically three types of hooks: pedicle, transverse process, and laminar. The pedicle hooks are designed for secure fixation in the thoracic spine by insertion into the facet with impingement on the thoracic pedicle. Pedicle hooks are used in an upgoing direction at T10 or higher. The laminar hooks can be used in the thoracic and lumbar spine. These can be placed around either the superior or inferior edge of the lamina according to the desired direction and point of application of forces. Transverse process hooks typically are used at the cranial end of a construct to provide a "soft landing" or more flexible transition between the mobile spine cranially and the rigid instrumented spine caudally. These are placed around the superior aspect of the transverse process and can provide only compression and not distraction.

PEDICLE HOOK IMPLANTATION

TECHNIQUE 8.11

- The pedicle hook is inserted in an upgoing direction from T1 to T10.
- The facet capsule is removed, and a portion of the inferior facet process is removed to facilitate insertion of the hook (Fig. 8.60A).

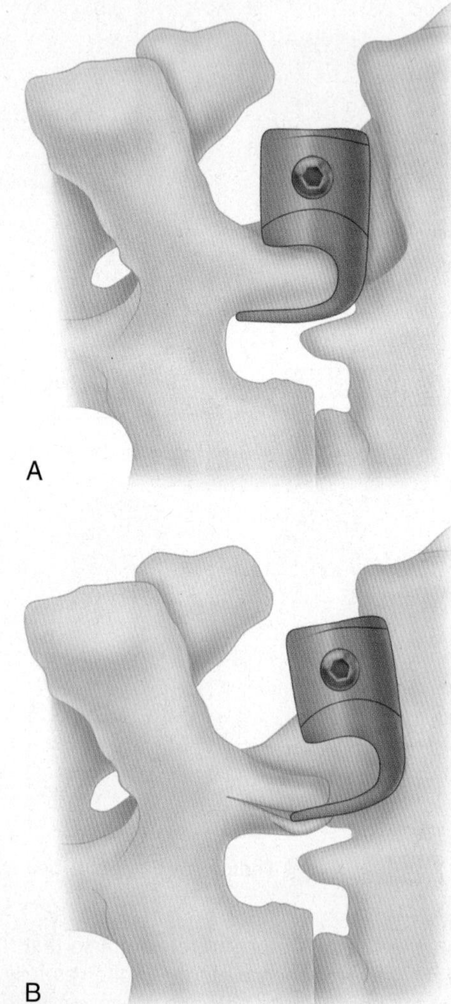

FIGURE 8.61 Pedicle hook implantation. **A,** Correct placement of the hook. **B,** Incorrect placement of the hook. **SEE TECHNIQUE 8.11.**

- After removal of the portion of the inferior facet process, use a curet to decorticate the facet joint.
- Introduce the pedicle finder into the facet joint and push gently against the pedicle (Fig. 8.60B). Take care in using this instrument that it is introduced into the intraarticular space and not into the bone of the inferior articular facet. It must find its way, sliding along the superior articular facet.
- Once the pedicle finder is in place, check the position by a laterally directed force applied to the finder. If the vertebra moves laterally when the pedicle finder is translated, the pedicle finder is in the correct place.
- Insert the pedicle hook with a hook inserter and holder if needed. Again, be certain that the horns of the bifid hook remain within the facet joint and do not hook into the remaining bone of the inferior facet (Fig. 8.61).

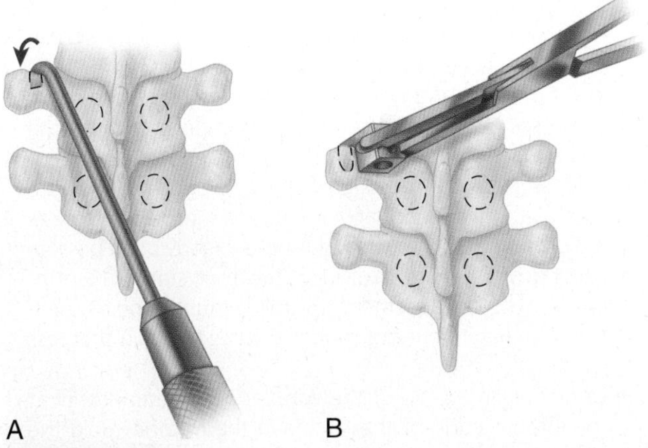

FIGURE 8.62 Area along superior edge of transverse process prepared using transverse process elevator. (Redrawn from Winter RB, Lonstein JW, Denis F, Smith MD, editors: Atlas of spine surgery, Philadelphia, 1995, WB Saunders, p 263.) **SEE TECHNIQUE 8.12.**

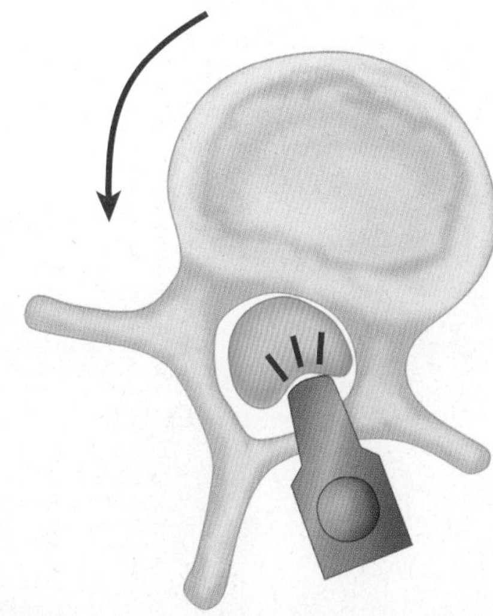

FIGURE 8.63 Laminar hook should be chosen carefully to match shape of lamina and to obtain closest possible fit to prevent hook impingement on spinal canal. **SEE TECHNIQUE 8.13.**

TRANSVERSE PROCESS HOOK IMPLANTATION

TECHNIQUE 8.12

- Prepare the area along the superior edge of the transverse process, using a transverse process elevator to separate the ligamentous attachment between the undersurface of the transverse process and the posterior arch of the rib medial to the rib transverse joint (Fig. 8.62).
- With use of a transverse process hook holder, insert the hook around the superior edge of the transverse process.

LAMINAR HOOK IMPLANTATION

TECHNIQUE 8.13

- Place laminar hooks around either the superior or inferior edge of the lamina, according to the desired direction of applied force. Carefully match the type of laminar hook to the shape of the lamina and obtain the closest possible fit to avoid the possibility of hook impingement on the spinal canal (Fig. 8.63).
- To insert the supralaminar hook, remove the ligamentum flavum with Kerrison rongeurs and curets (Fig. 8.64A). In the lumbar area, enough room generally exists between the vertebrae to allow implantation of the hook without removal of bone. In the thoracic area, however, the spinous process of the superior vertebra must be removed first.
- After the canal is open, obtain lateral extension of the area by excising the medial portion of the inferior articular facet of the superior vertebra. This will allow sufficient room for insertion of the thoracic laminar hook.
- When the infralaminar hook is inserted, partially remove the ligamentum flavum or separate it from the inferior surface of the lamina. If necessary, remove a piece of the inferior border of the lamina to allow proper seating of the hook on the lamina (Fig. 8.64B). Take care to preserve the lateral wall of the inferior facet to avoid lateral dislodgment of the hook.
- When the inferiormost laminar hook is inserted, preserve the interspinous ligament and facet capsule to prevent kyphosis distal to the rods.

SUBLAMINAR WIRES

Sublaminar wires generally are not used alone as anchors at the upper or lower instrumented vertebrae because they provide no axial stability. They are useful, however, in and around the apex of curves to aid in the translation maneuver, in which the spine can be pulled to a precontoured rod, thus minimizing the need for derotational maneuvers. The more rigid the curve is, the more helpful these sublaminar wires or cables are (Fig. 8.65). While sublaminar wires are simple and cost-effective, they have been replaced in many centers with sublaminar cables or tape because of increased safety, better load distribution, and the ability in some cases to attach directly to the rod and provide some measure of axial stability.

TECHNIQUE 8.14

- Expose the spine as described in Technique 8.6.
- With a needle-nose rongeur, gradually thin the ligamentum flavum until the midline cleavage plane is visible. In

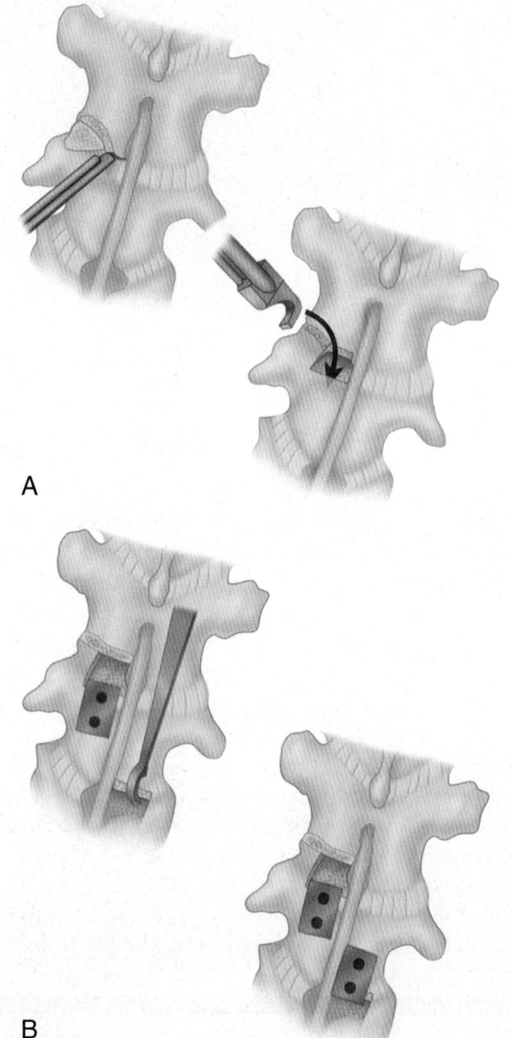

FIGURE 8.64 **A, Supralaminar hook insertion**. This insertion applies to lower two concave hooks in single thoracic curve instrumentation. Laminotomy is kept as small as possible to minimize risk of deep penetration into spinal canal during rod insertion. Tight fit is necessary, and thoracic laminar hook is used if laminar thickness is too small to allow lumbar laminar hook to be stable in anteroposterior plane. **B, Infralaminar hook insertion**. Lower convex hook in right thoracic curve is inserted in this manner. Ligamentum flavum is dissected off underside of lamina. Small inferior laminotomy provides horizontal purchase site for hook. Adjacent facet capsule should be spared because it is not included in fusion. **SEE TECHNIQUE 8.13.**

the thoracic spine, the spinous processes slant distally and must be removed before the ligamentum flavum can be adequately seen (Fig. 8.66). Once the midline cleavage is visible, carefully sweep a Penfield No. 4 dissector across the deep surface of the ligamentum flavum on the right and left sides (Fig. 8.67). Use a Kerrison punch to remove the remainder of the ligamentum flavum (Fig. 8.68). Take care during this step to avoid damaging the dura or epidural vessels.

- Johnston et al. showed that wire penetration into the neural canal during wire passage is substantial (up to 1 cm). Because the depth of penetration is less when a semicircular wire is used, shape the wire as shown in Figure 8.69. The largest diameter of the bend should be slightly larger than the lamina. Always pass the wire in the midline and not laterally and remove the spinous processes before wire passage. It is important that both the surgeon and the assistant be completely prepared for each step before passage of the wire and that they are careful about sudden movements and inadvertent touching or hitting of the wires that have already been passed.
- Passing of the wire is divided into four steps: (1) introduction, (2) advancement, (3) roll-through, and (4) pull-through. Pass the more cephalad wires first and progress caudally.
- Gently place the tip of the wire into the neural canal at the inferior edge of the lamina in the midline. Hold the long end of the doubled wire in one hand and advance the tip with the other. Rest the hand that is advancing the tip firmly on the patient's back. Lift the tails of the wire slightly, pulling them to keep the wire snugly against the undersurface of the lamina (Fig. 8.70A).
- Once the wire has been introduced, advance it 5 to 6 mm. Beginning roll-through too soon will cause the tip of the wire to strike the inferior portion of the vertebral arch, and the wire can be pushed more deeply into the neural canal (Fig. 8.70B).
- After advancement, roll the tip of the wire so that it emerges on the upper end of the lamina (Fig. 8.70C). As the tip of the wire emerges, use a nerve hook to pull the end farther up from the lamina to allow enough room for a needle holder, wire holder, or Kocher clamp to be placed into the loop of the wire by the assistant. Take the clamp from the assistant and pull the wire with the clamp until it is positioned beneath the lamina, with half its length protruding above and half below the lamina. As the clamp is pulled, gently feed the wire superiorly from the long end. This must be a coordinated maneuver and must be done by the surgeon.
- Once the wire has been pulled through, cut off the tip of the wire and place one length of the wire on the right side and the other length on the left side of the lamina.
- As an alternative, leave double wires on one side and pass another wire so that double wires are present on both sides.
- Crimp each wire into the surface of the lamina to prevent any wire from being pushed accidentally into the neural canal (Fig. 8.71).
- As more wires are passed, it becomes more likely that the other wires will be accidentally hit, and care must be taken to prevent this.

SUBLAMINAR CABLES/BANDS

The use of sublaminar cables or bands instead of monofilament stainless steel wire has become more popular because of wire breakage and migration, which have been serious complications of sublaminar wiring. The flexibility of sublaminar cables/bands, which are inserted in a similar fashion, prevents repeated contusions to the spinal cord that can occur during insertion of the rod and tightening of the wire. Sublaminar banding systems (OrthoPediatrics, Warsaw, IN) offer the advantage of a wider surface area for load sharing and the

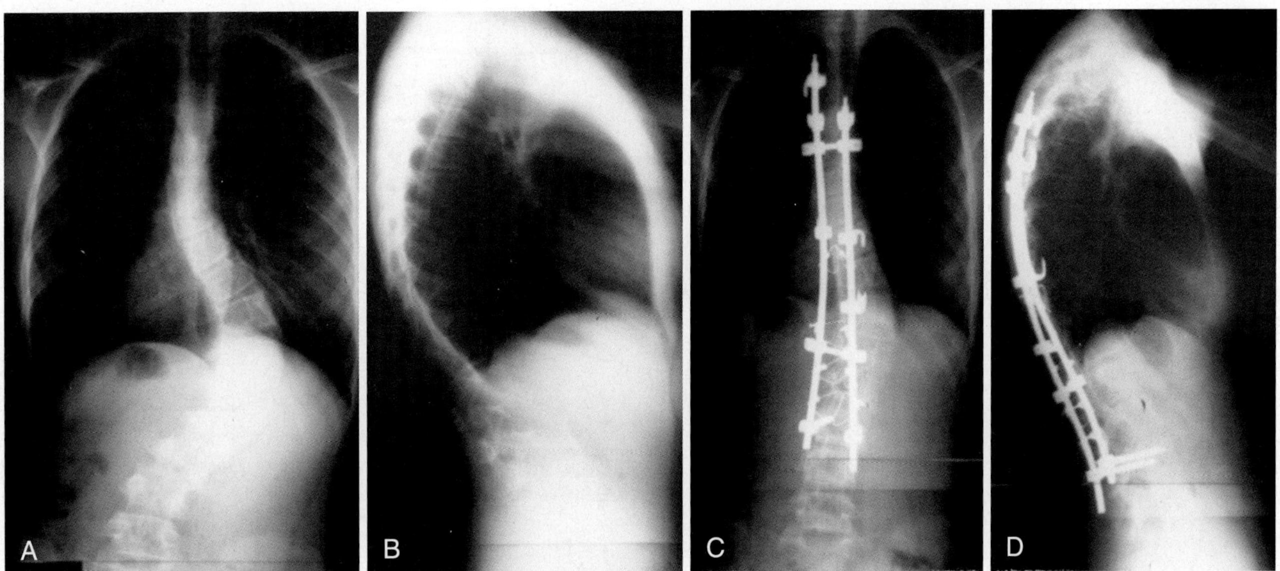

FIGURE 8.65 **A** and **B,** Preoperative anteroposterior and lateral standing scoliosis films. Thoracolumbar curve measures 77 degrees. **C** and **D,** Postoperative correction by hooks with sublaminar cables, correcting thoracolumbar curve to 22 degrees. **SEE TECHNIQUE 8.13.**

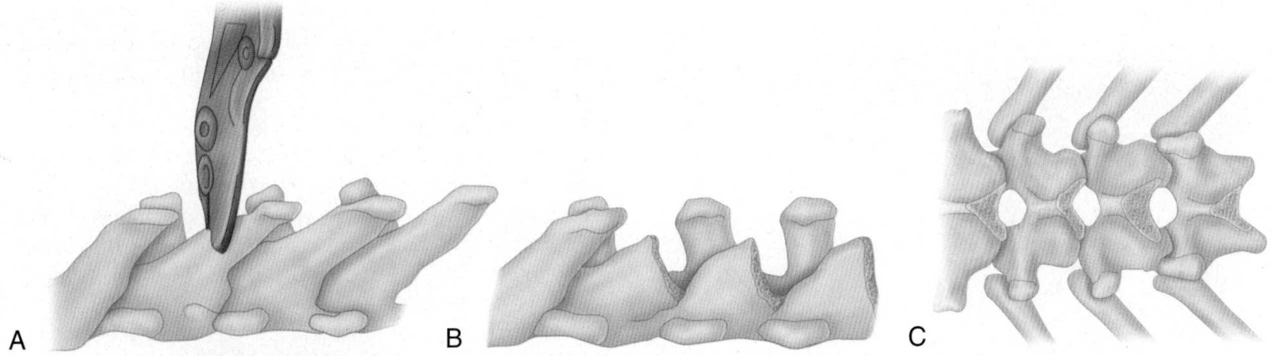

FIGURE 8.66 **A-C,** Removal of caudally slanting spinous processes to expose ligamentum flavum. **SEE TECHNIQUE 8.14.**

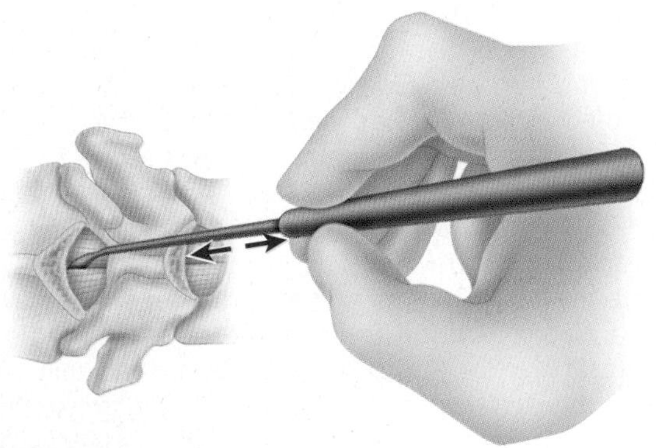

FIGURE 8.67 Penfield No. 4 dissector for freeing deep surfaces of ligamentum flavum. **SEE TECHNIQUE 8.14.**

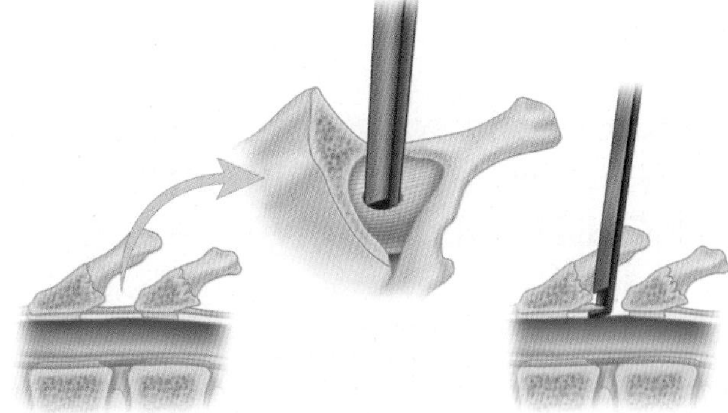

FIGURE 8.68 Spinous processes removed. Kerrison rongeur used for removal of remainder of ligamentum flavum. **SEE TECHNIQUE 8.14.**

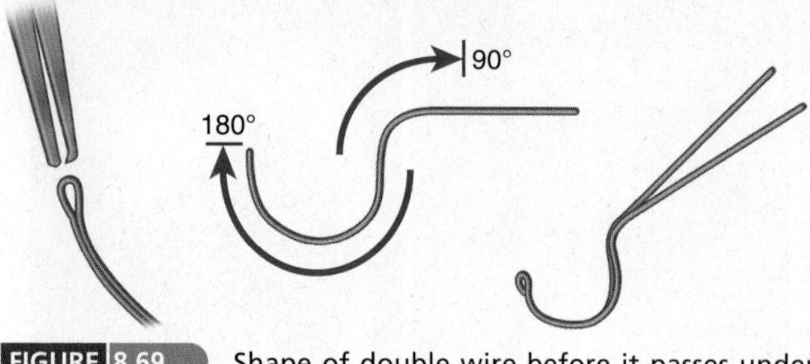

FIGURE 8.69 Shape of double wire before it passes under lamina.

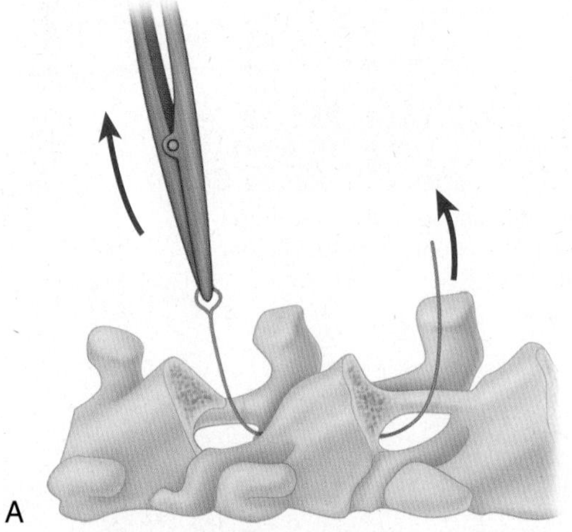

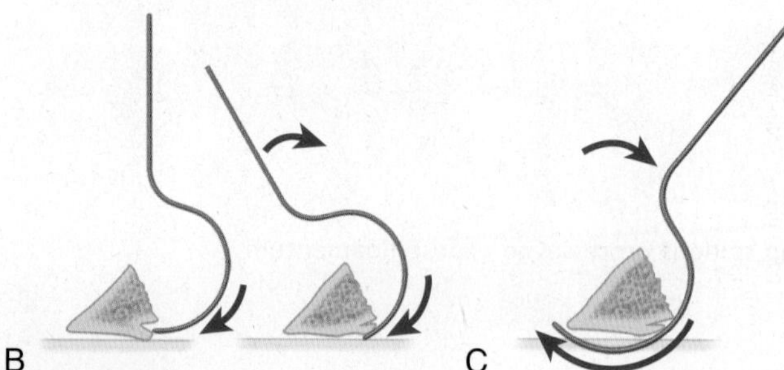

FIGURE 8.70 A-C, Passage of segmental wire beneath lamina. **SEE TECHNIQUE 8.14.**

ability to directly connect to the rod providing some axial stability (Fig. 8.72).

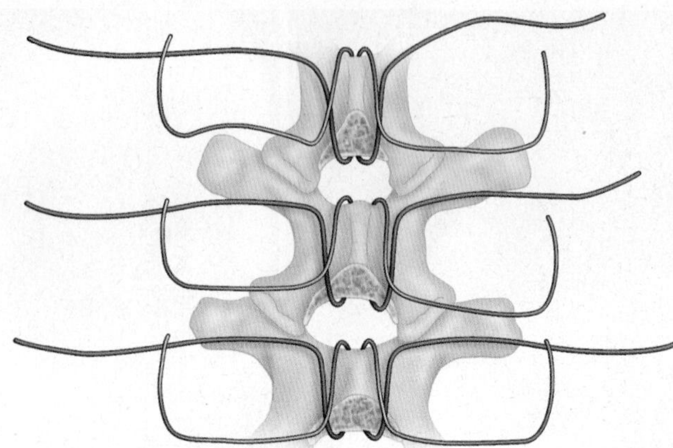

FIGURE 8.71 After division, wire placed on laminar surface of each side of spinous process.

INSTRUMENTATION SEQUENCE IN TYPICAL LENKE 1A CURVE

The following is a typical instrumentation sequence for a Lenke 1A curve. Multiple systems are available to accomplish this, and readers are referred to the system-specific technique manual for further details of the system that best fits their practice.

TECHNIQUE 8.15

- Place instrumentation at the appropriate levels based on the patient's anatomy and the desired arthrodesis levels. At this point, cut the correction rod that will be placed on the concave side to the appropriate length, which generally is 2 to 3 cm longer than the overall cranial-to-caudal anchor length.
- Bend the rod to achieve correct sagittal plane contour. In some cases, a slight "over-bend" is helpful in restoring the sagittal plane from hypokyphosis to normal kyphosis. This is accomplished with small, incremental steps by use of the French bender. The use of pre-contoured rods can also be helpful.
- Place the contoured rod into the implants. This can be started from either the superior or inferior anchors. Place the set screws into the first hooks where the rod seats perfectly. After the rod is inserted into the first one or two anchors, it then becomes necessary to use one of several methods to facilitate rod reduction and fully seat the rod into the saddle of the implants.
- The "forceps rocker" method is effective for seating the rod into the implant when there is only a slight height difference between the rod and the implant saddle. To use the rocker, grasp the sides of the implant with a rocker cam above the rod and the forceps tips facing the same direction as the hook blade. Lever the rocker backward over the rod to seat the rod into the saddle of the implant. The set screw is then inserted into the hook.
- In situations in which the difference between the hook and rod is such that the rocker cannot be used, a rod reducer can be used. Slowly close the reducer by squeezing the handles together, allowing the attached sleeve to slide down and seat the rod into the saddle of the implant.
- Place a set screw through the set screw tube of the reducer, using the provisional driver.
- Once the contoured rod and all of the set screws have been placed, perform the rod rotation maneuver. Because of the corrective forces placed on the spine, a mean arterial pressure of at least 70 mm Hg is essential to maintain spinal cord perfusion. It also is helpful to obtain a baseline motor-evoked potential measurement before any reduction maneuver for comparison once the maneuvers have been performed. This is done slowly, and it is essential to watch all of the anchors because

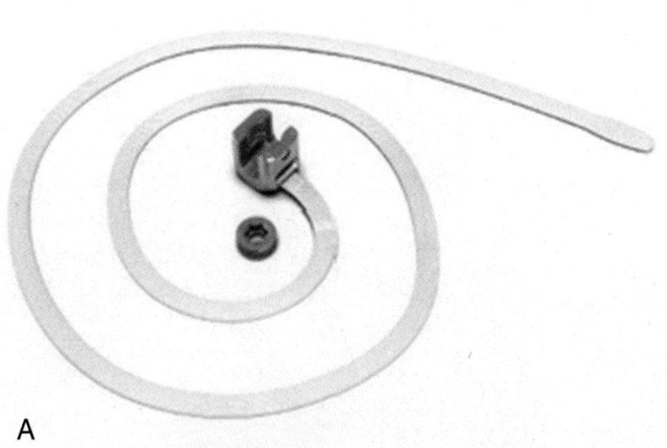

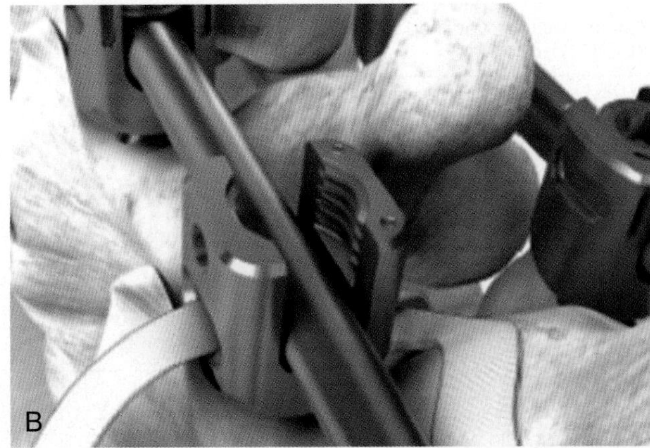

FIGURE 8.72 Polyester sublaminar tape with hook (**A**) that allows direct fixation to rod and axial control (**B**).

they can sometimes be dislodged during this rotational maneuver. The anchors at the curve apex are those most likely to back out during rod rotation. Using two rod holders, rotate the rod to translate the apex of the curve toward the midline. If the hooks begin to dislodge, place one of the rod grippers next to the hook and reseat the hook by use of a distractor. Once the rod rotation is complete, tighten the set screws.

- In situ benders are then used for correction and final adjustment of the rod in the sagittal plane. Bend the rod in small, incremental steps by use of the two bender tips positioned near each other on the rod.
- Once the contouring has been completed, if hook fixation has been used, perform distraction or compression to seat the hooks in their final positions. It is recommended to use a rod gripper as a stop for distraction maneuvers rather than any portion of the implant. Compression maneuvers generally are carried out on two hooks. Take care that these instruments are placed against the implant body and not against the set screw.
- Rod derotation maneuvers can now be performed if axial rotational correction is desired.
- After these maneuvers are complete, tighten the set screws further. Place the convex stabilizing rod, measure the length, and cut the rod to length. With use of the French bender, contour the rod according to the curvature of the spine in the residual position of alignment from the correction rod. Place the contoured rod into the hooks and provisionally secure the rods with set screws.
- Once the rod is secured to the implants, apply distraction and compression as necessary at the cranial and caudal ends of the construct to balance the spine and level the shoulders.
- Place the countertorque instrument over the implant and rod. Place the break-off driver through the cannulated countertorque.
- Perform decortication with either a power burr or Cobb gouge.
- Apply bone graft.
- Close the wound in the routine manner.

POSTOPERATIVE CARE There has been considerable interest in accelerated discharge protocols using multimodal pain management with early feeding and Foley catheter and drain removal, as well as aggressive mobilization. Fletcher et al. published their results with an accelerated discharge pathway that was associated with a 31% decrease in hospital days (2.9 vs. 4.3), 33% decrease in hospital room charges, and 11% decrease in physical therapy costs. With modern rigid segmental instrumentation systems, patients are allowed to ambulate immediately after surgery, and bracing rarely is used. A recent consensus best practice guideline regarding postoperative management of adolescent idiopathic scoliosis patients made 19 recommendations for the postoperative management of patients following posterior spinal fusion for adolescent idiopathic scoliosis (Fig. 8.73).

DEFORMITY CORRECTION BY DIRECT VERTEBRAL ROTATION

TECHNIQUE 8.16

- In this technique, bilateral pedicle screws are inserted at every level to be fused in the thoracic spine. The direct vertebral rotation is opposite to that of the vertebral rotation in the thoracic curve; apical and juxtaapical vertebrae are rotated clockwise for right thoracic curves in the transverse plane.
- Because of the corrective forces placed on the spine, a mean arterial pressure of at least 70 mm Hg is essential to maintain spinal cord perfusion. It is also helpful to obtain a baseline motor-evoked potential measurement before any reduction maneuver for comparison once the maneuvers have been completed.

1. Patients may be admitted to a general floor rather than the PICU.
2. A PCA pump should be used postoperatively.
3. An epidural is not necessary for management of postoperative pain.
4. Primary transition to oral narcotics should occur on a target date (*i.e.,* POD#1) rather than based on a clinical threshold (*i.e.,* passing flatus).
5. Muscle spasm, medications (*i.e.,* diazepam) should be used postoperatively.
6. Gabapentin should be used in the perioperative period.
7. Ketorolac should be used to minimize narcotic needs.
8. Clear liquids can be started as tolerated postoperatively.
9. A bowel regimen should be used beginning on POD#1.
10. Antiemetics should be given postoperatively.
11. A drain should be used postoperatively.
12. The patient may begin sitting on the side of the bed on POD#1.
13. The patient may begin ambulating on POD#1.
14. Physical therapy should see the patient twice daily beginning POD#1.
15. Chewing gum may be used to increase gastric motility.
16. Intraoperative, without postoperative radiographs, may suffice to evaluate implant placement and location.
17. Patients may be discharged before having a bowel movement.
18. Hospital discharge may occur on postoperative 2 or 3 assuming that pain is controlled on oral medications, the patient has cleared PT, and is tolerating a regular diet, regardless of whether the patient has had a bowel movement.
19. The patient should be contacted about their progress in the first week after surgery.

FIGURE 8.73 Best Practice Consensus Guidelines for postoperative care after posterior spinal fusion for adolescent scoliosis. (From Fletcher ND, Glotzbecker MP, Marks M, et al: Development of consensus-based best practice guidelines for postoperative care following posterior spinal fusion for adolescent idiopathic scoliosis, *Spine (Phila Pa 1976)* 42:E547, 2017.)

- Insert screw derotators onto the pedicle screws of the juxtaapical vertebrae on both the concave and convex sides and derotate the vertebrae as much as possible. This can be done most commonly in an en bloc fashion with multiple levels rotated simultaneously or in some cases each level at a time (Fig. 8.74).
- During rod derotation, push down on the convex screws and pull up on the concave screws simultaneously. An assistant should apply downward pressure on the convex apical ribs to aid in derotation as well.
- After completion of the derotation, lock the rod into position by tightening the set screws fully. This process can be repeated multiple times until the desired correction is obtained.

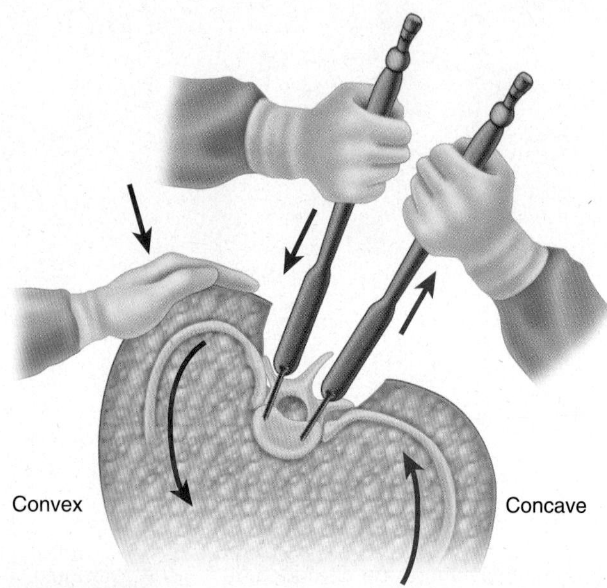

FIGURE 8.74 Direct vertebral rotation. (Redrawn from Newton PO, O'Brien MF, Sufflebarger HL, et al, editors: *Idiopathic scoliosis: the Harms Study Group treatment guide*, New York, 2010, Thieme.) **SEE TECHNIQUE 8.16.**

- If the curve is rigid, we have found that often little rod derotation is possible, and other techniques, such as rod bending, should be considered.

COMPLICATIONS AND PITFALLS IN SEGMENTAL INSTRUMENTATION SYSTEMS

In addition to the complications inherent in any spinal arthrodesis, segmental instrumentation systems have several potential pitfalls, most of which can be avoided by choosing the appropriate arthrodesis levels using criteria such as the Lenke classification, which helps determine which curve(s) to instrument and avoid ending instrumentation in the middle of a structural curve. One coronal plane problem that can occur is decompensation with selective fusion of the thoracic curve (Fig. 8.75). If the curve is severely rotated clinically, it probably will need to be incorporated in the fusion. If a selective thoracic fusion is performed, the lower instrumented vertebra should at least touch the center sacral line on the standing posteroanterior preoperative radiograph.

In addition, there has been considerable interest recently in sagittal plane abnormalities, most commonly hypokyphosis, in adolescent idiopathic scoliosis. With the use of rigid posterior fixation, it is important to avoid ending instrumentation at the apex of the sagittal plane abnormality, which can lead to a proximal or distal junctional kyphosis (Fig. 8.76).

Another common strategic mistake is failure to recognize the significance of the upper thoracic curve preoperatively. If the upper thoracic curve does not correct on supine bending films to the predicted correction of the lower thoracic curve, elevation of the left shoulder and an unsightly deformity will occur (Fig. 8.77). This mistake is prevented by carefully evaluating the clinical appearance

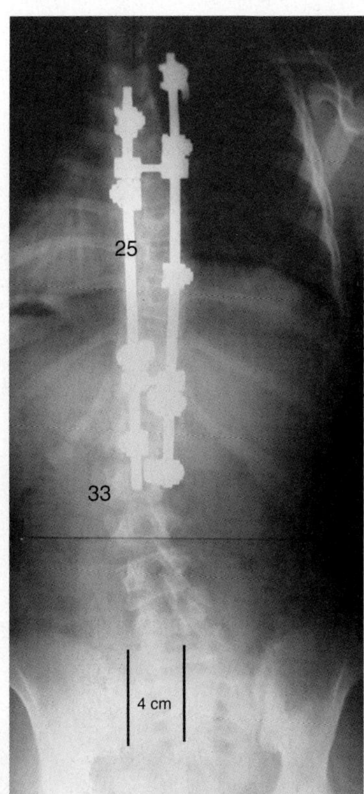

FIGURE 8.75 Decompensated lumbar curve after fusion of thoracic curve only.

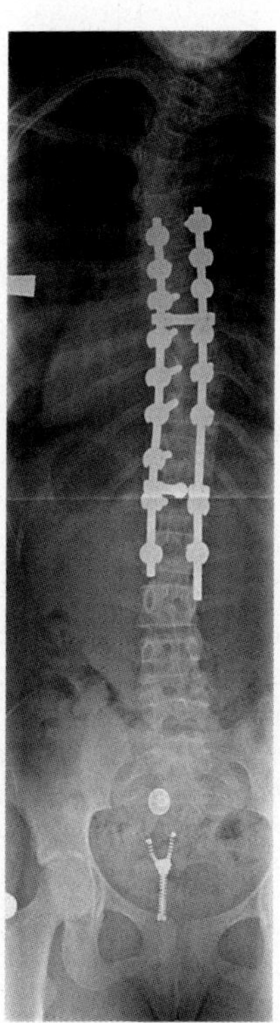

FIGURE 8.77 Elevation of shoulder caused by undercorrection of upper thoracic curve.

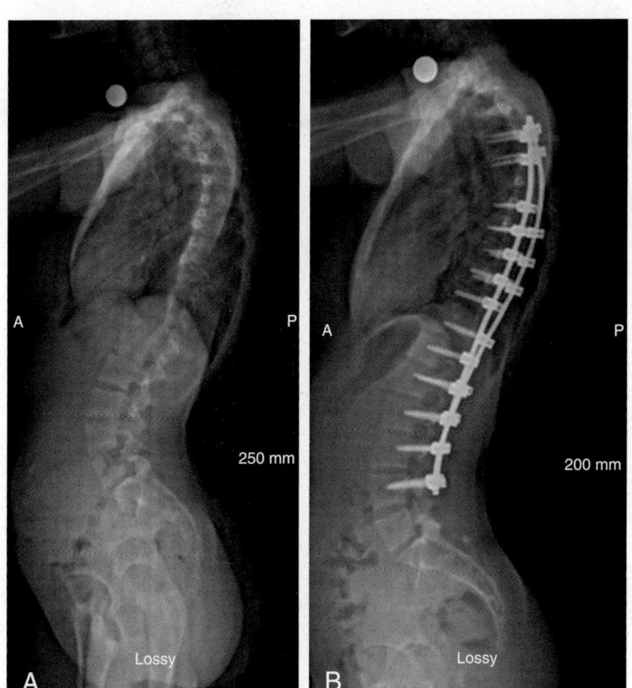

FIGURE 8.76 Proximal junctional kyphosis. Preoperative (**A**) and postoperative (**B**) images of 13-year-old girl who had posterior spinal fusion for adolescent idiopathic scoliosis. Postoperative proximal junctional kyphosis is +9 degrees, and the patient remains asymptomatic.

of the shoulders and the bending films, as well as the standing radiographs, with special attention to this upper curve. Useful measurements from standing radiographs are the T1 tilt angle, the clavicle angle, and the radiographic shoulder height. The T1 tilt angle is measured by the intersection of a line drawn along the T1 cephalad endplate and a line parallel to the horizontal reference line (Fig. 8.78). The clavicular angle is measured by the intersection of a line touching the two highest points of the clavicle and a line parallel to the horizontal reference line (Fig. 8.79). The radiographic shoulder height is determined by the difference in the soft-tissue shadow directly superior to each acromioclavicular joint on a standing posteroanterior radiograph (Fig. 8.80). A proximal thoracic curve should be considered structural if (1) the curve size is more than 30 degrees and remains more than 20 degrees on side-bending radiographs; (2) there is more than 1 cm of apical translation from the C7 plumb line; (3) there is a positive T1 tilt; and (4) clinical elevation of either shoulder (most commonly the left for right thoracic curves) is noted, depending on the curve type.

MANAGEMENT OF RIGID CURVES

HALO-GRAVITY TRACTION

Rigid curves of the spine in adolescents have historically been treated with halo traction as an adjunct to surgery. This allows gradual correction of up to 35% of large spinal deformities and allows preoperative nutritional and pulmonary optimization. Often, posterior releases and instrumentation can be done at the time of halo placement to improve correction in traction. Gradual weight progression to 30% to

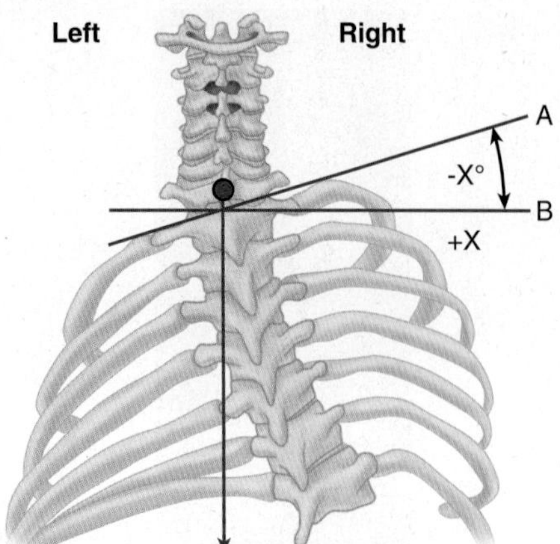

FIGURE 8.78 When right edge of vertebral body is up, tilt angle is defined as negative. When left edge of vertebral body is up, tilt angle is defined as positive. (Redrawn from O'Brien MF, Kuklo TR, Blanke KM, Lenke LG, editors: *Spinal deformity study group radiographic measurement manual*, Memphis, TN, 2004, Medtronic Sofamor Danek, p 55.)

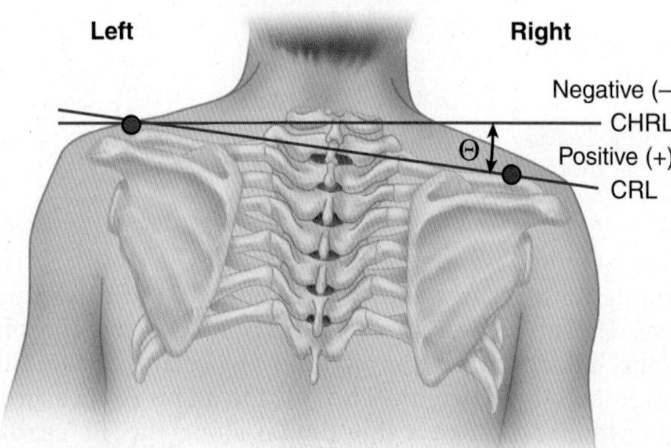

FIGURE 8.79 Clavicular angle. *CHRL*, Clavicle horizontal reference line; *CRL*, clavicle reference line. (Redrawn from O'Brien MF, Kuklo TR, Blanke KM, Lenke LG, editors: *Spinal deformity study group radiographic measurement manual*, Memphis, TN, 2004, Medtronic Sofamor Danek, p 56.)

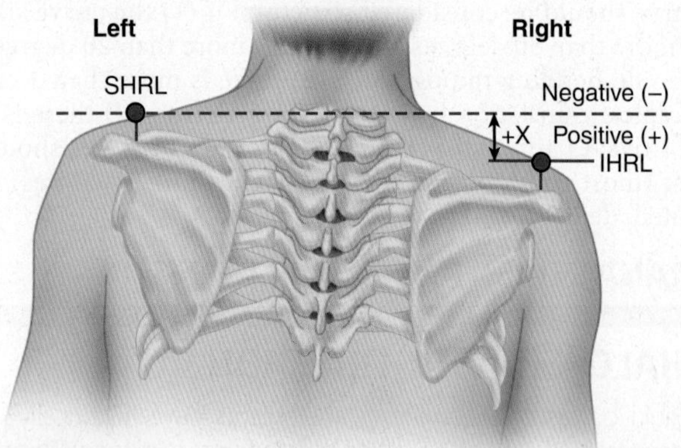

FIGURE 8.80 Radiographic shoulder height. *IHRL*, Inferior horizontal reference line; *SHRL*, superior horizontal reference line. (Redrawn from O'Brien MF, Kuklo TR, Blanke KM, Lenke LG, editors: *Spinal deformity study group radiographic measurement manual*, Memphis, TN, 2004, Medtronic Sofamor Danek, p 57.)

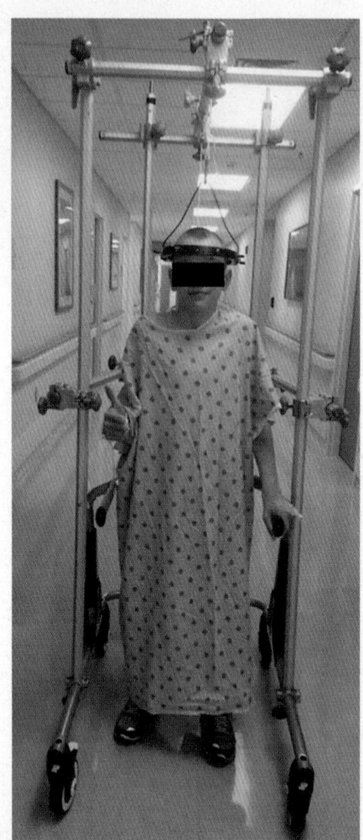

FIGURE 8.81 Child in halo-gravity traction. **SEE TECHNIQUE 8.17.**

50% of the patient's body weight is recommended, with at least daily neurologic assessments including the cranial nerves. Most commonly, hospitalization is required for this, with most correction being obtained in 3 to 4 weeks (Fig. 8.81).

TECHNIQUE 8.17

(SPONSELLER AND TAKENAGA)

- Sedation and local anesthesia should be used for this procedure.
- Place the halo just below the equator of the skull, above the eyebrows and pinnae of the ears.
- Six to eight pins are used in children younger than 6 years of age and tightened to 4 in-lb of torque. In older children or adults (if there is normal bone density), the pins are tightened to 8 in-lb. Place the anterior pins lateral to the midportion of the eyebrows to avoid the supraorbital nerves and ensure that the patient's eyes will close after pin placement. Place the posterior pins diametrically opposite the anterior pins. Retighten the pins after 24 to 48 hours. If there is loosening after this, the pin should be relocated.
- Begin traction immediately with 5 lb of weight for young children and 10 lb for children close to maturity.
- Gradually increase the traction weight by 2 to 3 lb/day as tolerated, with the goal being a weight of 33% to 50% of the patient's body weight. Incline the bed downward caudally.

- Inspect the patient's skin regularly because pressure sores from bony prominences are common, especially in patients who have trouble turning themselves.
- Continue traction throughout the day. Patients should be upright in a halo wheelchair or walker for part of the day. The goal is to suspend the patient's trunk as much as possible. Traction also can be applied when the patient is standing in a specially designed walker. Decrease the traction weight when the patient is sleeping, especially when the weight is near its maximum.
- Check the patient's neurologic status including cranial nerve function in the upper and lower extremities. If changes occur, immediately decrease or remove the weight and reassess the patient.
- The duration of preoperative halo-gravity traction may range from 2 to 12 weeks depending on the severity of the curve, its response to traction, and the overall condition of the patient.
- Obtain radiographs approximately every week to assess the improvement obtained.
- Longer periods of traction may help to optimize nutrition and minimize pulmonary problems in those with borderline pulmonary or nutritional reserve.

TEMPORARY DISTRACTION ROD

The use of temporary internal distraction rods in advance of the corrective surgical procedure has been described as an alternative to halo traction for severe rigid curves. Improved curve correction and restoration of sagittal and coronal contours have been cited as advantages to this technique. Placement of one or two temporary rods, soft-tissue releases, and osteotomies are performed usually 1 week before the permanent final implants are placed and fusion performed. The time between procedures can be longer than 1 week if necessary.

Before surgery, standard anteroposterior and lateral plain radiographs of the spine should be obtained with the patient standing or sitting, depending on the neurologic status. Traction films are helpful in predicting the amount of correction that can be obtained with a temporary rod. In addition, MRI and CT of the cervical, thoracic, and lumbar spine should be obtained to evaluate the precise spinal anatomy. Preoperative antibiotics should be administered.

TECHNIQUE 8.18

(BUCHOWSKI ET AL.)

- Position the patient on a Jackson table in routine fashion; Gardner-Wells tongs can be helpful to provide additional traction. The goal when positioning the patient on the table is to obtain as much correction of body alignment as possible to lessen the force required to achieve intraoperative correction, and neuromonitoring is essential because a distraction force will be placed on the spine.
- Place pedicle screws in a standard fashion in the one or two vertebral bodies that are not intended to be the final cephalad fixation due to loosening that may occur. Alternatively, spinal hooks or ribs can be used as temporary cephalad anchor points.
- For placement of the caudal anchors, use standard lumbar pedicle screws, placing two screws (or more, depending on bone quality) at adjacent vertebrae. Alternatively, sublaminar hooks can be used. Again, the vertebrae cephalad to the end vertebrae of the final construct should be chosen because some loosening of the temporary anchor points is expected to occur with distraction.
- If the pelvis is used for anchoring points, expose the iliac spine. Place an iliac screw in the posterior superior iliac crest close to (but not entering) the sciatic notch. It should be placed parallel and at least 2 cm lateral to where the permanent iliac screw will be placed. Alternatively, an S-shaped hook may be used, and this may be easier to connect to the distraction rod with a side-to-side connector.
- Although there are several possibilities for placement of internal distraction rod constructs (Fig. 8.82A-C), the simplest is to attach one distraction rod to the cephalad anchor points and a second rod to the caudal anchor points, connecting them in a side-to-side connector with overlap of the rods (Fig. 8.82B). In some patients with extreme deformity, it may be necessary to attach two short rods (one attached cephalad and one caudal) to a third distraction rod using multiaxial crosslink connectors (Fig. 8.82A).
- Apply distraction across these two rods serially by loosening and tightening the side-to-side connector. Careful attention should be given to spinal cord function during the distraction process. If a depression in the spinal cord signal is noticed, the amount of correction should be decreased and a wake-up test performed.
- Once the temporary rod or rods have been placed, expose the rest of the spine subperiosteally. Perform releases and osteotomies as necessary to allow additional correction of the spine. Although technically more difficult, additional anchor points can be placed after releases and osteotomies if necessary.
- Small amounts of distraction should be performed throughout the procedure to allow maximal correction with minimal stress. With time, soft-tissue release, facetectomies, and osteotomies, additional correction can be obtained with the goal at the end of surgery to have correction greater than that shown on the supine traction film with 50% or more correction in the Cobb angle. Bone graft is not used at this time but can be stored in a paraspinal muscle pouch for the final procedure.
- Closure may be difficult because substantial soft-tissue lengthening occurs with distraction and the rods usually are lateral to the transverse processes. If necessary, raise thick local flaps including the paraspinal muscles to make closure possible. Use closed suction drains in the space created during the closure.

STAGE II DEFINITIVE SURGERY

- Reexpose the spine. Leaving the temporary rod(s) in place if feasible, create the anchor points for the final construct. There should be a substantial increase in the ability to cor-

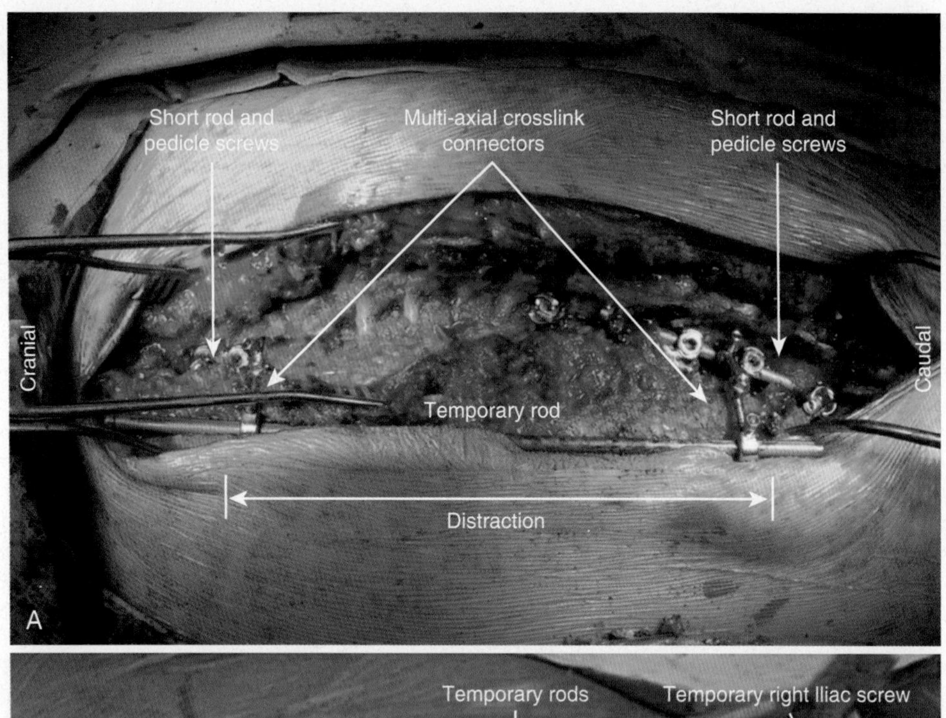

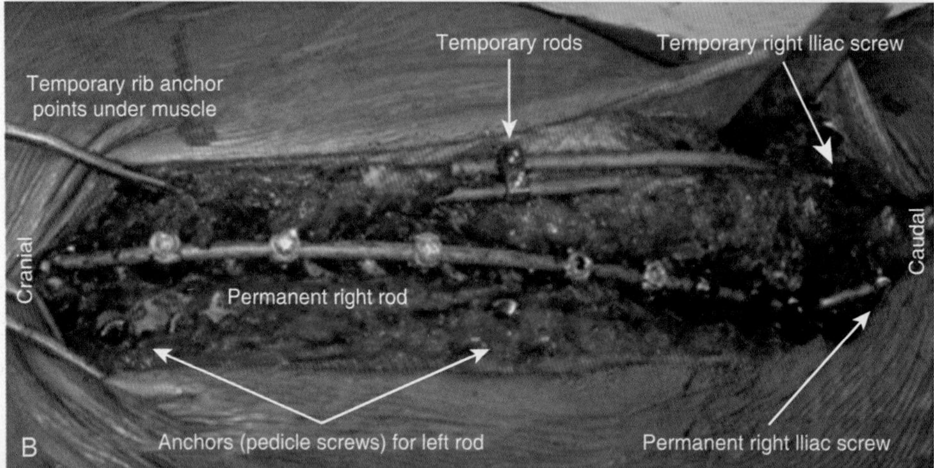

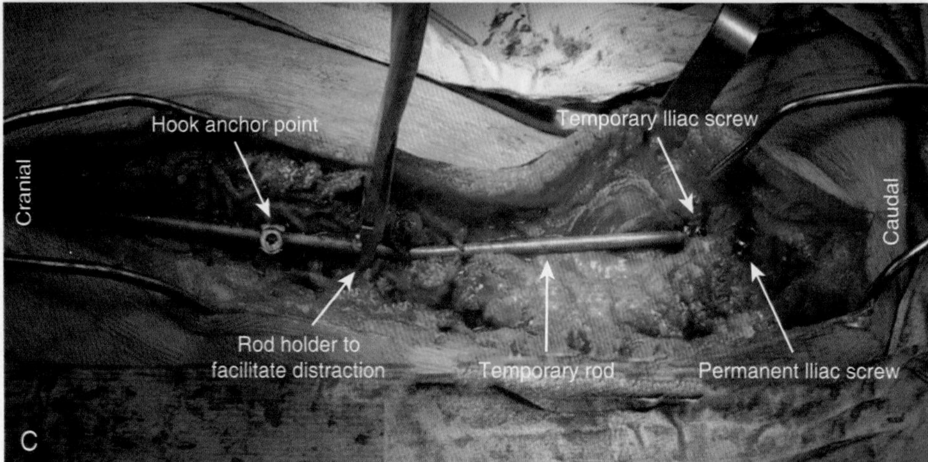

FIGURE 8.82 **A,** Two short rods (one at cephalad end, the other at caudad end, of construct) are connected to third distraction rod with multiaxial crosslink connectors. Distraction is applied across third rod, length of which spans deformity. **B,** Single temporary distraction rod is attached to spine with rib anchor points at cephalad end and lumbar pedicle screws and temporary iliac at caudal end. Permanent rod is then attached with pedicle screws and permanent iliac screw. **C,** Single temporary distraction rod, attached to spine with thoracic hook at cephalad end and temporary iliac screw at caudal end, is used to allow distraction between thoracic hook and rod holder to correct coronal deformity and pelvic obliquity. (From Buchowski JM, Skaggs DL, Sponseller PD: Temporary internal distraction as an aid to correction of severe scoliosis. Surgical technique, *J Bone Joint Surg Am* 89 [Suppl 2, Part 2]:297, 2007.)

rect the spine at this point, and it may be possible to gain additional distraction.
- Remove the temporary instrumentation and insert the final implants.
- Perform repeat pulsed irrigation and drainage and close the wound.

POSTOPERATIVE CARE Between the first and second stages, parenteral nutrition is recommended until the patient can optimize oral intake. Sitting, standing, and walking are encouraged to avoid pulmonary complications. Casting or bracing is not required.

ANTERIOR RELEASE

Complete anterior release of the thoracic or lumbar spine, or both, allows improved mobilization of a curve and correction of deformity; however, the benefits of this must be weighed against increased surgical time and potential complications. Anterior release can be done through an open thoracotomy, thoracoscopically, or in conjunction with anterior instrumentation. With the increased correction seen with posterior instrumentation systems, the use of anterior release alone continues to decrease. It is still useful in patients with large and/or stiff deformities.

TECHNIQUE 8.19

(LETKO ET AL.)
- In the thoracic spine, resect the convex rib heads and attempt to rupture the concave costovertebral joints.
- In both the thoracic and lumbar spine, remove the disc and posterior annulus. Release the posterior longitudinal ligament.
- Resect the convex inferior endplate with or without resection of the convex superior endplate to allow mobilization and correction in the coronal plane. By shortening the anterior column, hypokyphosis in the thoracic sagittal profile can be corrected to normal.
- Anterior structural support of the lumbar spine and thoracolumbar junction is recommended to prevent kyphosis.
- After complete anterior release, anterior instrumentation can be performed if the curve is not too rigid or large.

OSTEOTOMY IN COMPLEX SPINAL DEFORMITY

Spinal osteotomy should be considered for patients with large, stiff curves for whom instrumentation alone cannot correct the deformity or restore balance. The Smith-Petersen and Ponte osteotomies are the most straightforward, with the Ponte osteotomy being the most used dorsal column shortening osteotomy. The difference between the Smith-Petersen osteotomy and the Ponte osteotomy is that, while both shorten the dorsal column, the Smith-Petersen osteotomy opens the anterior column, placing stretch on the great vessels, where the Ponte osteotomy does not. The classic indication for Ponte osteotomies, which allows the posterior column of the spine to shorten, was a long rounded kyphosis as in Scheuermann kyphosis; however, it is a versatile procedure that can be performed safely to aid in the gradual correction of rigid scoliotic curves. If soft-tissue releases are insufficient in obtaining correction, proceeding to osteotomy is the next step. The Ponte osteotomy is performed for scoliosis of more than 70 to 75 degrees that does not bend down to less than 40 degrees or for kyphosis that corrects to greater than 40 to 50 degrees in hyperextension. The use of Ponte osteotomies in patients with adolescent idiopathic scoliosis is associated with high rates of blood loss and neuromonitoring events. A multicenter study of 2210 patients found the rate of neurologic complications (0.37% vs. 0.17%) and neuromonitoring events (7.6% vs. 4.2%) were higher in patients who had Ponte osteotomies compared to those who did not. The cause of this is multifactorial but should be kept in mind when considering the use of Ponte osteotomies. In general, 1 mm of resection equals 1 degree of correction, with a possible correction of 5 to 10 degrees per level. Multiple levels can be resected to obtain more correction. A collapsed or immobile disc may be a contraindication to this technique. The choice of osteotomy depends on the apex of the deformity.

TECHNIQUE 8.20

Figure 8.83

(PONTE OSTEOTOMY)
- After exposing the spine as described in Technique 8.6, perform complete facetectomies for complete exposure.
- Develop the screw tracks for subsequent pedicle screw placement (without placing the screws) to help guide the osteotomy.
- Remove the lamina, ligamentum flavum, and superior and inferior articular processes bilaterally, and resect the spinous process of the vertebra just cephalad to the osteotomy site.
- Create a wedge-shaped osteotomy 7 to 10 mm in width and carry it laterally to the intervertebral notch with small Kerrison rongeurs. An ultrasound bone scalpel, which provides excellent hemostasis and safety, can also be used. The point should be oriented distally. Both limbs of the wedge should be symmetric unless some coronal plane correction is desired. Take care to avoid the pedicles above and below the osteotomy and the nerve roots. If there is significant rotational deformity, open the osteotomy to a larger degree on the convex side.
- Remove the more superior facet to help prevent impingement of the superior nerve root.
- At this point, instrumentation can be added as indicated to achieve necessary correction.

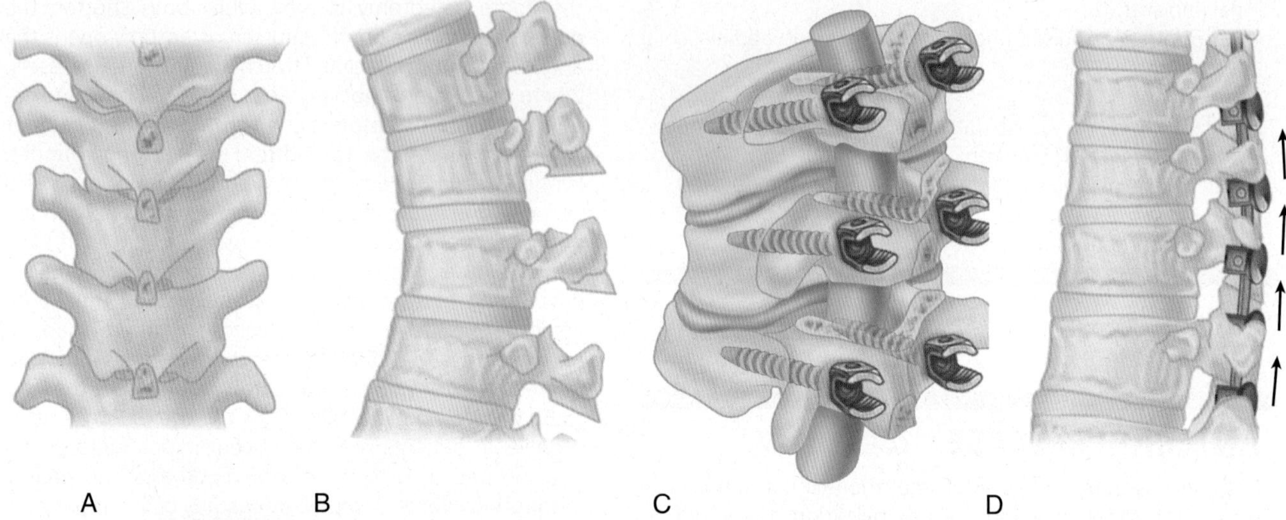

FIGURE 8.83 Ponte osteotomies for correction of kyphosis. **A** and **B**, Wedge-shaped osteotomies. **C** and **D**, Placement of rod for correction. (Redrawn from Geck MJ, Macagno A, Ponte A, Shufflebarger HL: Posterior only treatment of Scheuermann's kyphosis using segmental posterior shortening and pedicle screw instrumentation, *J Spinal Disord Tech* 20:586, 2007.) **SEE TECHNIQUE 8.20.**

POSTERIOR THORACIC VERTEBRAL COLUMN RESECTION

Vertebral column resection is indicated for patients with complex, rigid, spinal deformities that cannot be corrected by less aggressive osteotomies. Circumferential access is provided to the vertebral column and neural elements for decompression and stabilization. This procedure is quite challenging and should be done by surgeons with specialized training and experience. It entails resection of one or more entire vertebral segments, including the posterior elements, vertebral body, and adjacent discs. Patients with cardiopulmonary comorbidities may not be suitable candidates.

TECHNIQUE 8.21

(POWERS ET AL.)

- Position the patient on a Jackson table with adjustable pads. Intraoperative halo-gravity traction can be used. Neuromonitoring is essential for this procedure.
- Subperiosteally expose the spine out to the tips of the transverse process (Fig. 8.84A).
- Place pedicle screws using a freehand technique at the preplanned levels of fusion, a minimum of three levels above and three below the vertebral column resection (Fig. 8.84C). The spine is considered unstable from the time resection begins until final correction is achieved. A minimum of six points of fixation, both cephalad and caudal to the resection, is recommended. Multiaxial reduction screws can be placed at the apical concave regions of severe scoliosis or at the proximal or distal regions of severe kyphoscoliosis or kyphosis. In the lumbar spine, they should be placed in the concavity of the lumbar region.
- Expose 4 to 5 cm of the medial ribs corresponding with the level of resection. Remove the ribs by cutting each laterally and then disarticulating the costovertebral joints, or resect the transverse process at the level of the resection bilaterally to weaken the attachment of the rib head. The removal of the ribs and transverse process allows access to the lateral pedicle wall and vertebral body and can be used as a graft to fill the laminectomy defect later.
- After bilateral costotransversectomy, dissect the vertebral body wall anteriorly until the anterior vertebral body is exposed. Protect the thoracic sympathetic chain, anterior and posterior vessels, and pleura with a retractor.
- Perform bilateral laminectomies and facetectomies at the levels to be resected and complete the posterior decompression by removing the lamina cephalad to the pedicles above the resection and caudal to the pedicles below the resection (Fig. 8.85A). Posterior column exposure should be 5 to 6 cm to allow access to the spinal cord and to prevent dural buckling or impingement. Ligate the corresponding nerve roots medial and dorsal to the root ganglion.
- Once the osteotomies are complete, insert a temporary stabilizing rod and fix with two or three pedicle screws above and below the vertebral column resection (Fig. 8.85B,C). Depending on the deformity, one or two rods can be used to prevent subluxation of the spine.
- Identify the pedicles to be resected and enter through their lateral wall to gain access to the vertebral body. Complete the corpectomy by curetting the cancellous bone out of the vertebral body. Save this bone for later bone grafting. Most of the vertebral body removed should be from the

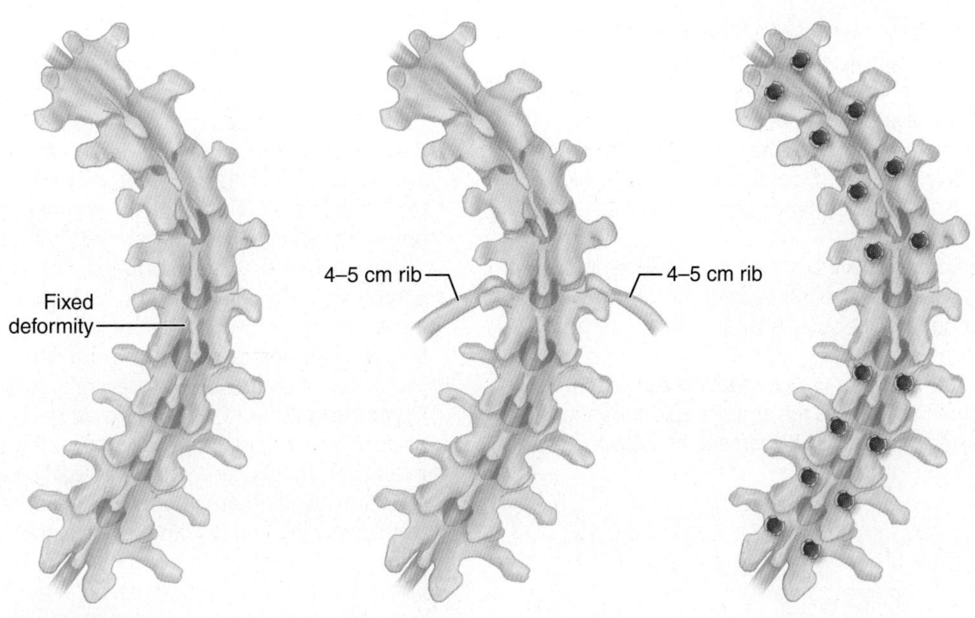

FIGURE 8.84 **A,** Posterior thoracic vertebral column resection. Spine exposed to tips of transverse processes. **B,** Medial 4 to 5 cm of ribs attached to vertebra excised to base of vertebral body. **C,** Pedicle screws placed segmentally, periadjacent to planned vertebrectomy site. (Redrawn from Powers AK, O'Shaughnessy BA, Lemke LG: Posterior thoracic vertebral column resection. In Wang JC, editor: *Advanced reconstruction: spine*, Rosemont, IL, 2011, American Academy of Orthopaedic Surgeons, p 265.) **SEE TECHNIQUE 8.21.**

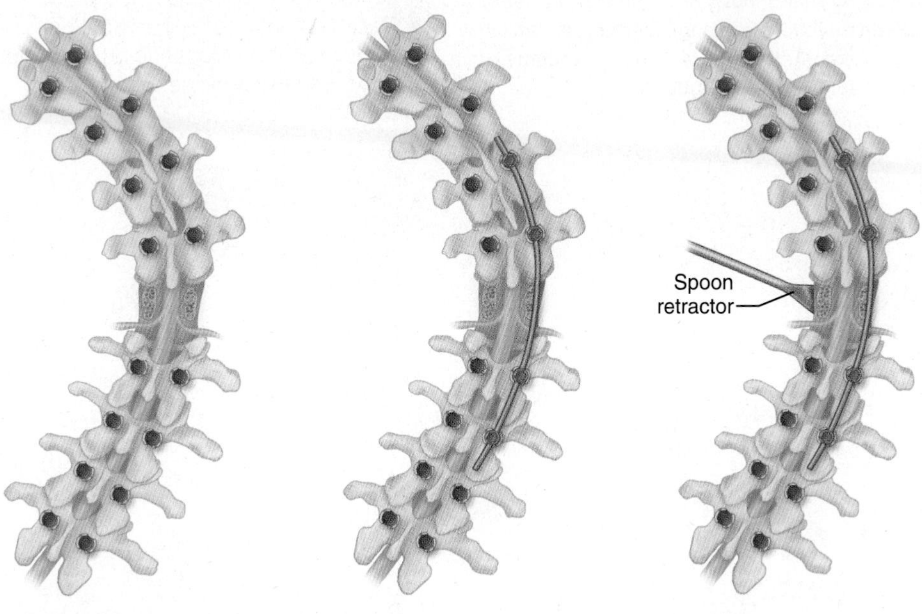

FIGURE 8.85 **A,** Complete laminectomy performed from inferior pedicles of level above to superior pedicles of level below planned resection. **B,** Temporary rod placed either unilaterally or bilaterally, depending on amount of instability anticipated. **C,** Vertebral body exposed superperiosteally or subperiosteally laterally and then anteriorly. Spoon retractor placed anterior to body. (Redrawn from Powers AK, O'Shaughnessy BA, Lemke LG: Posterior thoracic vertebral column resection. In Wang JC, editor: *Advanced reconstruction: spine*, Rosemont, IL, 2011, American Academy of Orthopaedic Surgeons, p 265.) **SEE TECHNIQUE 8.21.**

convexity of the deformity. Powers preferred to perform resection from the concave side before the convex side removal to minimize bleeding and to remove some tension from the concave side before proceeding. Except for the anterior shell, remove the entire vertebral body. Keep a thin rim of bone intact on the anterior longitudinal ligament for fusion. Thin the anterior bone if it is thick and cortical.

- Perform discectomies above and below the resected body to expose the adjacent vertebral body endplates; however, avoid violating these because this can lead to interbody cage subsidence (Fig. 8.86).
- For removal of the posterior wall, inspect the dura and free it of any attachments, such as the anterior epidural venous plexus, the posterior longitudinal ligament, or osteophytes.

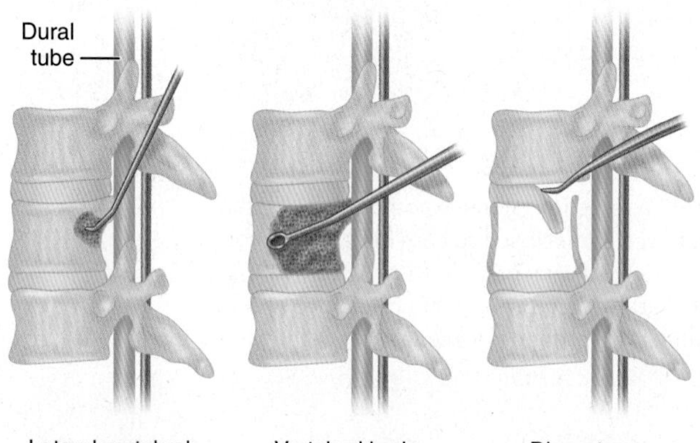

FIGURE 8.86 Vertebral body corpectomy and discectomy. (Redrawn from Powers AK, O'Shaughnessy BA, Lemke LG: Posterior thoracic vertebral column resection. In Wang JC, editor: *Advanced reconstruction: spine*, Rosemont, IL, 2011, American Academy of Orthopaedic Surgeons, p 265.) **SEE TECHNIQUE 8.21.**

Control epidural bleeding, which can be significant, with bipolar electrocautery. Once the dura is freed, the thin posterior vertebral body can be tamped away from the spinal cord into the corpectomy defect (Fig. 8.87A). Inspect the dura after posterior vertebral body removal and remove any points of attachment or compression.

- Once the resection is complete, closure of the defect and deformity correction are performed. In this procedure, the spinal column is always shortened, not lengthened, with compression. Obtain correction with pedicle screws or using a construct-to-construct closure method performed by placing a construct rod above and one below to distribute forces of correction over several pedicle screw levels. Compression should proceed slowly because subluxation or dural impingement may occur (Fig. 8.87B).
- In any deformity with a degree of kyphosis, Powers et al. recommend using an anterior structural cage to prevent overshortening and to help provide extra kyphosis correction.
- Once the vertebral column resection has been completed, place a permanent contralateral rod and remove the temporary rod. Then place a second permanent rod on the ipsilateral side and perform appropriate correction compression or distraction maneuvers as necessary.
- Confirm alignment by intraoperative radiographs (Fig. 8.88) and perform a final circumferential dural inspection.
- Place split-thickness rib autograft over the laminectomy defect and secure it to the rods using sutures or a cross-link.
- Irrigate the wound with saline. Decorticate the posterior spine and facet joints with a high-speed burr and place copious amounts of bone graft.
- Place subfascial and suprafascial Hemovac drains through separate stab incisions and close the wound in layers with interrupted absorbable sutures.

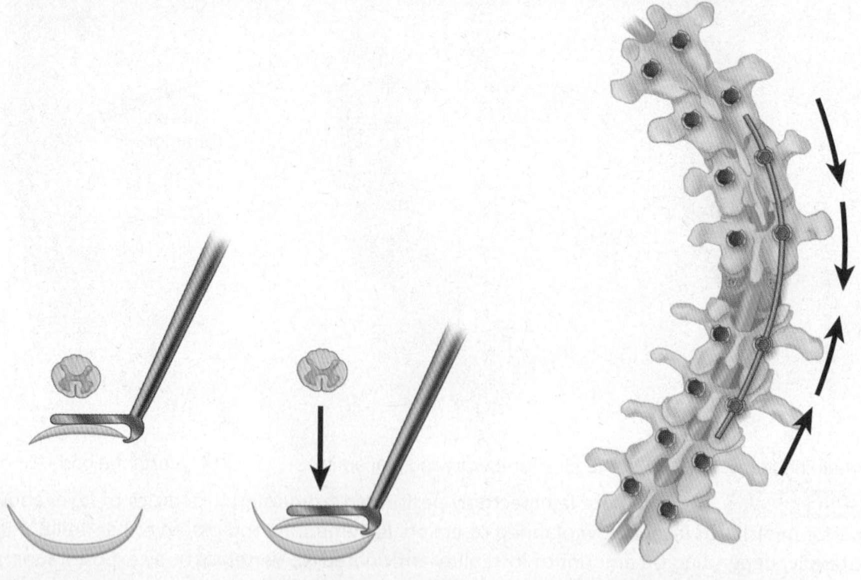

FIGURE 8.87 **A,** Impaction of posterior wall of vertebral body into defect created. **B,** Correction of deformity using compression. (Redrawn from Powers AK, O'Shaughnessy BA, Lemke LG: Posterior thoracic vertebral column resection. In Wang JC, editor: *Advanced reconstruction: spine*, Rosemont, IL, 2011, American Academy of Orthopaedic Surgeons, p 265.) **SEE TECHNIQUE 8.21.**

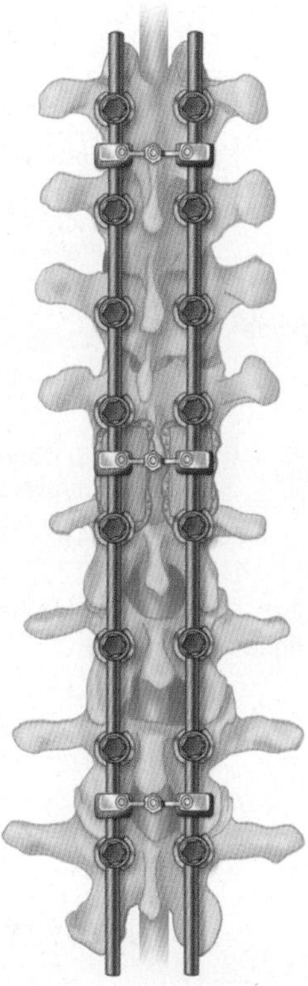

FIGURE 8.88 Permanent rods with rib bridge graft. (Redrawn from Powers AK, O'Shaughnessy BA, Lemke LG: Posterior thoracic vertebral column resection. In Wang JC, editor: *Advanced reconstruction: spine*, Rosemont, IL, 2011, American Academy of Orthopaedic Surgeons, p 265.) **SEE TECHNIQUE 8.21.**

POSTOPERATIVE CARE The suction drain is removed once the drainage is less than 50 mL per 8-hour shift or at 48 hours postoperatively. Most patients will develop a postoperative ileus. Food or liquids are begun slowly and advanced as tolerated. Most patients also develop a postoperative atelectasis and temperature elevation. This is managed with routine "pulmonary toilet" and incentive spirometer. Intravenous antibiotics are administered for 24 hours. If the patient is old enough, a patient-controlled pain medication pump is used. Postoperative continuous epidural analgesia using local anesthetic agents or opioids, or both, can be used in appropriate situations. The patient is gradually gotten out of bed as allowed by pain tolerance. A postoperative brace or no immobilization may be used depending on the stability of the instrumentation construct. When the temperature has subsided and the patient is relatively independently ambulatory and tolerating food and liquid intake, the patient is discharged. At the 6-month checkup, if the fusion appears solid, most limitations are lifted. We generally advise against contact sports after this type of spinal surgery.

COMPLICATIONS OF POSTERIOR SCOLIOSIS SURGERY

EARLY COMPLICATIONS

The Scoliosis Research Society morbidity and mortality database showed that for scoliosis surgery the overall complication rate was 10%, with a 0.7% new neurologic deficit rate for pedicle screw instrumentation and a 0.02% mortality rate for idiopathic scoliosis. A review of 2005 patients from the National Surgical Quality Improvement Program (NSQIP) database found a 10% complication rate at 30 days, which was higher in neuromuscular patients than in adolescent idiopathic scoliosis patients. Risk factors for readmission include cognitive delays, increased ASA class, and longer surgical time. The frequency of 2-year unplanned return to surgery for modern pedicle screw constructs is 3.5%, which increases to 7.5% at 5 years. The most common causes of reoperation include infection, symptomatic implants, and misplaced pedicle screws.

NEUROLOGIC INJURY

The most feared and unpredictable complication in scoliosis surgery remains neurologic injury. For patients undergoing spinal fusion for adolescent idiopathic scoliosis, the incidence of neurologic injury is relatively low, between 0.32% and 0.69%. Causative factors include unrecognized spinal cord tethers, ischemia secondary to spinal cord stretch, and direct injury from surgical instruments, often combined with intraoperative hypotension. Ponte osteotomies have been associated with increased rates of neuromonitoring alerts.

Management of an intraoperative neurologic deficit begins with a series of corrective actions that should be planned for by the surgical team, including nursing and anesthesia personnel, well in advance of the event. A recent expert consensus-based best practice guideline for neuromonitoring changes has been published (Fig. 8.89) and should be placed on the wall of the operating room and followed if neurologic changes occur. (Spinal cord monitoring and the wake-up test are discussed in the section on intraoperative considerations for operative treatment of adolescent idiopathic scoliosis.)

INFECTION

Perioperative wound infection is the most common cause of readmission for adolescent idiopathic surgical patients, with a rate of approximately 1%, although there is variability between centers. The rarity of postoperative infections in adolescent idiopathic scoliosis patients makes randomized clinical trials difficult, if not impossible. Best practice guidelines from high-risk patients, including neuromuscular and early-onset scoliosis patients, can be extrapolated to adolescent idiopathic patients. In neuromuscular patients, the most important factor was timely dosing of antibiotics within 1 hour of the start of the procedure. The use of vancomycin powder and dilute betadine irrigation at the end of the procedure were also believed to be helpful. A recent multicenter report found that obesity was the only factor that predicted a sevenfold increased infection rate in adolescent idiopathic scoliosis patients in high-volume centers.

There are two types of infections: immediate perioperative and delayed. The first is obvious because a high fever develops, usually within 2 to 5 days after surgery, and the wound almost always appears infected. In the second type, the temperature is elevated only slightly or moderately and the wound appears relatively normal. Diagnosis of this latter type of wound infection may be difficult. Patients often have postoperative temperature elevation of up to 102°F, which should decline gradually during the first 4 postoperative days. Any spike of temperature above 102°F should strongly suggest a deep wound infection, especially if the patient's general condition does not steadily improve. The appearance of

Checklist for the response to intraoperative neuromonitoring changes in patients with a stable spine

Gain control of room

- ❑ Intraoperative pause: stop case and announce to the room
- ❑ Eliminate extraneous stimuli (e.g. music , conversations, etc.)
- ❑ Summon ATTENDING anesthesiologist, SENIOR neurologist or neurophysiologist, and EXPERIENCED nurse
- ❑ Anticipate need for intraoperative and/or perioperative imaging if not readily available

Anesthetic/systemic

- ❑ Optimize mean arterial pressure (MAP)
- ❑ Optimize hematocrit
- ❑ Optimize blood pH and pCO_2
- ❑ Seek normothermia
- ❑ Discuss POTENTIAL need for wake-up test with ATTENDING anesthesiologist

Technical/neurophysiologic

- ❑ Discuss status of anesthetic agents
- ❑ Check extent of neuromuscular blockade and degree of paralysis
- ❑ Check electrodes and connections
- ❑ Determine pattern and timing of signal changes
- ❑ Check neck and limb positioning; check limb position on table especially if unilateral loss

Surgical

- ❑ Discuss events and actions just prior to signal loss and consider reversing actions:
  - ❑ Remove traction (if applicable)
  - ❑ Decrease/remove distraction or other corrective forces
  - ❑ Remove rods
  - ❑ Remove screws and probe for breach
- ❑ Evaluate for spinal cord compression, examine osteotomy and laminotomy sites
- ❑ Intraoperative and/or perioperative imaging (e.g. O-arm, fluoroscopy, x-ray) to evaluate implant placement

Ongoing considerations

- ❑ REVISIT anesthetic/systemic considerations and confirm that they are optimized
- ❑ Wake-up test
- ❑ Consultation with a colleague
- ❑ Continue surgical procedure versus staging procedure
- ❑ IV steroid protocol: Methylprednisolone 30 mg/kg in first hr, then 5.4 mg/kg/hr for next 23 hrs

FIGURE 8.89 Checklist for the response to intraoperative neuromonitoring changes in patients with a stable spine. (From Vitale MG, Skaggs DL, Pace GI, et al: Best practices in intraoperative neuromonitoring in spine deformity surgery: development of an intraoperative checklist to optimize response, *Spine Deform* 2:333, 2014.)

the wound can be deceiving, with no significant erythema or tenderness. Prompt aspiration of the wound in several sites is recommended. Urgent thorough irrigation and debridement with retention of implants, if possible, should be performed in conjunction with consultation with infectious disease experts for long-term antibiotic therapy. A recent multicenter review found that with aggressive treatment, patients with early postoperative infections can retain their implants 76% of the time. Delayed wound infections (>6 months after index procedure) are more common than acute deep wound infections and usually are caused by indolent skin flora organisms such as *Propionibacterium acnes* or *Staphylococcus epidermidis*. The rate of late infection may be decreasing due to the fact that the risk of delayed infection is higher with stainless steel implants than with other metals now in use. In these infections, implant removal usually is necessary to eradicate the infection.

ILEUS

Ileus is a common complication after both anterior and posterior spinal fusion. Oral feedings are resumed slowly after surgery. A multimodal approach to decreasing the rate of gastrointestinal complications, including early mobilization, decreased narcotic usage, epidural catheters, and early feeding, have been helpful. Malnutrition is uncommon in teenagers with idiopathic scoliosis, but patients requiring a two-stage corrective procedure may become malnourished as a result of the limited oral calorie intake and increased caloric requirements associated with closely spaced surgical procedures, and nutritional consultation and supplementation including parenteral nutrition should be considered.

SUPERIOR MESENTERIC ARTERY SYNDROME

Superior mesenteric artery syndrome can present 1 to 2 weeks after surgery as abdominal pain and distention and vomiting. It is due to compression of the duodenum between the superior mesenteric artery and the aorta that can occur after spinal deformity correction (Fig. 8.90). Risk factors include thin habitus and spinal lengthening that occurs during scoliosis correction. Prompt recognition, bowel rest and intravenous hydration, and gradual post-pyloric feeding are essential for a good outcome, which can take several weeks. General surgical and nutritional consultation are helpful.

ATELECTASIS

Atelectasis is a common cause of fever after scoliosis surgery. Frequent turning of the patient and the use of incentive spirometry and deep breathing and coughing usually

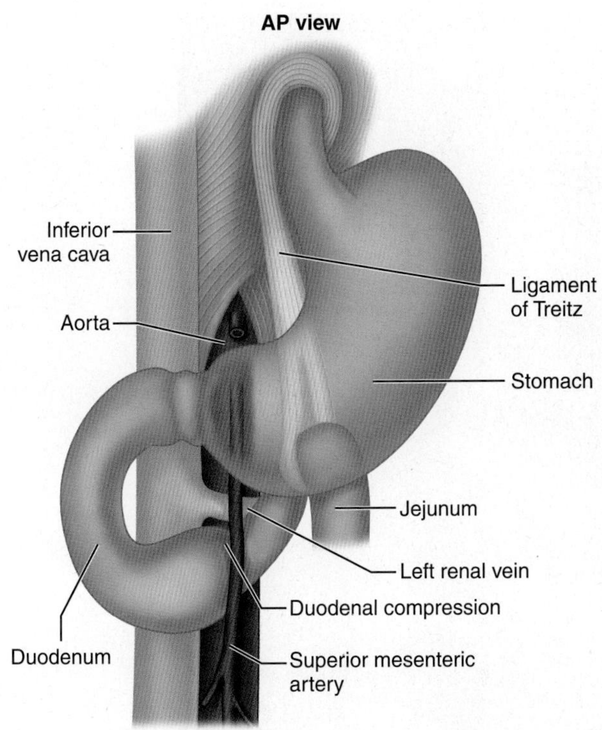

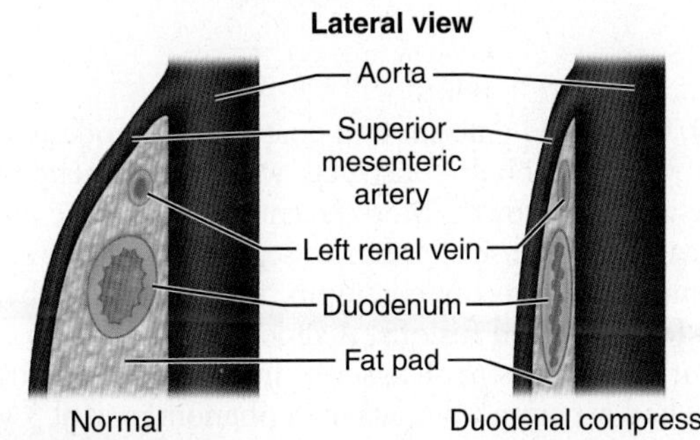

FIGURE 8.90 **Superior mesenteric artery syndrome. Relationship between superior mesenteric artery and duodenum.** (From Lam, DJ, Lee JZ, Chua JH, et al: Superior mesenteric artery syndrome following surgery for adolescent idiopathic scoliosis: a case series, review of the literature, and algorithm for management, *J Pediatr Orthop B* 23:312, 2014.)

control or prevent serious atelectasis. Inhalation therapy with intermittent positive-pressure breathing may be beneficial in cooperative patients. With current emphasis on early patient rehabilitation, significant atelectasis has become less common.

PNEUMOTHORAX

At the time of subperiosteal posterior spine exposure, the pleura may be entered inadvertently, most commonly between the transverse processes on the concave side of the scoliosis. If a thoracoplasty is done at the same time, a pneumothorax is more likely to occur. Observation of the pneumothorax is probably appropriate if it is less than 20%, but chest tube insertion is needed for larger pneumothoraces. A Valsalva maneuver in conjunction with the anesthesia team should be performed intraoperatively if a pneumothorax is suspected so that a chest tube can be placed.

DURAL TEAR

If a dural tear occurs during removal of the ligamentum flavum or insertion of a hook or wire, repair should be attempted. The laminotomy often must be enlarged to allow access to the ends of the dural tear. If repair is not done, drainage of the cerebrospinal fluid through the wound can cause problems postoperatively. Larger or non-repairable tears can be managed with soft-tissue, usually muscle or fascia, patches. When large tears are repaired or patched, the patient should be left supine for 24 hours before gradual sitting to decrease intraspinal pressure.

WRONG LEVELS

Care should be taken in the operating room to identify the correct vertebral levels as there are normal variants in the number of ribs and segmentation at the lumbosacral junction. In most instances, an intraoperative radiograph with use of a marker on the vertebra is the best way to accurately identify the appropriate spinal level.

URINARY COMPLICATIONS

The syndrome of inappropriate antidiuretic hormone secretion develops in the immediate postoperative period in up to one third of patients undergoing spinal fusion. This causes a decline in urinary output and is maximal 36 hours after surgery. If the serum osmolality is diminished and the urine osmolality is elevated, this syndrome should be considered and fluid overload should be avoided. The urinary output gradually increases in the next 2 to 3 days after surgery.

VISION LOSS

Postoperative loss of vision has an incidence of 0.02% to 0.2%. In a review of a nationwide database including over 40,000 patients under the age of 18 who had surgery for idiopathic scoliosis, De la Garza-Ramos et al. found that vision loss was reported in 0.16%. Prone positioning, particularly in the Trendelenburg position, has been noted to increase intraocular pressure. This is thought to be a risk factor for postoperative loss of vision as the result of decreased perfusion of the optic nerve. Other suggested risk factors include a younger age, a history of iron deficiency anemia, and long-segment fusions. The loss of vision manifests itself during the first 2 postoperative days. Most deficits are permanent.

LATE COMPLICATIONS

PSEUDARTHROSIS

In adolescents with idiopathic scoliosis, the pseudarthrosis rate is approximately 1%, which is lower than that in patients with neuromuscular scoliosis. The most common areas of pseudarthrosis are at the thoracolumbar junction and at the distally fused segment. With more rigid and stronger implants, the pseudarthrosis may not be apparent for years. In a review of cases of nonunion with segmental instrumentation, the average time to presentation of nonunion was 3.5 years. In 23% of patients with nonunion, implant failure was detected 5 to 10 years postoperatively. The diagnosis of pseudarthrosis usually is made by oblique radiographs, a broken implant, tomograms, CT, or bone scanning (Fig. 8.91). After successful posterior fusion, the disc height anteriorly should diminish as the vertebral body continues to grow at the expense of the disc space. A large disc space anteriorly may indicate a posterior pseudarthrosis. Often, however,

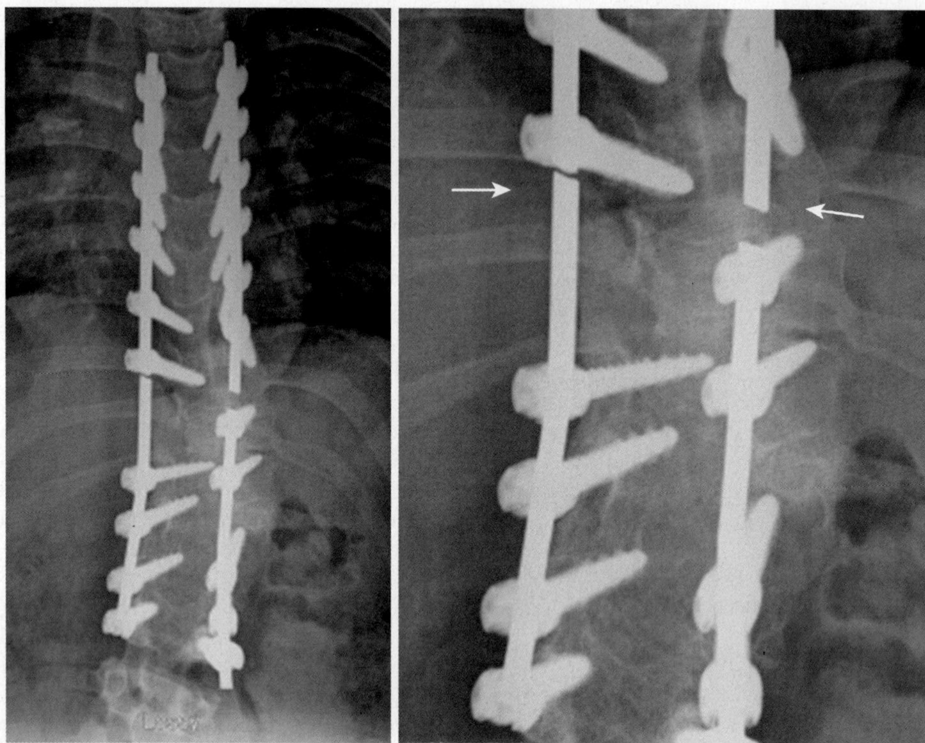

FIGURE 8.91 Pseudarthrosis with rod fracture *(arrows)* 4 years after posterior spinal fusion in 18-year-old male.

the pseudarthrosis cannot be confirmed even with the most sophisticated radiographic evaluation and can be detected only by surgical exploration.

If a pseudarthrosis does not cause pain or loss of correction, surgery may not be necessary. Asymptomatic pseudarthrosis is more common in the distally fused segments. A pseudarthrosis at the thoracolumbar junction is more likely to cause loss of correction and pain.

During surgical exploration, the cortex is smooth and firm over the mature and intact areas of the fusion mass and the soft tissues strip away easily. Conversely, at a pseudarthrosis, the soft tissues usually are adherent and continuous into the defect; however, a narrow pseudarthrosis may be difficult to locate, especially if motion is slight. In this instance, decortication of the fusion mass in suspicious areas is indicated and a search always should be made for several pseudarthroses. An extremely difficult type of pseudarthrosis to determine is a solid fusion mass posteriorly that is not well adherent to the underlying spine and lamina. Once the pseudarthrosis has been identified, it is cleared of fibrous tissue, and the curve is reinstrumented by the application of compression over the pseudarthrosis. If this is not done, kyphotic deformity may worsen because of incompetent spinal extensor muscles from the previous surgical exposure. The pseudarthroses are treated as ordinary joints to be fused: their edges are freshened and decorticated, and autogenous bone graft is applied in addition to the instrumentation.

CRANKSHAFT PHENOMENON

If posterior fusion alone is done in patients with a significant amount of anterior growth remaining, a crankshaft phenomenon can occur (see section on treatment of juvenile idiopathic scoliosis). Combined anterior and posterior arthrodesis with posterior wire and hook constructs were recommended to eliminate anterior growth. More recent reports in the literature indicate that the use of posterior segmental pedicle screw instrumentation with three-column fixation may obviate the need for combined fusions. A report of 46 patients with interval or continuous pedicle screw instrumentation found that none had experienced crankshaft phenomenon at 3-year follow-up.

POSTERIOR THORACOPLASTY

Of all the deformities caused by idiopathic scoliosis, the posterior rib prominence generally is the patient's main concern. With thoracic pedicle instrumentation and derotation techniques, we now rarely find it necessary to perform a thoracoplasty. Chen et al. found that posterior instrumentation in combination with thoracoplasty led to a significant decrease in pulmonary function at 3 months. Eventually, the function returned to normal at 1 year postoperatively. Approximately 75% of patients have a pleural effusion on chest radiograph. If necessary for cosmetic reasons, resection of the convex ribs can improve the postoperative cosmetic result of this surgery. With the advances in posterior correction techniques and convex rib resection at the time of spinal fusion, the use of delayed thoracoplasty has fallen out of favor.

CONCAVE RIB OSTEOTOMIES

Concave rib osteotomies can be used to help increase flexibility for very stiff curves. Cadaver studies have shown an average increase in deflection of 53%. Flexibility increased most when five or six ribs were resected. The addition of concave rib osteotomies to instrumentation and fusion procedures increases the risk of pulmonary morbidity and should

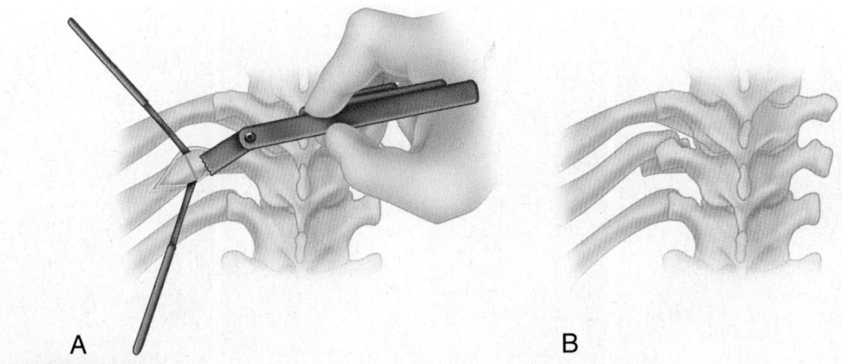

FIGURE 8.92 Rib osteotomy. **A,** Rib is exposed subperiosteally 1 cm lateral to transverse process. Osteotomy is completed with microsagittal saw. **B,** Overlap of lateral rib segment. **SEE TECHNIQUE 8.22.**

be used sparingly because of the increased power of modern instrumentation systems and high complication rate associated with their use.

OSTEOTOMY OF THE RIBS

TECHNIQUE 8.22

(MANN ET AL.)

- Approach the concave ribs through the midline incision used for the instrumentation and spinal fusion.
- Retract the paraspinous muscles lateral to the tips of the concave transverse processes. When needed, use electrocautery to incise overlying tissue along the rib axis.
- Incise the periosteum along the rib axis for 1.5 cm lateral to the transverse process and use small elevators to expose the rib periosteally.
- Protect the pleura with the elevators and use a rib cutter to section the rib approximately 1 cm lateral to the transverse process (Fig. 8.92A).
- Lift the lateral rib segment with a Kocher clamp and allow it to posteriorly overlap the medial segment (Fig. 8.92B).
- Rongeur any jagged ends and place a small piece of thrombin-soaked Gelfoam between the rib and pleura for protection and hemostasis.
- Make four to six osteotomies over the apical concave vertebrae.
- Approximate the paraspinous muscles with an absorbable suture.
- Complete the instrumentation and fusion and insert a chest tube.

ANTERIOR INSTRUMENTATION FOR IDIOPATHIC SCOLIOSIS

Anterior instrumentation and fusion for idiopathic scoliosis is a well-accepted procedure for certain thoracolumbar and lumbar curves, although with newer segmental posterior instrumentation systems, the use of anterior arthrodesis and instrumentation has declined dramatically. A Lenke type 4 curve pattern in which the thoracolumbar or lumbar curve is the structural component and the main thoracic or proximal thoracic curves are nonstructural is the ideal situation for this type of procedure. Anterior instrumentation can provide derotation and correction of the curve in the coronal plane. The child must be old enough for the vertebrae to be large enough to allow screw fixation, and caution is advised in using these systems in children younger than 9 years. In general, the lowest instrumented vertebra is the lower end vertebra of the Cobb measurement. The proximal level usually is the neutral vertebra. The fusion should not extend into the compensatory thoracic curve above. On the convex bending film, the disc below the lowest instrumented vertebra should open up on both sides. This indicates that the lower vertebra selected can be made horizontal with the anterior approach.

The anterior approach for thoracolumbar and lumbar curves has several potential disadvantages: chylothorax; injury to the ureter, spleen, or great vessels; retroperitoneal fibrosis; and prominent instrumentation that must be carefully isolated from the great vessels. Without careful attention to detail, a kyphosing effect can occur even with solid-rod and dual-rod anterior instrumentation systems. The attachment to the spine is through relatively cancellous vertebral bodies, and proximal screw dislodgement also is a risk. Many orthopaedic surgeons require the assistance of a thoracic or general surgeon with anterior approaches.

Anterior instrumentation and fusion can also be used in the treatment of thoracic curves but has generally been replaced by posterior techniques because of the potential disadvantages of this approach, including chest cage disruption, need for a chest tube, effects on pulmonary function, the need for the assistance of a thoracic surgeon, an increased risk of progressive kyphosis because of posterior spinal growth in skeletally immature patients (Risser grade 0), and smaller vertebrae and less secure fixation, especially of the proximal screw (Fig. 8.93). The aorta can be very close to the screw tips if bicortical fixation is achieved (Fig. 8.94). A comparison of curve correction by posterior spinal fusion and thoracic pedicle screws with anterior spinal fusion by single-rod instrumentation in Lenke type 1 curves found that posterior spinal fusion by thoracic pedicle screw instrumentation provided superior instrumented correction of the main thoracic

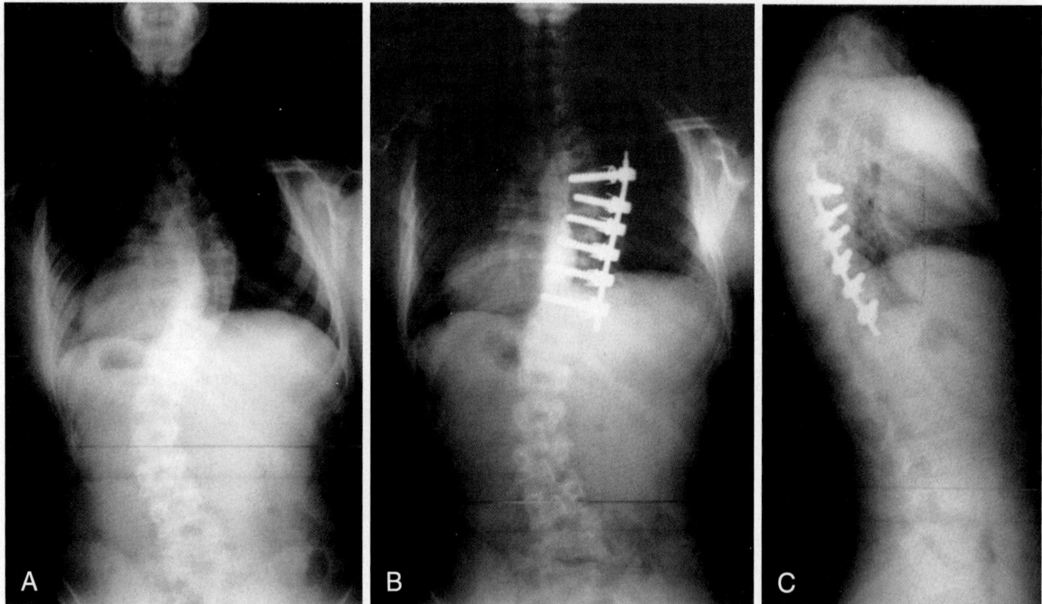

FIGURE 8.93 **A,** Standing posteroanterior radiograph of patient with idiopathic scoliosis. With posterior approach, this patient would require fusion well down into the lumbar spine. **B and C,** Postoperative posteroanterior and lateral radiographs after anterior instrumentation. Although some loss of fixation of proximal screw is noted, patient achieved satisfactory correction and well-balanced spine in both coronal and sagittal planes by instrumentation of only thoracic spine deformity.

curves and spontaneous correction of the thoracolumbar and lumbar curves, as well as improved correction of thoracic torsion and rotation.

If the curve to be instrumented is a thoracolumbar curve, a thoracoabdominal approach is required. If the curve is purely lumbar, a lumbar extraperitoneal approach can be used.

THORACOABDOMINAL APPROACH

TECHNIQUE 8.23

- Place the patient in the lateral decubitus position with the convex side of the curve elevated.
- Make a curvilinear incision along the rib that is one level higher than the most proximal level to be instrumented. This generally is the ninth rib in most thoracolumbar curves. Make the incision along the rib and extend it distally along the anterolateral abdominal wall just lateral to the rectus abdominis muscle.
- Expose and excise the rib.
- Enter the chest and retract the lung.
- Identify the diaphragm as a separate structure; it tends to closely approximate the wall of the thoracic cage. The diaphragm can be removed in two ways. We prefer to remove it from the chest cavity and then continue with retroperitoneal dissection distally. Alternatively, the retroperitoneum can be entered below the diaphragm, and then the diaphragm can be divided. To remove the diaphragm from the chest cavity, enter the chest cavity transpleurally through the bed of the rib. Then use electrocautery to divide the diaphragm close to the chest wall. Leave a small tag of diaphragm for reattachment.
- Once the diaphragm has been reflected, expose the retroperitoneal space.
- Dissect the peritoneal cavity from underneath the internal oblique muscle and the abdominal musculature.
- Split the internal oblique and the transverse abdominal muscles in line with the skin incisions and extend the exposure distally as far as necessary.
- Identify the vertebral bodies and carefully dissect the psoas muscle laterally off the vertebral disc spaces. The psoas origin usually is at about L1.
- Divide the prevertebral fascia in the direction of the spine.
- Identify the segmental arteries over the waist of each vertebral body and isolate and ligate them in the midline.
- Expose the bone extraperiosteally.
- The exposure from T10 to L2 or L3 with this approach is simple; but more distally the iliac vessels overlie the L4 and L5 vertebrae, and exposure in this area requires more meticulous dissection and displacement of these vessels.

LUMBAR EXTRAPERITONEAL APPROACH

TECHNIQUE 8.24

- Place the patient in the lateral decubitus position with the convex side up.

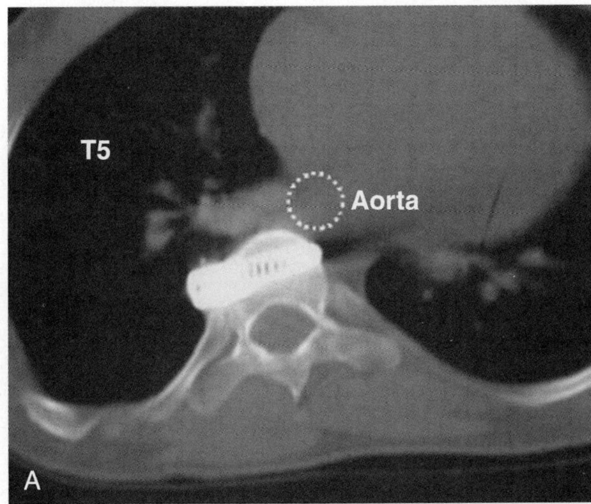

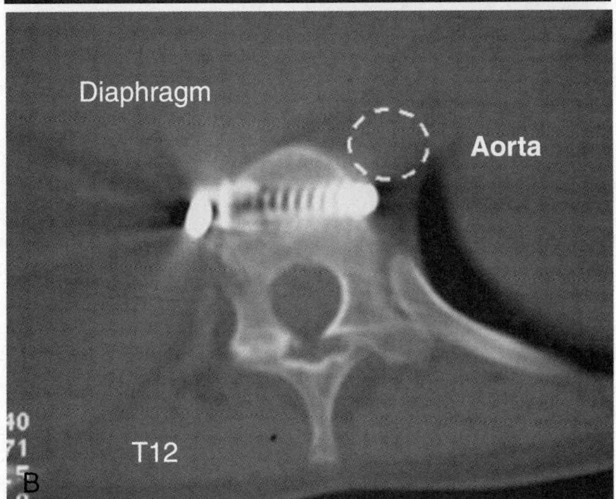

FIGURE 8.94 A, CT image at T5 showing good screw position. B, With descending aorta at 2-o'clock position, 26% of distal screw was thought to be adjacent to aorta at 2 mm or less. (From Kuklo TR, Lehman RA Jr, Lenke LG: Structures at risk following anterior instrumented spinal fusion for thoracic adolescent idiopathic scoliosis, *J Spinal Disord Tech* 18:S58, 2005.)

- Make a midflank incision from the midline anteriorly to the midline posteriorly (Fig. 8.95A).
- Divide the abdominal oblique muscles in line with the incision (Fig. 8.95B,C).
- As the dissection leads laterally, identify the latissimus dorsi muscle as it adds another layer: the transversalis fascia and the peritoneum. The transversalis fascia and the peritoneum diverge posteriorly as the transversalis fascia lines the trunk wall, and the peritoneum turns anteriorly to encase the viscera. Posterior dissection in this plane allows access to the spine without entering the abdominal cavity.
- Repair any inadvertent entry into the peritoneum immediately because it may not be identifiable later.
- Reflect all the fat-containing areolar tissue back to the transverse fascia and the lumbar fascia, reflecting the ureter along with the peritoneum (Fig. 8.95D).
- Locate the major vessels in the midline, divide the lumbar fascia, and carefully retract the great vessels.
- Divide the segmental arteries and veins as they cross the waist of the vertebra in the midline and ligate them to control hemorrhage.
- The skin incision must be placed carefully to ensure that the most cephalad vertebra to be instrumented can be easily seen.

DISC EXCISION

TECHNIQUE 8.25

- Once the anterior portion of the spine has been exposed, the discs can be felt as soft, rounded, protuberant areas of the spine compared with the concave surface of the vertebral body.
- Divide the annulus sharply with a long-handled scalpel (Fig. 8.96) and remove it.
- Remove the nucleus pulposus with rongeurs and curets. It is not necessary to remove the anterior or posterior longitudinal ligaments.
- Once the disc excision has been completed, remove the cartilaginous endplates with use of either ring curets or an osteotome. The posterior aspects of the cartilaginous endplates often are more easily removed with angled curets.
- Obtain hemostasis with Gelfoam soaked in thrombin unless a cell saver is in use.
- Significant correction of the curve usually occurs during the discectomies, and it becomes more flexible and more easily correctable.

ANTERIOR INSTRUMENTATION OF A THORACOLUMBAR CURVE

TECHNIQUE 8.26

- After exposure of the spine and removal of the discs, staples and screws are inserted into each vertebral body, beginning proximally and working distally.
- Place an appropriate-sized staple on the lateral aspect of the vertebral body, being sure to be posterior enough to allow placement of the anterior screw. Various staple lengths are available to accommodate different-sized patients. Normally, in the lower thoracic spine, the staple is placed just anterior to the rib head.
- Impact the staple into the vertebral body (Fig. 8.97A,B). Make a pilot hole with an awl in the vertebral body, which eliminates the need to tap the screws.

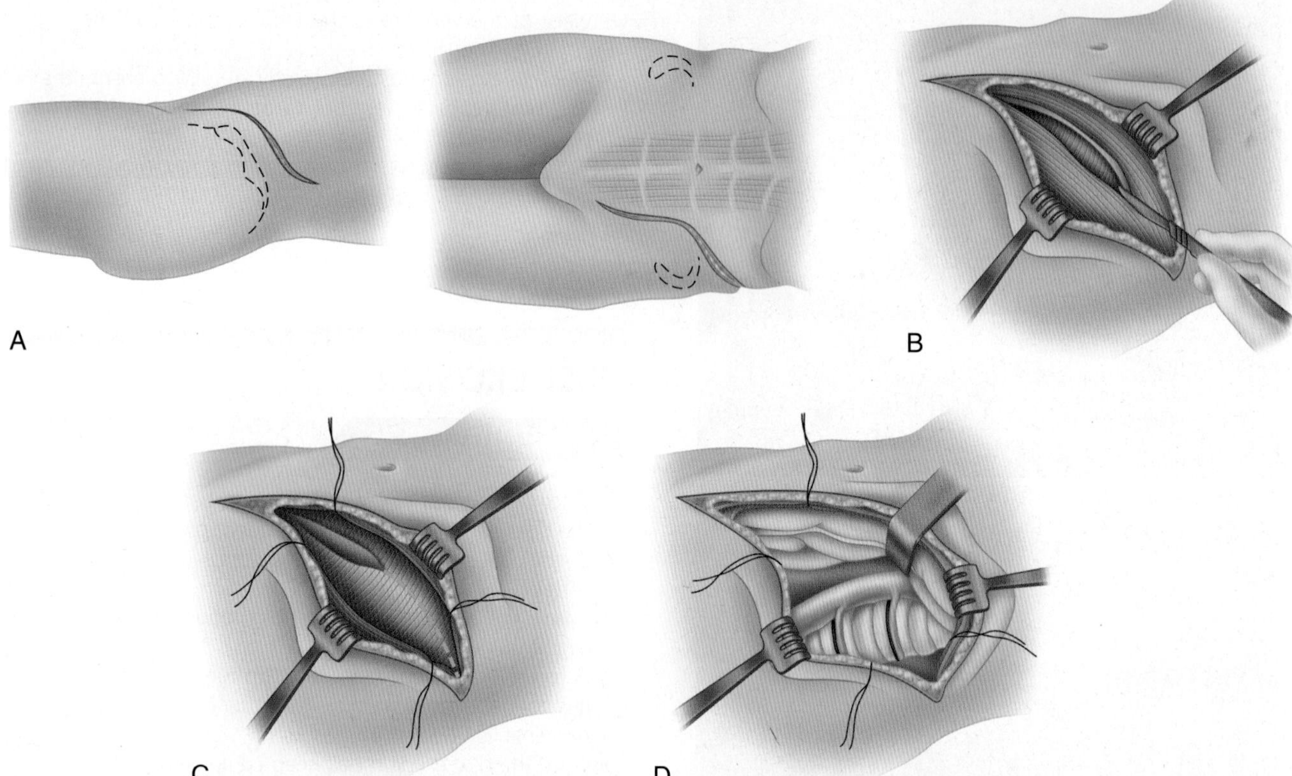

FIGURE 8.95 **A,** Skin incision for extraperitoneal approach to lumbar and lumbosacral spine. **B,** Incision of fibers of external oblique muscle. **C,** Incision into fibers of internal oblique muscle. **D,** Exposure of spine before ligation of segmental vessels. **SEE TECHNIQUE 8.24.**

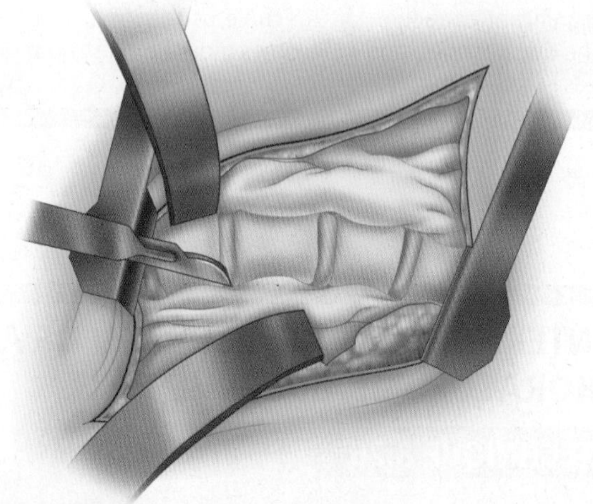

FIGURE 8.96 Disc excision. Annulus is divided with long-handled scalpel and removed. **SEE TECHNIQUE 8.25.**

- In the posterior hole, insert a screw of appropriate diameter and length angled approximately 10 degrees posterior to anterior, perpendicular to the base of the staple. Leave the screw slightly elevated off the staple surface until the anterior screw is fully seated to prevent tilting of the staple (Fig. 8.97C).
- Place the anterior screws in a neutral but slightly anterior to posterior angular position. Once again, the goal is to place the screw perpendicular to the base of the staple (Fig. 8.97D). Bicortical purchase is required at the ends of the construct and is suggested in the intermediate levels as well. Figure 8.97E shows the staples and screws inserted from T11 to L3 before rod insertion.
- Decorticate the endplates before graft placement.
- Place intervertebral structural grafts beginning in the most caudal disc and working in a proximal direction. Structural grafts are placed in the anterior aspect of the disc to facilitate lordosis (Fig. 8.97F). Posteriorly, autogenous morselized rib graft is placed against the decorticated endplates.
- Perform appropriate biplanar bending of the posterior rod.
- Engage the posterior rod proximally and cantilever it into the distal screws. Capture the rod at each level with set screws (Fig. 8.97G). The orientation of the posterior rod is shown in Figure 8.97H prior to the rod rotation maneuver.
- Place the rod grippers onto the rod and rotate it 90 degrees from posterior to anterior. This will facilitate both scoliosis correction and the production of sagittal lordosis (Fig. 8.97I).
- Perform intervertebral compression across the posterior screws after locking the apical screw and compressing from the apex to both ends (Fig. 8.97J).
- Place the anterior rod sequentially into the screws and seat and lock it with mild compression forces. This is just a stabilizing rod, and no further correction is attempted. Correction in the coronal and sagittal planes can be determined on intraoperative anteroposterior radiographs.

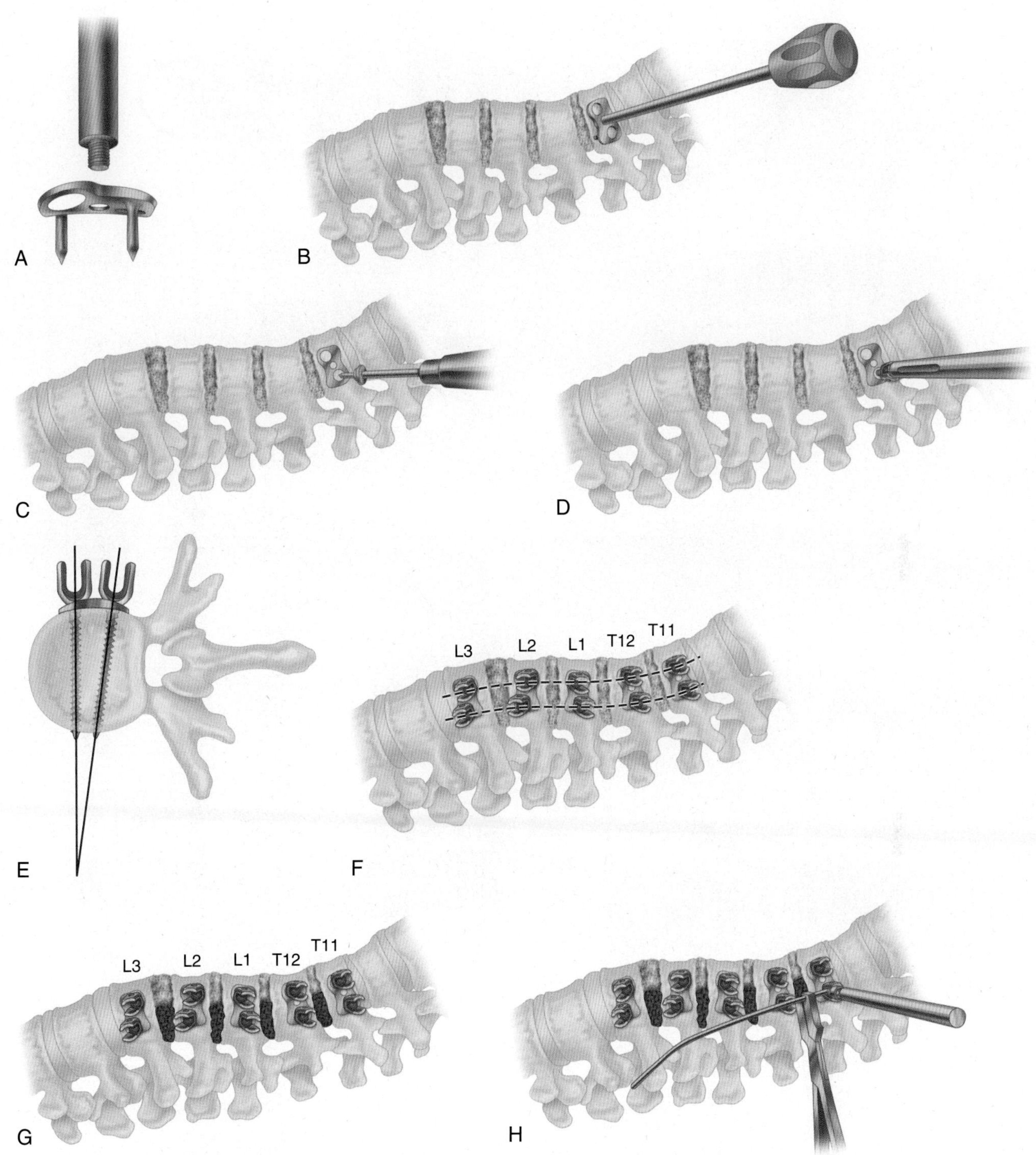

FIGURE 8.97 **A-Q,** Anterior instrumentation of thoracolumbar curve with dual-rod instrumentation. See text for description. (Medtronic Sofamor Danek.) **SEE TECHNIQUE 8.26.**

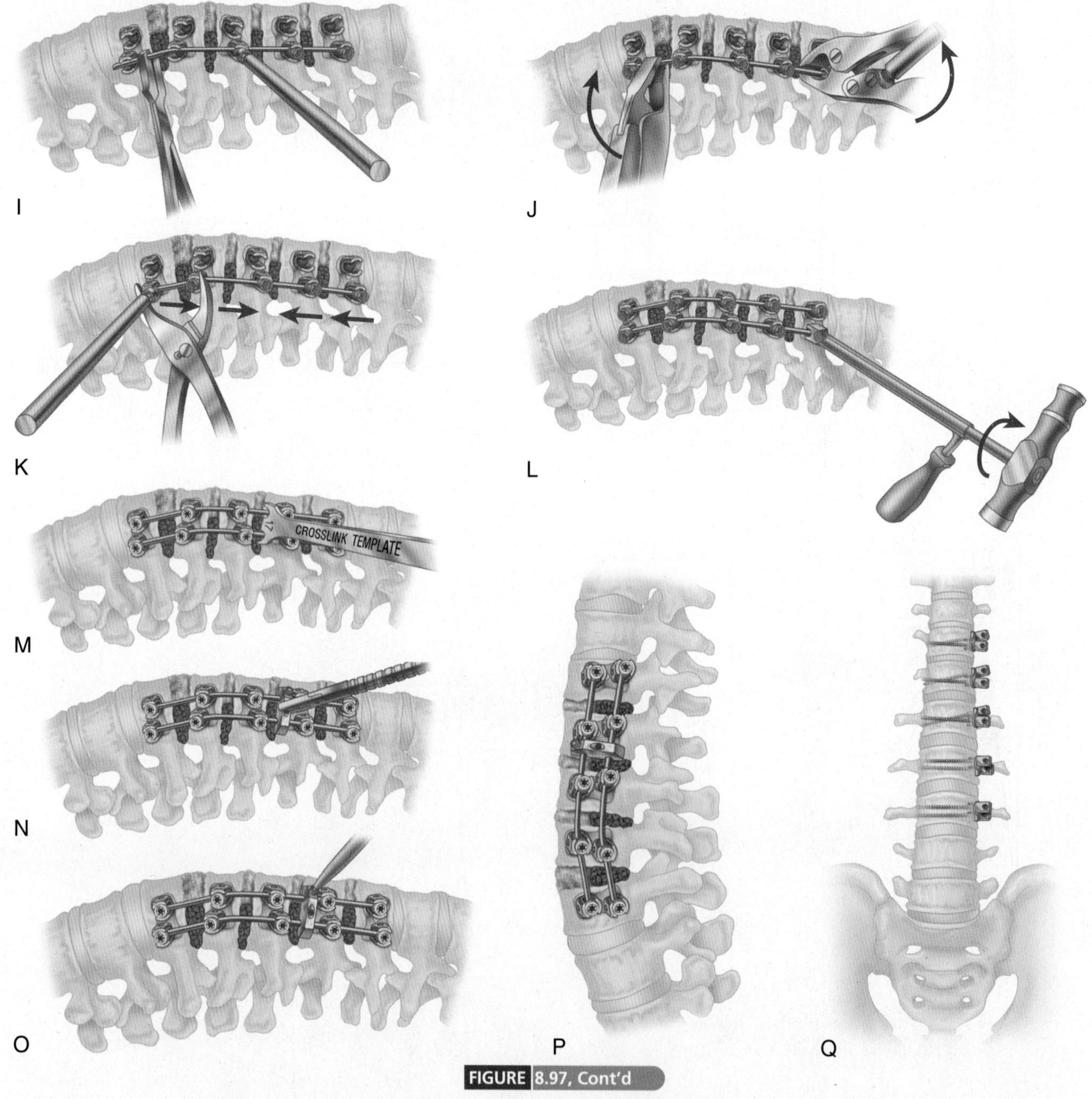

FIGURE 8.97, Cont'd

- Once the final position is confirmed, break off the set screws with the counterforce device (Fig. 8.97K).
- Place one or two crosslink plates to create a rectangular construct, which increases rigidity of the system. Use the crosslink plate measuring tools to determine the required implant size (Fig. 8.97L) and then grasp the appropriate-sized crosslink and place it on the rods (Fig. 8.97M and N).
- The lower profile of this anterior instrumentation (Fig. 8.97O,P) allows the closure of the pleura distally to the junction of the pleura and the diaphragm.
- Complete the closure procedure. Close the diaphragm, deep abdominal layers, chest wall (after chest tube placement), muscle layers, subcutaneous tissues, and skin.

POSTOPERATIVE CARE The patient is allowed up on the first postoperative day. The chest tube usually is left in place for 48 to 72 hours and is removed when the drainage decreases to less than 50 mL for two consecutive 8-hour periods. A TLSO can be used for immobilization, but if the screws have good purchase, no postoperative immobilization is used. A Foley catheter is necessary to monitor urine output because urinary retention is common. An ileus is to be expected after anterior surgery and usually lasts 2 to 3 days. Temperature elevation consistent with atelectasis is common and usually responds to pulmonary therapy and ambulation as soon as the patient is capable (Fig. 8.98).

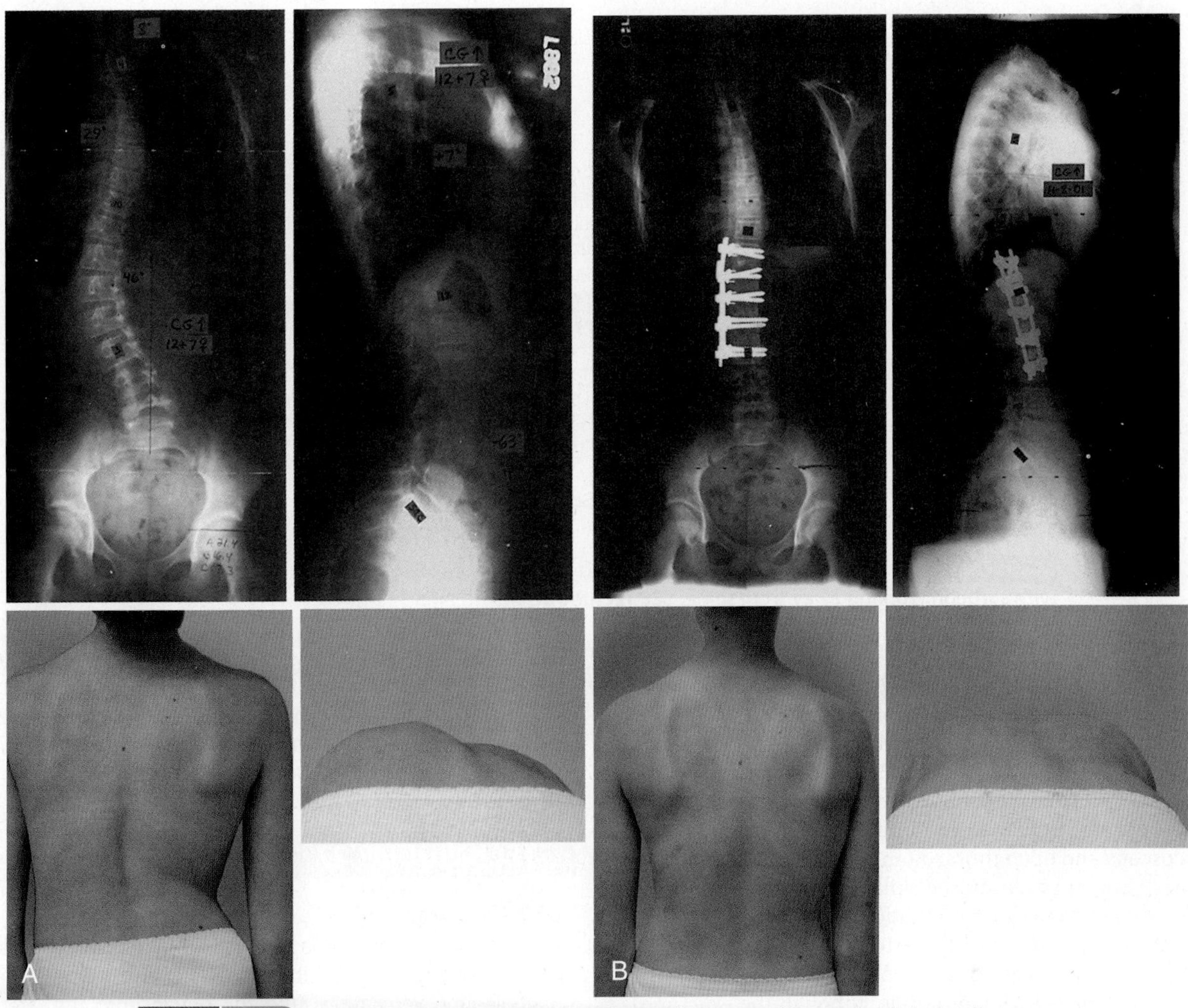

FIGURE 8.98 **A,** Preoperative clinical and radiographic views of 12-year-old, skeletally immature patient. **B,** Clinical and radiographic views after anterior spinal fusion and instrumentation from T11 to L3. (From Lenke LG: *CD Horizon Legacy Spinal System anterior dual-rod surgical technique manual*, Memphis, TN, 2002, Medtronic Sofamor Danek.) **SEE TECHNIQUE 8.26.**

COMPLICATIONS AND PITFALLS OF ANTERIOR INSTRUMENTATION

Pitfalls and complications may be related to poor patient selection, poor level selection, or instrument technical difficulties. A common technical problem is failure of the most proximal screw (see Fig. 8.93), which can be prevented by watching this screw carefully during the derotation maneuver. At any sign of screw loosening, the correction maneuver should be stopped. Another technical problem is encountered if the screw heads are not aligned properly and one screw head is offset from the others. If one screw is off just slightly, rod placement can be difficult. Variable-angle screws or polyaxial screws allow some adjustment to account for this offset.

A number of studies have emphasized the potential complications associated with an anterior approach to the spine, including respiratory insufficiency requiring ventilatory support, pneumonia, atelectasis, pneumothorax, pleural effusion, urinary tract infection, prolonged ileus, hemothorax, splenic injury, retroperitoneal fibrosis, and partial sympathectomy.

Neurologic injury can occur during discectomy or screw insertion. The screws should be placed parallel to the vertebral endplates. When the segmental vessels are ligated, the anastomosis at the intervertebral foramina should be avoided to minimize the chance of injury to the vascular supply of the spinal cord. A scoliotic deformity is approached from the convex side of the curve, and because the great vessels are inevitably on the concave side of the curve, the risk of injury to them is low. To increase purchase of the screws, however, the opposite cortex of the vertebra should be engaged by the screw, and care must be taken to be certain that the screw is not too prominent on the concave side.

VIDEO-ASSISTED THORACOSCOPY

Video-assisted thoracoscopic surgery in the treatment of pediatric spinal deformity can be used for anterior release and instrumentation; however, it rarely is used due to similar issues related to anterior arthrodesis, a steep learning curve, and advances in posterior arthrodesis and instrumentation. Advantages of thoracoscopic surgery over open thoracotomy, in addition to better illumination and magnification at the site of surgery, include less injury to the latissimus muscle and chest wall with less long-term pain, decreased blood loss,

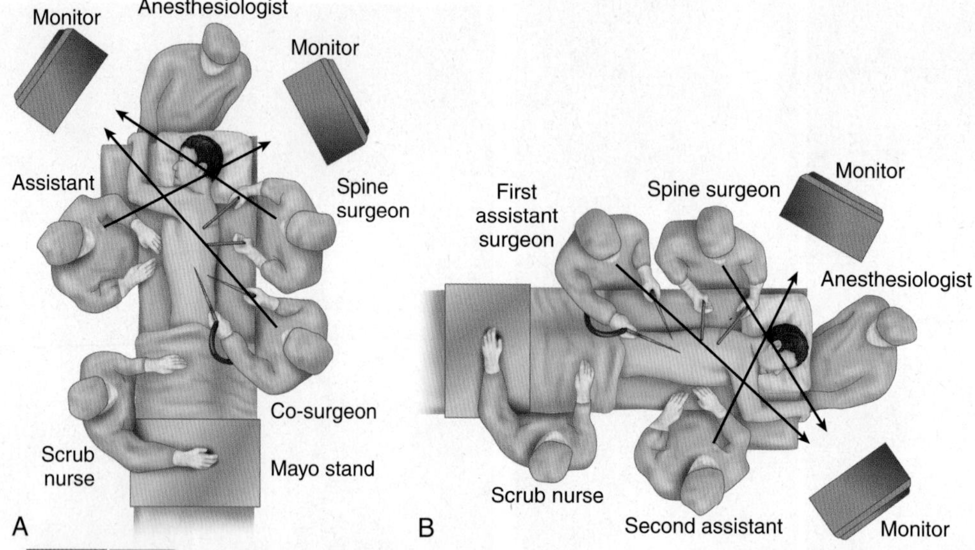

FIGURE 8.99 **A,** Conventional setup for video-assisted thoracoscopic spinal surgery. **B,** Setup with surgeon working away from spine. **SEE TECHNIQUE 8.27.**

better cosmesis, shorter recovery time, improved postoperative pulmonary function, and potentially shorter hospital stays. The primary disadvantages of thoracoscopy are related to a steep learning curve and the technical demands of the procedure. Specialized equipment is required for these procedures. A general, pediatric, or thoracic surgeon familiar with thoracoscopy and open thoracotomies should be present, and the anesthesiologist should be skilled in the use of double-lumen tubes and one-lung ventilation.

With the introduction of vertebral body tethering and spinal growth modulation, there has been renewed interest in thoracoscopic spinal approaches, although the exact indications and expected outcomes for vertebral body tethering remain unknown; they are a topic of active investigation.

Contraindications to the thoracoscopic spinal procedure include the inability to tolerate single-lung ventilation, severe or acute respiratory insufficiency, high airway pressures with positive-pressure ventilation, emphysema, and previous thoracotomy.

VIDEO-ASSISTED THORACOSCOPIC DISCECTOMY

Some surgeons prefer to work facing the patient with the patient in a lateral decubitus position (Fig. 8.99A), whereas others prefer to work from behind the patient, therefore working away from the spinal cord (Fig. 8.99B). Two monitors are positioned so that they can be seen from each side of the table. Because the traditional setup for most endoscopic procedures requires members of the surgical team to be on opposite sides of the patient, and because working opposite the camera image can lead to disorientation, Horton described turning the assistant's monitor upside down. The monitor on the posterior aspect of the patient is inverted, and once the visualization port for the camera is established, the scope is inserted into the camera and rotated 180 degrees on the scope mount so that the camera is upside down. The assistant holding the inverted camera views the inverted monitor, which projects a normal monitor image as would be seen in an open thoracotomy (Fig. 8.100).

TECHNIQUE 8.27

(CRAWFORD)

- After general anesthesia is obtained by either a double-lumen endotracheal tube or a bronchial blocker for single-lung ventilation, turn the patient into the lateral decubitus position. Prepare and drape the operative field as the anesthesiologist deflates the lung. About 20 minutes is required for complete resorption atelectasis to be obtained.
- Place the upper arm on a stand with the shoulder slightly abducted and flexed more than 90 degrees to allow placement of portals higher into the axilla. Use an axillary roll to take pressure off the axillary structures.
- Identify the scapular borders, 12th rib, and iliac crest, and outline them with a marker.
- Place the first portal at or around the T6 or T7 interspace in the posterior axillary line (Fig. 8.101A).
- Make a skin incision with a scalpel and then continue with electrocautery through the intercostal muscle to enter the chest cavity. To avoid damage to the intercostal vessels and nerves, make the incision over the top of the rib. Insert a finger to be sure the lung is deflated and that it is away from the chest wall so it will not be injured when the trocar is inserted.
- Insert flexible portals through the intercostal spaces with a trocar (Fig. 8.101B,C).
- Insert a 30-degree angled, 10-mm rigid thoracoscope. Prevent fogging of the endoscope by prewarming it with warm irrigation solution and wiping the lens with a sterile fog-reduction solution. Wipe the endoscope lens intermittently with this solution to optimize visibility. Some endoscopes have incorporated irrigating and

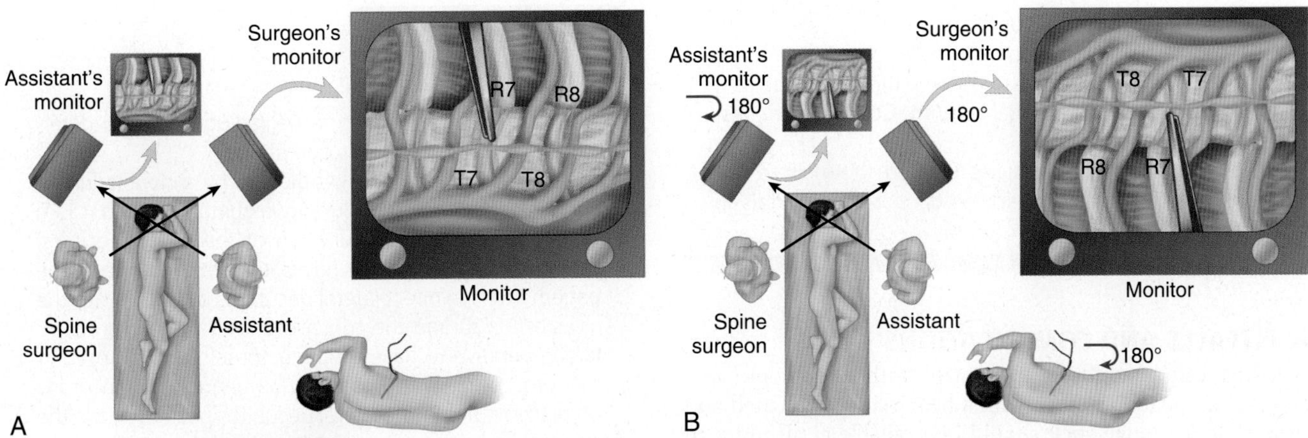

FIGURE 8.100 **A,** Thoracoscopic traditional technique. **B,** Thoracoscopic inversion technique. **SEE TECHNIQUE 8.27.**

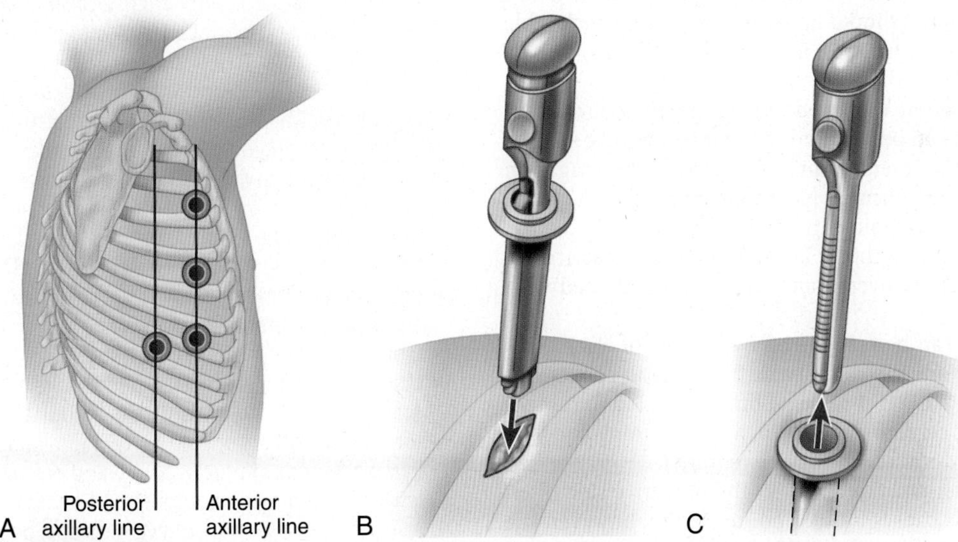

FIGURE 8.101 **A,** First portal for anterior thoracoscopic release of spine created along posterior axillary line between T6 and T8 intercostal spaces. Subsequent portals are created along anterior axillary line. **B,** Technique of portal insertion. Fifteen- to 20-mm incision is made parallel to superior surface of rib. Flexible portal is inserted with trocar. **C,** Trocar is removed, leaving flexible portal in place. **SEE TECHNIQUE 8.27.**

windshield-like cleaning mechanisms to further simplify the procedure.

- Evaluate the intrathoracic space to determine anatomy, as well as possible sites for other portals. The superior thoracic spine usually can be seen without retraction of the lung once the lung is completely deflated; however, some retraction usually is necessary below T9-T10 because the diaphragm blocks the view.
- Once the spinal anatomy has been identified, continue to identify levels. The first rib usually cannot be seen, and the first visually identifiable rib is the second rib. Count the ribs sequentially to identify the levels to be released. Insert a long, blunt-tipped needle into the disc space and obtain a radiograph to confirm the levels intraoperatively.
- Select other portal sites after viewing from within. View the trocars with the endoscope as they are inserted. Take care on inserting the inferior portal to avoid perforation of the diaphragm. Use a fan retractor to retract the diaphragm, but take care not to lacerate the lung.
- Divide the parietal pleura with an endoscopic cautery hook.
- Place the hook in the parietal pleura in the region of the disc, midway between the head of the rib and the anterior spine.
- Pull the pleura up and cauterize in successive movements proximally and distally, avoiding the segmental vessels.
- Identify the intervertebral discs as elevations on the spinal column and the vertebral bodies as depressions.
- For a simple anterior release, do not ligate the segmental vessels because of the risk of tearing. Bleeding can be difficult to control endoscopically. Crawford recommended coagulation of any vessels that appear to be at risk for bleeding.
- Vertebral body tethering instrumentation can be placed at this time.

- The pleura can be closed or left open.
- Place a chest tube through the most posterior inferior portal. Use the endoscope to observe the chest tube as it is placed along the vertebral column. Connect the chest tube to a water seal.
- Once the anesthesiologist has inflated the lung to determine whether an air leak exists, close the portals in routine fashion.

PITFALLS AND COMPLICATIONS

Bleeding can be difficult to control with endoscopic surgery. A radiopaque sponge with a heavy suture attached and loaded on a sponge stick should be available at all times to apply pressure. The suture allows later retrieval of the sponge. After application of direct pressure, electrocautery should be used for hemostasis. If necessary, endoscopic clip appliers or another hemostatic agent should be used. Instrumentation for open thoracotomy should be set up on a sterile back table to avoid delays or confusion if an immediate thoracotomy is needed to control bleeding.

Lung tissue can be damaged during the procedure. If an air leak occurs, it can be repaired with an endoscopic stapler. Cloudy fluid in the intervertebral disc space after irrigation and suctioning may indicate a lymphatic injury, which can be closed with an endoscopic clip applier. The thoracic duct is especially vulnerable to injury at the level of the diaphragm. If a chylothorax is discovered after closure, it is treated with a low-fat diet.

A dural tear can be recognized by leakage of clear cerebrospinal fluid from the disc space. Hemostatic agents can sometimes seal small cerebrospinal fluid leaks. If a dural tear continues to leak cerebrospinal fluid, a thoracotomy and vertebrectomy with dural repair may be required.

The sympathetic nerve chain on the operative side often is transected. This causes little or no morbidity; however, the surgeon needs to inform the patient and family members of the possibility of temperature and skin color changes below the level of the surgery.

Postoperative pulmonary problems often involve the downside lung, in which mucous plugs can form. The anesthesiologist should suction both lungs before extubation.

ENDOSCOPIC ANTERIOR INSTRUMENTATION OF IDIOPATHIC SCOLIOSIS

As experience with video-assisted thoracoscopy has increased, techniques have been developed for anterior instrumentation of the thoracic spine through a thoracoscopic approach. While the initial goal was to allow thoracoscopic anterior discectomy, fusion, and instrumentation, the most common use is now for the placement of vertebral body tethers.

THORACOSCOPIC VERTEBRAL BODY INSTRUMENTATION FOR VERTEBRAL BODY TETHER

TECHNIQUE 8.28

(PICETTI)

- Obtain appropriate preoperative radiographs and determine the fusion levels by Cobb angles.
- After general anesthesia is obtained by a double-lumen intubation technique (children weighing less than 45 kg may require selective intubation of the ventilated lung) and one-lung ventilation has been achieved, place the patient into the direct lateral decubitus position, with the arms at 90/90 and the concave side of the curve down. It is imperative to have the lung completely collapsed in this procedure. If the patient's oxygen saturation drops on placement into the lateral decubitus position, have the anesthesiologist readjust the tube.
- Tape the patient's hips and the shoulders to the operating table. Have a general or thoracic surgeon assist in the first part of the procedure if necessary.
- With the use of C-arm intensification, identify the vertebral levels and portal sites. A straight metallic object is used as a marker to identify the vertebral levels and portal sites. The superior and inferior access incisions are the most critical because the vertebrae at these levels are at the greatest angle in relation to the apex of the curve.
- View the planes with a C-arm in the posteroanterior plane and make sure the endplates are parallel and well defined. Rotate the C-arm until it is parallel to the vertebral body endplates, not perpendicular to the table.
- Position the marker posterior to the patient and align with every other vertebral body.
- Obtain a C-arm image at each level.
- Once the marker is centered and parallel to the endplates, make a line on the patient at each portal site in line with the marker. Marks should be two interspaces apart to allow placement of portals above and below the rib at each level and to provide access to two levels through a single skin incision. Use three to five incisions, depending on the number of levels to be instrumented.
- Once marks are made at all portal sites, rotate the C-arm to the lateral position. Place the marker end on each line and adjust the marker position until the C-arm image shows the end of the marker at the level of the rib head on the vertebrae. Place a cross mark on the previous line. This is the location of the center of the portals and will show the degree of rotation of the spine.
- The spine surgeon's position at the patient's back allows all of the instruments to be directed away from the spinal cord.

EXPOSURE AND DISCECTOMY

- Prepare and drape the patient, including the axilla and scapula.
- Check positioning to confirm that the patient has remained in the direct lateral decubitus position. This orientation provides a reference to gauge the anteroposterior and lateral direction of the guidewires and the screws.
- Make a modified thoracotomy incision at the central mark. The incision can be smaller because it is used only for the central discectomies, screw placement, and viewing. The other discectomies and screw placements are done through the access portals because they provide better alignment to the end disc spaces and vertebral bodies.

- After the lung has been deflated completely, make the initial portal in the sixth or seventh interspace by use of the alignment marks made previously. Make sure that the portal is in line with the spine and positioned according to the amount of spinal rotation. Insertion of the first portal at this level will avoid injury to the diaphragm, which normally is more caudal.
- Once the portal is made, use a finger to confirm that the lung is deflated and make sure there are no adhesions.
- Place 10.5- to 12-mm access portals under direct observation at the predetermined positions. Count the ribs to ensure that the correct levels are identified on the basis of preoperative plans.
- Incise the pleura longitudinally along the entire length of the spine to be instrumented.
- Place a Bovie hook on the pleura over a disc and make an opening. Insert the hook under the pleura and elevate it and incise along the entire length. Use suction to evacuate the smoke from the chest cavity.
- Dissect the pleura off the vertebral bodies and discs. Continue pleural dissection anteriorly off the anterior longitudinal ligament and posteriorly off the rib heads by use of a peanut or endoscopic grasper.
- Place a Kirschner wire into the disc space and confirm the level with C-arm intensification.
- With electrocautery, incise the disc annulus.
- Remove the disc in standard fashion with use of various endoscopic curets and pituitary, Cobb, and Kerrison rongeurs. If necessary, use endoscopic shavers and rasps to assist in discectomy.
- Once the disc is completely removed, thin the anterior longitudinal ligament from within the disc space with a pituitary rongeur. Thin the ligament to a flexible remnant that is no longer structural but will contain the bone graft.
- Remove the disc and annulus posteriorly back to at least the rib head. Use a Kerrison rongeur to remove the annulus posterior to the rib heads. Leave the rib head intact at this point because it will be used to guide screw placement.
- Once the disc has been evacuated, remove the endplate completely and inspect the disc space directly with the scope. Pack the disc space with Surgicel to control endplate bleeding.

GRAFT HARVEST (IF NECESSARY)

- Use an Army-Navy retractor to stabilize the rib.
- With a rib cutter, make two vertical cuts through the superior aspect of the rib and perpendicular to the rib extending halfway across it. Use an osteotome to connect the two cuts while the retractor supports the rib.
- Remove and morselize the rib section.
- Remove three or four other rib sections in a similar fashion until enough bone graft has been obtained.
- If a rib is removed through an access incision, retract the portal anteriorly as far as possible. Dissect the rib subperiosteally and carry posterior dissection as far as the portal can be retracted. This technique yields an adequate amount of graft and preserves the integrity of the rib, thus protecting the intercostal nerve and decreasing postoperative pain.
- If the patient has a large chest wall deformity, perform thoracoplasties and use rib sections for grafting.
- Do not remove the rib heads at this time because they function as landmarks for screw placement.

SCREW PLACEMENT

- Position the C-arm at the most superior vertebral body to be instrumented. It is imperative to have the C-arm parallel to the spine to give an accurate image.
- The vessels are located in the depression or middle of the vertebral body and serve as an anatomic guide for screw placement.
- Grasp the segmental vessels and coagulate at the mid–vertebral body level with the electrocautery. Hemoclip and cut larger segmental vessels if necessary.
- Check positioning again to ensure that the patient is still in the direct lateral decubitus position.
- Place the Kirschner guidewire onto the vertebral body just anterior to the rib head. Check this position with the C-arm to verify that the wire will be parallel to the endplates and in the center of the body.
- Check the inclination of the guide in the lateral plane by examining the chest wall and the rotation. The guide should be in a slight posterior to anterior inclination, directing the wire away from the canal. If there is any doubt or concern about the anterior inclination, obtain a lateral C-arm image to verify position.
- Once the correct alignment of the guide has been attained, insert the Kirschner wire into the cannula of the Kirschner guide that is positioned centrally on the vertebral body.
- Drill the guidewire to the opposite cortex, ensuring that it is parallel to the vertebral body.
- Confirm the position with the C-arm as the wire is inserted. Take care not to drill the wire through the opposite cortex because this can injure the segmental vessels and the lung on the opposite side.
- The most superior mark on the guidewire represents a length of 50 mm, and the etched lines are at 5-mm increments. The length of the Kirschner wire in the vertebral body can be determined by these marks. Start at the 50-mm mark and subtract 5 mm for each additional mark that is showing. For example, if there are four marks in addition to the 50-mm mark, the length of the Kirschner wire would be 30 mm.
- Remove the guide and place the tap over the Kirschner wire onto the vertebral body. To maximize fixation strength, use the largest-diameter tap that will fit in the vertebral bodies, based on the preoperative radiographs. Grasp the distal end of the wire with a clamp and hold it as the tap is inserted so that the wire will not advance. This is important to avoid a pneumothorax in the opposite chest cavity. Tap only the near cortex. Use the C-arm to monitor tap depth and Kirschner wire position.
- Place the appropriate-sized screw, based on the Kirschner wire measurement and tap diameter, over the wire with the Eclipse screwdriver and advance it. To ensure bicortical fixation, select a screw that is 5 mm longer than the width of the vertebral body as measured with the Kirschner wire. Grasp the wire again to avoid advancement while the screw is inserted.
- Remove the wire when the screw is approximately halfway across the vertebral body.

- Check the screw direction with the C-arm as it is advanced and seated against the vertebral body. The screw should penetrate the opposite cortex for bicortical fixation.
- Instrument all Cobb levels.
- Use each rib head as a reference for subsequent screw placement to help ensure that the screws are in line and will produce proper spinal rotation when the rod is inserted. With the screws properly aligned, the screw heads form an arc that can be verified with a lateral image.
- Adjust the side walls of the screws (saddles) to be in line for insertion of the rod. If a screw is sunk more than a few millimeters deeper than the rest of the screws, reduction of the rod into the screw head may be difficult. The C-arm image can confirm depth of screw placement as the screws are inserted.
- Once all the screws have been placed, remove the Surgicel and use the graft funnel and plunger to deliver the graft into the disc spaces. Fill each disc space all the way across to the opposite side.

ROD MEASUREMENT AND PLACEMENT

- Determine the rod length with the rod length gauge. Place the fixed ball at the end of the measuring device into the saddle of the inferior screw. Then guide the ball at the end of the cable through all of the screws with a pituitary rongeur to the most superior screw and insert it into the saddle. Pull the wire tight and take a reading from the scale. The scale is in centimeters.
- Cut the 4.5-mm-diameter rod to length and insert it into the chest cavity through the thoracotomy. The rod has slight flexibility, so do not bend it before insertion.
- Apply anterior compression to obtain kyphosis in the thoracic spine.
- Do not cut the rod longer than measured because the total distance between the screws will be reduced with compression.
- Manipulate the rod into the inferior screw with the rod holder. The end of the rod should be flush with the saddle of the screw to prevent the rod from protruding and irritating or puncturing the diaphragm.
- Once the rod is in place, remove the portal and place the plug introduction guide over the screw to guide the plug and to hold the rod in position.
- Place the obturator in the tube to assist in the insertion through the incision if necessary.
- Load a plug onto the plug-capturing T25 driver. Insert the plug with the flat side and the laser etching up.
- Once the plug is placed on the driver, turn the sleeve clockwise to engage the plug with the sleeve.
- Place the plug through the plug introduction guide and insert it into the screw. Do not place the plug without using the introduction guide and the plug inserter.
- To ensure proper threading, turn the sleeve once counterclockwise before advancing the plug.
- Once the plug has been correctly started, hold the locking sleeve to prevent any further rotation. This will disengage the plug from the inserter as the plug is placed into the screw.
- Remove the driver and introduction guide and torque the screw with the torque-limiting wrench. This is the only plug that is tightened completely at this time.
- Sequentially insert the rod into the remaining screws with use of the rod pusher. Place the rod pusher on the rod several screws above the screw into which the rod is being placed.
- Apply the plugs through the plug introduction guide as described. To allow compression, do not fully tighten the plugs at this time.
- Once the rod has been seated and all the plugs are inserted into the screws, apply compression between the screws.

COMPRESSION: RACK AND PINION

- Insert the compressor through the thoracotomy incision. Once it is in the thoracic cavity, manipulate it by holding the ball-shaped attachment with the compressor holder. The rack and pinion compressor fits over two screw heads on the rod; turning the compressor driver clockwise compresses the two screws. Start compression at the inferior end of the construct with the most inferior screw's plug fully tightened.
- Once satisfactory compression has been obtained on a level, tighten the superior plug with the plug driver through the plug introduction guide.
- Apply compression sequentially superiorly until all levels have been compressed, then torque each plug to 75 in-lb with the torque-limiting wrench. The construct is complete at this point.

COMPRESSION: CABLE COMPRESSOR

- Insert each end of the cable through one of the distal holes on the side of the guide (not the larger central hole). The actuator should be in the position closest to the compressor body.
- Form a 3-inch loop at the end of the guide, with the two cable ends passing through the actuator body.
- Engage the lever arm by use of one of the plug drivers through the cam mechanism.
- Place the end of the compressor through the distal portal. With the portal removed, place a plug introduction guide through the adjacent incision, through the loop, and over the next screw to be compressed.
- Place the foot of the compressor over the rod and against the inferior side of the end screw.
- Fully tighten the plug in the end screw. Squeeze the handle of the compressor several times to compress.
- Once satisfactory compression has been obtained at a level, tighten the superior plug with the plug driver through the plug introduction guide.
- To disengage the compressor, tilt it toward the superior screw until the foot disengages from the inferior screw.
- Turn the actuator mechanism 90 degrees to disengage the ratchet.
- With the cable loop still around the plug introduction guide that is on the superior screw, pull the compressor until the actuator is next to the compressor body.
- Repeat the steps described on subsequent screws. Apply compression sequentially until all levels have been compressed and then torque each plug to 75 in-lb with the torque-limiting wrench. The construct is complete at this point.
- Place a 20-French chest tube through the inferior portal and close the incisions. Obtain anteroposterior and lateral

radiographs before the patient is transferred to the recovery room.

POSTOPERATIVE CARE The chest tube is left in until drainage is less than 100 mL every 8 hours. Patients can be ambulatory after the first postoperative day, and they can be discharged from the hospital the day after the chest tube is removed. A brace should be worn for 3 months.

NEUROMUSCULAR SCOLIOSIS

The specific causes of neuromuscular scoliosis are unknown, but several contributing factors are well known. Loss of muscle strength or voluntary muscle control and loss of sensory abilities, such as proprioception, in the flexible and rapidly growing spinal column of a juvenile patient are believed to be factors in development of these curves. As the spine collapses, increased pressure on the concave side of the curve results in decreased growth of that side of the vertebral body and wedging of the vertebral body itself. The vertebrae also can be structurally compromised by malnutrition or disuse osteopenia.

The SRS has established a classification for neuromuscular scoliosis (Box 8.5).

Neuromuscular curves develop at a younger age than do idiopathic curves, and a larger percentage of neuromuscular curves are progressive. Unlike idiopathic curves, even small neuromuscular curves may continue to progress beyond skeletal maturity. Many neuromuscular curves are long, C-shaped curves that include the sacrum, and pelvic obliquity is common. Hip subluxation or dislocation often is associated with the pelvic obliquity. Patients with neuromuscular scoliosis also may have pelvic obliquity from other sources, such as hip joint and other lower extremity contractures, all of which can affect the lumbar spine. Progressing neurologic or muscular disease also can interfere with trunk stability. These patients generally are less tolerant of orthotic management than are patients with idiopathic scoliosis, and brace treatment often is ineffective in preventing curve progression. Spinal surgery in this group is associated with increased bleeding and less satisfactory bone stock; longer fusions, often to the pelvis, are needed.

Many neuromuscular spinal deformities require operative intervention. The goal of treatment is to maintain a spine balanced in the coronal and sagittal planes over a level pelvis. The basic treatment methods are similar to those for idiopathic scoliosis: observation, orthotic treatment, and surgery.

NONOPERATIVE TREATMENT

OBSERVATION

Not all neuromuscular spinal deformities require immediate treatment. Small curves of less than 20 to 25 degrees can be observed carefully for progression before treatment is begun. Similarly, large curves in severely involved patients in whom the curve is not causing any functional disability or hindering nursing care can be observed. If progression of a small curve is noted, orthotic management may be considered if the patient can tolerate this form of treatment. If the functional ability of severely impaired patients is compromised by increasing curvature, treatment may be instituted.

BOX 8.5

Scoliosis Research Society Classification of Neuromuscular Spinal Deformity

- Primary neuropathies
- Upper motor neuron neuropathies
  - Cerebral palsy
  - Spinocerebellar degeneration
    - Friedreich ataxia
    - Roussy-Levy disease
    - Spinocerebellar ataxia
  - Syringomyelia
  - Spinal cord tumor
  - Spinal cord trauma
- Lower motor neuron pathologies
  - Poliomyelitis
  - Other viral myelitides
  - Traumatic
  - Charcot-Marie-Tooth disease
  - Spinal muscular atrophy
    - Werdnig-Hoffmann disease (SMA type 1)
    - Kugelberg-Welander disease (SMA type 3)
  - Dysautonomia
    - Riley-Day syndrome
  - Combined upper and lower pathologies
    - Amyotrophic lateral sclerosis
    - Myelomeningocele
    - Tethered cord
- Primary myopathies
  - Muscular dystrophy
    - Duchenne muscular dystrophy
    - Limb-girdle dystrophy
    - Facioscapulohumeral dystrophy
  - Arthrogryposis
  - Congenital hypotonia
  - Myotonia dystrophica

ORTHOTIC TREATMENT

Progressive neuromuscular scoliosis in a very young patient can be treated with an orthosis. The scoliosis often continues to progress despite orthotic treatment, but the rate of progression can be slowed, and further spinal growth can occur before definitive spinal fusion. The brace also can provide patients with trunk support, allowing the use of the upper extremities.

A custom-molded TLSO usually is required for these children because their trunk contours do not accommodate standard braces. Most patients with neuromuscular scoliosis lack voluntary muscle control, normal righting reflexes, and the ability to cooperate with an active brace program; therefore, passive-type orthotics have been more successful in our experience in managing these neuromuscular curves. Patients with severe involvement and no head control frequently require custom-fabricated seating devices combined with orthoses or head-control devices.

A more malleable type of spinal brace, the soft Boston orthosis, is fabricated from a soft material that is well tolerated by patients, yet it is strong enough to provide good trunk support. The major complaint with the use of this brace has been heat retention.

Because of problems with brace treatment of neuromuscular patients, growing rods and rib-based techniques have been successfully used to control progressive neuromuscular curves. Several authors have reported improvement in the Cobb angle and pelvic obliquity with these techniques, but a deep wound infection rate of 30% also has been reported.

OPERATIVE TREATMENT

The goal of surgery in patients with neuromuscular scoliosis is to produce solid arthrodesis of the spine, balanced in both the coronal and sagittal planes and over a level pelvis. In doing so, the surgery should maximize function and improve the quality of life. To achieve this goal, a much longer fusion is necessary than usually is indicated for idiopathic scoliosis. Because of a tendency for cephalad progression of the deformity when fusion ends at or below the fourth thoracic vertebra, fusion should extend to T4 or above. The decision on the distal extent of the fusion generally is whether to fuse to the sacrum or to attempt to stop short of it. On occasion, the fusion can exclude the sacrum if the patient is an ambulator who requires lumbosacral motion, has no significant pelvic obliquity, and has a horizontal L5 vertebral body. Many of these patients, unfortunately, are nonambulators with a fixed spinopelvic obliquity. If the spinopelvic obliquity is fixed on bending or traction films (>10 to 15 degrees of L4 or L5 tilt relative to the interiliac crest line), the caudal extent of the fusion usually is the sacrum or the pelvis. Maintaining physiologic lordosis in the lumbar spine is important in insensate patients who require fusion to the pelvis. This permits body weight to be distributed more equally beneath the ischial tuberosities and the posterior region of the thigh, reducing the risk of pressure sores over the coccyx and ischium. Bone-bank allograft usually is used to obtain a fusion.

■ PREOPERATIVE CONSIDERATIONS

Patients with neuromuscular scoliosis must have complete medical evaluations, including cardiac, pulmonary, and nutritional status. In a literature review, Legg et al. reported that the complication rate after scoliosis surgery in neuromuscular patients varied from 10% to as high as 70%, with a mortality rate between 2.18% and 19%; when only the most recent studies were included, the mortality rate was 5%. The respiratory complication rate ranged from 26% to 57% and the infection rate from 2.5% to 56%. McCarthy et al. cited an overall complication rate between 44% and 80%, a mortality rate between 0 and 7%, major pulmonary complication rate of 21%, and wound problem rate of 8.7%. They also noted significant gastrointestinal and instrument or pseudarthrosis problems. Watanabe et al. reported three intraoperative cardiac arrests in their series of 84 patients, highlighting the fragility of these patients.

The treating surgeon also should assess hospital services and support services that are available during and after surgery. Toovey et al. reported that the mean ICU stay after neuromuscular scoliosis surgery was 4.4 days (range, 1.7 to 6.7) and mean hospital stay was 16.9 days (range, 8.7 to 24.5). To improve the complication rate to an acceptable rate less than 10%, ICU stay of less than 24 hours, and hospital stay less than 7 days, a care team is needed to assess risk factors and take steps to decrease them before any surgery, including discussions with the medical providers, treating surgeon, patient, and caregivers. Shrader et al. reported decreased complication rates, surgical time, and length of hospitalization if an experienced second surgeon was present during the surgery.

Most patients with neuromuscular scoliosis, especially those with cerebral palsy, have diminished pulmonary function, and careful preoperative evaluation is essential. Nickel et al. found that patients with vital capacities of less than 30% of predicted normal required respiratory support postoperatively, and those with a similar decrease of vital capacity and without a voluntary cough reflex required tracheostomy. The pulmonary service should be actively involved in preoperative and postoperative care to minimize the risk of pulmonary complications. Khirani et al. reported that noninvasive pulmonary techniques and coaching before surgery decreased respiratory complications and decreased the need for prolonged intubation.

Patients often are malnourished, and their nutritional status should be improved preoperatively. Jevsevar and Karlin found an increase in complications if albumin was less than 35 g/L and total blood lymphocyte count was less than 1.5 g/L. The endocrine service should be involved to ensure optimized bone health in patients who often have significantly decreased bone mineral because of non–weight bearing and poor nutritional support. Optimizing bone health preoperatively will allow better fixation of the implants used to correct scoliosis and potentially less implant failure.

Many neurologic conditions, such as Duchenne muscular dystrophy and Friedreich ataxia, are associated with cardiac involvement, and the patient's cardiac status should be evaluated. Gastrointestinal and general surgery consultation may be needed for possible gastrostomy-tube placement and management and evaluation of the need for a gastric fundoplication to prevent or decrease the risk of reflux and aspiration. Otolaryngology evaluation for management of excessive drooling also may decrease the risk of aspiration.

Neurology specialists should be involved for seizure management. Valproic acid has been shown to increase bleeding times and interfere with clotting, and an alternative seizure medication may be needed before surgery. Having the assistance of a plastic surgeon to aid in wound closure has been shown to decrease wound complications. Ambulatory status should be evaluated carefully before surgery. Often a patient with marginal ambulation capabilities and progressive scoliosis may not walk again after spinal surgery. The patient and parents must understand this before surgery.

Techniques to minimize blood loss intraoperatively should be available, including electrocautery, hypotensive anesthesia, hemodilution techniques, and a cell saver. Use of antifibrinolytics has been shown to decrease intraoperative blood loss during posterior spinal fusion and instrumentation in neuromuscular scoliosis surgery. Dhawale et al. reported that tranexamic acid was more effective than epsilon-aminocaproic acid in decreasing blood loss in neuromuscular patients. Most patients with neuromuscular disease have insufficient autogenous bone; allograft bone usually is used to obtain fusion and is an acceptable alternative.

As in other types of scoliosis surgery, the fusion levels and instrumentation must be determined preoperatively. The source of pelvic obliquity must be determined (Fig. 8.102). Several methods have been described for radiographic measurement of pelvic obliquity, including those devised by Maloney (Fig. 8.103A), O'Brien (Fig. 8.103B), Osebold

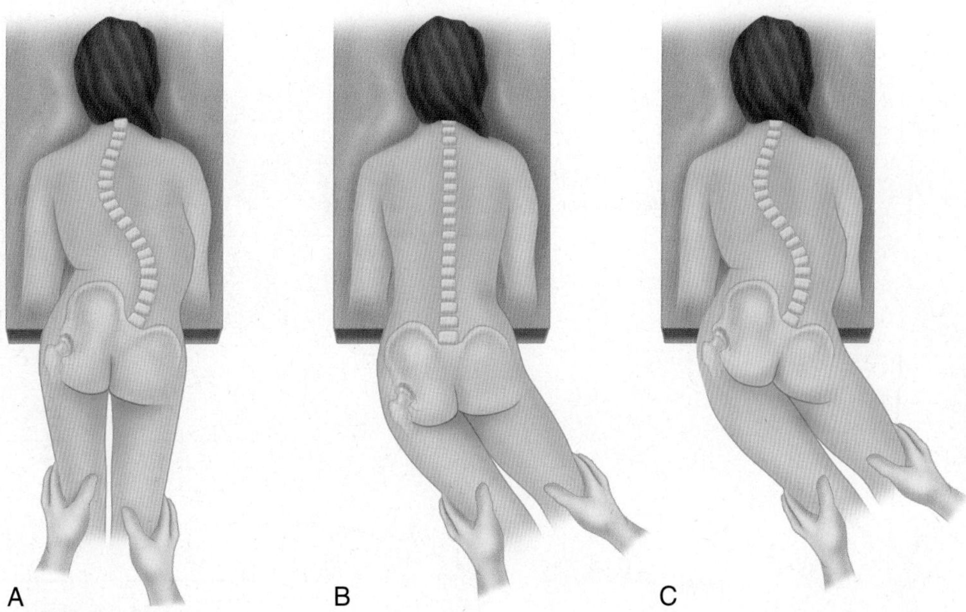

FIGURE 8.102 **A,** Pelvic obliquity. **B,** If pelvic obliquity is eliminated by abduction or adduction of hips, pelvic-femoral muscle contracture is cause. **C,** If obliquity persists despite abduction or adduction of hips, fixed spinal-pelvic deformity exists. (From Shook JE, Lubicky JP: Paralytic scoliosis. In Bridwell KH, DeWald RL, editors: *The textbook of spinal surgery*, ed 2, Philadelphia, 1997, Lippincott-Raven.)

(Fig. 8.103C), Lindseth (Fig. 8.103D), and Allen and Ferguson (Fig. 8.103E). Shrader et al. compared these measurement techniques and determined that the Maloney method was the most reliable method of measuring pelvic obliquity on a frontal view radiograph.

Ko et al. reported that more than half of cerebral palsy patients had more than 10 degrees of asymmetry in the transaxial plane between right and left sides of the pelvis. There was greater asymmetry in patients with windswept hips. Combined anterior and posterior arthrodeses may be required for severe pelvic obliquity. Other indications for a combined anterior and posterior approach include necessity for an anterior release for further correction of severe kyphosis, severe and rigid scoliosis that cannot be corrected by bending or traction to less than 60 degrees, and deficient posterior elements, such as those in patients with myelomeningocele. With the use of pedicle screws the need for anterior surgery has decreased. Most neuromuscular deformities can be treated with a posterior surgery with segmental instrumentation using pedicle screw fixation and supplemented with sublaminar cables as needed. Several authors have compared results of posterior-only surgery with those of anterior and posterior surgery and found similar correction, less surgical time, shorter hospitalizations, and fewer complications.

Finally, the patient's family should be clearly informed of the potential benefits and risks of any surgical procedure. With good preoperative planning and medical management, good results from scoliosis surgery in neuromuscular patients and improved quality of life for the patient with an acceptable risk of complications can be expected.

OPERATIVE CONSIDERATIONS

The potential for intraoperative complications in patients with neuromuscular scoliosis is great. Death can result from anesthesia problems, although more frequently it occurs from postoperative pulmonary deterioration. Relative hypothermia can easily occur in a lengthy spinal operation in which a large area of tissue is exposed and can cause myocardial depression and arrhythmias. Spinal surgery is associated with greater blood loss in patients with neuromuscular disease than in patients with idiopathic scoliosis. The anesthesiologist should be aware of both of these potential problems and should be prepared for them with an arterial line, a central venous pressure line, temperature probes, and careful management of urine output. Because the curves generally are larger, more rigid, and more difficult to instrument, neurologic complications can occur during surgery. Many patients with neuromuscular scoliosis are unable to cooperate with an intraoperative wake-up test. Spinal cord monitoring can be a valuable technique in these patients. Schwartz et al. and Salem et al. evaluated the safety of using transcranial motor-evoked potentials in neuromuscular patients. There were no episodes of seizures in any neuromuscular patients, including those with a history of epilepsy. The decision to use neuromonitoring for patients with a history of seizures should be a joint decision between the surgeon and the neuromonitoring team.

The surgical technique must include meticulous debridement of the soft tissue off the posterior elements of the spine. Ablation of the facet joints and a large amount of bone graft are necessary. The bone frequently is osteopenic, and appropriate stable segmental instrumentation should be used. Anterior release and fusion can be considered in patients with large curves with a fixed spinal pelvic obliquity or in patients with posterior element deficiencies. Anterior instrumentation in neuromuscular curves may be used if needed, but it is rarely used. A 29% failure rate has been reported with pelvic fixation in neuromuscular patients. Myung et al. recommended placing bilateral pedicle screws at L5 and S1, in addition to two iliac screws, to decrease the failure rate of pelvic fixation in neuromuscular patients. Lee

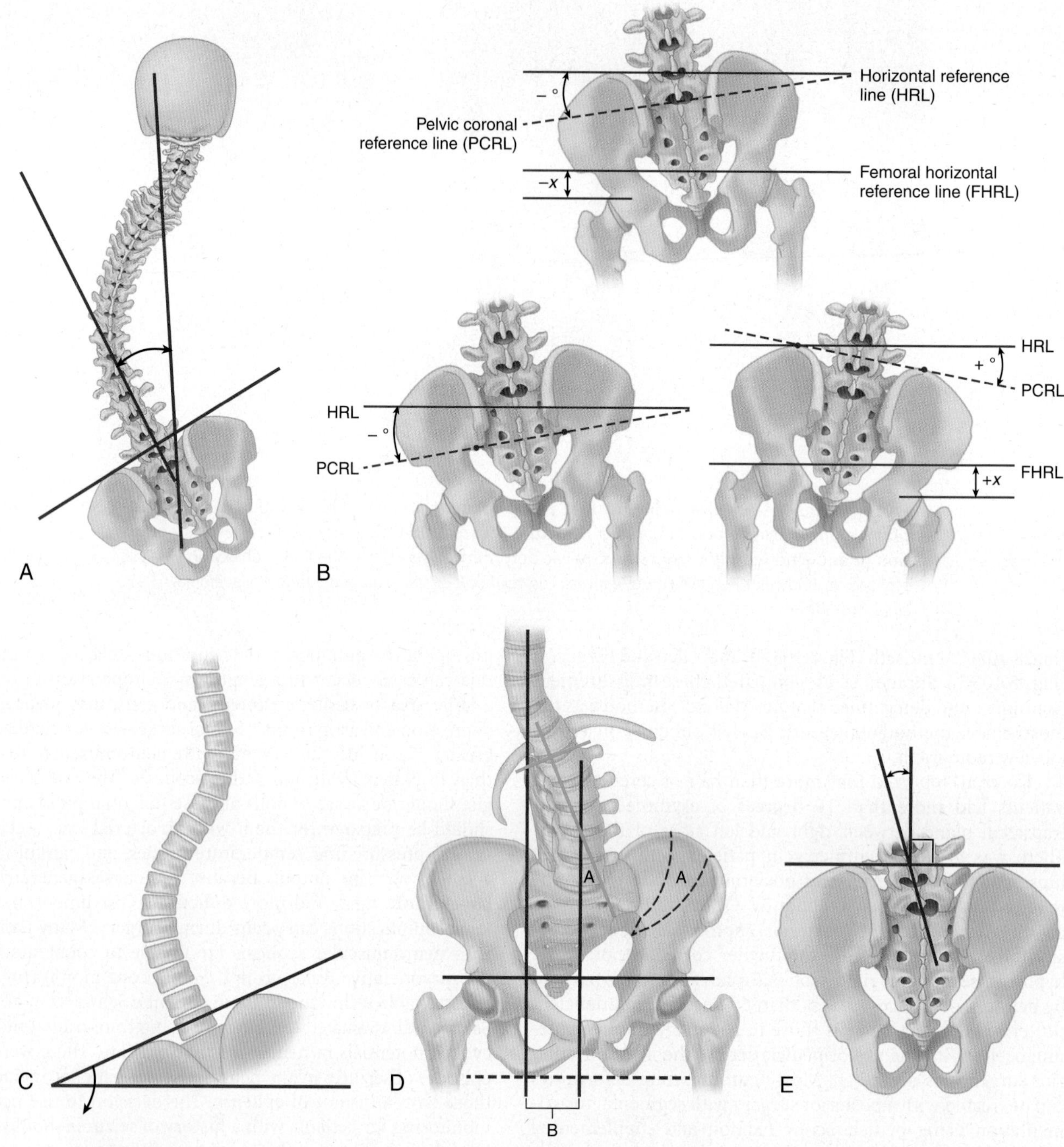

FIGURE 8.103 Radiographic measurement of pelvic obliquity. **A,** Maloney method. **B,** O'Brien method. **C,** Osebold method. **D,** Lindseth method. **E,** Allen and Ferguson method.

et al. and Shabtai et al. reported better results with the use of sacral alar screws than with traditional iliac screws.

POSTOPERATIVE CONSIDERATIONS

Pulmonary problems are the most likely complications in the immediate postoperative period, and the assistance of a pulmonary specialist is invaluable. Ventilatory support may be necessary, and such techniques as suctioning, spirometers, and intermittent positive-pressure breathing may be appropriate. Possibly the best measure to prevent postoperative pulmonary problems is a spinal construct strong enough to allow early mobilization.

Fluid balance must be monitored carefully. After spinal surgery, especially in patients with neuromuscular scoliosis, antidiuretic hormone levels may be increased, leading to oliguria. If fluids are increased to overcome the oliguria, fluid overload may occur. This is especially disastrous in patients with impaired renal function, pulmonary compromise, and cardiac difficulties.

The necessity for postoperative orthotic support must be determined for each patient. If a complication, such as extremely osteopenic bone, compromises spinal fixation, or if less than ideal instrumentation is used, the use of postoperative external support may be wise.

Infection is a frequent problem in patients with neuromuscular scoliosis, probably because of the metabolically compromised host and the lengthy spinal fusions necessary. Patients with myelomeningocele and cerebral palsy have the highest infection rates. A major source of postoperative infection is the urinary tract. Spinal infection is treated in the same manner as in patients with idiopathic scoliosis (see section on complications of posterior scoliosis surgery).

Pseudarthrosis with subsequent instrumentation failure is a potential late problem. If the pseudarthrosis causes pain or loss of correction, repair probably will be necessary, but asymptomatic pseudarthrosis without curve progression or pain can be observed.

LUQUE ROD INSTRUMENTATION WITH SUBLAMINAR WIRING

Eduardo Luque is credited with popularizing the use of long L-shaped rods and sublaminar wires in the surgical treatment of spinal deformity. The rods can be contoured, and the spine is corrected as the wires are tightened.

Wilber et al. noted neurologic changes in 17% of their patients with idiopathic scoliosis, but since surgeons have become more proficient with the technique, the incidence of neurologic injury has been much lower. The neurologic complications from sublaminar wires are of three types: cord injury, root injury, and dural tears. Root injuries are the most common and lead to hyperesthesia, but these generally resolve within 2 weeks. Although sublaminar wires or cables have potential risks, we have found that for neuromuscular curves, the advantages of this type of segmental instrumentation far outweigh the potential risks.

The original Luque rods were L-shaped rods that were contoured to appropriate sagittal contours. Appropriately sized alloy rods are contoured to the appropriate sagittal contours and are connected proximally and distally with crosslinks. Originally, stainless-steel wires in diameters of 16- and 18-gauge were used. We now usually use sublaminar cables as opposed to the wire (see Technique 8.17).

LUQUE ROD INSTRUMENTATION AND SUBLAMINAR WIRES WITHOUT PELVIC FIXATION

TECHNIQUE 8.29

- The spine is exposed posteriorly as described in Technique 8.6.
- Wires or cables are passed as described in Technique 8.14.
- Two rods are used for most scoliosis corrections, with the first rod applied either to the convex or concave side of the curve. Lumbar scoliosis generally is more easily corrected by the concave rod technique. And because most neuromuscular curves include the lumbar spine and pelvis, the concave rod technique is most frequently used.
- Bend the appropriate amount of lordosis and kyphosis into the rods with the rod benders.
- Place the initial rod with its short limb passing transversely across the lamina of the lowermost vertebra to undergo instrumentation on the concave side.
- Pass it through the hole at the base of the spinous process if possible.
- Tighten the inferior double wire or cable on the concave side to supply firm fixation at the distal level. Now tighten the wires or cables to the lamina of the vertebra above the curve.
- Loosely attach the convex rod proximally after the short end has been placed loosely under the long limb of the concave rod. Once the concave rod has been completely tightened, it often is difficult to pass this short limb under the long limb of the concave rod.
- Reduce the spine to the rod by manual correction and a wire or cable tightener. An assistant can apply appropriate manual correction by pressure on the trunk as the wires or cables are tightened beneath the apex of the curvature (Fig. 8.104).
- As each wire or cable is tightened, more correction is obtained, and the twisting maneuver must be repeated two or three times on each wire to ensure a tight fit.
- Securely fasten the convex rod, tightening wires or cables from cephalad to caudad.
- Once in position, both rods usually can be brought into firm contact with the lamina by squeezing them together with the rod approximator. As this is done, the concave wires or cables will again loosen and must be tightened.
- Trim the wires to about ½ inch in length and bend them toward the midline.
- With the internal fixation device in place, very little bone is exposed for decortication and facet excision. We prefer to excise the facets if at all possible.
- A large volume of bone graft is necessary, and cancellous bone is harvested from the posterior iliac crest. Because the instrumentation often includes the iliac crest (see Technique 8.36), allograft bone usually is necessary. Place the graft lateral to the rods on both sides of the spine and out to the tips of the transverse processes. If possible, place bone graft between the wires, along the laminae.

SACROPELVIC FIXATION

Many patients with neuromuscular problems require instrumentation and fusion to the sacrum. O'Brien described three fixation zones for sacropelvic fixation (Fig. 8.105). Examples of zone I fixation include S1 sacral screws and a McCarthy S-rod. Zone II fixation includes S2 screws and the Jackson intrasacral rod technique (see later section on combined anterior and posterior fusion for scoliosis in patients with myelomeningocele). Zone III fixation includes the Galveston L-rod technique and sacroiliac screws.

If fixation to the pelvis is necessary, an S-rod technique as described by McCarthy et al. can be useful (Fig. 8.106). The two rods are crosslinked at the lumbosacral junction and then fixed with a combination of hooks, pedicle screws, and

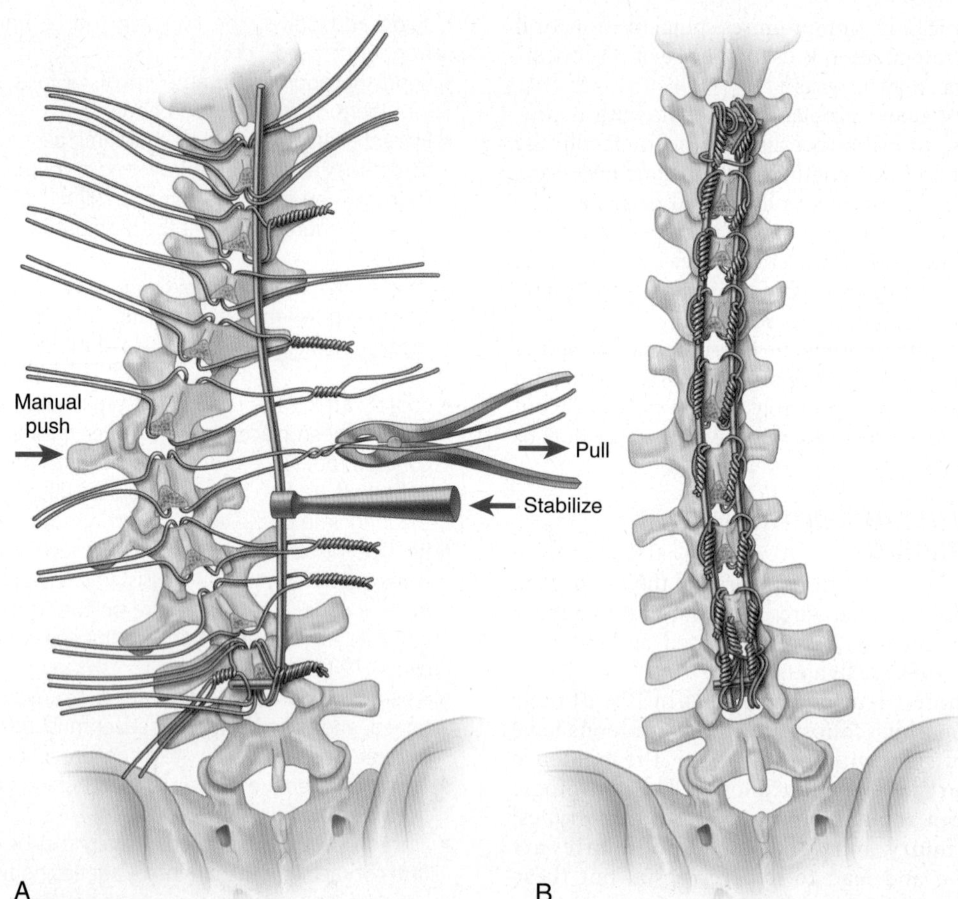

FIGURE 8.104 **A** and **B**, Concave rod technique for correction of lumbar scoliosis. (From *Segmental spinal fixation and correction using Richards' L-rod instrumentation*, Memphis, TN, Smith & Nephew Richards.) **SEE TECHNIQUE 8.29.**

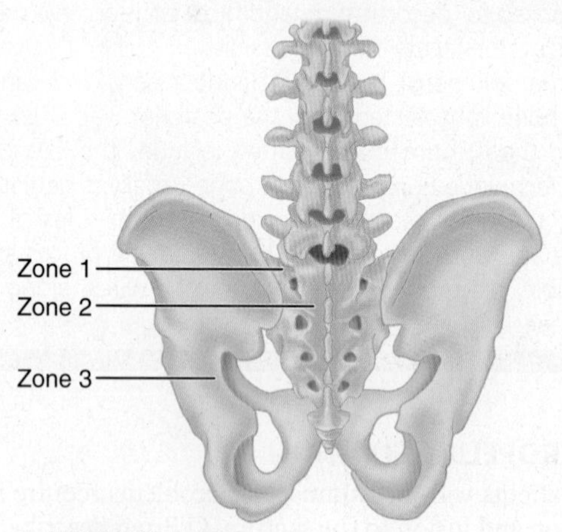

FIGURE 8.105 Sacropelvic fixation zones.

sublaminar wires or cables bilaterally throughout the lumbar and thoracic spine. The rods generally are crosslinked below the upper fixation to provide further stability against migration or rotation of the rods. We have found that if hooks or screws are not used at the upper end, wires alone provide no support against axial loading.

The advantages of the S-rod are that firm fixation is provided around the sacral ala without crossing the sacroiliac joint and that harvesting of bone graft from the ilium is not a problem because the ilium is not violated as it is when the Galveston technique is used. Prebent S-rods are available; complex bends cannot be done effectively at the time of surgery. The rods can be further contoured with a rod bender at the time of surgery to accommodate the size of the sacrum and to provide the appropriate sagittal plane correction.

SACROPELVIC FIXATION

TECHNIQUE 8.30

(MCCARTHY)

- Expose the spine posteriorly as described in Technique 8.8.
- Perform careful dissection of the sacral ala, using a curet to clean the superior edge. Use finger dissection ventrally.
- The rods come in different sizes and contours. In most instances, a 5.5-mm rod provides satisfactory fit to the sacral ala.
- Contour the rods to appropriate sagittal contours.
- Place the S-rod over the sacral ala from posterior to anterior in a position adjacent to the anterior border of the

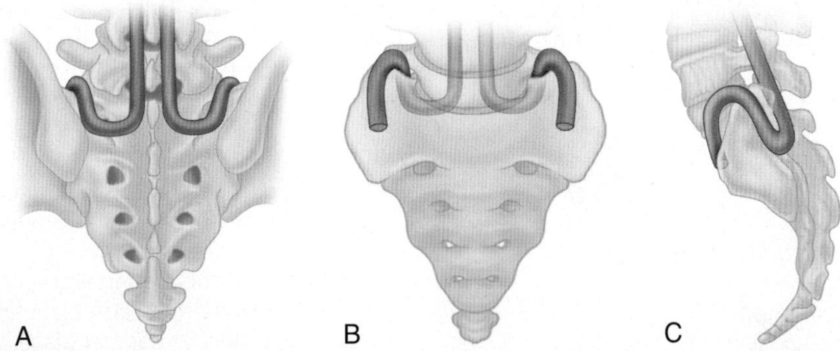

FIGURE 8.106 **A-C,** S-rods are manufactured as a pair to fit over the right and left sacral alae for fixation to the sacrum without crossing the sacroiliac joint. They are available in 3⁄16-inch and 1⁄4-inch rods.

sacroiliac joint. It lies posterior to the L5 nerve root and roughly parallel to it.

- Seat the S-portion of the rod firmly against the sacral ala by distraction between an L4-level hook or pedicle screw. The rods then can be used as a firm fixation point for translation or correction of scoliotic deformities or by placing the right and left rods simultaneously and cross-linking them, applying a strong cantilever corrective force for correction of pelvic obliquity. Crosslinking the two S-rods provides stability and eliminates the increased time and difficulty of insertion of rods into the ilium.
- Elevate the medial aspect of the iliac apophysis and rotate it over the top of the S-rod on the sacral ala.
- Provide bone graft to encase the S-rod into the sacrum.

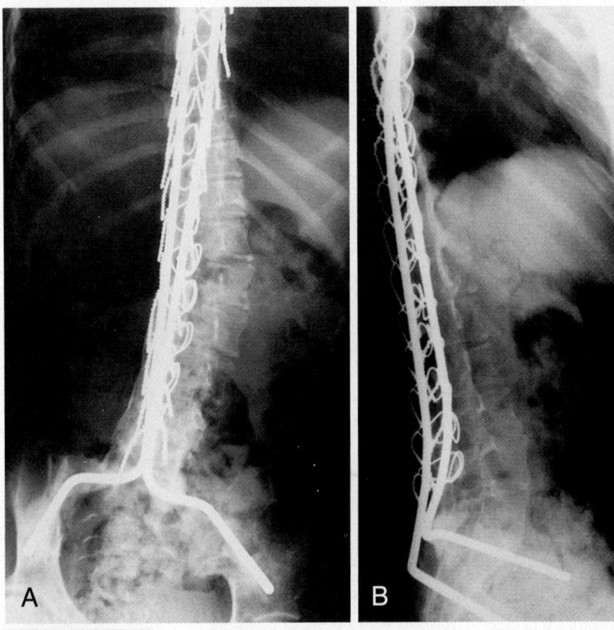

FIGURE 8.107 **A** and **B,** Stabilization of pelvis with Galveston technique. Segment of rod is driven into each ilium. **SEE TECHNIQUE 8.31.**

GALVESTON SACROPELVIC FIXATION

Another popular method for achieving sacropelvic fixation is the Galveston technique described by Allen and Ferguson in which the pelvis is stabilized by driving a segment of the L-rod into each ilium (Fig. 8.107). The rod is inserted into the posterior iliac crest and rests between the cortices above the sciatic notch. This fixation provides immediate firm stability and is biomechanically a stable construct. There are potential disadvantages, however, because the rod crosses the sacroiliac joint. It is postulated that motion in the sacroiliac joint is responsible for a "halo" that is often seen around the end of the Galveston rod in the iliac wing. Whether this radiographic phenomenon actually results in clinical problems is unknown.

TECHNIQUE 8.31

(ALLEN AND FERGUSON)

- Expose both iliac crests from the midline incision at the level of the posterior superior iliac spine. Expose the iliac crest to the sciatic notch. The area just proximal to the sciatic notch provides the most satisfactory fixation.
- Use a large, smooth Steinmann pin corresponding to the size of the rod diameter or a pedicle awl to create a tunnel for the rod. The insertion site is just posterior to the sacroiliac joint at the level of the posterior inferior iliac spine, distal to the posterior superior iliac spine, along the transverse bar of the ilium. The area for insertion often is difficult to identify, and the rod may be inserted too superiorly.
- Carefully identify the area for insertion and use a rongeur to carefully remove soft tissue and bone to expose the inner and outer tables of the ilium.
- Drill the Steinmann pin to a depth of 6 to 9 cm.
- Asher et al. described use of a pedicle awl for pin insertion. This allows tactile perception to determine whether the awl is perforating the cortex of the ilium.
- Use a rongeur to remove enough cartilage and cortical bone to create a 1 × 1-cm entry site into the inferior portion of the posterior superior iliac spine. This exposes the intramedullary space.
- Introduce a blunt-tipped pedicle awl into the intracortical space and advance it by gentle oscillating pressure on the handle of the awl.

- Direct the awl to 2 cm above the sciatic notch and advance it to the appropriate depth of the rod in the ilium (Fig. 8.108).

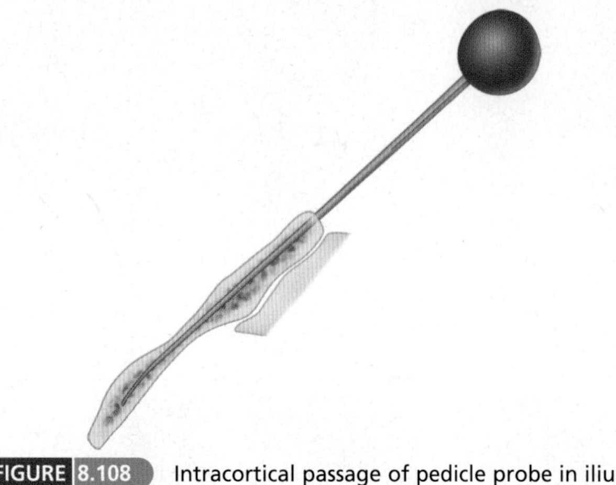

FIGURE 8.108 Intracortical passage of pedicle probe in ilium. **SEE TECHNIQUE 8.31.**

- Now use a flexible ball-tipped pedicle probe to ensure that the hole made by the blunt-tipped probe is completely intracortical. Place the smooth Steinmann pin into the iliac hole.

ROD CONTOURING (ASHER)

- Preparation of the rod is made easier by the use of a variable-radius bender set. To prepare the rod for iliac (Galveston) placement, four measurements are needed: (1) the length of the intrailiac portion of the rod (Fig. 8.109A), (2) the transverse plane angle of the iliac fixation site to the midsagittal plane (Fig. 8.109B), (3) the medial-lateral distance from the iliac entry site to the intended line of longitudinal passage of the rod along the spine (Fig. 8.109C), and (4) the length of the rod needed from the sacrum to the most cephalad instrumentation site.
- Lay suture along the spine line from the sacrum to the facet above the last instrumented vertebra; its length plus 1 cm is the usual length for this portion of the rod.

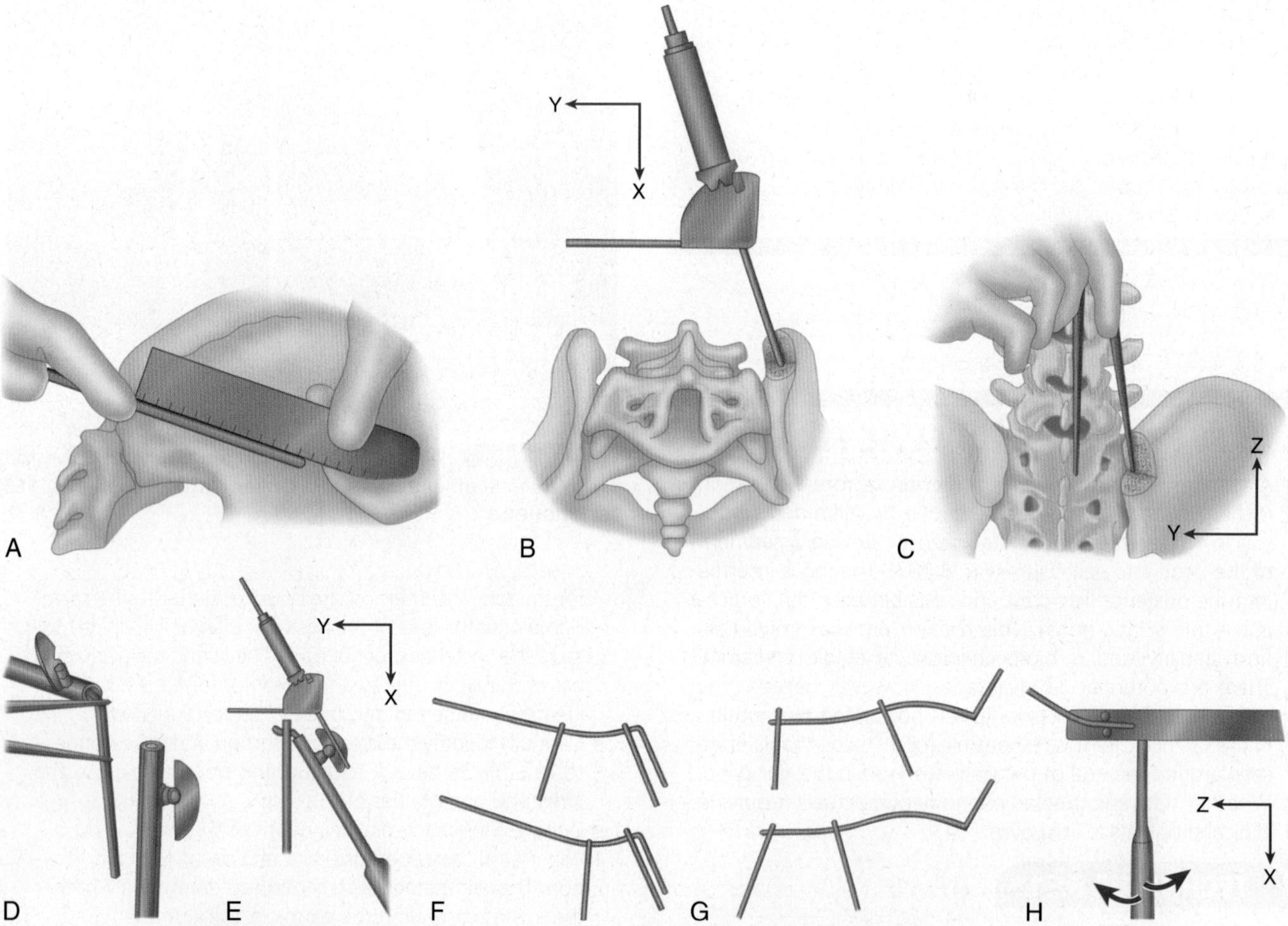

FIGURE 8.109 Technique of Asher. **A,** Length of intrailiac portion of rod. **B,** Transverse angle of iliac fixation site in midsagittal plane. **C,** Coronal plane distance from iliac entry site to intended line of longitudinal passage along spine. **D,** Right-angle bend. **E,** Iliosacral axial plane bend. **F,** Placement of long- and short-radius lordosis. **G,** Placement of long and short thoracic kyphosis. **H,** Sagittal plane iliac angle adjustment. (Redrawn from Boachie-Adjei O, Asher MA: Isola instrumentation for scoliosis. In McCarthy R, editor: *Spinal instrumentation techniques*, vol. 2, Rosemont, IL, 1998, Scoliosis Research Society.) **SEE TECHNIQUE 8.31.**

- Add the first and third measurements. A right-angle bend is placed at this distance from one end (Fig. 8.109D); this is the iliosacral portion of the rod.
- The medial-lateral distance (measurement 3) minus approximately 3 mm to allow for the bend is from the middle of the right-angle bend. Mark this at the iliosacral portion of the rod.
- After the right-left orientation is verified, place an angle identical to that of the iliac fixation site to the midsagittal plane at this second mark (Fig. 8.109E). This separates the iliosacral portion of the rod into the iliac and sacral portions.
- Add sagittal plane bends, beginning at L5-S1, thus leaving a straight portion over the sacrum. Because lordosis is not uniform but is greater in the lower lumbar spine, two contours are necessary. The contour for the entire lumbar spine is a long radius, whereas that for the lower lumbar spine is shorter (Fig. 8.109F).
- Add thoracic kyphosis, again by use of the flat benders (Fig. 8.109G).
- Attempt a trial placement to check whether the sagittal plane bend of the sacroiliac bend is correct. This can be determined by measuring the distance from the rod to the spine at the cephalad and caudal levels of the rod.
- Make final sagittal plane iliac angle adjustments with flat bender posts and a tube bender (Fig. 8.109H).
- The Galveston technique can be combined with a multiple-hook or pedicle screw segmental system with crosslinks if desired.

UNIT ROD INSTRUMENTATION WITH PELVIC FIXATION

When two unlinked L-rods are used, the rods may translate with respect to one another and compromise control of pelvic obliquity. In addition, twisting within the laminar wires can result in rotation of one rod relative to another. The ¼-inch rods generally used in neuromuscular patients are difficult to bend so that they can conform to the complex three-dimensional curves of the spine. In response to these problems, Bell et al. developed the unit rod. The unit rod is a single, continuous ¼-inch stainless-steel rod with a U bend at the top and "bullet-ended" pelvic legs for implantation into the pelvis. The three-dimensional preshaped kyphosis, lordosis, and pelvic legs were devised from a database of patients without spinal deformity. Eight lengths of rod are available, increasing in 20-cm increments from 310 to 450 cm. Right and left iliac guides facilitate drilling into the posterior ilia and subsequent introduction of the pelvic legs. The length of the iliac legs decreases proportionally as the rod shortens. The unit rod attempts to normalize body alignment in both the sagittal and coronal planes by establishing normal lordosis and kyphosis and correcting pelvic obliquity. We have not found the unit rod satisfactory for extremely rigid curves unless an anterior release or osteotomies are done to reduce the spinal stiffness. If, however, the curves seem relatively flexible on bending films or physical examination, correcting to less than 40 degrees, we have had excellent results with the use of the unit rod.

TECHNIQUE 8.32

- Expose the spine as described in Technique 8.6. Expose both iliac crests to the posterior superior iliac spine and down to the sciatic notch.
- Mark a ¼-inch drill with a marking pen at 15 mm longer than the sciatic notch if the child weighs more than 45 kg and at 10 mm if the child weighs less than 45 kg.
- Place the appropriate right or left drill guide into the sciatic notch. Keep the lateral handle of the drill guide parallel to the pelvis (Fig. 8.110A) and the axial handle of the drill guide parallel to the body axis (Fig. 8.110B).
- Start the drill hole as far inferiorly on the posterior superior iliac crest as possible (Fig. 8.110C).
- Drill a hole in the ilium to the marked depth and check the hole with a wire to make certain the cortex has not been penetrated.
- Use a similar technique on the opposite iliac crest.
- Pass the sublaminar wires.
- Measure the length of the rod by placing the rod upside down, with the corner of the rod at the drilled hole on the elevated side of the pelvis. If kyphosis is severe, choose one length shorter because the kyphotic spine shortens as it corrects. If pelvic obliquity is severe, test the length from both the high and low sides and choose an intermediate length. If the rod is placed and turns out to be too long, it may be necessary to cut off the superior end; the upper end then can be connected with a crosslink.
- Cross the legs of the appropriate-length rod and insert them first into the hole on the low side of the pelvic obliquity (Fig. 8.111A). Cross the rod so that the leg going into the low side is underneath the other leg.
- Insert approximately one half to three fourths of the leg length into the hole. Then insert the next leg by holding it with a rod holder and guiding it into the correct direction of the hole.
- Use the impactor and drive the rod leg in by alternately impacting each leg (Fig. 8.111B). Be certain that each rod leg is impacted in the exact direction of the hole or the cortex may be penetrated.
- Once the rod is firmly seated, use the proximal end of the rod as a "rudder" to bring the distal end of the rod to the spine (Fig. 8.111C).
- Do not push the rod down completely into the wound in one move because this may pull the legs out of the pelvis or fracture the ilium. Instead, push the rod to line it up with the L5 lamina only and tie these wires down with a jet wire twister.
- Now push the rod to the L4 vertebra, twist the wires, and cut them off.
- Tighten the wires from caudad to cephalad one level at a time. Do not relax the push on the rod between the levels of the major curve or too much load may be applied to the end vertebra. Do not use the wires themselves to pull the rod down to the lamina or the wires will cut through the lamina.
- After all the wires have been tightened, go back and verify that all previously tightened wires are well seated.

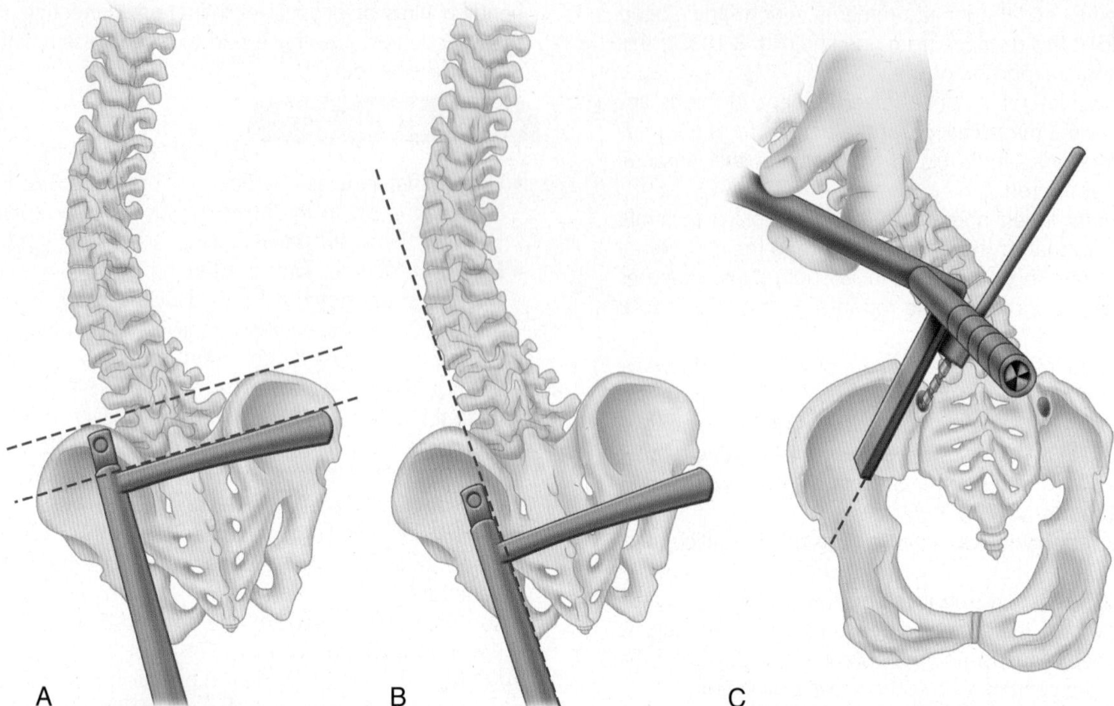

FIGURE 8.110 **A and B,** Unit rod for neuromuscular scoliosis developed by Bell, Moseley, and Koreska. Single, continuous ¼ -inch stainless steel rod has U-shaped bend at top and bullet-shaped ends for insertion into pelvis. **SEE TECHNIQUE 8.32.**

- Cut the wires at 10- to 15-mm lengths.
- Bend all wires into the midline of the rod and direct them caudally (Fig. 8.111D).
- Apply bone graft. Bank bone usually is needed because the iliac crest is used for pelvic fixation.

ILIAC FIXATION WITH ILIAC SCREWS

Iliac screws provide secure and rigid pelvic fixation, which has the advantage of not having prefixed angles for pelvic fixation. The disadvantage is the need for a lateral connector for attachment to the rod.

TECHNIQUE 8.33

- After the spine is exposed, dissect laterally underneath the spinal fascia to reach the medial aspect of the iliac wing at its very distal aspect.
- Identify the posterior superior iliac spine. The starting point for screw placement is 1 cm inferior to the posterior superior iliac spine and 1 cm proximal to the distal edge of the posterior superior iliac spine (Fig. 8.112A). If required, expose the lateral aspect of the iliac wing to help with the trajectory of the pathway down the iliac bone (Fig. 8.112B).
- With a 4-mm burr, create a medial cortical defect at the appropriate starting point.
- By use of an iliac probe or pedicle probe with the tip facing medially and the trajectory 45 degrees caudal and lateral, tunnel down between the cortices of the ilium (Fig. 8.112C). It is more likely to exit laterally than medially. That is the reason for the probe to face medially. The ideal placement of the screw will be just cephalad to the superior gluteal notch, which is the thickest part of the ilium.
- Once the tunnel has been formed with the probe, use a flexible ball-tip sounding probe to palpate the intraosseous borders of the ilium to confirm intraosseous placement of the screw. Tap the tunnel if necessary.
- Various angles are available on the screw heads to allow easier placement of the connector rods. Screw trials are used to determine which type of screw best fits the patient's anatomy. Select an appropriate-sized screw.
- Insert the screw with the screwdriver. If angled screw heads are used, each angle screw has its own screwdriver. Once the screw is placed snuggly into the ilium, it is important that the top of the screw head rest below the top of the posterior superior iliac spine (Fig. 8.112D). This ensures that the screw will not be prominent postoperatively.
- Position the screw head facing directly medial to allow the lateral connector to engage and thus keep the rod vertical in its orientation.
- Determine the length of the lateral connector after placing and aligning the more cephalad spinal instrumentation; the goal is a vertical rod with only sagittal plane and minimal coronal plane bending.
- Once the offset is determined, cut the lateral connector to length and insert it into the screw head and provisionally tighten the screw.

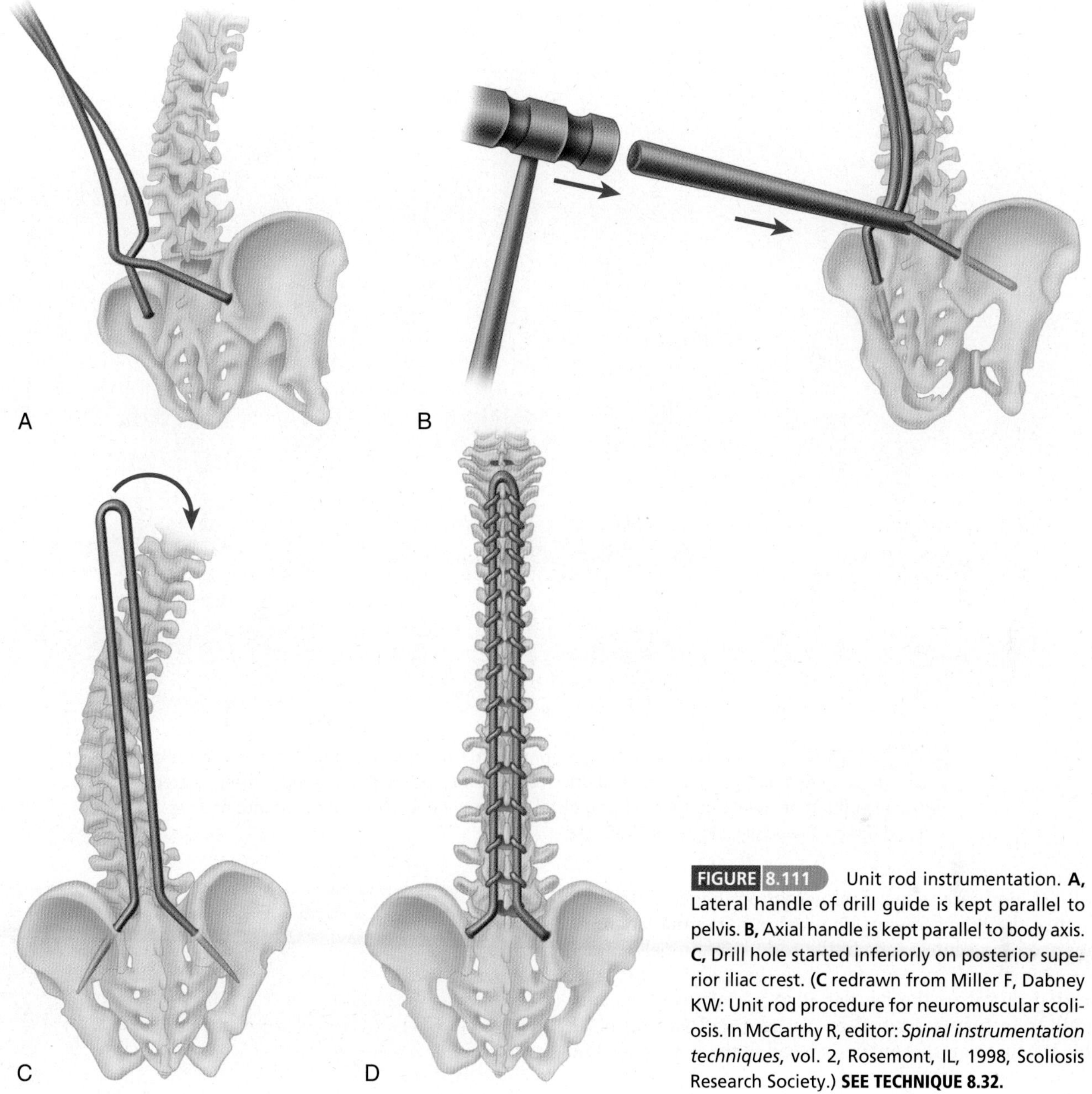

FIGURE 8.111 Unit rod instrumentation. **A,** Lateral handle of drill guide is kept parallel to pelvis. **B,** Axial handle is kept parallel to body axis. **C,** Drill hole started inferiorly on posterior superior iliac crest. (**C** redrawn from Miller F, Dabney KW: Unit rod procedure for neuromuscular scoliosis. In McCarthy R, editor: *Spinal instrumentation techniques*, vol. 2, Rosemont, IL, 1998, Scoliosis Research Society.) **SEE TECHNIQUE 8.32.**

- Insert the rod into the lateral connector and cantilever it down into the cephalad spinal instrumentation (Fig. 8.112E).
- Place the set screw for the lateral connector and provisionally tighten it.
- When all implants are securely in place, perform final tightening and break off the set screw head (Fig. 8.112F).

POSTOPERATIVE CARE Postoperative immobilization is not recommended after L-rod or unit-rod instrumentation. However, because neuromuscular curves frequently are associated with osteoporosis, spasticity, inability of the patient to cooperate, and severe curves, postoperative immobilization in a TLSO for 3 to 6 months may be needed if there is any question about stability of the instrumentation construct.

S2 ILIAC LUMBOPELVIC SCREW PLACEMENT

The screws in this technique do not require a separate skin or fascial incision, and average lengths of 70 to 100 mm are attainable. Additionally, this fixation does not interfere with aggressive iliac crest harvest. The advantages of

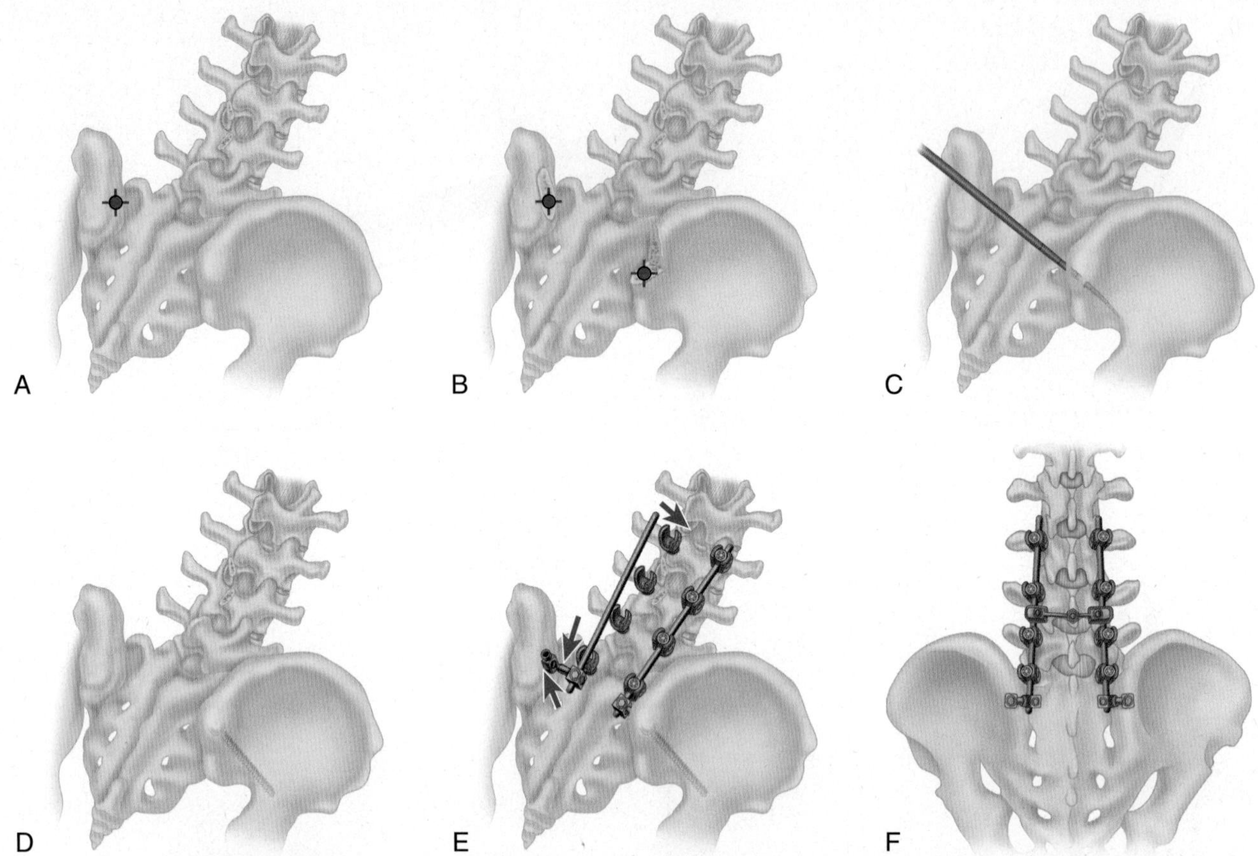

FIGURE 8.112 Unit rod instrumentation, *continued.* **A,** One leg of rod is placed into low side of pelvic obliquity first. **B,** Impactor is used to drive rod legs into pelvis. **C,** Once rod is firmly seated, proximal end can be used as rudder to bring distal end to spine. **D,** Wires are bent into midline of rod and directed caudally. **SEE TECHNIQUE 8.32.**

this technique are reduced implant prominence and placement of the iliac screw in line with other spinal anchors, thus avoiding acute bends in the rod to obtain pelvic fixation. Ramchandran et al. described the use of an alternate starting portal to the S2 alar iliac portal using an anatomic trajectory described by Vaccaro and Harrop et al. This starting portal is on medial wall of the iliac crest (Fig. 8.113).

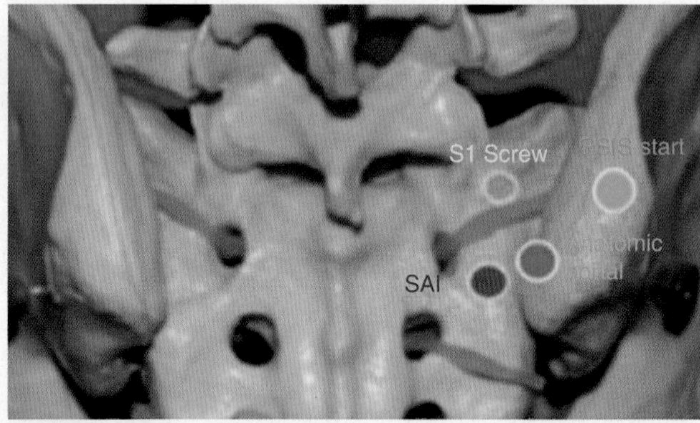

FIGURE 8.113 Model of pelvis and sacrum showing entry points for various iliac fixation methods: traditional iliac PSIS entry; SAI (S2-alar-iliac) screw entry; S1 pedicle screw entry; and anatomic trajectory portal for iliac screw. (Redrawn from Ramchandran S, George S, Asghar J, et al: Anatomic trajectory for iliac screw placement in pediatric scoliosis and spondylolisthesis: an alternative to S2-alar-iliac portal, *Spine* Deform 7:286, 2019.)

ILIAC AND LUMBOSACRAL FIXATION WITH SACRAL-ALAR-ILIAC SCREWS

TECHNIQUE 8.34

- Place the patient prone on a radiolucent table, ensuring that the pelvis is as neutral as possible with minimal rotation.
- Extend a midline skin incision to expose the dorsal foramina of the sacrum, specifically the S1 and S2 foramina. Additional lateral dissection to the iliac crest is not needed.
- Stand on the contralateral side of the patient to identify the starting point. Find the midpoint between the S1 and S2 dorsal foramina and the lateral border of the foramen; the starting point is where these two lines intersect (Fig. 8.114A). This starting point should be in line with the S1 pedicle screw.
- Be aware that the entry point may vary with the local anatomy of the patient. If the pelvis is asymmetric in the

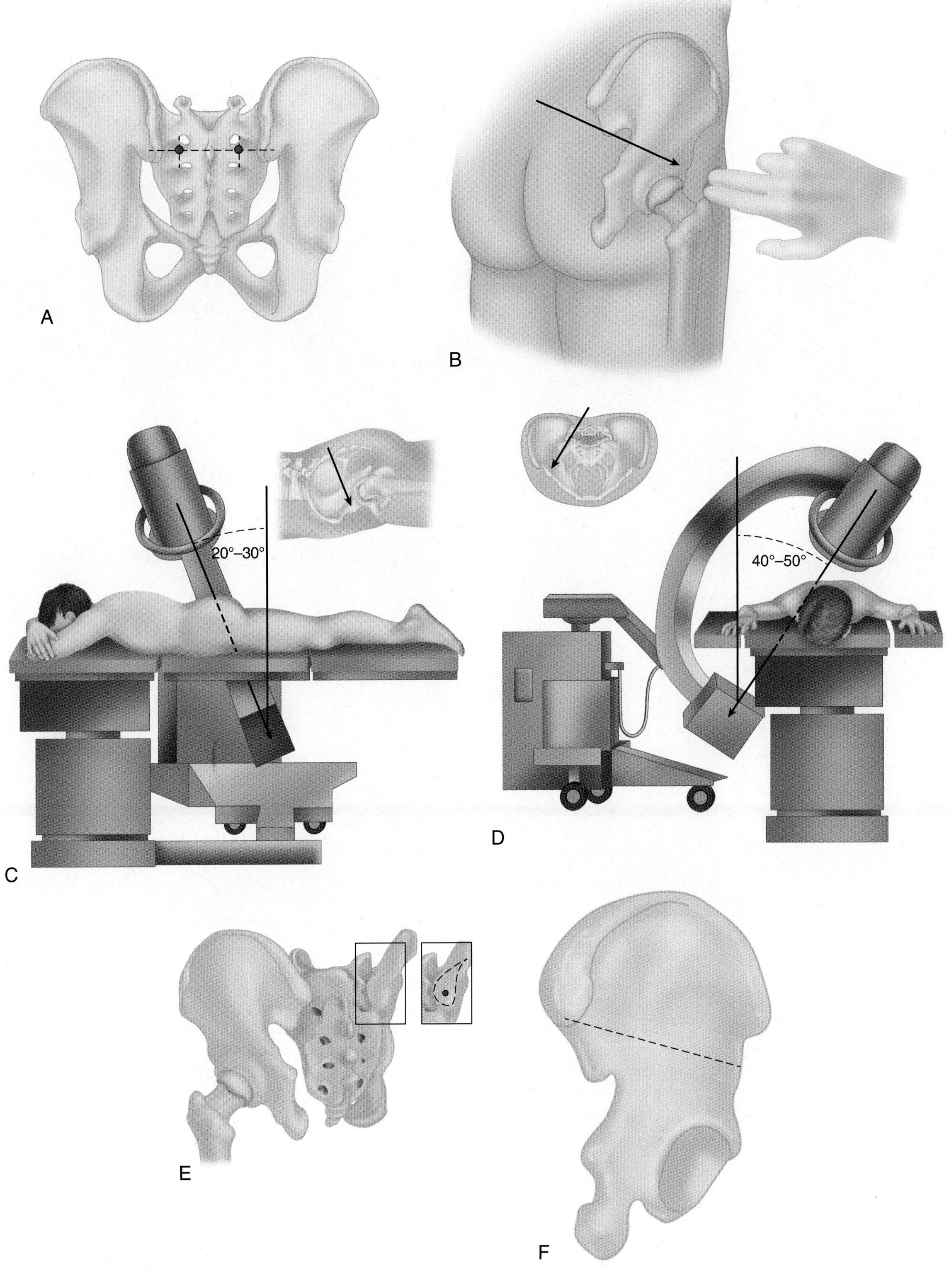

FIGURE 8.114 Iliac and lumbosacral fixation with sacral-alar-iliac screws. **A,** Starting point for screw insertion. **B,** Screw trajectory. **C** and **D,** Fluoroscopic confirmation of appropriate trajectory.

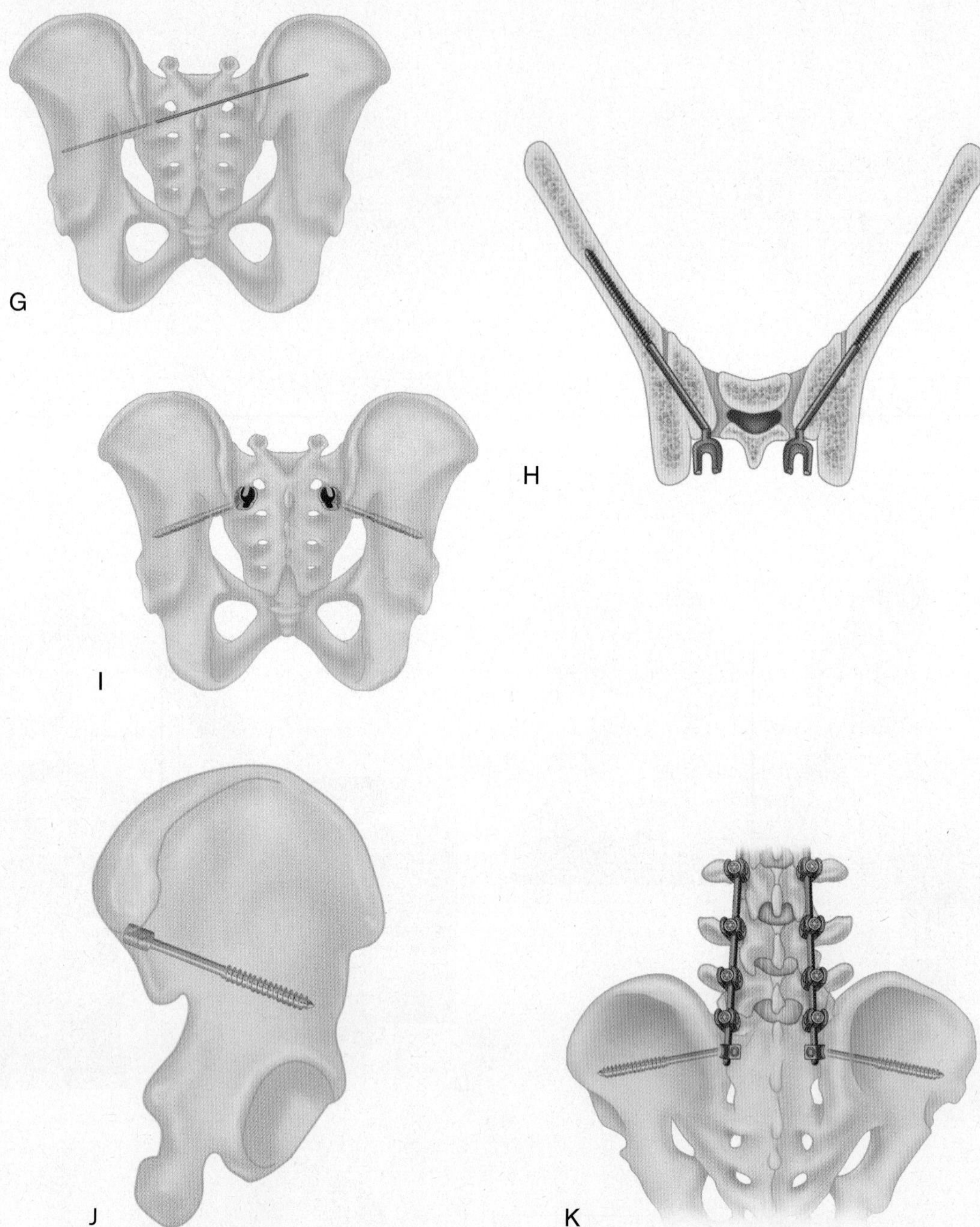

FIGURE 8.114, Cont'd **E,** With proper trajectory, iliac teardrop should be visible on anteroposterior image. **F,** Path of probe or drill within 20 mm of the greater sciatic notch and aimed toward the anterior inferior iliac spine. **G,** Guidewire placed through drilled hole. **H-J,** Fluoroscopic teardrop view to confirm screw placement. **K,** Final position of rods. (Courtesy DePuy Synthes Companies of Johnson & & Johnson.) **SEE TECHNIQUE 8.34.**

transverse plane, as is common in patients with genetic or neuromuscular disorders, the starting point may need to vary in the mediolateral plane.

- Determine the proper trajectory of the sacral-alar-iliac fixation. Aim for the anterior inferior iliac spine, which can be found by palpating the top of the greater trochanter (Fig. 8.114B). The trajectory should pass immediately above the sciatic notch.
- To use fluoroscopy to identify the appropriate trajectory, orient the C-arm in the intended trajectory and position it above the starting point. Then angle the C-arm 20 to 30 degrees caudal (Fig. 8.114C) and 40 to 50 degrees to the vertical plane (Fig. 8.114D), aiming for the anterior inferior iliac spine. With this trajectory, the iliac teardrop should be visible on the anteroposterior fluoroscopic image (Fig. 8.114E).
- Use an awl and probe or pelvic 2.5-mm drill bit to verify the correct trajectory. The path of the probe or drill should be within 20 mm of the greater sciatic notch and aiming toward the anterior inferior iliac spine (Fig. 8.114F). This trajectory may vary with pelvic obliquity and lumbar lordosis.
- If using a drill, feel for the bony end point after each advancement of the drill. Once the drill crosses the sacroiliac joint, use a 3.2-mm drill bit to avoid breaking the smaller bit in the ilium. Alternatively, an awl can be used in a dysplastic pelvis.
- Obtain a teardrop fluoroscopic image to ensure that the anterior-posterior trajectory is within the thickest part of the ilium, without a cortical breach.
- Use a ball-tipped probe to palpate the course of the screw and confirm the bony end point. Note the appropriate screw length as shown on the ball-tipped probe or on the tap.
- Place a guidewire through the probed or drilled hole to preserve the trajectory (Fig. 8.114G) and confirm its position with fluoroscopy.
- Tap the hole using the same-size pedicle tap as the intended screw diameter. Make sure that the guidewire does not advance during advancement of the tap.
- Insert the screw, aiming for the anterior inferior iliac spine with the trajectory within 20 mm above the greater sciatic notch. Before the screw is fully seated, remove the guidewire to prevent bending or breakage.
- Using the teardrop fluoroscopy view, confirm screw placement (Fig. 8.114H-J).
- Choose a rod length that will span the full length of the construct. Sagittally contour the rod before implanting it.
- Check to ensure that the sacral-alar-iliac screws are in line with the S1 screws and proximal screws in the construct. Rods can be inserted from caudal to cranial (most commonly) or from cranial to caudal in the case of severe proximal deformity.
- Insert the set screw to capture the rod. Tighten the rod to fix the rod to the distal screw and continue in a cephalad direction, capturing the rod with the rest of the screws in the construct (Fig. 8.115), and tighten the set screws.

CEREBRAL PALSY

Neuromuscular spinal deformities are most common in patients with cerebral palsy, and their risk of developing scoliosis has been related to disease severity. Children with severe spasticity and quadriplegic limb involvement have the highest risk of developing scoliosis. The Gross Motor Function Classification System (GMFCS) has been helpful in assessing the risk of developing scoliosis in patients with cerebral palsy. GMFCS I and II levels have almost no risk of developing scoliosis, while GMFCS levels IV and V have a 50% risk of developing moderate to severe spine deformity. Patients with GMFCS level IV and V classifications often have significant comorbidities that can make surgical correction of their scoliosis challenging; however, surgical correction of scoliosis has been reported to improve the quality of life in these patients, and patients and caregivers report high satisfaction rates after surgical correction of scoliosis, despite high complication rates. Although quality of life is improved and patient/caregiver satisfaction is high, it is the responsibility of the treating surgeon to accurately access the risks and benefits of surgery.

The greatest progression has been noted in patients who are unable to walk and have thoracolumbar or lumbar curves (average progression 0.8 degree per year in curves less than 50 and 1.4 degrees per year in curves more than 50 degrees).

Scoliosis in patients with cerebral palsy is best managed by early recognition and control of the curve before the deformity becomes severe. If the scoliosis is left untreated, function may be lost. If the patient is ambulatory, the trunk may become so distorted that standing erect becomes impossible. Sitting may become more difficult with increasing pelvic obliquity. If supplemental support by the hands is needed to sit, the patient will lose the ability to perform activities that require use of the upper extremity.

Bonnett et al. listed the following seven goals of scoliosis treatment in patients with cerebral palsy:

- Improvement in assisted sitting to make positioning and transfer easier for nursing attendants and family
- Relief of pain in the hips and back
- Increased independence because of a decreased need for assistance, both for the positioning required to relieve pain and to prevent pressure areas and for feeding
- Improvement in upper extremity function and table-top activities by eliminating the need to use the upper extremities for trunk support
- Reduction of the equipment needed, making possible the use of other equipment
- Placement of the patient in a different facility, one in which less care is provided
- Improved eating ability made possible by a change in position

Each patient must be evaluated individually to determine the potential for achieving these rehabilitation goals.

CLASSIFICATION

Lonstein and Akbarnia classified cerebral palsy curves into two groups (Fig. 8.116). Group I curves—double curves with both thoracic and lumbar components—occurred in 40% of their patients. These curves, which are similar to curves of idiopathic scoliosis, occurred more commonly

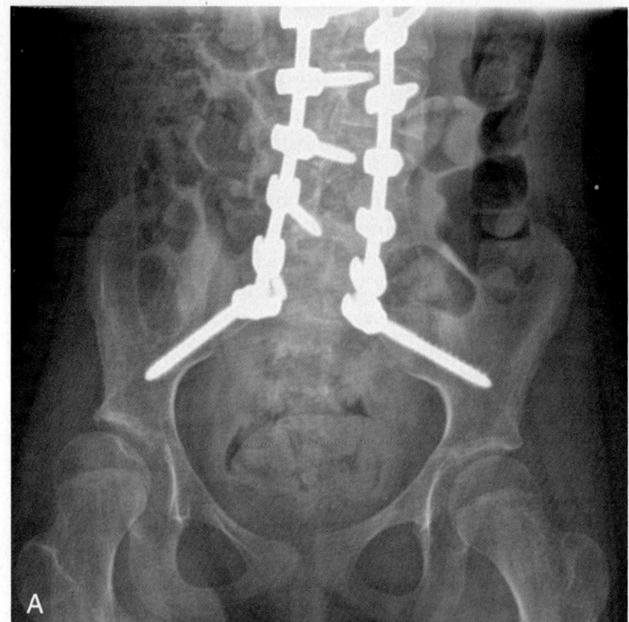

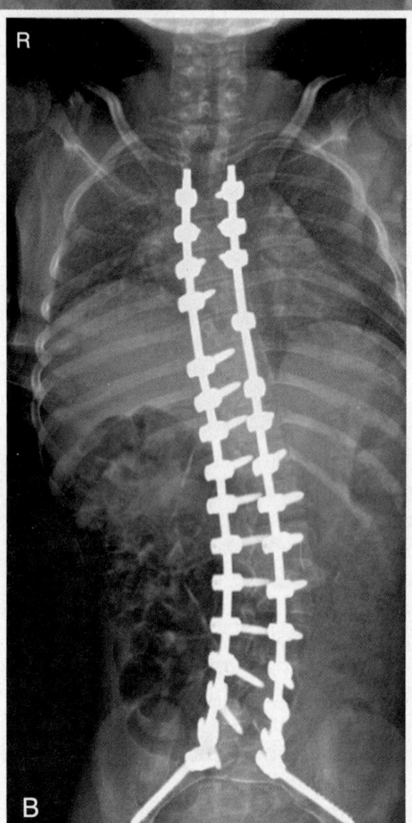

FIGURE 8.115 Alar-S2-iliac pedicle screw fixation. **SEE TECHNIQUE 8.35.**

in patients who were ambulatory and lived at home. Group II curves were present in 58% of patients. These curves were more severe lumbar or thoracolumbar curves that extended into the sacrum, with marked pelvic obliquity. Patients with these curves usually were nonambulatory with spastic quadriplegia, generally were not cared for at home, and were more likely to have the classic form of cerebral palsy.

NONOPERATIVE TREATMENT

If the curve is small, careful observation is indicated. If the curve progresses or is more than 30 degrees in a growing child who is an independent ambulator or sitter, treatment should be instituted. If a child is skeletally mature, bracing is not likely to be effective and surgery is indicated if the curve is 50 degrees or more.

Most nonambulatory patients with cerebral palsy do not have head or neck control during the first years of life. Custom seating may be effective in providing these patients with a straight spine and a level pelvis. Custom seating also can effectively accommodate severe spinal deformities and allow an upright posture in severely involved individuals.

If the curve is progressive, an orthotic device may be helpful as a temporizing device but will not provide permanent control of the curve. Orthoses generally are used for curve control during growth in a child who is ambulatory or who has independent sitting ability. The orthosis often provides enough trunk support to free the upper extremities for functional use. The orthosis of choice is a custom-molded total-contact TLSO.

OPERATIVE TREATMENT

The operative treatment of scoliosis in cerebral palsy is complex. Determining which type of surgery is needed, and even whether any surgical procedure is warranted, is difficult.

The surgical techniques available for scoliosis in patients with cerebral palsy have improved significantly. A pseudarthrosis rate of 20% has been reported in patients with posterior spinal fusion and Harrington instrumentation. Combined anterior and posterior procedures with anterior and posterior instrumentation result in adequate correction with a low incidence of pseudarthrosis. With pedicle screw instrumentation and posterior-only surgery, results are reported to be similar to those of anterior and posterior surgery. There probably is no one ideal technique for managing these complex curves. In general, we use pedicle screws, and pelvic fixation is preferred when possible. The rods can be crosslinked to increase stability. Our preference at this time for pelvic fixation is the iliac screw technique or S2 iliac screw technique (see Techniques 8.29 and 8.30). If the pelvis is too small to accept screw fixation, we use the McCarthy S-rod technique (see Technique 8.30) with crosslinking for pelvic fixation.

The type of surgery also depends on the type of scoliosis. According to Lonstein and Akbarnia, patients with group I curves usually require only a posterior fusion, with fusion to the sacrum rarely needed. Group II curves usually require a long fusion to the sacrum because the sacrum is part of the curve and pelvic obliquity is present. Traction radiographs should be obtained. If a level pelvis and balanced spine can be obtained, a one-stage posterior approach is indicated. However, if the traction radiograph shows significant residual pelvic obliquity, or if the torso is not balanced over the pelvis, a two-stage approach may be indicated, although with

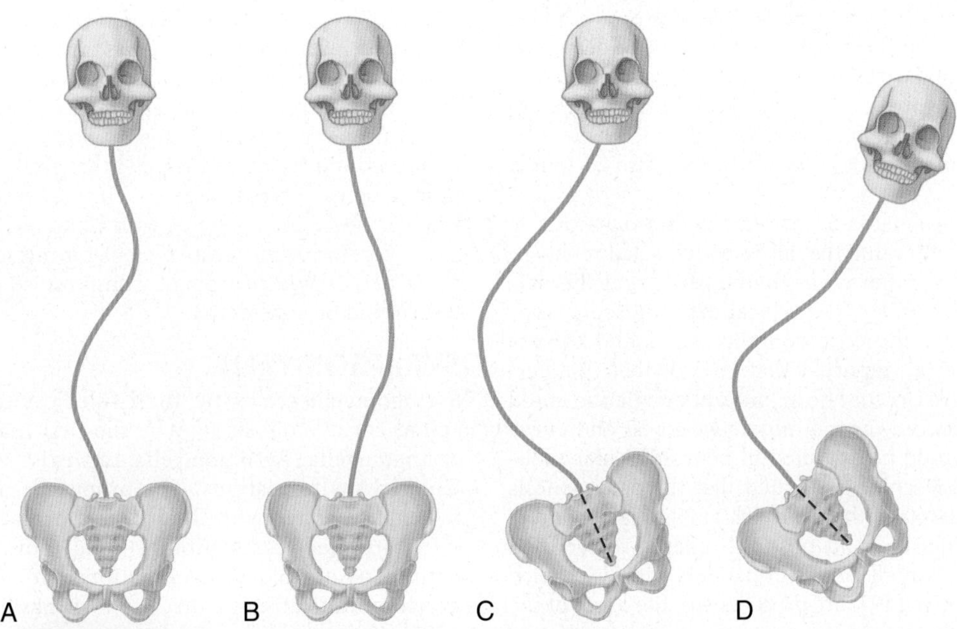

FIGURE 8.116 **A** and **B**, Group I double curves with thoracic and lumbar component and little pelvic obliquity. **C** and **D**, Group II large lumbar or thoracolumbar curves with marked pelvic obliquity.

current segmental instrumentation with pedicle screws, anterior and posterior procedures usually are not needed. Jackson et al. and LaMothe et al. reported that the use of intraoperative traction may decrease the need for anterior surgery and allow adequate correction with a posterior-only procedure.

Radiographic evaluation of patients with contractures around the hips can lead to erroneous conclusions. The radiograph often is made with the patient supine and the hips extended. If one hip has an adduction contracture and the opposite hip has an abduction contracture, it may appear that pelvic obliquity is present. An appropriate radiographic evaluation should include a supine view obtained with the hips in a relaxed position, whatever the contractures dictate. This allows the spine and pelvis to assume a neutral alignment without the influence of hip contractures. Kyphosis can be caused by tight hamstrings and should be evaluated carefully because if the hamstrings are not released, increased stress will be placed on the instrumentation.

Several technical points should be considered in instrumentation of patients with cerebral palsy. The most proximal level of the fusion should be above T4 to prevent junctional kyphosis above the instrumentation. Only small portions of the ligamentum flavum on either side of the superior interspinous space to be instrumented should be removed. If possible, the supraspinous and interspinous ligaments at the superior level should be preserved to prevent an increase in kyphosis above instrumentation. Pedicle hooks or screws are used for fixation at the most proximal level to add axial load support to the system.

With current instrumentation techniques, postoperative immobilization usually is not needed. If the bone is obviously osteopenic or instrumentation is less than ideal, postoperative external support may be necessary.

COMPLICATIONS

Improved techniques of instrumentation and preoperative and postoperative management have decreased complications, but a much higher complication rate should be expected after surgery for this type of scoliosis than after that for idiopathic curves. Complications in patients with cerebral palsy have been reported in up to 81%, including infection in 15% to 19%. Patients with cerebral palsy are believed to be at an increased risk for infection. Deep infections can be treated by irrigation and debridement, administration of systemic antibiotics, and delayed primary closure or closure over a suction drain.

Pulmonary complications often develop in these patients because they cannot cooperate in deep breathing and coughing exercises, and appropriate prophylactic pulmonary measures are needed.

If the upper limit of the fusion is not selected carefully (above T4), kyphosis cephalad to the upper limit of the fusion can occur. Pseudarthrosis is less frequent with newer instrumentation systems, but it still occurs and often results in implant failure. Other possible complications are those inherent in any spinal operation, such as urinary tract infection, ileus, and blood loss.

Although the complications can be significant in these patients, the functional improvement or prevention of deterioration of function may be worth the effort and the risks of surgery. Complications should be expected and planned for; prompt treatment will lessen their severity.

FRIEDREICH ATAXIA

Friedreich ataxia is a recessively inherited condition characterized by spinocerebellar degeneration. The genetic cause has been found to be a flaw within the frataxin gene on chromosome 9q13. The clinical onset takes place between the ages of 6 and 20 years. Primary symptoms include progressive ataxic gait, dysarthria, decreased proprioception or vibratory sense, muscle weakness, and lack of deep tendon reflexes. Secondary symptoms include pes cavus, scoliosis, and cardiomyopathy. Affected children frequently are wheelchair bound in the first or second decade of life. The cardiomyopathy often leads to death in the third or fourth decade of life.

Labelle et al. evaluated 56 patients with a diagnosis of Friedreich ataxia and found that all 56 patients had scoliosis. The most common pattern was double structural thoracic and lumbar curves (57%). The typical neuromuscular thoracolumbar curve with pelvic obliquity was found in only 14%. Milbrandt et al. reported that 63% of their patients developed scoliosis. Because no significant correlation could be established between overall muscle weakness and curve progression, as would be expected in neuromuscular scoliosis, Cady and Bobechko postulated that the pathogenesis of scoliosis in patients with Friedreich ataxia may be a disturbance of equilibrium and postural reflexes rather than muscle weakness. Not all curves in patients with Friedreich ataxia are progressive (49% are progressive); the onset of the disease at an early age and the presence of scoliosis before puberty have been found to be major factors in progression. Scoliosis appearing in the late teens or early 20s is less likely to be progressive.

Most authors have not found bracing to be useful for progressive curves in patients with Friedreich ataxia. The orthosis fails to control the curve, and by the time scoliosis develops, the patients often have a significant degree of ataxia and the restriction of a spinal orthosis makes ambulation more difficult. Curves of less than 40 degrees should be observed, curves of more than 60 degrees should be treated operatively, and curves of between 40 and 60 degrees should be observed or treated operatively, depending on the age of the patient, the onset of the disease, and such characteristics of the scoliosis as the patient's age when it is recognized and evidence of progression of the curve. If the curve is observed too long, cardiomyopathy may have progressed to the point that surgery is risky, if not impossible; early surgical treatment is therefore recommended for progressive curves.

Cardiology evaluation is mandatory before any surgery is considered in these patients. Prolonged bed rest postoperatively must be kept to a minimum, or weakness can increase rapidly. For these reasons, the ideal instrumentation for these patients is segmental spinal instrumentation with multiple fixation devices, such as hooks, sublaminar cables, or pedicle screws, that do not require external support postoperatively. In general, these patients require a long fusion with attention to sagittal contours to prevent later problems with thoracic kyphosis. Milbrandt recommended segmental instrumentation and fusion from T2 to the sacrum. The pelvis usually is not included in these fusions unless pelvic obliquity is significant. Spinal cord monitoring usually is not effective in these patients and plans for a wake-up test should be made preoperatively to evaluate the neurologic status after instrumentation and correction.

CHARCOT-MARIE-TOOTH DISEASE

Classic Charcot-Marie-Tooth disease is a demyelinating neuropathy. The condition is dominantly inherited, with considerable variation in severity. The reported incidence of spinal deformity in Charcot-Marie-Tooth disease varies from 10% to 26%. Some authors have found brace treatment to be well tolerated, whereas others have had little success, with curve progression reported in 71% and with 33% requiring instrumentation and fusion. The sagittal plane deformity accompanying this scoliosis most frequently is kyphosis, and fusion to the pelvis generally is not necessary unless pelvic obliquity exists. Intraoperative monitoring rarely is possible in patients with Charcot-Marie-Tooth disease; therefore, preoperative plans for intraoperative assessment of possible neurologic compromise with a wake-up test should be considered.

SYRINGOMYELIA

Syringomyelia is a cystic, fluid-filled cavitation within the spinal cord. Scoliosis may be the first manifestation of a syringomyelia. Syringomyelia can exist with or without Chiari I malformations. The proposed cause of syringomyelia associated with Chiari I malformation is disturbed or obstructed cerebrospinal fluid flow. Syringomyelia without associated Chiari I malformation is described as a noncommunicating syrinx. Scoliosis has been reported in 63% to 73% of children with syringomyelia. Physical findings that may indicate syringomyelia include neurologic deficits and pain associated with the scoliosis, intrinsic muscle wasting of the hands, cavus deformity, asymmetric muscle bulk, occipital and upper cervical headaches, and loss of superficial abdominal reflexes. Radiographic features suggestive of syringomyelia include Charcot changes in joints and a left thoracic curvature. Patients with syringomyelia and scoliosis have been found to have thoracic kyphosis (>40 degrees) instead of thoracic hypokyphosis seen with idiopathic scoliosis. Cervical lordosis also is increased in this patient population. If the diagnosis of syringomyelia is suspected, MRI should be done (Fig. 8.117). In obtaining the MRI study, care must be taken to include the craniocervical junction to rule out the presence of an Arnold-Chiari malformation.

The association of syringomyelia with scoliosis may have a significant influence on treatment. Paraplegia and rupture of a large cyst in the cord resulting in death have been reported in patients with syringomyelia who had instrumentation and fusion. Because of the possibility of these complications, surgery for scoliosis in patients with syringomyelia should be approached cautiously. The rate of progression of the neurologic deficit and the prognosis of the curve should be considered carefully before any extensive surgery is considered. Drainage of the cyst, followed by observation to determine if the subsequent curve stabilizes, has been recommended as initial treatment. In one study, improvement was noted in three of 15 patients, and progression did not occur in any patient. Another study showed that drainage of the syrinx delayed but did not prevent curve progression in immature patients; however, drainage of the syrinx did allow use of distraction-type instrumentation without complications. At our institution, the pediatric neurosurgeons believe that the syrinx usually is associated with Chiari I malformations. Their preferred management is decompression of the posterior fossa. If the curve continues to progress after posterior fossa decompression, surgery may be indicated. If instrumentation is necessary in these patients, distraction should be limited. This can be accomplished by either anterior instrumentation or posterior thoracic pedicle

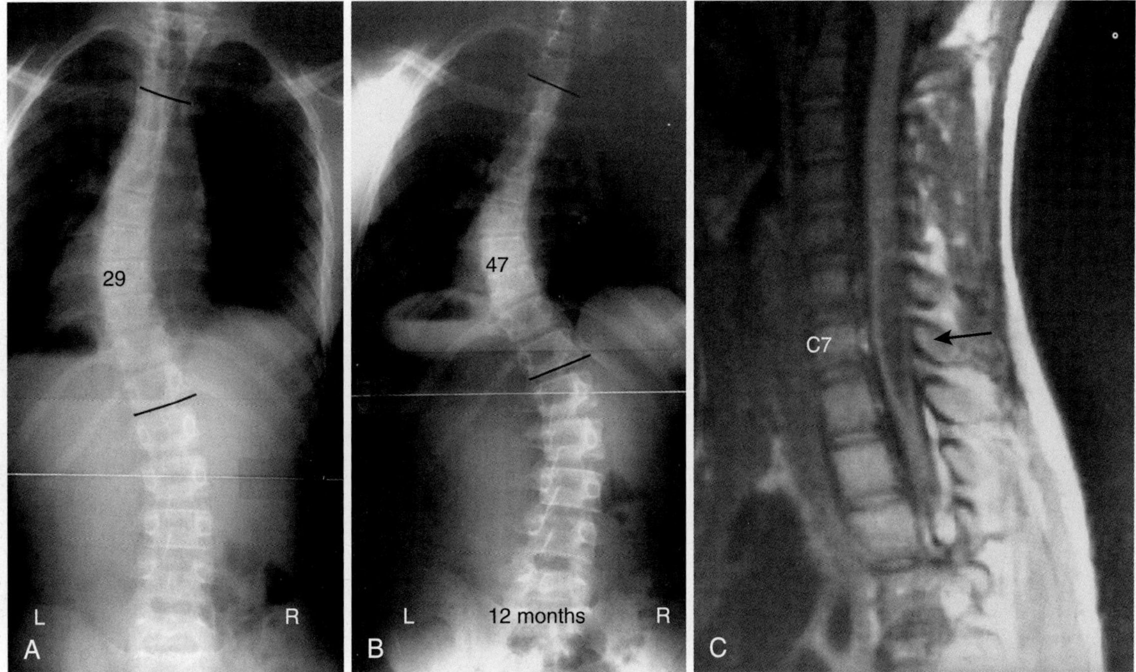

FIGURE 8.117 Progressive curve in patient with syringomyelia. **A,** Initial curve. **B,** One year later. **C,** MRI shows syrinx at C7 *(arrow)*.

instrumentation with a direct vertebral rotation technique. Direct communication with the neurosurgeon always is indicated preoperatively in these patients to minimize the possibility of spinal cord injury.

SPINAL CORD INJURY

Several series in the literature have reported an incidence of spinal deformity in 99% of children with spinal cord injuries before the adolescent growth spurt. Spinal deformity is much more common and the rate of curve progression much greater in preadolescents than in older patients.

Increasing curvature with pelvic obliquity in a child with a spinal cord injury can lead to a loss of sitting balance that requires the use of the upper extremities for trunk support rather than for functional tasks. Pressure sores may occur on the downside of the ischium, and hip subluxation can occur on the high side of the pelvic obliquity.

ORTHOTIC TREATMENT

Although some authors believe that alteration of the natural progression of scoliosis in these patients is impossible with devices such as braces and corsets, other authors indicated that orthotic treatment does have a place in the management of scoliosis in preadolescent patients with spinal cord injuries. Orthotic treatment is difficult because of potential skin problems, but effective slowing of progression has been noted. The use of an orthosis may delay the need for surgery in preadolescent patients until longitudinal growth of the spine is more complete. Orthotic treatment requires close cooperation among the physician, the family, and the patient. A custom-fitted, well-padded, plastic total-contact TLSO generally is used. Close attention must be paid to any evidence of pressure changes on the skin. The brace can be removed at night and used only during sitting.

OPERATIVE TREATMENT

Most preadolescent children with spinal cord injuries ultimately require surgical stabilization of their scoliosis (50% to 60%). If the curve progresses despite orthotic treatment, operative intervention is indicated. If the curve is more than 60 degrees when the child is first seen, surgery should be considered. Curves treated with an orthosis are considered for surgery if they progress beyond 40 degrees, and curves between 40 and 60 degrees are considered individually. In young children, growing constructs can be used to control the spinal deformity during growth.

The prevalence of pseudarthrosis in these patients reported in the literature ranges from 27% to 53%. Dearolf et al. found pseudarthrosis in 26% of their patients, and they attributed the lower figure to the use of segmental fixation in recent years. Segmental instrumentation allows more rigid fixation, and postoperative immobilization can be avoided (Fig. 8.118). Complete urinary tract evaluation should be done before surgery because urinary tract infections are common in patients with spinal cord injuries. Rapidly progressive curves in patients with spinal cord injury should be evaluated with MRI for the possibility of a posttraumatic syrinx.

If possible, surgery should be delayed until the patient weighs more than 100 lb. This allows the use of larger rods and more stable fixation. With the increased use of thoracic pedicle screws and lumbar pedicle screws, anterior release is becoming less necessary. For patients younger than 10 years with progressive curves of more than 50 degrees, growing rods can be used to control the curve during growth. If a definitive fusion is required in a young child at risk for future crankshaft problems, a first-stage anterior release and fusion should be considered, followed by posterior segmental spinal instrumentation and fusion. With the better correction in the coronal, sagittal, and axial planes provided by posterior

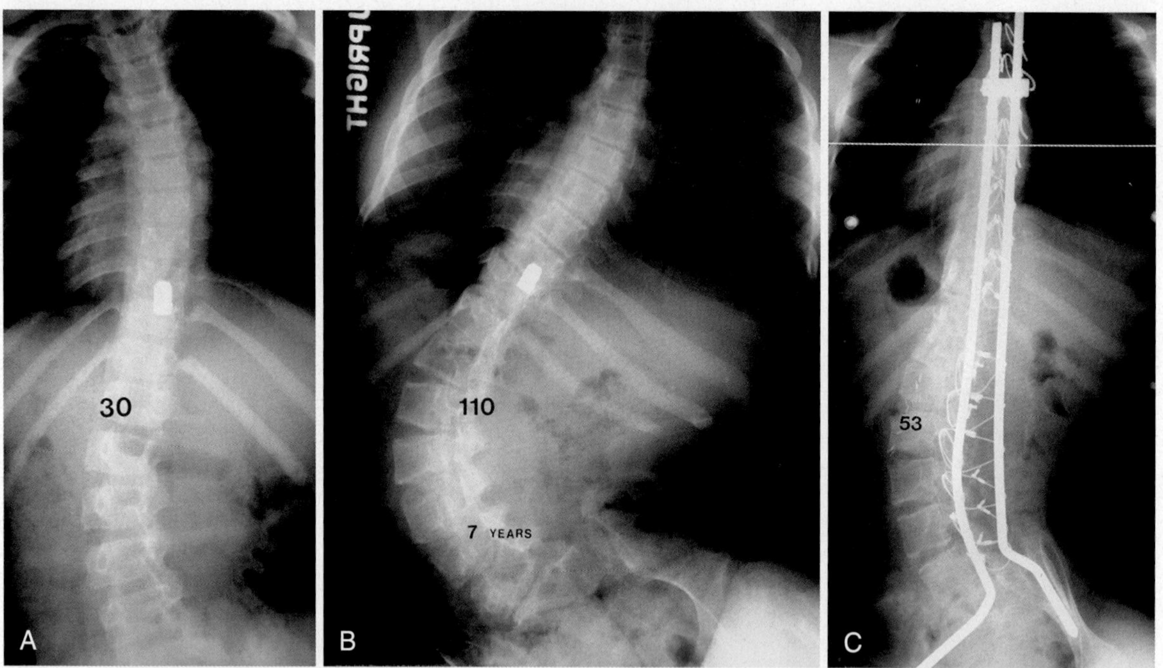

FIGURE 8.118 Progressive paralytic scoliosis after gunshot wound. **A,** Initial curve of 30 degrees. **B,** Seven years later, curve is 110 degrees. **C,** After fusion and segmental instrumentation, correction to 53 degrees.

pedicle screw instrumentation, anterior fusion may not be necessary even in these young children.

Dearolf et al. reported pseudarthroses in 3 of 10 preadolescent patients and in 1 mature patient who had fusion to the sacrum. They believed that if there was little residual pelvic obliquity, fusion to L4 or L5 would be sufficient. If, on the other hand, the pelvis was significantly involved in the curve, fusion probably should include the sacrum with pelvic instrumentation. For patients who are ambulators and in whom adequate correction can be obtained without involving the pelvis, an effort should be made to end the instrumentation above the pelvis. In carefully selected patients, Shook and Lubicky used short anterior spinal fusion with instrumentation alone. They reported that this provided excellent curve correction over a short segment and allowed a number of open disc spaces below the fused segment (Fig. 8.119).

If laminectomy was used to treat the initial spinal cord injury, an increased incidence of kyphosis can be expected.

POLIOMYELITIS

Because the Salk and Sabin vaccines have made poliomyelitis in children rare in the United States, most recent experience in treating postpolio spinal deformities is in adult patients. The basic principles of treatment, however, are no different from those of treatment of spinal deformities resulting from other neuromuscular diseases. Bonnett et al. outlined the indications for correction and posterior spine fusion in patients with poliomyelitis (Box 8.6).

As in any other neuromuscular curve, the length of fusion is much greater in patients with poliomyelitis than in those with idiopathic scoliosis. Segmental instrumentation is recommended. In evaluation of the distal extent of the fusion in a patient with poliomyelitis, it must be determined whether the pelvic obliquity is caused by the spinal curvature itself or by other factors, such as iliotibial band contractures.

SPINAL MUSCULAR ATROPHY

Spinal muscular atrophy is an autosomal recessive condition in which the anterior horn cells of the spinal cord, and occasionally the bulbar nuclei, atrophy. Spinal muscular atrophy can be classified into four types based on the severity of disease and the age of the patient at the time of clinical onset. Type I, or acute infantile Werdnig-Hoffmann disease, is the most severe form and is usually diagnosed within the first 6 months of life. The course of the disease is progressive, with most of these children dying within the first 2 to 3 years of life. Children with type 2 spinal muscular atrophy (chronic or intermediate form) manage to achieve normal motor milestones until 6 to 8 months of age. They often are very weak but can usually sit without support. Patients usually survive into the third or fourth decade. Type III, or Kugelberg-Welander disease, usually is seen after 2 years of age. It is more slowly progressive, and most patients are able to ambulate independently. Type IV presents in adolescence or early adulthood.

On clinical examination, children with spinal muscular atrophy have severe weakness of the trunk and limb muscles. Fasciculations of the tongue and tremors of the extremities are frequent. Reflexes are diminished. Most patients have normal intelligence, and the heart is unaffected by the disease process. Motor and sensory nerve conduction velocities are normal, but electromyography demonstrates denervation with fibrillation potentials. The cause of death usually

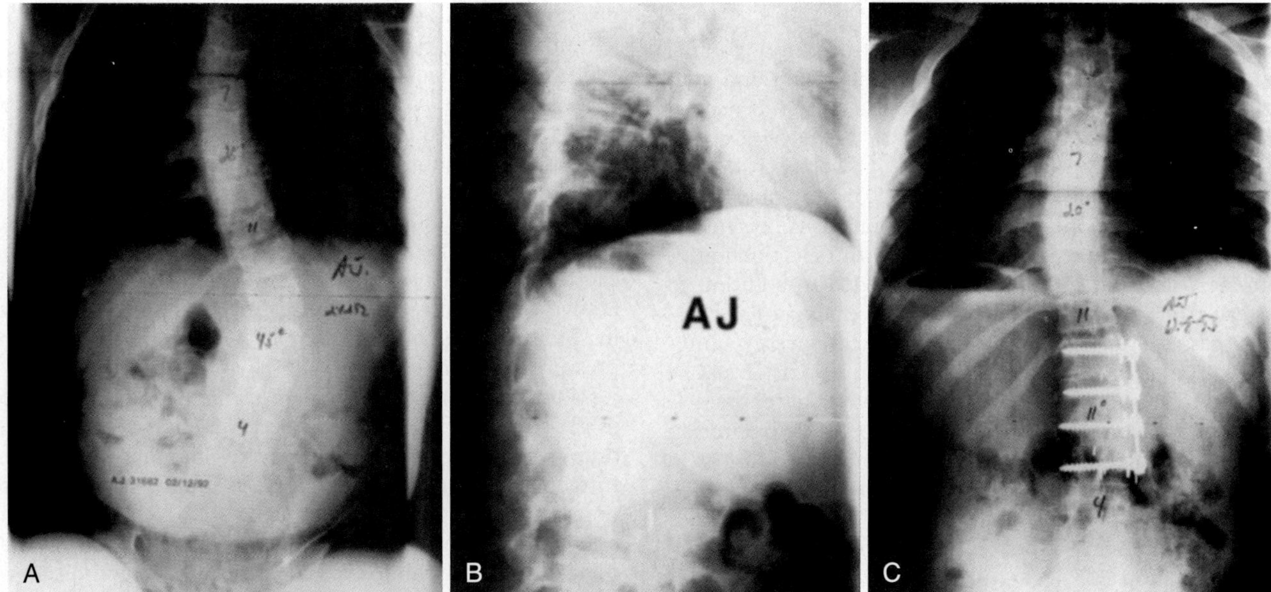

FIGURE 8.119 Fourteen-year-old boy who was paraplegic as result of gunshot wound to spine. **A** and **B**, Anteroposterior and lateral sitting thoracolumbar spine views showing 45-degree right lumbar curve with minimal pelvic obliquity. Lateral view shows thoracolumbar junction to be fairly straight. Because patient wanted to continue walking with braces, preservation of as many mobile segments below fusion was thought advantageous. Because of behavior of lumbar curve on side bending, it was thought that anterior fusion alone with instrumentation would provide correction of scoliosis and maintain sagittal contour. **C**, Anteroposterior sitting thoracolumbar spine view postoperatively shows excellent correction of scoliosis and preservation of sagittal contour. Anterior procedure was done with subperiosteal stripping of spine, and fusion healed rapidly within a few months. (From Shook JE, Lubicky JP: Paralytic scoliosis. In Bridwell KH, DeWald RL, editors: *The textbook of spinal surgery*, ed 2, Philadelphia, 1997, Lippincott-Raven.)

BOX 8.6

Indications for Correction and Posterior Spine Fusion in Patients with Poliomyelitis

- Collapsing spinal deformity because of marked paralysis
- Progressive spinal deformity that does not respond to nonoperative treatment
- Reduction of cardiorespiratory function associated with progressive restrictive lung disease
- Decreasing independence in functional activities because of spinal instability that necessitates use of the upper extremities for trunk support rather than for tabletop activities
- Back pain and loss of sitting balance associated with pelvic obliquity, which frequently causes ischial pain and pressure necrosis on the downside of the gluteal region

is pulmonary insufficiency. Ninety percent of these patients have scoliosis, and it is the most severe problem in those who survive childhood. Once patients with spinal muscular atrophy are wheelchair bound, their scoliosis develops rapidly. Aprin et al. noted that scoliosis usually is diagnosed between 6 and 8 years of age, and the more severe the disease, the more likely the curve is to be progressive. The scoliosis is a typical neuromuscular spinal deformity with a long C-shaped curve pattern. Thoracolumbar curves are seen in 80% of patients, and thoracic curves are noted in only 20% of patients.

Repeated injections of nusinersen have improved survival and motor development in infants with severe SMA. Nusinersen is administered intrathecally, so allowances must be made for continued injections if treatment of progressive scoliosis is planned.

ORTHOTIC TREATMENT

Bracing has been reported to slow progression of the curve and allows sitting for longer periods. However, patients treated in braces have been found to be less functional because of decreased flexibility of the spine and therefore tend to be noncompliant. When the scoliosis in a skeletally immature patient reaches 20 degrees in the sitting position, orthotic treatment can be considered, usually with a total-contact TLSO. This is used only during sitting to minimize progression of the curve and to provide an extremely weak child with a stable sitting support. Severe chest wall deformities can occur from bracing, and developing chest wall deformities are a contraindication to brace treatment. Although bracing may not eliminate the need for surgical stabilization, it may delay surgery until the child is closer to the end of growth. The use of a growing rod construct as an effective option in the treatment of scoliosis in patients with spinal muscular atrophy has been reported by several authors. This is the preferred option until a definitive posterior fusion can be done.

OPERATIVE TREATMENT

Surgical treatment of the spinal deformity is posterior spinal fusion with posterior segmental instrumentation and adequate bone grafting. Because fusion to the sacrum is needed for many of these patients, fixation to the pelvis can be obtained by the Galveston, iliac screw, or S2 alar screw technique (see Techniques 8.31, 8.33, and 8.35). Augmentation of the fusion with bone-bank allograft bone usually is necessary. For a severe fixed lumbar curve with pelvic obliquity, anterior release and fusion may be needed in addition to posterior instrumentation. It should be understood, however, that anterior surgery in patients with severe pulmonary compromise carries a great risk, and this risk must be evaluated carefully before surgery. With posterior pedicle screw instrumentation, which provides better correction in the coronal, sagittal, and axial planes, anterior fusion usually is not necessary. Preoperative traction can offer an excellent method to improve the flexibility of the spine and also improves pulmonary function before posterior fusion and instrumentation.

Complications should be expected in this group of patients (45%). Pseudarthrosis, atelectasis, pneumonitis, and death have been reported. Brown et al. reduced their complication rate from 35% to 15% with the use of Luque segmental instrumentation and the elimination of postoperative immobilization.

Frequent pulmonary complications in patients with spinal muscular atrophy require respiratory support for a longer than normal period after surgery and rapid mobilization when possible. Patients with spinal muscular atrophy may be especially sensitive to medications that depress the respiratory centers, and the use of these drugs in the postoperative period should be minimal. Lonstein and Renshaw found that patients with forced vital capacity of less than 20% of that predicted are at great risk for postoperative death. A vigorous preoperative and postoperative physical therapy program is mandatory.

The patient and the family should be warned of the possibility of some loss of function after spinal instrumentation and fusion. A flexible spine allows a weak trunk to collapse forward to increase the reach of the upper extremity. Also, flexibility of the spine and extremities allows the center of gravity to be placed where weak muscles have the best mechanical advantage. Spinal fusion creates a longer lever arm that weak hip muscles are unable to control. Gross motor activities, such as transfers, rolling, bathing, dressing, and toileting, have been noted to decline after spinal fusion. This loss of function, however, must be weighed against the predicted functional loss and pulmonary compromise from severe, untreated spinal deformity. During the long, progressive course of this disease, the advantages of a stable trunk far outweigh the disadvantages.

FAMILIAL DYSAUTONOMIA

Familial dysautonomia (Riley-Day syndrome), first described in 1949, is a rare autosomal recessive disorder found mostly in Jewish children of Eastern European extraction. Its clinical features include absence of overflow tears and sweating, vasomotor instability that often leads to hyperthermia, and relative indifference to pain. Other frequent findings include episodic hypertension, postural hypotension, transient blotching of the skin, hyperhidrosis, episodic vomiting, disordered swallowing, dysarthria, and motor incoordination. Death is caused most often by pulmonary disease. Scoliosis is the major orthopaedic problem in patients with this disease. The scoliosis may be progressive and may be large enough to contribute to early death because of kyphoscoliotic cardiopulmonary decompensation. Kyphosis also is a frequent sagittal plane deformity in these patients. If surgery for the scoliosis is considered, however, features of the syndrome such as vasomotor and thermal instability can cause troublesome and sometimes fatal operative or postoperative complications. Brace treatment, although beneficial in some patients, often is complicated by the tendency for pressure ulcers to develop.

Posterior spinal fusion with instrumentation was required in 13 of 51 patients in the Israeli series of Kaplan et al. All children undergoing surgery had severe pulmonary problems. Intraoperative and postoperative respiratory and dysautonomic complications were frequent. Because of osteopenic bone, only minor improvement of the spinal deformity was possible, and a small loss of correction was common; however, those surviving noted a marked decrease in the frequency of pneumonia and, for some reason, an improvement in the degree of ataxia.

One technical problem in instrumenting these curves is the frequent occurrence of severe kyphosis combined with weak bone. Anterior procedures should be approached with caution because of the frequency of respiratory problems. Despite the significant dangers and high complication rates in patients with familial dysautonomia, surgery can be done successfully with proper precautions and can improve the quality of life.

ARTHROGRYPOSIS MULTIPLEX CONGENITA

Arthrogryposis multiplex congenita is a syndrome of persistent joint contractures that are present at birth. A myopathic subtype is characterized by muscle changes similar to those found in progressive muscular dystrophy. In the neuropathic subtype, anterior horn cells are reduced or absent in the cervical, thoracic, and lumbosacral segments of the spinal cord. In the third subtype, joint fibrosis and contractures alone are the main problems.

Scoliosis is common in patients with arthrogryposis multiplex congenita (20% to 66%). A single thoracolumbar curve is the predominant curve pattern. The scoliosis usually is detected at birth or within the first few years of life. Brace treatment rarely is successful and should be used only with small, flexible curves (<30 degrees) in patients who were ambulators. In patients who are nonambulatory or have a curve of more than 30 degrees, the brace is ineffective in controlling the curve. Rib-based distraction using the VEPTR has been reported to be effective in controlling scoliosis and kyphosis and maintaining thoracic growth in patients with arthrogryposis.

The onset of pelvic obliquity is a serious problem. If treatment of the pelvic obliquity by release of the contractures in the hip area does not halt progression of the curve, spinal fusion to the sacrum may be necessary. The onset of thoracic lordosis also requires prompt treatment. Because of the severity and rigidity of the curves, postoperative complications are frequent. The connective tissue is tough, and the bones are osteoporotic. An average blood loss of 2000 mL has been reported, and Herron et al. obtained a

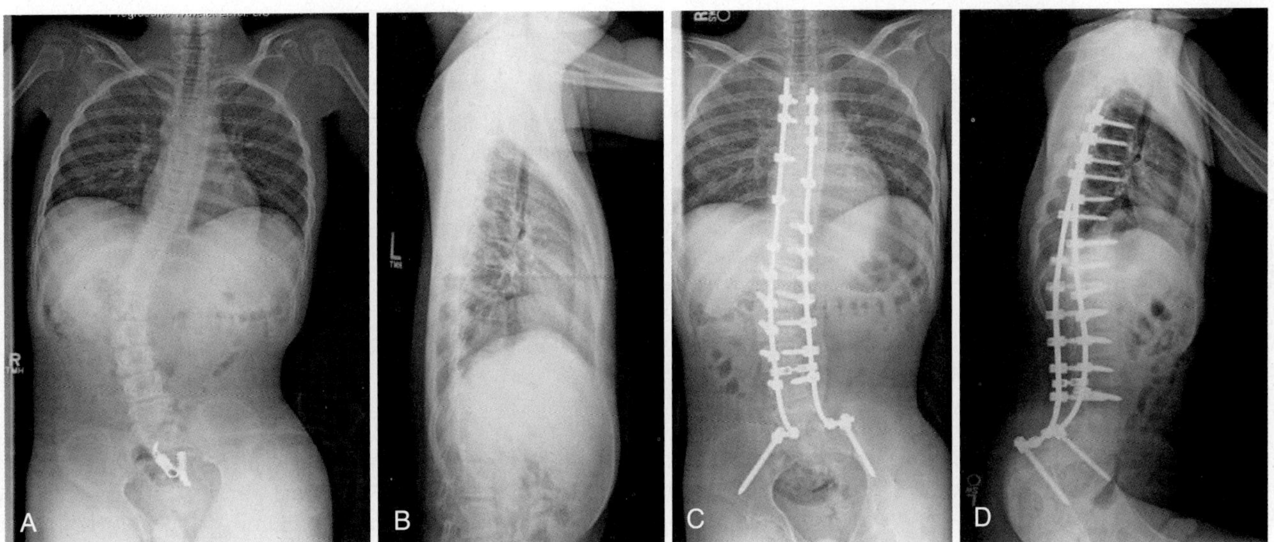

FIGURE 8.120 **A** and **B**, Progressive scoliosis in patient with Duchenne muscular dystrophy. **C** and **D**, After fusion with Luque rod instrumentation.

maximal correction of only about 25% with Harrington instrumentation and posterior fusion. Combined anterior and posterior spinal arthrodesis can be considered for these patients to allow better correction and circumferential arthrodesis, but posterior segmental instrumentation is preferred. If patients have less than 90 degrees of passive flexion of the hip, caution should be exercised in extending spinal arthrodesis to the pelvis because this is likely to make sitting difficult.

DUCHENNE MUSCULAR DYSTROPHY

Duchenne muscular dystrophy is an inherited X-linked recessive condition caused by a frameshift mutation in the dystrophin gene at the Xp21.2 locus of the X chromosome. The clinical course is one of progressive weakness, loss of the ability to walk at 10 to 14 years of age, and eventual wheelchair dependence. Death from pulmonary or cardiac compromise usually occurs in the second or third decade of life. Scoliosis develops in most patients with Duchenne muscular dystrophy, although the use of corticosteroids may decrease the development of spinal deformity in these patients. Before steroids were used in Duchenne patients, scoliosis developed in more than 90%; since steroid use began, the rate has fallen to only 10% to 20% (Fig. 8.120). A review of the Nationwide Inpatient Sample from 2001 to 2012 demonstrated a significant decrease in the rate of scoliosis surgery in patients with Duchenne muscular dystrophy. Lebel et al. reported that only 20% of their patients receiving steroids went on to undergo spinal fusion, but 90% of patients not receiving steroids had spinal fusions.

Spinal deformity usually occurs after the patient becomes confined to a wheelchair, although very early scoliosis has been detected in some ambulatory patients. The curves are predominantly long thoracolumbar curves with pelvic obliquity, the collapse of which is caused by absence of muscles and not by asymmetric muscle activity or contracture. Once a curve develops, it generally is progressive and cannot be controlled by braces or wheelchair seating systems. In patients with Duchenne muscular dystrophy, pulmonary function deteriorates approximately 4% each year after the age of 12 years. When the forced vital capacity decreases to less than 35%, surgery may result in significant pulmonary problems postoperatively. Patients with Duchenne muscular dystrophy have reduced cardiac function that may alter the anesthetic management. Hypotensive anesthesia to minimize blood loss may not be possible. Increased intraoperative blood loss is commonly seen in patients with Duchenne muscular dystrophy. This may be due to having to dissect through dystrophic and fibrotic muscle, loss of vasoconstriction of blood vessels from the absence of dystrophin, and altered platelet function.

Lonstein and Renshaw's indications for spinal fusion in patients with Duchenne muscular dystrophy are curves of more than 30 degrees, forced vital capacity of more than 30% of normal, and prognosis of at least 2 years of life remaining. Because the scoliosis invariably increases, many authors recommended spinal fusion at the onset of the deformity in patients who use a wheelchair full time even when the curves are as small as 20 degrees or less. In decision making, the patient's pulmonary function probably is just as important as the size of the curve. The vital capacity should be 40% to 50% of normal. If the curve is allowed to progress beyond 30 to 40 degrees, the forced vital capacity can be less than 40% of predicted normal. Most patients with Duchenne muscular dystrophy generally have a forced vital capacity of 50% to 70% of normal when they begin to use a wheelchair full time. Surgery is recommended during the first few years of full-time wheelchair use, when the patient almost always has a small, flexible curve and little or no pelvic obliquity but still has a forced vital capacity of 40% or more. Suk et al. found that surgery in patients who had Duchenne muscular dystrophy with scoliosis improved function and decreased the deterioration of forced vital capacity compared with patients treated conservatively; however, the muscle power and forced vital capacity continued to decrease in both groups.

Treatment of scoliosis in patients with Duchenne muscular dystrophy consists of segmental instrumentation with sublaminar wires or cables, hooks, or pedicle screws and fusion from T2 to the pelvis. In patients with smaller curves and no fixed pelvic obliquity, the fusion and instrumentation can end at L5. If fixed pelvic obliquity is more than 15 degrees, fusion to the pelvis with iliac screw or S-rod pelvic fixation is indicated. Correction of pelvic obliquity is reported to be more certain with instrumentation and fusion to the sacrum in larger curves (average, 61 degrees), and better maintenance of correction of pelvic obliquity has been reported in patients who had fusions that extended to the pelvis than in patients in whom the distal extent of fusion was in the lumbar spine. The fusion should extend to the high upper thoracic spine (T2), to prevent proximal or junctional kyphosis. The sagittal contours of the spine, especially lumbar lordosis, should be maintained for sitting balance and pressure distribution. Bone-bank allograft is needed because a large amount of bone graft will be necessary to obtain a solid fusion. Because of the pulmonary compromise in these patients, rapid postoperative mobilization is important. When segmental spinal instrumentation is used, postoperative bracing usually is not necessary.

Lonstein and Renshaw listed the following benefits of spinal fusion in patients with Duchenne muscular dystrophy: preserves sitting balance, prevents back pain, improves spinal decompensation, frees the arms of the necessity of trunk support, improves body image, and possibly slows the deterioration of pulmonary function. However, the rate of decline of forced vital capacity is not changed by preventing scoliosis with spinal fusion. The use of corticosteroids in patients with Duchenne muscular dystrophy has been shown to prolong the time that patients are able to walk. The use of corticosteroids also has a positive effect on the prevention of spinal deformity.

VARIANTS OF MUSCULAR DYSTROPHY OTHER THAN DUCHENNE TYPE

Spinal curvature in association with non–Duchenne muscular dystrophy is uncommon. The occurrence of scoliosis in patients with non–Duchenne muscular dystrophy depends on the specific type of dystrophic disease, and the prognosis is related to the severity of the primary problem. For instance, Siegel found that childhood dystrophia myotonica is not associated with spinal curvature. Facioscapulohumeral dystrophy is more rapidly progressive when the onset occurs in childhood. Frequently, it also is asymmetric in distribution, and structural scoliosis can occur. None of the 11 patients described by Daher et al. had pelvic obliquity. Thoracic lordosis was present in 36% of their patients, all of whom developed poor vital capacity and shortness of breath. The use of an orthosis during the juvenile years controlled the curve until the pubertal growth spurt, when progression occurred. The brace should not be used, however, when a thoracic lordosis exists. Spinal fusion is effective in maintaining correction and preventing curve progression in these patients.

CONGENITAL SCOLIOSIS

Congenital scoliosis is a lateral curvature of the spine caused by the presence of vertebral anomalies that result in an imbalance of the longitudinal growth of the spine.

BOX 8.7

Classification of Congenital Scoliosis

- Failure of formation
  Partial failure of formation (wedge vertebra)
  Complete failure of formation (hemivertebra)
- Failure of segmentation
  Unilateral failure of segmentation (unilateral unsegmented bar)
  Bilateral failure of segmentation (block vertebra)
- Miscellaneous

The prevalence rate of congenital scoliosis is thought to be approximately 1 in 1000 live births. The critical time in the development of the spine embryologically is the fifth to sixth week—the time of segmentation processes—and congenital anomalies of the spine develop during the first 6 weeks of intrauterine life. Some type of anomaly must be visible on the radiographs of the spine before a diagnosis of congenital scoliosis can be made. Because congenital scoliosis often is rigid and correction can be difficult, it is important to detect these curves early and to institute appropriate treatment while the curve is small rather than to attempt salvage-type procedures that are necessary when the deformity is severe.

A specific cause for congenital scoliosis has not been identified. Evidence suggests a role for both genetic and environmental factors such as hypoxia, alcohol use, valproic acid, and hyperthermia during the prenatal period. Researchers hypothesize that environmental factors affect the delivery of genetic instructions during the critical stages of development of the spine, resulting in vertebral anomalies. A family of genes referred to as the homeobox, or HOX, genes have been shown to direct and regulate the processes of embryonic differentiation and segmentation of the axial skeleton. Loder et al. suggested that environmental factors, such as low oxygen tension, may modulate the expression of the sonic hedgehog or homeobox genes that are involved in normal vertebral segmentation. However, the etiology of most congenital scoliosis cases cannot be determined by a history.

CLASSIFICATION

Classification of congenital scoliosis is based on the abnormal embryologic development of the spine and the type of vertebral anomaly. Then it is further classified by the site at which the anomaly occurs. The classification proposed by MacEwen et al. and later modified by Winter, Moe, and Eilers is the one most uniformly accepted (Box 8.7; Figs. 8.121 and 8.122). The vertebral anomalies may be caused by a failure of formation or a failure of segmentation, or by a combination of these two factors, resulting in a mixed deformity. The congenital curve also should be classified according to the area of the spine involved because this is indicative of the prognosis of the specific deformity. The areas generally distinguished are the cervicothoracic spine, thoracic spine, thoracolumbar spine, lumbar spine, and lumbosacral spine. The purpose of this classification is to distinguish curves with a poor prognosis that may require early intervention

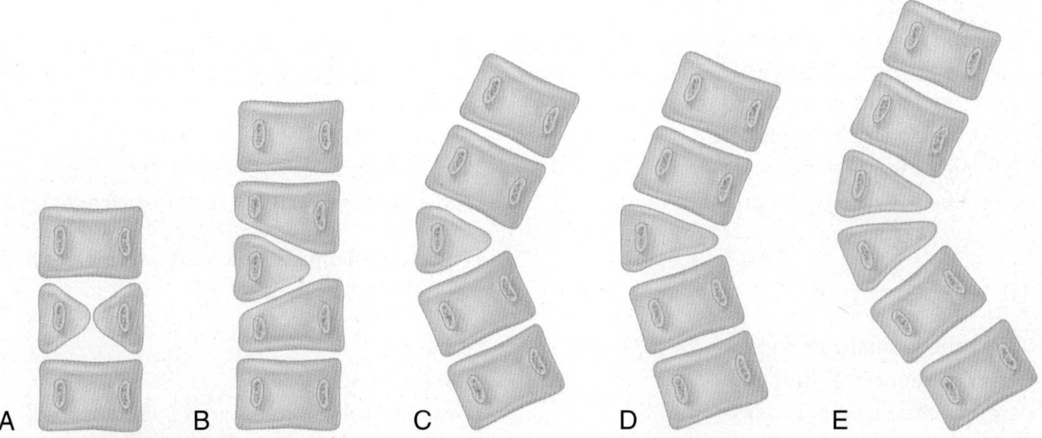

FIGURE 8.121 Defects of formation. **A,** Anterior central defect. **B,** Incarcerated hemivertebra. **C,** Free hemivertebra. **D,** Wedge vertebra. **E,** Multiple hemivertebrae.

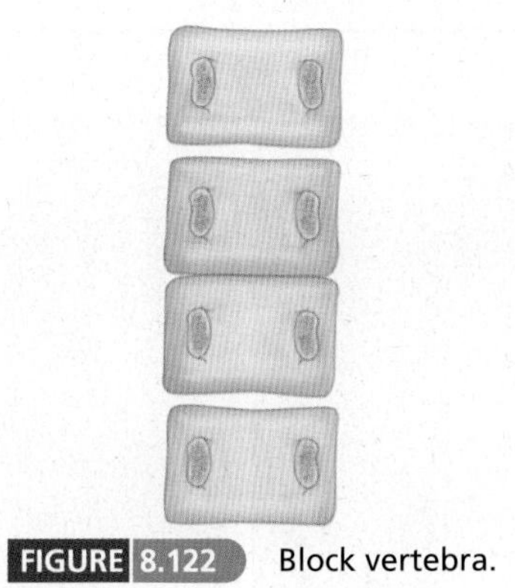

FIGURE 8.122 Block vertebra.

from curves that have a more benign natural history that may be observed. Kawakami et al. recommended a three-dimensional classification based on three-dimensional CT images. They found that congenital spinal deformity could be classified into four types: type I, solitary simple; type 2, multiple simple; type 3, complex; and type 4, segmentation failure (Table 8.6).

PATIENT EVALUATION

In addition to the routine spinal evaluation, some specific physical findings should be sought in patients with congenital scoliosis. The skin of the back should be carefully examined for signs such as hair patches, lipomas, dimples, and scars, which may indicate an underlying anomalous vertebra or spinal cord anomalies. The neurologic evaluation should be thorough. Evidence of neurologic involvement, such as clubfoot, calf atrophy, absent reflexes, and atrophy of one lower extremity compared with the other, should be noted carefully. Many children with congenital scoliosis have other anomalies.

Neural axis abnormalities are present in up to 35% of patients. Congenital heart disease has been reported to be present in 25% to 54% of patients with congenital scoliosis. Patients who are undergoing surgery for congenital scoliosis should have a screening echocardiogram and evaluation by a cardiologist. Genitourinary anomalies have been reported in 20% to 40% of patients with congenital scoliosis. A renal ultrasound remains the standard for urologic screening in these patients, but also may be evaluated on MRI if this is being obtained for other reasons. MacEwen, Winter, and Hardy emphasized the importance of a complete evaluation of the genitourinary system: 18% of their patients had urologic anomalies, including 2.5% who had obstructive disease that could be life-threatening. Other musculoskeletal anomalies also occur frequently in association with congenital spine anomalies (Figs. 8.123 and 8.124).

A high-quality series of routine radiographs is essential to evaluate the deformity. The congenital curve should be classified as a failure of segmentation or a failure of formation, and the radiographs should be examined carefully for any evidence of widening of the pedicles or midline bony defects that may indicate an underlying cord anomaly.

Probably more important than classification of the curve is an analysis of the growth potential of the curve to better determine the possibility of curve progression. All congenital curves should be carefully measured with the Cobb technique, including compensatory or secondary curves in seemingly normal parts of the spine. Measurements should include each end of the anomalous area, as well as each end of the entire curve generally considered for treatment. CT and MRI have allowed us to better study the spinal anatomy and to screen for spinal dysraphism (Fig. 8.124). There is a high risk of congenital intraspinal anomalies in patients with congenital scoliosis and a lack of cutaneous manifestations in a significant number of patients. MRI during infancy may help delineate the anatomic deformity, which may not be visible on plain radiographs, and also better delineates the physis. The prevalence rate of spinal dysraphism on MRI examination approaches 43% in patients with congenital spinal deformities.

NATURAL HISTORY

Progression of congenital scoliosis is dependent on the type and location of the vertebral anomaly. Curve progression occurs more rapidly during the first 5 years of life and during the adolescent growth spurt. These two periods represent the most rapid stages of spinal growth. Analysis of the growth status is the most important factor in predicting the possibility of progression of these congenital deformities. Dubousset et al.

TABLE 8.6

Algorithm for Evaluating Congenital Spinal Deformities

Step 1	Count the number of vertebral anomalies	Solitary or multiple
Step 2	Detect the abnormal formation	(+), (−), or (±)
Step 3	Determine the site of abnormal formation	Anterior or posterior, or both
Step 4	Determine the type of abnormal formation	Anterior: hemivertebra, anterior wedge, lateral wedge, butterfly Posterior: bilamina (wedged), incomplete bilamina, hemilamina Spina bifida
Step 5	Detect the mismatched formation	(+) or (−)
Step 6	Detect the abnormal formation	(+), (−), or (±)
Step 7	Determine the type of segmentation	Anterior: fully segmented, semisegmented, nonsegmented Posterior: fully segmented, semisegmented, nonsegmented
Step 8	Determine the site of abnormal segmentation	Anterior, unilateral, or posterior, or all
Step 9	Detect the discordant segmentation	(+) or (−)

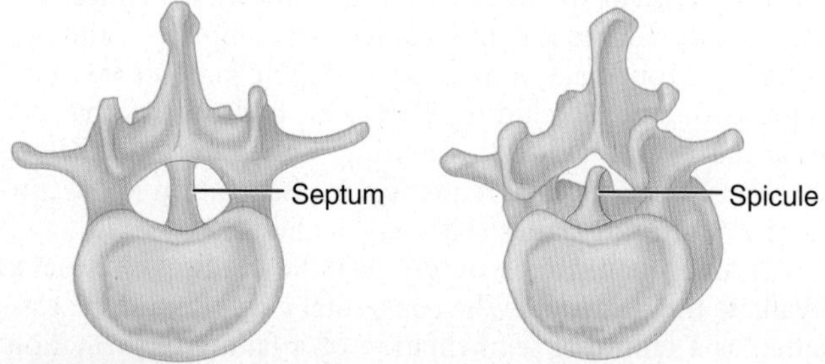

FIGURE 8.123 Diastematomyelia spicule invaginates dura and divides spinal cord, either partially or completely.

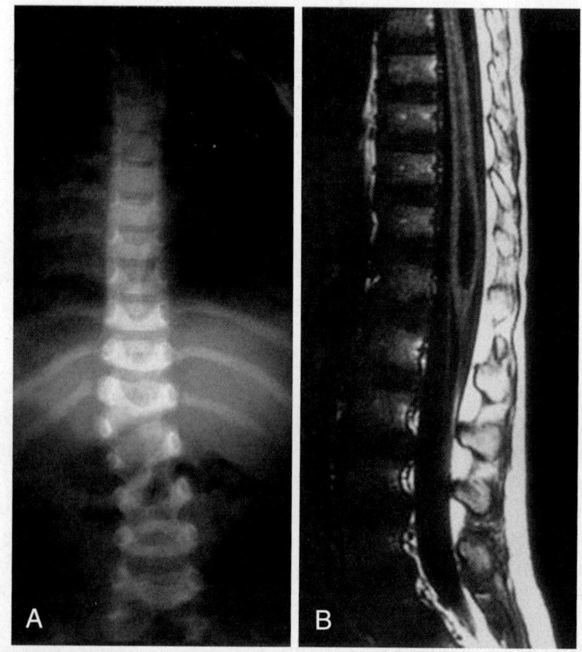

FIGURE 8.124 **A,** Congenital scoliosis with hemivertebrae. **B,** MRI shows occult syrinx extending from C4 to the conus. (From Prahinski JR, Polly DW Jr, McHale K, Ellenbogen RG: Occult intraspinal anomalies in congenital scoliosis, *J Pediatr Orthop* 20:59, 2000.)

emphasized the importance of considering growth of the spinal canal in three dimensions (Fig. 8.125). Analysis of the potential growth on both sides of the curve will help with the prognosis. For example, if normal convex growth is expected and deficient concave growth is likely, major deformity will occur (Fig. 8.126); however, if growth is deficient on both the convex and concave sides, progressive lateral deformity may not occur. If both sides are deficient in growth potential over many levels, shortening of the trunk may occur without lateral curvature.

The deformity produced by a failure of formation is much more difficult to predict than that caused by failure of segmentation. A hemivertebra produces scoliosis through an enlarging wedge on the affected side of the spine, whereas a unilateral unsegmented bar retards growth on the affected side. The growth imbalance in patients with hemivertebrae is not as severe as in those with unilateral unsegmented bars. A hemivertebra can exist tucked into the spine between adjacent normal vertebrae without causing a corresponding deformity. Winter called this an "incarcerated hemivertebra." When the hemivertebra is separated from either of the adjacent vertebrae by a disc, it is a segmented hemivertebra with two functioning physes on either side and is likely to cause a slowly progressive curve (Fig. 8.127). If the hemivertebra has only one adjacent disc and is fused to an adjacent vertebra, this is called a semisegmented hemivertebra, and if there are no adjacent discs associated with a hemivertebra, this is termed a nonsegmented hemivertebra and it has little growth potential.

Several excellent studies have outlined the natural history of congenital scoliosis and have found that the rate of deterioration and the ultimate severity of the curve depend on both the type of anomaly and the site at which it occurs. The most progressive of all anomalies is a concave, unilateral unsegmented bar with a convex hemivertebra (Fig. 8.128). The mean rate of curve progression is 6 to 7 degrees per year before 10 years of age. The majority of curves will exceed 50 degrees by 2 years of age. Second in severity is a unilateral unsegmented

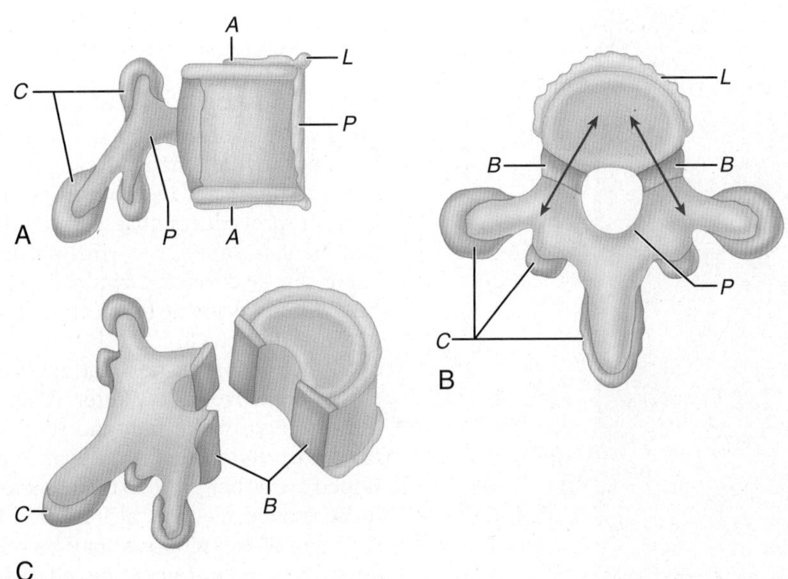

FIGURE 8.125 Vertebral growth. **A,** Body endplates (superior and inferior; labeled as *A*). **B,** Neurocentral cartilage (bipolar) fusion at age 7 or 8 years (labeled as *B*). **C,** Posterior elements cartilage (labeled as *C*). *L*, Ring apophysis (begins at age 7 to 9 years, closed at age 14 to 24 years); *P*, periosteum. (Redrawn from Dubousset J, Katti E, Seringe R: Epiphysiodesis of the spine in young children for congenital spinal deformations, *J Pediatr Orthop* B 1:123, 1993.)

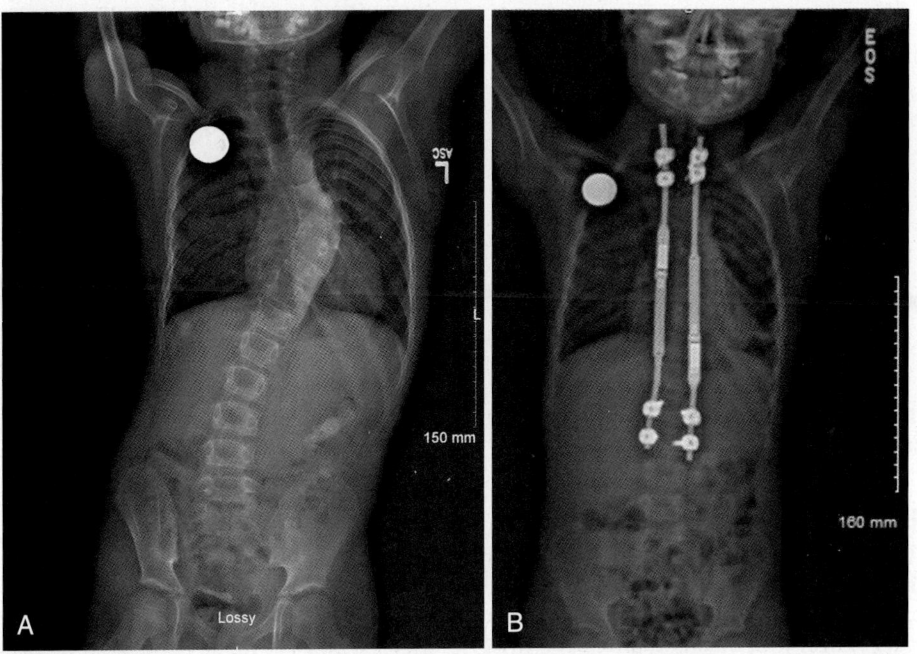

FIGURE 8.126 **A,** Eight-year-old boy with congenital scoliosis. Deficient concave growth has resulted in major deformity. **B,** After insertion of MAGEC growing rods.

bar. A mean of three vertebrae usually are affected. The mean rate of curve progression is 5 degrees per year, with the curve exceeding 50 degrees by 10 years of age and 70 degrees by skeletal maturity. Next in severity of risk of progression is a double convex hemivertebra. These curves usually progress at 3 to 4 degrees per year, with most exceeding 50 degrees by 10 years of age and exceeding 70 degrees by skeletal maturity. A fully segmented hemivertebra will progress relatively slowly, at 1 or 2 degrees per year. For each type of anomaly, the rate of deterioration usually is less severe if the abnormality is in the upper thoracic region, more severe in the thoracic region, and most severe in the thoracolumbar region (Fig. 8.129). The rate of deterioration of the curve is not constant, but if the curve is present before the patient is 10 years of age, it usually increases, especially during the adolescent growth spurt. The least severe scoliosis is caused by a block vertebra.

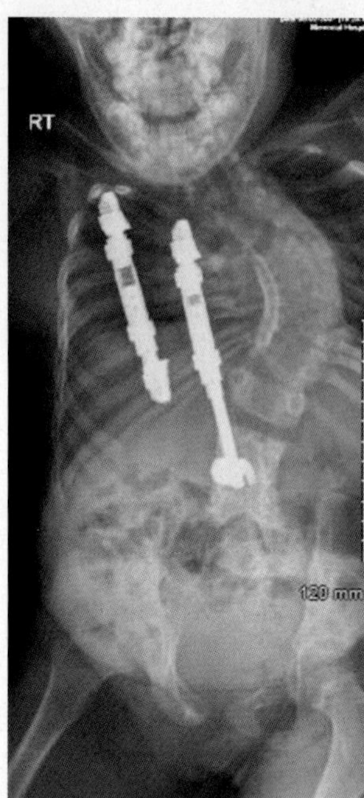

FIGURE 8.127 Progression of deformity in a 5-year-old girl with arthrogryposis and a large unsegmented bar treated with rib-based distraction.

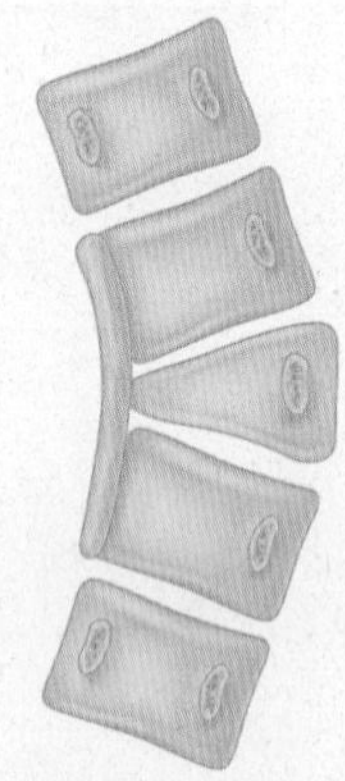

FIGURE 8.128 Unilateral and unsegmented bar with contralateral hemivertebra.

NONOPERATIVE TREATMENT

Nonoperative treatment is of limited value in patients with congenital scoliosis. Nonprogressive curves require regular observation during periods of rapid growth (0 to 5 years of age and 10 to 15 years of age) with quality radiographs twice a year. Observation also is helpful in patients with multiple anomalies in whom the prognosis is difficult to determine.

Bracing sometimes can be used to control secondary curves when the primary congenital curve is being treated nonoperatively. Also, bracing may prevent progression of a secondary curve that is causing balance problems. If orthotic treatment is elected, careful measurement and comparison of spine radiographs at 6-month intervals must be made. Because of the slow progression of some curves, it is important to compare current radiographs with all previous films, including the original films, to detect curve progression. Demirkiran et al. reported that serial derotational casting was a safe and effective time-buying strategy to delay surgical intervention in patients with congenital spine deformities.

OPERATIVE TREATMENT

Because 75% of congenital curves are progressive, surgery remains the fundamental treatment. Congenital spinal deformity can be treated by procedures that prevent further deformity or procedures that correct the present deformity. If treatment is aimed at correcting the present deformity, the curve can be corrected gradually or immediately. The surgical methods available for treatment of congenital scoliosis are outlined in Box 8.8.

Whether or not to treat any associated diastematomyelia is controversial. Winter et al. advocated resection of the osseous spicule first and reoperation in 3 to 6 months for deformity correction. Ayvaz et al. and Shen et al. questioned whether a diastematomyelic abnormality needs to be treated. Feng et al. reported that an osseous spur at the apex of the scoliosis may be related to a higher risk of developing a neurologic deficit, especially in patients with kyphotic deformity. When neurosurgical intervention is needed, the deformity correction can be safely performed simultaneously.

■ POSTERIOR FUSION WITHOUT INSTRUMENTATION

In situ fusion allows for stabilization of a curve that has shown documented progression or is predicted to progress. It is ideally done early for small curves to prevent the curve from becoming unacceptably large. A controversy with in situ fusion is whether a combined anterior and posterior fusion is required. Posterior fusion alone can control curve progression, but if there is significant anterior growth in the involved vertebra, progression of the deformity may occur in some young children owing to the crankshaft phenomenon. If anterior fusion is needed, then this may be performed either through an anterior open technique, thoracoscopically, or with a posterior approach through the pedicles. In situ fusion for unilateral unsegmented bars usually only includes the involved vertebra. One level cephalad and one level caudad to the involved vertebrae are included in the fusion.

The basic posterior spinal fusion technique is described in Technique 8.6. Postoperatively, a corrective cast or brace is used for immobilization. Smaller-sized implants that are appropriate for the patient's size can be used for stabilization of in situ fusion and decrease the time needed for a cast or brace.

■ POSTERIOR FUSION WITH INSTRUMENTATION

The advantages of instrumentation in congenital scoliosis are that slightly more correction can be obtained, the rate of pseudarthrosis can be reduced somewhat, and the need for a postoperative cast or brace is less. Congenital scoliosis is the condition in which paraplegia occurs most often after instrumentation. The risk of neurologic injury can be lowered but not eliminated with careful preoperative evaluation by myelography or MRI, by intraoperative spinal cord monitoring with somatosensory-evoked potentials and motor-evoked potentials, and by the routine use of the wake-up test. Instrumentation does not alter the length of the fusion or the necessity for facet fusion, decortications, or abundant bone graft (Box 8.9).

No treatment required
May require spinal fusion
Requires spinal fusion
* Too few or no curves

Site of curvature	Type of congenital anomaly					
	Block vertebra	Wedged vertebra	Hemivertebrae: Single	Hemivertebrae: Double	Unilateral unsegmented bar	Unilateral unsegmented bar and contralateral hemivertebrae
Upper thoracic	< 1° – 1°	* – 2°	1° – 2°	2° – 2.5°	2° – 4°	5° – 6°
Lower thoracic	< 1° – 1°	1° – 2°	2° – 2.5°	2° – 3°	5° – 6.5°	6° – 7°
Thoracolumbar	< 1° – 1°	1.5° – 2°	2° – 3.5°	5° – *	6° – 9°	> 10° – *
Lumbar	< 1° – *	< 1° – *	< 1° – 1°	*	> 5° – *	*
Lumbosacral	*	*	< 1° – 1.5°	*	*	*

FIGURE 8.129 Median yearly rate of deterioration without treatment for each type of single congenital scoliosis in each region of spine. Numbers on left in each column refer to patients seen before 10 years of age; numbers on right refer to patients seen at age 10 years or older.

BOX 8.8

Treatment of Congenital Scoliosis

- Prevention of future deformity
  In situ fusion
- Correction of deformity—gradual
  Hemiepiphysiodesis and hemiarthrodesis
  Growing rod nonfusion
  Vertical expandable prosthetic titanium rib
- Correction of deformity—acute
  Instrumentation and fusion
  Hemivertebra excision
  Vertebral column resection
  Osteotomy

BOX 8.9

Common Errors in Instrumentation in Patients with Congenital Scoliosis

- Use of rods in small children in whom the bone structure is not strong enough to add any stability
- Excessive distraction leading to paralysis
- Failure to preoperatively evaluate for a tethered cord or other intraspinal abnormalities
- Failure to do a wake-up test after rod insertion
- Failure to perform adequate fusion because of reliance on internal stability
- Failure to supplement the instrumentation with adequate external immobilization

COMBINED ANTERIOR AND POSTERIOR FUSIONS

The main indications for anterior and posterior fusions instead of isolated posterior fusion are to treat sagittal plane problems, to increase the flexibility of the scoliosis by discectomy, to eliminate the anterior physis to prevent bending or torsion of the fusion mass with further growth (crankshaft phenomenon), and to treat curves with a significant potential for progression. The anterior procedure consists of removal of the disc, cartilage endplates, and bony endplates. Bone graft in the form of bone chips is placed into the disc space for fusion. Anterior instrumentation usually is not used. The spine is exposed on the convex side, but the approach is dictated by the level of the curve. The anterior fusion can be done through an open anterior approach or thoracoscopically. After the anterior fusion, a posterior procedure is done, with or without instrumentation. The postoperative management is the same as after posterior fusion with or without instrumentation. Dubousset et al. recommended anterior and posterior fusions in young patients who are fused at the lumbar level before Risser grade 0 and who have significant residual deformity of 30 and 10 degrees of rotation. For thoracic curves, the amount of crankshaft effect that can be tolerated is weighed against the risks of the thoracotomy necessary to perform the anterior epiphysiodesis.

TRANSPEDICULAR CONVEX ANTERIOR HEMIEPIPHYSIODESIS AND POSTERIOR ARTHRODESIS

King et al. described a technique of transpedicular convex anterior hemiepiphysiodesis combined with posterior arthrodesis for treatment of progressive congenital scoliosis. In effect, a combined anterior and posterior fusion can be done through a single posterior approach. These authors reported arrest of curve progression in all nine of their patients after this procedure. The average age of patients at surgery was 9 years. Their technique is based on the work of Michel and Krueger, who described a transpedicular approach to the vertebral body, and Heinig, who described the "eggshell" procedure, so called because the vertebral body is hollowed out until it is eggshell thin before it is collapsed. King et al. found the pedicle dimensions to be adequate for this technique even in infants; however, they recommended preoperative CT through the center of each pedicle to be included in the epiphysiodesis.

TECHNIQUE 8.35

(KING)

- Position the patient prone on a radiolucent operating table, with a frame or chest rolls. After preparation and draping, obtain a radiograph over a skin marker to identify the appropriate level for the incision.
- Make a single midline posterior incision and retract the paraspinous muscles on both sides of the curve as far as the tips of the costotransverse processes in the thoracic spine and lateral to the facet joints in the lumbar spine.
- Remove the cortical bone in the area of the pedicle to be mined caudad to the facet joint and at the base of the costotransverse process in the thoracic spine.
- Use the curet to remove the cancellous bone. The medullary cavity of the pedicle can now be seen. The cortex medially indicates the boundary of the spinal canal, and caudally and cranially it indicates the margins of the intervertebral neural foramina. Use progressively larger curets until only the cortical rim of the pedicle remains (Fig. 8.130A). The pedicle margins then expand into the vertebral body.
- Remove cancellous bone, creating a hole in the lateral half of the vertebral body, and use curved curets to remove cancellous bone from the vertebral body in the cephalad and caudal directions until the endplate bone, the physis, and the intervertebral disc are encountered. Brisk bleeding may occur, and the surgeon should be prepared for it.
- For a single hemivertebra, mine the pedicle of the hemivertebra itself, along with that of the adjacent vertebrae in the cephalad and caudal directions (Fig. 8.130B). Communication with each pedicle hole across the physis and disc space is readily achieved (Fig. 8.130C).
- Pack autogenous bone from the iliac crest down the pedicles and across the vertebral endplates and discs.
- Posteriorly, excise the convex and concave facet joints and pack with cancellous bone. Carry out decortication bilaterally.
- Use autologous iliac crest bone graft or allograft bone graft.
- If internal fixation is needed, a wire, compression device, or pedicle screw device can be used.

POSTOPERATIVE CARE The patient is placed in a TLSO for 4 to 6 months. After that, no further immobilization is used.

COMBINED ANTERIOR AND POSTERIOR CONVEX HEMIEPIPHYSIODESIS (GROWTH ARREST)

Gradual correction of congenital scoliosis may be obtained through the use of a convex hemiepiphysiodesis. This technique is used for curves that are the result of failure of formation. There is no role for this technique in failures of segmentation. Correction of deformity relies on the future growth of the spine on the concave side. In deformities caused by failure of segmentation, there is really no growth potential on the concave side. This technique is best for treating a single hemivertebra that has not resulted in a large curve at the time of surgery. This technique is appropriate in children younger than 5 years who meet certain criteria: a documented progressive curve, a curve of less than 50 degrees, a curve of six segments or fewer, concave growth potential, and no pathologic congenital kyphosis or lordosis. Even if the concave side ceases to grow, the anterior and posterior fusions obtain a good result as far as stabilizing the curve. Epiphysiodesis of the entire curve, not merely the apical segment, should be done. Rigid spinal immobilization is used until the fusions are solid, usually at least 6 months after surgery.

Preoperative planning is important. Each vertebra should be considered a cube divided into four quadrants, with each quadrant growing symmetrically around the spinal canal (Fig. 8.131). When growth is unbalanced, the zones that must be fused to reestablish balanced growth are determined preoperatively. King et al. noted a true epiphysiodesis effect after transpedicular convex anterior hemiepiphysiodesis (see Technique 8.37) in four of their nine patients, all four of whom had a single hemivertebra. On the basis of these results, they recommended transpedicular hemiepiphysiodesis with posterior hemiarthrodesis in selected patients with a single hemivertebra. Demirkiran et al. reported that a convex growth arrest could be obtained with a posterior fusion and pedicle screw instrumentation at each involved level, with results similar to those of an anteroposterior convex hemiepiphysiodesis.

CONVEX ANTERIOR AND POSTERIOR HEMIEPIPHYSIODESES AND FUSION

TECHNIQUE 8.36

(WINTER)

- Place the patient in a straight lateral position with the convexity of the curve upward. Prepare and drape the back and side in the same field. The anterior approach technique varies according to the level to be fused (see Techniques 8.23 and 8.24). The posterior approach is a standard subperiosteal exposure (see Technique 8.6) but is always only on the convex side of the curve.
- Once the curve has been exposed, insert needles or other markers both anteriorly and posteriorly so that both are visible on one cross-table radiograph. Failure to place the fusion precisely in the proper area can lead to a poor result.

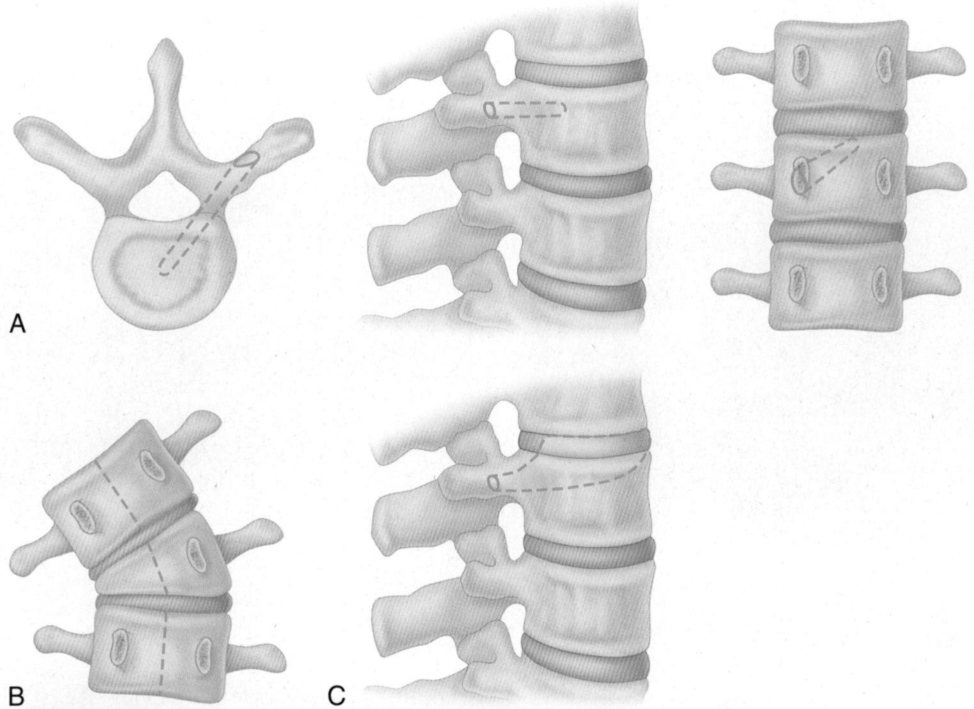

FIGURE 8.130 **A,** How pedicles are curetted. **B,** Anterior view of bone removed during "eggshell" procedure. **C,** Bone is almost completely hollowed out, and endplates and discs have been removed. **SEE TECHNIQUE 8.35.**

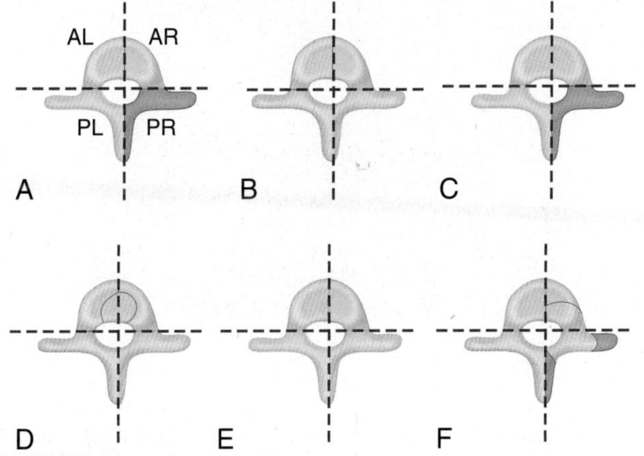

FIGURE 8.131 **A,** Vertebral growth on horizontal plane, four segments: *AL*, Anterior left; *AR*, anterior right; *PL*, posterior left; and *PR*, posterior right. **B,** Congenital posterior bar involving PL and PR; level of epiphysiodesis must be AL and AR. **C,** Anterior defect involving AL and AR; epiphysiodesis must involve PL and PR. **D,** Anterior excess of growth potential involving both AR and AL; epiphysiodesis must involve both AR and AL above and below. **E,** Congenital posterolateral bar involving PL only; epiphysiodesis must involve only AR. **F,** Excess (hemivertebra) growth involving only AR and part of PR; hemiepiphysiodesis must involve AR and PR. (Modified from Dubousset J, Katti E, Seringe R: Epiphysiodesis of spine in young children for congenital spinal deformation, *J Pediatr Orthop B* 1:23, 1992.)

- Once the proper area has been identified, incise the periosteum of the anterior vertebral bodies and peel it forward to the lateral edge of the anterior longitudinal ligament and backward to the base of the pedicle (Fig. 8.132A).
- Incise the annulus of the disc at its superior and inferior margins and remove the superficial portion of the nucleus pulposus.
- Carefully remove the cartilaginous endplates, which are thick in children, taking at least one third of the physes but never more than half.
- Once the cartilaginous endplates have been removed, remove the cortical bony endplate with a curet.
- Make a trough in the lateral side of the vertebral bodies (Fig. 8.132B) and lay the autogenous rib graft in the trough. Use cancellous bone to augment the autogenous rib graft. If autogenous rib is not available, use iliac or bone-bank bone.
- The posterior procedure consists of a standard, unilateral, subperiosteal exposure of the area to be fused (Fig. 8.132C).
- Excise the facet joints, remove any facet cartilage, decorticate the entire area, and apply a bone graft.
- Apply a corrective Risser cast while the child is still under anesthesia to avoid having to use a second anesthetic.

POSTOPERATIVE CARE Casting is continued for 6 months, and the cast is changed as frequently as necessary. Follow-up must be continued until the end of growth. Results may appear excellent for years but can deteriorate during the adolescent growth spurt.

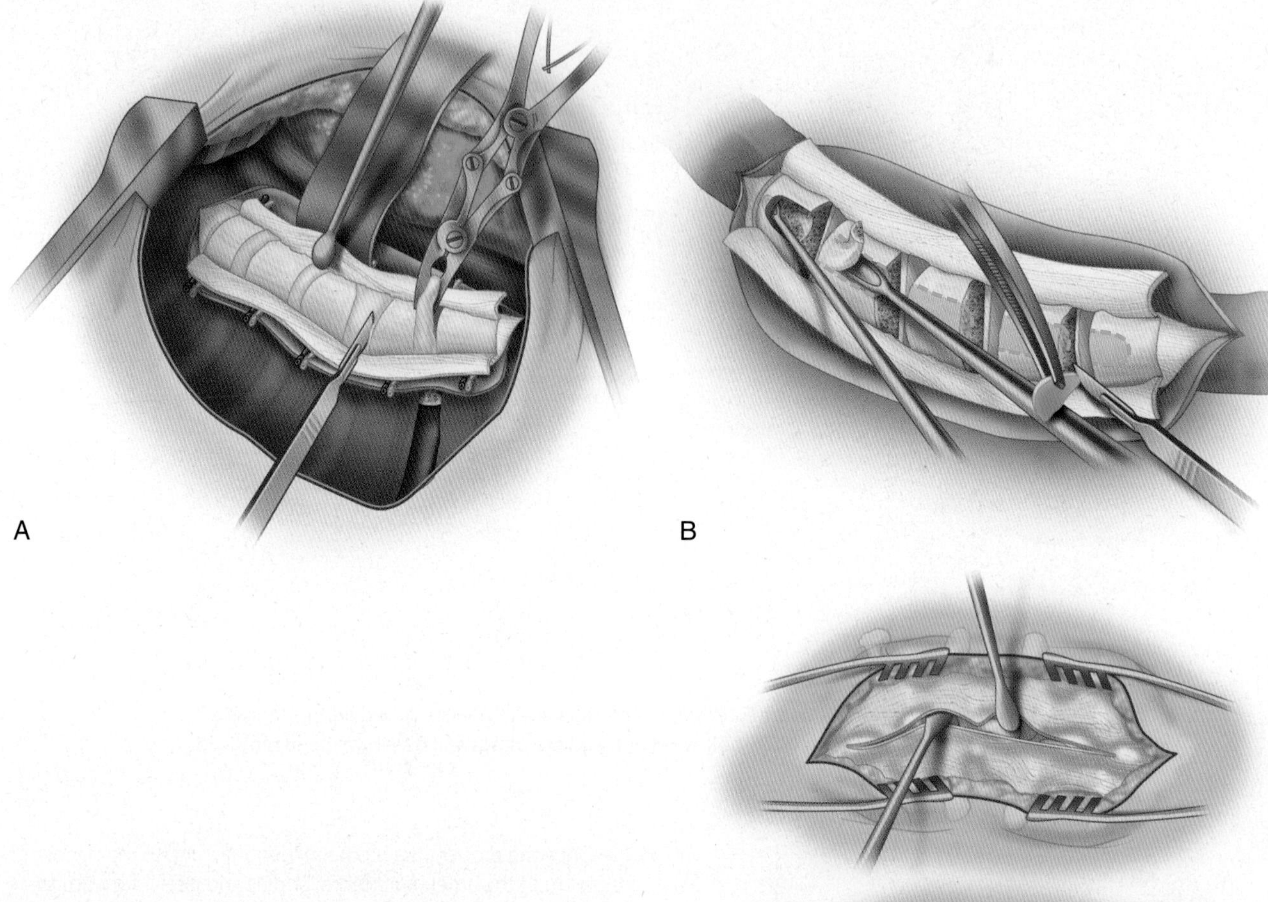

FIGURE 8.132 Combined anterior and posterior convex hemiepiphysiodesis. **A,** Periosteum of anterior vertebral bodies incised and peeled forward and backward. **B,** Trough created in lateral side of vertebral bodies. Autogenous rib graft placed in trough. **C,** Area to be fused exposed through standard, unilateral, subperiosteal exposure. Area is decorticated, and bone graft is applied. **SEE TECHNIQUE 8.36.**

Growing rods and VEPTR instrumentations that have been used to treat early-onset scoliosis also have been used for gradual correction and stabilization of progressive congenital curves. Several authors have reported good results with these techniques, with acceptable complication rates. The growing rod technique is suggested for patients with primary vertebral anomalies (Fig. 8.133); patients with rib fusion or associated thoracic insufficiency syndrome with congenital scoliosis usually are treated with a VEPTR.

HEMIVERTEBRA EXCISION

Hemivertebra excision can produce immediate correction of a congenital spine deformity. This technique will remove the cause of and prevent further worsening of the deformity. Hemivertebra excision usually is reserved for patients with pelvic obliquity or with fixed, lateral translation of the thorax that cannot be corrected by other means. At the lumbosacral area, excision of the hemivertebra can improve trunk imbalance. The L3, L4, or lumbosacral level, below the level of the conus medullaris, is the safest level at which to excise a hemivertebra. Hemivertebra excision in the thoracic area has more risk because this area of the spinal canal is the narrowest and has the least blood supply, but with spinal cord monitoring (somatosensory-evoked potentials and motor-evoked potentials) the excision can still be performed.

The curves best managed by hemivertebra excision are angular curves in which the hemivertebra is the apex. This technique has been reported mostly in lumbosacral hemivertebrae that produce lateral spinal decompensation in patients for whom curve-stabilizing techniques cannot achieve adequate alignment. Hemivertebra resection can be done at any age, but the optimal indication of hemivertebra resection is a patient younger than 5 years with a thoracolumbar, lumbar, or lumbosacral hemivertebra that is associated with truncal imbalance or a progressive curve. Chang et al. recommended early resection before structural changes occur above and below the hemivertebra. They also found that if resection was done before 6 years of age, the patients had significantly better

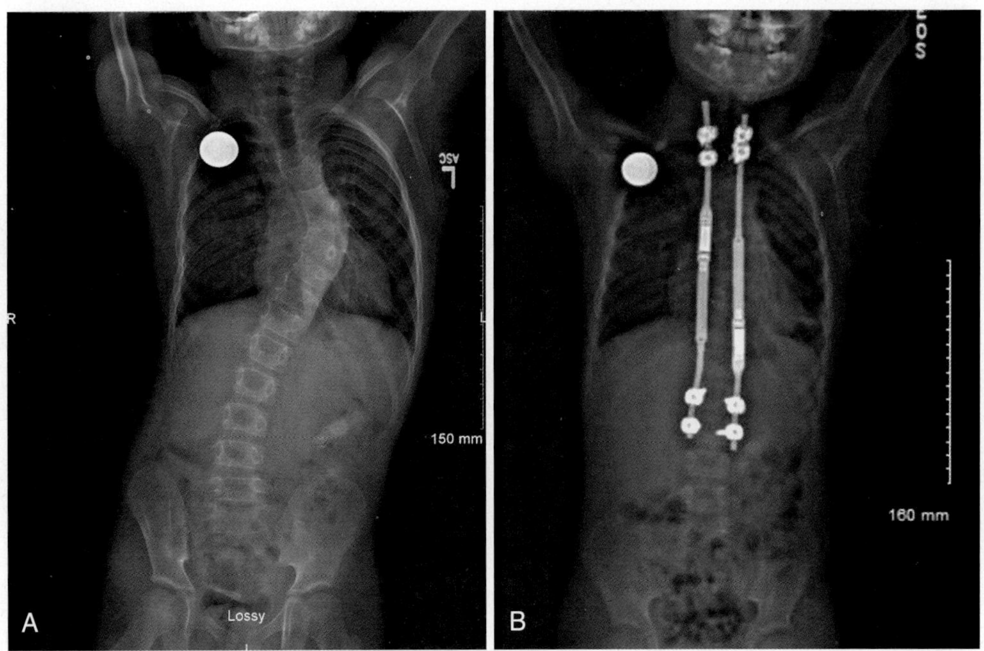

FIGURE 8.133 A, Eight-year-old boy with congenital scoliosis. B, After correction and insertion of MAGEC growing rods. **SEE TECHNIQUE 8.36.**

deformity correction and did not have any negative effects on the growth of the vertebral body or spinal canal compared with patients treated after 6 years of age. Yaszay et al. found that while hemivertebra resection had a higher complication rate than either hemiepiphysiodesis/in situ fusion or instrumented fusion without resection, posterior hemivertebra resection in younger patients resulted in a better percentage of correction than the other two techniques.

Hemivertebra excision should be considered a convex osteotomy at the apex of the curve. The entire curve front and back must be fused. Neurologic risk is inherent in hemivertebra excision because the spinal canal is entered both anteriorly and posteriorly.

Leatherman and Dickson recommended a two-stage procedure in which the vertebral body is removed through an anterior exposure; then, in a second stage, the posterior elements are removed and fusion is done. Other authors have reported acceptable results with one-stage anterior and posterior hemivertebra resection. The hemivertebra can be excised from a posterior-only technique as described by Ruf and Harms or through a costotransversectomy as described by Smith. In general, postoperative cast or brace immobilization is prescribed for 6 months. The use of instrumentation will give adequate fixation and may permit a brace to be worn rather than a cast, but the bone stock must be adequate to accept the instrumentation or a postoperative cast will be needed.

Heinig described a decancellation procedure done with curets through the pedicle. Lubicky recommended both internal fixation and external immobilization with this technique. He found that the amount of immediate correction from this technique was unpredictable, but it did generally lead to a hemiepiphysiodesis when it was combined with a convex posterior fusion at the same level. He recommended that the technique be done with C-arm control (Figs. 8.134A, B). Heinig and Lubicky advised leaving the hemilamina in place until the vertebral body resection is complete to protect the neural tube while the curet is used. This technique can be useful if the hemivertebra is located posteriorly next to the spinal canal, where seeing the hemivertebra from anteriorly can be difficult.

Hedequist, Emans, and Proctor described hemivertebra excision through a posterior approach (see Technique 8.6). With a discrete hemivertebra, the spinal cord or lumbar nerve roots are toward the concavity of the curve, while the hemivertebra is toward the convexity, placing the majority of the operation at a distance from the neural elements. Pedicle screw fixation may be tenuous in the thoracic spine of young children, and standard lumbar hooks should be placed on the rib above and below the excised hemivertebra, just lateral to the transverse process. These hooks are then attached with a rod and compressed across the ribs to achieve closure of the osteotomy while avoiding any compromise of the pedicle screws. The final rod can then be placed across the pedicle screws, and the temporary rib-to-rib rod removed.

HEMIVERTEBRA EXCISION: ANTEROPOSTERIOR APPROACH

TECHNIQUE 8.37

(HEDEQUIST AND EMANS)

- Place the patient in the lateral decubitus position for the simultaneous anteroposterior approach. The anterior approach is on the convex side and should be marked before surgery (Fig. 8.135A).
- For the anterior procedure, approach the spine through a standard transthoracic, transthoracic-retroperitoneal, or retroperitoneal approach, depending on the location

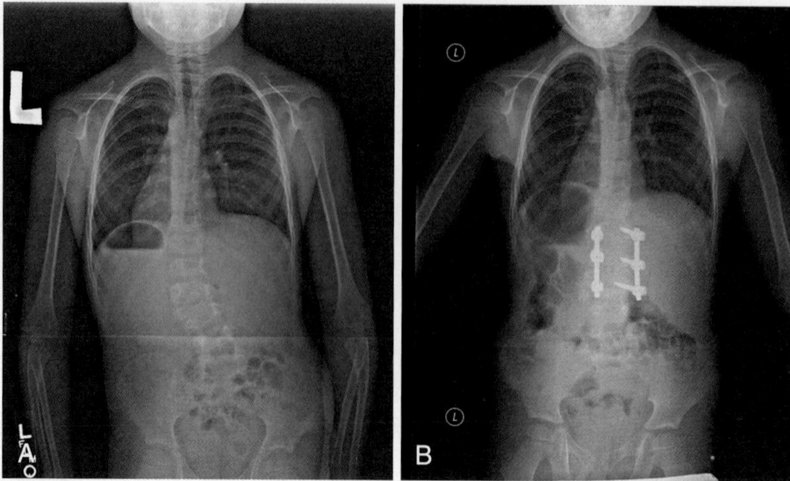

FIGURE 8.134 **A,** Congenital scoliosis in a 7-year-old boy. **B,** After hemivertebra excision and fusion with short-segment rods and pedicle screws.

of the hemivertebra. The only exposure needed is of the hemivertebra and the discs above and below it.

- For the posterior approach, make a standard posterior midline incision and carry the dissection out to the tips of the transverse process, taking care when dissecting over the areas of laminar deficiency.
- After the dissection is complete, obtain a spot radiograph or fluoroscopic view to confirm the appropriate level.

HEMIVERTEBRA EXCISION

- Begin the excision by dissecting over the edge of the transverse process and down the lateral wall of the body with a Cobb elevator and a curve-tipped device. Place a curved retractor. If the hemivertebra is in the thoracic region, resect the rib head first to obtain access.
- Resect the cartilaginous surfaces of the concave facet to encourage fusion.
- With a Kerrison rongeur, begin resection in the midline with the ligamentum flavum followed by resection of the hemilamina (Fig. 8.135B). Extend the resection over to the facet, protecting the nerve roots above and below the hemivertebra. Resect the transverse process and cortical bone over the pedicle until cancellous bone of the pedicle and cortical outlines of its walls are seen. Once again, take care to avoid nerve roots. Gelfoam and cottonoids can be used to protect the dura during resection.
- Develop the subperiosteal plane down the lateral wall of the pedicle and body with the use of a Cobb elevator to facilitate retraction and protection. The dural contents can be protected with a nerve root retractor. Blood loss can be controlled by bipolar sealing of the epidural vessels. Use a diamond-tipped burr to continue resection to the pedicle and into the hemivertebral body to protect against unwanted injury to the soft tissues. Work stepwise within the walls of the pedicle and confines of the body to make removal of the cortical shells easier (Fig. 8.135C). Resect the walls of the pedicle and the remaining walls of the hemivertebral body. Generally, the dorsal cortex of the vertebral body is removed last. The resection is wedge shaped and includes the discs above and below, as well as the concave area of the disc.
- While protecting the dura and its contents, remove the disc material with a pituitary rongeur and curet. Do not remove the disc material above or below or correction will be limited. Proceed with wedge closure and deformity correction.

CLOSURE OF WEDGE RESECTION

- Place resected vertebral cancellous bone and allograft chips into the wedge resection site anteriorly.
- Closure of the wedge resection is achieved with the use of laminar hooks and external three-point pressure on the body.
- Place a downgoing supralaminar hook at the superior level and an upgoing infralaminar hook on the inferior level.
- To close the resection site, insert the rod, using compression to obtain correction. Using the rod avoids having to place large compression forces across the pedicle screws and allows the screws to maintain correction without plowing of the screws into the immature bone. The compression should be slow and controlled. Observe the dura to make sure it does not get caught in the closure of the posterior elements (Fig. 8.135D). If insufficient correction is obtained, resect further along the edges of the laminae.
- Place two additional rods on either side of the spine connected to the corresponding screws. Apply a crosslink if possible.
- Decorticate the spine and place vertebral corticocancellous allograft.

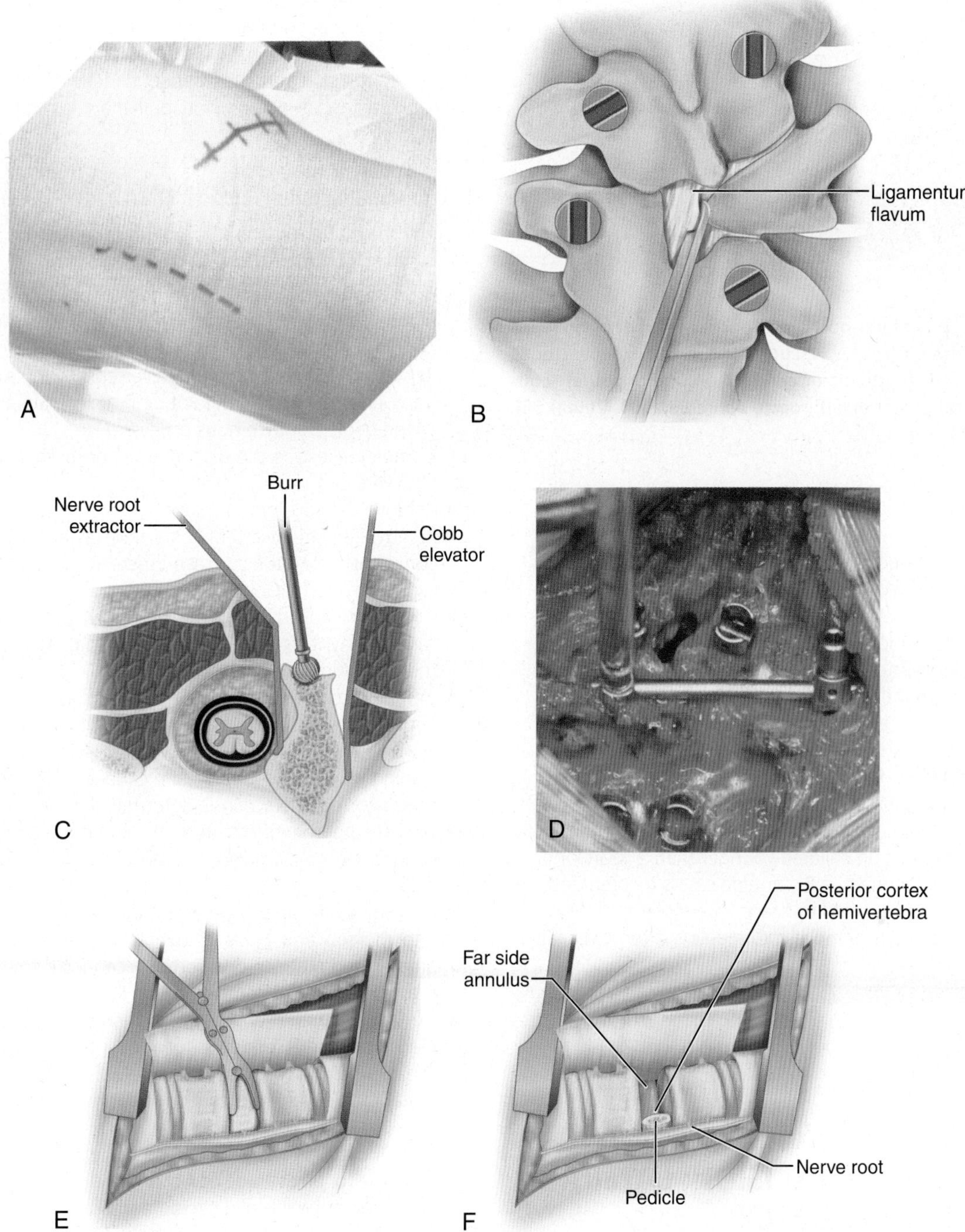

FIGURE 8.135 Hemivertebra excision. **A,** Patient positioning for anteroposterior excision. **B** and **C,** Resection of posterior hemilamina with Kerrison rongeur. **D,** Compression of laminar hooks with closure of excision site. **E,** Anterior resection. **F,** Resection carried back to pedicle. (From Hedequist DJ, Emans JB: Hemivertebra excision. In Wiesel SW, editor: *Operative techniques in orthopaedic surgery*, Philadelphia, 2011, Wolters Kluwer/Lippincott Williams & Wilkins, p 1466.) **SEE TECHNIQUE 8.37.**

ANTEROPOSTERIOR EXCISION

- If anteroposterior excision is performed, place the posterior implant anchors before resection. Once complete exposure has been performed, place the posterior screws.
- Create a full-thickness subperiosteal flap over the hemivertebra after localization is confirmed (Fig. 8.135E).
- Starting at the inferior endplate of the adjacent superior body and the superior endplate of the adjacent inferior body, create longitudinal full-thickness cuts in the periosteum, working anteriorly to the contralateral side. Then move posteriorly until the hemivertebral pedicle is seen.
- Resect the discs above and below the hemivertebra all the way posterior to the posterior longitudinal ligament.
- Resect the hemivertebral body back to the posterior cortical wall of the body with rongeurs and a diamond-tipped burr. The posterior wall can be resected off the posterior longitudinal ligament starting at the level of the disc re-

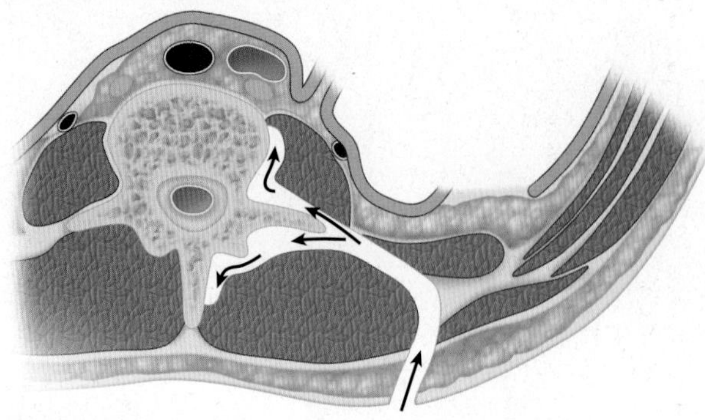

FIGURE 8.136 Lateral-posterior approach for hemivertebra resection. (Redrawn from Li X, Luo Z, Li X, et al: Hemivertebra resection for the treatment of congenital lumbar spinal scoliosis with lateral-posterior approach, *Spine* 33:2001, 2008.) **SEE TECHNIQUE 8.38.**

sections. The part of the pedicle that can be seen can be resected.

- For posterior resection, start with the hemilamina and proceed to the pedicle (Fig. 8.135F). With both incisions open and fields exposed, the pedicle can be resected though both incisions.
- Once the hemivertebra has been resected, wedge closure and correction of the deformity can proceed as described earlier.

POSTOPERATIVE CARE Postoperative care is similar to that for other spinal correction procedures. If fixation is adequate, patients can be placed in a custom-molded TLSO for 3 months. In children younger than 2 years or if fixation is not adequate, a Risser type cast is recommended for 2 months followed by brace wear for 6 months. It may be necessary to remove the implants after a year if prominence is a problem.

HEMIVERTEBRA EXCISION: LATERAL-POSTERIOR APPROACH

Li et al. described a lateral-posterior approach for hemivertebra resection that gave a safe and stable resection through a single incision (Fig. 8.136).

TECHNIQUE 8.38

(LI ET AL.)

- After administration of general anesthesia, place the patient in a lateral decubitus position, with the convex side of the curve up. Prepare and drape the flank in routine fashion.
- Use an L-shaped lateral-posterior approach to expose the hemivertebra (Fig. 8.137A). Make a straight longitudinal incision about 3.5 cm lateral to the spinous process from one segment cephalad to one segment caudad to the hemivertebra, and then turn to the lateral.
- Carry the dissection down to the lumbodorsal fascia and retract the skin and subcutaneous tissue on either side.
- Make a fascial incision and pull the sacrospinal muscle medially.
- Expose the lumbar transverse processes, facet joints, lamina, and spinous process subperiosteally.
- After pulling the psoas major laterally, proceed with dissection directly anteriorly on the pedicle to the vertebral body.
- After segmental vessels have been ligated, the hemivertebra and the appendage, which have been identified radiographically, are exposed (Fig. 8.137B).
- Remove the lamina of the hemivertebra with its attached transverse process, facet joint, and the remaining portion of the pedicle and spinous process.
- Completely excise the disc material on both sides of the hemivertebra.
- Remove the vertebral physes.
- Remove the hemivertebra, starting dissection from the convex aspect to the concave aspect. If the dura has been exposed, place a Gelfoam sponge over it.
- Cut the removed hemivertebral body into morsels and carefully lay it as a graft in the gap that was created by the resection.
- Carry out compression and stabilization on the convex side with short-segmental instrumentation (Cotrel-Dubousset Horizon, Medtronic Sofamor Danek, Memphis, TN), including vertebrae cephalad and caudad to the hemivertebra to correct the scoliosis deformity (Fig. 8.137D).
- Decorticate the facets and the laminae cephalad and caudad to the hemivertebra on the convex side of the curve.
- Cut any bone that is removed during the laminectomy into morsels and place it as graft material through the area extending from one vertebra cephalad to one vertebra caudad to the hemivertebra (Fig. 8.137E).
- Control bleeding with thrombin-soaked Gelfoam and place thrombin-soaked Gelfoam over the dural sac. Close the wound in a routine manner.
- Obtain radiographs to confirm curve correction.

POSTOPERATIVE CARE A rigid brace is worn full time or part time for an average of 4 months, depending on when the fusion appears solid on radiographs.

HEMIVERTEBRA EXCISION: POSTERIOR APPROACH

TECHNIQUE 8.39

(HEDEQUIST, EMANS, PROCTOR)

- Place the patient prone with good fluoroscopic imaging of the hemivertebra verified.

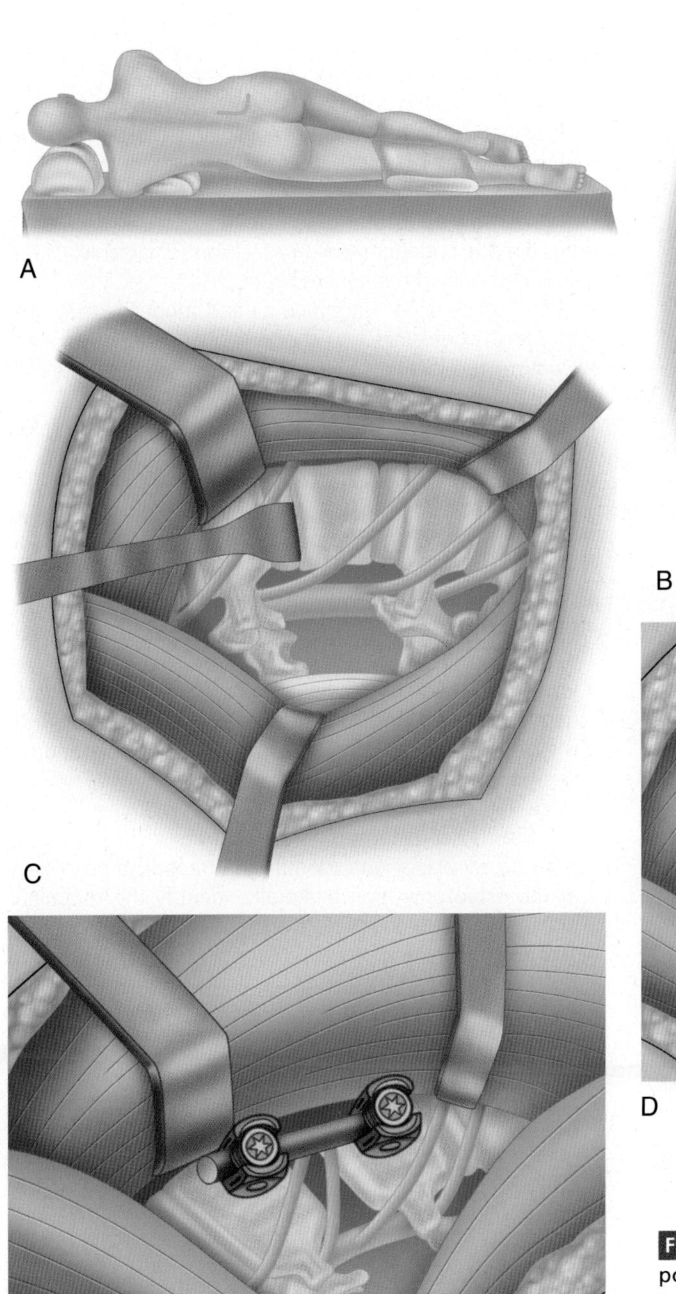

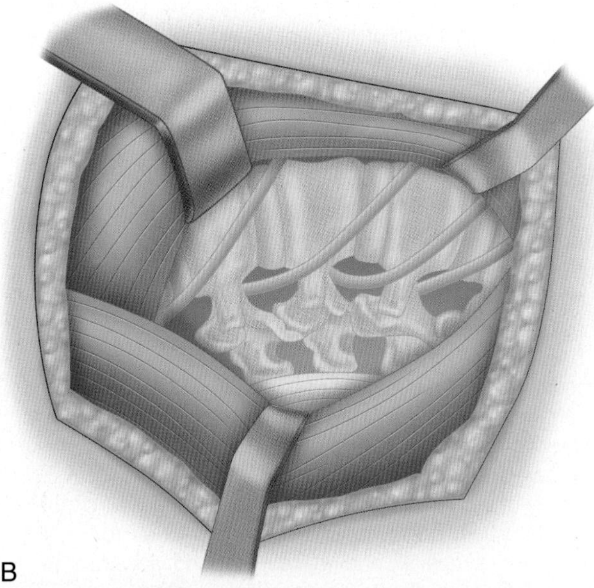

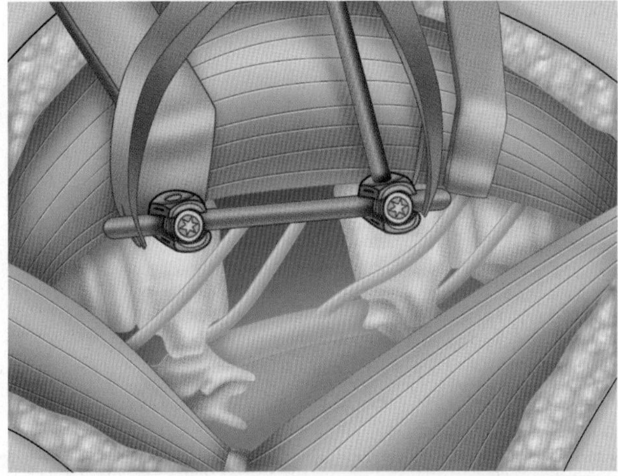

FIGURE 8.137 Hemivertebra excision through lateral-posterior approach. **A,** Patient positioning. **B,** Exposure of hemivertebra. **C,** Resection of hemivertebra. **D,** Compression and stabilization. **E,** Fusion. (Redrawn from Li X, Luo Z, Li X, et al: Hemivertebra resection for the treatment of congenital lumbar spinal scoliosis with lateral-posterior approach, *Spine* 33:2001, 2008.) **SEE TECHNIQUE 8.38.**

- Remove the hemilamina and surrounding ligamentum flavum.
- Place pedicle screws in the vertebrae above and below the hemivertebra that is to be removed. Enter the pedicle with a pedicle probe and expand this track with a series of enlarging curets (Fig. 8.138A).
- In the thoracic region, remove about 4 cm of the attached rib and remove the transverse process. The rib head can be removed or left in place and later pushed out laterally during closure of the osteotomy.
- Using a series of straight and downgoing curets, remove the cancellous portion of the vertebral body in its entirety. Frequent use of bone wax on cancellous bone limits bleeding and improves visualization.
- In young children, a layer of cartilage and/or periosteum remains intact and separates the excised vertebra from struc-

tures anterior and lateral to the vertebral body. Take care to leave the medial wall of the pedicle and the posterior wall of the vertebra intact (Fig. 8.138B). This is key from a safety standpoint: as long as the medial pedicle wall and posterior vertebral cortex are intact, the neural structures are protected.

- Remove the discs above and below the isolated hemivertebra, including the physes.
- If needed to maximize correction, remove bone above and below the vertebra. At this stage, it is not unusual to encounter threads of the pedicle screw in the inferior vertebral body, confirming that more than enough tissue has been removed.
- The challenge at this point usually is to dissect sufficiently medially across the midline of the spine; fluoroscopy with the curet in place may help confirm the medial extent of dissection. Remove tissue up to, but not including, the concave annulus.
- During this part of the dissection, the lateral wall of the pedicle usually breaks open, allowing the curet to be directed more medially and providing a good view into the cavity with a headlamp.
- With a pituitary rongeur or curet, remove the medial wall of the pedicle, while gently retracting nerve root and dura from this area. Bipolar cautery is helpful to separate the dural sac from the bone to be removed.
- Push the thinned-out posterior cortex of the vertebral body anteriorly to complete hemivertebra excision.
- Close the opening wedge, making certain that no bone or tissue buckle into the spinal canal.
- Fill any gaps with bone graft.

POSTOPERATIVE CARE If fixation is secure, a TLSO can be used for 3 months. If there is trunk imbalance or a substantial curve above or below the resection, bracing should be extended for as long as needed until the spine seems balanced.

TRANSPEDICULAR EGGSHELL OSTEOTOMIES WITH FRAMELESS STEREOTACTIC GUIDANCE

Mikles et al. described a technique for transpedicular eggshell osteotomies for congenital scoliosis with frameless stereotactic guidance. This technique is recommended in older patients who have congenital scoliosis with multiplanar spinal abnormalities. The guidance system was used to locate the pedicles intraoperatively for accurate screw placement. They thought that screw placement was difficult because of the abnormal anatomy, and they found the use of the guidance system to be helpful in obtaining screw placement proximally and distally and, therefore, a rigid instrumentation construct.

TECHNIQUE 8.40

(MIKLES ET AL.)

- Obtain an operative CT scan with 1-mm cuts from one level above to one level below the spinal deformity, with use of the appropriate protocol for the frameless stereotactic guidance system. Three-dimensional reconstructions are assimilated. With newer fluoroscopic image guidance systems, CT may not be necessary.
- Determine the level of the osteotomy before surgery. This usually corresponds with an eggshell osteotomy of the hemivertebra but is individualized for each patient.
- Monitor spinal cord and cauda equina function by somatosensory-evoked potentials.
- Position the patient prone on a Jackson spinal table. Carefully pad bony prominences.
- Make a midline posterior incision and subperiosteally dissect to the deformity.
- Confirm the location and identification of the vertebral elements by plain radiographs.
- Place an appropriate reference arc on the upper thoracic spinous processes.
- Register numerous skeletal sites by paired-point and surface-matching techniques. Registration points are determined for only two levels above and below the osteotomy site.
- By use of the guidance system, locate the pedicles with the digitized probe, a digitized drill guide, or a digitized pedicle tap.
- Probe the pedicle with a pedicle probe to the appropriate depth and angle. Insert a digitized ball-tipped probe into the pedicle hole to check the length of the hole and to verify the intrapedicular position.
- Place the screws approximately two levels above and below the chosen osteotomy site.
- After screw placement, identify the transverse processes at the osteotomy level bilaterally; identify the foramina above and below the pedicle and check with fluoroscopy.
- Trim the midline region down carefully with a burr until a thin layer of lamina is left.
- Perform a central laminectomy at the chosen level, including any overhanging lamina from the levels above or below.
- Start the posterior decancellation osteotomy on the side of the most accurately detailed anatomy. Identify the pedicle circumferentially and remove it with its transverse process while visual protection of the nerve root is maintained.
- Identify the pedicle opposite the proposed osteotomy and perform a similar exposure.
- After pedicle removal, expose the vertebral body and inferior floor of the spinal canal.
- Elevate the dura off the posterior wall of the vertebral body and begin the decancellation of the body through the pedicle remnants. Use angled curets to remove the cancellous bone from the vertebral body. Remove the disc spaces if necessary. Push the floor of the canal into the created space with reverse curets and subsequently remove it. Complete vertebrectomy is attempted but not always achieved. This allows the best correction of the curve.
- After completion of the osteotomy, apply gentle pressure to the posterior spine with extension of the hips to close the osteotomy site. Spinal cord monitoring is followed carefully during this time. The dura and nerve roots are continuously viewed to prevent entrapment. Titanium instrumentation is used. Some additional coronal correction is obtained with compression and distraction of the

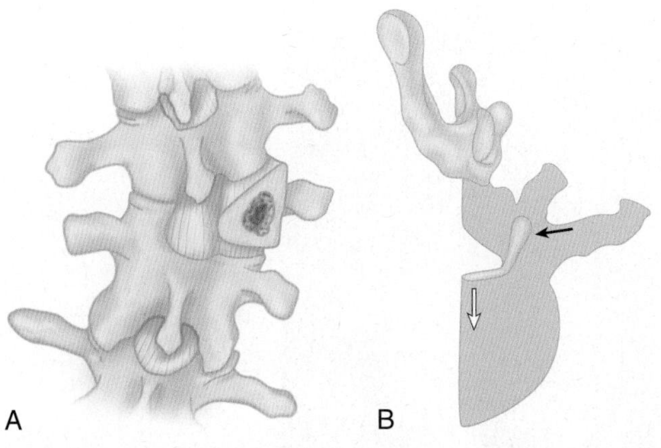

FIGURE 8.138 Hemivertebra excision. **A,** Pedicle is entered with standard pedicle probe and expanded with series of increasing sized curets; this often creates a hole large enough to see into. **B,** Cross-section of hemivertebra. Medial wall of pedicle *(black arrow)* is second-to-last thing to be removed. Posterior wall of vertebral body is last thing to be removed by pushing anteriorly, away from neural elements *(white arrow)*. In this case, not only are inferior disc and endplate removed, but also some of vertebral body is removed to maximize correction. (From Hedequist DJ, Emans JB: Hemivertebra excision. In Rhee J, Wiesel SW, Boden SD, et al, editors: *Operative techniques in spine surgery*, Philadelphia, 2013, Lippincott Williams & Wilkins, pp 367-375.) **SEE TECHNIQUE 8.39.**

osteotomy site. Additional lordosis can be obtained with in situ contouring.

- Place two crosslinks and local autogenous bone graft, which was harvested from the vertebral body, laterally along the decorticated transverse processes of the instrumented segment.
- Close the deep fascial layer and place a suction drain subcutaneously.
- Perform a Stagnara wake-up test in the operating room.

POSTOPERATIVE CARE The patient is fitted with a well-molded TLSO, which is worn for 12 weeks, starting on the second postoperative day.

THORACIC INSUFFICIENCY SYNDROME

Growing rod techniques can be used to treat congenital deformities involving long sections of the spine or deformities with large compensatory curves in normally segmented regions above and below a congenital deformity. Thoracic insufficiency syndrome may be associated with congenital scoliosis and fused ribs. When this occurs, it is best managed during growth by expansion thoracostomy and insertion of expandable VEPTR devices.

Campbell defined thoracic insufficiency syndrome as the inability of the thorax to support normal respiration or lung growth. This condition occurs in patients with hypoplastic thorax syndromes, such as Jeune and Jarcho-Levin syndromes, progressive infantile scoliosis with reductive distortion of the thoracic volume from spinal rotation, and congenital scoliosis associated with fused ribs on the concave side

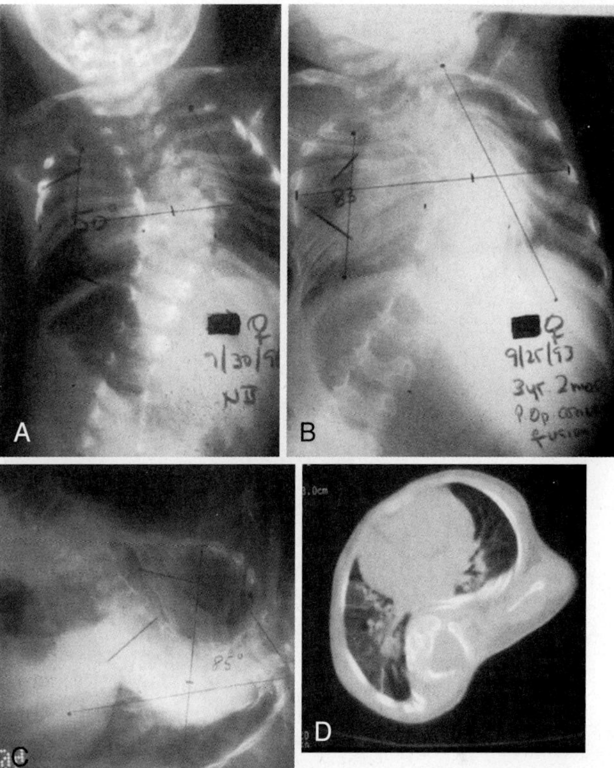

FIGURE 8.139 **A,** Birth radiograph of girl with 50-degree congenital scoliosis due to multiple vertebral anomalies. **B,** Curve had increased to 83 degrees by age 3 years. She underwent anterior convex spinal fusion and developed respiratory insufficiency 6 months after surgery, requiring supplemental nasal oxygen. **C,** "False" lateral decubitus view, better showing changes in dimensions of thorax in addition to spinal curvature. **D,** CT scan shows extreme hypoplasia of chest and underlying lungs. (From Campbell RM: Congenital scoliosis due to multiple vertebral anomalies associated with thoracic insufficiency syndrome, *Spine: State of the Art Reviews* 14:210, 2000.)

of the curve. In a hypoplastic thorax associated with congenital scoliosis, "extrinsic" restrictive lung disease can be caused by volume restriction of the underlying growing lungs and motion restriction of the ribs with reduction of the secondary breathing mechanism, as well as altered diaphragmatic mechanics. Thoracic and, therefore, lung volume increases to 30% of adult size by the age of 5 and to 50% of adult size by the age of 10.

Lung growth is limited to the anatomic boundaries of the thorax, so any spine or rib cage malformation that reduces the thoracic volume early in life may adversely affect the size of the lungs at skeletal maturity (Fig. 8.139). Maximizing thoracic height and volume is especially important in very young patients because lung growth between birth and the age of 8 years is related to increases in alveolar number and size and because growth of the lung between 8 years and maturity is primarily a result of increases in alveolar size.

Patients with early-onset scoliosis have been shown to have a higher mortality rate from respiratory failure than those with adolescent idiopathic scoliosis. A review of the literature found that young patients treated with thoracic fusions had a high rate of revision surgery (24% to 39%) and

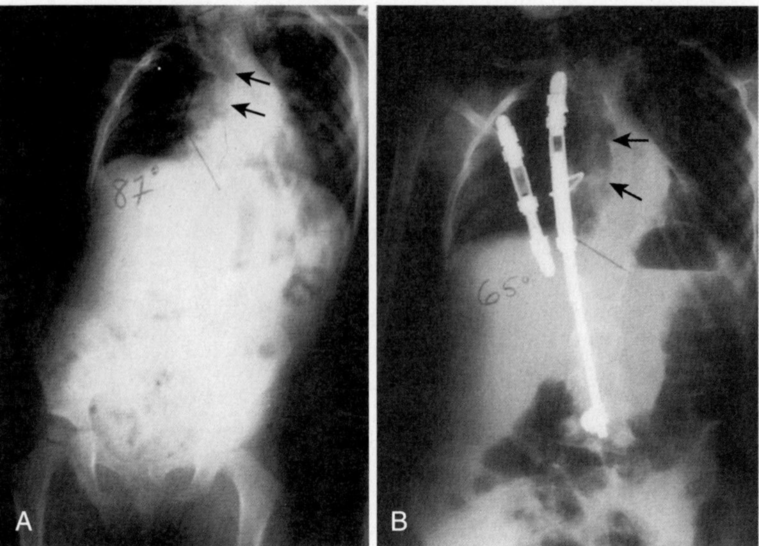

FIGURE 8.140 **A,** Multiple congenital anomalies of thoracic spine, including hemivertebra on convex side of curve and long unilateral unsegmented bar on concave side *(arrows),* in 2½-year-old girl with 87-degree scoliosis. **B,** At 6-year follow-up, curve is corrected to 65 degrees. Length of large central, unilateral segmented bar from T5 to T11 on concave side of curve *(arrows)* compared preoperatively and postoperatively suggests growth on concave side of curve. (From Campbell RM: Congenital scoliosis due to multiple vertebral anomalies associated with thoracic insufficiency syndrome, *Spine: State of the Art Reviews* 14:210, 2000.)

restrictive lung disease (43% to 64%), with those patients having upper thoracic fusions being at the highest risk. Long thoracic fusions by limiting thoracic and lung growth in young patients should be avoided to prevent the development of iatrogenic thoracic insufficiency.

Because of the inability of traditional spinal correction techniques to increase the dimensions of the thorax, Campbell developed a technique to directly treat chest wall deformity with indirect correction of the congenital scoliosis. This procedure treats the total global deformity of the thorax, allowing the spine to grow undisturbed by surgical intervention, with increased height of the thoracic spine and the thorax.

Gruca described a technique of operative compression of the ribs to obtain correction of idiopathic scoliosis on the convex side of the curve; however, concerns exist about this limiting thoracic and therefore lung growth. Campbell developed rib distraction instrumentation techniques for treatment of primary hemithorax constriction in severe spinal deformity in young children. He postulated that indirect correction of scoliosis could be obtained by surgical expansion of the chest through rib distraction on the concave side of the curve. He compared this technique with an opening wedge osteotomy of a malunion of a long bone. In this technique, the thoracic deformity is corrected by an "opening wedge thoracostomy" in the center of the deformity of the concave constricted hemithorax. Once the constricted hemithorax is lengthened, the thorax is equilibrated, with indirect correction of the scoliosis. Correction is maintained with an expandable titanium rib prosthesis. A substantial correction of the hemithorax deformity, an average curve correction of approximately 20 degrees, and the continued growth of the spine were noted as well. Elongation of unilateral unsegmented bars over time in patients treated with chest wall distraction techniques also has been noted (Fig. 8.140). The advantages of this technique are that it directly treats the anatomic causes of thoracic insufficiency syndrome and does not interfere with any subsequent spinal procedures that may be needed later in life.

Campbell treated 34 patients who had progressive congenital scoliosis associated with fused ribs of the concave hemithorax with expansion thoracoplasty and a titanium rib prosthesis. He recommended consideration of spinal growth-sparing techniques, such as growth rods and expansion thoracoplasty, for patients with multiple levels of malformation in the thoracic spine (jumbled spine) with associated areas of either rib deletion or fusion (jumbled thorax). Patients treated with rib-based distraction have been shown to have improvement in their coronal and sagittal spine deformities, pulmonary status, hemoglobin levels, and nutritional status. Although Cobb angle correction with this technique is well described, it has been shown to correlate poorly with pulmonary function and so the exact method(s) of physiologic improvement remain unknown.

Since the initial reports, rib-based distraction has now been used in the treatment of thoracic insufficiency and scoliosis in other conditions such as neuromuscular scoliosis and myelomeningocele. Because this is a posterior-based distraction technique, there is a potential for the development of increased kyphosis, especially in patients with increased preoperative kyphosis. Increased kyphosis may also play a role in proximal rib anchor failure. Longer constructs from the pelvis to ribs have been used to prevent excessive kyphosis; however, these should be avoided in ambulatory patients because of the increased incidence of postoperative crouch gait caused by changes in the lumbosacral mechanics. Intraoperative neuromonitoring is recommended for all initial insertions and in lengthening in which patients have neurologic changes at the time of their initial insertion. The role of its use in routine lengthenings in neurologically normal patients remains controversial. A large multicenter study found a rate of eight neurologic injuries in 1736 consecutive procedures (0.5%) of which five were at the time of initial implantation. When used, it should include monitoring of the upper extremities because the upper extremity was involved in six of eight cases, which may have been related to brachial plexus injury.

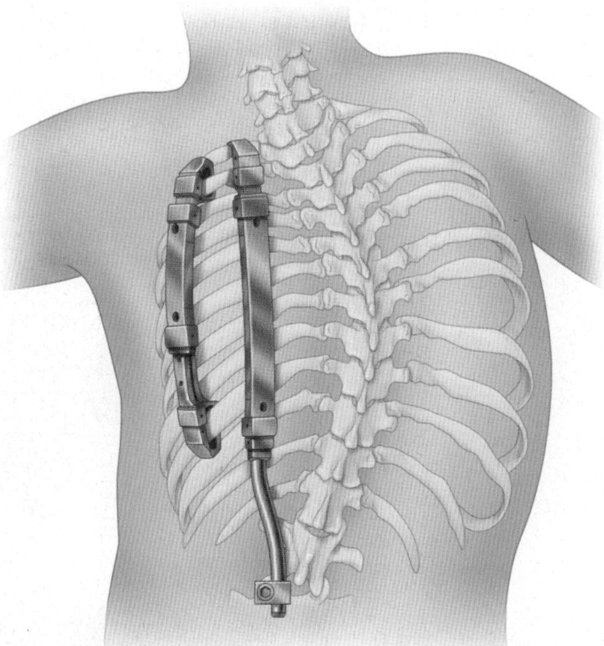

FIGURE 8.141 Expandable prosthetic rib device. (Redrawn from Campbell RM, personal communication.) **SEE TECHNIQUE 8.41.**

EXPANSION THORACOPLASTY

The VEPTR device comes in two forms. The device with a radius of 220 mm is most commonly used in the treatment of fused ribs and scoliosis. The titanium alloy permits the use of MRI postoperatively. There are three anchors available: rib, spine, and pelvis. The rib anchor consists of two C-shaped clamps that, when locked, form a loose encirclement around the rib to avoid vascular compromise of the underlying rib. Lateral stability is provided by the surrounding soft tissues. The spine anchor consists of a low-profile closed laminar hook. The pelvic anchor consists of an S-shaped modified McCarthy hook that is placed over the iliac crest. The central portion of the device consists of two sliding rib sleeves. The superior sleeve is attached to the cranial anchor, which is usually a rib, and the inferior sleeve is attached to the caudal anchor, which can be a rib, the spine, or the pelvis. The device is locked inferiorly by a peg-type lock through one of two holes, 5 mm apart in the distal rib sleeve, into partial-thickness holes in the inferior rib cradle post. This provides variable expandability for the device in increments of 5 mm. It is important to insert the device with the sleeves completely overlapped to maximize the excursion of the construct before revision is necessary (Fig. 8.141).

TECHNIQUE 8.41

(CAMPBELL)

- Place the patient in a lateral decubitus position with the concave side of the hemithorax upward. A small padded bolster can be placed at the apex of the curve to help with correction.
- Intraoperative spinal monitoring of both upper and lower extremities is used. Begin prophylactic intravenous antibiotics.
- Make a thoracotomy incision around the tip of the scapula and carry it anteriorly. Often in patients with fused ribs, the scapula is both hypoplastic and elevated proximally. In these patients, the skin incision may need to be brought more distal as it courses around the scapula.
- If a hybrid device is to be used, make a second incision 1 cm lateral to the midline over the proximal lumbar spine (Fig. 8.142A).
- Through the thoracotomy incision, elevate the muscle flaps and proximally identify the middle scalene muscle. Place devices on the second rib posterior to the scalene muscle. Anterior to the middle scalene muscle device, attachment is not done proximally because of the risk of impingement on the neurovascular bundle (Fig. 8.142B).
- Once exposure has been completed, identify the central rib fusion mass by the absence of intercostal muscles. This is the center of the apex of thoracic deformity where the concave hemithorax is most tightly constricted by rib fusion and is best seen on preoperative bending radiographs.
- Before the opening wedge thoracostomy is performed, prepare the rib prosthesis cradle sites proximally and distally. Make 1-cm incisions by use of an electrocautery in the intercostal muscles under the second rib, with a second 5-mm incision above it in the muscle.
- Use an elevator to carefully strip off only the anterior portion of the rib periosteum without violating the pleura (Fig. 8.142C).
- Insert a second elevator into the proximal intercostal muscle incision to encircle the rib.
- Prepare the inferior rib cradle site in the same fashion.
- Insert the rib cradle cap into the proximal intercostal muscle incision sideways and then turn it distally to encircle the rib, similar to insertion of a spinal laminar hook.
- Pass the superior rib cradle into the inferior intercostal muscle incision (Fig. 8.142D), mate it with the cradle cap, and lock it into place with pliers (Fig. 8.142E).
- The sites for the cradles should be just lateral to the transverse processes of the spine. The superior cradle site should be at the top of the area of the constricted hemithorax. If that site does not allow enough distance between the cradle sites for a device of sufficient length to have reasonable expansion capability, the site can be moved superiorly. In very flexible spines, however, care must be taken not to induce a large compensatory curve in the spine above the primary hemithorax constriction by placing the rib cradle too far superiorly. The inferior cradle site should be in a stable base of the area of the

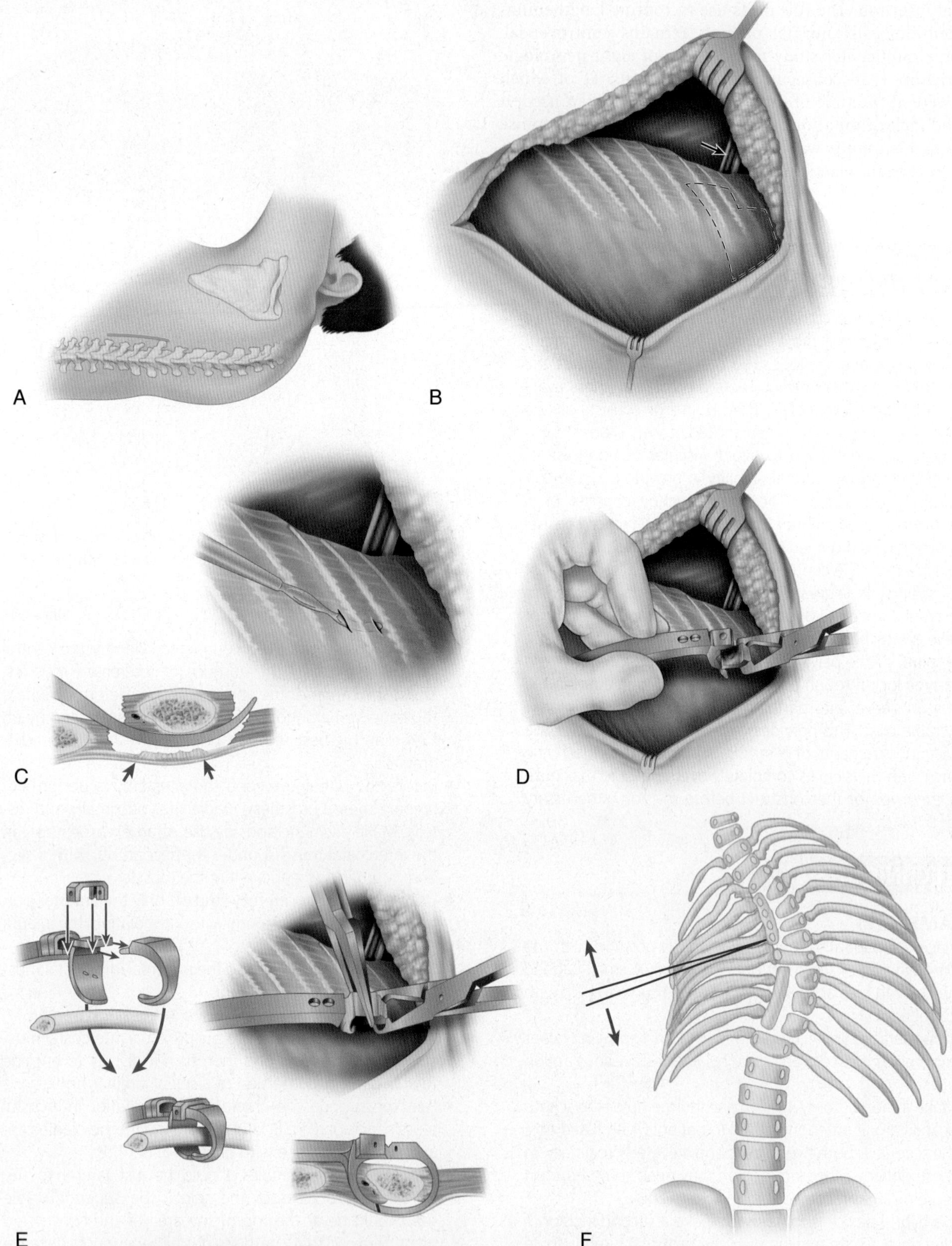

FIGURE 8.142 **A–J,** Campbell technique of expansion thoracoplasty. See text for description. (Redrawn from Campbell RM, personal communication, 2000.) **SEE TECHNIQUE 8.41.**

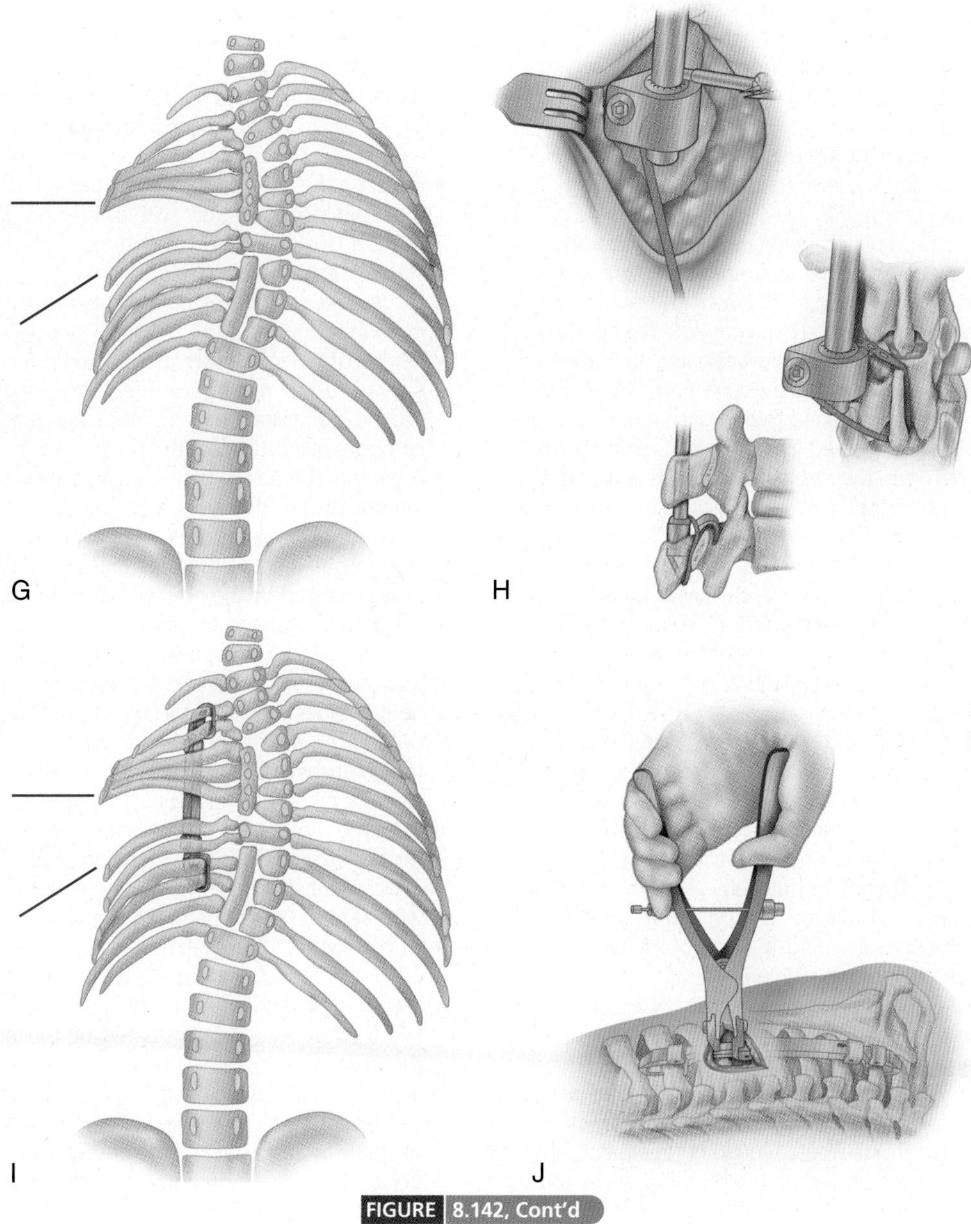

FIGURE 8.142, Cont'd

constricted hemithorax, below the line of the opening wedge thoracostomy, and usually encircling two fused ribs.

- Select the inferior rib cradle site by picking a rib of attachment that is clinically stable, as horizontal as possible, and at the inferior edge of the thoracic constriction. Avoid unstable rib attachments distally (vestigial rib) because of the high loads placed on the device in the expansion of a fused chest wall.
- Insert the superior cradle before the opening wedge thoracostomy is made. The inferior cradle is not placed at this point because the size of the device required to hold acute hemithorax correction is not known until the hemithorax is lengthened by the opening wedge thoracostomy.
- The deformity of the concave hemithorax is corrected by an opening wedge thoracostomy (Fig. 8.142F). This corrects the "angulated thorax," similar to the use of an opening wedge osteotomy to correct malunion of a long bone.
- Place the thoracostomy in the apex of the thoracic constriction where it can best correct the concave hemithorax, lengthen the constricted segment, and flare out the superior ribs laterally to increase thoracic volume. In most patients, this line of correction passes not through the apex of the scoliosis but above it.
- To confirm the correct position, place metal markers on the chest wall and verify the location with C-arm radiographs and then compare with the preoperative plan.
- The line of cleavage for the primary opening wedge thoracostomy may be through a mass of fused ribs, an area of fibrous adhesions between two ribs, or vestigial intercostal muscle. If the chosen interval is osseous, use a rongeur and Kerrison punches to make the thoracostomy. Be careful not to reflect periosteum from the rib incision

site, which will devascularize the rib. Strip away the underlying periosteum with a No. 4 Penfield elevator. The line of the thoracostomy extends from the sternum, along the contours of the ribs, to the transverse processes of the spine posteriorly.

- Reflect the paraspinous muscles from lateral to medial. Take care not to expose the spine to minimize the risk of inadvertent fusion.
- Once exposure is completed, gently spread the thoracostomy interval apart with two vein retractors to allow a lamina spreader to be inserted between the ribs in the midaxillary line of the thorax. Then complete the opening wedge thoracostomy by gradually widening the lamina spreader about 5 mm every 3 minutes (Fig. 8.142G) until the thoracic interval is widened to approximately 1 cm.
- If the ribs are easily distracted and there is at least 0.5 cm of soft tissue between the ribs as they articulate with the spine medially, no further resection is necessary.
- If rib distraction is difficult, additional rib fusion mass probably requires resection medially. If further resection is needed, cut a 1-cm wide channel medially at the posterior apex of the opening wedge thoracostomy, resecting the remaining fused rib anterior to the transverse process and following it down to the vertebral body for complete removal.
- Expose the bone to be removed a few millimeters at a time by subperiosteal dissection with a Freer elevator.
- Use a rongeur to remove the exposed bone. Take care to resect only visible bone, avoiding the spinal canal posteriorly and the esophagus and great vessels anteriorly. Preserve anomalous segmental vessels.
- Disarticulate the last 5 mm of fused rib from the spine with an angled curet, avoiding the neuroforamen, until the cartilage articular disc is visible.
- Secure hemostasis with bipolar cautery.
- Place bone wax over any raw bone surfaces.
- If the maximal thoracostomy interval distraction is 2 cm or less, the underlying pleura generally stretches and remains intact. If distraction is more than 2 cm, the pleura may begin to tear. Small tears in the pleura require no treatment, but substantial defects are treated with a Gore-Tex sheet (WL Gore and Assoc., Newark, DE) sutured to the edges of the intact pleura. Avoid attaching it to rib, muscle, or periosteum because it will become a tether. A Gore-Tex sheet of 0.6-mm thickness is used for small defects, and a 2-mm sheet is used for larger defects. The Gore-Tex sheet usually is placed after the device has been implanted to allow accurate sizing of the sheet needed for maximal thoracic volume. The surface of the sheet is brought outward to maximize volume.
- After the chest is expanded by the lamina spreader, measure the distance between the superior and inferior cradle sites to determine the size of the device needed. The inferior rib cradle and the rib sleeve should be of compatible sizes. An inferior rib cradle that is substantially shorter than the rib sleeve will reduce the device's ability for later expansion and require more frequent change-outs.
- Assess the orientation of the device and cradle after acute thoracostomy expansion so that they conform best to the corrected anatomy.
- After the device is sized and the orientation for the inferior cradle is chosen, relax the lamina spreader to ease access to the cradle sites.
- Insert the cradle cap inferiorly, implant the inferior cradle, and lock the components together with a cradle lock.
- If a hybrid device is used to span down to the lumbar spine, place this in a supralaminar position by resecting the intraspinous ligament and ligamentum flavum using a Kerrison rongeur.
- Place a bone graft on the lamina down to the hook to further stabilize a construct with a one-level fusion. Alternatively, a two-level claw construct can be used to increase stability, especially in older patients.
- If the superior cradle has not been previously inserted, implant it now.
- Reinsert the lamina spreader between medial ribs at the apex of the opening wedge thoracostomy. Reexpand the interval, expanding the thorax by bringing the device components out to length.
- Assemble the device by threading the rib sleeve over the inferior cradle and levering the rib sleeve in line with the superior rib cradle by the device wrenches. The acute correction obtained by the opening wedge thoracostomy is now stabilized by the rib device (Fig. 8.142H).
- For primary thoracic scoliosis in children younger than 18 months, only a single thoracic device is placed posteriorly, adjacent to the transverse processes of the spine. If a patient is older than 18 months and has adequate lumbar canal size and laminae, more support of the thoracostomy can be provided by a hybrid device and a second thoracic prosthesis added posterolaterally.
- Place the thoracic prosthesis in the posterior axillary line to further expand the constricted hemithorax, with proximal attachment just posterior to the middle scalene muscle with at least 0.5 cm between the superior rib cradles.
- Once assembled, tension both devices by expanding them 0.5 cm to fit snugly without excessive distraction pressure and then place two distraction locks on the rib sleeve.
- If the chest wall defect created by the opening wedge thoracostomy is larger than 2 cm, potential chest wall instability will need to be considered. A chest wall defect up to 3 cm wide is well tolerated proximally because of the splinting effect of the scapula posteriorly and the pectoralis muscle anteriorly. A distal chest wall defect of more than 2 cm and a proximal defect of more than 3 cm may need augmentation to provide chest wall stability by centralization of surgically created "pseudoribs" in the defect, addition of more devices, or implantation of a Gore-Tex sheet (2 mm thick) over the defect.
- In the first technique, called transport centralization, separate a single rib or pseudorib of two or three fused ribs away from the superior border of the opening wedge thoracostomy and rotate it downward, like a "bucket handle," to lie centrally in the chest wall defect. The goal of this technique is to divide the chest wall defect into a series of smaller defects, none larger than 2 cm. If the defect is too large for a single rib, separate another rib or pseudorib from the inferior border of the open wedge thoracostomy and bring it into the defect, dividing the larger defect into three smaller ones. Take care to preserve all soft-tissue attachments to avoid devascularization of the rib.
- The second method of augmentation is to add additional devices if transport centralization is not feasible or bone stock is inadequate. This method is practical only in larger

patients with adequate soft tissue for device coverage, and usually three devices are the maximum that can be used safely.

- Finally, a 2-mm Gore-Tex sheet can be used to supplement either of the other two methods. When the scoliosis extends from the thorax into the lumbar spine, use a lumbar hybrid rod extension. This lumbar extension can be used only in patients with adequate lumbar spinal canal size for hook placement, and generally the patient should be at least 18 months of age. Preoperatively assess the width of the canal by CT. The usual site of distal insertion is at either L1 or L2; but if the scoliosis extends well distally into the lumbar spine, L3 can be used. Avoid more distal insertion sites on the spine if possible.
- Spinal dysraphism of the proximal lumbar spine may require that the laminar hook be placed in the distal lumbar spine or that a modified McCarthy hook for the pelvis be coupled to the hybrid lumbar extension.
- Through a separate skin incision over the lumbar spine, insert the hybrid distraction device and pass it percutaneously from proximal to distal through the paraspinal muscles. Because of the kyphosis of the thorax, if the device is passed in a proximal direction, it may inadvertently penetrate the chest. Size the device similar to the all-thoracic technique and complete the opening wedge thoracostomy.
- Implant the superior cradle with an empty rib sleeve sized to extend to the inferior border of the thorax at the 12th rib.
- Size a hybrid rod lumbar extension to match the rib sleeve and select for implantation.
- Insert the inferior hook sublaminar. Size a hybrid rod lumbar extension to match the rib sleeve.
- With a lamina spreader in place to maintain the correction obtained with the opening wedge thoracostomy, use in situ benders to bend the hybrid rod into a slight kyphosis proximally and slight valgus and lordosis distally to best fit the lamina hook. The length of the rod should allow it to extend 1 cm distal to the hook.
- With a Kelly clamp, create a tunnel from the proximal incision through the paraspinal muscles, moving proximally to distally, with a finger in the lumbar incision to palpate the tip of the clamp as it exits the muscle. Use the Kelly clamp to grasp a small chest tube and pull it into the proximal incision.
- Attach the hybrid device to the tube and, by use of the tube, thread it proximally to engage the rib cradle and then into the hook.
- Distract the rib and tighten the hook.
- Place bone graft over the laminae.
- A large amount of correction may push the anterior portion of the proximal fused ribs proximally into the brachial plexus. To check for acute thoracic outlet syndrome, bring the scapula back into position while the anesthesiologist monitors pulses and ulnar nerve function is monitored by somatosensory potentials. If both are normal, close the muscle flaps with absorbable suture and close the skin in standard fashion with absorbable subcutaneous sutures.
- If either the pulse or ulnar nerve function is abnormal, retract the scapula and subperiosteally resect 2 cm of the proximal two ribs that are anterior under the brachial plexus.
- Bring the scapula back into position and check somatosensory potentials again. If they are normal, close the incision.

POSTOPERATIVE CARE The patient is placed in the intensive care unit until extubation, which will depend on the severity of the preoperative pulmonary compromise. In general, we leave our uncomplicated thoracostomy patients intubated overnight and wean respiratory support as tolerated. No bracing is used postoperatively to avoid constriction of chest wall growth. At intervals of approximately 6 months after the initial implantation, the device is expanded in an outpatient procedure. Prophylactic intravenous antibiotics are administered, and the distal end of the device is exposed with an incision through the thoracostomy incision if possible. Once the underlying muscle is exposed, it is split along its fibers or cut vertically either on the medial or lateral side of the device to form a thick muscle flap. Incisions directly over the device(s) should be avoided owing to the potential for skin breakdown and implant infection. The distraction lock over the device is removed, and distractor pliers are inserted to lengthen the device (Fig. 8.142I,J). The prosthesis is lengthened slowly, approximately 2 mm every 3 minutes, to avoid fracture. Once maximal reactive pressure is reached, the device is locked in place with a new distraction lock. Lengthening usually is a minimum of 0.5 cm and up to 1.5 cm. Once the device has exhausted its expandability, a change-out operative procedure is done through small proximal and distal transverse incisions. The sleeves are removed and replaced with larger components (implants). Devices that extend well under the scapula may be difficult to exchange and often require opening of a large portion of the old thoracotomy incision to change the components.

KYPHOSIS

In the sagittal plane, the normal spine has four balanced curves: the cervical spine is lordotic; the thoracic spine is kyphotic (20 to 50 degrees), with the curve extending from T2 or T3 to T12; the lumbar region is lordotic (31 to 79 degrees); and the sacral curve is kyphotic. On standing, the thoracic kyphosis and lumbar lordosis are balanced. Normal sagittal balance is defined as a plumb line dropped from C7 and intersecting the posterosuperior corner of the S1 vertebra (Fig. 8.143). Positive sagittal balance occurs when the plumb line falls in front of the sacrum, and negative sagittal balance occurs when the plumb line falls behind the sacrum.

In the upright position, the spine is subjected to the forces of gravity, and several structures maintain its stability: the disc complex (nucleus pulposus and annulus), the ligaments (anterior longitudinal ligament, posterior longitudinal ligament, ligamentum flavum, apophyseal joint ligaments, and intraspinous ligament), and the muscles (the long spinal muscles, short intrinsic spinal muscles, and abdominal muscles). Kyphosis of 50 degrees or more in the thoracic spine usually is considered abnormal. Kyphotic deformity may occur if the anterior spinal column is unable to withstand compression, causing shortening of the anterior column. Disruption of the

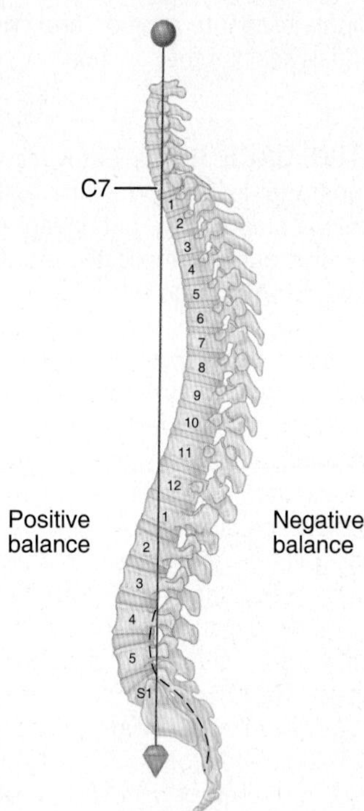

FIGURE 8.143 Plumb line is dropped from middle of C7 vertebral body to posterosuperior corner of S1 vertebral body. (Redrawn from Bernhardt M: Normal spinal anatomy: normal sagittal plane alignment. In Bridwell KH, DeWald RL, editors: *The textbook of spinal surgery*, ed 2, Philadelphia, 1997, Lippincott-Raven.)

posterior column and inability to resist tension can lead to relative lengthening of the posterior column and kyphosis (Fig. 8.144).

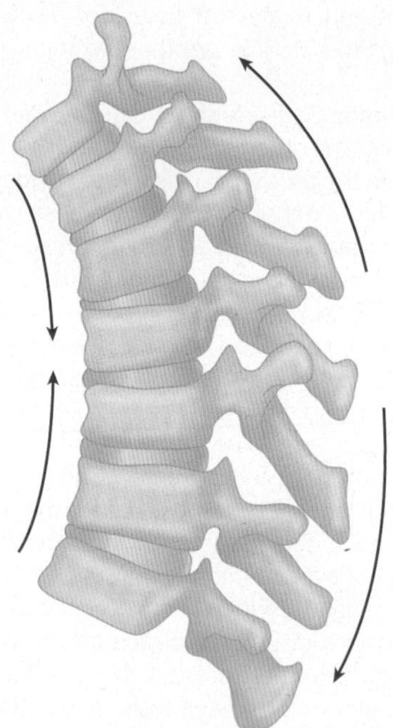

FIGURE 8.144 Forces that contribute to kyphotic deformity of thoracic spine. Anterior vertebral bodies are in compression, and posterior vertebral elements are in tension.

SCHEUERMANN DISEASE

Scheuermann originally described a rigid juvenile kyphosis in 1920. Scheuermann disease is a structural kyphosis of the thoracic or thoracolumbar spine that occurs in 0.4% to 8.3% of the general population. It occurs slightly more often in males. The age at onset usually is during the prepubertal growth spurt, between 10 and 12 years of age.

CLASSIFICATION

Scheuermann disease is divided into two distinct groups: a typical form and an atypical form. These two types are determined by the location and natural history of the kyphosis, including symptoms occurring during adolescence and after growth is completed. Typical Scheuermann disease usually involves the thoracic spine. This classic form of Scheuermann kyphosis has three or more consecutive vertebrae, each wedged 5 degrees or more, producing a structural kyphosis. In contrast, atypical Scheuermann disease usually is located in the thoracolumbar junction or the lumbar spine. It is characterized by vertebral endplate changes, disc space narrowing, and anterior Schmorl nodes but does not necessarily have three consecutively wedged vertebrae of 5 degrees. Thoracic Scheuermann disease is the most common form.

ETIOLOGY

The cause of Scheuermann disease is probably multifactorial. Scheuermann thought that the kyphosis resulted from osteonecrosis of the ring apophysis of the vertebral body. However, the ring apophysis lies outside the true cartilaginous physis and contributes nothing to the longitudinal growth of the body; therefore, a disturbance in the ring apophysis should not affect growth of the vertebra or cause vertebral wedging. In 1930, Schmorl suggested that the vertebral wedging is caused by herniation of disc material into the vertebral body; these herniations now are known as Schmorl nodes. Schmorl theorized that as the disc material is extruded into the vertebral body the height of the intervertebral disc is diminished, which causes increased pressure anteriorly and disturbances of enchondral growth of the vertebral body and subsequent wedging. However, Schmorl nodes are relatively common and frequently occur in patients with no evidence of Scheuermann disease. Ferguson implicated the persistence of anterior vascular grooves in the vertebral bodies during preadolescence and adolescence. He suggested that these vascular defects create a point of structural weakness in the vertebral body, which leads to wedging and kyphosis.

Bradford and Moe and Lopez et al. found that osteoporosis may be responsible for the development of Scheuermann disease. However, a study of bone density in a group of trauma patients and teenagers with Scheuermann disease, as well as a cadaver study, found no evidence of osteoporosis in the vertebrae.

Mechanical factors are a likely cause of Scheuermann disease. Lambrinudi and others suggested that the upright posture and the tightness of the anterior longitudinal ligament of the spine contribute to the deformity. Scheuermann kyphosis is more common in patients who do heavy lifting or manual labor. The fact that some correction of the kyphosis can be obtained by bracing that relieves pressure on the anterior vertebral regions also indicates that mechanical factors are important. The kyphosis probably increases pressure on the vertebral endplates anteriorly, causing uneven growth of the vertebral bodies as a response to the law of Wolff.

A biochemical abnormality of the collagen and matrix of the vertebral endplate cartilage also has been suggested as an important factor in the cause. Abnormal collagen fibers and a decrease in the ratio between collagen and proteoglycan have been found in the matrix of the endplate cartilage in patients with Scheuermann disease.

Several authors have found support for a genetic basis for Scheuermann disease. A high familial predilection has been noted in several studies. The disease may be inherited in an autosomal dominant fashion. Additional support for a genetic basis is provided by Carr et al. in a report of Scheuermann disease occurring in identical twins. In summary, many causes have been suggested but none has been proved. Further research is required to better investigate the ultimate causes of Scheuermann disease.

CLINICAL FINDINGS

Scheuermann disease usually appears around the adolescent growth spurt. The presenting complaint is either pain in the middle or lower back or concern about posture. Frequently, the parents believe that the kyphosis is postural, so diagnosis and treatment are delayed. Pain usually is located in the area of the deformity or in the lower back, is made worse by activity, and typically improves with the cessation of growth. If pain is present in the lumbar area and the deformity is in the thoracic region, the possibility of spondylolysis should be considered.

Physical examination shows an angular thoracic or thoracolumbar kyphosis with compensatory hyperlordosis of the lumbar spine. The kyphosis is sharply angular and does not correct with the prone extension test (Fig. 8.145). The lumbar lordosis below the kyphosis usually is flexible and corrects with forward bending. Tight hamstrings and pectoral muscles are common. On forward bending, a small structural scoliosis may be present in as many as 30% of patients.

Physical findings in patients with atypical (lumbar) Scheuermann disease may differ from those in patients with thoracic deformity. These patients usually have low back pain, but, unlike patients with the more common form of Scheuermann disease, they may not have as noticeable a deformity. Pain with spinal movement is the primary symptom. The condition is especially common in males involved in competitive athletics and in farm laborers, suggesting that it represents an injury to the vertebral physes from repeated trauma rather than true Scheuermann disease.

Abnormal neurologic findings have been reported in 9% to 15% of patients with Scheuermann kyphosis; such findings emphasize the importance of a detailed neurologic examination. Spinal cord compression from kyphosis, thoracic disc herniation, epidural cysts, and epidural lipomatosis have been reported. If lower extremity weakness, hyperreflexia, sensory changes, or other neurologic findings are detected, MRI of the kyphotic area should be done.

RADIOGRAPHIC FINDINGS

Standing anteroposterior and lateral radiographs of the spine should be obtained. The amount of kyphosis is determined by the Cobb method on a lateral radiograph of the spine. The cranial and most caudal tilted vertebrae in the kyphotic deformity are selected. A line is drawn along the superior endplate of the cranial vertebra and the inferior endplate of the most caudal vertebra. Lines are drawn perpendicular to the line along the endplates, and the angle they form is the degree of kyphosis. The criteria for the diagnosis of typical Scheuermann disease are more than 5 degrees of wedging of at least three adjacent vertebrae at the apex of the kyphosis and vertebral endplate irregularities with a thoracic kyphosis of more than 50 degrees (Fig. 8.146). Bradford suggested that three wedged vertebrae are not necessary for the diagnosis but rather an abnormal, rigid kyphosis is indicative of Scheuermann disease. Flexibility and the structural nature of the deformity are determined by taking a lateral radiograph with the patient lying over a bolster placed at the apex of the deformity to hyperextend the spine. On a lateral radiograph, most patients will be in negative sagittal balance measured by dropping a plumb line from the center of the C7 vertebral body and measuring the distance from this line to the posterosuperior corner of the S1 vertebra. Scoliosis is evident on posteroanterior radiographs in approximately a third of patients. A lateral radiograph should be made with the patient in the hyperextended position over a bolster to determine the structural nature of the deformity.

Atypical Scheuermann disease of the lumbar spine is characterized by irregularity of the vertebral endplates, the presence of Schmorl nodes, and narrowing of the intervertebral discs, without wedging of the vertebral bodies or kyphosis.

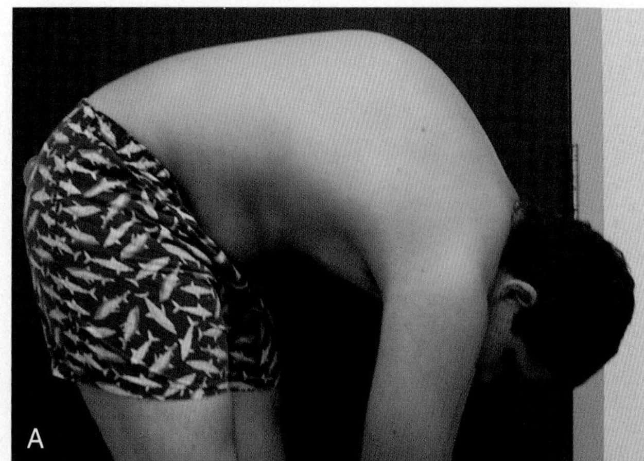

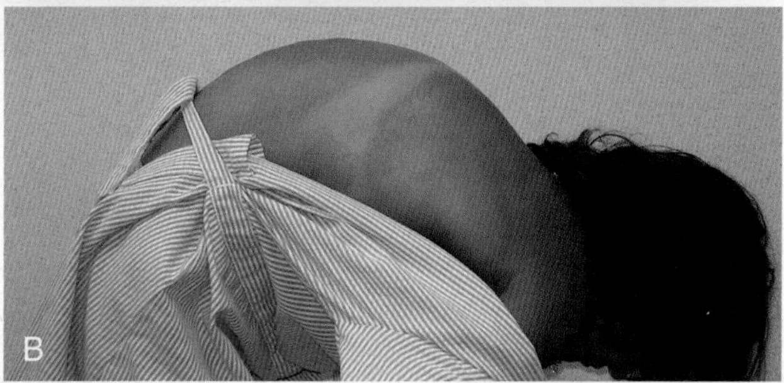

FIGURE 8.145 **A,** Scheuermann kyphosis. **B,** Postural kyphosis. (From Warner WC: Kyphosis. In Morrissy RT, Weinstein SL, editors: *Lovell and Winters pediatric orthopaedics*, ed 6, Philadelphia, 2006, Lippincott Williams & Wilkins, p 797.)

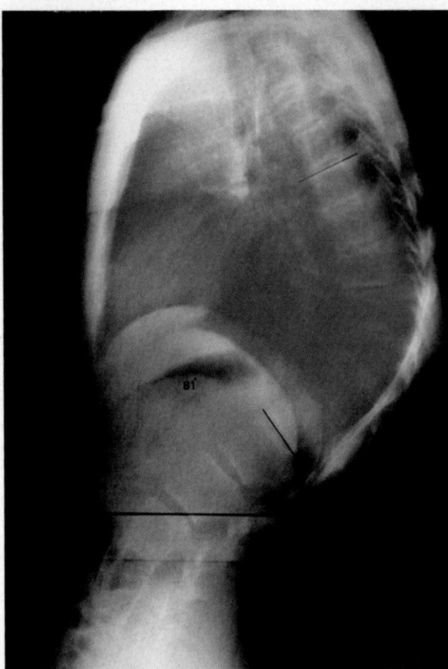

FIGURE 8.146 Scheuermann kyphosis. Kyphotic deformity of 81 degrees and Schmorl nodes.

NATURAL HISTORY

In most cases, Scheuermann disease results in minimal deformity and few symptoms. The kyphotic deformity can progress rapidly during the adolescent growth spurt. Back pain and fatigue are common complaints during adolescence but usually disappear with skeletal maturity. Factors that contribute to the risk of continued progression of kyphosis include the number of years of growth remaining and the number of wedged vertebrae. Neurologic symptoms have occasionally been reported in adolescents because of herniation of a thoracic disc, an epidural cyst, or the severe kyphotic deformity alone with subsequent compression of the cord.

The true natural history of untreated Scheuermann disease in adulthood is not well established. Travaglini and Conte found that the kyphosis increased during adulthood in 80% of their patients, although few developed severe deformity. During middle age, degenerative spondylosis is common, but radiographic findings do not always correlate with the presence or absence of back pain. If the kyphosis is less than 60 degrees, these changes usually do not occur in adulthood.

Patients with Scheuermann kyphosis were found in one study to have more intense back pain, jobs that tend to have lower requirements for activity, loss of extension of the trunk, and different localization of pain. However, the level of education, number of days absent from work because of back pain, pain that interfered with activities of daily living, self-esteem, social limitations, use of medication for back pain, or level of recreational activities were not significantly different from those without Scheuermann disease. Most patients reported little preoccupation with their physical appearances. Normal or above-normal averages of pulmonary function were found in patients in whom the kyphosis was less than 100 degrees. Patients who have Scheuermann kyphosis may have some functional limitation, but it does not significantly affect their lives. Patients who have not had surgery for the kyphosis adapt reasonably well to their condition.

Lumbar Scheuermann disease, which usually is associated with strenuous physical activity, generally becomes asymptomatic within several months after restriction of activities.

ASSOCIATED CONDITIONS

Mild-to-moderate scoliosis is present in about one third of patients with Scheuermann disease, but the curves tend to be small (10 to 20 degrees). Scoliosis associated with Scheuermann disease usually has a benign natural history. Deacon et al. divided scoliotic curves in patients with Scheuermann disease into two types on the basis of the location of the curve and the rotation of the vertebrae into or away from the concavity of the scoliotic curve. In the first type of curve, the apices of the scoliosis and kyphosis are the same and the curve is rotated toward the convexity. The rotation of the scoliotic curve is opposite to that normally seen in idiopathic scoliosis. They suggested that the difference in direction of rotation is caused by scoliosis occurring in a kyphotic spine, instead of the hypokyphotic or lordotic spine that is common in idiopathic scoliosis. In the second type of curve, the apex of the scoliosis is above or below the apex of the kyphosis and the scoliotic curve is rotated into the concavity of the scoliosis, more like idiopathic scoliosis. This type of scoliosis seen with Scheuermann kyphosis is the more common, and it rarely progresses or requires treatment.

Lumbar spondylolysis is frequently found in patients with Scheuermann kyphosis (Fig. 8.147). The suggested reason for the increased incidence of spondylolysis (50% to 54%) is that increased stress is placed on the pars interarticularis because of the associated compensatory hyperlordosis of the lumbar spine. This increased stress causes a fatigue fracture at the pars interarticularis, resulting in spondylolysis. Other conditions reported in patients with Scheuermann disease include endocrine abnormalities, hypovitaminosis, inflammatory disorders, and dural cysts.

DIFFERENTIAL DIAGNOSIS

The most common entity to be differentiated from Scheuermann disease is postural round-back deformity. This deformity characteristically produces a slight increase in thoracic kyphosis, which is mobile clinically and is easily correctable on the prone extension test. Radiographs show normal vertebral body contours without vertebral wedging. The kyphosis is more gradual than the angular kyphosis commonly seen in Scheuermann disease. A normal radiograph, however, may not rule out Scheuermann disease because radiographic changes may not be apparent until a child is 10 to 12 years of age.

If pain is a presenting symptom, infectious spondylitis must be considered. This usually can be excluded, however, by clinical and laboratory studies and by MRI, CT, or bone scan of the spine. On occasion, traumatic injuries can confuse the differential diagnosis, but usually the wedging caused by a compression fracture involves only a single vertebra rather than the three or more vertebrae involved in true Scheuermann kyphosis. Osteochondrodystrophies, such as Morquio and Hurler syndromes, as well as tumors and congenital deformities, especially congenital kyphosis, also must be considered. In young men, ankylosing spondylitis must be ruled out, and this may require an HLA-B27 blood test.

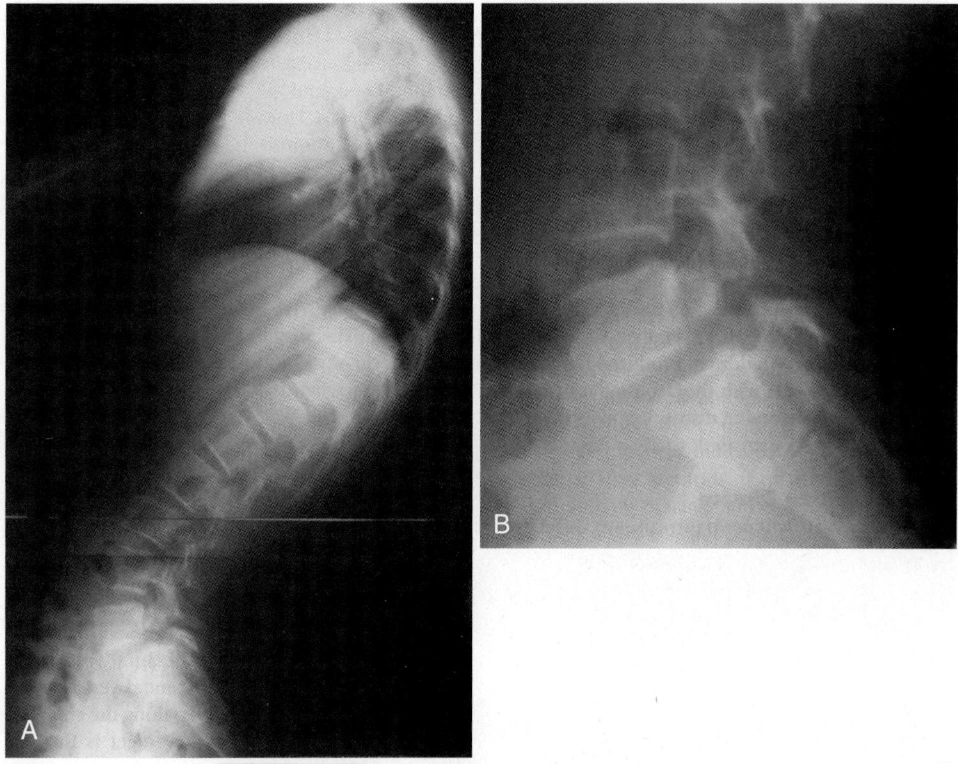

FIGURE 8.147 Spondylolisthesis with kyphosis.

TREATMENT

The indications for treatment of patients with Scheuermann kyphosis can be grouped into five general categories: pain, progression of deformity, neurologic compromise, cardiopulmonary compromise, and cosmesis. Treatment options include observation, conservative methods, and surgery.

NONOPERATIVE TREATMENT

OBSERVATION

Adolescents with mildly increased kyphosis of less than 50 degrees without evidence of progression can be evaluated with repeated standing lateral radiographs every 4 to 6 months. Exercises alone have not been shown to provide any correction of the deformity in patients with Scheuermann disease. An exercise program, however, can help maintain flexibility, correct lumbar lordosis, and strengthen the extensor muscles of the spine and may improve any postural component of the deformity. Stretching exercises should be prescribed for patients with associated tightness of the hamstring or pectoralis muscles. Patients with lumbar Scheuermann disease and back pain should avoid heavy lifting and should be prescribed an exercise program for the lower back.

ORTHOTIC TREATMENT

The Milwaukee brace has been recommended for the treatment of Scheuermann disease but has been replaced with more low-profile braces. The brace acts as a dynamic three-point orthosis that promotes extension of the thoracic spine. Indications for brace treatment are at least 1 year of growth remaining in the spine, some flexibility of curve (40% to 50%), and kyphosis of more than 50 degrees. The brace is worn full time for the first 12 to 18 months. If the curve has stabilized and no progression is noted, then a part-time brace program can be used until skeletal maturity. An improvement in lumbar lordosis of 35% and in thoracic kyphosis of 49% has been reported in teenagers with Scheuermann kyphosis treated in this manner. Overall, at long-term follow-up, some loss of correction had occurred, but 69% of patients had improvement from the initial kyphosis. Others have reported less correction (30% initially), with the final kyphosis correction averaging only 10%.

Although the Milwaukee brace has been shown to effectively prevent kyphosis progression and offers some modest permanent correction, full-time brace wear often is resisted by adolescents. Gutowski and Renshaw found that the Boston lumbar kyphosis orthosis was satisfactory for correction of curves of less than 70 degrees and had better compliance. They recommended the Boston lumbar orthosis as an acceptable alternative to the Milwaukee brace in patients with flexible kyphotic curves of less than 70 degrees and in whom compliance may be a problem. The rationale for the Boston lumbar orthosis is that reduction of the lumbar lordosis will cause the patient to dynamically straighten the thoracic kyphosis to maintain an upright posture. This presupposes a flexible kyphosis, a normal neurovestibular axis, and the absence of hip flexion contractures.

Lowe used a modified underarm TLSO with padded anterior, infraclavicular outriggers for patients with thoracolumbar-pattern Scheuermann disease (apex T9 and below) and found that it was as effective as the Milwaukee brace and was cosmetically more acceptable to patients. This is now the more popular bracing method.

Hyperextension casting has been used with excellent results in Europe, but this method is associated with frequent problems with the skin, restrictions of physical activity, and the need for frequent cast changes.

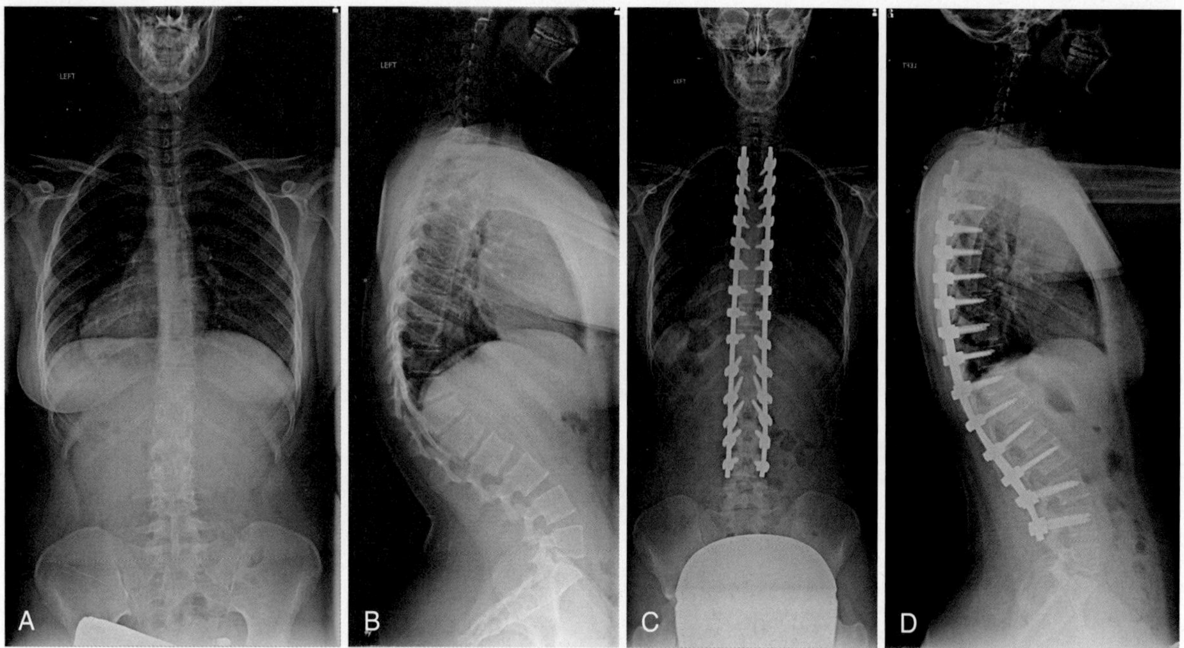

FIGURE 8.148 **A** and **B,** Scheuermann kyphosis. **C** and **D,** After correction and posterior fusion.

OPERATIVE TREATMENT

The indications for surgery in patients with Scheuermann kyphosis are a progressive kyphosis of more than 70 degrees and significant kyphosis associated with pain that is not alleviated by conservative treatment methods. The biomechanical principles of correction of kyphosis include lengthening the anterior column (anterior release), providing anterior support (interbody fusion), and shortening and stabilizing the posterior column (compression instrumentation and arthrodesis). Surgical correction can be achieved by a posterior approach, an anterior approach, or a combined anterior and posterior approach. The combined anterior and posterior approach has been the most frequently recommended, but with the development of pedicle screw fixation and posterior spinal osteotomy techniques, such as the Ponte procedure, posterior-only surgery has become the preferred approach. A posterior procedure without osteotomy can be considered if the kyphosis is flexible and can be corrected to, and maintained at, less than 50 degrees while a posterior fusion occurs (Fig. 8.148). Historically, the use of Harrington compression rods was common, but these have been replaced by segmental hook and pedicle screw instrumentation.

When a combined anterior and posterior procedure is used for Scheuermann disease, the anterior release and fusion are done first. The anterior release can be done through an open anterior procedure or by thoracoscopy. Herrera-Soto et al. showed good sagittal correction, with no loss of correction or junctional kyphosis, with a thoracoscopic technique. Interbody cages have been used in an effort to improve sagittal correction; however, Arun et al. found no difference in outcomes between patients with anterior fusion using interbody cages and those with anterior fusion using autogenous rib grafting. The posterior fusion and instrumentation can be done on the same day as the anterior release and fusion or as a staged procedure. Segmental instrumentation systems using multiple hooks or pedicle screws are used for the posterior spinal fusion.

Other instrumentation techniques have been used for correction of Scheuermann kyphosis. Sturm, Dobson, and Armstrong reported good results with posterior fusion alone by use of large, threaded Harrington compression rods rather than small ones.

The use of posterior spinal osteotomies such as the Ponte osteotomy allows for relative shortening of the posterior column and greater correction of the kyphosis. Several studies have shown similar sagittal correction with combined anterior and posterior procedures and posterior-only procedures with Ponte osteotomies. Posterior fusion and instrumentation should include the proximal vertebra in the measured kyphotic deformity and the first lordotic disc distally. If the fusion and instrumentation end in the kyphotic deformity, a junctional kyphosis at the end of the instrumentation may occur. Cho et al. reported the occurrence of distal junctional kyphosis despite inclusion of the first lordotic disc. They recommended inclusion of the lumbar vertebral body bisected by a vertical line drawn from the posterosuperior corner of the sacrum to prevent distal junctional kyphosis.

Junctional decompensation has been reported to occur in as many as 30% of patients. Overcorrection of the deformity should be avoided to prevent junctional kyphosis. No more than 50% of the preoperative kyphosis should be corrected, and the final kyphosis should not be less than 40 degrees. Lowe found that patients with Scheuermann disease tend to be in negative sagittal balance and become further negatively balanced after surgery, which may predispose them to develop a junctional kyphosis. Lonner et al. found that the pelvic incidence may be related to the amount of proximal junctional kyphosis and that distal junctional kyphosis was related to fusion that ended cranial to the neutral sagittal vertebra. Denis et al. suggested that the incidence of proximal junctional kyphosis can be minimized by the appropriate selection of the upper end vertebra and avoiding disruption of the junctional ligamentum flavum. They also recommended incorporation of the first lordotic disc into the fusion construct.

ANTERIOR RELEASE AND FUSION

TECHNIQUE 8.42

- The levels of the anterior release are those with the most wedging and the least flexibility on hyperextension lateral views. This region generally includes seven or eight interspaces centered on the apex of the kyphosis.
- Select the appropriate anterior approach for the levels to be fused. If there is no associated scoliosis, make the approach through the left side. If there is a concomitant scoliosis, approach the spine on the convexity of the scoliosis.
- Release the anterior longitudinal ligament and excise the entire disc and cartilaginous endplate, leaving only the posterior portion of the annulus and the posterior longitudinal ligament.
- Curet the bony endplates but do not remove them completely.
- Use a laminar spreader to loosen or to mobilize each joint.
- Pack each disc space temporarily with Gelfoam or Surgicel to minimize blood loss.
- Perform an interbody fusion with use of the morselized rib graft.
- Anterior instrumentation can be used to aid in correction of the deformity and stabilization until a solid fusion occurs.

POSTERIOR MULTIPLE HOOK AND SCREW SEGMENTAL INSTRUMENTATION

With multiple hook and screw segmental instrumentation systems, several techniques are available for reduction of kyphosis. The cantilever method (Fig. 8.149) consists of inserting the precontoured rod into the pedicle–transverse process claws or thoracic pedicle screws above the apex of the kyphosis. With the apex of the deformity as a fulcrum, the distal end of the rod is pushed into the lower hood or pedicle screws at the caudal end of the deformity by a cantilever maneuver. The disadvantage of this method is that the correction is a three-point cantilever maneuver and the correction is therefore somewhat abrupt and forces are concentrated at the ends of the construct. Reduction pedicle screws and instruments can be used to make this reduction maneuver more gradual. Another method for correction is an apical compression technique using multisegmental hooks or pedicle screw constructs on either side of the apex. A combination of the cantilever and compression techniques also can be used. These two techniques often are combined with a posterior column shortening procedure, allowing gradual correction of the kyphosis. Rigid posterior instrumentation systems can be combined with posterior column shortening (Ponte osteotomies) to correct the kyphosis without the need for anterior release and fusion.

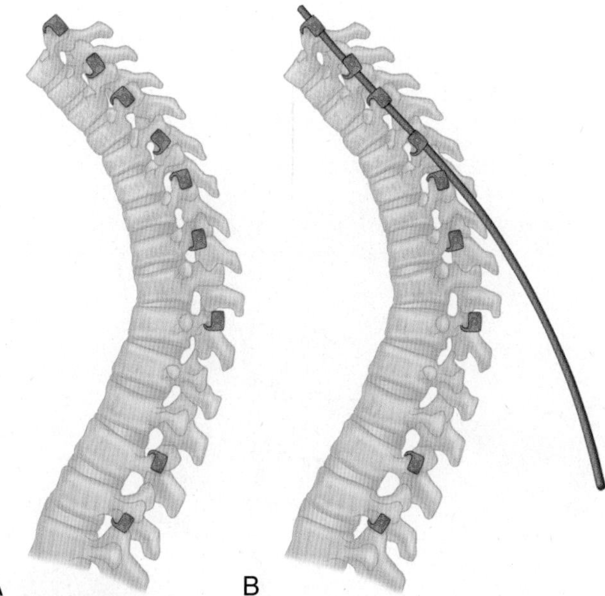

FIGURE 8.149 Reduction of kyphosis, standard method. **A,** Insertion of hooks. Note three sets of pedicle-transverse claws above apex of kyphosis. **B,** Rod passed through hooks of proximal segment and distal end of rod pushed to lower spine with rod pusher. Note that lower tip bend in rod facilitates hook insertion under distal lamina. **SEE TECHNIQUE 8.43.**

TECHNIQUE 8.43

(CRANDALL)

- Place the patient prone on a Jackson frame. The spine is approached posteriorly. The instrumentation frequently extends proximally to T2 to T3.
- Determine the apex of the kyphosis on preoperative radiographs.
- Use at least two sets of pedicular-transverse process claws or thoracic pedicle screws above the apex if the curve is flexible. In very large patients with rigid curves, extra fixation sites may be needed. A third set of fixation points may be used. Below the apex, reduction pedicle screws are used. At least three sets of screws are recommended.
- Debride the facet joints at each level to allow posterior column compression and to provide a bony surface for fusion.
- Perform osteotomies if necessary.
- Bend both rods above the kyphosis to approximate the normal spinal contour. Proper rod contouring is important. Leave the distal rods uncontoured.
- Insert the upper end of both rods into the proximal points. If hooks are being used, compress each claw construct to ensure that each hook claw remains seated. Tighten the threaded plugs to hold the upper hooks or pedicle screws securely in the rod.

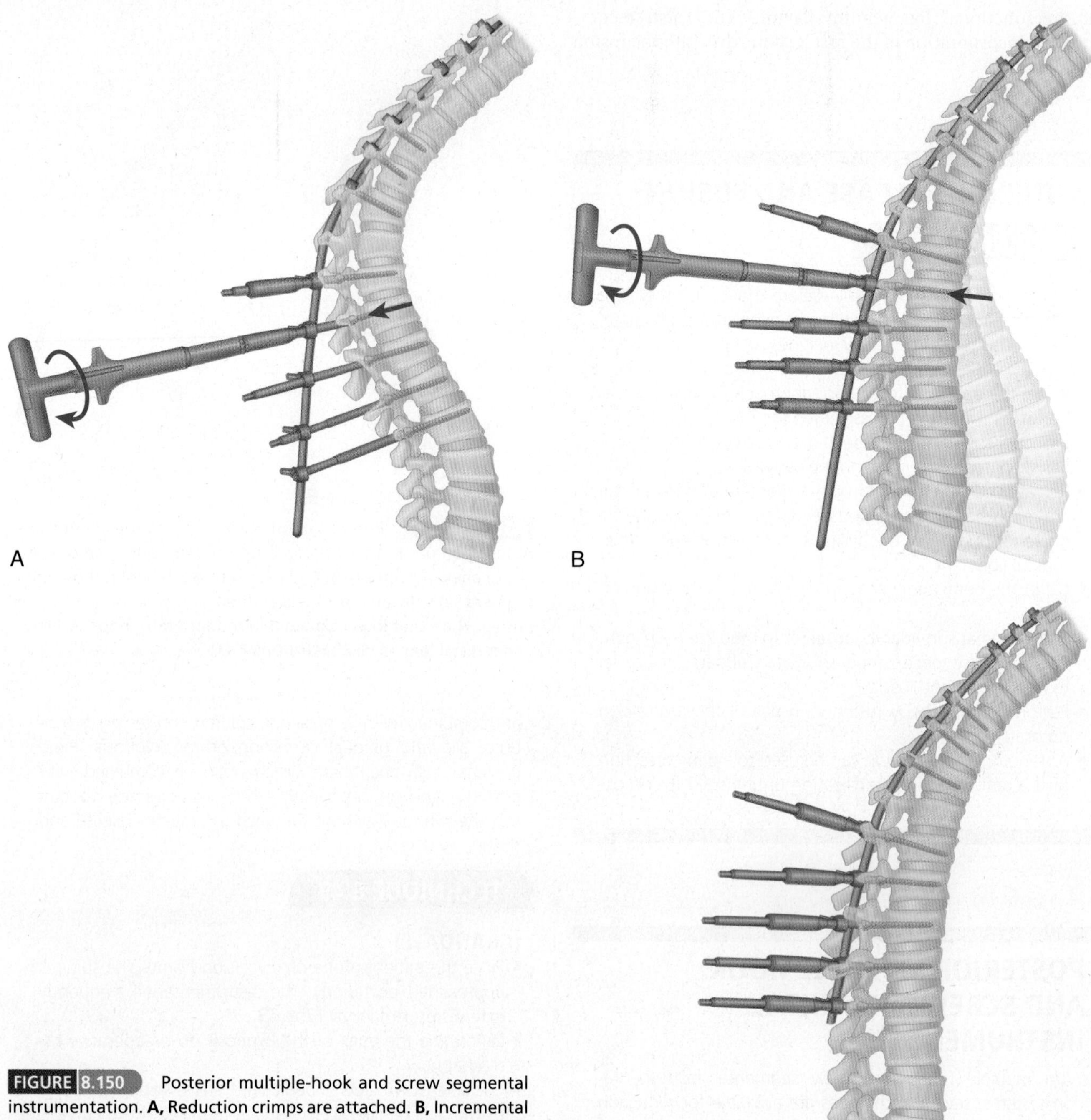

FIGURE 8.150 Posterior multiple-hook and screw segmental instrumentation. **A,** Reduction crimps are attached. **B,** Incremental reduction. **C,** Distal end of rod cut to appropriate length. **SEE TECHNIQUE 8.43.**

- After all the rods are in the proximal fixation points, place a crosslink plate on the rods. Attach the distal ends of both rods into the reduction screws (Fig. 8.150A).
- Begin the incremental reduction process with all reduction screws to pull the spine up to the rod (Fig. 8.150B).
- Cut the distal ends of the rods to the appropriate length (Fig. 8.150C).
- As the intermediate points of fixation come in contact with the rod, lock them to the rod and compress them to the proximal points of fixation. Gradual, repeated tightening, a few turns at a time with "two-finger" force on the driver, will bring the spine up in a safe and controlled fashion (Fig. 8.151). The spine is directly translated to the rod from any direction, achieving simultaneous correction in both the coronal and sagittal plane. Importantly, this correction should not proceed too quickly. A gradual reduction allows the spine to stretch the soft-tissue structures contracted in the kyphosis and allows the least amount of stress on the construct and spinal cord.

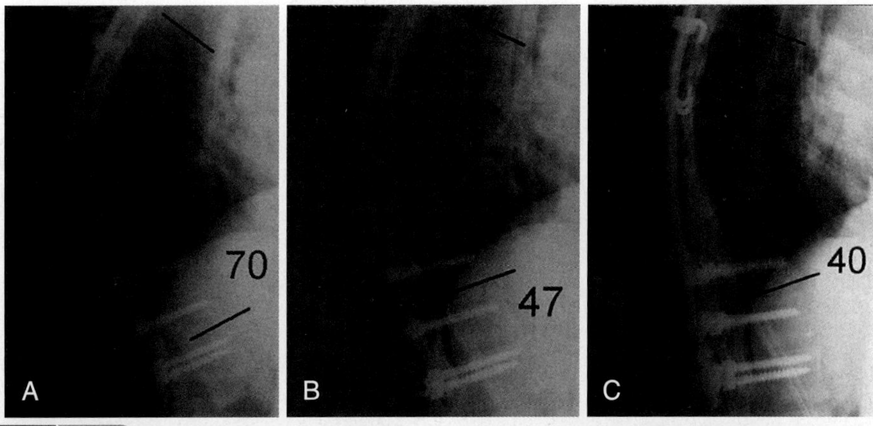

FIGURE 8.151 **A,** Beginning of correction, 70 degrees of kyphosis. **B,** Midpoint of correction, 47 degrees of kyphosis. **C,** Final construct, 40 degrees of kyphosis. **SEE TECHNIQUE 8.43.**

- After full kyphosis correction, fully compress the posterior column and lock it into position. Place a crosslink plate distally and proximally (Fig. 8.152).
- During tightening of the reduction crimps (every 3 to 5 minutes), harvest bone graft and decorticate the spine and facets.
- At the completion of the instrumentation, add abundant autogenous bone graft.

POSTOPERATIVE CARE Unless the bone quality is poor and fixation is tenuous, postoperative bracing is not required. If there is any concern about fixation, an extension orthosis, such as a Jewett brace, can be used until the fusion begins to consolidate, usually in 3 to 6 months. Ambulation is started as soon as possible. All patients start isometric and isotonic back exercise programs when the fusion appears solid. In adolescents, the fusion generally is solid in approximately 6 months. The patient generally is allowed to sit up on the second or third day postoperatively.

POSTERIOR COLUMN SHORTENING PROCEDURE FOR SCHEUERMANN KYPHOSIS

Ponte, Gebbia, and Eliseo described a posterior column shortening technique for the correction of Scheuermann kyphosis. The potential advantages of this technique include that it is a single-stage posterior procedure; the posterior spine is shortened rather than the anterior spine lengthened, thereby increasing safety; a gradual correction is obtained; there are no complications from a thoracotomy or thoracoscopy; and there is no surgical interference with anterior blood supply to the spinal cord.

TECHNIQUE 8.44

(PONTE ET AL.)

- A posterior midline approach is performed.
- Expose the spine subperiosteally to include one vertebra above and one vertebra below the fusion levels. The proximal extent of the fusion may need to include T1 to minimize the risk of cranial junctional kyphosis. The caudal limit must always be included and is determined by the first lordotic disc (open anteriorly) on lateral standing films.
- Resect the spinous processes and perform wide facetectomies and partial laminectomies of both the inferior and superior laminar borders at every intersegmental level of the fusion area. Ideally, gaps of 4 to 6 mm should be obtained (Fig. 8.153A). A generous resection of the facet joints as far as the pedicles is an essential step of this technique.
- Remove the ligamentum flavum entirely at all levels. The gaps extend uniformly over the entire width of the posterior spine (Fig. 8.153B-D).
- Insert the rods into the supralaminar hooks. If closed hooks are used, preload the hooks onto the rod and insert it as a unit. Pass the rod through the hooks just proximal to the apex. If open hooks are used, use appropriate set screws to hold the rod in the hooks or screws above the apex of the kyphosis.
- Leave the apical vertebra uninstrumented (Fig. 8.153D-H).
- Apply minimal compression force to keep the hooks in place. Any corrective tightening at this point would narrow the gaps and make placement of the hooks for the second rod difficult.
- Repeat the same sequence for the second rod. Apply compressive forces, beginning with the two opposing hooks facing the apex and then continuing sequentially to the cranial and caudal ends (see Fig. 8.153G).
- Repeat these maneuvers alternately on both sides and several times, always beginning at the apex. As compression proceeds, the rods will gradually straighten out and the intersegmental gaps will close. Creating small notches for the hook blades will prevent their interference with the closure of the gaps.
- Obtain an intraoperative radiograph to assess the magnitude of the correction. Fine-tuning is performed as needed to obtain a harmonious distribution of intersegmental correction.
- Secure two transverse connectors if they are needed for additional stability.

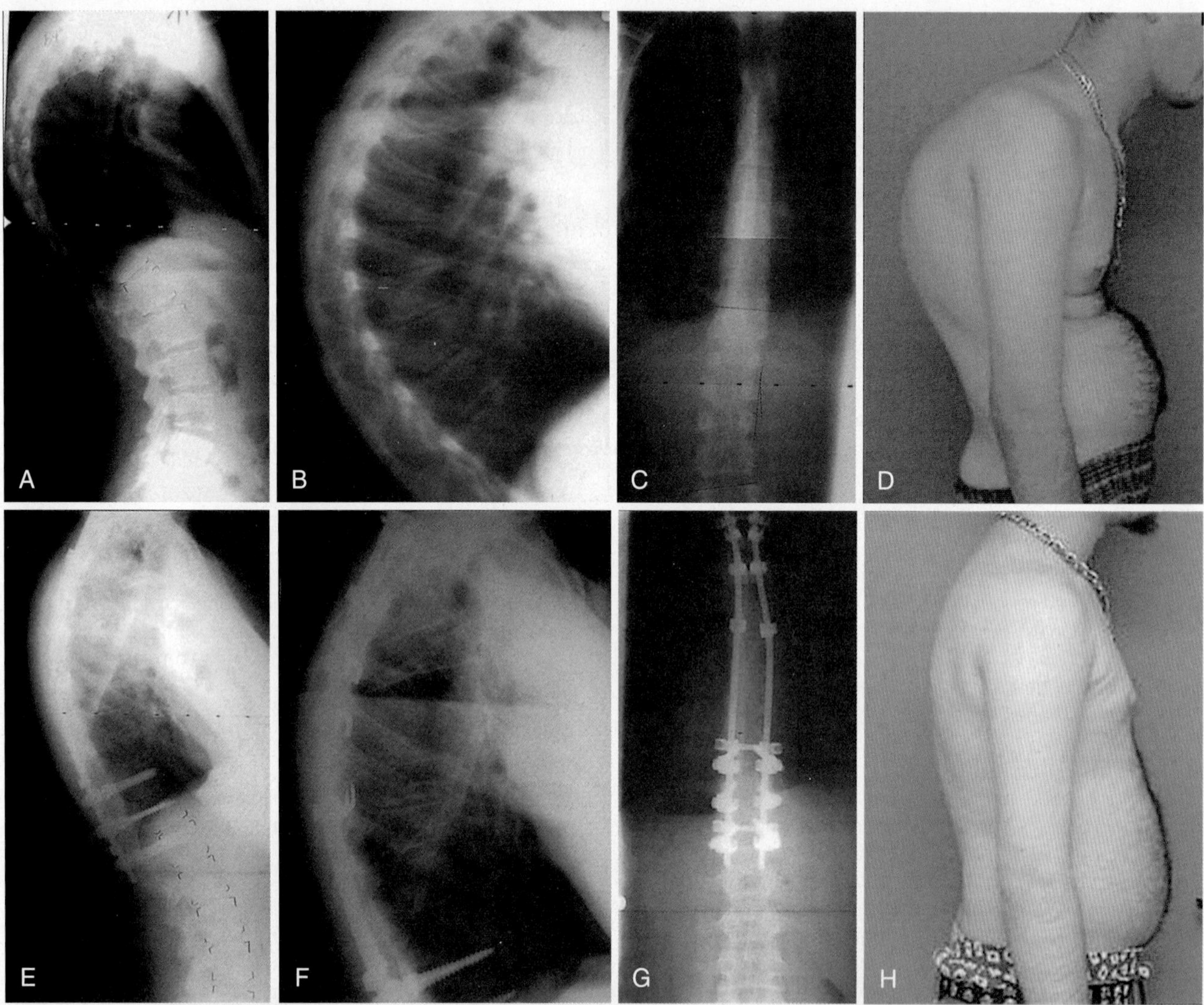

FIGURE 8.152 **A-C,** Preoperative radiographs of patient with Scheuermann kyphosis. **D,** Preoperative clinical photograph. **E-G,** Postoperative radiographs. **H,** Postoperative photograph. **SEE TECHNIQUE 8.43.**

- Perform decortication and add morselized bone graft.
- The same principle, with Ponte osteotomies, can be used with different instrumentation, including pedicle screws. Pedicle screws provide secure fixation without the problem of multiple hooks within the spinal canal and without the problem of the hooks potentially blocking the closure of the osteotomies. Gradual reduction-type pedicle screws can be used distally to allow a more gradual correction of the kyphosis.

POSTOPERATIVE CARE The patient is allowed to sit out of bed on the first postoperative day. There is no need for external support, such as bracing. Physical activities, such as sports or lifting of more than 5 or 10 lb, are restricted for 3 to 6 months. Radiographic assessment of the fusion at 6 months is performed, and if the fusion appears solid, gradual return to full activities is then allowed. Patients with an osteopenic spine or who are overweight or noncompliant may require a brace until the fusion is solid.

COMPLICATIONS

Complications are more frequent after the operative treatment of Scheuermann kyphosis than adolescent idiopathic scoliosis; in the case of major complications, Lonner et al. reported that they were four times more likely in Scheuermann kyphosis. Proximal junctional kyphosis has been reported to be present in as many as 30% and distal junctional kyphosis in 12% of surgically treated patients. To decrease the risk of junctional kyphosis, Denis et al. suggested that the fusion should include all vertebrae involved in the kyphosis, disruption of the ligamentous complex at the ends of the fusion should be avoided, and the fusion should extend distally to include the vertebra below the first lordotic disc. Distal and proximal implant failure is caused by the increased stresses placed on the instrumentation.

CONGENITAL KYPHOSIS

Congenital kyphosis is an uncommon deformity, but neurologic deficits resulting from this deformity are frequent. Congenital kyphosis occurs because of abnormal

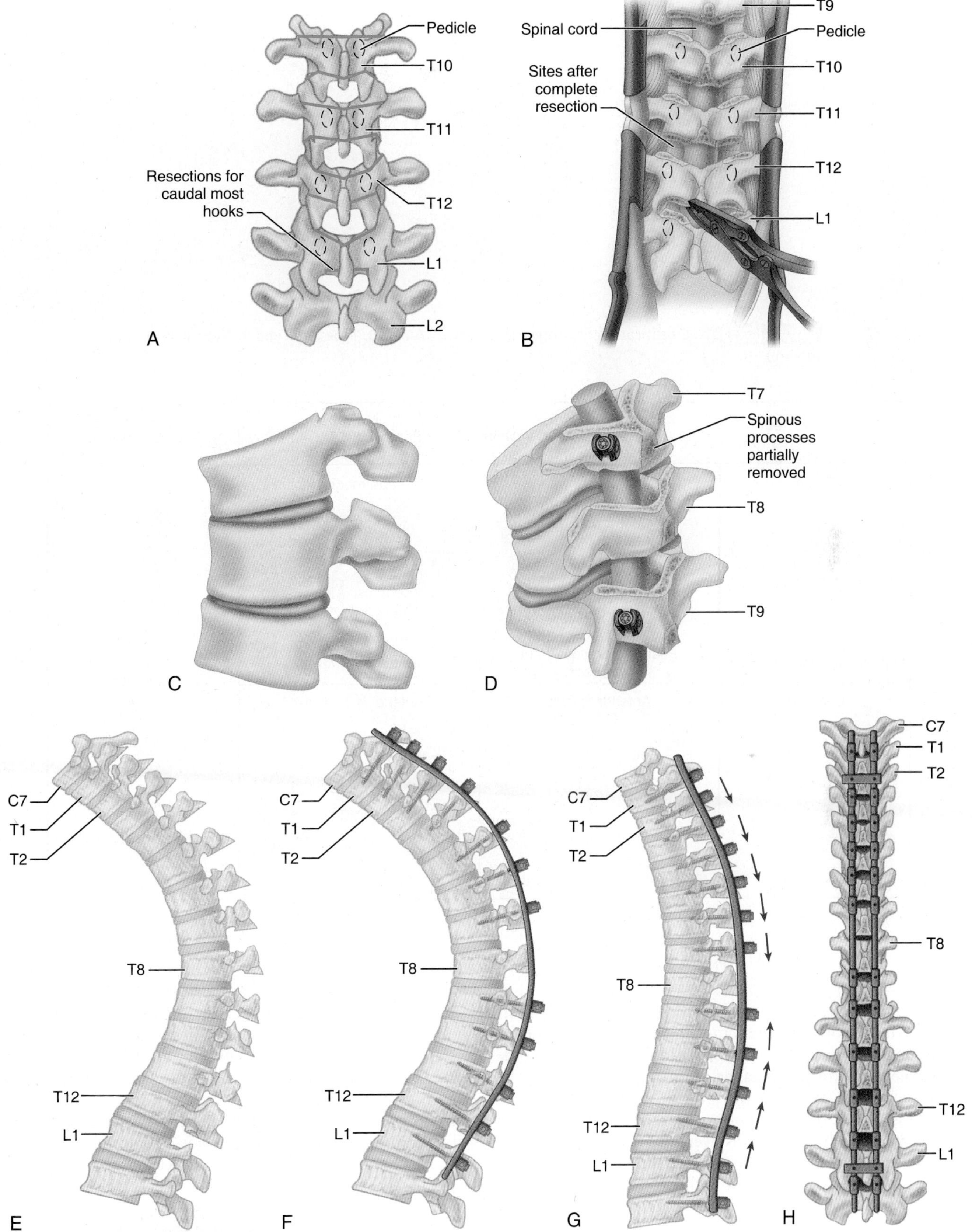

FIGURE 8.153 Posterior column shortening for Scheuermann kyphosis. **A,** Broad posterior resection *(shaded parts)* at every intersegmental level of entire area of fusion and instrumentation. **B,** Posterior view showing levels of completed resections. **C,** Lateral view showing gaps from osteotomies. Correction is achieved by closing gaps. **D,** Oblique view showing three apical vertebrae after completion of bone resections. Apical vertebra is left uninstrumented. **E-H,** Schematic representation of reduction of kyphosis. (Redrawn from Ponte A: Posterior column shortening for Scheuermann's kyphosis. An innovative one-stage technique. In Haher TR, Merola AA, editors: *Surgical techniques for the spine*, New York, 2003, Thieme.) **SEE TECHNIQUE 8.44.**

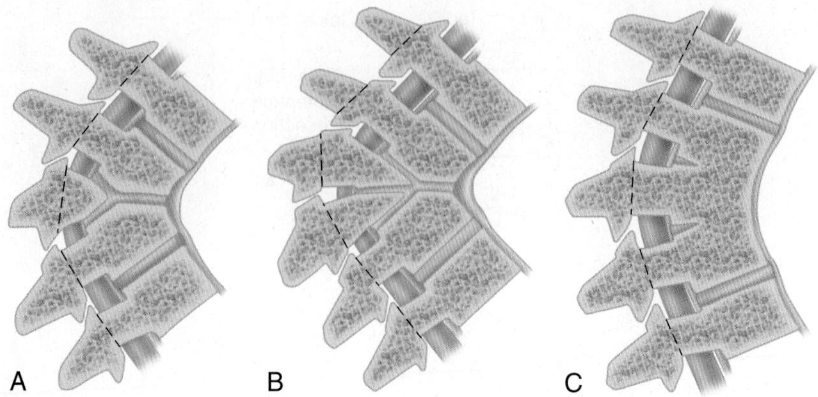

FIGURE 8.154 Classification of congenital kyphosis. **A** and **B**, Type I. **C**, Type II. (Type III is not shown.)

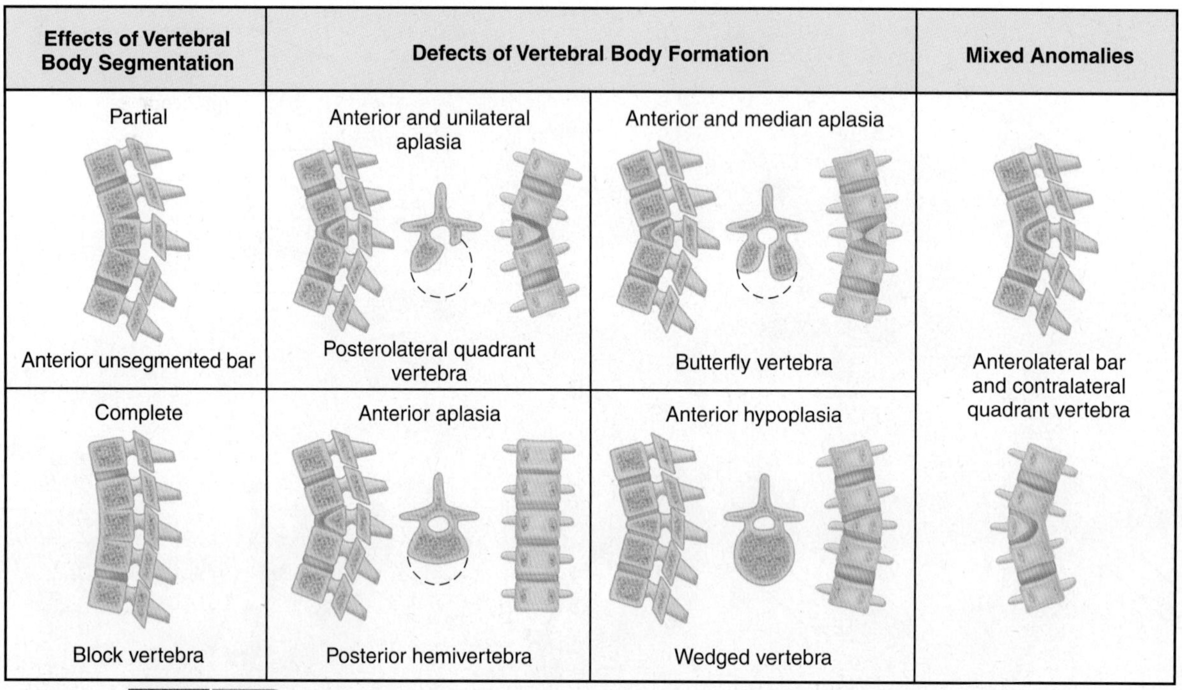

Effects of Vertebral Body Segmentation	Defects of Vertebral Body Formation		Mixed Anomalies
Partial Anterior unsegmented bar	Anterior and unilateral aplasia Posterolateral quadrant vertebra	Anterior and median aplasia Butterfly vertebra	Anterolateral bar and contralateral quadrant vertebra
Complete Block vertebra	Anterior aplasia Posterior hemivertebra	Anterior hypoplasia Wedged vertebra	

FIGURE 8.155 **Different types of vertebral anomalies that produce congenital kyphosis or kyphoscoliosis.** (From McMaster MJ, Singh H: Natural history of congenital kyphosis in kyphoscoliosis: a study of 112 patients, *J Bone Joint Surg* 81A:1367, 1999.)

development of the vertebrae consisting of a failure of formation or failure of segmentation of the developing segments. The spine may be either stable or unstable, or it may become unstable with growth. Spinal deformity in congenital kyphosis usually will progress with growth, and the amount of progression is directly proportional to the number of vertebrae involved, the type of involvement, and the amount of remaining normal growth in the affected vertebrae. Winter et al. described 130 patients with congenital kyphosis of three types. Type I is congenital failure of vertebral body formation. Type II is failure of vertebral body segmentation (Fig. 8.154). Type III is a combination of both of these conditions. McMaster and Singh further subdivided type I congenital kyphosis into posterolateral quadrant vertebrae, posterior hemivertebrae, butterfly (sagittal cleft) vertebrae, and anterior or anterolateral wedged vertebrae (Fig. 8.155). This classification is important in predicting the natural history of these congenital kyphotic deformities. Dubousset and Zeller et al. added a rotatory dislocation of the spine, and Shapiro and Herring further divided type III displacement into type A (sagittal plane only) and type B (rotatory, transverse, and sagittal planes). Any classification can be further subdivided into deformities with or without neurologic compromise.

The natural history of congenital kyphosis is well known and based on the type of kyphosis. Type I deformities are more common than type II deformities and occur more commonly in the thoracic spine and at the thoracolumbar junction. They are extremely rare in the cervical spine. In the series of McMaster and Singh, progression was most rapid in type III kyphosis, followed by type I. Kyphosis caused by two adjacent type I vertebral anomalies progressed more rapidly and produced a more severe deformity than did a single anomaly. Approximately 25% of patients with type I deformities had neurologic deficits, and deformities in the upper thoracic spine were more likely to be associated with neurologic problems. No patient in whom the apex of the kyphosis was at or caudad to the 12th thoracic vertebra had neurologic abnormalities. However, type I kyphosis progressed relentlessly during growth and usually accelerated during the adolescent growth spurt before stabilizing at skeletal maturity. An anterior failure of vertebral body formation produces a sharply angular kyphosis that is much more deforming and potentially dangerous neurologically than a curve with a similar Cobb measurement, owing to an anterior failure of segmentation that affects several adjacent vertebrae and produces a smooth, less obvious deformity.

Type II deformities (failure of segmentation) are less common. An absence of physes and discs anteriorly in one or more vertebrae results in the development of an anterior unsegmented bar. The amount of kyphosis produced is proportional to the discrepancy between the amounts of growth in the anterior and posterior portions of the defective vertebral segments. Mayfield et al. reported that these deformities progress at an average rate of 5 degrees a year and are not as severe as type I deformities. Paraplegia usually is not reported in patients with type II kyphosis; however, low back pain and cosmetic deformities are significant and early treatment is warranted.

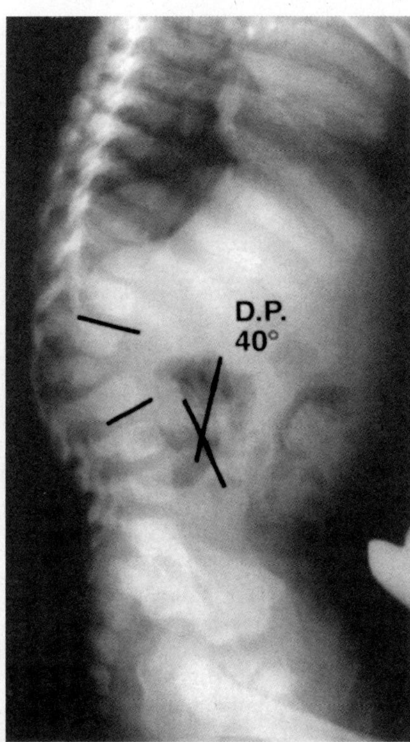

FIGURE 8.156 Two-year-old child with type I congenital kyphosis measuring 40 degrees. Radiograph shows failure of formation of anterior portion of first lumbar vertebra. (From Warner WC: Kyphosis. In Morrissy RT, Weinstein SL, editors: *Lovell and Winter's pediatric orthopaedics*, ed 6, Philadelphia, 2006, Lippincott Williams & Wilkins.)

CLINICAL AND RADIOGRAPHIC EVALUATION

The diagnosis of a congenital spine problem usually is made by a pediatrician before the patient is seen by an orthopaedist. The deformity may be detected before birth on a prenatal ultrasound examination or noted as a clinical deformity in a neonate. If the deformity is mild, congenital kyphosis can be overlooked until a rapid growth spurt makes the condition more obvious. Some mild deformities are found by chance on radiographs that are obtained for other reasons. Clinical deformities seen in the neonate tend to have a worse prognosis than those discovered as an incidental finding on plain radiographs.

Physical examination usually reveals a kyphotic deformity at the thoracolumbar junction or in the lower thoracic spine. A detailed neurologic examination should be done to look for any subtle signs of neurologic compromise. Associated musculoskeletal and nonmusculoskeletal anomalies should be sought on physical examination. High-quality, detailed anteroposterior and lateral radiographs provide the most information in the evaluation of congenital kyphosis (Fig. 8.156). Failure of segmentation and the true extent of failure of formation may be difficult to detect on early films because of incomplete ossification. Flexion and extension lateral radiographs are helpful in determining the rigidity of the kyphosis and possible instability of the spine. CT with three-dimensional reconstructions can identify the amount of vertebral body involvement and can determine whether more kyphosis or scoliosis might be expected (Fig. 8.157). CT can only identify the nature of the bony deformity and the size of the cartilage anlage; it does not show the amount of growth potential in the cartilage anlage and therefore only estimates the possible progression. An MRI study should be obtained in most patients because of the significant incidence of intraspinal abnormalities. In addition, the location of the spinal cord and any areas of spinal cord compression caused by the kyphosis can be seen on MRI. The cartilage anlage will be well defined by MRI in patients with failure of formation (Fig. 8.158).

Genitourinary abnormalities, cardiac abnormalities, Klippel-Feil syndrome, and intraspinal abnormalities are frequent in these patients. Cardiac evaluation and renal ultrasonography should be done. Myelograms have been used for documenting spinal cord compression but generally have been replaced by MRI.

OPERATIVE TREATMENT

The natural history of this condition usually is one of continued progression and an increased risk of neurologic compromise. Therefore surgery is the preferred method of treatment. If the diagnosis is uncertain or the deformity is mild, close observation may be an option. Unless compensatory curves are being treated above or below the congenital kyphosis, bracing has no role in the treatment of congenital kyphosis because it neither corrects the deformity nor stops the progression of kyphosis.

Surgery is recommended for congenital kyphosis. The type of surgery depends on the type and size of the deformity, the age of the patient, and the presence of neurologic deficits. Procedures include posterior fusion, anterior fusion, combined anterior and posterior fusion, anterior osteotomy with posterior fusion, posterior column shortening and fusion, and vertebral body resection. Fusion can be done with or without instrumentation.

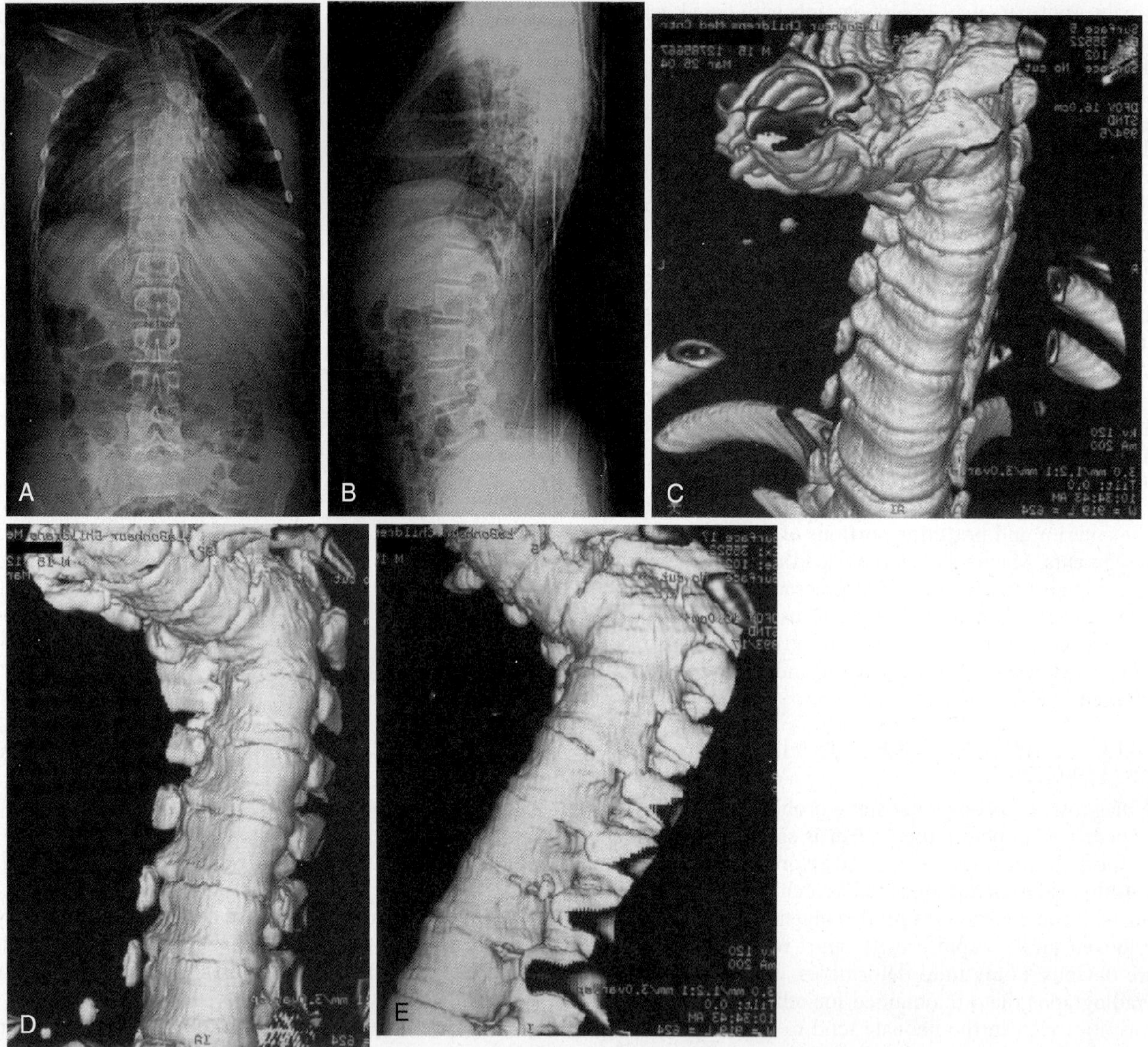

FIGURE 8.157 Congenital kyphosis. **A** and **B,** Anteroposterior and lateral radiographs. Note inadequate detail of kyphosis on lateral radiograph of spine. **C-E,** CT three-dimensional reconstruction views that clearly show bony anatomy of congenital kyphosis. (From Warner WC: Kyphosis. In Morrissy RT, Weinstein SL, editors: *Lovell and Winter's pediatric orthopaedics*, ed 6, Philadelphia, 2006, Lippincott Williams & Wilkins.)

TREATMENT OF TYPE I DEFORMITY

The treatment of type I deformity depends on the stage of the disease. For type I deformity, the best treatment is early posterior fusion. In a patient younger than 5 years old with a deformity of less than 50 or 55 degrees, posterior fusion alone, extending from one level above the kyphotic deformity to one level below, is recommended. This allows for some improvement because growth continues anteriorly from the anterior endplates of the vertebrae one level above and below the kyphotic vertebrae that are included in the posterior fusion. Although McMaster and Singh reported 15 degrees of correction in most patients treated with this technique, Kim et al. reported that correction of kyphosis occurred with growth only in patients younger than 3 years of age with type II and type III deformities. In curves of more than 60 degrees, anterior and posterior spinal fusions at least one level above and one level below the kyphosis are indicated. This halts the progression of the kyphotic deformity, but because the anterior physes are ablated, there is no possibility of correction with growth.

Posterior fusion alone may be successful if the kyphosis is less than 50 to 55 degrees in older patients with type I kyphotic deformity. If the deformity is more than 55 degrees, anterior and posterior fusion produces more reliable results. Anterior fusion alone will not correct the deformity, and anterior strut grafting with temporary distraction and posterior fusion, with or without posterior compression instrumentation, is necessary for deformity correction (Fig. 8.159). Posterior instrumentation may allow for some correction of the kyphosis but should be regarded more as an internal stabilizer than as a correction device. Although instrumentation has been reported to decrease the occurrence of pseudarthrosis, it should be used with caution in rigid, angular curves because of the high incidence of neurologic complications.

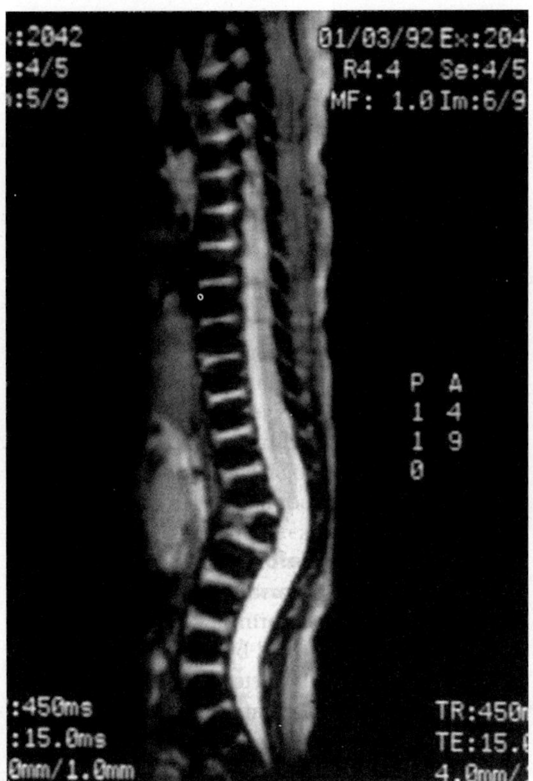

FIGURE 8.158 MRI of type I congenital kyphosis. Failure of formation of anterior vertebral body is shown, but growth potential of involved vertebra cannot be determined. Note pressure on dural sac. (From Warner WC: Kyphosis. In Morrissy RT, Weinstein SL, editors: *Lovell and Winter's pediatric orthopaedics*, ed 6, Philadelphia, 2006, Lippincott Williams & Wilkins.)

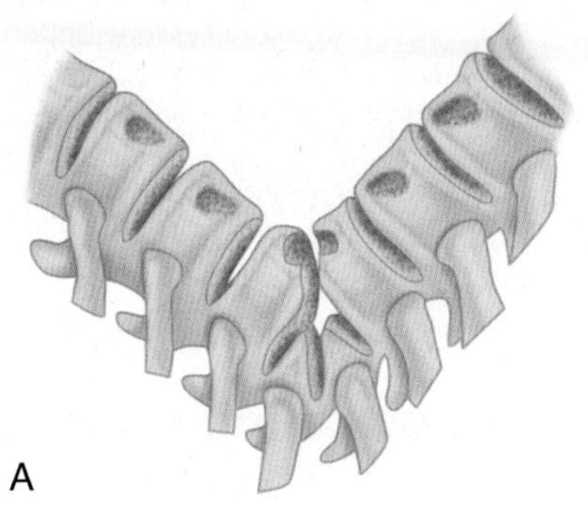

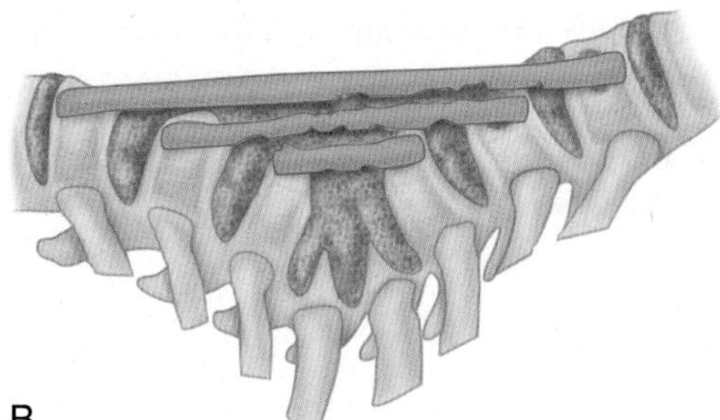

FIGURE 8.159 **A,** Preparation of tunnels for strut grafts. **B,** Insertion of strut grafts into prepared tunnels with cancellous bone graft in disc spaces.

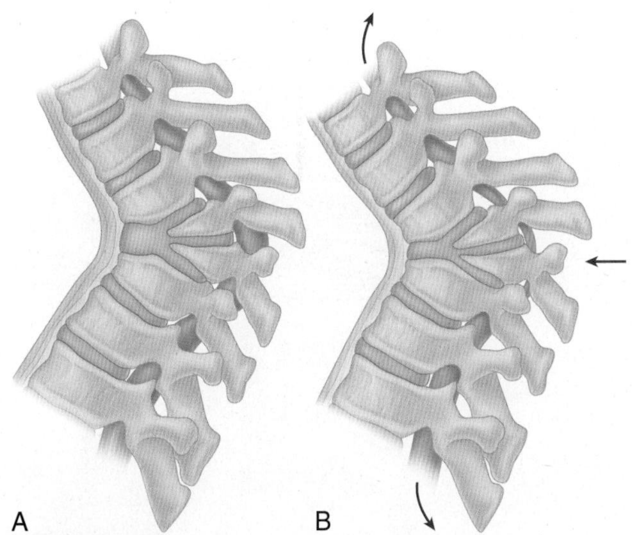

FIGURE 8.160 Effect of traction on rigid congenital kyphosis. **A,** Apical area does not change with traction, but adjacent spine is lengthened. **B,** As spine lengthens, so does spinal cord, producing increased tension in cord and aggravating existing neurologic deficits.

If anterior strut grafting is done, the strut graft should be placed anteriorly under compression. If the goal of surgery is to stop the progression of deformity without correction, an anterior interbody fusion with a posterior fusion can be done. Simultaneous anterior and posterior approaches through a costotransversectomy that allows resection of the posterior hemivertebra and correction of the kyphosis with posterior compression instrumentation have been described. After removal of the hemivertebra, correction can be obtained safely and the thecal sac observed during correction. Use of skeletal traction (halo-pelvic, halo-femoral, or halo-gravity) to correct the deformity is tempting but is not recommended because there is a risk of paraplegia (Fig. 8.160). Traction pulls the spinal cord against the apex of the rigid kyphosis, which can lead to neurologic compromise in a patient with a rigid gibbus deformity.

Late treatment of a severe congenital kyphotic deformity that is accompanied by spinal cord compression is difficult; laminectomy has no role in the treatment of this condition. If there is an associated scoliosis, the anterior approach for decompression may need to be on the concavity of the scoliosis to allow the spinal cord to move both forward and into the midline after decompression. After adequate decompression, the involved vertebrae are fused with an anterior strut graft. Posterior fusion, with or without posterior stabilizing instrumentation, is then performed. Postoperative support using a cast, brace, or halo cast may be required. Posterior vertebral column resection or decompression and subtraction osteotomy, followed by stabilizing instrumentation, also can be used. Chang et al. described circumferential decompression and cantilever bending correction with posterior instrumentation.

TREATMENT OF TYPE II DEFORMITY

If a type II kyphosis is mild (<50 degrees) and detected early, posterior fusion using compression instrumentation can be done. All the involved vertebrae plus one vertebra above

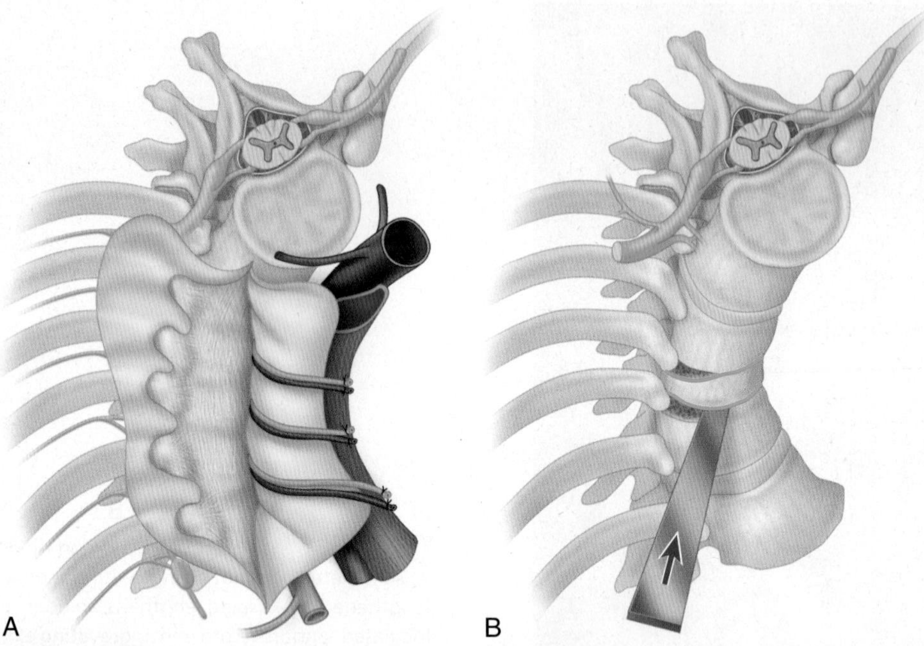

FIGURE 8.161 **A,** Anterolateral exposure of spine in preparation for anterior osteotomy. **B,** Completion of osteotomy with osteotome. **SEE TECHNIQUE 8.45.**

and one vertebra below the congenital kyphosis should be included in the posterior fusion.

Because the kyphosis is rounded and affects several segments in type II deformity, instead of being sharply angular as in type I, compression instrumentation can be safely used. If the deformity is severe and detected late, correction can be obtained only with anterior osteotomies and fusion, followed by posterior fusion and compression instrumentation.

ANTERIOR OSTEOTOMY AND FUSION

TECHNIQUE 8.45

(WINTER ET AL.)

- Expose the spine through an appropriate anterior approach.
- Ligate the segmental vessels and expose the spine by subperiosteal stripping (Fig. 8.161A). The anterior longitudinal ligament usually is thickened and must be divided at one or more levels. Make sure that a circumferential exposure is made all the way to the opposite foramen before beginning the osteotomy.
- Divide the bony bar with a sharp osteotome or high-speed burr. Start the division anteriorly and work posteriorly until the remaining disc material is entered.
- Once the remaining disc material is seen, use a laminar spreader and excise the disc material back to the level of the posterior longitudinal ligament (Fig. 8.161B). If the bony bar is complete, make the osteotomy all the way through the posterior cortex at the level of the foramina. Take care in the area of the posterior longitudinal ligament because the ligament may be absent.
- Once the osteotomies have been completed, insert strut grafts, slotting them into bodies above and below the area of the kyphos. Hollow out the cancellous bone of each body with a curet. With rib, fibula, or iliac crest grafts of sufficient length, insert the upper end of the graft into the slot first. As manual pressure is applied posteriorly against the kyphos, use an impactor to tap the lower end of the graft into place. Place additional grafts in the disc space defects and close the pleura over them if possible. More than one strut graft may be necessary, depending on the severity of the curve. The grafts should be placed as far anterior to the axis of the flexion deformity as possible.
- Winter et al. found that failures of anterior fusion in their patients generally were associated with strut grafts that were too short or placed too close to the apex of the kyphosis or with inadequate removal of the intervertebral discs in the fusion area.

ANTERIOR CORD DECOMPRESSION AND FUSION

TECHNIQUE 8.46

(WINTER AND LONSTEIN)

- Expose the spine through an appropriate anterior approach.
- Identify the apical vertebra and the site of compression and remove the intervertebral disc completely on each side of the vertebral body or bodies.

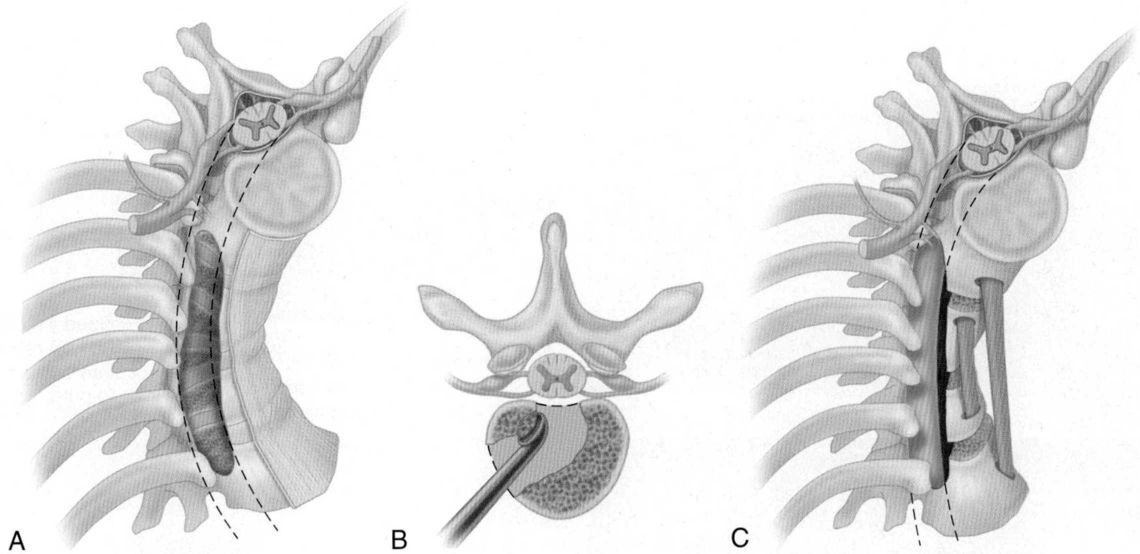

FIGURE 8.162 **A,** Anterolateral exposure of spine and partial removal of apex of kyphosis. **B,** Posterior cortex is removed, allowing decompression of spinal cord. **C,** Cord is decompressed and strut grafts are in place. **SEE TECHNIQUE 8.45.**

- Remove the vertebral body laterally at the apex of the kyphosis with curets, rongeurs, or high-speed burrs.
- Remove the cancellous bone back to the posterior cortex of the vertebral body from pedicle to pedicle, removing a wedge-shaped area of bone (Fig. 8.162A).
- Beginning on the side away from the surgeon, use angled curets to remove the posterior cortical shell. Removal of the bone farthest away first prevents the spinal cord from falling into the defect and blocking vision on the far side (Fig. 8.162B).
- Next, remove the closest bony shell, working toward the apex. Control epidural bleeding with thrombin-soaked Gelfoam.
- Once the cord has been decompressed, perform an anterior strut graft fusion (Fig. 8.162C).
- Close and drain the incision in the routine manner.
- At a second stage, a posterior fusion with or without instrumentation is done.

ANTERIOR VASCULAR RIB BONE GRAFTING

Bradford et al. noted frequent fracture of strut grafts when the grafts were not in contact with the vertebral bodies and simply spanned an open area between vertebrae. A rib or fibular graft may take up to 2 years for replacement, and it is weakest approximately 6 months after surgery. To prevent graft fracture, Bradford developed a technique of vascular pedicle bone graft for the treatment of severe kyphosis when the strut must be placed more than 4 cm from the spine. He credited Rose et al. with first describing the technique in 1975.

TECHNIQUE 8.47

(BRADFORD)

- Plan the thoracotomy to remove enough rib to bridge the kyphosis. For a severe kyphotic deformity from T6 to T12, a vascularized fifth rib would be used to strut the deformity.
- Make a skin incision as in the routine transthoracic exposure. Take care to identify the appropriate rib and avoid the use of electrocautery over the rib periosteum.
- Divide the intercostal muscles sharply off the cranial portion of the rib. This rib dissection is always extraperiosteal. Divide the rib distally to provide enough length to span the area of deformity.
- At the level of the distal rib osteotomy, ligate the intercostal vessels and sharply cut the intercostal nerve and allow it to retract. The intercostal muscles attached to the caudal portion of the rib should remain attached to provide protection for the intercostal vessels that will perfuse the rib.
- At the level for the proximal rib osteotomy, mobilize the periosteum away from the rib.
- Once the osteotomy is completed, the rib is connected only to the caudal intercostal muscle and its intercostal vascular pedicle. Carefully divide the intercostal vessels below the rib in the direction of the costovertebral joint, retaining the muscle around the intercostal pedicle. Do not dissect out the intercostal artery and vein.
- If the rib and muscle are poorly perfused, dissect the vascular pedicle away from the intercostal vessels (Fig. 8.163).
- Mobilize the rib with its intact intercostal musculature and artery and vein complex (Fig. 8.164A).
- Carefully peel back the periosteum on the rib graft for 2 or 3 mm on each end to provide bone-to-bone contact without soft-tissue intervention when the graft is rotated into position.

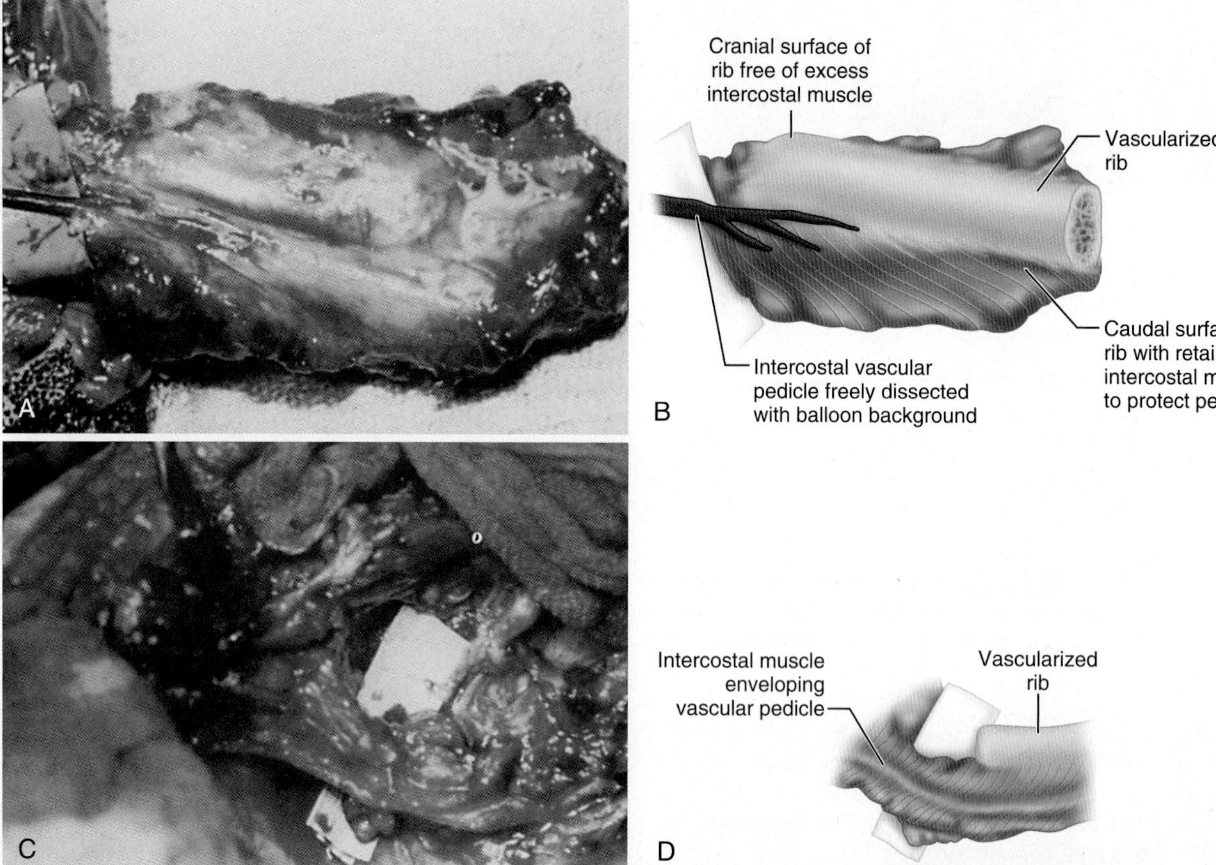

FIGURE 8.163 **A** and **B,** Background balloon placed behind intercostal vascular pedicle. Ordinarily, it is not necessary to dissect out vascular pedicle. **C** and **D,** Retaining portion of intercostal muscle with vessel as shown here reduces likelihood of pedicle injury during harvest. (From Shaffer JW, Bradford DS: The use of and techniques for vascularized rib pedicle grafts. In Bridwell KH, DeWald RL, editors: *The textbook of spinal surgery*, ed 2, Philadelphia, 1997, Lippincott-Raven.) **SEE TECHNIQUE 8.47.**

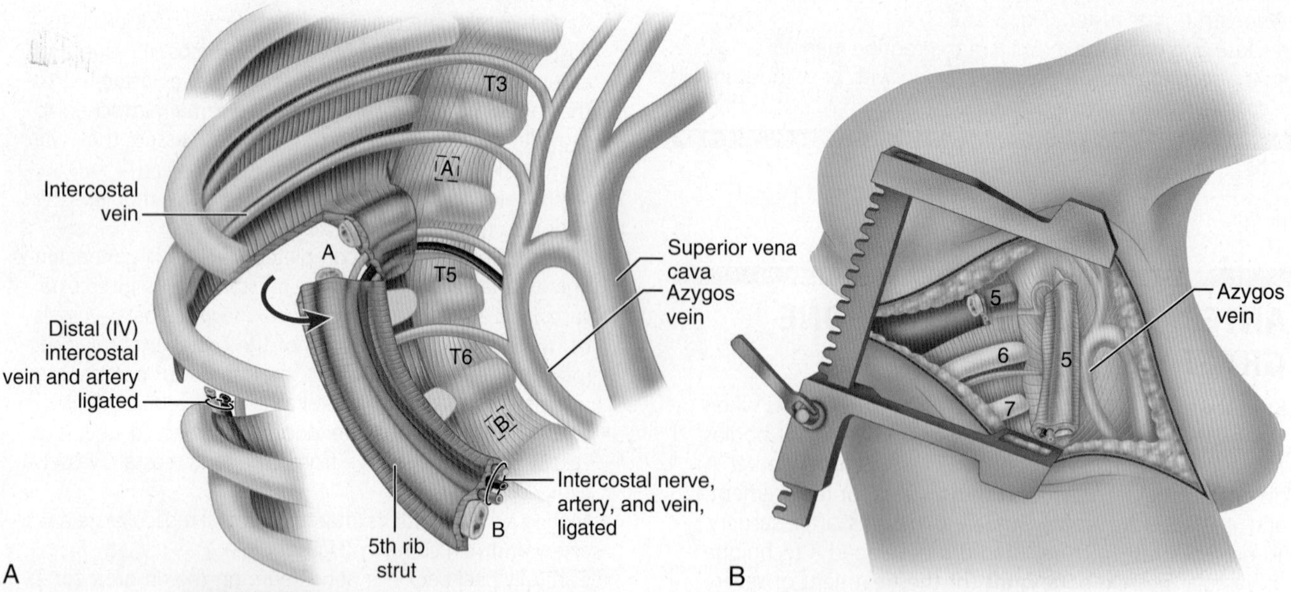

FIGURE 8.164 Thoracotomy. **A,** Wide margin of intercostal muscle left attached to rib to ensure intact blood supply. **B,** Rib graft rotated 90 degrees on its axis and keyed into vertebral bodies over length of kyphosis to be fused. **SEE TECHNIQUE 8.47.**

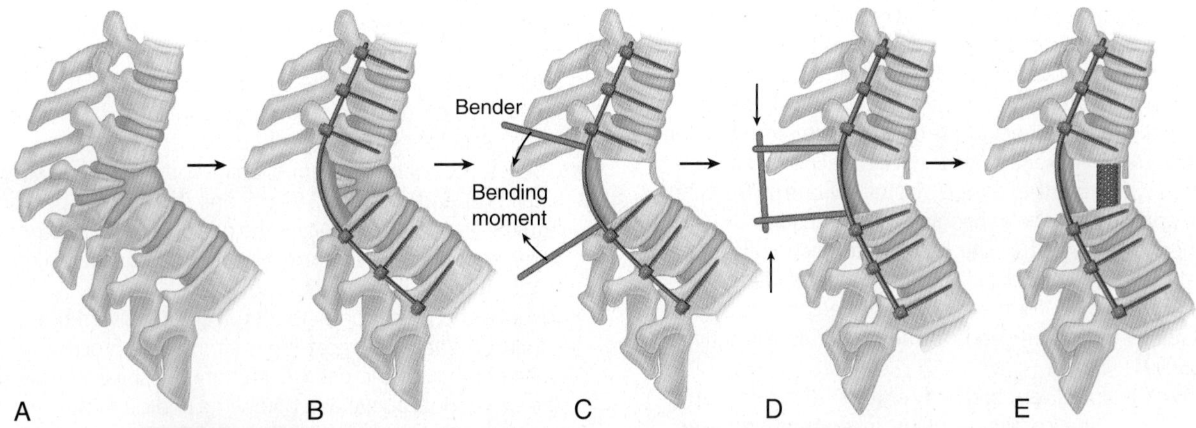

FIGURE 8.165 Hinge technique for correction of severe, rigid kyphotic deformity. **A,** Severe angular kyphosis. **B,** Laminectomy, pediculectomy, and rods placed on same plane as the cord. **C,** Complete circumferential decompression and placement of rod benders. **D,** Cantilever bending to correct kyphosis. **E,** Insertion of mesh cage to provide anterior support. (Redrawn from Chang KW, Cheng CW, Chen HC, Chen TC: Correction hinge in the compromised cord for severe and rigid angular kyphosis with neurologic deficits, *Spine* 34:1040, 2009.) **SEE TECHNIQUE 8.48.**

- Identify the vertebral bodies proximally and distally to be included in the fusion.
- Make a hole in the anterior aspect of the vertebral body above and below to accept the ends of the rib graft.
- Trim the rib so that the ends will match the length of the spine to be fused.
- Rotate the rib on its axis approximately 90 degrees and wedge it into the vertebrae above and below (Fig. 8.164B).
- Close the chest in a routine fashion over chest tubes.
- Immobilization of the spine after vascular grafting is the same as after nonvascular graft procedures.

CIRCUMFERENTIAL DECOMPRESSION AND CANTILEVER BENDING

TECHNIQUE 8.48

(CHANG ET AL.)

- With the patient prone and somatosensory-evoked potential monitoring initiated, make a straight posterior midline incision.
- After subperiosteal dissection, expose three to five vertebrae (depending on the bone quality) above and below the apex to the tips of the transverse process.
- Insert pedicle screws segmentally except at the levels of circumferential decompression, where at least three segments of fixation are made at either end of the decompression.
- Carry dissection out laterally, exposing the ribs corresponding to the levels of circumferential neurologic decompression as determined by preoperative radiographic analysis (most often at the apex of the kyphotic deformity).
- Remove the transverse process and the corresponding ribs on both sides of the neurologic decompression to expose the lateral wall of the pedicle.
- Deepen the subperiosteal dissection, following the lateral wall of the vertebral body, until a comfortable working space for neurologic decompression is evident beneath the compromised cord.
- Take care to avoid damaging segmental vessels during the exposure. Injured segmental vessels should be clamped, ligated, and cut under spinal cord monitoring to ensure that there are no changes in somatosensory-evoked potentials.
- Carry out total laminectomy and facetectomy at the apex to expose the compromised neural tissue. In thoracic vertebrae, cut the nerve roots to facilitate thorough neurologic decompression; in the lumbar vertebrae, keep the nerve roots intact.
- Remove the pedicle to expose the lateral portion of the compromised dural tube.
- Connect pedicle screws on both sides by two rods contoured to the shape of the deformity to facilitate rigid fixation.
- Because of the marked angular change in segments around the apex, the rods can be situated nearly on the same coronal plane as the compromised cord by adjusting the protruding height of the screw heads at the levels immediately cephalad and caudad to the apex (the level of circumferential neurologic decompression) and properly precontouring the rods (Fig. 8.165A).
- Create a tunnel beneath the compromised cord by penetrating a blunt-end cage trial from one side of the apical vertebral body to the other. Enlarge the tunnel and use rongeurs, curets, and pituitary forceps to remove the portion of the apical vertebral body above the tunnel and adjacent to the anterior compromised dural tube (including the posterior vertebral wall).

- After completion of this neurologic decompression, check to ensure that the canal is clear of any residual compression at the resection margins. Use a curet to remove cancellous bone within the portion of the apical vertebral body; deepen the tunnel to the depth of the anterior vertebral cortex. Weaken the cortex at several points by penetration with a blunt-end cage trial to facilitate its fracture while applying cantilever bending for correction.
- Connect one pair of in situ benders to each contoured rod at the levels immediately cephalad and caudad to the apex (Fig. 8.165B). Fix the position of the benders by using wire to tie the free ends at the desired location (Fig. 8.165C).
- Fracture the apical vertebral body anterior to the cord and open it with the correction hinge in the compromised cord.
- Slowly increase the bending force. If resistance is felt, stop the correction and fix.
- After correction, perform a wake-up test.
- Measure the height of the anterior interbody gap. Fill a titanium mesh with bone chips and insert it into the anterior gap, and place an autogenous iliac bone graft around the titanium mesh. Insert the mesh cage from the lateral side to fit on the cephalad and caudal bone base.
- Confirm proper cage position by direct observation and fluoroscopy. Make sure there is ample space between the cage and the cord before releasing the benders and locking the cage in place (Fig. 8.165D).
- Connect two transverse links to the rods at the cephalad and caudad levels to the level of neurologic decompression.
- Perform posterior fusion at all instrumented levels.
- Close the wound in the usual fashion over suction drains.

POSTOPERATIVE CARE Patients are fitted with a custom-made, plastic thoracolumbosacral orthosis and are allowed out of bed 72 hours after surgery. The orthosis is worn for 6 months.

POSTERIOR HEMIVERTEBRA RESECTION WITH TRANSPEDICULAR INSTRUMENTATION

TECHNIQUE 8.49

(RUF AND HARMS)

- Carefully expose the posterior elements of the spine at the affected levels, including the lamina, transverse processes, and facet joints, and, in the thoracic spine, the surplus rib head on the convex side.
- Mark the entry points for the pedicle screws with a fine needle and check their position with image intensification in an anteroposterior view. In the lumbar region, the entry point is the base of the transverse process at the lateral border of the superior articular facet. In the thoracic region, the entry point is at the superior margin of the transverse process, slightly lateral to the lower lateral edge of the articular facet. On image intensification, the tips of the cannulas should project onto the oval of the pedicles, ideally slightly lateral to the center.
- Open the bone at the entry point with a sharp awl or small burr and advance a 2-mm drill through the pedicle into the vertebral body. Mark the drill holes with Kirschner wires and check their correct position with fluoroscopy. After tapping, insert the screws.
- Remove the posterior elements of the hemivertebra, including the lamina, facet joints, transverse process, and posterior part of the pedicle. Identify the spinal cord and the nerve roots above and below the pedicle of the hemivertebra. In the thoracic spine, resect the rib head and the proximal part of the surplus rib at the convex side also.
- After resection of the transverse process and the rib head, expose the lateral-anterior part of the hemivertebra by blunt dissection; this exposure is retroperitoneal in the lumbar spine and extrapleural in the thoracic spine.
- Remove the remnants of the pedicle and expose the posterior aspect of the vertebral body of the hemivertebra; this is made easier by the fact that the hemivertebra lies far laterally on the convex side, whereas the spinal cord usually is shifted to the concave side.
- Cut the discs adjacent to the hemivertebra and mobilize and remove the body of the hemivertebra, using a blunt spatula to protect the anterior structures.
- Completely remove the remaining disc material of the upper and lower disc spaces and debride the endplates down to bleeding bone. Make sure that disc removal reaches the contralateral side.
- Complete the instrumentation and apply compression on the convex side until the gap left after resection is closed completely. If a void remains, fill it with cancellous bone.
- When kyphosis is present, anterior column support can be added to create a fulcrum to achieve lordosis. The neural structures must be controlled and protected at all times during the resection and during the corrective maneuver.
- If there is a single hemivertebra without bars, rib synostosis, or other major structural changes of the neighboring vertebrae, only the two vertebrae adjacent to the resected hemivertebra are fused. If major structural changes are present in the adjacent vertebrae or there is a more severe kyphotic deformity, one or two additional segments may be included in the fusion.
- For contralateral bar formation and rib synostosis, the synostosed rib heads on the concave side are removed and the bar is cut. The fusion is extended with segmental instrumentation over the whole length of the bar formation to the adjacent vertebrae.

POSTOPERATIVE CARE Postoperative management is as described for Technique 8.48.

Zeng et al. described pedicle subtraction osteotomy and posterior vertebral column resection (Fig. 8.166) in 23 patients with kyphosis or kyphoscoliosis. Overall, satisfactory correction was obtained in 91%, with comparable complications.

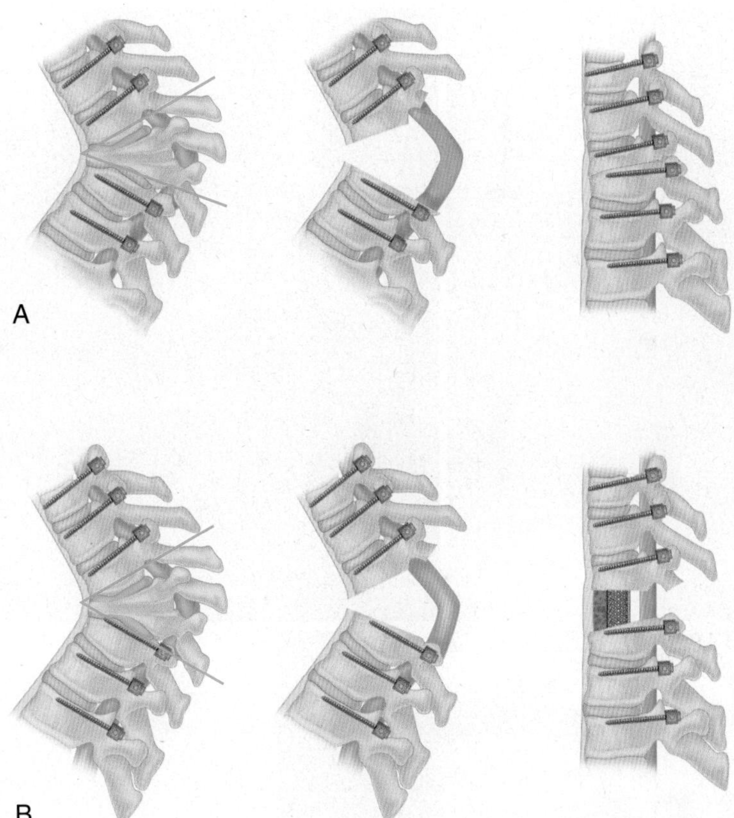

FIGURE 8.166 Pedicle subtraction osteotomy and posterior vertebral column resection for congenital kyphosis. **A,** Pedicle subtraction osteotomy. **B,** Posterior vertebral column resection. (Redrawn from Zeng Y, Chen Z, Qi Q, et al: The posterior surgical correction of congenital kyphosis and kyphoscoliosis: 23 cases with minimum 2 years follow-up, *Eur Spine J* 22:372, 2013.) **SEE TECHNIQUE 8.49.**

COMPLICATIONS OF OPERATIVE TREATMENT

Some of the more frequent complications of treatment of congenital kyphosis are pseudarthrosis, progression of kyphosis, and paralysis. Pseudarthrosis and progression of the kyphotic deformity can be minimized by performing anterior and posterior fusions for deformities of more than 50 degrees. The posterior fusion should extend from one level above to one level below the involved vertebra.

Paralysis is perhaps the most feared complication of spinal surgery. The risk of this complication can be lessened by not attempting to maximally correct the deformity with instrumentation. Instrumentation should be used more for stabilization of rigid deformities rather than correction unless there has been an anterior decompression or vertebral column resection. Halo traction in rigid congenital kyphotic deformities has been associated with an increased risk of neurologic compromise. Another long-term problem, occurring in approximately 38% of patients with kyphosis, is low back pain caused by increased lumbar lordosis that is needed to compensate for the kyphotic deformity.

PROGRESSIVE ANTERIOR VERTEBRAL FUSION

Progressive anterior vertebral fusion is an uncommon cause of kyphosis in children that may be confused with type II congenital kyphosis if it is discovered late. However, it is distinguishable from type II congenital kyphosis in that the disc spaces and vertebral bodies are normal at birth and later become anteriorly fused. Knutsson first described progressive anterior vertebral fusion in 1949, and fewer than 100 cases have since been reported. The cause is unknown, and it is probably a distinct clinical condition; however, it may possibly represent a delayed type II congenital kyphosis.

Certain forms of type II congenital kyphosis (failure of segmentation) can be inherited with failure of segmentation and delayed fusion of the anterior vertebral elements, which are not visible on radiographs until 8 or 10 years of age. Familial occurrence has been reported by several authors. Associated anomalies, including hearing defects, tibial agenesis, foot deformities, Klippel-Feil syndrome, Ito syndrome, pulmonary artery stenosis, and hemisacralization of L5, also have been reported.

Neurologic deficits usually do not occur in patients with progressive anterior vertebral fusion, but spinal cord compression resulting from an acutely angled kyphosis has been reported.

Van Buskirk et al. described five stages of progressive anterior vertebral fusion: stage 1, disc space narrowing that occurs to a greater extent anteriorly than posteriorly; stage 2, increased sclerosis of the vertebral endplates of the anterior and middle columns; stage 3, fragmentation of the anterior vertebral endplates; stage 4, fusion of the anterior and sometimes the middle columns; and stage 5, development of a kyphotic deformity.

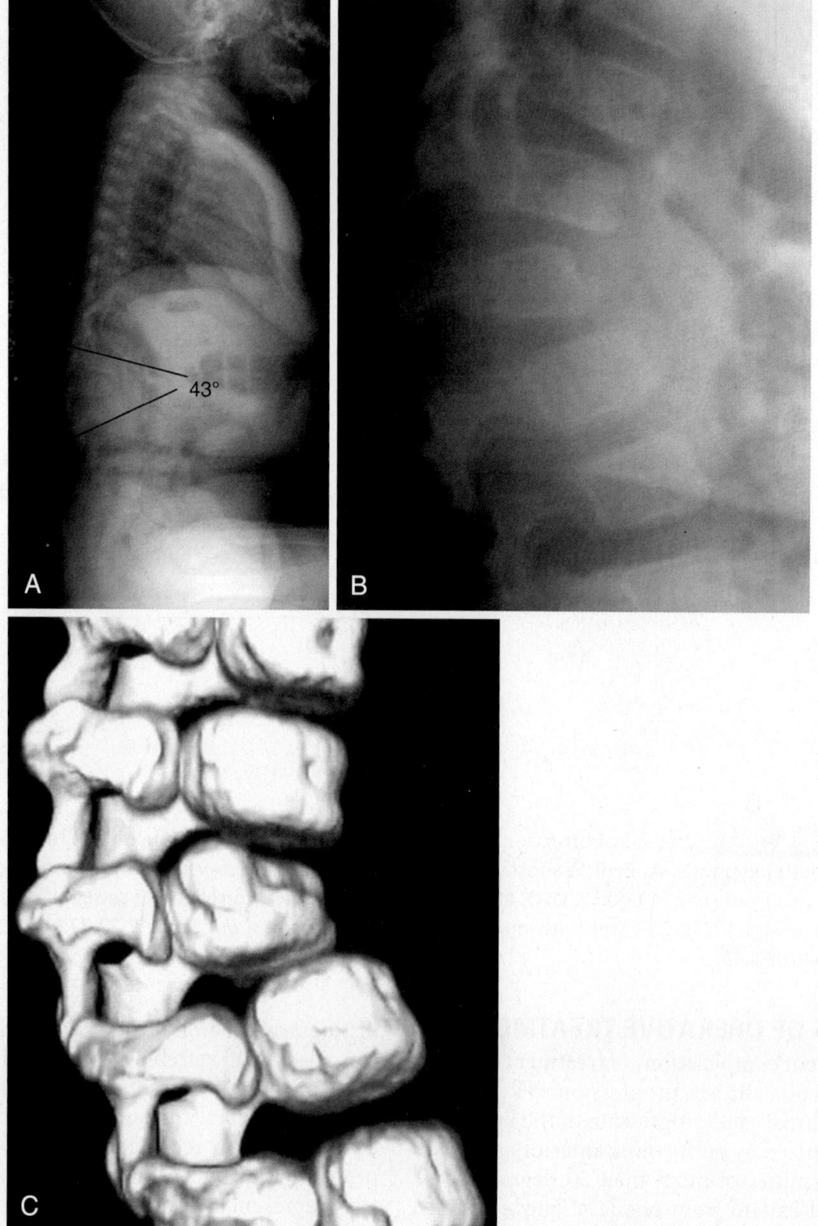

FIGURE 8.167 **A and B, L2 hypoplasia in patient with spontaneous resolution. Note beaked vertebra at L2. C, Three-dimensional CT showing beaked L2 vertebra.** (From Campos MA, Fernandes P, Dolan LA, Weinstein SL: Infantile thoracolumbar kyphosis secondary to lumbar hypoplasia, *J Bone Joint Surg* 90A:1726, 2008.)

Kyphosis that occurs in the last stage of progressive anterior vertebral fusion is the result of the anterior disc space fusing while the posterior disc space remains open. Growth continues in the posterior disc space and the posterior column. Patients with thoracic progressive anterior vertebral fusion have a better prognosis than those with lumbar involvement. This is probably because of the normal kyphotic posture of the thoracic spine. Nonoperative treatment is recommended for most thoracic progressive anterior vertebral fusion deformities. If it occurs in the lumbar spine, a posterior spinal fusion is indicated for stage 1 through stage 3 deformity. For stages 4 and 5, the kyphotic deformity has already occurred in a normal lordotic lumbar spine and posterior fusion will only stop progression of the deformity. An anterior osteotomy with posterior fusion and instrumentation is necessary to obtain normal sagittal alignment.

INFANTILE LUMBAR HYPOPLASIA

Thoracolumbar kyphosis secondary to lumbar hypoplasia was reported by Campos et al. in seven normal infants in whom the thoracolumbar kyphosis resolved spontaneously with growth. It began improving with walking age and corrected to normal by 6 years of age. The average initial kyphosis was 34 degrees. The patients had a clinically apparent kyphotic deformity during the first year of life, and on radiographs they had a relatively sharply angled kyphosis, with the apex at the affected vertebra (Fig. 8.167A). The affected vertebra was wedge shaped with an anterosuperior indentation, giving

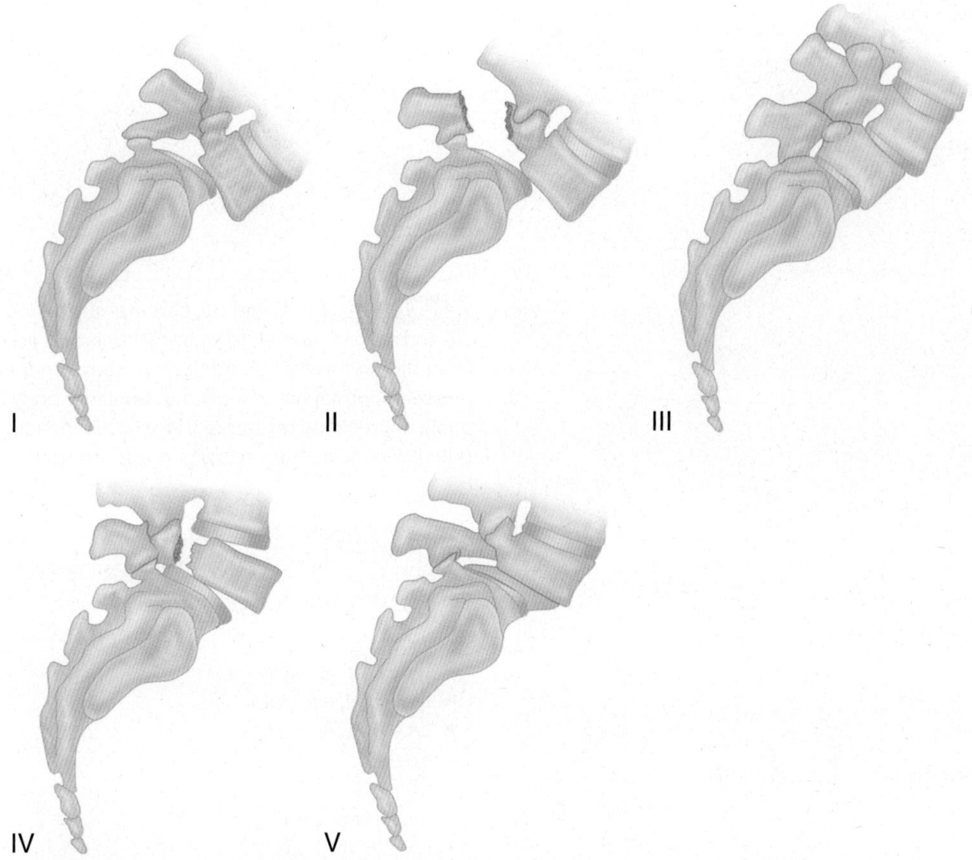

FIGURE 8.168 **Five types of spondylolisthesis: type I, dysplastic; type II, isthmic; type III, degenerative; type IV, traumatic; type V, pathologic.** (Redrawn from Hensinger RN: Spondylolysis and spondylolisthesis in children, *Instr Course Lect* 32:132, 1983.)

it the appearance of a beak (Fig. 8.167B,C). Only one vertebra was involved in all seven infants, either L1 or L2. Campos et al. recommended an initial period of observation to get a better assessment of the deformity as ossification progresses and to avoid overtreatment of lumbar hypoplasia that will improve with growth.

SPONDYLOLYSIS AND SPONDYLOLISTHESIS

Herbiniaux, a Belgian obstetrician, noted a bone prominence in front of the sacrum that caused problems in delivery. He generally is credited with having first described spondylolisthesis. The term *spondylolisthesis* was used by Kilian in 1854 and is derived from the Greek *spondylos,* meaning "vertebra," and *olisthenein,* meaning "to slip." Spondylolisthesis is defined as anterior or posterior slipping of one segment of the spine on the next lower segment. Spondylolysis is a unilateral or bilateral defect of the pars interarticularis.

CLASSIFICATION

Wiltse, Newman, and Macnab's classification of spondylolisthesis is illustrated in Figure 8.168 and Box 8.10. Marchetti and Bartolozzi suggested that the classification of Wiltse et al. is based on a mixture of etiologic and topographic criteria, that it is difficult to predict progression or response to surgery with this classification, and that it also is difficult to identify the type of spondylolisthesis precisely. They therefore attempted to further classify spondylolisthesis by

BOX 8.10

Classification of Spondylolisthesis (Wiltse et al.)

- Type I, dysplastic—Congenital abnormalities of the upper sacral facets or inferior facets of the fifth lumbar vertebra that allow slipping of L5 on S1. No pars interarticularis defect is present in this type.
- Type II, isthmic—Defect in the pars interarticularis that allows forward slipping of L5 on S1. Three types of isthmic spondylolistheses are recognized:
  Lytic—a stress fracture of the pars interarticularis
  An elongated but intact pars interarticularis
  An acute fracture of the pars interarticularis
- Type III, degenerative—This lesion results from intersegmental instability of a long duration with subsequent remodeling of the articular processes at the level of involvement.
- Type IV, traumatic—This type results from fractures in the area of the bony hook other than the pars interarticularis, such as the pedicle, lamina, or facet.
- Type V, pathologic—This type results from generalized or localized bone disease and structural weakness of the bone, such as osteogenesis imperfecta.

BOX 8.11

Classification of Spondylolisthesis (Marchetti and Bartolozzi)

Developmental
- High dysplastic
  With lysis
  With elongation
- Low dysplastic
  With lysis
  With elongation

Acquired
- Traumatic
  Acute fracture
  Stress fracture
- Postsurgery
  Direct surgery
  Indirect surgery
- Pathologic
  Local pathology
  Systemic pathology
- Degenerative
  Primary
  Secondary

From DeWald RL: Spondylolisthesis. In Bridwell KH, DeWald RL, editors: *The textbook of spinal surgery*, ed 3, Philadelphia, 2011, Lippincott Williams & Wilkins.

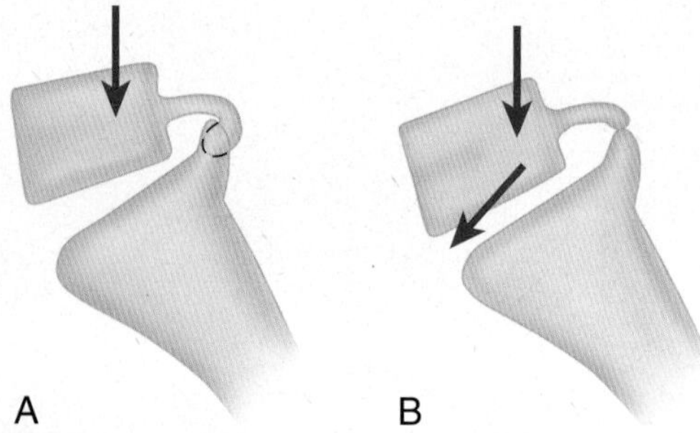

FIGURE 8.169 **A,** Pedicle, pars interarticularis, inferior facets of L5, and sacral facets all form bony hook that prevents L5 vertebra from sliding forward along slope of sacral endplate. **B,** Difference between normal bony hook and dysplastic bony hook that is incapable of providing resistance to forward slippage of the L5 vertebra under weight-bearing stresses in upright spine.

BOX 8.12

Classification of Spondylolisthesis and Spondylolysis (Herman and Pizzutillo)

- Type I—Dysplastic
- Type II—Developmental
- Type III—Traumatic
  Acute
  Chronic
    Stress reaction
    Stress fracture
    Spondylolytic defect
    Nonunion of pars
- Type IV—Pathologic

From Herman MJ, Pizzutillo PD: Spondylolysis and spondylolisthesis in the child and adolescent, *Clin Orthop Relat Res* 434:46, 2005.

dividing the condition into developmental and acquired forms (Box 8.11). Their classification removes the isthmic or lysis part of spondylolisthesis from the primary role in causation and emphasizes the developmental and dysplastic aspects. In analyzing the spondylolisthesis, the surgeon must first decide if the condition is developmental or acquired. If it is developmental, the degree of dysplasia must be determined as high (severe) or low (mild) by evaluation of the quality of the posterior bony hook (Fig. 8.169). The degree of lordosis and the position of the gravity line also are important; the farther anterior the gravity line is, the more likely the spondylolisthesis is to increase. The competency of the disc at the level of the spondylolisthesis also is important; MRI may be required to determine this. Indications of an unstable situation include a significant localized kyphosis (high slip angle) of the slip. Bony changes, such as a trapezoid-shaped L5 vertebral body and a dome-shaped sacrum, also are indicative of instability and significant dysplasia. The implications of the classification system are that the more dysplastic and unstable the situation is, the more aggressive the surgical procedure should be to solve the problem.

Herman and Pizzutillo proposed a new classification for spondylolysis and spondylolisthesis in children and adolescents that uses pertinent elements of the Wiltse et al. and the Marchetti and Bartolozzi classifications. This four-part classification was based on clinical presentation and morphology of the spinal abnormality. Type I is a dysplastic spondylolysis and spondylolisthesis similar to the Wiltse et al. dysplastic category. Type II is referred to as developmental spondylolysis and spondylolisthesis. This type usually is an incidental finding. Type III refers to traumatic spondylolysis and spondylolisthesis and is subdivided into acute and chronic types. The chronic type is further subdivided into (1) stress reaction, (2) stress fracture, and (3) spondylolytic defect or nonunion of pars. Type IV is pathologic spondylolysis and spondylolisthesis (Box 8.12).

Hollenberg et al. described an MRI classification system for spondylolysis: grade 0, normal; grade 1, bone edema and intact cortices compatible with stress reaction; grade 2, incomplete fracture; grade 3, complete active fracture with accompanying bone edema; and grade 4, complete fracture without accompanying bone marrow edema.

Developmental spondylolisthesis and the acquired stress fracture type of spondylolysis are the focus of this section. Acquired degenerative spondylolisthesis is discussed in chapter 4.

ETIOLOGY AND NATURAL HISTORY

The prevalence of spondylolisthesis in the general population is 5% to 8%. The male-to-female ratio for this condition is 2:1. Developmental spondylolisthesis with lysis is considered to be the result of a fatigue fracture caused by repetitive mechanical stresses on the lower lumbar spine in children with a genetic predisposition for the defect. During flexion and extension, the load on the posterior bony arch increases considerably from L1 to L5, with the highest mechanical stress concentrated at the pars interarticularis of L5. The defect has not been noted at birth or in chronically bedridden patients. Wiltse et al. postulated that lumbar lordosis is accentuated by the normal flexion contractures of the hip in childhood and that this posture places the weight-bearing forces on the pars interarticularis. Letts et al. suggested that shear stresses are greater on the pars interarticularis when the lumbar spine is extended. Cyron and Hutton found that the pars interarticularis is thinner and the vertebral disc is less resistant to shear in children and adolescents than in adults. It also is more common in certain types of sporting activities with repetitive hyperextension and rotational loads applied to the lumbar spine. Adequate separation between the adjacent articular facets allows the posterior elements to overlap one another during hyperextension. As reported by Ward et al., a lack of sufficient interfacetal distance in the cranial to caudal direction is likely to pinch the L5 lamina between the inferior facets of L4 and the superior facets of S1 during repetitive hyperextension of the lumbar spine, leading to the development of a spondylolytic defect. The prevalence of spondylolysis and spondylolisthesis increases in children and adolescents who are active in sports that involve repetitive hyperextension of the lumbar spine, such as gymnastics, weightlifting, swimming, wrestling, and rowing. The incidence can vary from 11% to 30% but has been reported to be as high as 47% in elite athletes who participate in high-risk sports such as diving and gymnastics. These observations indicate that the condition is acquired rather than congenital. However, as many as 50% of the Inuit population are reported to have spondylolisthesis, whereas only 6% to 7% of white males and 1.1% of adult black women have the condition, indicating a definite genetic predisposition.

Beutler et al. followed up on a prospective study started in the early 1950s by Dr. Daniel Baker to determine the incidence and natural history of spondylolysis and spondylolisthesis. From 1955 to 1957, radiographs were taken of all first-grade children in a northern Pennsylvania town, a study population of 500 children. A lytic defect of the pars interarticularis was found in 4.4%. By adulthood, lumbar lytic lesions had developed in additional subjects, bringing the total incidence to 6%. Four decades later, all subjects with a pars defect were observed. Subjects with unilateral defects never experienced slippage during the course of the study. Progression of spondylolisthesis slowed with each decade. There was no association of slip progression and low back pain. There was no statistically significant difference between the SF-36 scores of the study population and those of the general population of the same age. Their findings indicated a benign course for the first 50 years of life. Only a small percentage of subjects developed symptomatic slippage progression in long-term follow-up studies. Their findings confirm that there is no justification for advising children and adolescents with spondylolysis and low-grade spondylolisthesis not to participate in competitive sports.

Progression of spondylolisthesis is uncommon if it is less than 30%. If increased slipping occurs, it usually occurs between the ages of 9 and 15 years and seldom after the age of 20 years. Harris and Weinstein, in a long-term follow-up of untreated patients with grade III and grade IV spondylolistheses, found that 36% of patients were asymptomatic, 55% had mild symptoms, and only one patient had significant symptoms. All patients led active lives, and all had required only minor adjustments in their lifestyles. None of the patients was dissatisfied with his or her appearance, and none stated that it had interfered with social or business relationships. In a similar group of patients treated with in situ posterior interlaminar arthrodeses, 57% were asymptomatic and 38% had mild symptoms.

CLINICAL FINDINGS

Patients with spondylolysis and spondylolisthesis usually present with symptoms of mechanical low back pain that is aggravated by high activity levels or competitive sports. Pain is diminished with activity restriction and rest. Often no symptoms will be present and the patient seeks medical evaluation because of a postural deformity or gait abnormality. Pain most often occurs during the adolescent growth spurt and is predominantly backache, with only occasional leg pain. Symptoms are aggravated by high activity levels or competitive sports and are diminished by activity restriction and rest. The back pain probably results from instability of the affected segment, and the leg pain usually is related to irritation of the L5 nerve root.

Back pain on lumbar hyperextension is a common clinical finding. Pain can be reproduced by performing the one-leg hyperextension test or "stork test." This usually reproduces pain on the affected side. Buttock pain radiating into the posterior thighs is common during walking or standing. A neurologic deficit affecting the L5 or S1 nerve root is present in 15% of patients. With a significant slip, a step-off at the lumbosacral junction is palpable, motion of the lumbar spine is restricted, and hamstring tightness is evident on straight-leg raising. Tightness of the hamstrings is present in 80% of symptomatic patients. As the vertebral body is displaced anteriorly, the patient assumes a lordotic posture above the level of the slip to compensate for the displacement. The sacrum becomes more vertical, and the buttocks appear heart shaped because of the sacral prominence. With more severe slips, the trunk becomes shortened and often leads to complete absence of the waistline. These children walk with a peculiar gait, described as a "pelvic waddle" by Newman, because of the hamstring tightness and the lumbosacral kyphosis. Children, unlike adults, seldom have objective signs of nerve root compression, such as motor weakness, reflex change, or sensory deficit. Tight hamstrings often are the only positive physical finding.

Scoliosis is relatively common in younger patients with spondylolisthesis and is of three types: (1) sciatic, (2) olisthetic, or (3) idiopathic. Sciatic scoliosis is a lumbar curve caused by muscle spasm. Usually, this is not a structural curve, and it resolves with recumbency or relief of symptoms. Olisthetic scoliosis is a torsional lumbar curve with rotation that blends with the spondylolytic defect and results from asymmetric slipping of the vertebra. These lumbar curves generally resolve after treatment of the spondylolisthesis. Severe curves, however, may become structural, and treatment is more complicated. Fusion of the lumbosacral area has been found to have no corrective effect on thoracic or thoracolumbar curves. When idiopathic scoliosis and spondylolisthesis occur together, they should be treated as separate problems.

RADIOGRAPHIC FINDINGS

The key to diagnosis of spondylolysis and spondylolisthesis lies in routine radiographs. The initial evaluation should include anteroposterior views, standing lateral views, and a Ferguson coronal view. The lateral view should be taken with the patient standing because a 26% increase in slipping has been noted on standing films compared with recumbent films. In spondylolysis without slippage, the pars interarticularis defect often is difficult to see. Oblique views of the lumbar spine can put the pars area in relief apart from the underlying bony elements, making viewing of the defect easier. A recent study has called into question whether routine oblique radiographs are useful and needed in the evaluation of a patient with spondylolysis or spondylolisthesis. A bone scan may be indicated in children in whom an acquired pars defect is believed to be present but cannot be confirmed by plain films. The bone scan may detect the stress reaction stage before the fracture occurs. Isotope imaging with single-photon emission computed tomography (SPECT) is considered an extremely sensitive technique for early diagnosis of acute spondylolysis. Unfortunately, SPECT is nonspecific, detects only 17% of chronic lesions, and cannot distinguish between stress reactions and complete fractures.

CT has long been considered the gold standard for detecting pars interarticularis fractures. Limitations of CT, however, include low accuracy in distinguishing between a recent active fracture or a stress reaction and a chronic nonunion. Another drawback is the increased radiation exposure associated with CT scanning.

MRI can identify stress reactions and fractures in the pars; however, it is technique dependent, and T2-weighted fat-suppressed images in the oblique and sagittal planes are needed to evaluate bone marrow edema in acute lesions. MRI is useful for evaluation of disc pathology and any nerve root compression. Disadvantages are cost, availability, and need for an experienced radiologist in reading the image. Hollenberg et al. described an MRI classification system for spondylolysis: grade 0, normal; grade 1, bone edema and intact cortices compatible with a stress reaction; grade 2, incomplete fracture; grade 3, complete active fracture with accompanying bone edema; and grade 4, complete fracture without accompanying bone marrow edema.

The most commonly used radiographic grading system for spondylolisthesis is that of Meyerding. In this system, the slip grade is calculated by determining the ratio between the anteroposterior diameter of the top of the first sacral vertebra and the distance the L5 vertebra has slipped anteriorly (Fig. 8.170). Grade I spondylolisthesis is displacement of 25% or less; grade II, between 25% and 50%; grade III, between 50% and 75%; and grade IV, more than 75%. A grade V spondylolisthesis represents the position of L5 completely below the top of the sacrum. This also is termed *spondyloptosis.*

Bourassa-Moreau et al. emphasized the importance of standardizing the measurement techniques for determining slip severity in spondylolisthesis. They used two measurement techniques: technique 1 used a line drawn from the posteroinferior corner of the L5 vertebra that is perpendicular to the S1 vertebral endplate, and technique 2 used a line tangential to the posterior wall of the L5 vertebra that intersects the S1 vertebral endplate (Fig. 8.171). They found a significant difference between the two measurement techniques, highlighting the need to standardize and specify the measurement techniques used to plan and assess any intervention in spondylolisthesis (Fig. 8.172).

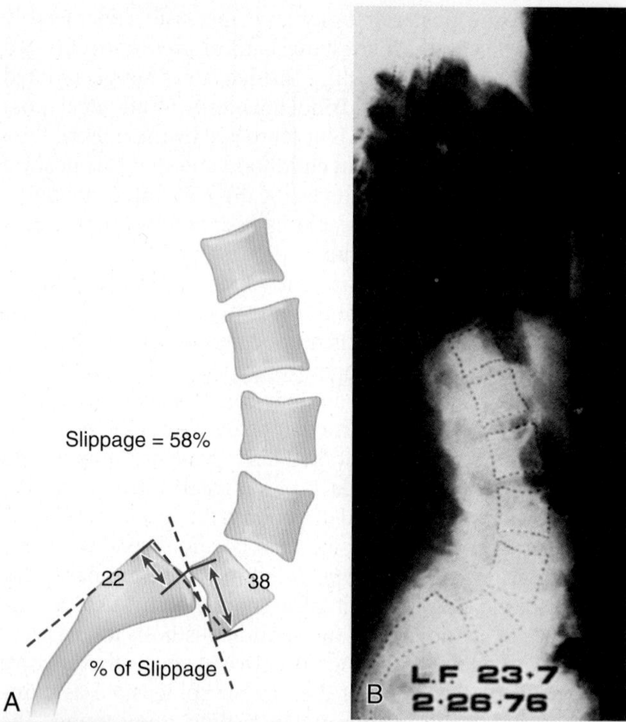

FIGURE 8.170 **A** and **B,** Percentage of slipping calculated by measurement of distance from line parallel to posterior portion of first sacral vertebral body to line parallel to posterior portion of body of L5; anteroposterior dimension of L5 inferiorly is used to calculate percentage of slipping.

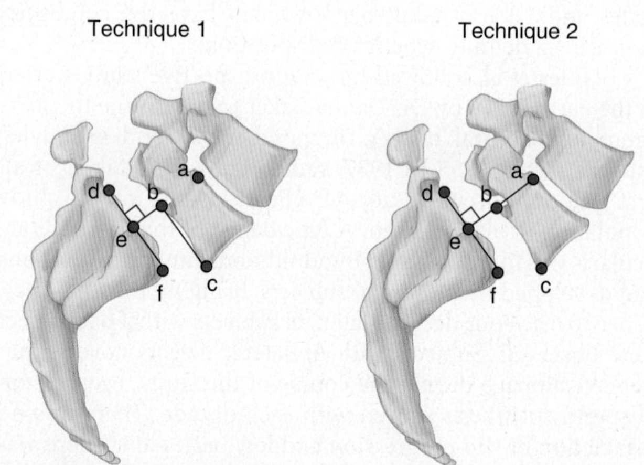

FIGURE 8.171 Two techniques for spondylolisthesis measurement. Technique 1 uses b-f line perpendicular to S1 endplate (line e-d); technique 2 uses tangent to L5 posterior wall, line a-b. These lines indicate position of L5 on S1 in point f. (Redrawn from Bourassa-Moreau E, Mac-Thiong JM, LaBelle H: Redefining the technique for the radiologic measurement of slip in spondylolisthesis, *Spine* 35:1401, 2010.)

DeWald recommended a modification of the Newman system to better define the amount of anterior roll of L5 (Fig. 8.173). The dome and the anterior surface of the sacrum are divided into 10 equal parts. The scoring is based on the position of the posterior inferior corner of the body of the fifth lumbar vertebra with respect to the dome of the sacrum. The second number indicates the position of the anterior

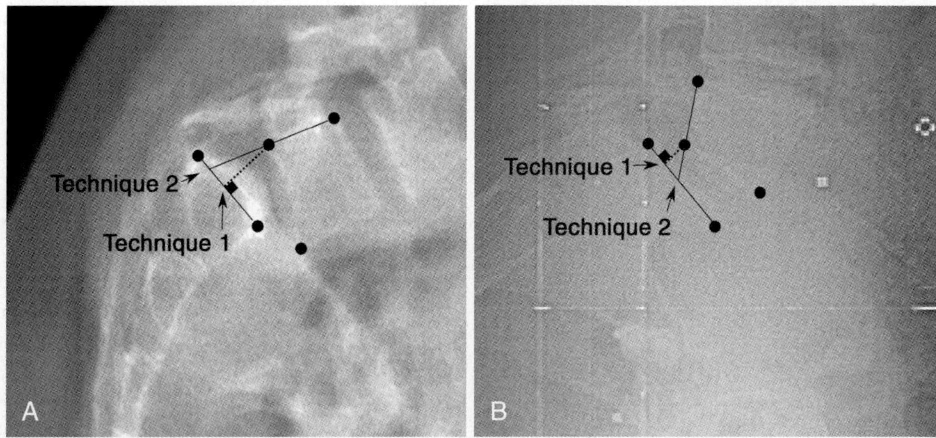

FIGURE 8.172 Two clinical cases illustrating how differences between technique 2 and technique 1 (see Fig. 8.171) vary with respect to orientation of L5 over S1. **A,** In kyphotic alignment (high LSA), technique 2 underestimates value obtained. **B,** In lordotic alignment (low LSA), technique 2 overestimates technique 1 value. These cases illustrate negative correlation between LSA and technique 2 difference. *LSA,* Lumbosacral angle. (From Bourassa-Moreau E, Mac-Thiong JM, LaBelle H: Redefining the technique for the radiologic measurement of slip in spondylolisthesis, *Spine* 35:1401, 2010.)

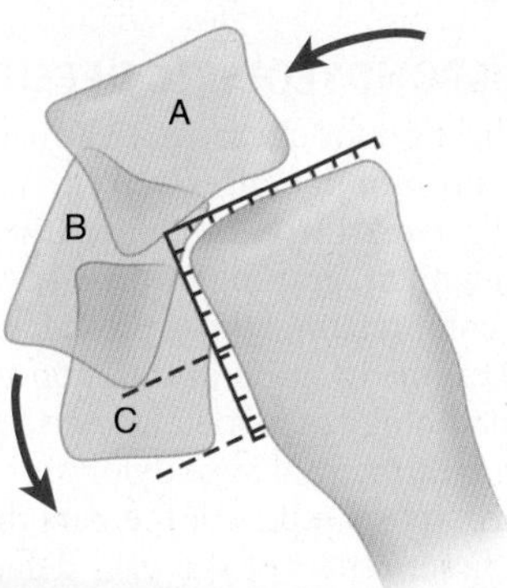

FIGURE 8.173 Modified Newman spondylolisthesis grading system. Degree of slip is measured by two numbers, one along sacral endplate and second along anterior portion of sacrum: A = 3 + 0; B = 8 + 6; and C = 10 + 10.

inferior corner of the body of the L5 vertebra with respect to the anterior surface of the first sacral segment.

The angular relationships are the best predictors of instability or progression of the spondylolisthesis deformity. These relationships are expressed as the slip angle, which is formed by the intersection of a line drawn parallel to the inferior or superior aspect of the L5 vertebra and a line drawn perpendicular to the posterior aspect of the body of the S1 vertebra (Fig. 8.174). The normal slip angle in a patient without spondylolisthesis should be lordotic. With a high-grade spondylolisthesis, the angle is commonly kyphotic. The degree of kyphosis may become large, representing a severe form of segmental kyphosis at L5-S1. Boxall et al. found an association between a high slip angle (>55 degrees) and progression of the deformity.

Restoration of spinopelvic balance is important in the treatment of spondylolisthesis. Hresko et al. described two patterns of deformity in patients with a high-grade spondylolisthesis, based on the alignment of the sacrum and pelvis. The first group was classified as balanced, and the sacral slope and pelvic tilt were similar to those of patients without spondylolisthesis in this balanced group. The second group was classified as unbalanced and had marked retroversion of the sacropelvic complex. The balanced group is characterized by a high sacral slope and low pelvic tilt. The unbalanced group has a vertical sacrum, a low sacral slope, and a high pelvic tilt (Fig. 8.175).

TREATMENT OF ACQUIRED SPONDYLOLYSIS

Treatment of acquired spondylolysis from a stress fracture in children and adolescents depends on whether the spondylolysis is acute or chronic. Micheli, Jackson et al., and Rabushka et al. described children and adolescents in whom acute spondylolytic defects healed with cast or brace immobilization. Typically, these children have an acute onset of symptoms and the episode of injury is clearly documented. Often they are participating in a sport, such as gymnastics, that causes repetitive hyperextension of the spine. A SPECT scan or MRI can be helpful in determining whether the process is acute or chronic. If the SPECT scan detects an abnormality or MRI shows edema in the pedicle, a CT scan of the suspected area can be obtained to distinguish between a stress reaction and an acute stress fracture. CT scanning is the most helpful radiographic technique for determining the presence or absence of healing.

Nonoperative treatment will return most adolescents to normal activities. The spectrum of nonoperative treatment recommendations ranges from rest and restriction of activities to bracing and a structured rehabilitation program. Treatment begins with rest and restriction of activities; however, El Rassi et al. found that there was only a 42% compliance rate with restriction of activities. This finding highlights the need for participation by the patient, parents, and coaches in the treatment plan. Brace treatment has been controversial because of the inability of a standard TLSO to completely immobilize the lumbosacral junction. A brace will give some global restriction of

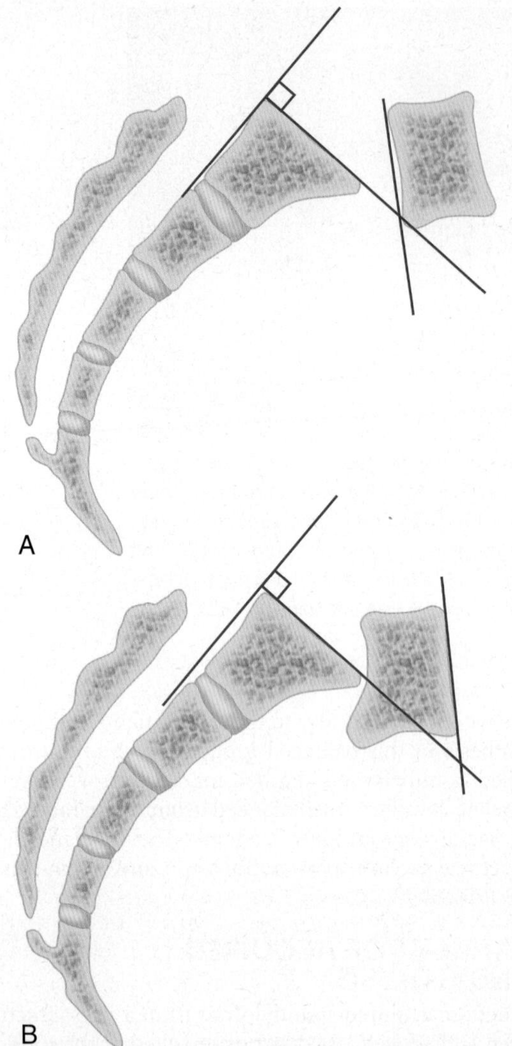

FIGURE 8.174 Schematic representation of slip angle or kyphotic malalignment of lumbosacral junction present in high-grade isthmic dysplastic spondylolisthesis. **A**, Standard method of measurement. **B**, Method used when inferior L5 endplate is irregularly shaped.

motion of the lumbar spine but is probably most effective in forcing restriction of activities. Electrical stimulation has been used with varied results in attempts to heal an acute pars fracture.

A structured rehabilitation program is essential to return the patient to sports. This program has four phases: (1) acute, (2) subacute, (3) pre-sport, and (4) sport-conditioning. The acute phase focuses on relief of pain and inflammation and rehabilitation of the lumbopelvic stabilizers. The subacute phase emphasizes core strengthening and restoration of trunk range of motion. Nonimpact cardio activities can be begun during this stage. The therapist initiates sports-simulated movements to increase the patient's strength and endurance during the pre-sport phase. In the final sports-conditioning phase, sport-specific drills and impact cardio training are begun with the goal of returning the patient to his or her desired sport. The nonoperative treatment and structured rehabilitation program usually requires 12 weeks to complete. Patients with a stress reaction may progress faster, but some patients may require 4 to 5 months of rehabilitation before they are ready to return to sports.

Children and adolescents in whom the spondylolysis is of long duration are treated with routine nonoperative measures. Activities are restricted, and back, abdominal, and core-strengthening exercises are prescribed. If the symptoms are more severe, a brief period of brace immobilization may be required. Once the pain has improved and the hamstring tightness has lessened, the child is allowed progressive activities. Yearly examinations with standing spot lateral radiographs of the lumbosacral spine are advised to rule out the development of spondylolisthesis. If the patient remains asymptomatic, limitation of activities or contact sports is not necessary. Most children with spondylolysis have excellent relief of symptoms or only minimal discomfort at long-term follow-up. If a child does not respond to conservative measures, other causes of back pain, such as infection, tumor, osteoid osteoma, and herniated disc, should be ruled out. Special attention should be paid to children whose symptoms do not respond to bed rest or who have objective neurologic findings. A very small percentage of children with spondylolysis who do not respond to conservative measures and in whom the other possible causes of back pain have been eliminated may require operative treatment.

REPAIR OF SPONDYLOLYTIC DEFECT

The primary indication for operative treatment of spondylolysis is failure of a 6-month conservative treatment program. The principles of pseudarthrosis repair are the same as for any long bone: debridement, grafting of the site with autogenous bone graft, and compression across the fracture. The type of surgery is based on the location of the spondylolysis and any associated disc pathology or associated vertebral dysplasia.

The surgical treatment of spondylolysis can be either an intervertebral fusion or a repair of the pars defect. When the lesion is at L5, direct repair of the pars defect and an L5 to S1 fusion will give similar results. If there is associated disc pathology at L5 or S1 or any associated dysplasia, fusion is the preferred treatment. When the pars lesion is at L4 or L3, direct repair is recommended. Four repair techniques have been described: (1) Scott wiring, (2) Buck screw, (3) pedicle screw and hook, and (4) V-rod or U-rod technique. With all techniques, the rate of return to sports is reported to be 80% to 90%. The Scott technique places wires around the transverse process on each side and through the spinous process to compress the pars defect. This is the least rigid of all the fixation methods, but it nonetheless has a healing rate of nearly 80%. Direct intralaminar screw fixation of a pars defect, described by Buck in 1970 with good outcomes in 93%, offers a minimally invasive and motion-preserving technique. The use of pedicle screws and infralaminar hoods attached to a short rod allows compression of the pars defect along the rod to stabilize the defect. This is the most rigid construct. A similar technique uses a U-shaped rod placed inferior to the spinous process for stabilization and compression of the pars defect. Sairyo et al. described restoration of disc stresses to normal at the cranial and caudal levels of the pars defect after direct intralaminar screw fixation using the Buck technique. Several other studies also have shown a superior biomechanical advantage of the Buck technique relative to other common fixation techniques; however, according to a biomechanical study of the four different techniques, all of which restored

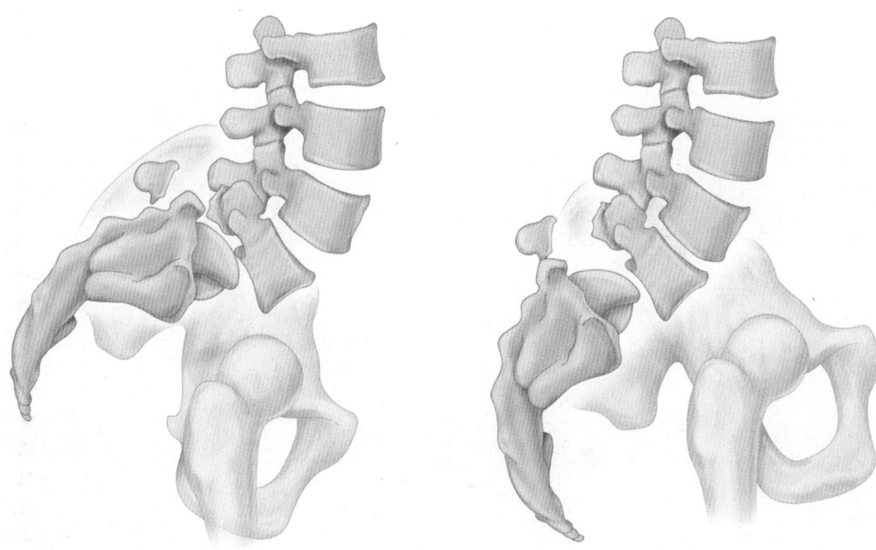

FIGURE 8.175 **Sagittal view of spinopelvic alignment in high-grade spondylolisthesis.** (From Hresko MT, LaBelle H, Roussouly P, Berthonnaud E: Classification of high-grade spondylolistheses based on pelvic version and spine balance, *Spine* 32:2208, 2007.)

normal intervertebral rotation, the Scott and Buck constructs were found to be less stable than the screw-hook or U-rod constructs. Mihara et al. found that the Buck screw technique restored more normal motion at the involved level and adjacent level.

Kakiuchi reported successful union of pars defects with the use of a pedicle screw, laminar hook, and rod system. A pedicle screw is placed in the pedicle above the pars defect. The pars defect is bone grafted. A rod is placed in the pedicle screw and then into the caudal laminar hook, and compression is applied. This gives a more stable construct than that afforded by wire techniques. A second surgery for removal of prominent implants after healing may be necessary.

SPONDYLOLYSIS REPAIR

TECHNIQUE 8.50

(KAKIUCHI)

- Place the patient prone on a Hall frame.
- Expose the involved vertebra, including the defect of the pars interarticularis, through a midline posterior incision. Remove the fibrous tissue in and behind the defect with a Cobb elevator, rongeur, or curet. To maintain the length of the pars interarticularis, do not remove the sclerotic bone on both sides of the defect.
- Clean the lateral aspect of the inferior half of the superior articular process and the medial third of the posterior aspect of the transverse process of soft tissue without interfering with the capsule of the facet.
- Decorticate the posterior aspect of the pars interarticularis and adjoining portion of the lamina with use of a small chisel (Fig. 8.176A). Do not decorticate the lateral and inferior aspects of the superior articular process to maintain the strength of the osseous structures for pedicle screw placement.
- If nerve root decompression is indicated, remove the bone spurs over the nerve root with an osteotome (Fig. 8.176B). Bury free fat tissue in the defect created above the nerve root to prevent bone graft from falling onto the nerve root.
- To achieve a wider area for bone grafting, make the starting point for the insertion of the pedicle screw is near the intersection of a vertical line through the center axis of the pedicle and a horizontal line at the superior border of the pedicle (Fig. 8.176C).
- Direct the screw slightly caudally so that it enters the vertebral body at the center axis of the pedicle.
- After insertion of the pedicle screw, take strips of cancellous bone from the posterior aspect of the ilium through the same incision in the skin.
- Pack the cancellous bone as an onlay graft from the medial third of the transverse process to the decorticated portion of the lamina to form a sheet of bone about 1 cm thick (see Fig. 8.176C).
- If the multifidus muscle is too tight for pedicle screw insertion through this midline approach (which is more common at L5 than more cephalad levels), the starting point for insertion of the pedicle screw on the superior articular process should be exposed through the paraspinal approach over the pedicle through the same midline incision in the skin and additional small fascial incisions made 2 to 3 cm lateral to the midline (Fig. 8.176D). Insert a finger through the natural cleavage plane between the multifidus and longissimus muscles to the insertion point over the pedicle.

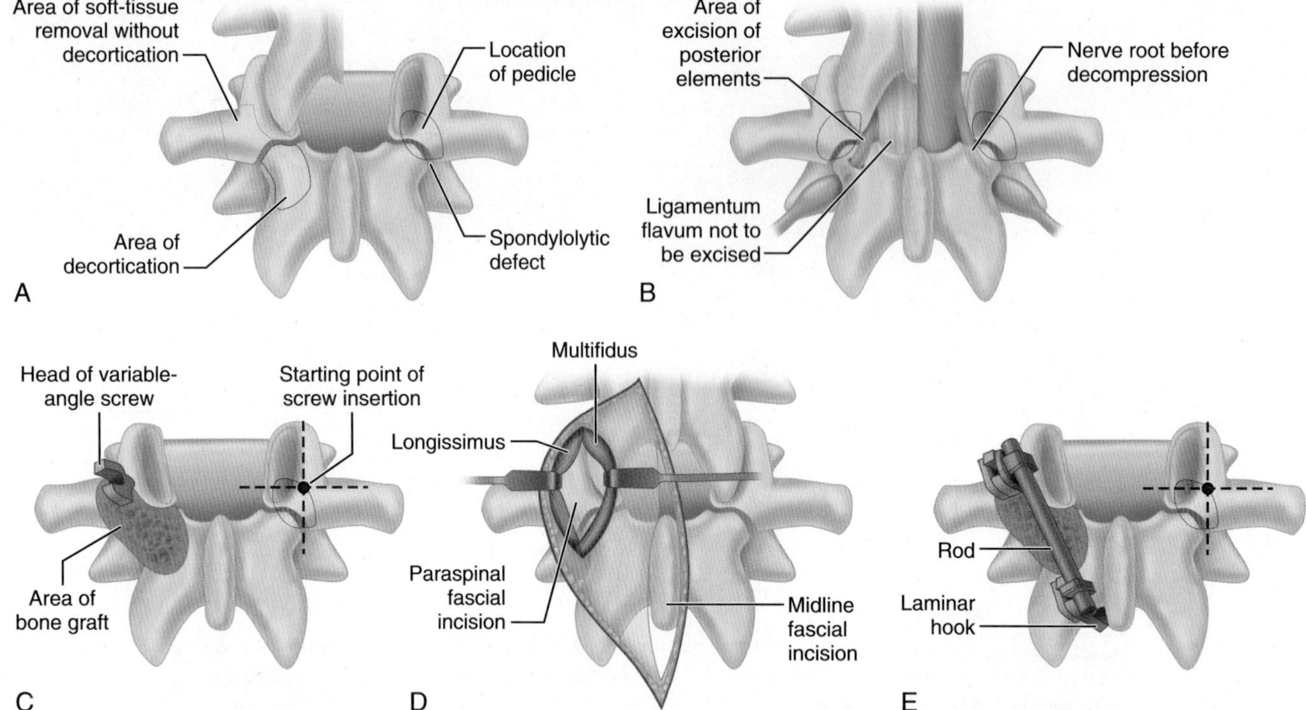

FIGURE 8.176 **A,** Recipient bed prepared for autogenous cancellous bone graft. **B,** Posterior elements overlying affected nerve root are excised. **C,** Variable-angle pedicle screw and bone graft inserted. **D,** Paraspinal approach can be used when the multifidus muscle is too tight for pedicle screw insertion through the midline. **E,** Rod attached to head of screw with variable-angle eyebolt. Laminar hook attached to rod. (From Kakiuci M: Repair of the defect in spondylolysis, *J Bone Joint Surg* 79A:818, 1997.) **SEE TECHNIQUE 8.50.**

- Cut the rod to the appropriate length and attach it to the head of the variable-angle screw. Insert a laminar hook to the inferior edge of the lamina and attach it to the rod (Fig. 8.176E).
- To reduce the size of the defect of the pars interarticularis, apply a mild compression force between the hook and the head of the screw with the hook compressor before tightening the locknut in the eyebolt.
- Repeat the procedure on the contralateral side.

POSTOPERATIVE CARE Usually patients are allowed to stand and walk on the second or third postoperative day. A hard lumbosacral corset is worn for 2 months, but its use should be determined on an individual basis. Patients are allowed unrestricted activity after 6 months.

MODIFIED SCOTT REPAIR TECHNIQUE

Van Dam reported success in 16 patients with a modification of the Scott repair technique. In 26 direct pars repairs, union was achieved in 22.

TECHNIQUE 8.51

(VAN DAM)

- Approach the lumbar spine posteriorly.
- Identify and debride the area of the pars pseudarthrosis.
- Place a 6.5-mm cancellous screw approximately two thirds of the way into the ipsilateral pedicle.
- Loop an 18-gauge wire around the screw head and pass the wire through a hole at the base of the spinous process.
- Pass the ends of the wire through a metal button and tighten the wire loop around the screw head.
- Twist the wire ends tightly against the metal button and cut the excess wire away.
- Place autogenous cancellous bone in and around the debrided pars defect.
- Fully seat the screw to accomplish final tightening of the wire (Fig. 8.177).
- Taddonio described the use of pedicle screws attached to Cotrel-Dubousset rods and offset laminar hooks to accomplish the same mechanical stability as in the Buck technique and Bradford technique. Roca et al. described the use of a titanium variable-angle pedicular-laminar hook-screw especially designed for direct spondylolysis repair.

POSTOPERATIVE CARE The patient should use a lumbosacral orthosis for a minimum of 3 months and up to 6 months after surgery. Healing of the pars is ascertained by follow-up CT scan.

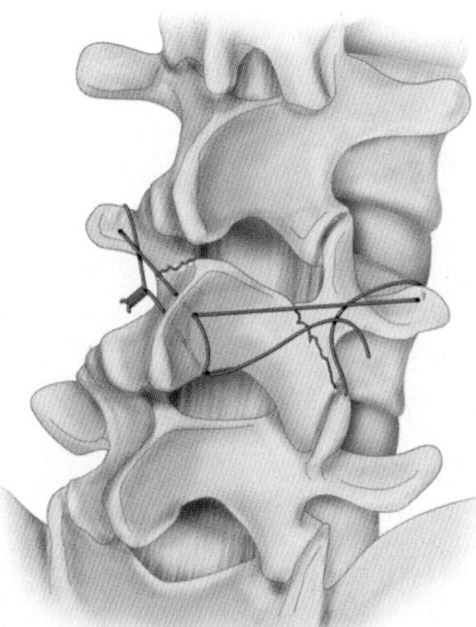

FIGURE 8.177 Scott wiring technique. (Redrawn from Rechtine G II: Spondylolysis repair. In Vaccaro A, Albert TJ, editors: *Spine surgery tricks of the trade*, New York, 2003, Thieme.) **SEE TECHNIQUE 8.51.**

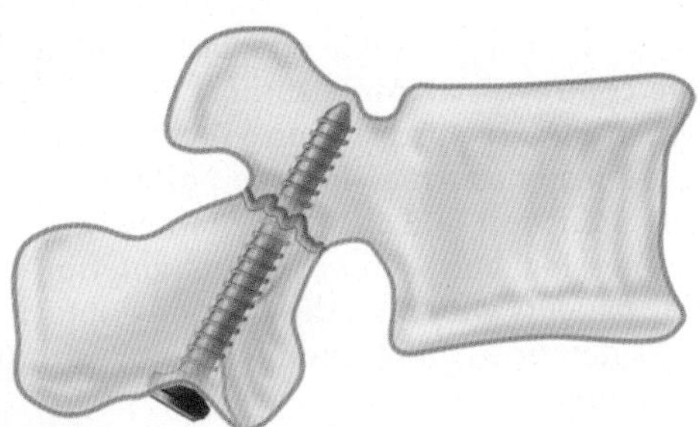

FIGURE 8.178 Technique of Buck screw fixation of pars defect. **SEE TECHNIQUE 8.52.**

INTRALAMINAR SCREW FIXATION OF PARS DEFECT (BUCK SCREW TECHNIQUE)

TECHNIQUE 8.52

PARS SCREW FIXATION

- With the patient prone in a position to minimize lordosis, use fluoroscopy to localize the level of the defect.
- Make a midline incision approximately 5 cm long lateral to the corresponding spinous process to expose the lamina and the defect.
- Use a curet to clean the defect.
- Under fluoroscopy, and alternating between anteroposterior and lateral views, make a percutaneous stab wound with a 4.5-mm cannulated screw guidewire.
- Drill the wire through the caudal laminar surface, bisecting the pedicle to the superior cortex of the pedicle and traversing the pars defect (Fig. 8.178).
- Use a 3.2-mm cannulated drill to drill over the guidewire.
- Remove the wire and use a ball-tipped probe to feel the cortices.
- Measure and tap the screw length.
- If the lamina is large enough, overdrill it distally.
- Insert a solid (rather than cannulated) 4.5-mm screw of the appropriate size, with compression as needed.
- Through the same incision, harvest a posterior iliac crest bone graft and place the cancellous graft in the defect. Overlay a corticocancellous strip from the lamina to the transverse process.

SPONDYLOLYSIS REPAIR WITH U-ROD OR V-ROD

TECHNIQUE 8.53

(SUMITA ET AL.)

- With the patient prone, make a midline incision and elevate the paraspinal musculature laterally to expose the lamina, pars, and base of the transverse process. Take care not to injure the capsule of the facet joint.
- Expose the defect in the pars and use a curet to remove the fibrocartilage.
- Use a burr to decorticate the defect and the corresponding lamina and transverse process.
- Using anatomic landmarks and fluoroscopy, determine the starting point for the pedicle screw.
- Create the starting hole with a burr and use a pedicle finder to enter the pedicle.
- Assess the walls and floor with a ball-tipped probe and tap the hole for a 5-mm pedicle screw.
- Harvest bone graft from the iliac crest, place it in the defect, and impact it before insertion of the screw.
- After the screws are placed, contour a rod into a U shape or V shape (Fig. 8.179) and place it just caudal to the interspinous ligament of the affected level; attach the rod to each pedicle screw, and tighten the screws to compress the defect.
- Confirm correct placement of the screw and rod with fluoroscopic imaging.

POSTOPERATIVE CARE Intravenous antibiotics are administered until the wound is dry. The patient is mobilized without a brace.

POSTEROLATERAL FUSION

Posterolateral fusion is the conventional operative treatment of symptomatic spondylolysis at L5 unresponsive to conservative treatment. Pedicle instrumentation and fusion often are done to avoid the necessity of postoperative bracing. If no internal fixation is used, the patient is immobilized in a TLSO. A pantaloon cast or a TLSO with a thigh extension also may be used for greater immobilization. Fusion rates of approximately 90% have been reported with similar percentages of

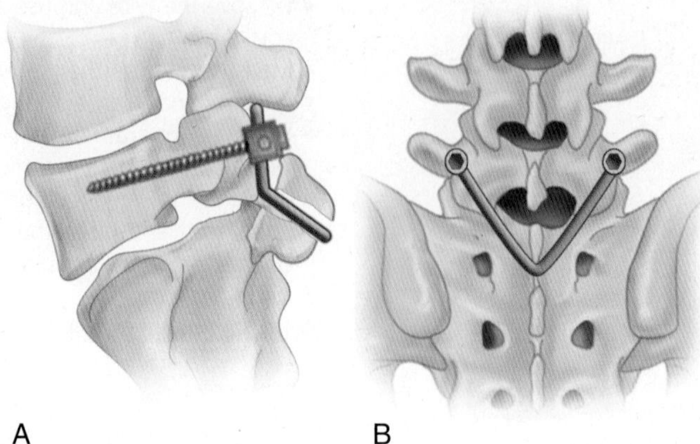

FIGURE 8.179 Sagittal **(A)** and axial **(B)** position of the pedicle screw instrumentation for V-rod fixation. **SEE TECHNIQUE 8.53.**

relief of symptoms after fusion of L5 to the sacrum. Extension of the fusion to L4 is not necessary. The Gill procedure or a wide laminectomy in a child is not necessary.

TREATMENT OF DEVELOPMENTAL SPONDYLOLISTHESIS

NONOPERATIVE TREATMENT

Surgery is not always necessary for spondylolisthesis. Restriction of the patient's activities, muscle rehabilitation (spinal, abdominal, and trunk), and other nonoperative measures, including the intermittent use of a rigid back brace, often are sufficient if the symptoms are minimal and the slippage is mild. If symptoms improve, progressive increases in activity are permitted. Activity restrictions are unnecessary for patients with mild degrees of spondylolisthesis. For symptom-free patients with slips of more than 25% but less than 50%, contact sports and activities that carry a high probability of back injury should be avoided. Standing spot lateral radiographs of the lumbosacral junction are made every 6 to 12 months until the completion of growth.

OPERATIVE TREATMENT

Indications for surgery include persistent symptoms despite conservative treatment for 6 months to 1 year, persistent tight hamstrings, abnormal gait, and pelvic-trunk deformity. Development of a neurologic deficit is an indication for operative intervention, as is progression of the slip, which is indicative of a severe dysplasia. Early surgery may prevent more difficult or risky surgeries at a later time. If a patient is asymptomatic and has a slip of more than 50%, severe dysplasia (high dysplastic spondylolisthesis) is likely and surgery is indicated.

A posterolateral fusion between L5 and the sacrum is recommended for slips of less than 50% in children and adolescents whose symptoms persist despite conservative treatment. This degree of slippage has a mild dysplasia (low dysplastic type), usually without a significant slip angle. These patients usually do well with a posterolateral fusion in situ or with a partial reduction. Unless there is significant lumbosacral kyphosis, there is no need for anatomic reduction. Instrumentation with pedicle screw fixation will avoid the need for postoperative immobilization. Extremely tight hamstrings, decreased Achilles tendon reflexes, and even footdrop may improve after a solid arthrodesis. Laminectomy as an isolated technique in a growing child is contraindicated because further slipping will occur.

TREATMENT OF SEVERE (HIGH DYSPLASTIC) SPONDYLOLISTHESIS

Operative treatment of high dysplastic spondylolisthesis is more controversial. Most authors agree that slippage of more than 50% requires fusion. The operative options, however, are many and may include posterior fusion with or without reduction and instrumentation, with or without decompression, and with or without anterior interbody fusion. For patients with a grade V spondyloptosis, Gaines and Nichols described an L5 spondylectomy with fusion of L4 to the sacrum.

Lenke et al. found that 21% of 56 in situ bilateral transverse process fusions for spondylolisthesis were definitely not fused, but despite this low fusion rate, overall clinical improvement was noted in more than 80% of patients. Other authors recommended combined anterior fusion and reduction with posterior spinal instrumentation for high dysplastic slips because of problems with the healing of a posterior arthrodesis alone. In addition to improving the appearance, the reduction of spondylolisthesis with instrumentation improves the chance of fusion (Fig. 8.180). Johnson and Kirwan and Wiltse et al. reported excellent results in patients with slips of more than 50% treated with bilateral lateral fusions. Freeman and Donati found similar results after in situ fusion in patients observed for an average of 12 years (Fig. 8.181). Poussa et al. compared the results of in situ fusion of spondylolisthesis of more than 50% with results of reduction by a transpedicular system and found no differences between the groups in functional improvement or pain relief. In situ fusion gave a satisfactory cosmetic appearance; reduction procedures were associated with increased operative time, complications, and reoperations. Other reports have recorded an increased rate of nonunion and delayed neurologic complications when posterolateral fusion in situ has been performed in high-grade slips.

Instrumentation with pedicle screws has been used in an attempt to prevent further deterioration of the spondylolisthesis with in situ fusion. The goal of surgical treatment in patients with a high-grade spondylolisthesis is to restore the global sagittal balance of the spinopelvic complex. The degree of reduction of the translatory displacement in high-grade

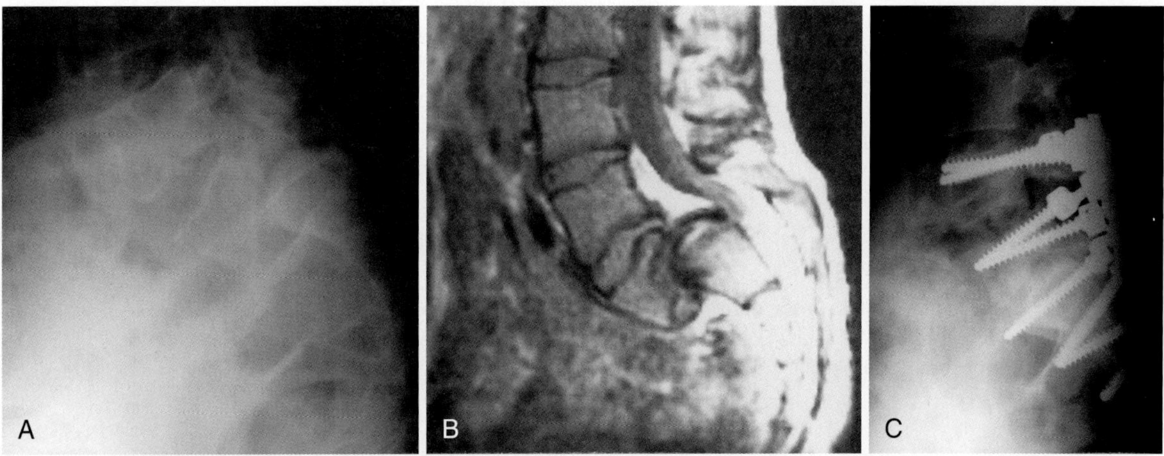

FIGURE 8.180 A, Severe spondylolisthesis. B, MR image shows slip. C, After anterior and posterior reduction and fusion with posterior instrumentation.

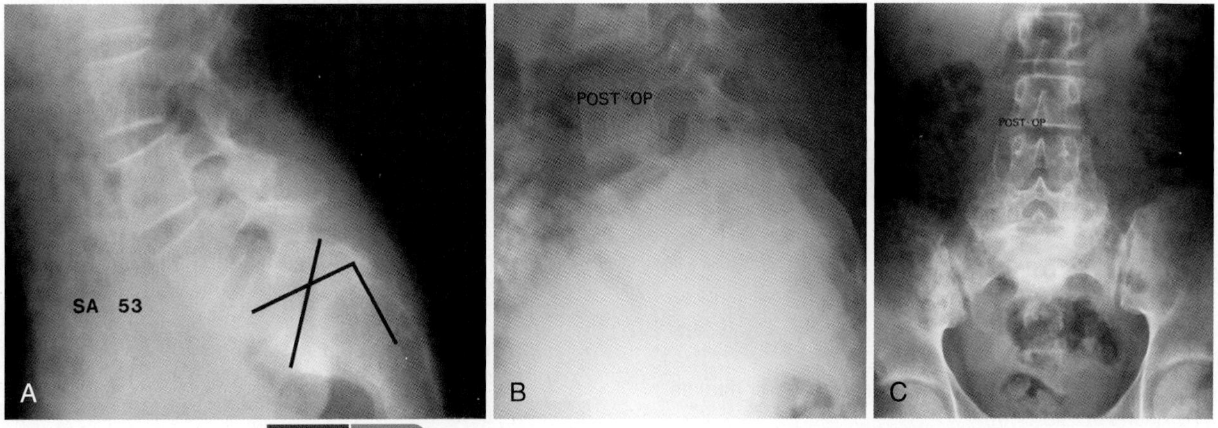

FIGURE 8.181 A, Severe spondylolisthesis. B and C, After in situ fusion.

slips is less important than improving the lumbosacral kyphosis and restoring sagittal imbalance. In severe cases, the fusion may need to be extended to L4. The advantages of reduction of high-grade spondylolisthesis include reduction of the slip angle (lumbosacral kyphosis), which improves the sagittal lumbosacral orientation and places the fusion mass in more compression, and improves the global sagittal balance and the cosmetic appearance. Direct neural decompression also is allowed with this procedure. Disadvantages are that more extensive surgery is required, an additional anterior procedure often is needed, and there is an increased risk for neurologic injury.

Cauda equina injuries may occur after in situ fusions. In severe spondylolisthesis, the sacral roots are stretched over the back of the body of S1 and are sensitive to any movement of L5 on S1. It has been postulated that muscle relaxation after general anesthesia and the surgical dissection may lead to additional slippage that further stretches these sacral roots. Patients most at risk have an initial slip angle of more than 45 degrees. Thorough neurologic evaluation before and after in situ arthrodesis is recommended in all patients with grade III or grade IV spondylolisthesis. Examination should include clinical assessment of perineal sensation, function of the bladder, and rectal tone. If a patient has a detectable neurologic deficit preoperatively, decompression of the cauda equina at the time of the arthrodesis with removal of the posterior superior lip of the sacrum (Fig. 8.182) can be done. Because this decompression causes additional instability, segmental instrumentation with pedicle screws is required. Alternatively, decompression of the cauda equina can be combined with reduction of the forward slip with posterior pedicle segmental instrumentation. If injury to the cauda equina is evident after an otherwise uneventful in situ arthrodesis, prompt decompression with removal of the posterior aspect of S1 is recommended. In situ pedicle segmental instrumentation should be considered to further stabilize the area.

There are no definite guidelines regarding the appropriate surgical treatment of children and adolescents with high dysplastic spondylolisthesis. Intuitively, it seems that the more dysplastic and unstable the spine is, the more justifiable is some type of reduction and instrumentation. Boachie-Adjei et al. proposed a technique of partial reduction of the lumbosacral kyphosis, decompression of the nerve roots, posterolateral fusion, and pedicle screw transvertebral fixation of the lumbosacral junction. This technique has the advantage of providing three-column fixation by the lumbosacral transfixation, yet it is performed through a single posterior approach. It also allows interbody grafting to be done if necessary without a formal anterior procedure. Lenke and Bridwell also

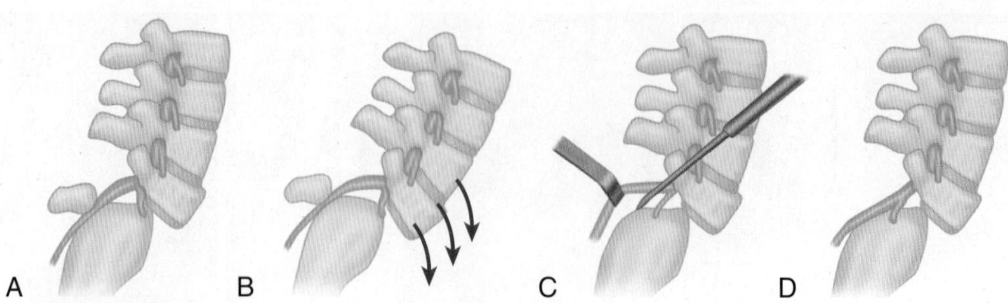

FIGURE 8.182 **A,** Severe spondylolisthesis. **B,** Increase that may occur intraoperatively. **C,** Operative decompression of cauda equina with sacroplasty. **D,** Appearance of sacrum after excision of posterior superior aspect.

found that this approach provided the best fusion rates and clinical outcomes with acceptable complication rates.

POSTEROLATERAL FUSION AND PEDICLE SCREW FIXATION

TECHNIQUE 8.54

(LENKE AND BRIDWELL)

- Place the patient prone on a radiolucent table. Initially, the patient can be positioned with the knees and hips flexed to facilitate decompression.
- Approach the spine through a standard posterior midline lumbosacral incision.
- Perform a Gill laminectomy and bilateral L5 and S1 nerve root decompressions. It is extremely important to decompress the L5 nerve roots widely past the tips of the L5 transverse processes.
- Place pedicle screws at L5 and S1. For additional sacropelvic fixation points, use bilateral distal iliac wing screws. In high-grade slips, instrumentation to L4 may be needed.
- Apply mild distraction to the L5-S1 segment and perform a sacroplasty to shorten the sacrum and decrease the stretch of the L5 nerve roots.
- At this point, if the hips and knees are flexed, extend them to flex the pelvis to meet the L5 segment.
- Attempt to access the L5-S1 disc space from the posterior approach. If this can be done, remove the disc and use morselized bone graft or place structural cages in the L5 disc.
- Contour the rod and place it into the distal fixation segment; flex the sacrum with the rod to meet the L5 segment.
- Place the graft anterior just before locking the instrumentation into place.
- Review the intraoperative anteroposterior and lateral radiographs.
- Perform a formal wake-up test to assess bilateral foot and ankle movement.
- Place iliac crest bone graft harvested proximal to the iliac screw site over the decorticated transverse process and sacral ala bilaterally (Fig. 8.183).
- If an adequate anterior spinal fusion could not be performed posteriorly, the patient is brought back 5 to 7 days later for an anterior procedure.
- Depending on the degree of reduction obtained, a formal discectomy with structural grafts or metallic cages is used with the anterior iliac crest graft for fusion.
- If the slip angle and translation correction have not been enough to allow access to the L5 disc anteriorly, ream over a Kirschner wire that is placed from the midportion of the L5 through the L5-S1 disc and into the proximal sacrum and insert the fibular allograft.

POSTOPERATIVE CARE Depending on the security of the fixation obtained, a single pantaloon brace or TLSO may be needed. The brace can be discontinued when it appears that the fusion is solid enough to safely do so, usually at 3 to 4 months postoperatively.

INSTRUMENTED REDUCTION

In high dysplastic spondylolisthesis, reduction and fusion with internal fixation and a sagittally aligned spine can eliminate the complication of progression of the deformity that can occur after in situ fusion. Lumbar root pain or deficit may require decompression of the L5 symptomatic roots and internal fixation. Internal fixation makes it possible to decompress these roots fully without fear of residual instability or progressive slipping (Fig. 8.184). Sacral radiculopathy caused by stretching of the sacral roots over the posterosuperior corner of the sacrum theoretically can be relieved by restoring the lumbar spine to its proper position over the sacrum. This relieves the anterior pressure from the sacral roots, shortens their course, and relaxes the cauda equina. Correction of the slip angle (kyphosis) greatly reduces the bending moment and tensile stress that works against the posterior lumbosacral graft. When normal biomechanics are restored by correction of the deformity, it may be possible to fuse fewer lumbosacral segments. Theoretically, restoring body posture and mechanics to normal may lessen future problems in the proximal areas of the spine. Physical appearance is a concern of adoles-

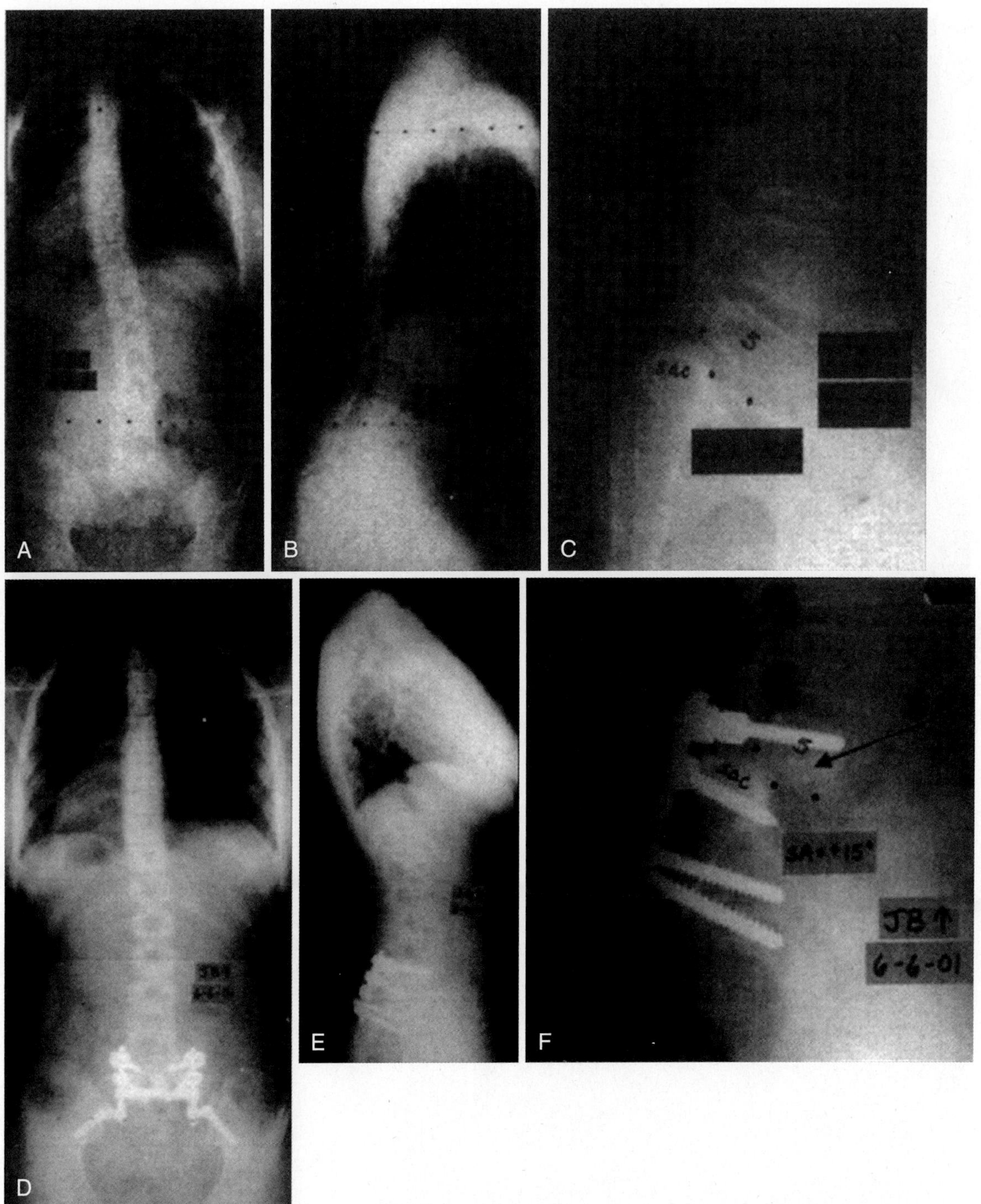

FIGURE 8.183 Radiographs of 12-year-old girl with high-grade IV isthmic dysplastic spondylolisthesis. Patient has small amount of sciatic scoliosis on coronal view (**A** and **B**). Sacrum is vertical on sagittal radiograph **(C)**, and she is positioned with her trunk anterior to her pelvis, showing anterior sagittal imbalance. Patient had posterior decompression, partial reduction, sacral dome osteotomy, and posterolateral fusion with instrumentation from L5 to sacrum. One week later, she had anterior fibular dowel graft placement from L5 to sacrum. Radiographs **D** to **F** show improved position of L5 on sacrum and excellent alignment in overall coronal **(D)** and sagittal **(E)** radiographs. **F,** *Arrow* points to anterior edge of fibular graft. (From Lenke LG, Bridwell KH: Evaluation and surgical treatment of high-grade isthmic dysplastic spondylolisthesis, *Instr Course Lect* 52:525, 2003.) **SEE TECHNIQUE 8.54.**

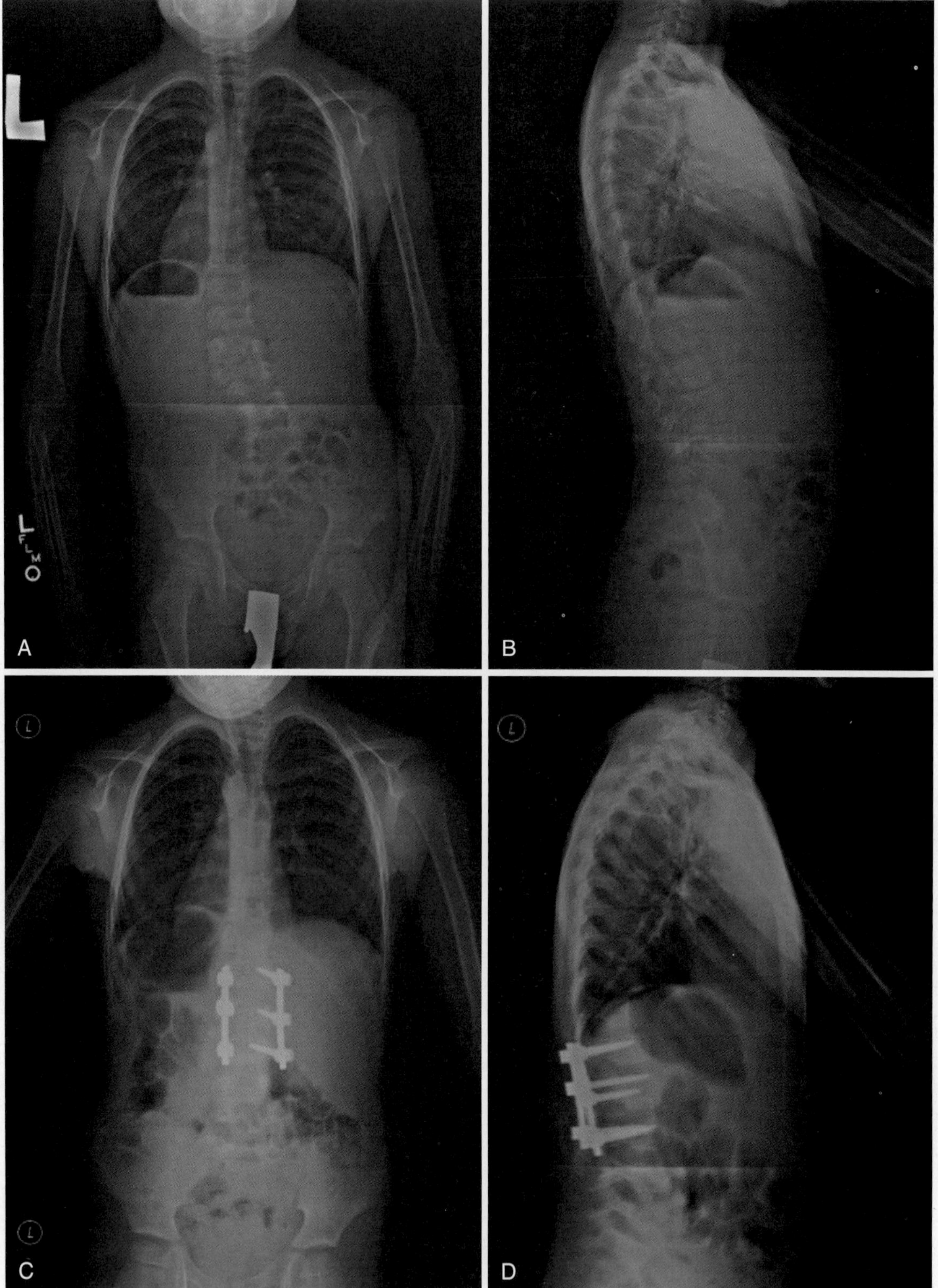

FIGURE 8.184 In high dysplastic spondylolisthesis (**A** and **B**), lumbar root pain or deficit may require decompression of the L5 symptomatic roots and internal fixation. **C** and **D**, Internal fixation makes it possible to decompress these roots fully without fear of residual instability or progressive slipping.

cents with high-grade spondylolisthesis, and this can be improved with reduction of the deformity.

These advantages, however, should be weighed against the potential risks of the surgery. These procedures are technically demanding and carry with them a significant risk of nerve root injury. As techniques are evolving, these risks are decreasing but are still present. Numerous techniques to obtain complete reduction of high-grade dysplastic spondylolisthesis have been described. The following technique is just one of those described.

TECHNIQUE 8.55

(CRANDALL)

- After general anesthesia is obtained, place the patient prone on a radiolucent table.
- Use a routine midline approach to the lumbosacral spine.
- Perform a full L5 laminectomy, inferior facetectomy, and nerve root decompression. A discectomy at L5-S1 will also make L5 more mobile for reduction.
- Prepare and tap the pedicles at L5-S1 and insert long post screws bilaterally at L5.
- Screws also should be placed bilaterally at S1.
- For high-grade spondylolisthesis, a distal point of fixation is needed to form a strong and stable base from which L5 can be pulled into position. Options include iliac screws (Fig. 8.185A) and S2 alar screws (Fig. 8.185B,C).
- Aim the S2 multiaxial screws laterally into the beak of the sacral ala.
- After all screws are placed, select a rod of the appropriate length and diameter, along with the corresponding three-dimensional connectors, and preassemble the construct.
- Place screw extenders on the post of the S1 screws to ease insertion.
- Slide the preassembled construct down the screw extenders at S1 and the threaded post of the long post screw at L5 and into the multiaxial screw heads at S2.
- Repeat the same process on the contralateral side of the spine.
- Once the connectors are in place, temporarily secure them at S1 with a lock screw. When the construct is in place, each rod creates a "diving board" over L5 (Fig. 8.185D).
- Place a low-profile crosslink plate between the S1 and S2 levels of the construct. If iliac screws are used, this is not necessary.
- Place the provisional reduction crimps on both the long post three-dimensional screws at L5 (Fig. 8.185E). Place the crimp driver on the threaded posts of the screws. Advance the driver down the threaded post to the provisional reduction crimp. Sequentially tighten the driver by rotating clockwise and pushing down on the reduction crimps (Fig. 8.185F). By use of the provisional reduction crimps, the spine is brought into its correct anatomic position in a gradual and highly controlled way (Fig. 8.185G,H).
- If the L5 connector "bottoms out" onto the screw head before full reduction is achieved (Fig. 8.185I), there are two options for getting the last few millimeters of correction.
- Contour the rod with more lordosis at L5 to increase the reduction distance for L5 to be pulled back (Fig. 8.185J), or place the connector at S1 at the very top of the post, which creates more reduction distance (Fig. 8.185K).
- Once the spondylolisthesis is fully corrected, compress L5 to S1 with the compressor to make the alignment as stable as possible. The correction is more likely to be maintained if bone or a small cage is placed into the disc space through a posterior lumbar interbody fusion or transforaminal lumbar interbody fusion before L5 is compressed to S1.
- Place lock screws in the three-dimensional connectors at L5 and S1 (Fig. 8.185L) and tighten all four lock screws. As the tightening occurs, the break-off portion of the set screw will shear off and remain in the sleeve of the driver.
- Use a "cutter" to cut the long post flush with the assembly (Fig. 8.185M,N).

REDUCTION AND INTERBODY FUSION

Satisfactory results have been reported with reduction and posterior interbody fusion for the management of high-grade spondylolisthesis in pediatric and adult patients. Reduction can be augmented with an anterior fusion using morselized bone graft or a structural cage in the L5 disc. Placement of a transsacral fibular graft or direct placement of sacral screws across the L5 disc into the L5 vertebral body also can be used to augment a partial reduction and fusion, as described by Smith et al.

TECHNIQUE 8.56

(SMITH ET AL.)

- Place the patient prone on a four-poster frame. Neuromonitoring is strongly recommended for this technique, including an intraoperative wake-up test in adult patients.
- Perform standard subperiosteal dissection of the posterior elements from L2 to the sacrum. Perform decompression and sacral laminectomies of S1 and S2.
- Place a temporary distracting rod from the inferior aspect of the lamina of L2 to the sacral ala, allowing distraction with concomitant extension moment applied by extension of the thighs. If distraction prevents reduction of the slip angle, the primary reduction maneuver is extension of the hip joints.
- If the sacral dome is thought to cause significant anterior impingement of the dural sac, perform partial sacral dome resection to decompress the neural elements further.
- Sweep the dural sac toward the midline in the vicinity of the S1-S2 disc.
- While protecting the neural elements under fluoroscopic control, advance a guidewire through the body of S1, across the L5-S1 disc space, and up to the anterior cortex of L5.
- Overream the guidewire under fluoroscopic guidance, beginning at 6 mm and increasing by 2 mm increments, usually up to 12 mm.

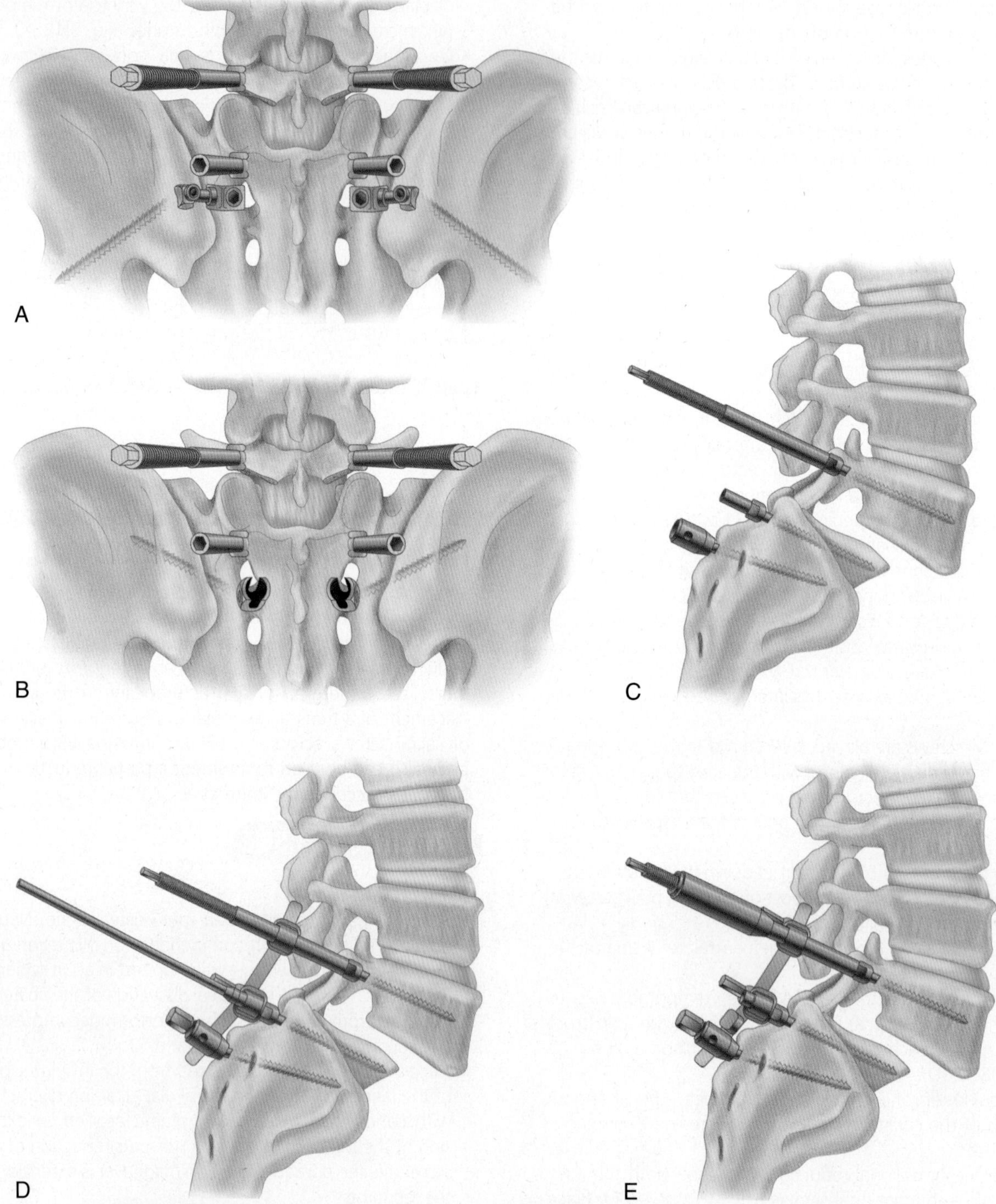

FIGURE 8.185 **A-N,** Reduction and fusion in high dysplastic spondylolisthesis with internal fixation. See text for description. (Redrawn from Crandall D: *TSRH-3D Plus MPA spinal instrumentation-deformity and degenerative, surgical technique manual*, Memphis, TN, 2005, Medtronic Sofamor Danek.) **SEE TECHNIQUE 8.55.**

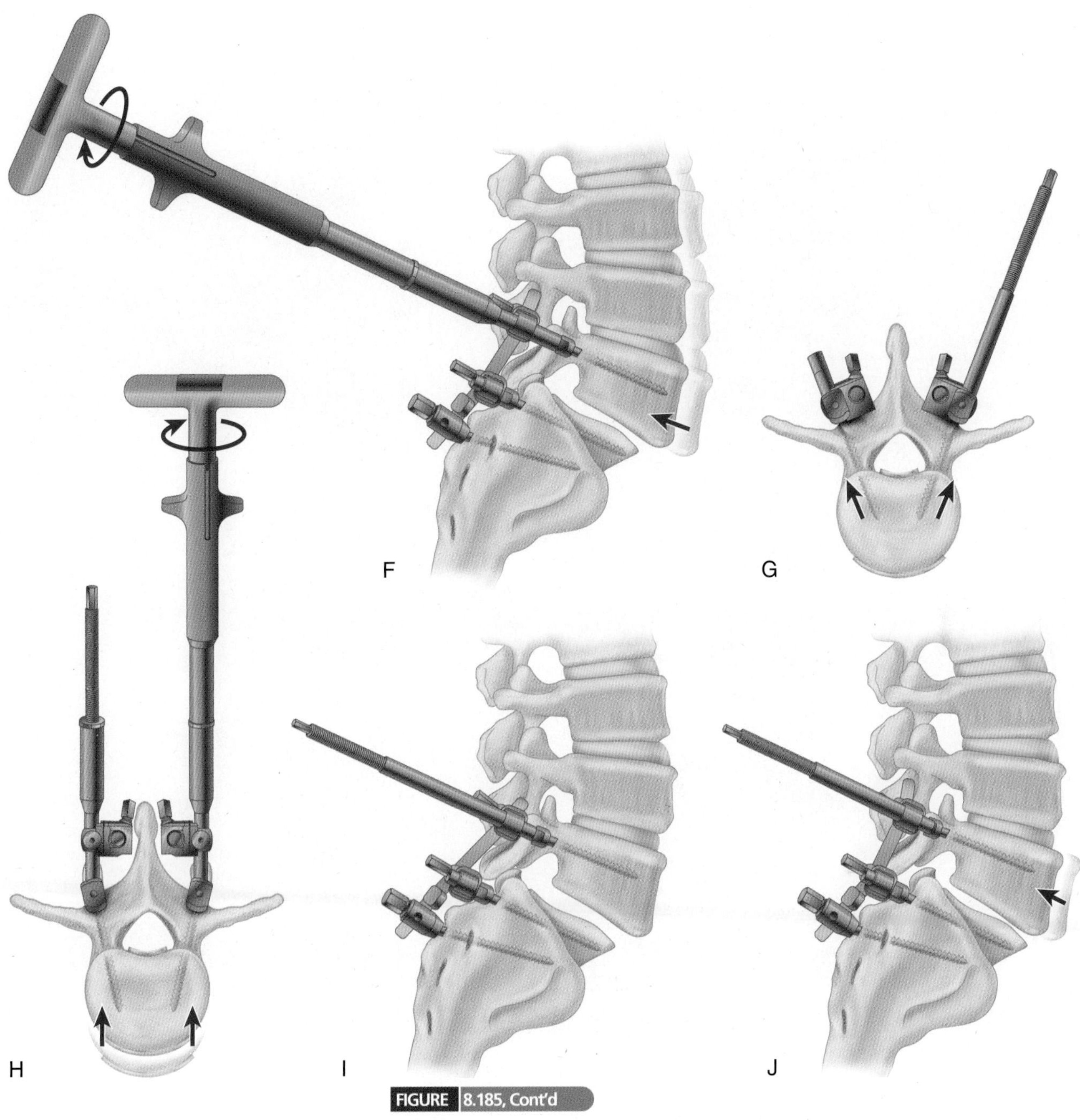

FIGURE 8.185, Cont'd

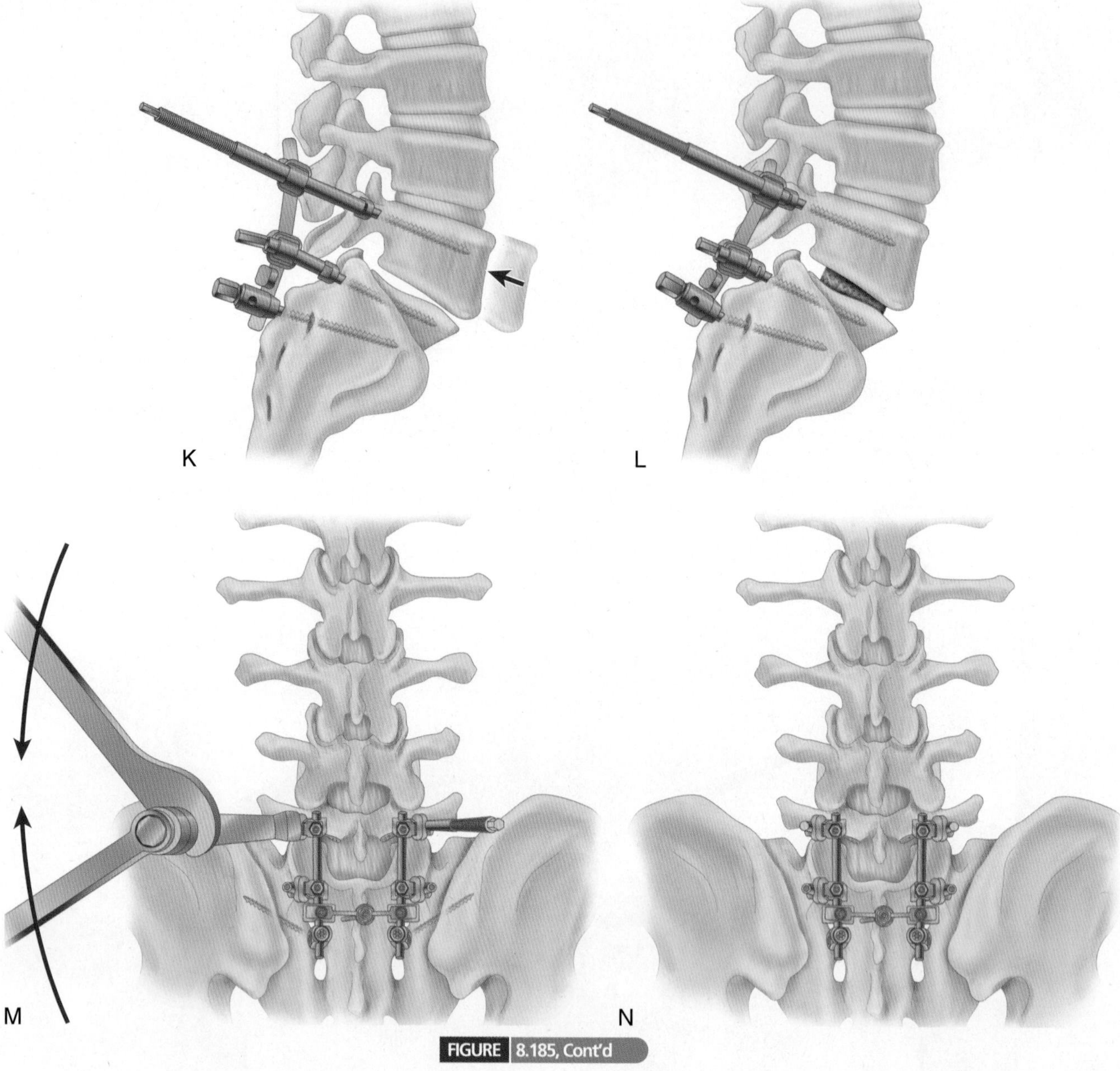

FIGURE 8.185, Cont'd

- Measure a single fibular allograft. Cut it and impact it into position. Remove the temporary distraction rod.
- To augment the transsacral fibula, place pedicle screw fixation in L4 and transsacral pedicle screws capturing L5. Direct the sacral screws along the same sagittal trajectory as the fibula to capture L5 with subsequent placement of rods connecting the pedicle screws (Fig. 8.186).
- Perform a posterolateral fusion from L4 to the sacral ala after harvest of iliac crest bone graft.

POSTOPERATIVE CARE Postoperative care is the same as that after the one-stage decompression and posterolateral interbody fusion.

ONE-STAGE DECOMPRESSION AND POSTEROLATERAL INTERBODY FUSION

TECHNIQUE 8.57

(BOHLMAN AND COOK)

- Place the patient prone, with the right leg draped free as the graft donor site.
- Approach the spine through a standard midline incision from the third lumbar level to the second sacral level. Subperiosteally strip muscle to the tip of the transverse process and sacral ala on each side.

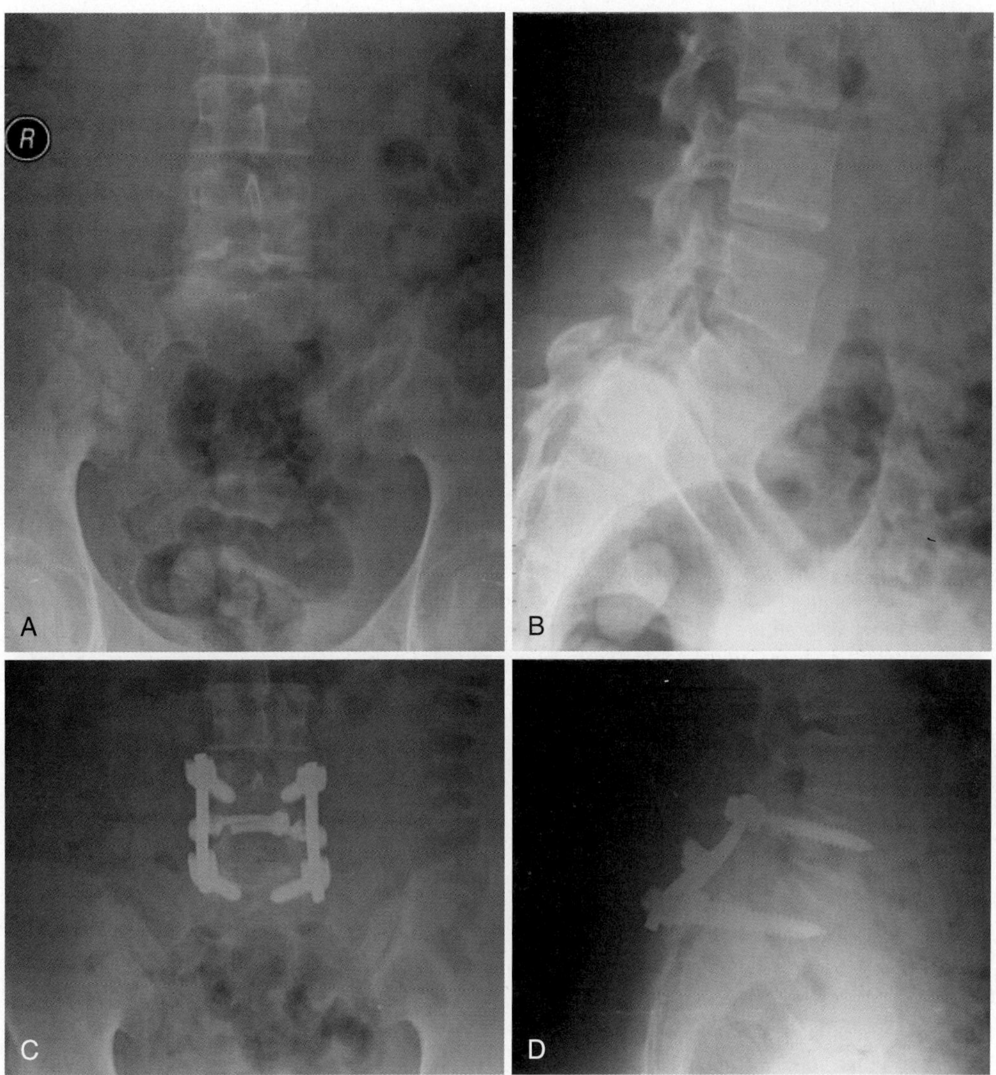

FIGURE 8.186 To augment the transsacral fibula, place pedicle screw fixation in L4 and transsacral pedicle screws capturing L5. Direct the sacral screws along the same sagittal trajectory as the fibula to capture L5 with subsequent placement of rods connecting the pedicle screws.

- Remove the posterior elements of the fifth lumbar and first sacral vertebrae (and fourth lumbar vertebra if necessary).
- Perform a wide foraminotomy to decompress the fifth lumbar and first sacral nerve roots.
- Gently free the dura from the posterosuperior prominence of the first sacral vertebral body with a Penfield elevator. Osteotomize the sacral prominence with a curved osteotome to create a ventral trough for the dura and to eliminate all pressure on the dura (Fig. 8.187A).
- Introduce a guide pin between the fifth lumbar and first sacral nerve roots on each side. Each pin is approximately 1 cm lateral to the midline and is directed through the first sacral vertebral body anteriorly. Confirm the proper position of each guidewire with radiographs.
- Drill a ⅜-inch epiphysiodesis bit over each guide pin to the appropriate depth, being careful not to violate the anterior cortex of the fifth lumbar vertebra (≈5 cm).
- Obtain a fibular graft from the right leg and divide it longitudinally. Insert one half of the graft into each hole and countersink it 2 mm so as not to impinge on the dura (Fig. 8.187B).
- Perform a standard bilateral, posterolateral transverse process fusion from the third or fourth lumbar vertebra to the sacral ala using iliac crest grafts (Fig. 8.187B,C).
- Close the wound over a drain.

POSTOPERATIVE CARE The patient is kept at bed rest for 7 to 10 days and then is mobilized in a lumbosacral orthosis. The drain is removed in 48 hours.

UNINSTRUMENTED CIRCUMFERENTIAL IN SITU FUSION

Circumferential in situ fusion has been used for the treatment of high-grade spondylolisthesis in chil-dren with

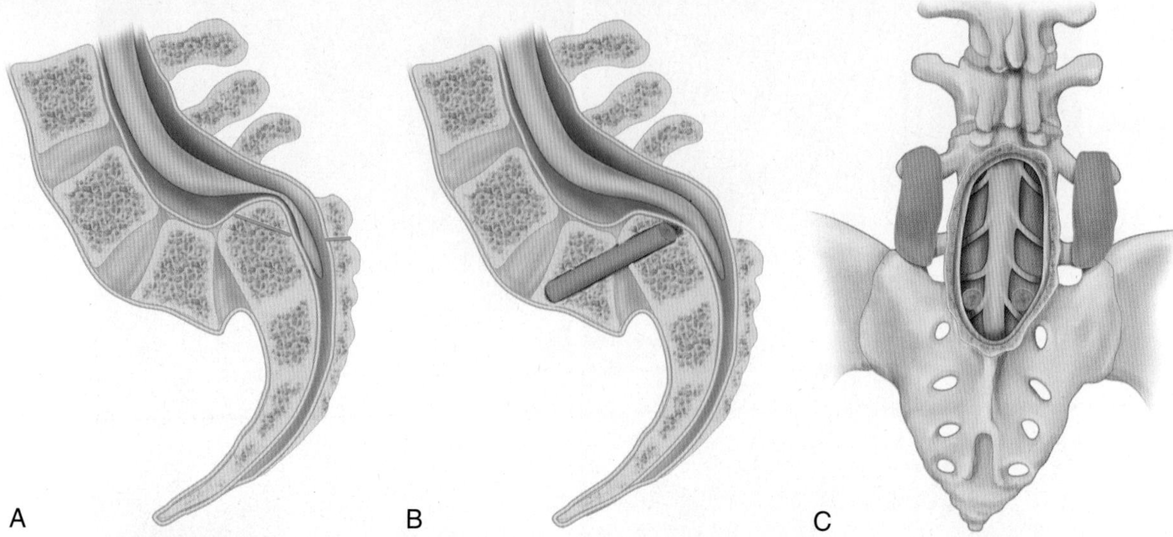

FIGURE 8.187 **A,** Amount of first sacral vertebral body resected to decompress dura *(blue line)*. **B,** Insertion of interbody fibular graft and posterior decompression. **C,** After posterior decompression and fusion. *Colored area* represents posterolateral fusions. Ends of two fibular grafts are shown just above first sacral nerve roots. (From Bohlman HH, Cook SS: One-stage decompression and posterolateral and interbody fusion for lumbosacral spondyloptosis through a posterior approach, *J Bone Joint Surg* 64A:415, 1982.) **SEE TECHNIQUE 8.57.**

better long-term results reported than after posterolateral or anterior fusion alone. The SRS recommends that if reduction is performed, circumferential fusion with instrumentation should be done at the time of reduction.

TECHNIQUE 8.58

(HELENIUS ET AL.)

- Place the patient prone on a four-poster Relton frame.
- Make a posterior midline skin incision and develop the space bilaterally through the erector spinae muscles, 3 cm from the midline. Identify the L5 transverse process, the L5-S1 facet joint, and the sacral ala.
- Expose the posterior iliac wing through the same incision and obtain corticocancellous bone graft material.
- Open the L5-S1 facet joint with an osteotome and decorticate and curet the L5 transverse process and sacral ala. Place autogenous graft over the decorticated bone and impact it into the L5-S1 facet joint space.
- Close the fasciae on both sides as well as the subcutaneous tissues and skin with running absorbable suture.
- Place the patient supine, with both hips extended and the lower extremities spread apart. Place a small bolster under the lumbar spine to obtain lumbar lordosis. A Trendelenburg position of the table helps to keep the abdominal contents cephalad to the operating area.
- Make a longitudinal midline incision from just caudal to the umbilicus to just cephalad to the symphysis pubis.
- Open the fascia over the rectus abdominis muscle and develop the internervous plane between the abdominal muscles.
- After opening the peritoneum, extend the approach cephalad by cutting through the linea alba and packing the abdominal contents superiorly. Take care not to enter the dome of the bladder caudally.
- Open the posterior peritoneum (Fig. 8.188A) and assess the anatomy of the iliac vessels. Usually, the presacral intervertebral disc can be approached between the great vessels. Protect the left iliac vein across the L5 vertebral body and caudal to the aortic bifurcation.
- With forceps, use blunt dissection to expose the L5-S1 disc.
- Identify the anterior longitudinal ligament and ligate the middle sacral artery. To help retract the iliac vessels, two Steinmann pins can be inserted on either side of the L5 vertebral body. Try to preserve all the parasympathetic nerve fibers in this area by approaching the disc space in the midline.
- Open the anterior longitudinal ligament horizontally, just cephalad to the L5-S1 disc space (Fig. 8.188B). The lower anterior lip of the L5 vertebra can be resected along the anterior longitudinal ligament to better expose the disc space.
- Carefully remove all intervertebral disc material up to the posterior longitudinal ligament, as well as the ring apophysis on both sides. Prepare the endplates with curettage.
- Obtain two to three tricortical wedge-shaped bone grafts (15 mm anterior and 10 mm posterior dimension) from either anterior iliac wing. The length of this graft is approximately 20 mm but may vary some. The grafts must fit into the disc space as prepared (Fig. 8.188C). A moderate increase in disc height and proper patient positioning reduce the spondylolisthesis and lumbosacral kyphosis. Using three structural autogenous grafts provides the best stability.
- In slips of nearly 100%, it may be necessary to increase the area for anterior spinal fusion. In these cases, an osteotomy of the sacrum may be necessary. Continue the release of the anterior ligament inferiorly, producing an osteoperiosteal flap over the S1 vertebral body. Apply corticocancellous bone grafts beneath this flap to increase the area for anterior intervertebral fusion.

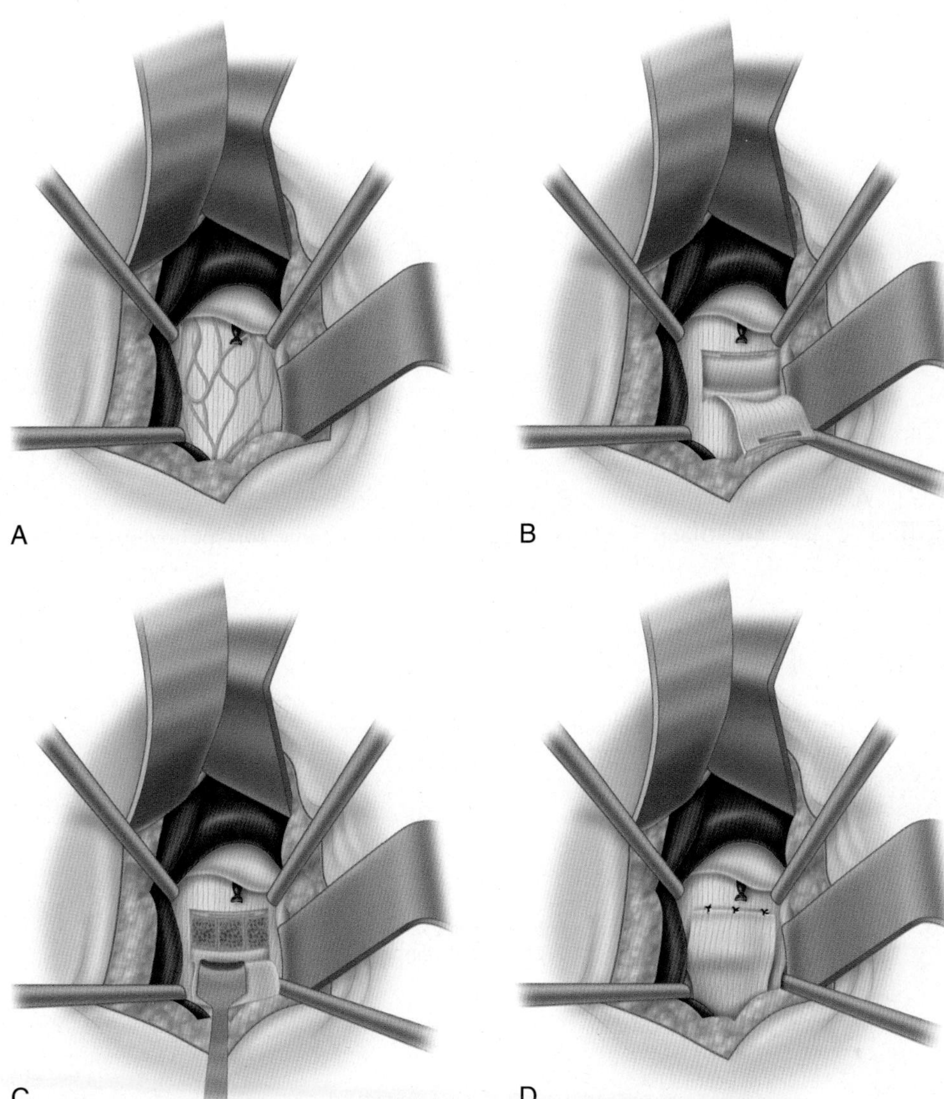

FIGURE 8.188 **A,** Posterior peritoneum opened and middle sacral artery ligated. **B,** Anterior longitudinal ligament opened, and small piece of bone removed from lower lip of L5. **C,** After discectomy, structural autogenous grafts placed. **D,** Anterior longitudinal ligament reattached through osseous channels and posterior peritoneal and laparotomy incisions are subsequently closed. (From Helenius I, Remes V, Poussa M: Uninstrumented in situ fusion for high-grade childhood and adolescent isthmic spondylolisthesis: long-term outcome, *J Bone Joint Surg* 90A:145, 2008.) **SEE TECHNIQUE 8.58.**

- Reattach the anterior longitudinal ligament with absorbable sutures through osseous channels in the L5 vertebra.
- Close the posterior peritoneal and laparotomy incision (Fig. 8.188D).

POSTOPERATIVE CARE A postoperative custom-molded TLSO is worn, and the patient is allowed to mobilize 2 to 3 days after surgery. Bending, lifting, and sports are restricted for 3 to 6 months or until a solid fusion is obtained.

TREATMENT OF SPONDYLOPTOSIS

L5 VERTEBRECTOMY

Spondyloptosis exists when the entire body of L5 on a lateral standing radiograph is totally below the top of S1. Gaines popularized a two-stage L5 vertebrectomy procedure for this difficult problem (Fig. 8.189). The objective is to restore sagittal plane balance to avoid nerve root damage from cauda equina and nerve root stretching during reduction. This is a challenging procedure and should be done only by surgeons experienced in the surgical treatment of patients with high-grade isthmic dysplastic spondylolisthesis.

TECHNIQUE 8.59

(GAINES)

- This technique is performed in two stages, during either a single anesthetic or two separate anesthetic procedures.
- In the first stage, perform an L5 vertebrectomy and totally remove the L4-L5 and L5-S1 discs through a transverse abdominal incision (Fig. 8.190A).

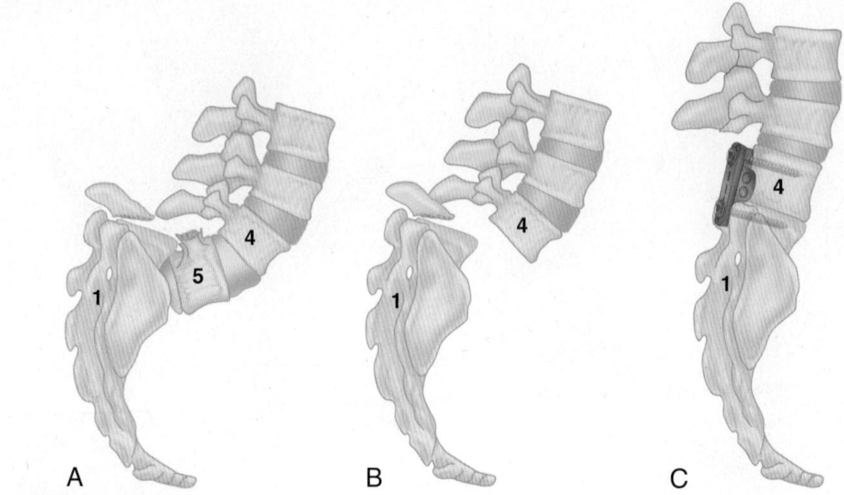

FIGURE 8.189 **A-C,** Diagram of two-stage L5 vertebrectomy for spondyloptosis. **SEE TECHNIQUE 8.59.**

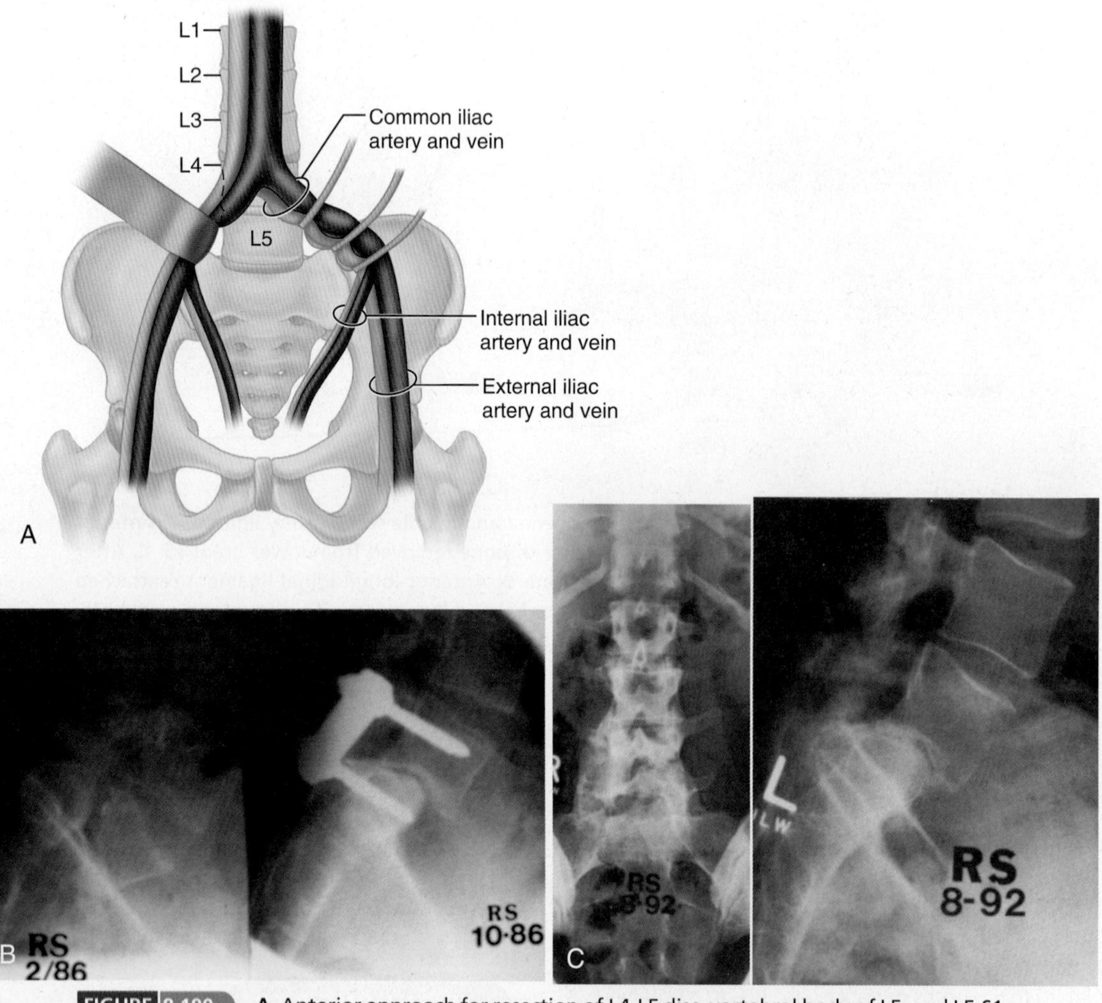

FIGURE 8.190 **A,** Anterior approach for resection of L4-L5 disc, vertebral body of L5, and L5-S1 disc is made through incision extending transversely across both rectus abdominis muscles. Great vessels are mobilized laterally after being carefully identified, and structures to be resected are seen between bifurcation of vena cava and aorta. **B,** Preoperative and postoperative lateral radiograph. **C,** Radiographs of same patient 7 years later. Solid intertransverse fusion and interbody fusion are shown. Reconstructed L4-S1 intervertebral foramen is wide open on lateral radiograph. (**A** redrawn from and **B** and **C** from Gaines RW Jr: The L5 vertebrectomy approach for the treatment of spondyloptosis. In Bridwell KH, DeWald RL, editors: *The textbook of spinal surgery*, ed 2, Philadelphia, 1997, Lippincott-Raven.) **SEE TECHNIQUE 8.59.**

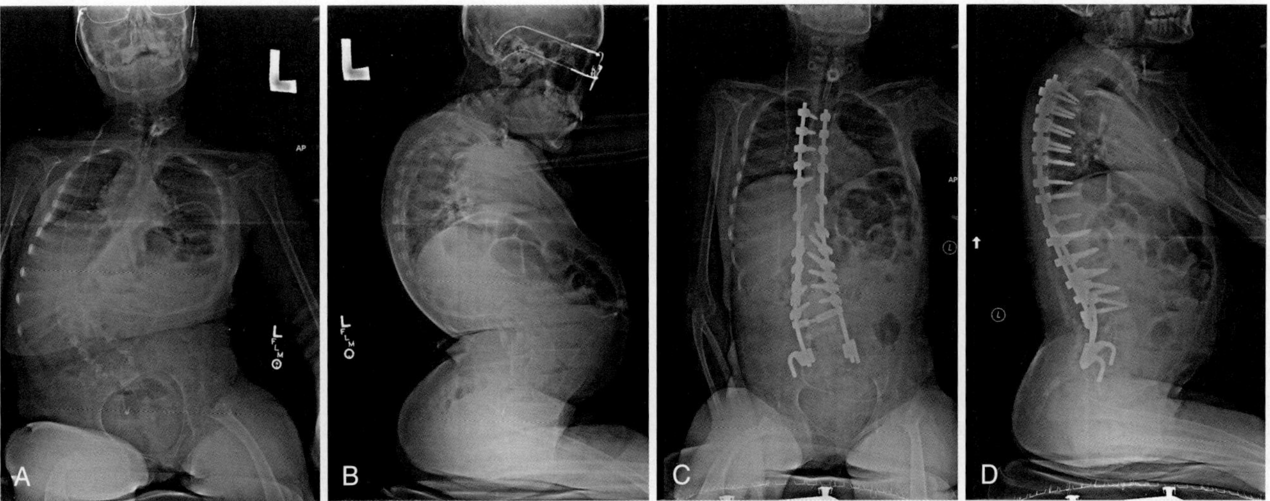

FIGURE 8.191 A and B, Scoliosis in patient with myelomeningocele; note C-shaped curve. C and D, After posterior fusion and instrumentation.

- Excise the L5 body back to the base of the pedicles and control epidural bleeding with Gelfoam.
- Do not attempt reduction of the deformity at this time.
- Remove the caudal cartilage endplate of L4 after the L5 vertebrectomy is completed.
- For the second stage, place the patient prone.
- Through a posterior approach, remove the L5 pedicles, facets, and laminar arch bilaterally.
- Place the pedicle screws into L4 and S1.
- Clean the upper surface of the sacrum of the cartilage endplate but preserve the cortical endplate for docking with the inferior endplate of L4. Bone from the vertebrectomy is left between the L4 and S1 screws posterolaterally (Fig. 8.190B,C). L4 must touch S1 directly after the reduction, and the L5 and S1 nerve roots must both be free. Direct exposure of the L5 nerve roots and dural tube is the most important way to avoid serious iatrogenic injury to the cauda equina.

KYPHOSCOLIOSIS

MYELOMENINGOCELE

Treatment of patients with myelomeningocele spinal deformities is the most challenging in spine surgery. It requires a team effort, with cooperation of consultants in several subspecialties. These children often have multiple system dysfunctions that influence the treatment of their spinal deformity.

INCIDENCE AND NATURAL HISTORY

Scoliosis and kyphosis with secondary adaptive changes are common in patients with myelomeningocele. Spinal deformity may be the result of developmental deformities that are acquired and related to the level of paralysis or congenital deformities that are the result of vertebral malformation. Developmental and congenital forms of spinal deformity may exist concurrently in patients with myelomeningocele. These deformities often are progressive and can lead to significant disabilities. The incidence of scoliosis increases with increasing age and neurologic level. Trivedi et al. found the prevalence of scoliosis to be 93%, 72%, 43%, and less than 1%, respectively, in patients with thoracic, upper lumbar, lower lumbar, and sacral motor levels. Congenital scoliosis in myelomeningocele is associated with structural disorganization of the vertebrae with asymmetric growth and includes all of the congenital anomalies associated with scoliosis: hemivertebrae, unilateral unsegmented bars, and various combinations of the two. Congenital scoliosis occurs in 15% to 20% of patients with myelomeningocele, and most curves in myelomeningocele patients are paralytic. In these patients, the spine is straight at birth and gradually develops a progressive curvature because of the neuromuscular problems. These generally are long, C-shaped curves with the apex in the thoracolumbar or lumbar spine (Fig. 8.191). These paralytic curves often extend into the lumbosacral junction and often are associated with pelvic obliquity. In these children, spinal curvatures often develop at a younger age than in children with idiopathic scoliosis, beginning at 3 to 4 years of age, and can become severe before the patient is 10 years old. Future trunk growth and final trunk height are considerations in treatment, although Lindseth noted that children with myelomeningocele have slow growth because of growth hormone deficiency and mature earlier than usual, often by 9 to 10 years in girls and 11 to 12 years in boys.

CLINICAL EVALUATION

Thorough evaluation is critical for determining the appropriate management of patients with myelomeningocele and spinal deformity. The following areas are closely investigated: presence of hydrocephalus, any operative procedures for shunting, bowel and bladder function, frequency of urinary tract infections, use of an indwelling catheter or intermittent catheterization, possible latex allergies, current medications, mental status, method of ambulation, level of the defect, any noticeable progression of the curve, and any lower extremity contractures. The spine is examined to determine the type and flexibility of the deformity and to detect any evidence of pressure sores or lack of sitting balance. In patients with progressive paralytic scoliosis, hydromyelia, disturbed ventricular shunts, syringomyelia, tethered cord, or compression from an Arnold-Chiari syndrome may contribute to the progression of scoliosis. Most patients with myelomeningocele have radiographic tethering of the spinal cord at the site of the sac closure, but the mere presence of radiographic tethering does not necessarily imply traction on the cord. Other clinical signs and symptoms of cord tethering should be observed, including back pain, new or increased spasticity, changes in muscle strength, difficulty with gait, changes in bowel or bladder function, and the appearance of lower extremity deformities.

Careful evaluation of any pelvic obliquity is necessary. Because patients with myelomeningocele are prone to development of contractures around the hips, careful physical examination of the hip adductors, extensors, and flexors is important in evaluating the cause of pelvic obliquity. Lubicky noted a difficult but unusual problem in some patients with myelomeningocele and extension contractures of the hips. In these patients, flexion through the thoracolumbar spine was needed for them to sit upright. Spinal fusion would make sitting impossible and would place significant mechanical stresses on the instrumentation. Physiologic hip flexion should be restored in these patients before spinal instrumentation and fusion are undertaken.

RADIOGRAPHIC FINDINGS

Radiographs should be taken with the patient upright and supine. If the patient can ambulate, standing films should be made. If the patient is nonambulatory, sitting films should be made. The upright films allow better evaluation of the actual deformity of the spine and will demonstrate the contribution of the paralytic component to the spine deformity. Supine films show better detail of various associated spinal deformities. The flexibility of the curves is determined with traction or bending films.

Radiographic evaluation of the pelvic obliquity should include a supine view obtained with the hips in the "relaxed" position. In this view, the hips are flexed and abducted or adducted as dictated by the contractures. Alternatively, radiographs can be made with the patient prone and the hips off the edge of the radiographic table and placed in abduction or adduction.

Various specialized radiographs are helpful. Myelography and MRI are useful for evaluating such conditions as hydromyelia, tethered cord (Fig. 8.192), diastematomyelia, and Arnold-Chiari malformation. CT with reconstruction views will give better bone detail for associated congenital spine anomalies. Renal ultrasound or intravenous pyelography should be done at regular intervals, according to the urologist's recommendation.

SCOLIOSIS AND LORDOSIS IN MYELOMENINGOCELE

ORTHOTIC TREATMENT

Although the natural history of paralytic curves in patients with myelomeningocele is not changed by orthotic treatment, bracing may be useful to delay spinal fusion until adequate spinal growth has occurred. Bracing may accomplish this in paralytic curves but does not affect congenital curves. The brace also can improve sitting balance and free the hands for other activities. Custom-fitted braces are used but require close and frequent observation by the parents. The skin must be examined frequently for pressure areas; any sign of pressure requires immediate brace adjustment. Bracing usually is not instituted until the curve is beginning to cause clinical problems, and generally it is worn only when the patient is upright. If the curve fails to respond to bracing or if bracing becomes impossible because of pressure sores or noncompliance, surgery is indicated. The patient and the parents need to understand that the brace is not the definitive treatment of these curves.

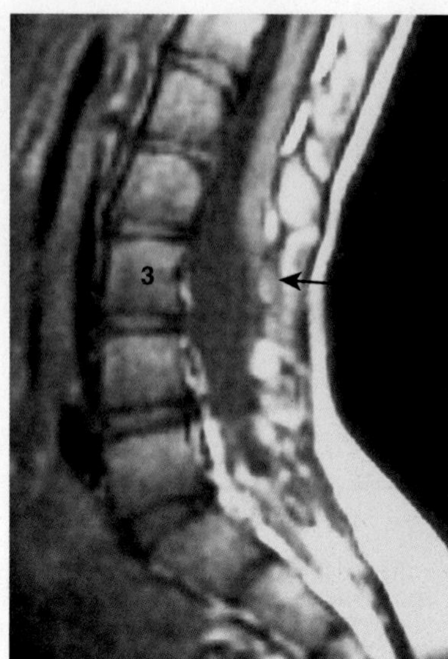

FIGURE 8.192 MRI shows tethered cord at L3 in patient with kyphoscoliosis.

Flynn et al. reported that VEPTR is a reasonable treatment option for spinal deformity in immature, nonambulatory myelomeningocele patients for correcting spinal deformity, allowing spinal growth, and maintaining adequate respiratory function until definitive fusion is needed.

OPERATIVE TREATMENT

Several authors have indicated that surgery on the myelomeningocele spine is accompanied by potentially serious complications. Although the operative procedures varied considerably in these reports, some observations could be made. Because of densely scarred and adherent soft tissue, spinal exposure often is lengthy and hemorrhagic. The deformity often is rigid, and correction may be limited. The quality of the bone often provides poor fixation for instrumentation systems, and the inadequacy of the posterior bone mass provides a poor bed for bone grafting. The lack of normal posterior vertebral elements makes instrumentation and achieving a solid fusion difficult. The abnormal placement of the paraspinal muscles results in the lack of usual soft-tissue coverage of the spine and instrumentation systems. Newer techniques of surgery and instrumentation, bank bone, and prophylactic antibiotics have lessened but not eliminated these problems. The parents must be aware of these potential problems before surgery and must accept these as inherent in the operative treatment.

Emans et al. called attention to the problem of latex allergy in patients with myelomeningocele. Repeated exposures to latex during daily catheterization and multiple operations most likely accounts for sensitization of these patients to natural latex. The allergy is to the residual plant proteins in natural latex products and is an immunoglobulin E–mediated, immediate type of hypersensitivity. Anaphylaxis may occur intraoperatively and easily can be confused with other intraoperative emergencies. Patients with myelomeningocele should be closely questioned about any preoperative reactions to latex. Latex allergy testing can now be performed. We routinely treat all patients with myelomeningocele as if they have a latex allergy.

Congenital abnormalities that cause scoliosis in patients with myelomeningocele are treated in the same manner as in other patients with congenital scoliosis with early operative intervention. Paralytic scoliosis is more common than congenital scoliosis, and lordoscoliosis is the most common type. The combined anterior and posterior fusion method provides the best chance to achieve a durable fusion. Stella et al. also reported that the best correction was obtained in patients who had instrumented anterior and posterior fusions. High pseudarthrosis rates have been reported in patients with myelomeningocele and are related to the surgical approach, type, and presence of instrumentation or the use of a posterior-only approach. The reported pseudarthrosis rates are 0 to 50% for anterior fusion, 26% to 76% for isolated posterior fusion, and 5% to 23% for combined anterior and posterior fusions. Infection rates have approached 43% and are highest when surgery is performed with concurrent urinary tract infections. Preoperative urinary cultures are mandatory, as is treatment with antibiotics preoperatively and postoperatively. Prophylactic antibiotic use has reduced the infection rate to 8%.

Selection of Fusion Levels. The levels of fusion depend on the age of the child, location of the curve, level of paralysis, ambulatory status, and presence or absence of pelvic obliquity. Spinal fusion generally should extend from neutral vertebra to neutral vertebra, with the end vertebra of the scoliotic curve located within the stable zone. Paralytic curves often tend to be fused too short, especially proximally. In deciding whether to stop the fusion short or long, the longer fusion usually is safer. In the past, instrumentation was extended to the pelvis because deficient posterior elements of the lumbar spine made adequate fixation impossible. With pedicle screw fixation, fusion and instrumentation sometimes can be stopped short of the pelvis. Mazur et al. and Müller et al. showed that spinal fusion to the pelvis in ambulatory patients diminished their ambulatory status. They therefore recommended fusion short of the pelvis, if possible, in ambulatory patients. Ending the fusion above the pelvis eliminates the stresses on the instrumentation and fusion areas at the lumbosacral junction and allows some motion for adjustment of lordosis in those who have mild hip flexion contractures. In nonambulatory patients, unless the lumbar curve can be corrected to less than 20 degrees and the pelvic obliquity to less than 10 to 15 degrees, the scoliosis will continue to progress if the lumbosacral junction is not fused.

Attention to the sagittal contour is extremely important. Even in a nonambulatory patient, maintenance of lumbar lordosis is important. If the lumbar lordosis is flattened, the pelvis rotates and much of the sitting weight is placed directly on the ischial tuberosities; this can result in the development of pressure sores.

Anterior-Only Fusion. Sponseller et al. recommended anterior fusion and instrumentation alone in selected patients with myelomeningocele and paralytic scoliosis. Their indications for this procedure include thoracolumbar curves of less than 75 degrees, compensatory proximal curves of less than 40 degrees, no significant kyphosis in the primary curve, and no evidence of syrinx. Fourteen patients were treated with this technique. A rod and vertebral body screw construct was used most frequently anteriorly.

POSTERIOR INSTRUMENTATION AND FUSION

Posterior instrumentation and fusion alone has been reserved for flexible curves with most of the posterior elements intact so that adequate fixation can be obtained with pedicle screws. However, the curve must be flexible and correction must allow almost normal coronal and sagittal balance. Posterior-only instrumentation and fusion has been associated with the highest pseudarthrosis rates.

TECHNIQUE 8.60

- Place the patient prone on a radiolucent frame.
- Prepare and drape the back in a sterile manner.
- Make a midline incision from the area of the superior vertebra to be instrumented down to the sacrum.
- In the area of the normal spine, carry out subperiosteal dissection. An inverted-Y incision has been described to prevent exposure of the sac in the midline, but we have had difficulty with skin necrosis with use of this technique and have had better results with a midline incision that follows the scarred area of the skin posteriorly and careful dissection around the sac in the midline area.
- Make the skin incision carefully because the dural sac is just beneath the skin. If a dural leak is noted, repair it immediately.
- Carry the dissection laterally over the convex and concave facet areas and down to the ala of the sacrum to expose the area of normal spine to be fused and the bony elements in the region of the abnormal sac area.
- Hooks, pedicle screws, or sublaminar wires can be used to instrument the normal vertebra above the sac area.
- In the area of the defect, attempt to achieve segmental fixation. Pass a wire around a pedicle and twist it on itself to secure fixation. Pass wires on both the concave and the convex sides of the curve. Because these pedicles often are osteoporotic, take care in tightening the wires so that they do not "cut through."
- On the concave side of the curve, distraction can help correct pelvic obliquity.
- If the iliac wing is large enough to accept the Galveston fixation, make a Galveston bend in short rods and insert the short rods in the iliac crests. Alternatively, an iliac screw and/or an S2 alar screw can be used.
- An iliac screw with connectors can be used.
- Connect two longer rods to the spine with the segmental wires and connect the long rods to the Galveston-type rods with domino-type crosslinks (see Technique 8.31).
- Alternatively, if the iliac wings are too small, use the McCarthy technique (see Technique 8.30). Take care to preserve normal lumbar lordosis and secure the rods in place by tightening the segmental wires.

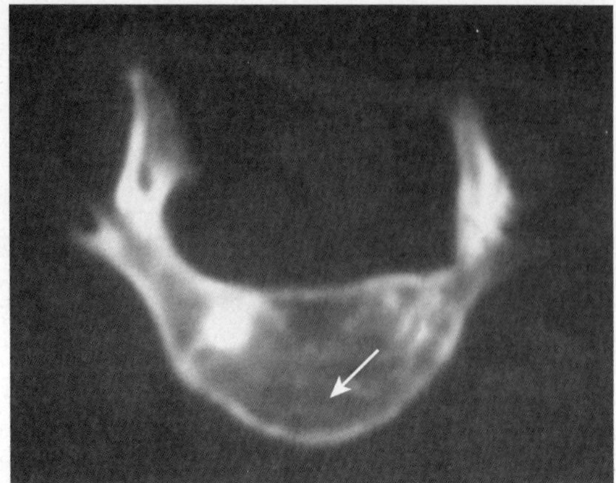

FIGURE 8.193 CT scan shows abnormal pedicle orientation in dysraphic vertebra. (From Rodgers WB, Frim DM, Emans JB: Surgery of the spine in myelodysplasia: an overview, *Clin Orthop Relat Res* 338:19, 1997.)

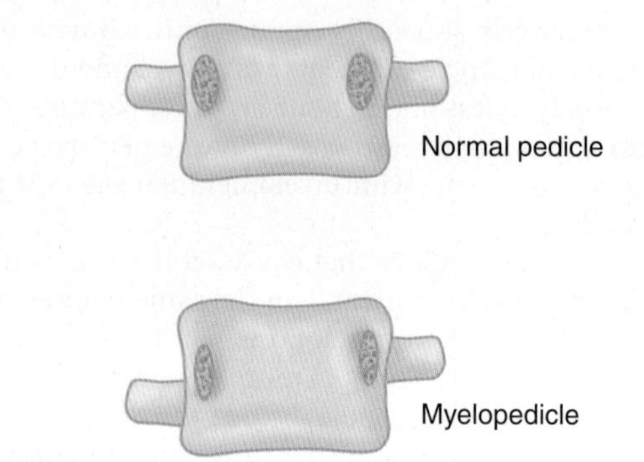

FIGURE 8.194 Diagram shows alteration in anatomic relationship of pedicle-transverse process.

- Apply copious bone-bank allograft to any areas of bony structures posteriorly.
- It is important to link the two rods with a crosslink system.

COMBINED ANTERIOR AND POSTERIOR FUSION

The most commonly required procedure for progressive scoliosis in patients with myelomeningocele combines anterior and posterior fusions with posterior instrumentation. Posterior instrumentation consists of a standard rod with hooks, pedicle screws, sublaminar wires, or cables, or a combination of these in the areas of normal posterior elements. The hooks and pedicle screws allow distraction or compressive forces to be applied, and the wires or cables allow a translational force to be applied.

The absence of posterior elements in the dysraphic portion of the spine makes fixation more of a problem, so various instrumentation systems need to be available (Fig. 8.193). Rodgers et al. noted that pedicle screws greatly improved fixation and correction of the dysraphic portion of the spine. In widely dysraphic vertebrae, the orientation and landmarks of the pedicle are altered (Fig. 8.194), and direct viewing of the pedicle is necessary to insert pedicle screws in these areas. The pedicle is exposed either by resection of a sufficient amount of facet or by dissection along the medial wall of the spinal canal and retraction of the meningocele sac to identify the medial wall of the pedicle. During probing of the pedicle, remaining within the cortices of the pedicle is imperative. The pedicle screws do not necessarily need to penetrate the anterior vertebral cortex. In the dysraphic spine, the pedicle screws often have to be inserted at an angle from lateral to medial (Fig. 8.195). This requires special attention to rod contouring to attach the rod to the screw because of the lateral position of the screw head. The small vertebral bodies and osteopenic bone often make the purchase of pedicle screws questionable.

Two other techniques for fixation of the dysraphic spine can be used. Drummond spinous process button wires can be passed through laminar remnants (Fig. 8.196), or segmental wires can be looped around each pedicle. When Drummond button wires are used, the dysraphic laminae are exposed and dissection is done between the sac and the adjacent laminae while the sac is carefully retracted medially. A hole is placed through the strongest available portion of the laminar remnant, and the wire is passed from medial to lateral, leaving the button on the inner surface of the lamina. Segmental wires can be looped around each pedicle by passing from one foramen around the pedicle and other posterior remnants medial to the pedicle and then back through the next foramen and back to the original wire. The passage of these wires usually is blind. The wires then attach to the rod. The wire also can be looped around a pedicle bone screw if it is difficult to contour the rod to easily fit in the screw.

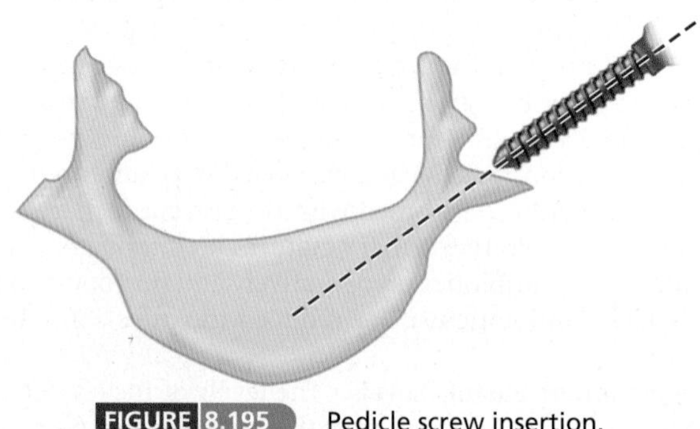

FIGURE 8.195 Pedicle screw insertion.

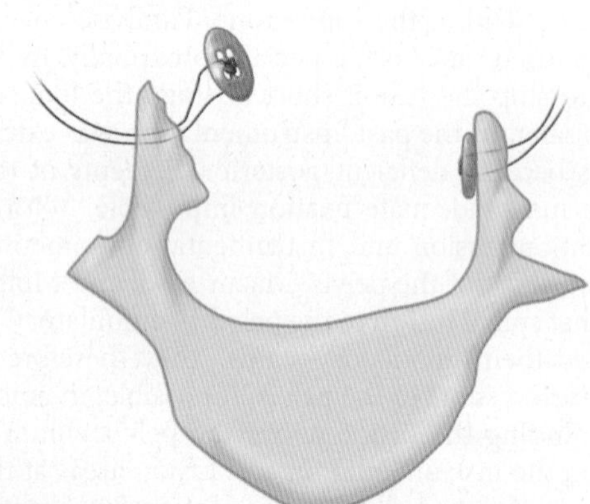

FIGURE 8.196 Diagram of Wisconsin button wire fixation of dysraphic vertebra.

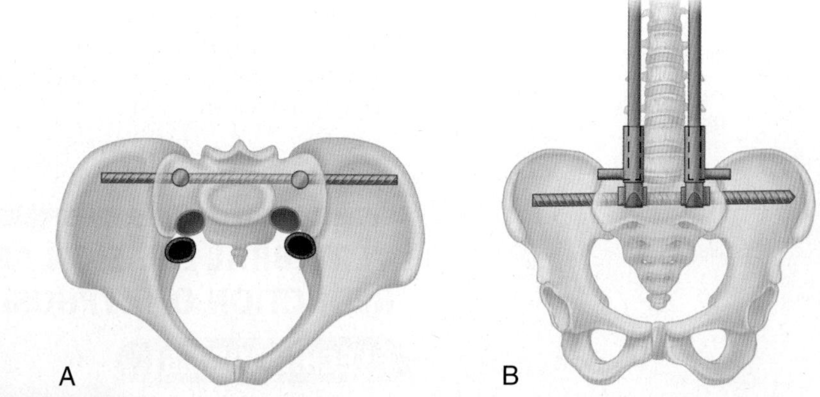

FIGURE 8.197 **A,** Correct passage of sacral bar through body of sacrum, posterior to great vessels and anterior to spinal canal. **B,** Connection between sacral bar and vertical rods.

Instrumentation to the pelvis frequently is necessary to correct associated pelvic obliquity in nonambulatory children. Fixation to the pelvis and sacrum is especially difficult in children with myelomeningocele because the bone often is osteoporotic and the pelvis is small, making secure instrumentation difficult. The stresses placed on distal fixation in scoliosis tend to displace sacral or sacropelvic instrumentation laterally. If there is associated kyphosis, these forces tend to displace sacral or pelvic instrumentation dorsally.

Several techniques have been described for extending fixation to the pelvis, including Galveston, Dunn-McCarthy, Jackson, Fackler, sacral bar, and pedicle screws. Our preferred technique for pelvic fixation in patients with paralytic scoliosis is the Galveston technique (see Technique 8.31). We believe this provides the most secure pelvic fixation for scoliotic curves. However, many patients with myelomeningocele have hypoplastic iliac crests, and in these patients, rods are fixed to the sacrum with the technique described by McCarthy (see Technique 8.30). This technique does not restrict lateral displacement as well as the Galveston intrapelvic fixation does, but crosslinking of the two rods may help decrease lateral displacement. Once the two rods are crosslinked, pelvic obliquity can be corrected by cantilevering the crosslinked rods. The Jackson intrasacral rod technique consists of inserting the rods through the lateral sacral mass and into the sacrum. The rod then penetrates the anterolateral cortex and usually is attached to a sacral screw, providing fixation in flexion and extension. The anatomy of the sacrum in patients with myelomeningocele makes this technique quite difficult. Widmann et al. described a technique using a sacral bar connected to standard Cotrel-Dubousset–like rods in 10 patients and found it to be effective (Fig. 8.197). Pelvic fixation by sacral pedicle screws is not reliable in these small osteopenic patients.

In patients who are treated with combined anterior and posterior fusion, the necessity for anterior instrumentation is controversial. One study found no statistical differences in fusion rate, curve correction, or change in pelvic obliquity with anterior and posterior instrumentation and fusion compared with anterior arthrodesis with only posterior instrumentation and fusion. However, other studies have reported better correction and a decrease in the rate of implant failure and postoperative loss of correction with instrumented anterior and posterior fusions. If anterior instrumentation is used, care must be taken to not cause a kyphotic deformity in the instrumented spine.

KYPHOSIS IN MYELOMENINGOCELE

INCIDENCE AND NATURAL HISTORY

Kyphosis in patients with myelomeningocele may be either developmental or congenital. Developmental kyphosis is not present at birth and progresses slowly. It is a paralytic kyphosis that is aggravated by the lack of posterior stability. Congenital kyphosis, which is a much more difficult problem, usually measures 80 degrees or more at birth. The level of the lesion usually is T12 with total paraplegia. The kyphosis is rigid and progresses rapidly during infancy. Children with severe kyphosis are unable to wear braces and often have difficulty sitting in wheelchairs because the center of gravity is displaced forward. An ulceration may develop over the prominent kyphosis and make skin coverage difficult. Progression of the kyphosis may lead to respiratory difficulty because of incompetence of the inspiratory muscles, crowding of the abdominal contents, and upward pressure on the diaphragm. Increased flexion of the trunk can interfere with urinary drainage and also may cause problems if urinary diversion or ileostomy becomes necessary.

Hoppenfeld described the anatomy of this condition and noted that the pedicles are widely spread and the rudimentary laminae actually are everted. The anterior longitudinal ligament is short and thick. The paraspinal muscles are present but are displaced far anterolaterally (Fig. 8.198); thus, all muscles act anterior to the axis of rotation, which tends to worsen the kyphosis.

OPERATIVE TREATMENT

Apical vertebral ostectomy, as proposed by Sharrard, makes closure of the skin easier in neonates but provides only short-term improvement, and the kyphotic deformity invariably recurs. Crawford et al. reported kyphectomies performed at the time of dural sac closure in the neonate. They found this to be a safe procedure with excellent initial correction. Eventual recurrence is expected despite the procedure. The recurrence, however, is a longer, more rounded deformity that is technically less demanding to correct. Lindseth and Selzer reported vertebral excision for kyphosis in children with myelomeningocele. Their most consistent results were obtained with partial resection of the apical vertebra and the proximal lordotic

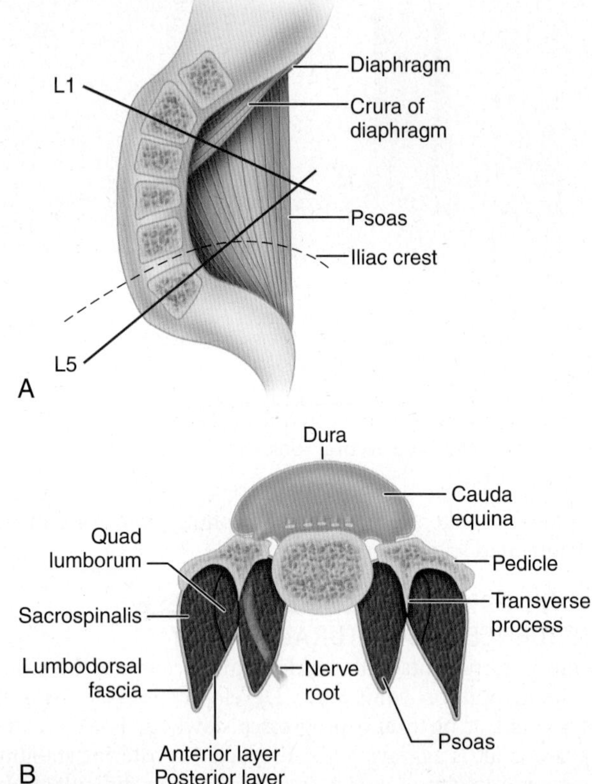

FIGURE 8.198 **A,** Sagittal diagram showing deforming effect of psoas muscle on kyphosis. **B,** Transverse section of lumbar spine and attached muscles in region of kyphosis. Pedicles and laminae of vertebrae are splayed laterally; erector spinae muscles enclosed in thoracolumbar fascia lie lateral to vertebral bodies and act as flexors.

curve. Others have found that the Warner and Fackler type of sacral anchoring (see Fig. 8.200) provides a rigid construct, good correction, and low-profile instrumentation. That has also been our experience and is our preferred method of sacral anchoring in kyphectomies. Other techniques using a Dunn-McCarthy technique, intrasacral fixation, and pedicle screws also have been described.

Although all severe congenital kyphoses in patients with myelomeningocele progress, not all patients require surgery. Kyphectomy is indicated to improve sitting balance or when skin problems occur over the apex. The trend is to delay surgery until the patient is 7 or 8 years of age, if possible. The surgery should be done before skeletal maturity, however. Delaying the surgery allows more secure internal fixation with less postoperative loss of correction.

Sarwark reported a subtraction osteotomy of multiple vertebrae at the apex, which creates lordosing osteotomies at each level. The vertebral body is entered and subtracted via the pedicles with a curet, distal to proximal. A closing osteotomy is done posteriorly to obtain correction. The spine is instrumented from the midthoracic level to the sacrum. The reported advantages include less blood loss, decreased morbidity, no need for cordotomy, and continued growth because the endplates are not violated.

Smith reported good results in the management of congenital gibbus deformity in the growing child with myelomeningocele using bilateral rib-based distraction instrumentation to the pelvis. He recommended intervening early while the gibbus was still flexible and before skin breakdown over the deformity. This technique effectively improved the gibbus deformity and avoided early vertebral column resection and fusion.

VERTEBRAL EXCISION AND REDUCTION OF KYPHOSIS

TECHNIQUE 8.61

(LINDSETH AND SELZER)

- Use a midline posterior incision (Fig. 8.199A), which can be varied somewhat, depending on local skin conditions.
- Expose subperiosteally the more normal vertebrae superiorly and the area of the abnormality, continuing the exposure past the lateral bony ridges.
- At this point, remove the sac.
- Dissect inside the lamina until the foramina are exposed on each side of the spine.
- Expose, divide, and coagulate the nerve, artery, and vein within each foramen, exposing the sac distally where it is scarred down and thin.
- At its distal level, cross-clamp the sac with Kelly clamps and divide it between the clamps (Fig. 8.199B).
- Close the scarred ends with a running stitch. Dissect the sac proximally.
- As this proximal dissection is done, large venous channels connecting the sac to the posterior vertebral body will be encountered; control the bleeding from the bone with bone wax and from the soft tissue with electrocautery.
- Dissect the sac up to the level of the dura that appears more normal (Fig. 8.199C).
- The sac can be transected at this point. If this is done, close the dura with a purse-string suture. Do not suture the cord itself shut but leave it open so that the spinal fluid can escape from the central canal of the cord into the arachnoid space.
- If the sac is not removed, it can be used at the completion of the procedure to further cover the area of the resected vertebra.
- Once the sac has been reflected proximally, continue dissection around the vertebral bodies, exposing only the area to be removed. If the entire kyphotic area of the spine is exposed subperiosteally, osteonecrosis of these vertebral bodies may occur.
- Remove the vertebrae between the apex of the lordosis and the apex of the kyphosis (Fig. 8.199D). Remove the vertebra at the apex of the kyphosis first by removing the intervertebral disc with a Cobb elevator and curets. Take care to leave the anterior longitudinal ligament intact to act as a stabilizing hinge.
- Once this vertebra has been removed, temporarily correct the spine to determine how many cephalad vertebrae should be removed. Remove enough vertebrae to correct the kyphosis as much as possible but not so many that approximation is impossible (Fig. 8.199E).

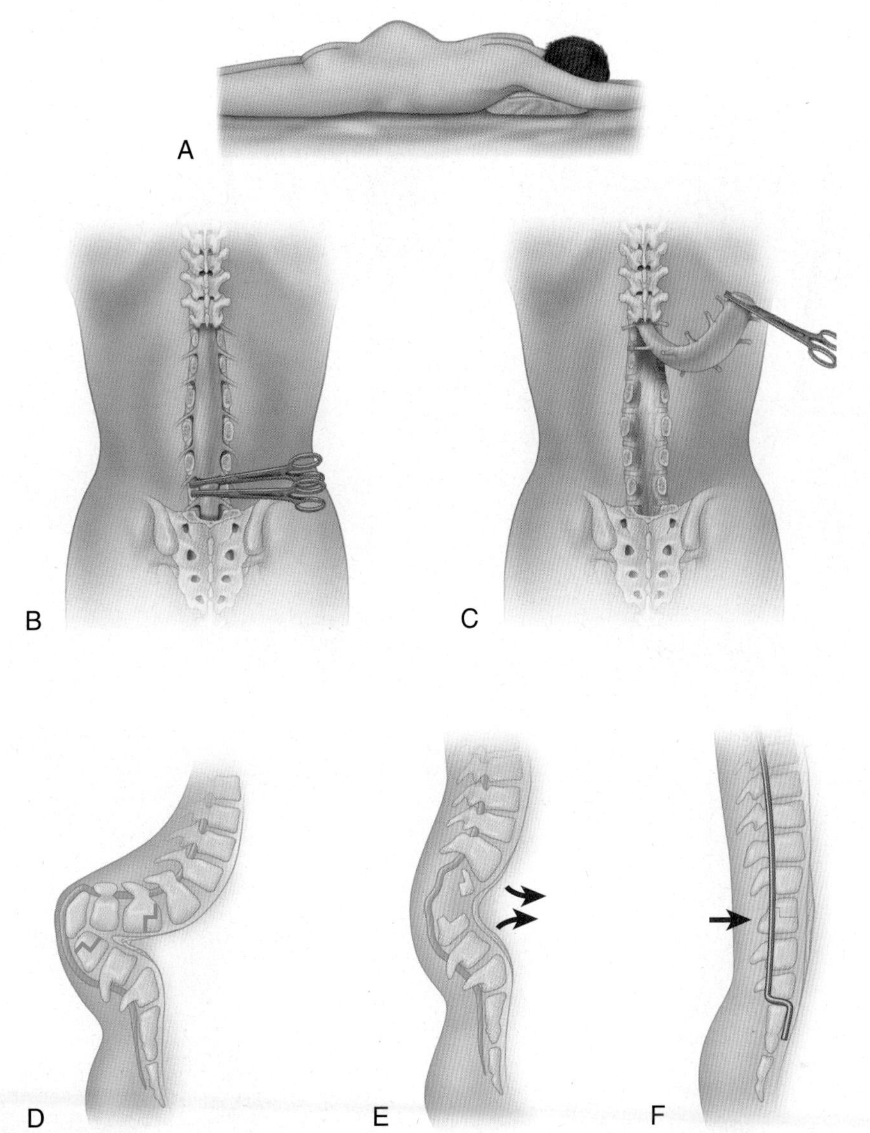

FIGURE 8.199 Technique of vertebral excision (Lindseth and Selzer). **A,** Patient positioning. **B,** Exposure of area of kyphosis and dural sac. **C,** Sac is divided distally and dissected proximally. **D,** Vertebrae between apex of lordosis and apex of kyphosis are removed. **E,** Kyphosis is reduced. **F,** Reduction is maintained with stable internal fixation (in this instance, with Luque rods and segmental wires). **SEE TECHNIQUE 8.61.**

- Morselization of these vertebral bodies provides additional bone graft.
- Many techniques have been described for fixation of the kyphotic deformity, but L-rod instrumentation to the pelvis with segmental wires is our preferred method (Fig. 8.199F). The distal end of the rod can be contoured. We prefer to use a prebent, right-angled rod and pass the bend through the S1 foramen rather than around the ala of the sacrum. This is the method of Warner and Fackler (Fig. 8.200).
- Move the distal segment to the proximal segment and tighten the segmental wires.

POSTOPERATIVE CARE If fixation is secure, the patient can be mobilized in a wheelchair as tolerated. Some patients in whom the bone is too osteoporotic and the stability of internal fixation is in doubt may be kept at bed rest or may require postoperative custom bracing. The fusion usually is solid in 6 to 9 months.

The postoperative care of these patients requires close observation by all subspecialty consultants involved. Postoperative infections, urinary tract problems, skin problems, and pseudarthrosis are frequent. The improved function, however, and the prevention of progression of the kyphosis make surgery worth the risks.

Paralytic kyphosis is treated with more standard techniques. When surgery becomes necessary, anterior fusion over the area of the apex and all levels of deficient posterior elements is done. This is followed by posterior fusion and instrumentation.

SACRAL AGENESIS

Sacral agenesis is a rare lesion that often is associated with maternal diabetes mellitus. Renshaw postulated that the condition is teratogenically induced or is a spontaneous genetic

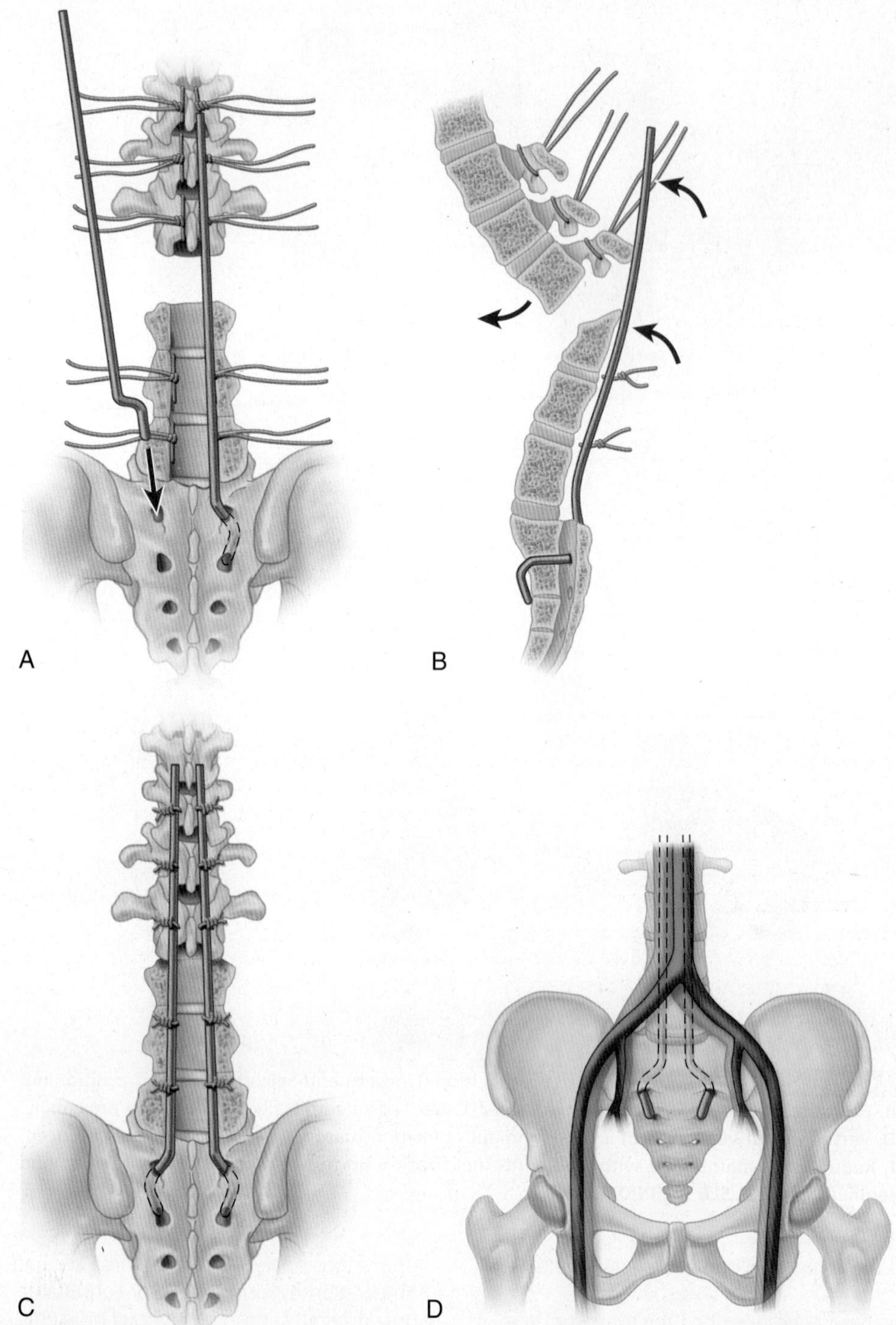

FIGURE 8.200 **A-D,** Anterior fixation of kyphotic deformity in patients with myelomeningocele. (From Warner WC Jr, Fackler CD: Comparison of two instrumentation techniques in treatment of lumbar kyphosis in myelodysplasia, *J Pediatr Orthop* 13:704, 1993.) **SEE TECHNIQUE 8.61.**

mutation that predisposes to or causes failure of embryonic induction of the caudal notochord sheath and ventral spinal cord. The dorsal ganglia and the dorsal (sensory) portion of the spinal cord continue to develop. The vertebrae and motor nerves are not subsequently induced, and the sacral agenesis results. Sensation remains relatively intact because the dorsal ganglia and the dorsal portion of the spinal cord have been derived from the neural crest tissue. This disturbance in the normal sequence of development explains the observation that the lowest vertebral body with pedicles corresponds closely to the motor level, whereas the sensory level is distal to the motor level.

Renshaw proposed the following classification: type I, either total or partial unilateral sacral agenesis (Fig. 8.201A); type II, partial sacral agenesis with partial but bilaterally symmetric defects and a stable articulation between the ilia and a normal or hypoplastic S1 vertebra (Fig. 8.201B); type III, variable lumbar and total sacral agenesis with the ilia articulating with the sides of the lowest vertebra present (Fig. 8.201C); and type IV, variable lumbar and total

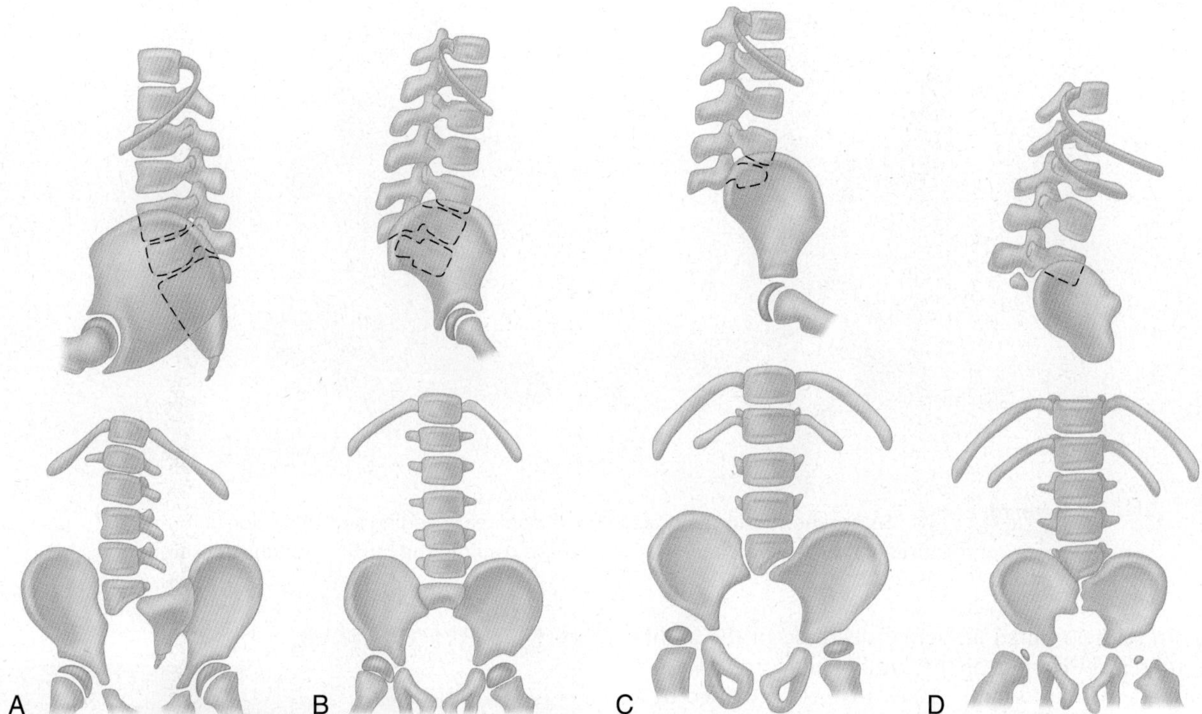

FIGURE 8.201 Types of sacral agenesis. **A,** Type I, total or partial unilateral sacral agenesis. **B,** Type II, partial sacral agenesis with partial, bilateral symmetric defects in stable articulation between ilia and normal or hypoplastic S1 vertebra. **C,** Type III, variable lumbar and total sacral agenesis; ilia articulate with lowest vertebra. **D,** Type IV, variable lumbar and total sacral agenesis; caudal endplate of lowest vertebra rests above fused ilia or iliac amphiarthrosis.

sacral agenesis with the caudal endplate of the lowest vertebra resting above either fused ilia or an iliac amphiarthrosis (Fig. 8.201D). Type II defects are most common, and type I are least common. Types I and II usually have a stable vertebral-pelvic articulation, whereas types III and IV produce instability and possibly a progressive kyphosis.

The clinical appearance of a child with sacral agenesis ranges from one of severe deformities of the pelvis and lower extremities to no deformity or weakness whatsoever. Those with partial sacral or coccygeal agenesis may have no symptoms. Those with lumbar or complete sacral agenesis may be severely deformed, with multiple musculoskeletal abnormalities, including foot deformities, knee flexion contractures with popliteal webbing, hip flexion contractures, dislocated hips, spinal-pelvic instability, and scoliosis. The posture of the lower extremities has been compared with a "sitting Buddha" (Fig. 8.202). Anomalies of the viscera, especially in the genitourinary system and the rectal area, are common. Inspection of the back reveals a bone prominence representing the last vertebral segment, often with gross motion between this vertebral prominence and the pelvis. Flexion and extension may occur at the junction of the spine and pelvis rather than at the hips.

Neurologic examination usually reveals intact motor power down to the level of the lowest vertebral body that has pedicles. Sensation, however, is present down to more caudal levels. Even patients with the most severe involvement may have sensation to the knees and spotty hypesthesia distally. Bladder and bowel control often is impaired.

TREATMENT

Phillips et al. reviewed the orthopaedic management of lumbosacral agenesis and concluded that patients with partial absence of the sacrum only (types I and II) have an excellent chance of becoming community ambulators. Management of more severe deformities (types III and IV) is more controversial.

Scoliosis is the most common spinal anomaly associated with sacral agenesis. No correlation has been found between the type of defect and the likelihood of scoliosis. Scoliosis may be associated with congenital anomalies, such as hemivertebra, or with no obvious spinal abnormality above the level of the vertebral agenesis. Progressive scoliosis or kyphosis requires operative stabilization as for similar scoliosis without sacral agenesis.

The treatment of spinal-pelvic instability is more controversial. Perry et al. noted that the key to rehabilitation of a patient with an unstable spinal-pelvic junction is establishment of a stable vertebral-pelvic complex around which lower extremity contractures can be stretched or operatively released. Renshaw also emphasized that patients with type III or type IV defects must be observed closely for signs of progressive kyphosis. If progressive deformity is noted, he recommended lumbopelvic arthrodesis as early as is consistent with successful fusion. In his series, fusion was done in patients 4 years of age or older. Ferland et al. reported successful spinopelvic fusion using vascularized rib grafts, with good outcomes in their patients. Phillips et al., however, found that spinal-pelvic instability was not a problem in 18 of the 20 surviving patients at long-term

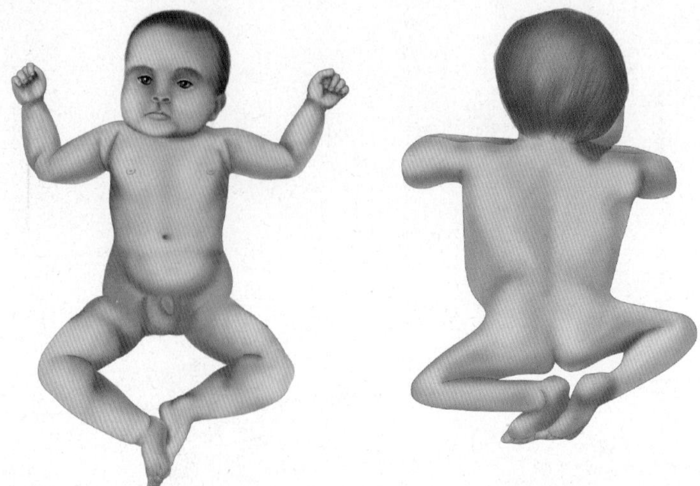

FIGURE 8.202 Severe knee flexion contractures with popliteal wedging and hip flexion deformities or contractures in children with lumbosacral agenesis result in the "sitting Buddha" position.

follow-up. Others noted an actual decrease in the ability to sit after stabilization of the lumbopelvic area. Proper care of patients with sacral agenesis is best provided by a treatment team, including an orthopaedic surgeon, urologist, neurosurgeon, pediatrician, physical therapist, and orthotist-prosthetist.

UNUSUAL CAUSES OF SCOLIOSIS

NEUROFIBROMATOSIS

Neurofibromatosis is a hereditary hamartomatous disorder of neural crest derivation. These hamartomatous tissues may appear in any organ system of the body. The most widely described clinical forms of neurofibromatosis are the peripheral (NF1) and central (NF2) types.

The classic neurofibromatosis (NF1) described by von Recklinghausen is an autosomal dominant disorder that affects approximately 1 in 4000 people. Patients with NF1 develop Schwann cell tumors and pigmentation abnormalities. Orthopaedic problems are frequent in patients with this type of neurofibromatosis, with spinal deformity being the most common.

Central neurofibromatosis (NF2) also is an autosomal dominant disorder; however, it is much less common. It is characterized by bilateral acoustic neuromas. NF2 usually does not have any bone involvement or orthopaedic manifestations.

The diagnosis of NF1 is based on clinical criteria (Box 8.13). Scoliosis is the most common osseous defect associated with neurofibromatosis. Studies have reported spinal disorders in 10% to 60% of patients with neurofibromatosis.

The spinal deformities of neurofibromatosis are of two basic forms: nondystrophic and dystrophic. Nondystrophic deformities mimic idiopathic scoliosis and behave accordingly; the neurofibromatosis seems to have little influence on the curve or its treatment. Scoliosis may also develop due to a leg-length discrepancy resulting from lower extremity hypertrophy or dysplasia of the long bones. Dystrophic scoliosis characteristically is a short-segment, sharply angulated curve with wedging of the vertebral bodies, rotation of the vertebrae, scalloping of the vertebral bodies, spindling of the transverse processes, foraminal enlargement, and rotation of the ribs 90 degrees in the anteroposterior direction that makes them appear abnormally thin. Rib penetration into the spinal canal has even been reported. Curves with significant sagittal plane deformity are common in dystrophic scoliosis. Dystrophic curves usually progress without treatment in patients with neurofibromatosis. Lykissas et al. found that the presence of three or more dystrophic features was highly predictive of curve progression and the need for operative stabilization (Fig. 8.203). Neurofibromatosis kyphoscoliosis is characterized by acute angulation in the sagittal plane and striking deformity of the vertebral bodies near the apex. Paraplegia has been reported in patients with this type of kyphoscoliosis. Severe thoracic lordoscoliosis also has been described in patients with neurofibromatosis.

BOX 8.13

Clinical Criteria for Diagnosis of Neurofibromatosis

For the diagnosis of neurofibromatosis to be made, two of the following features are necessary:

- A minimum of six café au lait spots larger than 1.5 cm in diameter in a postpubertal patient and larger than 5 mm in diameter in prepubertal patients
- Two or more neurofibromas of any type or one plexiform neurofibroma
- Freckling in the inguinal or axillary regions
- Optic glioma
- Two or more iris Lisch nodules by slit-lamp examination
- A distinctive osseous lesion
- A first-degree relative with a definitive diagnosis of neurofibromatosis

MANAGEMENT OF NONDYSTROPHIC CURVES

Nondystrophic curves have the same prognosis and evolution as do idiopathic curves, except for a higher risk of pseudarthrosis after operative fusion. Dystrophic vertebral body changes may develop over time in nondystrophic curves. A spinal deformity that develops before 7 years of age should

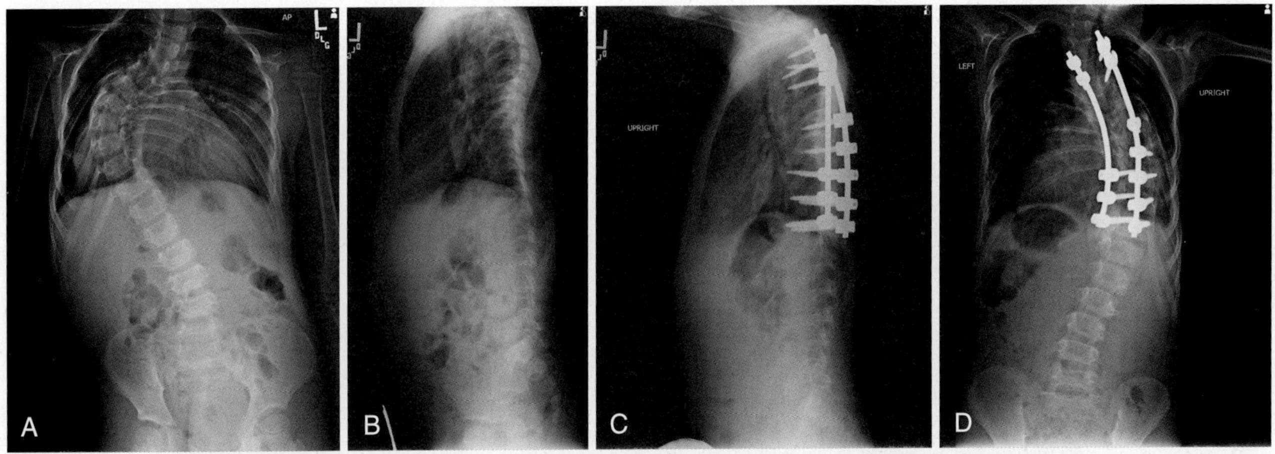

FIGURE 8.203 A and B, Dystrophic scoliosis. C and D, After posterior thoracic fusion and instrumentation.

be observed closely for potential evolving dystrophic features (modulation). If the curve then acquires either three penciled ribs or a combination of three dystrophic features, clinical progression is almost a certainty. The general guidelines for treating nondystrophic curves are the same as for idiopathic curves other than monitoring closely for any signs of modulation. Curves of less than 20 to 25 degrees are observed; if no dystrophic changes occur, a brace is prescribed when the deformity progresses to 30 degrees. If the deformity exceeds 40 to 45 degrees, a posterior spinal fusion with segmental instrumentation will produce results similar to those obtained in patients with idiopathic scoliosis. Also common in these patients are spinal canal neurofibromas, which may grow and cause pressure-induced dysplasia of the canal. MRI should be done before surgery to rule out the presence of any intraspinal canal neurofibroma.

MANAGEMENT OF DYSTROPHIC SCOLIOSIS

Brace treatment is probably not indicated for the typical dystrophic curve of neurofibromatosis. Appropriate operative treatment is determined by the presence or absence of a kyphotic deformity and by the presence or absence of neurologic deficits.

Before operative treatment of dystrophic curves in patients with neurofibromatosis, the presence of an intraspinal lesion, such as pseudomeningocele, dural ectasia, or intraspinal neurofibroma (dumbbell tumor), should be ruled out. Impingement of these lesions against the spinal cord has been reported to cause paraplegia after instrumentation of these curves. Routine neural axis MRI evaluation in patients with NF1 and spinal deformity should be performed, particularly if surgical intervention is planned.

SCOLIOSIS WITHOUT KYPHOSIS

Patients with dystrophic scoliosis without kyphosis should be observed at 6-month intervals if the curve is less than 20 degrees. As soon as the progression of the curve is noted, a posterior spinal fusion should be done. If this fusion is done before the curve becomes too large, anterior fusion may not be necessary. Traditionally, combined anterior and posterior fusion has been recommended unless there are contraindications to the anterior approach (e.g., patients with anterior neurofibromas, excessive venous channels, poor medical condition, or thrombocytopenia caused by splenic obstruction by a fibroma or peculiar anatomic configurations). However, more recent studies have suggested that posterior fusion alone can stabilize curves less than 90 degrees. Curves with kyphosis or with the apex below T8 should be considered for combined anterior and posterior fusion to decrease the rate of pseudarthrosis and curve progression. Segmental hook or screw instrumentation systems provide correction and permit ambulation with or without postoperative bracing. Sublaminar wires can be used to augment the instrumentation, particularly at the proximal end of the construction and across the apex of the curve. The fusion mass must be followed carefully. If there is any question as to the status of the fusion mass, the surgical area is explored 6 to 12 months after surgery and additional autogenous bone grafting is done. Similarly, if progression of more than 10 degrees occurs, the fusion mass is explored and reinforced. In younger patients, growing rods can be used to control the curve until definitive instrumentation and fusion can be done.

KYPHOSCOLIOSIS

Patients with dystrophic scoliosis and angular kyphosis have been shown to respond poorly to posterior fusion alone. Good results are obtained by combined anterior and posterior fusion. Reasons for fusion failure may include too little bone and too limited an area for fusion; therefore, the entire structural area of the deformity should be fused anteriorly. Ideally, all anterior grafts should be in contact throughout with other grafts or with the spine. Grafts surrounded by soft tissue tend to be resorbed in the midportion. Early diagnosis and treatment by combined anterior and posterior fusion with internal fixation, if possible, is recommended. If anterior fusion is necessary for kyphoscoliotic deformities, vascularized rib graft augmentation as described by Bradford (Fig. 8.204) may be considered.

However, some authors have questioned the necessity of an anterior approach in all dystrophic kyphoscoliotic curves. For smaller dystrophic scoliosis with kyphosis of less than 40 degrees, posterior spinal instrumentation with arthrodesis is considered as soon as possible. The fusion mass should be explored at 6 to 12 months after surgery or sooner if progression of more than 10 degrees occurs.

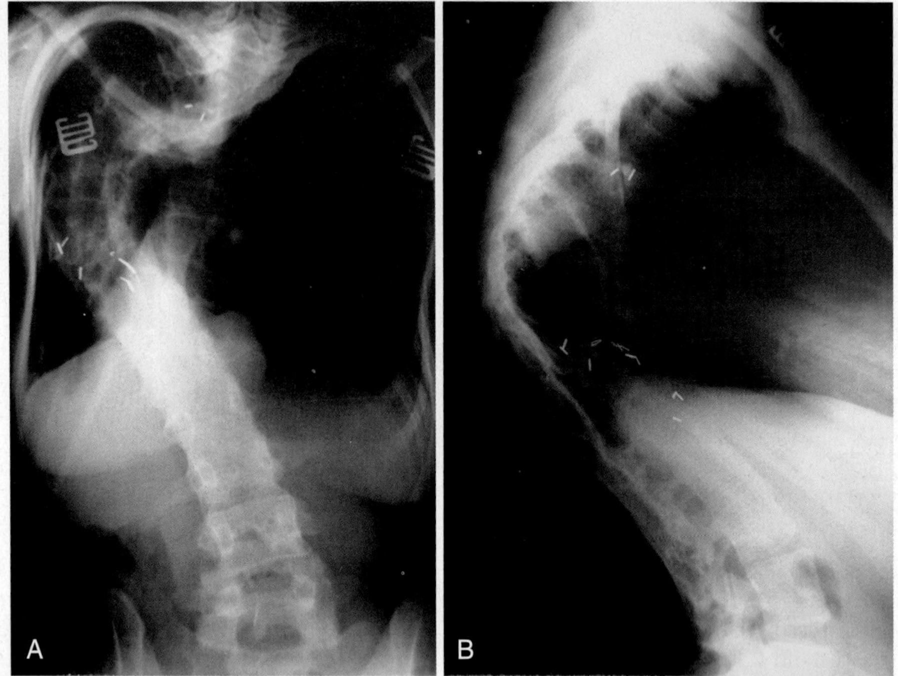

FIGURE 8.204 A and B, After anterior fusion with vascularized rib graft in patient with dystrophic kyphoscoliosis.

KYPHOSCOLIOSIS WITH SPINAL CORD COMPRESSION

Spinal cord or cauda equina compression caused by spinal angulation, rib penetration, or tumor has been described. Cord compression caused by an intraspinal lesion must be distinguished from kyphotic angular cord compression by MRI. Patients with severe scoliosis without significant kyphosis and with evidence of paraplegia should be assumed to have an intraspinal lesion until proved otherwise. If cord compression is caused by kyphoscoliotic deformity, laminectomy is contraindicated. Removal of the posterior elements adds to the kyphosis and also removes valuable bone surface for a posterior fusion. If spinal cord compression is minor and no intraspinal tumor is present, halo-gravity traction can be used. The patient's neurologic status must be monitored carefully even if the kyphosis is mobile. As the alignment of the spinal canal improves and the compression is eliminated, anterior and posterior fusions can be done without direct observation of the cord. However, significant cord compression in patients with severe structural kyphoscoliosis requires anterior cord decompression. If a tumor causes spinal cord compression anteriorly, anterior excision, spinal cord decompression, and fusion are indicated. If the lesion is posterior, a hemilaminectomy with tumor excision may be necessary. Instrumentation and fusion should be done at the time of decompression to prevent a rapidly increasing kyphotic deformity and neurologic injury.

POSTOPERATIVE MANAGEMENT

Patients with nondystrophic curves are managed the same as those with idiopathic curves. If, however, the instrumentation is tenuous, casting or bracing is used. However, patients with dystrophic scoliosis should be considered for immobilization in a cast or brace until fusion is evident on anteroposterior, lateral, and oblique radiographs. Exploration of the fusion mass at 6 to 12 months after surgery may be necessary in dystrophic curves, and prolonged immobilization often is needed. Even after the fusion is solid, the patient should be observed annually to be certain that no erosion of the fusion mass is occurring.

COMPLICATIONS OF SURGERY

In addition to the complications inherent in any major spinal surgery, several complications are related to the neurofibromatosis. Plexiform venous anomalies can be present in the soft tissues surrounding the spine and can impede the operative approach to the vertebral bodies, leading to excessive bleeding. The increased vascularity of the neurofibromatous tissue itself also may increase blood loss. The apical bodies may have subluxed into bayonet apposition or be so rotated that they no longer are in alignment with the rest of the spine. Anterior strut grafts are no longer commonly used. Pheochromocytoma, a tumor arising from chromaffin cells, can be associated with neurofibromatosis and can create an anesthetic challenge. Patients with neurofibromatosis have a general tendency for decreased bone mineral density and osteopenia, possibly increasing the challenge of obtaining stable implant fixation to the spine.

Many patients with neurofibromatosis and scoliosis have cervical spine abnormalities (Fig. 8.205). Deformities of the cervical spine that cause cord compression and paraplegia have been reported in patients with neurofibromatosis. Cervical lesions associated with scoliosis or kyphoscoliosis have been classified into two groups: abnormalities of bone structure and abnormalities of vertebral alignment. Cervical anomalies are most common in patients with short kyphotic curves or thoracic or lumbar curves that measure more than 65 degrees. These patients are more likely to require anesthesia,

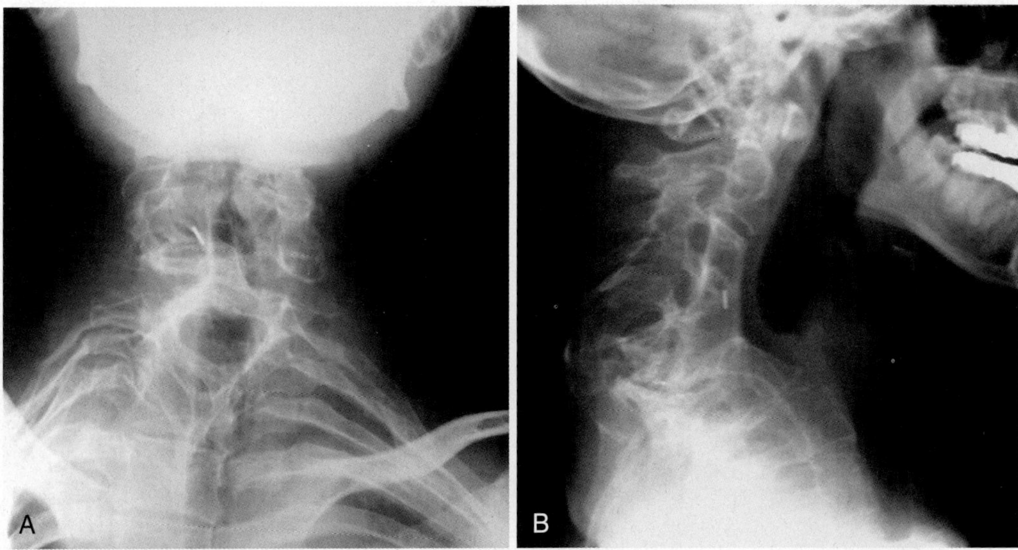

FIGURE 8.205 **A** and **B**, Cervical spine deformity in patient with neurofibromatosis.

traction, and operative stabilization of the spine. Routine radiographic evaluation of the cervical spine is recommended in all patients with neurofibromatosis before anesthesia for any reason and before traction for treatment of the scoliosis. High-grade spondylolisthesis of the lower lumbar spine also has been reported in association with neurofibromatosis. The entire spinal column must be carefully assessed for cervical and lumbosacral abnormalities.

Postoperative paralysis caused by contusion of the spinal cord by the periosteal elevator during exposure has been reported in two patients with unsuspected areas of laminar erosion because of dural ectasia. A total-spine MRI study can alert the surgeon to this before surgery. The most dangerous situation for neurologically intact patients with neurofibromatosis is instrumentation and distraction of the spine in the presence of unrecognized intraspinal lesions.

MARFAN SYNDROME

Marfan syndrome is a disorder of connective tissue inherited as an autosomal dominant trait. It occurs in 1 to 2 per 10,000 persons and affects males and females equally. Sporadic occurrences reportedly account for 25% of patients. In most cases, a mutation in the fibrillin-1 *(FBN1)* gene has been implicated, resulting in abnormalities in a protein essential to proper formatting of elastic fibers found in connective tissue.

DIAGNOSIS

In addition to genetic testing, the diagnosis of Marfan syndrome relies on physical findings, which have traditionally been divided into two categories: major and minor signs. Major signs include ectopia lentis, aortic dilation, severe kyphoscoliosis, and pectus deformity. Minor signs include myopia, tall stature, mitral valve prolapse, ligamentous laxity, and arachnodactyly. Newer diagnostic criteria place greater weight on cardiovascular manifestations; therefore, in the absence of a family history, the presence of both aortic root aneurysm and ectopia lentis is sufficient for the unequivocal diagnosis of Marfan syndrome. Screening tests for the Marfan phenotype in the orthopaedic examination include the thumb sign (the thumb extends well beyond the ulnar border of the hand when it is overlapped by the fingers) and the wrist sign (the thumb overlaps the fifth finger as the patient grasps the opposite wrist). The diagnosis of Marfan syndrome frequently is delayed because cardiovascular involvement is a major diagnostic criterion and may not be evident until adolescence or adulthood. Scoliosis is reported to occur in 40% to 60% of patients with Marfan syndrome. These curves develop in patients with multiple major signs (definite diagnosis of Marfan), as well as those with only minor signs (Marfan phenotype). Marfan curves of less than 40 degrees in adults tend not to progress, whereas curves of more than 40 degrees progress (an average of 2.8 degrees a year in a study by Sponseller et al.); the curve patterns of scoliosis in Marfan syndrome are similar to those in idiopathic scoliosis. Double major curves are more frequent, and the scoliosis progresses more frequently in younger patients. Disabling back pain is more frequently a presenting complaint in patients with scoliosis associated with Marfan syndrome than in patients with idiopathic scoliosis. Sagittal plane deformities are common (Fig. 8.206). A thoracolumbar kyphosis can be found in patients with Marfan syndrome (Fig. 8.207). Characteristic vertebral anomalies also are found in these patients, including narrow pedicles, wide transverse processes, and vertebral scalloping. Spondylolisthesis associated with Marfan syndrome also has been reported in one study. Cervical spine abnormalities also are common in patients with Marfan syndrome, but clinical problems from these abnormalities are rare. Basilar impression and focal cervical kyphosis are the most commonly reported cervical spine abnormalities. The focal cervical kyphosis usually is associated with a lordotic thoracic spine.

NONOPERATIVE TREATMENT

OBSERVATION

For young patients with small curves of less than 25 degrees, observation every 3 to 4 months is indicated. The family should be made aware, however, that many of these curves progress.

ORTHOTIC TREATMENT

Brace treatment is less successful in patients with Marfan syndrome than in those with idiopathic scoliosis. Sponseller et al.

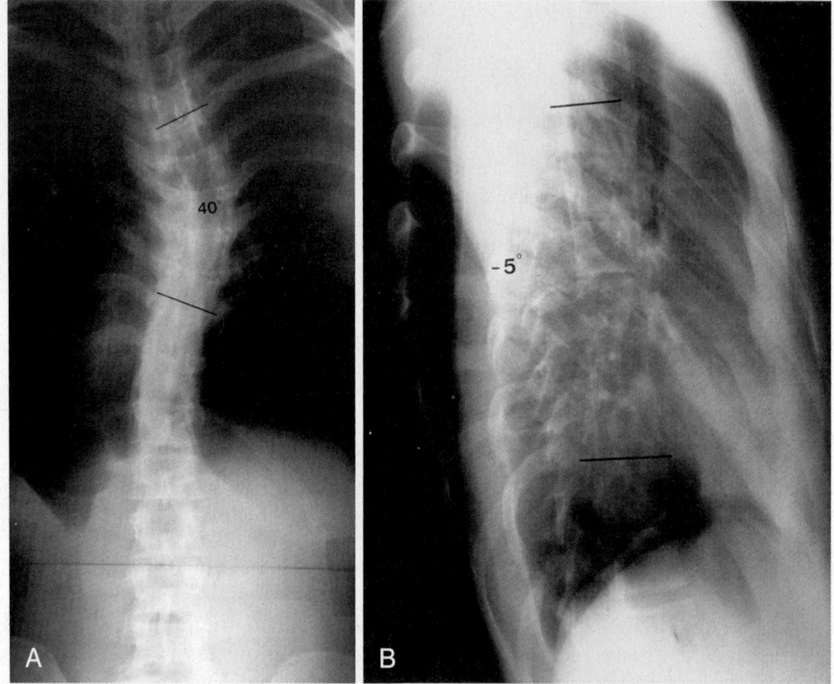

FIGURE 8.206 **A and B,** Thoracic lordosis in patient with Marfan syndrome.

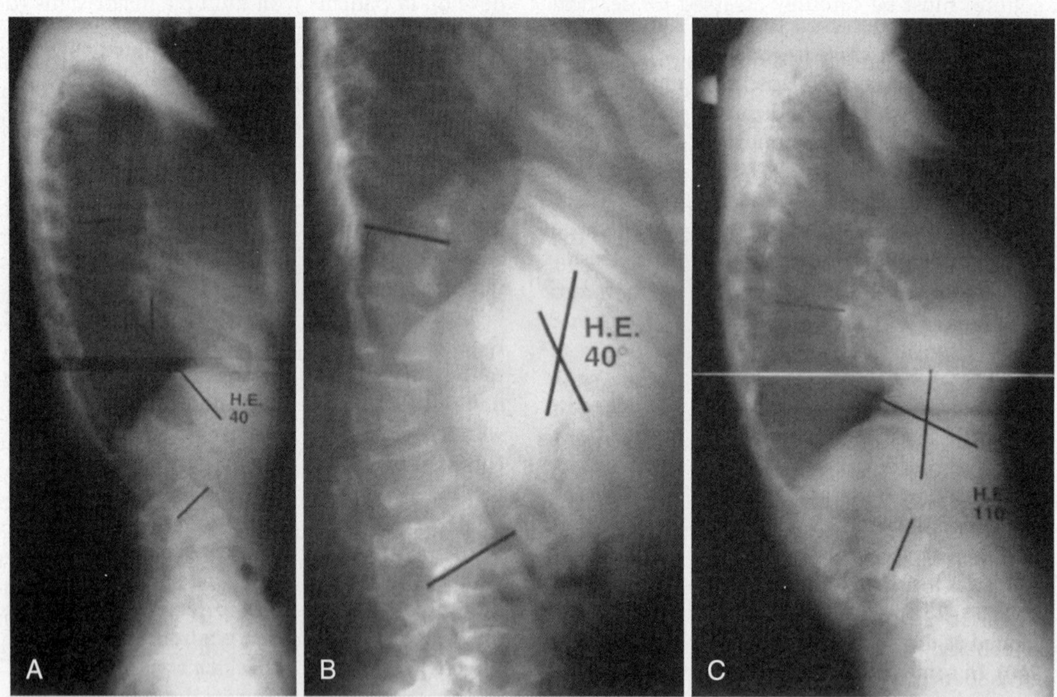

FIGURE 8.207 **A and B,** Lateral radiographs of 17-year-old child with Marfan syndrome and 40-degree progressive thoracolumbar kyphosis. **C,** Lateral radiograph of same patient 3 years later shows that thoracolumbar kyphosis has progressed to 110 degrees. (From Warner WC: Kyphosis. In Morrissy RT, Weinstein SL, editors: *Lovell and Winter's pediatric orthopaedics*, ed 6, Philadelphia, 2006, Lippincott Williams & Wilkins.)

reported successful brace treatment in 4 of 22 patients. Chest wall deformity, with narrowing of the inferior portion of the thoracic cage, also has been noted with the use of an underarm TLSO. Bracing should be considered for patients with flexible progressive curves between 25 and 40 degrees who do not have associated thoracic lordosis or lumbar kyphosis. Bracing is not indicated for large, rigid curves or curves associated with thoracic lordosis.

OPERATIVE TREATMENT

If progression occurs despite bracing or if the curve exceeds 40 degrees, spinal fusion is recommended. If nonoperative treatment is continued too long, cardiovascular involvement may progress to the point of making surgery dangerous, if not impossible. Before operative intervention is considered, a complete cardiovascular evaluation is mandatory. Aortic dilation can develop in these patients at any time from childhood to late adolescence or adulthood. Echocardiography is recommended to evaluate for aortic root dilation. Any evidence of aortic dilation should be treated medically or operatively before treatment of the spinal deformity.

Scoliosis in patients with Marfan syndrome can be corrected similar to the way it is corrected in idiopathic scoliosis, and solid fusion and maintenance of correction can be anticipated; however, Jones et al. and Gjolaj et al. found that the number of surgical complications was higher in patients with Marfan syndrome. Complications included increased blood loss, pseudarthroses (10%), dural tears (8%), infection (10%), and failure of fixation (21%). The development of scoliosis or kyphosis at the upper or lower fusion levels (adding on) can occur after surgery. Jones et al. found this complication to occur in the coronal plane in 8% of their patients and in the sagittal plane in 21%.

Large bone grafts, secure segmental internal fixation, and careful postoperative observation for pseudarthrosis are required in these patients. In general, the technique of instrumentation and selection of hook or screw levels are the same as for idiopathic scoliosis, but selection of the lowest instrumented vertebrae is ideally the neutral and stable vertebra in both the coronal and sagittal planes. Jones et al. recommended that any curve of more than 30 degrees should be included in the arthrodesis. As with all scoliotic deformity correction, care must be taken in determining the distal extent of the fusion to avoid junctional kyphosis.

Thoracic lordosis is relatively common in patients with Marfan syndrome and spinal deformity, and sagittal plane balance must be obtained in addition to improvement of the coronal plane deformity. Segmental instrumentation systems using hooks and pedicle screws or all pedicle screws are effective in correcting this problem. Surgical treatment should provide a more normal anteroposterior diameter of the chest, because this frequently is narrow.

Growing rod constructs have been used with success for patients with Marfan syndrome with early-onset scoliosis for which definitive spinal fusion is not possible because of skeletal immaturity. Dual rod constructs are recommended. Because these children will require multiple lengthening procedures, careful monitoring of the cardiovascular manifestations of Marfan syndrome is essential.

Severe spondylolisthesis associated with Marfan syndrome has been reported. It has been postulated that the spondylolisthesis may be more likely to progress because of poor musculoligamentous tissues.

VERTEBRAL COLUMN TUMORS

Because of their variable presentation, tumors of the vertebral column often present diagnostic problems. A team composed of a surgeon, a diagnostic radiologist, a pathologist, and often a medical oncologist and radiotherapist is necessary for treatment of the spectrum of tumors that involve the spine. The discussion in this section is on the most common primary tumors of the vertebral column in children.

CLINICAL FINDINGS

A complete history is the first step in the evaluation of any patient with a tumor. The initial complaint of patients with tumors involving the spine generally is pain. The exact type and distribution of pain vary with the anatomic location of the pathologic process. In general, pain caused by a neoplasm is not relieved by rest and often is worse at night. On occasion, constitutional symptoms such as anorexia, weight loss, and fever may be present. The age and sex of the patient may be important in the differential diagnosis.

Physical examination should include a general evaluation in addition to careful examination of the spine. The tumor may produce local tenderness, muscle spasm, scoliosis, and limited spine motion. Painful scoliosis can be the result of a spinal tumor. In such cases, the tumor is usually located at the concavity of the curve. Spine deformity also may be secondary to vertebral collapse or muscular spasms caused by pain. More than 50% of patients with malignant tumors of the spine present with neurologic symptoms. A careful neurologic examination is essential.

Laboratory studies should include a complete blood cell count, urinalysis, and sedimentation rate, as well as determination of serum calcium, phosphorus, and alkaline phosphatase concentrations. Alkaline phosphatase may be elevated two to three times normal in patients with osteosarcoma. Lactate dehydrogenase is a reliable indicator of the tumor burden in patients with Ewing sarcoma. An elevated white blood cell count with thrombocytopenia is characteristic of leukemia. Further laboratory studies may be indicated based on the clinical course.

RADIOGRAPHIC EVALUATION AND TREATMENT

Radiographs of the spine should be made in at least two planes at 90-degree angles. The radiographs should be evaluated for the presence of scoliosis, kyphosis, loss of lumbar lordosis, destruction of pedicles, congenital vertebral anomalies, lytic lesions, altered size of neural foramina, abnormal calcifications, and soft-tissue masses. If a scoliotic curve is present, the curve usually shows significant coronal decompensation. There is an absence of the usual compensatory balancing curve above or below the curve containing the lesion. The scoliosis lacks the usual structural characteristics associated with idiopathic scoliosis, such as vertebral rotation and wedging. Curves with these characteristics should raise the index of suspicion for an underlying cause of the scoliosis.

Bone scanning is helpful in certain tumors of the spine, especially osteoid osteoma. CT has greatly improved evaluation of the extent of the lesion and the presence of any spinal canal compromise; sagittal and coronal reformatted images are necessary to define the exact anatomic location and extent of the lesion. MRI is useful in evaluating the extent of soft-tissue involvement of the tumor and for determining the level

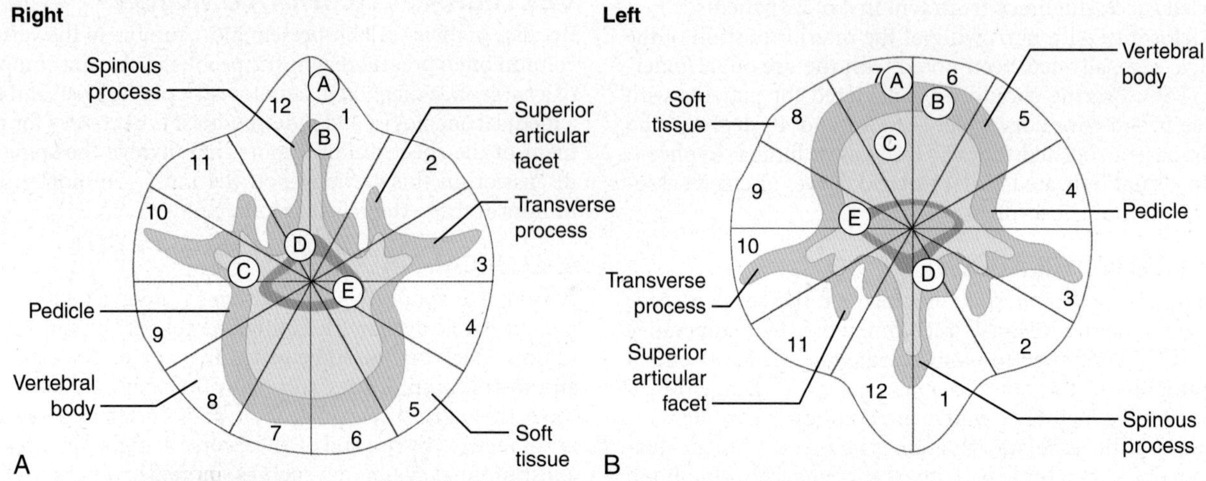

FIGURE 8.208 **A,** Weinstein-Boriani-Biagini tumor classification system. Vertebra is divided into 12 radiating zones that are numbered clockwise, beginning at one half of spinous process. Concentric layers are lettered sequentially from extraosseous soft tissues to intradural space. **B,** The Spine Oncology Study Group modified classification by numbering radial zones in counterclockwise fashion, beginning at left half of spinous process to allow for more anatomic orientation of diagram for ease of use. Circled letters: *A,* extraosseous soft tissues; *B,* intraosseous (superficial); *C,* intraosseous (deep); *D,* extraosseous (extradural); *E,* extraosseous (intradural). (**A** redrawn from Boriani S, Weinstein JN, Biagini R: Primary bone tumors of the spine: terminology and surgical staging, *Spine* 22:1036, 1997. **B** redrawn from Chan P, Boriani S, Fourney DR, et al: An assessment of the reliability of the Enneking and Weinstein-Boriani-Biagini classifications for staging of primary spinal tumors by the Spine Oncology Study Group, *Spine* 34:384, 2009.)

and extent of neurologic compromise in patients with a neurologic deficit.

Arteriography may be indicated to evaluate the extent of the tumor and to localize major feeder vessels.

Surgical staging classification systems specific to spine tumors have been designed to guide treatment and aid in defining the prognosis. The surgical staging systems proposed by Boriani et al. and Tomita et al. were devised to aid in surgical planning and are used to delineate the margins of the tumor. The Weinstein-Boriani-Biagini (WBB) classification is an alphanumeric system that can be used to evaluate the extent of a lesion in the axial plane by dividing the vertebrae into 12 radial zones and five concentric layers with a designation for the presence of metastasis (Fig. 8.208). The Spine Oncology Study Group modified this system by orienting the diagram to correspond to the orientation of the vertebrae on axial tomograms. The tumor is reported according to the spinal level or levels affected in the cephalocaudal dimension. The method of surgical excision is based on the zone or zones that the tumor occupies. Tomita et al. classified tumors based on their anatomic location in the axial and sagittal planes using a numeric system that reflects the most common progression of tumor growth (Figs. 8.209 and 8.210); this classification is used to guide surgical management.

BIOPSY

Certain tumors, such as osteochondroma and osteoid osteoma, generally can be diagnosed by their clinical presentation and radiographic appearance. Other benign tumors, such as osteoblastoma, aneurysmal bone cyst, and giant cell tumors, often are difficult to diagnose preoperatively. Biopsy is the ultimate diagnostic technique for evaluating neoplasms. The biopsy may be incisional (removal of a small portion of the tumor) or excisional (removal of the entire tumor).

Percutaneous CT-guided needle biopsy is an excellent diagnostic tool. Ghelman et al. obtained histologic diagnoses in 85% of 76 biopsy specimens, and Kattapuram, Khurana, and Rosenthal obtained accurate diagnoses in 92%. Metastatic diseases were most often diagnosed accurately (95%), and benign primary tumors were diagnosed least often (82%). Fine-needle cytologic aspirates are satisfactory for diagnosis of metastatic disease and most infections, but large-core biopsy specimens are preferable for primary bone tumors.

OPEN BIOPSY OF THORACIC VERTEBRA

If the needle biopsy is not diagnostic, an open biopsy or transpedicular biopsy will yield more tissue. Care must be taken that the open biopsy does not interfere with the definitive surgery if total resection is anticipated.

TECHNIQUE 8.62

(MICHELE AND KRUEGER)

- With the patient prone, make an incision over the side of the spinous process of the involved vertebra.
- Retract the muscles and expose the transverse process.
- Perform an osteotomy at the base of the transverse process at its junction with the lamina (Fig. 8.211A).

- By depressing or retracting the transverse process, expose the isthmus of the vertebra, revealing the cancellous nature of its bone structure. Radiographic verification of the level is important.
- Insert a 3/16-inch trephine with ¼-inch markings through the fenestra and guide it downward with slight pressure so that a mere twisting action leads the trephine into the pedicle and finally into the body (Fig. 8.211B). Remove the trephine repeatedly and in each instance check that the contents consist of cancellous bone, which indicates that the trephine is in the medullary substance of the pedicle and has created a channel from the posterior elements directly into the vertebral body.
- Remove the pathologic tissue with a small blunt curet.
- Alternatively, after the osteotomy of the base of the transverse process, expose the vertebral body by retracting the transverse process and depressing the adjacent rib to expose the junction of the pedicle and the body.
- Use the trephine to penetrate this junction at an angle of 45 degrees toward the midline and remove the material with a curet (Fig. 8.211C).

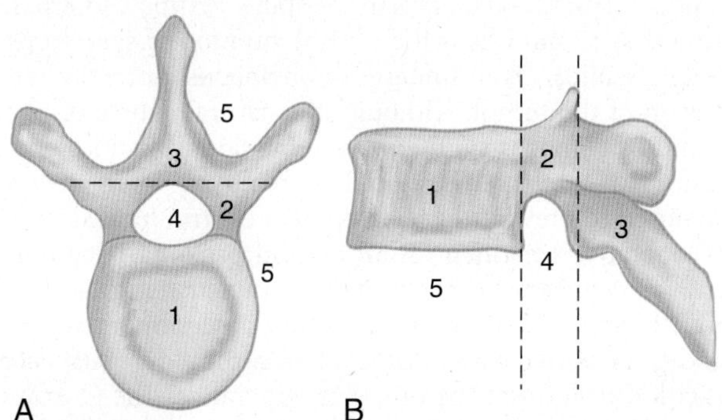

FIGURE 8.209 Axial **(A)** and lateral **(B)** illustrations of Tomita anatomic classification of primary spinal malignant tumors. Lesions are classified by their location on vertebra using numeric scheme that reflects most common progression of tumor growth: 1, vertebral body; 2, pedicle; 3, lamina and transverse and spinous processes; 4, spinal canal and epidural space; and 5, paravertebral space. (Redrawn from Tomita K, Kewahara N, Baba H, et al: Total en bloc spondylectomy: a new surgical technique for primary malignant vertebral tumors, *Spine* 22:324, 1997.)

BENIGN TUMORS OF THE VERTEBRAL COLUMN

The most common benign tumors of the vertebral column in children are osteoid osteoma, osteoblastoma, aneurysmal bone cyst, eosinophilic granuloma, and hemangioma.

OSTEOID OSTEOMA

Osteoid osteoma is a benign growth that consists of a discrete osteoid nidus and reactive sclerotic bone thickening around the nidus. No malignant change of these tumors has ever been documented. The lesion occurs more frequently in males than in females. Spinal lesions occur predominantly in the posterior elements of the spine, especially the lamina and the pedicles. Osteoid osteoma of the vertebral body has been reported but is rare. The lumbar spine is the most frequently involved area.

Typically, patients with spinal osteoid osteoma have pain that is worse at night and relieved by aspirin. The pain increases with activity and often is localized to the site of the lesion. Radicular symptoms are especially common with lesions of the lumbar spine. Lesions in the cervical spine can produce radicular-type symptoms in the shoulders and arms, but the results of the neurologic examination usually are normal.

Physical examination reveals muscle spasm in the involved area of the spine. The patient's gait may be abnormal

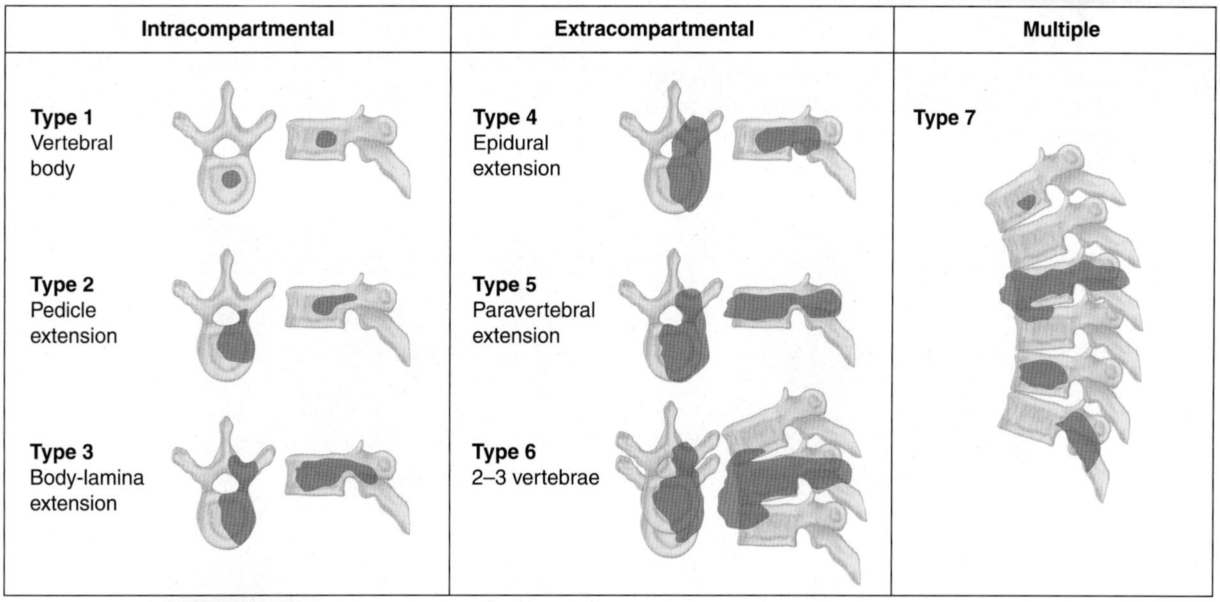

Intracompartmental	Extracompartmental	Multiple
Type 1 Vertebral body	**Type 4** Epidural extension	**Type 7**
Type 2 Pedicle extension	**Type 5** Paravertebral extension	
Type 3 Body-lamina extension	**Type 6** 2–3 vertebrae	

FIGURE 8.210 Tomita surgical classification of spinal tumors. Tumor types are categorized based on the number of vertebral areas affected. (Redrawn from Tomita K, Kewahara N, Baba H, et al: Total en bloc spondylectomy: a new surgical technique for primary malignant vertebral tumors, *Spine* 22:324, 1997.)

because of pain, and localized tenderness over the tumor may be moderate to severe.

Osteoid osteoma is the most common cause of painful scoliosis in adolescents. The scoliosis associated with osteoid osteoma usually is described as a C-shaped curve, but only 23% to 33% of patients have this classic curve pattern. The osteoid osteoma usually is located on the concave side of the curve and in the area of the apical vertebra.

When the osteoid osteoma is visible on plain radiographs, its appearance is diagnostic—a central radiolucency with a surrounding sclerotic bony reaction; however, the lesion often is not visible on plain films. Technetium bone scanning should be considered in any adolescent with painful scoliosis (Fig. 8.212A). False-negative bone scans have not been reported in patients with osteoid osteoma of the spine. MRI scans will show increased signal changes. CT with very narrow cuts will precisely define the location of the tumor and the extent of the osseous involvement (Fig. 8.212B).

Patients with spinal tumors and scoliosis reach a critical point after which the continuation of a painful stimulus results in structural changes in the spine. Pettine and Klassen found that 15 months is the critical duration of symptoms if antalgic scoliosis is to undergo spontaneous correction after excision of the tumor. Although the natural course of many osteoid osteomas is spontaneous remission, spinal lesions in children or adolescents should be removed when they are diagnosed to prevent the development of structural scoliosis. The operative treatment of an osteoid osteoma is complete removal; recurrence is likely after incomplete removal. If pain and deformity persist after removal of the lesion, incomplete removal or perhaps a multifocal lesion should be suspected. Exact localization of the tumor is imperative. The O-arm or intraoperative navigation will allow intraoperative localization of the lesion.

Excision of these lesions usually does not require spinal fusion, but if removal of a significant portion of the facet joints and pedicles makes the spine unstable, spinal fusion can be done at the time of tumor removal. Surgical navigation systems such as the O-arm can be used intraoperatively to evaluate the adequacy of resection. This is the preferred method if it is available in the treating institution. Radiofrequency ablation of osteoid osteoma of the spine is not recommended.

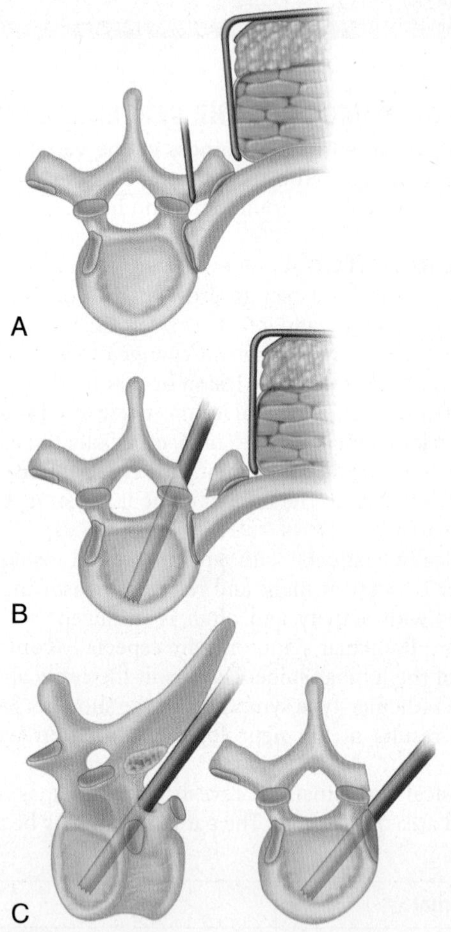

FIGURE 8.211 **A,** Transverse osteotomy at base of thoracic transverse process. **B,** Trephine through fenestra of isthmus, into pedicle and body. **C,** Trephine inserted into body at junction of pedicle. **SEE TECHNIQUE 8.62.**

OSTEOBLASTOMA

Most authors believe that osteoid osteoma and osteoblastoma are variant manifestations of a benign osteoblastic process, resulting in an osteoid nidus surrounded by sclerotic bone. The lesions are histologically similar. The primary difference is the tendency of the osteoblastoma to form a less sclerotic

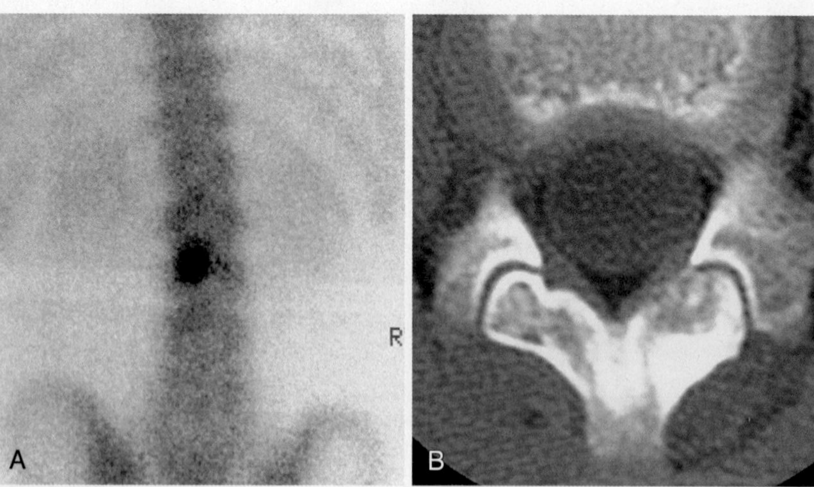

FIGURE 8.212 Bone scan **(A)** and CT scan **(B)** of patient with spinal osteoid osteoma.

but more expansile mass. Lesions larger than 1.5 cm in diameter are defined as osteoblastomas and those less than 1.5 cm as osteoid osteomas.

Benign osteoblastoma is an uncommon primary bone tumor that accounts for less than 1% of all bone tumors. Of these reported tumors, however, 40% have been located in the spine and more than one half were associated with scoliosis. The presenting symptom for most patients is pain; however, often the nonspecificity of symptoms may contribute to a delay in diagnosis. In one study, pain was present for an average of 16 months before the diagnosis was made, and scoliosis was present in 50% of patients with osteoblastomas involving the thoracic or lumbar spine. The osteoblastomas were always located in the concavity of the curve, near its apex.

In contrast to osteoid osteoma, plain radiographs often are sufficient to confirm the diagnosis of osteoblastoma. CT scans, MRI, and bone scans (Fig. 8.213), however, can be helpful for a cross-sectional evaluation and localization of the tumor before operative excision. Osteoblastoma of the spine involves predominantly the posterior elements (66%) or the posterior elements and vertebral bodies (31%). A neoplasm involving only a vertebral body is unlikely to be an osteoblastoma. Spinal osteoblastomas are typically expansile with a scalloped or lobulated contour, well-defined margins, and frequently a sclerotic rim.

The treatment of osteoblastoma of the spine is complete operative excision. Recurrences after incomplete curettage are not rare, and malignant change has been reported after incomplete curettage; complete excision is therefore advised whenever possible. Because of the possibility of late sarcomatous changes, irradiation of this lesion is not recommended. The scoliosis associated with vertebral column osteoblastoma usually is reversible after excision if the diagnosis is made early and treatment is undertaken at that time.

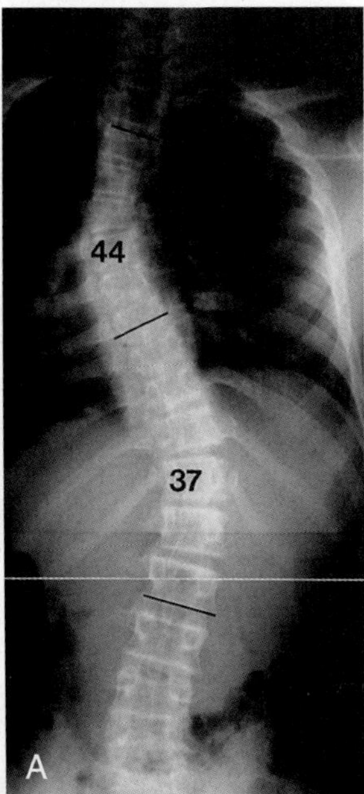

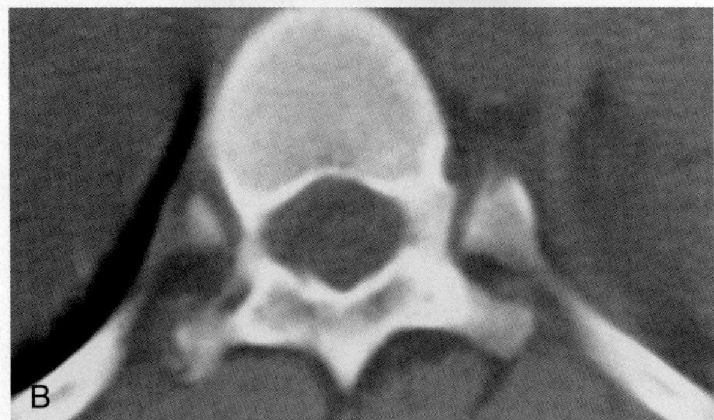

FIGURE 8.213 Radiograph **(A)** and CT scan **(B)** of patient with osteoblastoma on right side of spine that caused left thoracic curve.

ANEURYSMAL BONE CYSTS

An aneurysmal bone cyst is a nonneoplastic, vasocystic tumor originating on either a previously normal bone or a preexisting lesion. It is most common in children and young adults, and vertebral involvement is common. Its radiographic appearance is characteristic—an expansile lesion confined by a thin rim of reactive bone. The lesion can occur in the vertebral body but is more commonly seen in the posterior elements of the spine. An aneurysmal bone cyst is the only benign tumor that can cross the disc and involve more than one spinal level. Pain is the most common symptom, and radicular symptoms may be caused by cord compression.

Treatment is operative excision whenever possible. The tumors can be quite vascular, and if operative resection is contemplated, preoperative embolization should be considered. Embolization should be done in addition to the operative excision, and vessels supplying important segments of the spinal cord or brain should not be embolized. The indications for embolization are benign vascular tumors in central locations. In one study, three of the four tumors that were embolized were aneurysmal bone cysts. Contraindications include avascular tumors and tumors supplied by vessels that also supply important segments of the spinal cord because embolization of these vessels may infarct the spinal cord. Good clinical results have been reported after arterial embolization; however, the major disadvantage is the need for repeated procedures and repeated CT scans and angiography. Radiation therapy should be used only in those lesions that cannot be operatively excised.

Many patients with aneurysmal bone cysts of the vertebral column have neurologic symptoms (30%), including complete or incomplete paraplegia or root signs or symptoms. When these neurologic symptoms occur, complete excision of the aneurysmal bone cyst with decompression of the spinal canal is indicated. The approach, whether anterior, posterior, or combined anterior and posterior, is dictated by the location of the lesion.

EOSINOPHILIC GRANULOMA

Eosinophilic granuloma in childhood usually is a solitary lesion. The cause of this lesion, which may not represent a true neoplasm, is unknown. Approximately 10% involve the spine. Eosinophilic granuloma may produce varying degrees of vertebral collapse, including the classic picture of a vertebra plana (Fig. 8.214). Considerable collapse of the vertebral body may occur without neurologic compromise, and significant reconstitution in height may occur after treatment (Fig. 8.215). Bone scan may show increased uptake. A lytic radiographic image without vertebra plana with normal bone scan uptake probably is a benign lesion, but biopsy must still be done. The differential diagnoses include aneurysmal bone cyst, acute leukemia, metastatic neuroblastoma, Ewing

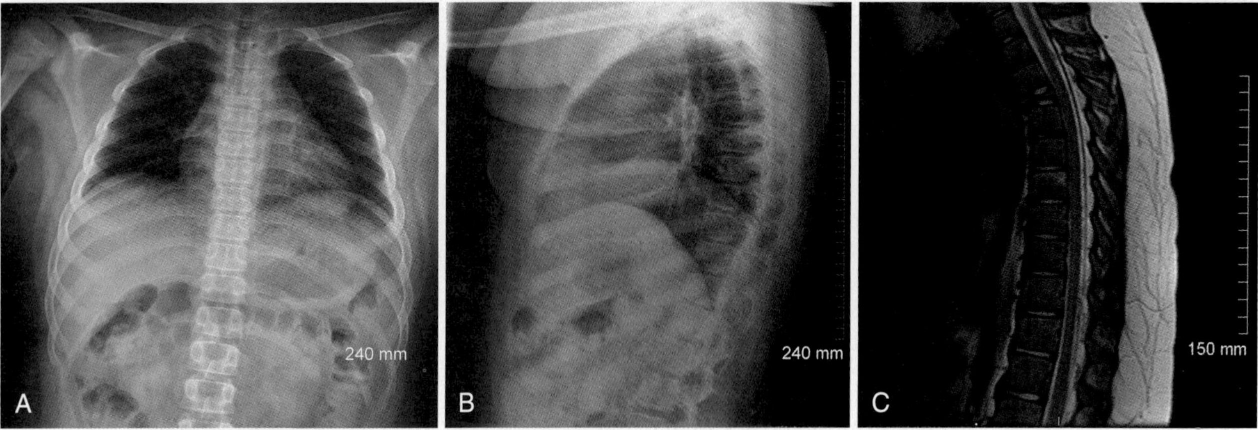

FIGURE 8.214 Eosinophilic granuloma in a 10-year-old child resulting in vertebra plana at T4. **A** and **B,** Radiographic appearance. **C,** Appearance on sagittal MRI.

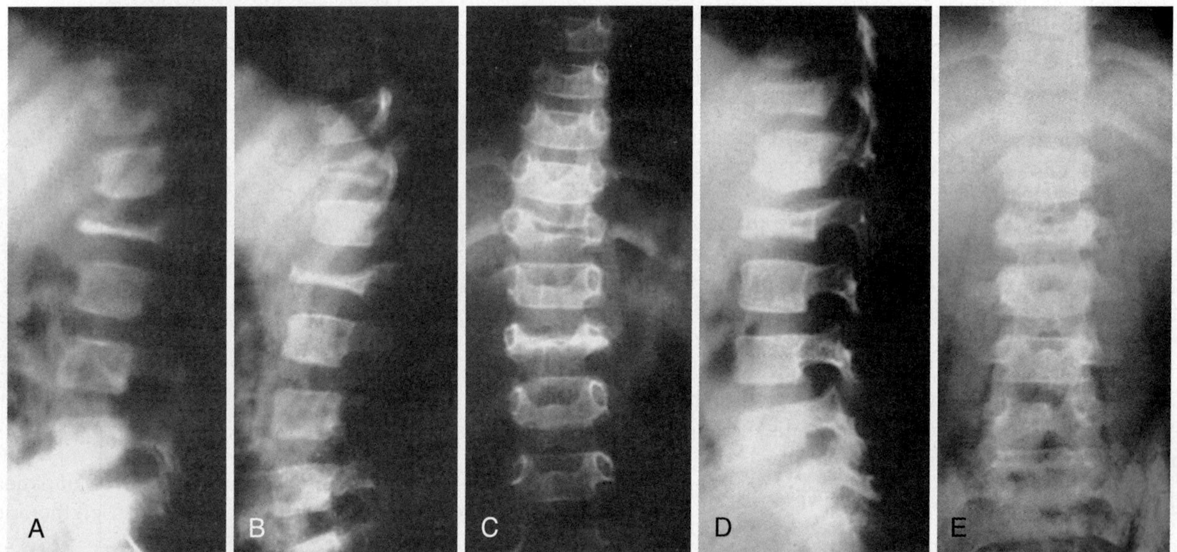

FIGURE 8.215 **A,** Eosinophilic granuloma of spine in 3½-year-old patient. **B,** Sudden collapse of T12 3 weeks later, in addition to vertebra plana at L2. **C,** Collapse of T12 and L2. **D** and **E,** Considerable reconstitution of the vertebral height of T12 and L2 16 months later. (From Seiman LP: Eosinophilic granuloma of the spine, *J Pediatr Orthop* 1:371, 1981.)

sarcoma, or multifocal osteomyelitis. MRI can be helpful in distinguishing eosinophilic granuloma from a malignant neoplasm. Eosinophilic granuloma will most often not have a prominent soft-tissue mass associated with the vertebral collapse. A malignant tumor, such as Ewing sarcoma, often has extensive soft-tissue involvement. The treatment of vertebra plana generally focuses on relief of symptoms. The usual result is spontaneous healing. Spinal deformity may be minimized by the use of an appropriate orthosis. Other reported treatment alternatives include curettage and bone grafting, radiotherapy, and interlesional instillation of corticosteroids, but they rarely are needed.

HEMANGIOMA

Hemangioma is the most common benign vascular tumor of bone. Most hemangiomas involve the vertebral bodies or skull, and involvement of other bones is rare. Vertebral involvement usually is an incidental finding and requires surgery only when neurologic function is compromised (Fig. 8.215C). Hemangioma has been reported in as many as 12% of spines studied by autopsy. The lesion usually produces a characteristic, vertical, striated appearance (Fig. 8.216A,B). Laredo et al. divided vertebral hemangiomas into three subcategories. The most common is the asymptomatic vertebral hemangioma; the second is a compressive vertebral hemangioma that compresses the cord or cauda equina; and the third is the rare vertebral hemangioma that causes clinical symptoms (symptomatic vertebral hemangioma). Six radiographic criteria were noted that were indicative of vertebral hemangioma leading to compressive problems: thoracic location (from T3 to T9), entire vertebral body involvement, neural arch (particularly pedicles) involvement, irregular honeycomb appearance, expanded and poorly defined cortex, and swelling of the soft tissue. It was suggested in patients with vertebral hemangioma and back pain of uncertain origin that the presence of three or more of these signs may indicate a potentially symptomatic vertebral hemangioma. Laredo et al. also compared MRI findings in asymptomatic and symptomatic vertebral hemangiomas. They found that vertebral hemangiomas with low-signal intensity on T1-weighted images

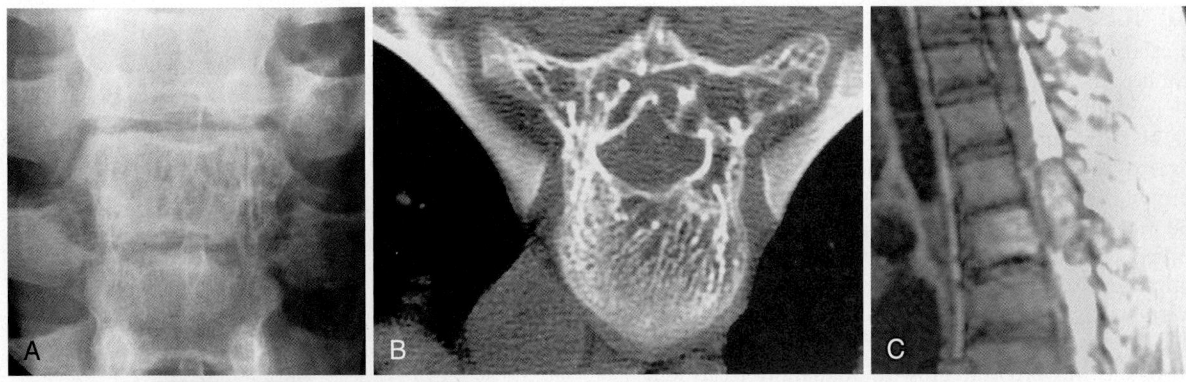

FIGURE 8.216 Radiograph **(A)**, CT scan **(B)**, and MRI **(C)** of patient with spinal hemangioma with canal compromise.

had a significant vascular component, which might have been a major contributing factor to the patient's symptoms. Most vertebral hemangiomas contained predominant fat attenuation values on CT and showed high-signal intensity on T1-weighted imaging, indicating a predominantly fatty content. These researchers emphasized, however, as has been our experience, that most vertebral hemangiomas are not symptomatic and are an incidental finding. If neurologic dysfunction and anterior collapse occur, operative excision of the lesion, perhaps with adjuvant embolization as described by Dick et al., is recommended.

PRIMARY MALIGNANT TUMORS OF THE VERTEBRAL COLUMN

Primary malignant tumors of the vertebral column are uncommon. In children, the most common are Ewing sarcoma and osteogenic sarcoma.

EWING SARCOMA

Ewing sarcoma is a relatively rare, primary malignant tumor of bone. The tumor occurs most frequently in males in the second decade of life. All bones, including the spine, may be affected. The tumor most commonly begins in the pelvis or long bones and rapidly metastasizes to other skeletal sites, including the spine, especially the vertebral bodies and pedicles.

The currently recommended treatment of Ewing sarcoma is radiotherapy and adjuvant chemotherapy. On occasion, surgery may be necessary to stabilize the spine because of compression of the neural elements and bony instability. If decompression of the neural elements is necessary, stabilization usually is needed at the same time.

OSTEOGENIC SARCOMA

Osteogenic sarcoma is the most common primary malignant bone tumor, excluding multiple myeloma, but less than 2% originate in the spine. It is a malignant tumor of bone in which tumor cells form neoplastic osteoid or bone, or both. Classic osteogenic sarcoma is more common in boys 10 to 15 years of age. This is a rapidly progressive malignant neoplasm, and multiple metastatic lesions to the vertebral column are more common than primary involvement (Fig. 8.217). The role of surgery for vertebral involvement is based on whether the spinal lesion is solitary, primary, or metastatic. If decompression of the spinal cord becomes necessary, or if structural integrity of the vertebral column is compromised, stabilizing procedures usually are required. If aggressive operative debridement is required, the neural structures limit the margin of the resection, making it impossible to achieve as wide a margin of resection as in the extremities.

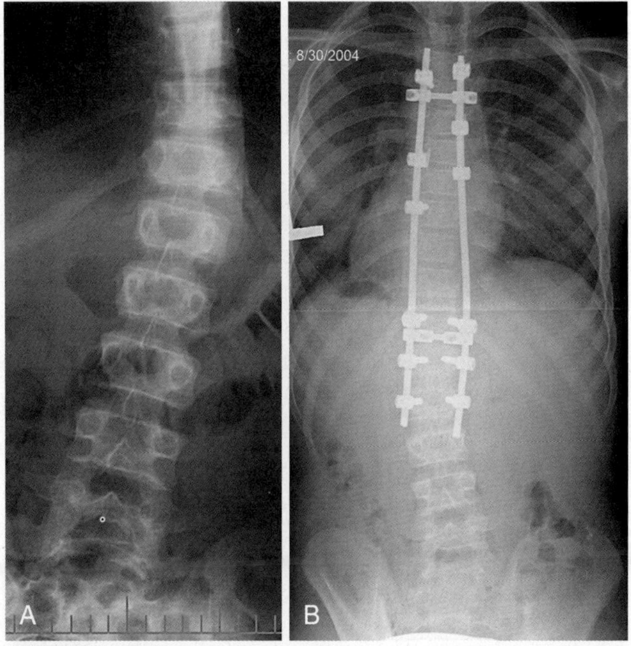

FIGURE 8.217 **A,** Osteogenic sarcoma in a 14-year-old child. **B,** After tumor resection and stabilization.

POSTIRRADIATION SPINAL DEFORMITY

Perthes in 1903 first described inhibition of osseous development by irradiation. Later studies indicated that the physis is particularly sensitive to radiation. A physis exposed to 600 rad or more showed some growth retardation, and complete inhibition of growth was produced by doses of more than 1200 rad. The longitudinal growth of a vertebral body takes place by means of true physeal cartilage, similar to the longitudinal growth of the metaphysis of the long bones. The three most common solid tumors of childhood for which radiation therapy is part of the treatment regimen and in which the vertebral column is included in the radiation fields are neuroblastoma, Wilms tumor, and medulloblastoma.

INCIDENCE

Mayfield et al. studied spinal deformity in children treated for neuroblastoma, and Riseborough et al. studied spinal deformity in children treated for Wilms tumor. Several principles can be summarized from these studies. A direct relationship seems to exist between the amount of radiation and the severity of the spinal deformity. In general, a dose of less than 2000 rad is not associated with significant deformity, a dose between 2000 and 3000 rad is associated with mild scoliosis, and a dose of more than 3000 rad is associated with more severe scoliosis. Irradiation in younger children, especially those 2 years of age or younger, produces the most serious disturbance in vertebral growth. Radiation treatment in children older than 4 years is less frequently associated with spinal deformity. Asymmetric irradiation is associated with significant spinal deformity. Progression usually occurs during the adolescent growth spurt. Scoliosis is a common deformity, and the direction of the curve usually is concave toward the side of the irradiation. Kyphosis may occur in association with the scoliosis, or kyphosis alone may be present, most frequently at the thoracolumbar junction. Children who require a laminectomy because of epidural spread of tumor are especially prone to the development of moderate-to-severe spinal deformity. Similarly, those children whose disease causes paraplegia also are prone to rapid progression of the deformity. Without these two complicating features, most radiation-induced scoliotic deformities remain small and do not require treatment. Because progression of these curves generally occurs during the adolescent growth spurt, any child undergoing radiation therapy to the spine should have orthopaedic consultation and regular follow-up until skeletal maturity.

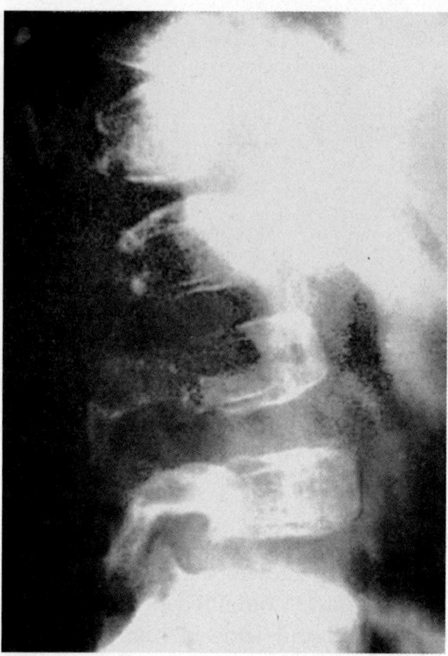

FIGURE 8.218 "Bone-in-bone" appearance of irradiated spine, equivalent of growth arrest line in long bone. (From Katzman H, Waugh T, Berdon W: Skeletal changes following irradiation of childhood tumors, *J Bone Joint Surg* 51A:825, 1969.)

RADIOGRAPHIC FINDINGS

Neuhauser et al. described the radiographic changes in previously irradiated spines, and Riseborough et al. divided the radiographic findings into four groups. The earliest noted changes were alterations in the vertebral bodies within the irradiated section of the spine, which are expressions of irradiation impairment of physeal enchondral growth at the vertebral endplates. The most obvious features of these lesions were growth arrest lines that subsequently led to the bone-in-bone picture (28%) (Fig. 8.218). Endplate irregularity with an altered trabecular pattern and decreased vertebral body height were seen most frequently (83% of patients). Contour abnormalities, causing anterior narrowing and beaking of the vertebral bodies, such as those seen in Morquio disease (Fig. 8.219), were present in 20% of patients. Asymmetric or symmetric failure of vertebral body development was apparent on the anteroposterior radiographs of all 81 patients studied. The second group of radiographic changes included alterations in spinal alignment. Scoliosis was present in 70% of patients and kyphosis in 25%. The third group of radiographic findings included skeletal alterations in bones other than the vertebral column, the most common of which were iliac wing hypoplasia (68%) and osteochondroma (6%). The fourth group consisted of patients with no evidence of deformity of the axial skeleton (27%).

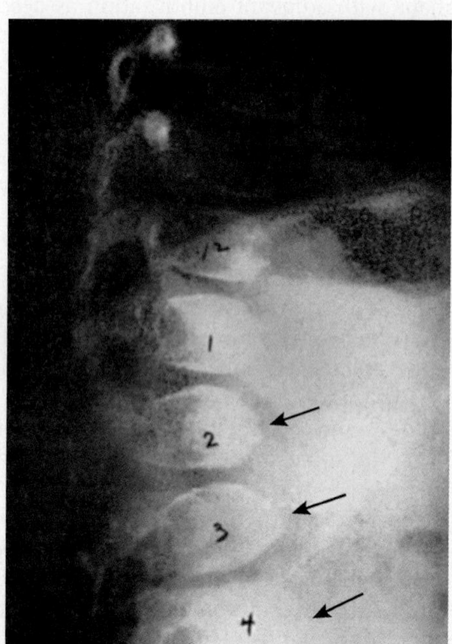

FIGURE 8.219 Contour abnormalities of vertebral bodies after radiotherapy for Wilms tumor in 8-month-old patient. (From Katzman H, Waugh T, Berdon W: Skeletal changes following irradiation of childhood tumors, *J Bone Joint Surg* 51A:825, 1969.)

TREATMENT

Most studies indicate that the curves usually remain slight until the adolescent growth spurt, when progression can be severe and rapid. Orthoses for treatment of postirradiation spinal deformity may or may not (50%) improve or stop progression of the deformity, especially if severe changes in the architecture of the vertebrae and excessive soft-tissue scarring are present. The indications for operative treatment are a scoliosis of more than 40 degrees and a thoracolumbar kyphosis of more than 50 degrees. Patients with progression despite brace treatment also are considered candidates for operative intervention. Riseborough et al. outlined the difficulties in obtaining adequate correction and fusion of these curves, which frequently are rigid. Extensive soft-tissue scarring may further complicate the surgery. Many patients requiring operative treatment have a kyphoscoliotic deformity, and many also have had previous laminectomies, which will inhibit solid fusion. Healing can be prolonged, and pseudarthrosis is common.

Combined anterior and posterior fusions with an anterior strut graft or anterior interbody fusion and posterior instrumentation should be considered for patients with kyphotic deformities of more than 40 degrees. Because of the unpredictable nature of the irradiated anterior bone stock, anterior instrumentation may not be possible. Segmental hook or screw instrumentation systems, with their ability to apply both compression and distraction, are ideal for posterior instrumentation in these patients. If irradiation was for a tumorous process, consideration should be given to titanium implants, which would allow better follow-up MRI, if necessary. The fusion area is selected by the same criteria as for idiopathic curves (see earlier section on fusion levels and hook site placement). A large quantity of bone from the nonirradiated iliac crest should be used. Ogilvie suggested exploration of the fusion 6 months after surgery for repeated bone grafting of any developing pseudarthrosis. Because of problems with bone stock, postoperative immobilization in a TLSO often is indicated until complete fusion is obtained.

COMPLICATIONS AND PITFALLS

Pseudarthrosis, infection, and neurologic injury are more frequent after spinal fusion for radiation-induced deformity than for other spinal deformities. The increase in pseudarthrosis is attributed to poor bone quality, decreased bone vascularity, kyphotic deformity, and absence of posterior bone elements after laminectomy. Poor vascularity and skin quality have been associated with an increased infection rate. Severe scarring sometimes is present in the retroperitoneal space, making the anterior exposure more difficult. Because viscera can be damaged by radiation, bowel obstruction, perforation, and fistula formation may occur after spinal fusion. This can be difficult to differentiate from postoperative cast syndrome. Paraplegia also has been reported in patients who had radiation treatment for neuroblastoma and surgical correction. It is believed that they had a subclinical form of radiation myelopathy and that spinal correction compromised what little vascular supply there was to the cord. The surgeon should be aware of this possibility and avoid overcorrection of these kyphotic deformities.

OSTEOCHONDRODYSTROPHY

DIASTROPHIC DWARFISM

Diastrophic dwarfism is inherited as an autosomal recessive disease. The diagnosis usually can be made at birth on the basis of clinical features and, for families at risk, before birth by ultrasound examination and molecular genetic testing. Clinical and radiographic findings are short limbs, short stature, multiple joint contractures, and early degeneration of joints. Spinal deformities, including cervical kyphosis, scoliosis, and exaggerated lumbar lordosis, often are seen. Remes et al. found scoliosis in 88% of patients with diastrophic dwarfism. They subdivided the scoliotic curves into three subtypes: early progressive, idiopathic-like, and mild nonprogressive. The early progressive type resembled the progressive form of infantile idiopathic scoliosis, with early onset, rapid progression, and severe outcome. Patients with the idiopathic-like scoliosis had features similar to patients with adolescent idiopathic scoliosis.

The indications for treatment of scoliosis in diastrophic dwarfism have not been fully established. Patients with diastrophic dwarfism already have many abnormalities in their appearance. The benefits of surgical treatment should therefore be evaluated critically. Brace treatment has been found to be useful only for small curves in these patients. If the curve cannot be braced successfully, the spinal deformity can progress to a severe scoliosis causing imbalance of the trunk. This can lead to difficulties in gait and a reduction in the already short standing height. The most important factors to be considered are the rate of progression and the time at onset: the earlier the time at onset, the more rapid and severe the progression and curve type. The early progressive type of scoliosis virtually always develops into a severe deformity unless surgery is performed. In very young children, growth rod–type instrumentation can be considered. However, because growth is limited, repeated surgeries to lengthen the rods are done at 15- to 18-month intervals instead of the usual 4- to 6-month interval. If a significantly progressive curve is noted in a very young child not appropriate for growing rods, combined anterior and posterior fusion should be considered. If a growth rod can be successfully used, by the age of 10 years, most of the spinal growth in a diastrophic dysplastic patient is complete and definitive fusion is then done.

Cervical kyphosis occurs commonly, and although it usually resolves with age, it can cause quadriplegia. Radiographic evaluation of the cervical spine is mandatory in these patients. If the cervical kyphosis worsens, surgical treatment is necessary. If the kyphosis is mild, posterior fusion alone, combined with a halo brace, should be considered. In an older child with a more severe kyphosis, combined anterior and posterior fusion should be considered. If the kyphosis is causing neurologic problems, decompression anteriorly at the apex of the kyphosis is needed along with anterior and posterior fusion.

SPONDYLOEPIPHYSEAL DYSPLASIA

Orthopaedic aspects of spondyloepiphyseal dysplasia are discussed in other chapter.

The spinal problems most commonly associated with this condition are scoliosis, kyphoscoliosis, and odontoid hypoplasia with atlantoaxial instability (Fig. 8.220). If the scoliosis and kyphoscoliosis are progressive, orthotic treatment sometimes is useful for delaying the fusion until the patient is older. Kopits found a 30% to 40% incidence of atlantoaxial instability in patients with spondyloepiphyseal dysplasia. In children with this condition who are not walking by 2 to 3 years of age, the most likely explanation is spinal cord compression at the upper cervical region. Flexion-extension lateral cervical spine radiographs should be obtained. If ossification delay in vertebral bodies makes accurate determination of movement at this level impossible, a flexion-extension lateral MRI study is indicated. Once the instability is diagnosed, the treatment is surgical fusion.

If the scoliotic curve continues to progress despite bracing, surgical fusion is considered. Unlike in achondroplasia, spinal stenosis generally is not present in patients with spondyloepiphyseal dysplasia.

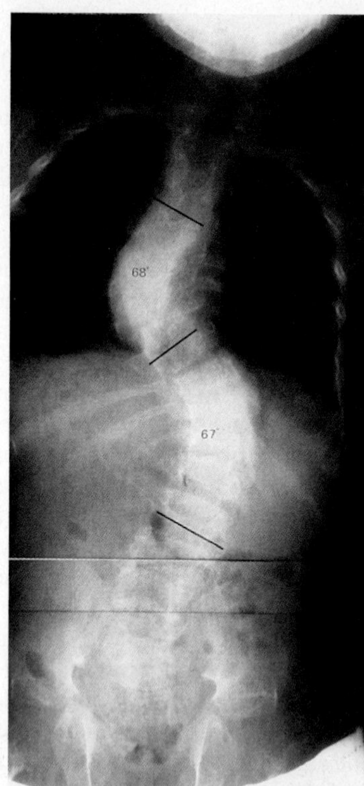

FIGURE 8.220 Spinal deformity in patient with spondyloepiphyseal dysplasia.

OSTEOGENESIS IMPERFECTA

Patients with osteogenesis imperfecta have abnormal collagen production that results in defective bone and connective tissue. Other orthopaedic aspects of osteogenesis imperfecta are described in other chapter.

The reported incidence of spinal deformity in patients with osteogenesis imperfecta ranges from 40% to 90%. Hanscom et al. developed a classification system based on the degree of bone involvement and the likelihood of development of a spinal deformity. Patients with type A disease have mild bony abnormalities with normal vertebral contours. Patients with type B disease have bowed long bones and wide cortices with biconcave vertebral bodies and a normal pelvic contour. Patients with type C disease have thin, bowed long bones and protrusio acetabuli, which develop around the age of 10 years. Patients with type D disease have deformities similar to type C, with the addition of cystic changes around the knee by the age of 5 years. Patients with type E disease are totally dependent functionally. Scoliosis occurred in 46% of their patients with type A disease and in all patients with types C and D. Benson et al., in a review of 100 patients with osteogenesis imperfecta, also concluded that the severity of the disease correlates with the risk of development and the severity of the scoliosis. Anissipour et al. reviewed 157 patients with osteogenesis imperfecta and scoliosis. Using the modified Sillence classification, they were able to follow patients having mild (type I), intermediate (type IV), and severe (type III) disease. There were high rates of scoliosis progression in types II and IV osteogenesis imperfecta, with a benign course in type I patients. Ishikawa et al. described biconcave vertebrae as a predictive factor for development of future scoliotic deformity. Patients with 6 or more biconcave vertebral fractures had a 93% prevalence of severe scoliosis (curve larger than 50 degrees). Patients with fewer than six biconcave vertebrae were not at risk to develop severe scoliosis. The age at which a child achieves motor milestones is associated with later development of spinal deformities. Bisphosphonate therapy has been shown to reduce and prevent vertebral deformity, but its effect on scoliosis and curve progression remains unclear. Bisphosphonates should be stopped 6 months before spinal fusion and not resumed until 6 months following surgery.

The natural history of scoliosis in patients with osteogenesis imperfecta is continued progression. Scoliosis present at a young age almost always is progressive, and progression may continue into adulthood. Severe and disabling spinal deformities have been found in many adults with osteogenesis imperfecta.

■ ANESTHESIA PROBLEMS

There are several areas of concern in the administration of anesthesia for a patient with osteogenesis imperfecta. The primary concern is the risk of fractures. Extreme care must be taken in handling these patients, including positioning on the operating table with adequate padding and care in transfer. Care also should be taken in establishment of the intravenous line or application of a blood pressure cuff because both can result in fracture. Intubation and airway control also can be problematic because these patients have large heads and short necks, as well as tongues that often are disproportionately large. Extension of the head to facilitate intubation could cause a cervical spine fracture or a mandibular fracture. Because many patients with osteogenesis imperfecta have thoracic deformities, poor respiratory function should be expected.

A tendency for hyperthermia to develop in patients with osteogenesis imperfecta also has been noted. This does not appear to be a malignant type, however, and it may be related to elevated thyroid hormone levels, which are found in at least half of the patients with osteogenesis imperfecta. Hyperthermia can be induced by various anesthetic agents, as well as by atropine, and atropine should be avoided in these patients. If hyperthermia occurs, it is controlled with cooling, supplemental oxygen, sodium bicarbonate, cardiovascular stimulants, and dantrolene sodium. Libman suggested preoperative treatment with dantrolene sodium to perhaps prevent hyperthermia. He also recommended minimizing fasciculations associated with succinylcholine chloride. If possible, other agents should be used. If succinylcholine chloride is necessary, the fasciculations may be minimized by prior administration of a nondepolarizing muscle relaxant.

■ ORTHOTIC TREATMENT

Most authors agree that bracing does not control progressive scoliosis in patients with severe osteogenesis imperfecta. Brace treatment has been found to be ineffective in stopping progression of scoliosis in patients with osteogenesis imperfecta even if the curves are small, although Hanscom et al. suggested that orthotic treatment under carefully controlled circumstances may be a reasonable alternative to operative intervention in patients with type A or type B osteogenesis imperfecta. It is doubtful whether any effective forces from an orthosis can be transmitted to the spine of a patient with preexisting deformity of the chest wall, fragile ribs, and deformed vertebral bodies.

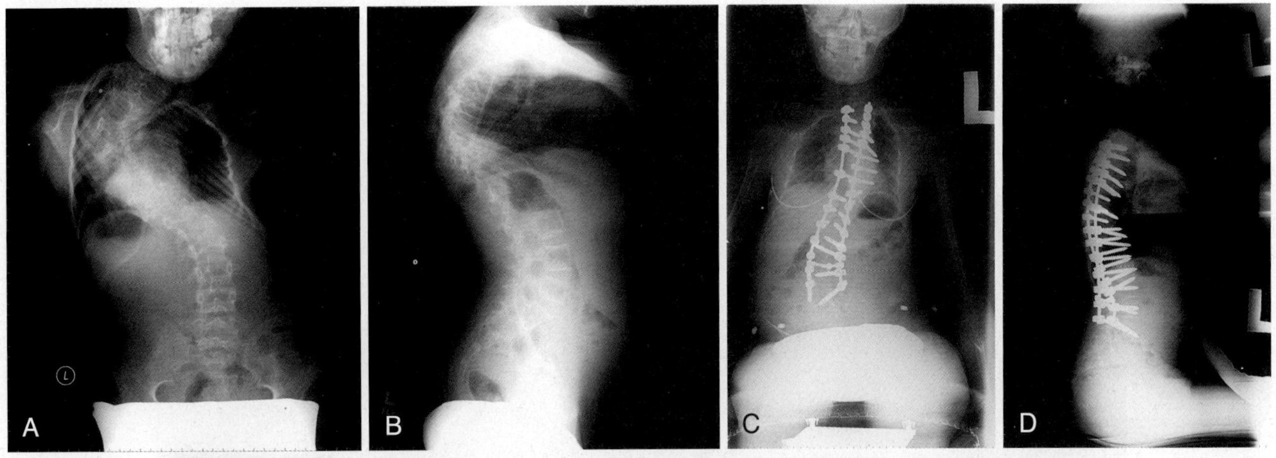

FIGURE 8.221 A and B, Spinal deformity in patient with osteogenesis imperfecta. C and D, Postoperative radiographs after posterior fusion and instrumentation.

OPERATIVE TREATMENT

Spinal fusion is recommended for curves of more than 50 degrees in patients with osteogenesis imperfecta, regardless of the age of the patient, provided there are no medical contraindications (Fig. 8.221). The decision to fuse the spine should depend on the extent of the curvature and the presence of progression rather than on the age of the patient. The upper instrumented level usually is T2 to reduce the risk of proximal junctional kyphosis. The lower instrumented level usually is between L3 and L5, with the goal of leveling the inferior endplate to the pelvis.

Segmental hook or screw instrumentation systems can be considered in patients with type A osteogenesis imperfecta. Patients with the milder form of the disease can be treated in the same manner as patients with idiopathic scoliosis, although significant correction of the curve should not be attempted. Bone graft should be obtained from the iliac crest, but often the amount of bone available is inadequate and allograft is required for a supplement. If the patient is small, pediatric instrumentation may be needed. The rod must be bent carefully to conform to the contours of the spine in both the coronal and sagittal planes to prevent excessive pull-out forces on the hooks.

In patients with more severe disease (type C or type D), segmental instrumentation with hooks and screws can be used. Segmental wires also can be used for fixation. Great care in tightening these wires should be taken to prevent a wire from pulling through the lamina posteriorly. An alternative is to use Mersilene tapes. Cement augmentation for pedicle screw fixation has been described by Yilmaz et al., who used cement augmentation at the 3 to 4 vertebral levels at the cranial and caudal ends of the spine to establish strong foundations at either end of the construct. For severe deformity, preoperative halo traction can be used to obtain preoperative correction instead of relying on fixation in poor quality bone. Anterior procedures should not be necessary if spinal deformities are stabilized before they become too severe.

Because of poor bone quality, immobilization in a two-piece TLSO often is necessary for 6 to 9 months after surgery until the fusion is solid.

UNUSUAL CAUSES OF KYPHOSIS

POSTLAMINECTOMY SPINAL DEFORMITY

Laminectomies most often are done in children for the diagnosis and treatment of spinal cord tumors, although they also may be needed in other conditions, such as neurofibromatosis and syringomyelia. Several authors reported the frequency of spinal deformities after laminectomy in children. The incidence of spinal deformity ranged from 33% to 100%.

Kyphosis is the most common deformity that occurs after multiple-level laminectomies (Fig. 8.222). Spinal deformity after laminectomy has been found to be more frequent in children younger than 15 years; also noted was the higher the level of the laminectomy, the greater the likelihood of spinal deformity or instability. All cervical or cervicothoracic laminectomies were followed by deformity in two studies. Lonstein et al. described two basic types of kyphosis, depending on the status of the facet joints posteriorly: sharp and angular or long and gradually rounding.

Scoliosis also may occur after laminectomy and generally is in the area of the laminectomy and associated with the kyphotic deformity. Scoliosis may occur at levels below the laminectomy, but this is usually caused by the paralysis from the cord tumor or its treatment rather than by the laminectomy.

The causes of instability of the spine after multiple laminectomies include skeletal and ligamentous deficiencies, neuromuscular imbalance, progressive osseous deformity, and radiation therapy. Increased wedging or excessive motion has been noted in children rather than subluxation as occurs in adults, possibly because, after laminectomy, pressure is increased on the cartilaginous endplates of the vertebral bodies anteriorly and, with time, cartilage growth is decreased and vertebral wedging occurs (Fig. 8.223). Panjabi et al. showed that the loss of posterior stability caused by removal of interspinous ligaments, spinous processes, and laminae allows the normal flexion forces to produce a kyphosis. Lonstein et al. emphasized the importance of the facet joints posteriorly in these deformities. They showed that when the facet joints are completely removed at one level, gross instability results, with maximal angulation at that level causing a sharp, angular kyphos, enlargement of the intervertebral foramen, and opening of the disc space posteriorly (Fig. 8.224). If complete removal is on one side only, the angular kyphosis is accompanied by a sharp scoliosis with the apex at the same level. If all the facets are preserved, a gradual rounding kyphos results in the area of the laminectomy.

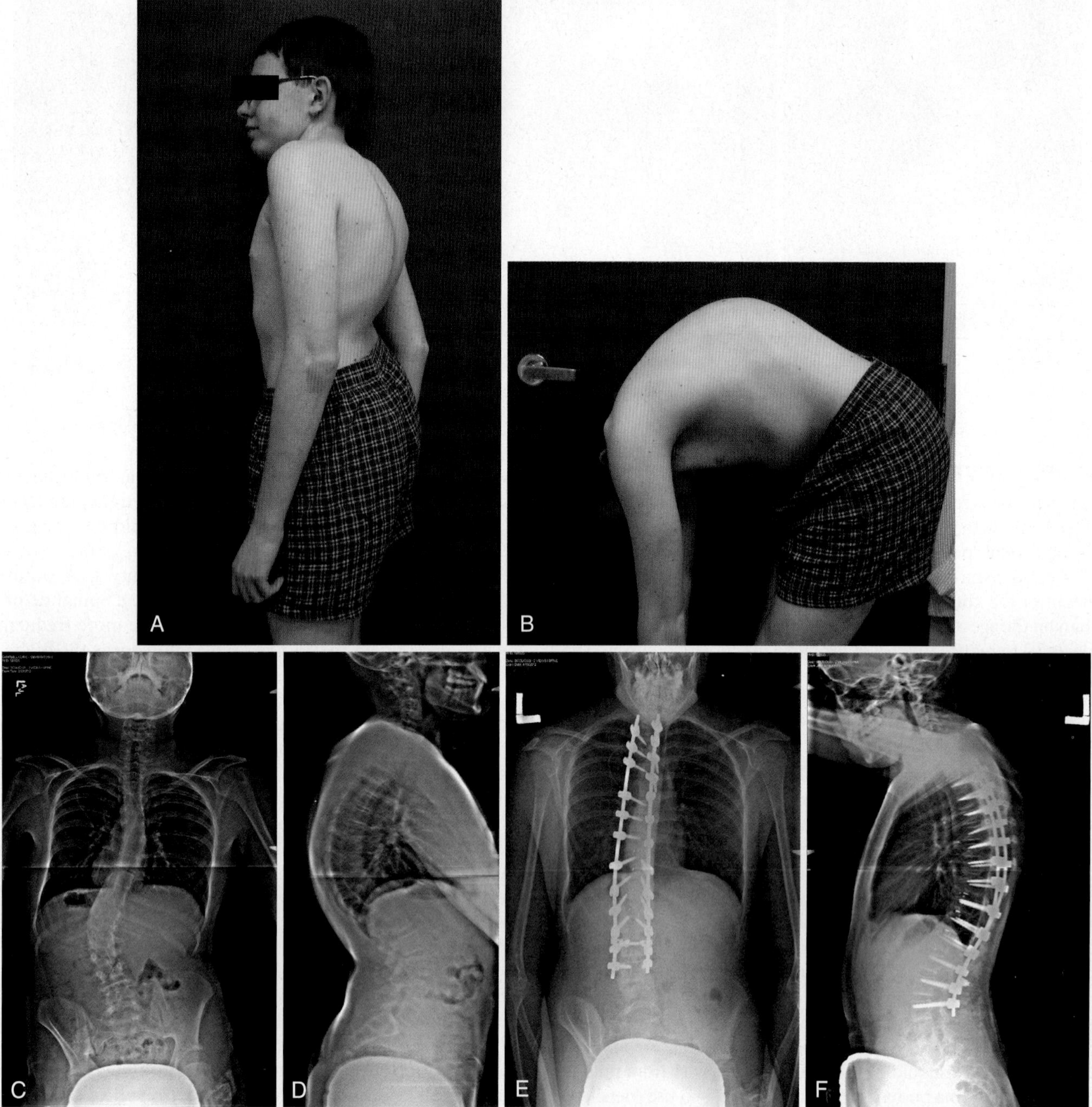

FIGURE 8.222 Postlaminectomy kyphosis. **A** and **B**, Clinical appearance. **C** and **D**, Radiographic appearance. **E** and **F**, After posterior fusion with pedicle screw instrumentation.

Many authors have reported extremely high incidences of spinal deformity in children younger than 10 years with complete paralysis. Children with extensive laminectomies and paralysis as a result of spinal cord tumors or their treatment are likely to have increasing spinal deformities. Radiation therapy, used to treat many spinal tumors, has been associated with injury to the vertebral physis and subsequent spinal deformity (see Postirradiation Spinal Deformity, earlier). The cause of postlaminectomy spinal deformity is therefore multifactorial.

TREATMENT

The treatment of postlaminectomy kyphosis is difficult, and, if at all possible, it is best to prevent the deformity from occurring. When laminectomy is necessary, the facet joints should be preserved whenever possible. Localized fusion at the time of facetectomy or laminectomy may help prevent progression of the deformity, but because of the loss of bone mass posteriorly, localized fusion may not produce a large enough fusion mass to prevent kyphosis. The surgical technique of laminoplasty to expose the spinal cord may lessen the chance of progressive deformity. This approach involves suturing the laminae back into place after removal or removing just one side of the laminae and allowing them to hinge open like a book to expose the spinal cord and then suturing that side of the lamina back in place. This procedure may provide a fibrous tether connecting the laminae to the spine, and Mimatsu has shown a decreased incidence

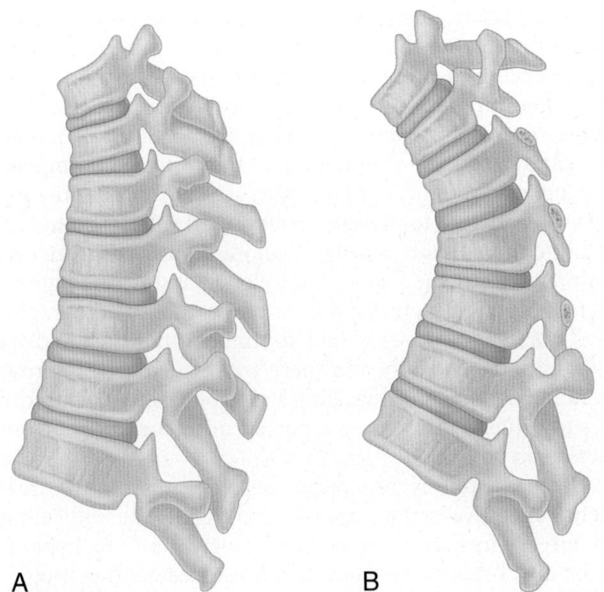

FIGURE 8.223 Drawings of thoracic spine before and after repeated laminectomy show effects on growth of vertebral bodies. **A,** Before laminectomy, anterior vertebral bodies are rectangular in configuration. **B,** Spine that has had multiple laminectomies will have increased compression anteriorly because of loss of posterior supporting structures. This compression results in less growth in anterior portion of vertebral body than in posterior portion. In time, this will result in wedging of vertebral bodies, causing kyphotic deformity.

of postlaminectomy kyphosis when it has been used. After surgery in which the laminae have been removed, the child should be examined regularly by an orthopaedic surgeon. If a spinal deformity is detected, brace treatment can be considered. The patient's long-term prognosis, however, should be considered before definitive treatment plans are made. If the prognosis for survival is poor, spinal fusion may not be appropriate. With modern treatment protocols and improved survival rates for tumors, fusion usually is indicated for progressive deformity.

Most authors recommend combined anterior and posterior fusions for this condition because of the small amount of bone surface posteriorly after a wide laminectomy. Also, many of these deformities have a kyphotic component and anterior spinal fusion is more successful biomechanically than posterior fusion. Anteriorly, the fusion mass is under compression rather than distraction forces. Of 45 patients treated for postlaminectomy scoliosis, Lonstein reported pseudarthroses in 33% with posterior fusion alone, in 22% with anterior fusion alone, and in 9.5% with combined anterior and posterior fusion. At the first stage, anterior fusion is done by removal of all of the disc material, taking special care to remove the entire disc back to the posterior longitudinal ligament to prevent growth in the posterior aspect of the vertebral endplate with increasing kyphotic deformity. Additional bone obtained locally from the vertebral bodies or ilium or remaining rib should be packed into the open disc spaces. Posterior fusion and instrumentation

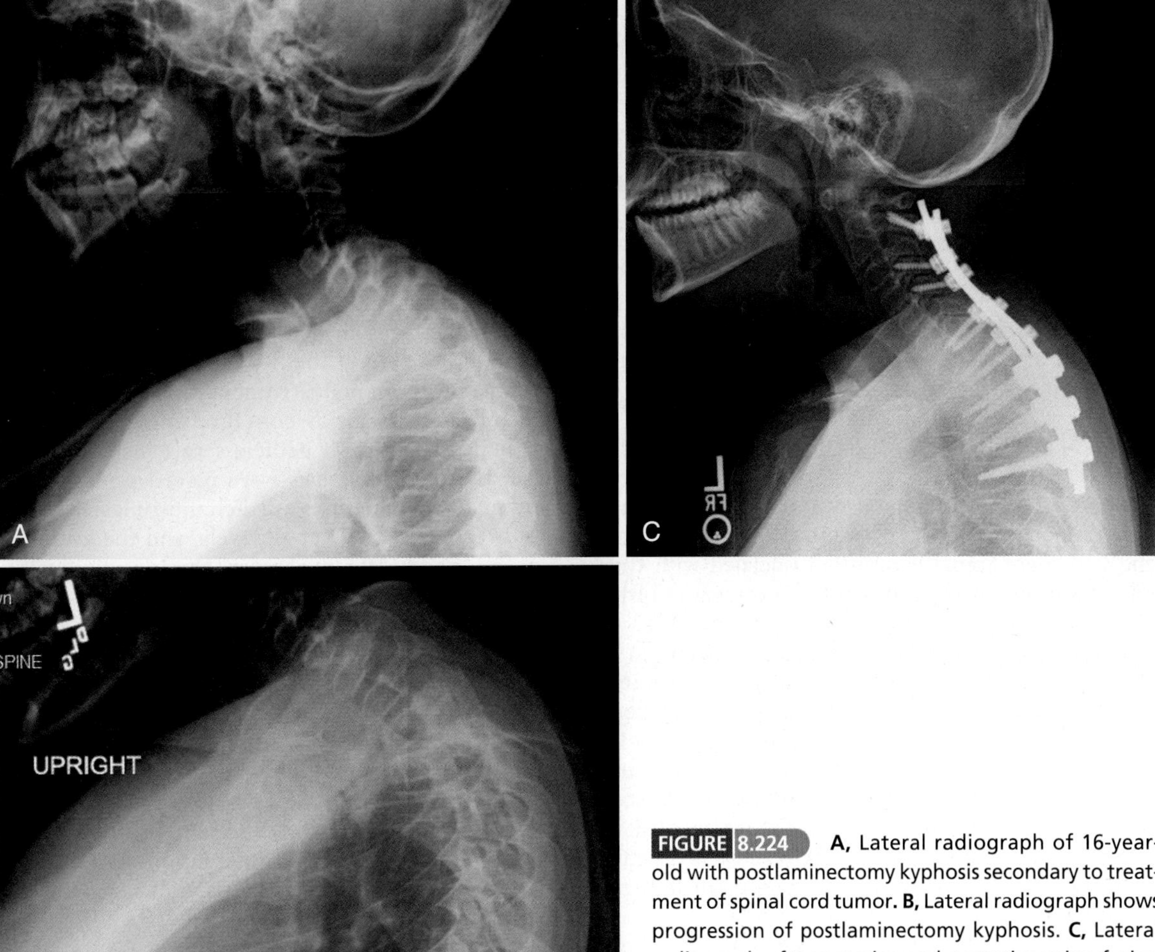

FIGURE 8.224 **A,** Lateral radiograph of 16-year-old with postlaminectomy kyphosis secondary to treatment of spinal cord tumor. **B,** Lateral radiograph shows progression of postlaminectomy kyphosis. **C,** Lateral radiograph after anterior and posterior spine fusion and instrumentation.

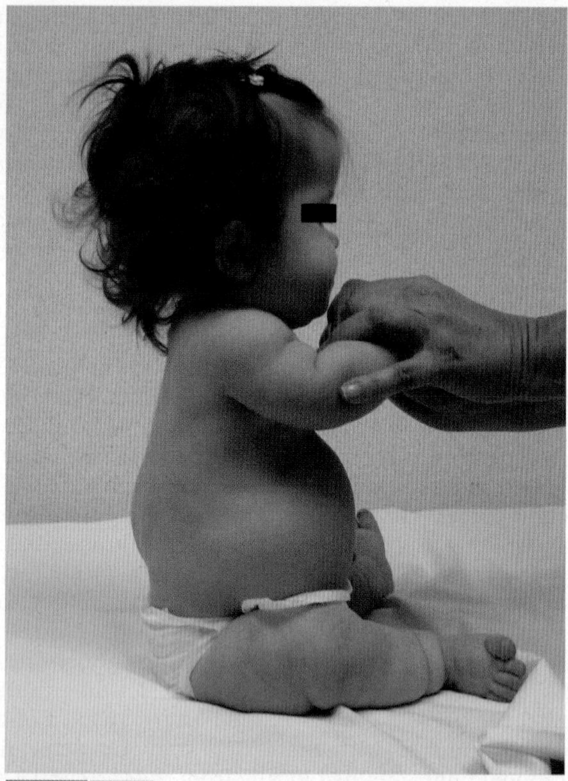

FIGURE 8.225 Kyphosis in infant with achondroplasia.

are done either immediately or a week after the anterior fusion. Because of the absence of the posterior elements, instrumentation of the involved spine is desirable but not always possible. Pedicle screw fixation has been helpful in allowing the use of posterior instrumentation for postlaminectomy kyphosis and scoliosis. This procedure provides secure fixation while the spinal fusion is maturing. The use of titanium rod instrumentation has been recommended at the time of laminectomy. The instrumentation provides stability postoperatively, and the titanium rods allow postoperative MRI to evaluate spinal cord tumors. Often, the extent of the deformity and the absence of the posterior elements make instrumentation impossible, and a halo cast or vest may be necessary in these patients after surgery.

SKELETAL DYSPLASIAS

ACHONDROPLASIA

Achondroplasia, the most common of the bony dysplasias, is caused by a mutation of fibroblast growth factor receptor 3. The most frequent spinal deformity associated with this condition is thoracolumbar kyphosis that is present at birth (Fig. 8.225). The frequency of kyphosis in achondroplasia is 87% from age 1 to 2 years, 39% from age 2 to 5 years, and 11% from age 5 to 10 years. As muscle tone develops and walking begins, the kyphotic deformity usually resolves, although persistent kyphosis has been reported and can become severe in some patients. This kyphosis is poorly tolerated by the patient with achondroplasia because of the decreased size of the spinal canal related to a marked decrease in the interpedicular distance in the lower lumbar region and to shortened pedicles, which cause a reduction in the anteroposterior dimensions of the spinal canal.

It is important to be aware of the possibility of persistent or progressive thoracolumbar kyphosis in these patients. Early bracing to prevent progression and correction of any associated hip flexion contractures to prevent hyperlordosis below the kyphosis are recommended. Pauli et al. showed the efficacy of early prohibition of unsupported sitting and bracing in a series of 66 infants with achondroplasia. The parents were advised to prevent unsupported sitting and to keep young children from sitting up more than 60 degrees even with support. If the kyphosis developed and became greater than 30 degrees (as measured on prone lateral radiographs), TLSO bracing was begun and continued until the child was walking independently and there was evidence of improvement in vertebral body wedging and kyphosis. With this form of early intervention, they reported no recurrences of progressive kyphosis.

If the kyphosis progresses despite conservative treatment, operative stabilization is indicated. The indications for surgery include a documented progression of a kyphotic deformity, kyphosis of more than 50 degrees, and neurologic deficits relating to the spinal deformity. Unless the kyphosis is rapidly progressive or there are neurologic deficits, surgery is delayed until 4 years of age. Neurologic deficits can occur as a direct result of the kyphotic deformity and also as a result of the lumbar stenosis. Neurologic deficits in infants with achondroplasia may indicate narrowing of the foramen magnum and basilar impression. Evaluation of neurologic deficits therefore should include appropriate imaging studies of the foramen magnum and the occipitocervical junction. A thorough physical examination and diagnostic study, including a CT scan or MRI, may be necessary to determine the source of neurologic deficits.

Patients with progressive thoracolumbar kyphosis require combined anterior and posterior fusion. The traditional approach has been to avoid posterior instrumentation because of the small canal, but if pedicle screws can be placed and the kyphosis is flexible, then posterior instrumentation and fusion can be used to treat progressive kyphosis. Ain and Browne recommended an anterior approach when the pedicle was too small to accommodate screw instrumentation. Corpectomy to relieve anterior impingement was needed when hyperextension over a bolster failed to correct the kyphosis to less than 50 degrees. Patients in whom no instrumentation was used posteriorly had repeated posterior bone grafting 4 months after the original procedure. If pedicle screw instrumentation was used, the pedicle screws were placed under fluoroscopic guidance. In patients with achondroplasia, the pedicles are directed cranially at all levels, and the average pedicle length is nearly 10 mm shorter than in individuals without achondroplasia. In Ain and Browne's patients, all kyphotic segments were included in the fusion. If a concomitant decompression was done, the fusion was ended at least one level cephalad to the most superior level of laminectomy to avoid development of junctional kyphosis (Fig. 8.226). They found that pedicle instrumentation of the pediatric achondroplastic spine did not cause intraoperative neurologic monitoring difficulties or lead to postoperative neurologic deficits. Posterior column shortening with pedicle screws and posterior instrumentation also has been used to successfully treat neurologic deficits secondary to thoracolumbar kyphosis.

Symptomatic spinal stenosis usually does not occur until the third or fourth decade of life, but it may develop before adolescence. The reported incidence of symptomatic spinal stenosis ranges from 37% to 89%. The interpedicular distance typically decreases from L1 to L5 and the pedicle diameter increases in the same direction, resulting in a 40% reduction in size of the sagittal and coronal diameter of the spinal canal. Approximately one fourth of all patients with achondroplasia will require surgery for spinal stenosis. Surgical indications are progressive symptoms, urinary retention, severe claudication (symptoms after walking less than two city blocks), and neurologic symptoms at rest. Surgical management of spinal stenosis is a decompressive laminectomy. Laminectomy alone is not always sufficient for decompression, and the nerve root recesses on both sides should be explored because lateral stenosis usually is present. Because of the high risk of developing a postlaminectomy kyphosis, concurrent posterior instrumentation and fusion are recommended.

MUCOPOLYSACCHARIDOSES

Of the many types of mucopolysaccharidoses, Morquio, Hurler, and Maroteaux-Lamy syndromes are the types most commonly associated with structural changes of the spine. The spinal deformity commonly seen in children with these conditions is kyphosis, usually in the thoracolumbar junction (Figs. 8.227 and 8.228). The vertebral bodies of these patients are deficient anteriorly and are flattened, beaked, or notched. The intervertebral discs are thick and bulging, often larger than the bodies. Thus, in time, the thoracolumbar spine collapses into kyphosis. The kyphosis is flexible in childhood but with progression becomes increasingly rigid. Treatment of the condition depends on the degree of the deformity, as well as the child's prognosis (Fig. 8.229).

Morquio syndrome is the most common of the mucopolysaccharidoses. Children with this condition may well live into adult life and have normal mentality. Many authors, including Blaw and Langer, Kopits, Langer, and Lipson, have emphasized the frequent occurrence of atlantoaxial instability in patients with Morquio syndrome. The most common presenting symptom is reduced exercise tolerance, followed by progressive upper motor neuron deficits. Blaw and Langer stated that neurologic problems in the first two decades of life usually are related to odontoid abnormalities or atlantoaxial instability; later, symptoms primarily are caused by the kyphosis or gibbus. Posterior fusion of C1 to C2 is the recommended treatment of atlantoaxial instability as soon as any signs of a myelopathy are identified. Blaw and Langer recommended that the developing gibbus during childhood be treated with an appropriate spinal orthosis to prevent neurologic deficits. Dalvie et al. described the use of anterior discectomy and anterior instrumentation to correct the thoracolumbar gibbus in these patients. The advantages of this technique are the opportunity for anterior decompression by excision of the bulging disc before correction of the kyphosis; the number of levels included in the fusion is less than required posteriorly; the posterior elements in these children are not strong enough to hold instrumentation, and, furthermore, associated canal stenosis, because of soft-tissue deposition, makes intracanal instrumentation unsafe; the interbody fusion obtained is of excellent quality; and anterior surgery can be performed, dissecting fewer muscle planes. The primary difficulty with this technique is technical in nature. The vertebral bodies are very small, and great care must be taken to ensure central placement of the screws. If the correction maneuver places excess stress on the implants, they may cut through the bone. The corrective maneuver must therefore include an external corrective force. Good correction of the kyphosis was obtained and maintained throughout the follow-up period (Fig. 8.230).

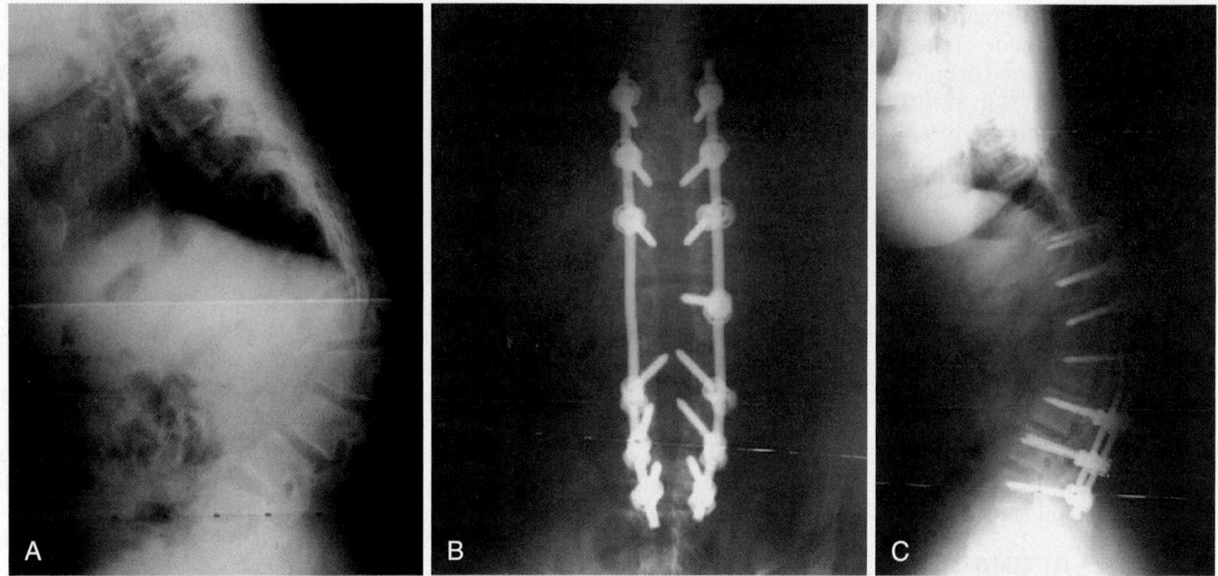

FIGURE 8.226 Spinal arthrodesis with instrumentation in pediatric achondroplasia. **A,** Preoperative lateral radiograph. **B,** Postoperative anteroposterior radiograph. **C,** Postoperative lateral radiograph. (From Ain MC, Browne JA: Spinal arthrodesis with instrumentation for thoracolumbar kyphosis in pediatric achondroplasia, *Spine* 29:2075, 2004.)

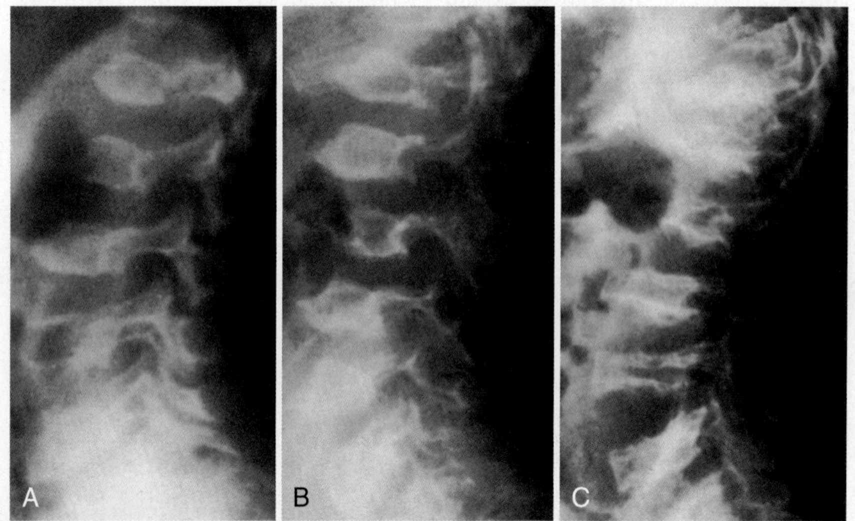

FIGURE 8.227 Spinal deformity in Morquio syndrome. **A,** Hook-shaped bodies in young child. **B,** Further anterior ossification in older child. **C,** Flattened, rectangular vertebral bodies in adult. (From Langer LO, Carey LS: The radiographic features of the KS mucopolysaccharidosis of Morquio, *Am J Roentgenol* 97:1, 1966.)

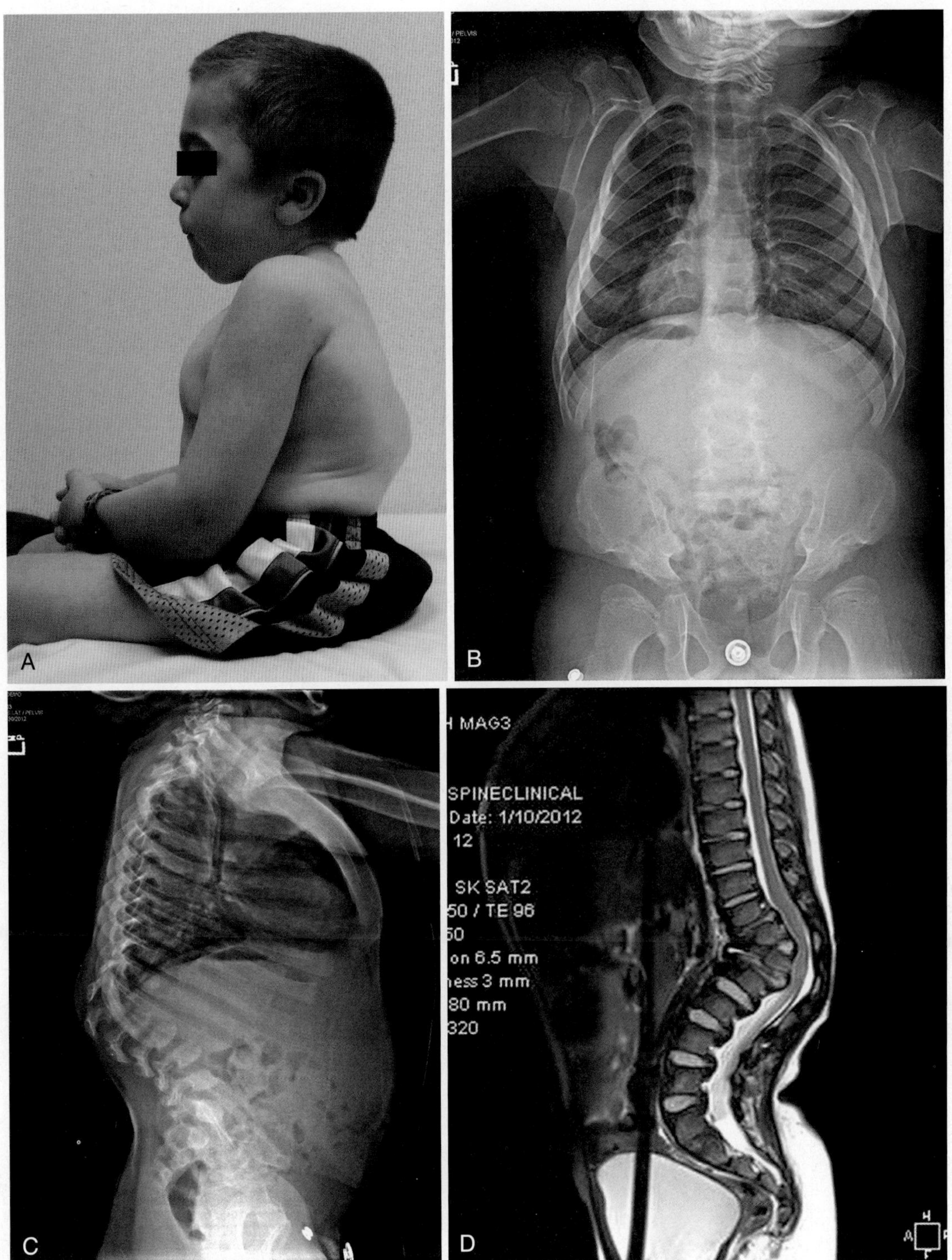

FIGURE 8.228 Kyphotic deformity in patient with mucopolysaccharidosis. **A,** Clinical appearance. **B** and **C,** Radiographic appearance. **D,** MRI.

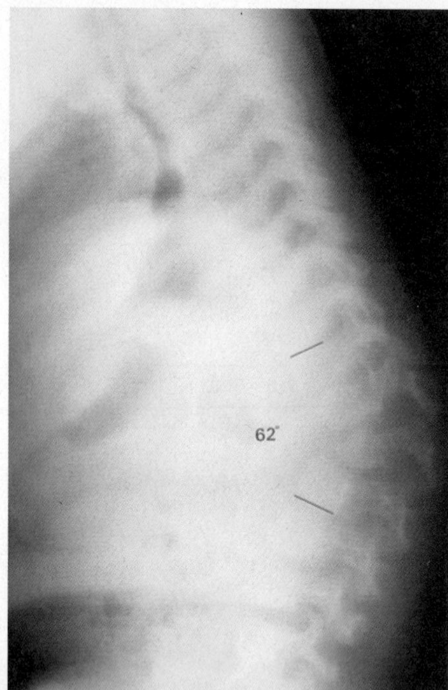

FIGURE 8.229 Kyphosis at thoracolumbar junction in patient with Hurler syndrome.

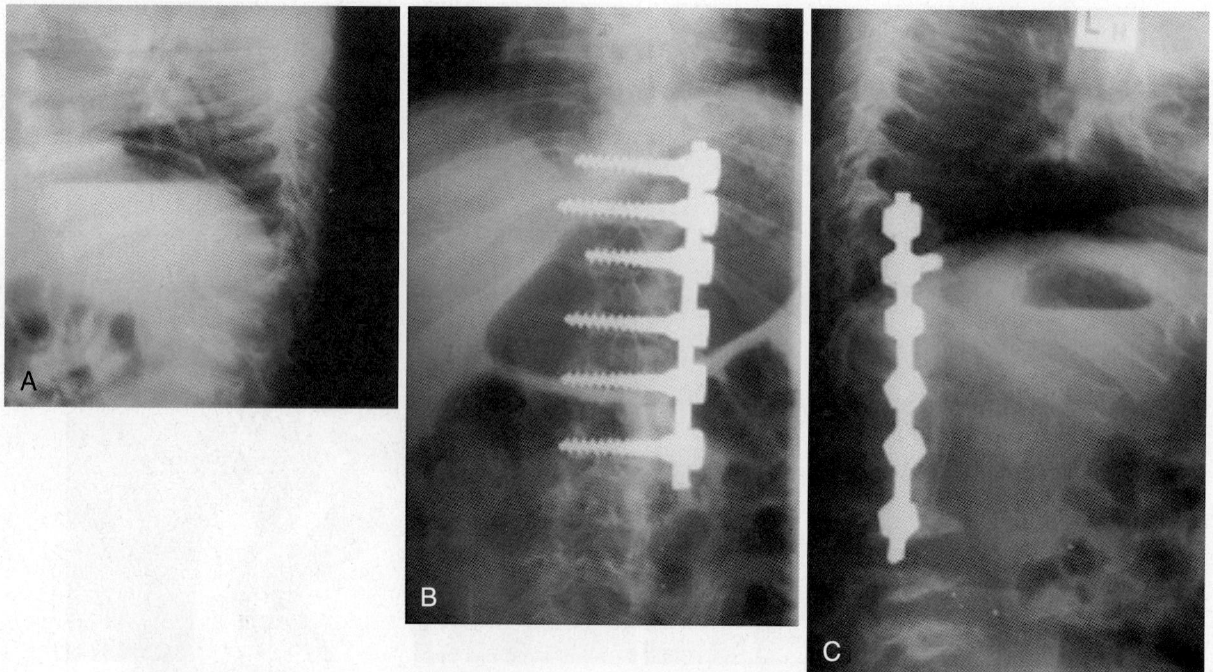

FIGURE 8.230 Anterior fusion for thoracolumbar kyphosis in mucopolysaccharidosis. **A,** Preoperative radiograph. **B,** Anteroposterior radiograph showing instrumentation in place. **C,** Radiograph at 3 years shows correction of gibbus with instrumentation and solid bony fusion. (From Dalvie SS, Noordeen MH, Vellodi A: Anterior instrumented fusion for thoracolumbar kyphosis in mucopolysaccharidosis, *Spine* 26:E539, 2001.)

REFERENCES

INFANTILE AND JUVENILE IDIOPATHIC SCOLIOSIS

Akbarnia BA: Management themes in early onset scoliosis, *J Bone Joint Surg* 89A:42, 2007.

Bess S, Akbarnia BA, Thompson GH, et al.: Complications of growing-rod treatment for early-onset scoliosis: analysis of one hundred and forty patients, *J Bone Joint Surg* 92A:2533, 2010.

Cahill PJ, Marvil S, Cuddihy L, et al.: Autofusion in the immature spine treated with growing rods, *Spine* 35:E1199, 2010.

Corona J, Sanders JO, Luhmann SJ, et al.: Reliability of radiographic measures for infantile idiopathic scoliosis, *J Bone Joint Surg* 94A:e86, 2012.

Crawford 3rd CH, Lenke LG: Growth modulation by means of anterior tethering resulting in progressive correction of juvenile idiopathic scoliosis: a case report, *J Bone Joint Surg* 92A:202, 2010.

Dede O, Demirkiran G, Bekmez S, et al.: Utilizing the "stable-to-be vertebra" saves motion segments in growing rods treatment for early-onset scoliosis, *J Pediatr Orthop* 36:336, 2016.

Flynn JM, Tomlinson LA, Pawelek J, et al.: Growing-rod graduates: lessons learned from ninety-nine patients who completed lengthening, *J Bone Joint Surg* 95A:1745, 2013.

Jain V, Lykissas M, Trobisch P, et al.: Surgical aspects of spinal growth modulation in scoliosis correction, *Instr Course Lect* 63:335, 2014.

Khoshbin A, Caspi L, Law PW, et al.: Outcomes of bracing in juvenile idiopathic scoliosis until skeletal maturity or surgery, *Spine* 40:50, 2015.

Lavelle WF, Samdani AF, Cahill PJ, Betz RR: Clinical outcomes of nitinol staples for preventing curve progression in idiopathic scoliosis, *J Pediatr Orthop* 31:S107, 2011.

McCarthy RE, Luhmann S, Lenke L, McCullough FL: The Shilla growth guidance technique for early-onset spinal deformities at 2-year follow-up: a preliminary report, *J Pediatr Orthop* 34:1, 2014.

McCarthy RE, McCullough FL: Shilla growth guidance for early-onset scoliosis: results after a minimum of five years of follow-up, *J Bone Joint Surg* 97A:1578, 2015.

Murray E, Tung R, Sherman A, et al.: Continued vertebral body growth in patients with juvenile idiopathic scoliosis following vertebral body stapling, *Spine Deform* 8:221, 2020.

Samdani AF, Ames RJ, Kimball JS, et al.: Anterior vertebral body tethering for idiopathic scoliosis: two-year results, *Spine* 39:1688, 2014.

Sankar WN, Skaggs DL, Yazici M, et al.: Lengthening of dual growing rods and the law of diminishing returns, *Spine* 36:806, 2011.

Schulz JF, Smith J, Cahill PJ, et al.: The role of the vertical expandable titanium rib in the treatment of infantile idiopathic scoliosis: early results from a single institution, *J Pediatr Orthop* 30:659, 2010.

Sucato DJ: Management of severe spinal deformity: scoliosis and kyphosis, *Spine* 35:2186, 2010.

Talmadge MS, Nielson SN, Heflin JA, et al.: Prevalance of hip dysplasia and associated conditions in children treated for idiopathic early-onset scoliosis—don't just look at the spine, *J Pediatr Orthop* 40:e49, 2020.

Yang JS, McElroy MJ, Akbarnia BA, et al.: Growing rods for spinal deformity: characterizing consensus and variation in current use, *J Pediatr Orthop* 30:264, 2010.

NATURAL HISTORY OF ADOLESCENT IDIOPATHIC SCOLIOSIS

Coillard C, Circo AB, Rivard CH: A prospective randomized controlled trial of the natural history of idiopathic scoliosis versus treatment with the SpineCor brace: sosort award 2011 winner, *Eur J Phys Rehabil Med* 50:479, 2014.

Grothaus O, Molina D, Jacobs C, et al.: Is is growth or natural history? Increasing spinal deformity after Sanders stage 7 in females with AIS, *J Pediatr Orthop* 40:e176, 2020.

Kruse LM, Buchan JG, Gurnett CA, Dobbs MB: Polygenic threshold model with sex dimorphism in adolescent idiopathic scoliosis: the Carter effect, *J Bone Joint Surg* 94A:1485, 2012.

Larson AN, Baky F, Ashraf A, et al.: Minimum of 20-year health-related quality of life and surgical rates after the treatment of adolescent idiopathic scoliosis, *Spine Deform* 7:417, 2019.

Ogilvie JW: Update on prognostic genetic testing in adolescent idiopathic scoliosis (AIS), *J Pediatr Orthop* 31(Suppl 1):S46, 2011.

Sitoula P, Verma K, Holmes Jr L, et al.: Prediction of curve progression in idiopathic scoliosis: validation of the Sanders Skeletal Maturity Staging System, *Spine* 40:1006, 2015.

Verma K, Errico T, Diefenbach C, et al.: The relative efficacy of antifibrinolytics in adolescent idiopathic scoliosis: a prospective randomized trial, *J Bone Joint Surg* 96A:e80, 2014.

Wang WJ, Yeung HY, Chu WC, et al.: Top theories for the etiopathogenesis of adolescent idiopathic scoliosis, *J Pediatr Orthop* 31(Suppl 1):S14, 2011.

Weinstein SL: The natural history of adolescent idiopathic scoliosis, *J Pediatr Orthop* 39(6 Suppl 1):S44, 2019.

PATIENT EVALUATION IN ADOLESCENT IDIOPATHIC SCOLIOSIS

Chen ZQ, Wang CF, Bai YS, et al.: Using precisely controlled bidirectional orthopedic forces to assess flexibility in adolescent idiopathic scoliosis: comparisons between push-traction film supine side bending suspension, and fulcrum bending films, *Spine* 36:1679, 2011.

Duchaussoy T, Lacoste M, Norberciak L, et al.: Preoperative assessment of idiopathic scoliosis in adolescent and young adult with three-dimensional T2-weighted spin-echo MRI, *Diagn Interv Imaging* 100:371, 2019.

Ilharreborde B, Steffen JS, Nectoux E, et al.: Angle measurement reproducibility using EOS three-dimensional reconstructions in adolescent idiopathic scoliosis treated by posterior instrumentation, *Spine* 36:E1306, 2011.

Johnston CE, Richards BS, Sucato DJ, et al.: Correlation of preoperative deformity magnitude and pulmonary function test in adolescent idiopathic scoliosis, *Spine* 36:1096, 2011.

Luk KD, Cheung WY, Wong Y, et al.: The predictive value of the fulcrum bending radiographs in spontaneous apical vertebral derotation in adolescent idiopathic scoliosis, *Spine* 37:E922, 2012.

Nault ML, Parent S, Phan P, et al.: A modified Risser grading system predicts the curve acceleration phase of female adolescent idiopathic scoliosis, *J Bone Joint Surg* 92A:1073, 2010.

NONOPERATIVE MANAGEMENT OF IDIOPATHIC SCOLIOSIS

Cheung JPY, Cheung PWH, Luk KDK: When should we wean bracing for adolescent idiopathic scoliosis? *Clin Orthop Relat Res* 477:2145, 2019.

Gammon SR, Mehlman CT, Chan W, et al.: A comparison of thoracolumbar orthoses and SpineCor treatment of adolescent idiopathic scoliosis patients using the Scoliosis Research Society standardized criteria, *J Pediatr Orthop* 30:531, 2010.

Guo J, Lam TP, Wong MS, et al.: A prospective randomized controlled study on the treatment outcome of SpineCor brace versus rigid brace for adolescent idiopathic scoliosis with follow-up according to the SRS standardized criteria, *Eur Spine J* 23:2650, 2014.

Gutman G, Benoit M, Joncas J, et al.: The effectiveness of the SpineCor brace for the conservative treatment of adolescent idiopathic scoliosis: comparison with the Boston brace, *Spine J* 16:626, 2016.

Harfouch BF, Weinstein SL: Intraoperative push-prone test: a useful technique to determine the lowest instrumented vertebra in adolescent idiopathic scoliosis, *J Spinal Disord Tech* 27:237, 2014.

Hawary RE, Zaaroor-Regev D, Floman Y, et al.: Brace treatment in adolescent idiopathic scoliosis: risk factors for failure—a literature review, *Spine J* 19:1917, 2019.

Katz DE, Herring JA, Browne RH, et al.: Brace wear control of curve progression in adolescent idiopathic scoliosis, *J Bone Joint Surg* 92A:1343, 2010.

Ohashi M, Watanabe K, Hirano T, et al.: Long-term impacts of brace treatment for adolescent idiopathic scoliosis on body composition, paraspinal muscle morphology, and bone mineral density, *Spine (Phil Pa 1976)* 44:E1075, 2019.

Ohrt-Nissen S, Hallager DW, Gehrchen M, Dahl B: Flexibility predicts curve progression in Providence nighttime bracing of patients with adolescent idiopathic scoliosis, *Spine (Phil Pa 1976)* 41:1724, 2016.

Pellios S, Kenanidis E, Potoupnis M, et al.: Curve progression 25 years after bracing for adolescent idiopathic scoliosis: long term comparative results between two matched groups of 18 versus 23 hours daily bracing, *Scoliosis Spinal Disord* 11:3, 2016.

Sponseller PD: Bracing for adolescent idiopathic scoliosis in practice today, *J Pediatr Orthop* 31(Suppl 1):S53, 2011.

Sponseller PD, Takenaga R: The use of traction in treating large scoliotic curves in idiopathic scoliosis. In Newton PO, O'Brien MF, Shufflebarger HL, et al., editors: *Idiopathic scoliosis: the Harms Study Group treatment guide*, New York, 2010, Thieme.

Watanabe K, Ohashi M, Hirano T, et al.: Health-related quality of life in non-operated patients with adolescent idiopathic scoliosis in the middle years: a mean 25-year follow-up study, *Spine (Phila Pa 1976)* 2019, [Epub ahead of print].

Weinstein SL, Dolan LA, Wright JG, Dobbs MB: Effects of bracing in adolescents with idiopathic scoliosis, *N Engl J Med* 369:1512, 2013.

OPERATIVE TREATMENT OF IDIOPATHIC SCOLIOSIS

Alzakri A, Vergari C, Van den Abbeele M, et al.: Global sagittal alignment and proximal junctional kyphosis in adolescent idiopathic scoliosis, *Spine Deform* 7:236, 2019.

Betz RR, Ranade A, Samdani AF, et al.: Vertebral body stapling: a fusionless treatment option for a growing child with moderate idiopathic scoliosis, *Spine* 35:169, 2010.

Baky FJ, Milbrandt T, Echternacht S, et al.: Intraoperative computed tomography-guided navigation for pediatric spine patients reduced return to operating room for screw malposition compared with freehand/fluoroscopic techniques, *Spine Deform* 7:577, 2019.

Bogunovic L, Lenke LG, Bridwell KH, et al.: Preoperative halo-gravity traction for severe pediatric spinal deformity: complications, radiographic correction and changes in pulmonary function, *Spine Deform* 1:33, 2013.

Buckland AJ, Moon JY, Betz RR, et al.: Ponte osteotomies increase the risk of neuromonitoring alerts in adolescent idiopathic scoliosis correction surgery, *Spine (Phila Pa 1976)* 44:E175, 2019.

Burton DC, Carlson BB, Place HM, et al.: Results of the scoliosis research society morbidity and mortality database 2009-2012: a report from the morbidity and mortality committee, *Spine Deform* 4:338, 2016.

Cahill PJ, Marvil SC, Cuddihy L, et al.: Autofusion of the skeletally immature spine treated with growing rod instrumentation, *Spine* 35:E1199, 2010.

Carlson BC, Milbrandt TA, Larson AN: Quality, safety and value in pediatric spine surgery, *Orthop Clin North America* 49:491, 2018.

de Kleuver M, Lewis SJ, Germscheid NM, et al.: Optimal surgical care for adolescent idiopathic scoliosis: an international consensus, *Eur Spine J* 23:2603, 2014.

de Mendonca RG, Sawyer JR, Kelly DM: Complications after surgical treatment of adolescent idiopathic scoliosis, *Orthop Clin North Am* 47:395, 2016.

Diab MG, Franzone JM, Vitale MG: The role of posterior spinal osteotomies in pediatric spinal deformity surgery: indications and operative treatment, *J Pediatr Orthop* 31:S88, 2011.

Diab M, Landman Z, Lubicky J, et al.: Use and outcome of MRI in the surgical treatment of adolescent idiopathic scoliosis, *Spine* 36:667, 2011.

Direito-Santos B, Queirós CM, Serrano P, et al.: Long-term follow-up of anterior spinal fusion for thoracolumbar/lumbar curves in adolescent idiopathic scoliosis, *Spine (Phila Pa 1976)* 44:1137, 2019.

Fletcher ND, Andras LM, Lazarus DE, et al.: Use of a novel pathway for early discharge was associated with a 48% shorter length of stay after posterior spinal fusion for adolescent idiopathic scoliosis, *J Pediatr Orthop* 37:92, 2017.

Fletcher ND, Shourbaji N, Mitchell PM, et al.: Clinical and economic implications of early discharge following posterior spinal fusion for adolescent idiopathic scoliosis, *J Child Orthop* 8:257, 2014.

Glotzbecker M, Troy M, Miller P, et al.: Implementing a multidisciplinary clinical pathway can reduce the deep surgical site infection rate after posterior spinal fusion in high-risk patients, *Spine Deform* 7:33, 2019.

Glotzbecker MP, Gomez JA, Miller PE, et al.: Management of spinal implants in acute pediatric surgical site infections: a multicenter study, *Spine Deform* 4:277, 2016.

Glotzbecker MP, St Hilaire TA, Pawelek JB, et al.: Best practice guidelines for surgical site infection prevention with surgical treatment of early onset scoliosis, *J Pediatr Orthop* 39, 2019:e602.

Helenius L, Diarbakerli E, Grauers A, et al.: Back pain and quality of life after surgicala treatment for adolescent idiopathic scoliosis at 5-year follow-up: comparison with healthy controls and patients with untreated idiopathic scoliosis, *J Bone Joint Surg Am* 101:1460, 2019.

Jain V, Kykissas M, Trobisch P, et al.: Surgical aspects of spinal growth modulation in scoliosis correction, *Instr Course Lect* 63:335, 2014.

Karol LA: Early definitive spinal fusion in young children: what we have learned, *Clin Orthop Relat Res* 469:1323, 2011.

Lam DJ, Lee JZ, Chua JH, et al.: Superior mesenteric artery syndrome following surgery for adolescent idiopathic scoliosis: a case series, review of the literature, and algorithm for management, *J Pediatr Orthop B* 23:312, 2014.

Larson AN, Polly Jr DW, Diamond B, et al.: Does higher anchor density result in increased curve correction and improved clinical outcomes in adolescent idiopathic scoliosis (AIS)? *Spine (Phila Pa 1976)* 39:571, 2014.

Letko L, Jensen RG, Harms J: The treatment of rigid idiopathic scoliosis: releases, osteotomies, and apical vertebral column resection. In Newton PO, O'Brien MF, Shufflebarger HL, et al., editors: *Idiopathic scoliosis: the harms study group treatment guide*, New York, 2010, Thieme.

Lonner BS, Ren Y, Asghar J, et al.: Antifibrinolytic therapy in surgery for adolescent idiopathic scoliosis: does Level 1 evidence translate into practice? *Bull Hosp Jt Dis* 76:165, 2013.

Lonner BS, Ren Y, Newton PO, et al.: Risk factors of proximal junctional kyphosis in adolescent idiopathic scoliosis-the pelvis and other considerations, *Spine Deform* 5:181, 2017.

Lonner BS, Toombs C, Parent S, et al.: Is anterior release obsolete or does it play a role in contemporary adolescent idiopathic scoliosis surgery? A matched pair analysis, *Pediatr Orthop*, 2019, [Epub ahead of print].

Marks MC, Newton PO, Bastrom TP, et al.: Surgical site infection in adolescent idiopathic scoliosis surgery, *Spine Deform* 1:352, 2013.

McCarthy KP, Chafetz RS, Mulcahey MJ, et al.: Clinical efficacy of the vertebral wedge osteotomy for the fusionless treatment of paralytic scoliosis, *Spine* 35:403, 2010.

McCarthy RE, Sucato D, Turner JL, et al.: Shilla growing rods in a caprine animal model: a pilot study, *Clin Orthop Relat Res* 468:705, 2010.

McNichol ED, Tzortzopoulou A, Schumann R, et al.: Antifibrinolytic agents in reducing blood loss in scoliosis surgery in children, *Cochrane Database Syst Rev* 19(9):CD006883, 2016.

Newton PO, Bastrom TP, Yaszay B: Patient-specific risk adjustment improves comparison of infection rates following posterior fusion for adolescent idiopathic scoliosis, *J Bone Joint J Am* 99:1846, 2017.

Newton PO, Upasani VV: Surgical treatment of the right thoracic curve pattern. In Newton PO, O'Brien MF, Shufflebarger HL, et al, editors: *Idiopathic scoliosis: the harms study group treatment guide*, New York, 2010, Thieme.

Powers AK, O'Shaughnessy BA, Lemke LG: Posterior thoracic vertebral column resection. In Wang JC, editor: *advanced reconstruction: spine*, Rosemont, IL, 2011, American Academy of Orthopaedic Surgeons, p 265.

Pugely AJ, Martin CT, Gao Y, et al.: The incidence and risk factors for short-term morbidity and mortality in pediatric deformity spinal surgery: an analysis of the NSQIP pediatric database, *Spine (Phila Pa 1976)* 39:1225, 2014.

Ramo B, Tran DP, Reddy A, et al.: Delay to surgery greater than 6 months leads to substantial deformity progression and increased intervention in immature adolescent idiopathic scoliosis (AIS) patients: a retrospective cohort study, *Spine Deform* 7:428, 2019.

Ramo BA, Richards BS: Repeat surgical interventions following "definitive" instrumentation and fusion for idiopathic scoliosis: five-year update on a previously published cohort, *Spine (Phila Pa 1976)* 37:1211, 2012.

Samdani AF, Belin EJ, Bennett JT, et al.: Unplanned return to the operating room in patients with adolescent idiopathic scoliosis: are we doing better with pedicle screws? *Spine (Phila Pa 1976)* 38:1842, 2013.

Sankar WN, Skaggs DL: Rib anchors in distraction-based growing spine implants. In Wang JC, editor: *Advanced reconstruction: spine*, Rosemont, IL, 2011, American Academy of Orthopaedic Surgeons.

Schulz JF, Smith J, Cahill P, et al.: The role of the vertical expandable titanium rib in the treatment of infantile idiopathic scoliosis: early results from a single institution, *J Pediatr Orthop* 30:659, 2010.

Smith JT: Bilateral rib-to-pelvis technique for managing early-onset scoliosis, *Clin Orthop Relat Res* 469:1349, 2011.

Sponseller PD, Jain A, Newton PO, et al.: Posterior spinal fusion with pedicle screws in patients with idiopathic scoliosis and open triradiate cartilage: does deformity progression occur? *J Pediatr Orthop* 36:695, 2016.

Sui WY, Ye F, Yang JL: Efficacy of tranexamic acid in reducing allogeneic blood products in adolescent idiopathic scoliosis surgery, *BMC Musculoskelet Disord* 17:187, 2016.

Tao F, Zhao Y, Wu Y, et al.: The effect of differing spinal fusion instrumentation on the occurrence of postoperative crankshaft phenomenon in adolescent idiopathic scoliosis, *J Spinal Disord Tech* 23:e75, 2010.

Trobisch PD, Ducoffe AR, Lonner BS, Errico TJ: Choosing fusion levels in adolescent idiopathic scoliosis, *J Am Acad Orthop Surg* 21:519, 2013.

Vitale MG, Moore DW, Matsumoto H, et al.: Risk factors for spinal cord injury during surgery for spinal deformity, *J Bone Joint Surg Am* 92:64, 2010.

White KK, Song KM, Frost N, Daines BK: VEPTR™ growing rods for early-onset neuromuscular scoliosis: feasible and effective, *Clin Orthop Relat Res* 469:1335, 2011.

NEUROMUSCULAR SCOLIOSIS (GENERAL)

Blumstein GW, Andras LM, Seehausen DA, et al.: Fever is common postoperatively following posterior spinal fusion: infection is an uncommon cause, *J Pediatr* 166:751, 2015.

Brooks JT: Sponseller PD: What's new in the management of neuromuscular scoliosis, *J Pediatr Orthop* 36:627, 2016.

Funk S, Lovejoy S, Mencio G, Martus J: Rigid instrumentation for neuromuscular scoliosis improves deformity correction without increasing complications, *Spine* 41:46, 2016.

Khirani S, Bersanini C, Aubertin G, et al.: Non-invasive positive pressure ventilation to facilitate the postoperative respiratory outcome of spine surgery in neuromuscular children, *Eur Spine J* 23(Suppl 4):S406, 2014.

LaMothe JM, Al Sayegh S, Parsons DL, et al.: The use of intraoperative traction in pediatric scoliosis surgery: a systematic review, *Spine Deform* 3:45, 2015.

Myung KS, Lee C, Skaggs DL: Early pelvic fixation failure in neuromuscular scoliosis, *J Pediatr Orthop* 35:258, 2015.

Patel J, Shapiro F: Simultaneous progression patterns of scoliosis, pelvic obliquity, and hip subluxation/dislocation in non-ambulatory neuromuscular patients: an approach to deformity documentation, *J Child Orthop* 9:345, 2015.

Salem KM, Goodger L, Bowyer K, et al.: Does transcranial stimulation for motor evoked potentials (TcMEP) worsen seizures in epileptic patients following spinal deformity surgery? *Eur Spine J* 25:3044, 2016.

Schwartz DM, Sestokas AK, Dormans JP, et al.: Transcranial electric motor evoked potential monitoring during spine surgery: is it safe? *Spine* 36:1046, 2011.

Shao ZX, Fang X, Lv QB, et al.: Comparison of combined anterior-posterior approach versus posterior-only approach in neuromuscular scoliosis: a systematic review and meta-analysis, *Eur Spine J* 27:2213, 2018.

Shirley E, Bejarano C, Clay C, et al.: Helping families make difficult choices: creation and implementation of a decision aid for neuromuscular scoliosis surgery, *J Pediatr Orthop* 35:831, 2015.

Sponseller PD, Zimmerman RM, Ko PS, et al.: Low-profile pelvic fixation with the sacral alar iliac technique in the pediatric population improves results at two-year minimum follow-up, *Spine* 35:1887, 2010.

Ward JP, Feldman DS, Paul J, et al.: Wound closure in nonidiopathic scoliosis: Does closure matter? *J Pediatr Orthop* 37:166, 2017.

White KK, Song KM, Frost N, Daines BK: VEPTR growing rods for early-onset neuromuscular scoliosis: feasible and effective, *Clin Orthop Relat Res* 469:1335, 2011.

CEREBRAL PALSY

Beckmann K, Lange T, Gosheger G, et al.: Surgical correction of scoliosis in patients with severe cerebral palsy, *Eur Spine J* 25:506, 2016.

Chong HS, Padua MR, Kim JS, et al.: Usefulness of noninvasive positive-pressure ventilation during surgery of flaccid neuromuscular scoliosis, *J Spinal Disord Tech* 28:298, 2015.

Crawford L, Herrera-Soto J, Ruder JA, et al.: The fate of the neuromuscular hip after spinal fusion, *J Pediatr Orthop* 37:403, 2017.

Dhawale AA, Shah SA, Sponseller PD, et al.: Are antifibrinolytics helpful in decreasing blood loss and transfusions during spinal fusion surgey in children with cerebral palsy scoliosis? *Spine* 37:E549, 2012.

Funk S, Lovejoy S, Mencio G, et al.: Rigid Instrumentation for neuromuscular scoliosis improves deformity correction without increasing complications, *Spine (Phila Pa 1976)* 41:46, 2016.

Hollenbeck SM, Yaszay B, Sponseller PD, et al.: The pros and cons of operating early versus late in the progression of cerebral palsy scoliosis, *Spine Deform* 7:489, 2019.

Jackson TJ, Yaszay B, Pahys JM, et al.: Intraoperative traction may be a viable alternative to anterior surgery in cerebral palsy scoliosis ≥100 degrees, *J Pediatr Orthop* 38:e278, 2018.

Ko PS, Jameson 2nd PG, Chang TL, Sponseller PD: Transverse-plane pelvic asymmetry in patients with cerebral palsy and scoliosis, *J Pediatr Orthop* 31:277, 2011.

McElroy MJ, Sponseller PD, Dattilo JR, et al.: Growing rods for the treatment of scoliosis in children with cerebral palsy: a critical assessment, *Spine* 37:E1504, 2012.

Miller DJ, Flynn JJM, Pasha S, et al.: Improving health-related quality of life for patients With nonambulatory cerebral palsy: who stands to gain from scoliosis surgery?, *J Pediatr Orthop*, 2019, [Epub ahead of print].

Ramchandran S, George S, Asghar J, et al.: Anatomic trajectory for iliac screw placement in pediatric scoliosis and spondylolisthesis: an alternative to S2-alar iliac portal, *Spine Deform* 7:286, 2019.

Shabtai L, Andras LM, Portman M, et al.: Sacral alar iliac (SAI) screws fail 75% less frequently than iliac screws in neuromuscular scoliosis, *J Pediatr Orthop* 37, 2017:e470.

Shrader MW, Andrisevic EM, Belthur MV, et al.: Inter- and intraobserver reliability of pelvic obliquity measurement methods in patients with cerebral palsy, *Spine Deform* 6:257, 2018.

Takaso M, Nakazawa T, Imura T, et al.: Segmental pedicle screw instrumentation and fusion only to L5 in the surgical treatment of flaccid neuromuscular scoliosis, *Spine (Phila Pa 1976)* 43:331, 2018.

Toovey R, Harvey A, Johnson M, et al.: Outcomes after scoliosis surgery for children with cerebral palsy: a systematic review, *Dev Med Child Neurol* 59:690, 2017.

Yousef MAA, Dranginis D, Rosenfeld S: Incidence and diagnostic evaluation of postoperative fever in pediatric patients with neuromuscular disorders, *J Pediatr Orthop* 38:e104, 2018.

INHERITABLE NEUROLOGIC DISORDERS—NEUROFIBROMATOSIS

Abdulian MH, Liu RW, Son-Hing JP, et al.: Double rib penetration of the spinal canal in a patients with neurofibromatosis, *J Pediatr Orthop* 31:6, 2011.

Carbone M, Vittoria F, Del Sal A: Treatment of early-onset scoliosis with growing rods in patients with neurofibromatosis-1, *J Pediatr Orthop B* 28:278, 2019.

Deng A, Zhang HQ, Tang MX, Liu SH, et al.: Posterior-only surgical correction of dystrophic scoliosis in 31 patients with neurofibromatosis Type 1 using the multiple anchor point method, *J Neurosurg Pediatr* 19:96, 2017.

Feldman DS, Jordan C, Fonesca L: Orthopaedic manifestation of neurofibromatosis type I, *J Am Acad Orthop Surg* 18:346, 2010.

Heflin JA, Cleveland A, Ford SD, et al.: Use of rib-based distraction in the treatment of early-onset scoliosis associated with neurofibromatosis type 1 in the young child, *Spine Deform* 3:239, 2015.

Jain VV, Berry CA, Crawford AH, et al.: Growing rods are an effective fusionless method of controlling early-onset scoliosis associated with neurofibromatosis type 1 (NF1): a multicenter retrospective case series, *J Pediatr Orthop* 37, 2017:e612.

Lykissas MG, Schorry EK, Crawford AH, et al.: Does the presence of dystrophic features in patients with type 1 neurofibromatosis and spine deformities increase the risk of surgery? *Spine* 38:1595, 2013.

Mao S, Shi B, Wang S, et al.: Migration of the penetrated rib head following deformity correction surgery without rib head excision in dystrophic scoliosis secondary to type 1 neurofibromatosis, *Eur Spine J* 24:1502, 2015.

Tauchi R, Kawakami N, Castro MA, et al.: Long-term surgical outcomes after early defnitive spinal fusion for early-onset scoliosis with neurofibromatosis type 1 at a mean follow-up of 14 years, *J Pediatr Orthop* 40:42, 2020.

Tsirikos AL, Smith G: Scoliosis in patients with Friedreich's ataxia, *J Bone Joint Surg* 94B:684, 2012.

Xu E, Gao R, Jiang H, et al.: Combined halo gravity traction and dual rod technique for the treatment of early onset dystrophic scoliosis in neurofibromatosis type 1, *World Neurosurg* 126:e173, 2019.

Yao Z, Li H, Zhang X, et al.: Incidence and risk factors for instrumentation-related complications after scoliosis surgery in pediatric patients with NF-1, *Spine (Phila Pa 1976)* 43:1719, 2018.

SPINAL MUSCULAR ATROPHY

Bekmez S, Dede O, Yataganbaba A, et al.: Early results of a management algorithm for collapsing spine deformity in young children (below 10-year old) with spinal muscular atrophy type II, *J Pediatr Orthop*, 2019, [Epub ahead of print].

Holt JB, Dolan LA, Weinstein SL: Outcomes of primary posterior spinal fusion for scoliosis in spinal muscular atrophy: clinical, radiographic, and pulmonary outcomes and complications, *J Pediatr Orthop* 37:e505, 2017.

Labianca L, Weinstein S: Scoliosis and spinal muscular atrophy in the new world of medical therapy: providing lumbar access for intrathecal treatment in patients previously treated or undergoing spinal instrumentation and fusion, *J Pediatr Orthop B* 28:393, 2019.

Lenhart RL, Youlo S, Schroth MK, et al.: Radiographic and respiratory effects of growing rods in children with spinal muscular atrophy, *J Pediatr Orthop* 37, 2017:e500.

Lorenz HM, Badwan B, Hecker MM, et al.: Magnetically controlled devices parallel to the spine in children with spinal muscular atrophy, *JB JS Open Access* 2:e0036, 2017.

McElroy MJ, Shaner AC, Crawford TO, et al.: Growing rods for scoliosis in spinal muscular atrophy: structural effects, complications, and hospital stays, *Spine* 36:1305, 2011.

Rosenfeld S, Schlechter J, Smith B: Achievement of guided growth in children with low-tone neuromuscular early-onset scoliosis using a segmental sublaminar instrumentation technique, *Spine Deform* 6:607, 2018.

Strauss KA, Carson VJ, Brigatti KW, et al.: Preliminary safety and tolerability of a novel subcutaneous intrathecal catheter system for repeated outpatient dosing of nusinersen to children and adults with spinal muscular atrophy, *J Pediatr Orthop* 38, 2018:e610.

Wijngaarde CA, Brink RC, de Kort FAS, et al.: Natural course of scoliosis and lifetime risk of scoliosis surgery in spinal muscular atrophy, *Neurology* 93:e149, 2019.

SYRINGOMYELIA

Godzik J, Holekamp TF, Limbrick DD, et al.: Risks and outcomes of spinal deformity surgery in Chiari malformation, type 1, with syringomyelia versus adolescent idiopathic scoliosis, *Spine J* 15:2015, 2002.

Li Z, Lei F, Xiu P, et al.: Surgical treatment for severe and rigid scoliosis: a case-matched study between idiopathic scoliosis and syringomyelia-associated scoliosis, *Spine J* 19:87, 2019.

Sha S, Qiu Y, Sun W, et al.: Does surgical correction of right thoracic scoliosis in syringomyelia produce outcomes similar to those in adolescent idiopathic scoliosis? *J Bone Joint Surg* 98A:295, 2016.

Shen J, Tan H, Chen C, et al.: Comparison of radiological features and clinical characteristics in scoliosis patients with Chiari I malformation and idiopathic syringomyelia: a matched study, *Spine (Phila Pa 1976)* 44:1653, 2019.

Strahle J, Smith BW, Martinez M, et al.: The association between Chiari malformation type I, spinal syrinx, and scoliosis, *J Neurosurg Pediatr* 15:607, 2015.

Zebala LP, Bridwell KH, Baldus C, et al.: Minimum 5-year radiographic results of long scoliosis fusion in juvenile spinal muscular atrophy patients: major curve progression after instrumented fusion, *J Pediatr Orthop* 31:480, 2011.

Zhang ZX, Feng DX, Li P, et al.: Surgical treatment of scoliosis associated with syringomyelia with no or minor neurologic symptoms, *Eur Spine J* 24:1555, 2015.

ARTHROGRYPOSIS MULTIPLEX CONGENITA

Astur N, Flynn JM, Flynn JM, et al.: The efficacy of rib-based distraction with VEPTR in the treatment of early-onset scoliosis in patients with arthrogryposis, *J Pediatr Orthop* 34:8, 2014.

Greggo T, Martikos K, Pipitone E, et al.: Surgical treatment of scoliosis in a rare disease: arthrogryposis, *Scoliosis* 5:24, 2010.

Komolkin I, Ulrich EV, Agranovice OE, et al.: Treatment of scoliosis associated with arthrogryposis multiplex congenital, *J Pediatr Orthop* 37(Suppl 1):S24, 2017.

Li Y, Sheng F, Xia C, et al.: Risk factors of impaired pulmonary function in arthrogryposis multiplex congenital patients with concomitant scoliosis: a comparison with adolescent idiopathic scoliosis, *Spine (Phila Pa 1976)* 43:E456, 2018.

Xu L, Chen Z, Qui Y, et al.: Case-matched comparative analysis of spinal deformity correction in arthrogryposis multiplex congenital versus adolescent idiopathic scoliosis, *J Neurosurg Pediatr* 23:22, 2018.

DUCHENNE MUSCULAR DYSTROPHY

Archer JE, Gardner AC, Roper HP, et al.: Duchenne muscular dystrophy: the management of scoliosis, *J Spine Surg* 2:185, 2019.

Cheuk DK, Wong V, Wraige E, et al.: Surgery for scoliosis in Duchenne muscular dystrophy, *Cochrane Database Syst Rev* (10):CD005375, 2015.

Choi YA, Shin HI, Shin HI: Scoliosis in Duchenne muscular dystrophy children is fully reducible in the initial stage, and becomes structural over time, *BMC Musculoskelet Disord* 20:277, 2019.

Chua K, Tan CY, Chen Z, et al.: Long-term follow-up of pulmonary function and scoliosis in patients with Duchenne's muscular dystrophy and spinal muscular atrophy, *J Pediatr Orthop* 36:63, 2016.

Garg S: Management of scoliosis in patients with Duchenne muscular dystrophy and spinal muscular atrophy: a literature review, *J Pediatr Rehabil Med* 9:23, 2016.

Lebel DE, Corston JA, McAdam LC, et al.: Glucocorticoid treatment for the prevention of scoliosis in children with Duchenne muscular dystrophy: long-term follow-up, *J Bone Joint Surg* 95A:1057, 2013.

Lee MC, Jarvis C, Solomito MJ, et al.: Comparison of S2-Alar and traditional iliac screw pelvic fixation for pediatric neuromuscular deformity, *Spine J* 18:648, 2018.

Raudenbush BL, Thirukumaran CP, Li Y, et al.: Impact of a comparative study on the management of scoliosis in Duchenne muscular dystrophy: are corticosteroids decreasing the rate of scoliosis surgery in the United States? *Spine* 41:E1030, 2016.

Scannell BP, Yaszay B, Bartley CE, et al.: Surgical correction of scoliosis in patients with Duchenne muscular dystrophy: 30-year experience, *J Pediatr Orthop* 37:e469, 2017.

Suk KS, Lee BH, Lee HM, et al.: Functional outcomes in Duchenne muscular dystrophy scoliosis: comparison of the differences between surgical and nonsurgical treatment, *J Bone Joint Surg* 96A:409, 2014.

CONGENITAL SCOLIOSIS

Ayvaz M, Akalan N, Yazici M, et al.: Is it necessary to operate all split cord malformations before corrective surgery for patients with congenital spinal deformities? *Spine (Phila Pa 1976)* 34:2413, 2009.

Chang DG, Kim JH, Ha KY, et al.: Posterior hemivertebra resection and short segment fusion with pedicle screw fixation for congenital scoliosis in children younger than 10 years: greater than 7-year follow-up, *Spine* 40:484, 2015.

Chang DG, Suk SI, Kim JH, et al.: Surgical outcomes by the age at the time of surgery in the treatment of congenital scoliosis in children under age 10 years, *Spine J* 15:1783, 2015.

Demirkiran HG, Bekmez S, Celilov R, et al.: Serial derotational casting in congenital scoliosis as a time-buying strategy, *J Pediatr Orthop* 35:43, 2015.

Feng F, Shen J, Zhang J, et al.: Characteristics and clinical relevance of the osseous spur in patients with congenital scoliosis and split spinal cord malformation, *J Bone Joint Surg Am* 98:2096, 2016.

Flynn JM, Emans JB, Smith JT, et al.: VEPTR to treat nonsyndromic congenital scoliosis: a multicenter, mid-term follow-up study, *J Pediatr Orthop* 33:679, 2013.

Furdock R, Brouillet K, Luhmann SJ: Organ system anomalies associated with congenital scoliosis: a retrospective study of 305 patients, *J Pediatr Orthop* 39, 2019:e190.

Imrie MN: A "simple" option in the surgical treatment of congenital scoliosis, *Spine J* 11:119, 2011.

Jalanko T, Rintala R, Puisto V, Helenius I: Hemivertebra resection for congenital scoliosis in young children, *Spine* 36:41, 2011.

Karaarslan UC, Gurel IE, Yucekul A, et al.: Team approach: contemporary treatment of congenital scoliosis, *JBJS Rev* 7:e5, 2019.

Li XF, Liu ZD, Hu GY, et al.: Posterior unilateral pedicle subtraction osteotomy of hemivertebra for correction of the adolescent congenital spinal deformity, *Spine J* 11:111, 2011.

Lonstein JE: Long-term outcome of early fusions for congenital scoliosis, *Spine Deform* 6:552, 2018.

Louis ML, Gennari JM, Loundou AD, et al.: Congenital scoliosis: a frontal plane evaluation of 251 operated patients 14 years old or older at follow-up, *Orthop Traumatol Surg Res* 96:741, 2010.

McMaster MJ, McMaster ME: Prognosis for congenital scoliosis due to a unilateral failure of vertebral segmentation, *J Bone Joint Surg* 95A:972, 2013.

Murphy RF, Moisan A, Kelly DM, et al.: Use of vertical expandable prosthetic titanium rib (VEPTR) in the treatment of congenital scoliosis without fused ribs, *J Pediatr Orthop* 36:329, 2016.

Pahys JM, Guille JT: What's new in congenital scoliosis? *J Pediatr Orthop* 38:e172, 2018.

Passias PG, Poorman GW, Jalai CM, et al.: Incidence of congenital spinal abnormalities among pediatric patients and their association with scoliosis and systemic anomalies, *J Pediatr Orthop* 39:e608, 2019.

Shen J, Wang Z, Liu J, et al.: Abnormalities associated with congenital scoliosis: a retrospective study of 226 Chinese surgical cases, *Spine* 38:814, 2013.

Shen J, Zhang J, Feng F, et al.: Corrective surgery for congenital scoliosis associated with split cord malformation: It may be safe to leave diastematomyelia untreated in patients with intact or stable neurological status, *J Bone Joint Surg Am* 98:926, 2016.

Wang S, Zhang J, Qiu G, et al.: Dual growing rods technique for congential scoliosis: more than 2 years outcomes: preliminary results of a single center, *Spine* 37:E1639, 2012.

Yaszay B, O'Brien M, Shufflebarger HL, et al.: Efficacy of hemivertebra resection for congenital scoliosis: a multicenter retrospective comparison of three surgical techniques, *Spine* 36:2052, 2011.

KYPHOSIS

SCHEUERMANN DISEASE

Abul-Kasim K, Schlenzka D, Selariu E, Ohlin A: Spinal epidural lipomatosis: a common imaging feature in Scheuermann disease, *J Spinal Disord Tech* 25:356, 2012.

Cho W, Lenke LG, Bridwell KH, et al.: The prevalence of abnormal preoperative neurological examination in Scheuermann kyphosis: correlation with X-ray, magnetic resonance imaging, and surgical outcome, *Spine* 39:1771, 2014.

Makurthou AA, Oei L, El Saddy S, et al.: Scheuermann disease: evaluation of radiological criteria and population prevalence, *Spine* 38:1690, 2013.

Polly Jr DW, Ledonio CGT, Diamond B, et al.: What are the indications for spinal fusion surgery in Scheuermann kyphosis, *J Pediatr Orthop* 39:217, 2019.

Toombs C, Lonner B, Shah S, et al.: Quality of life improvement following surgery in adolescent spinal deformity patients: a comparison between Scheuermann kyphosis and adolescent idiopathic scoliosis, *Spine Deform* 6:676, 2018.

Tsirikos AI, Jain AK: Scheuermann's kyphosis: current controversies, *J Bone Joint Surg* 93B:857, 2011.

Wood KB, Melikian R, Villamil F: Adult Scheuermann kyphosis: evaluation, management, and new developments, *J Am Acad Orthop Surg* 20:113, 2012.

Zeng Y, Chen Z, Qi Q, et al.: The posterior surgical correction of congenital kyphosis and kyphoscoliosis: 23 cases with minimum 2 years follow-up, *Eur Spine J* 22:372, 2013.

CONGENITAL KYPHOSIS

Alyvaz M, Olgun ZD, Demirkiran HG, et al.: Posterior all-pedicle screw instrumentation combined with multiple chevron and concave rib osteotomies in the treatment of adolescent congenital kyphoscoliosis, *Spine J* 14:11, 2014.

Atici Y, Sököcü S, Uzümcügil O, et al.: The results of closing wedge osteotomy with posterior instrumented fusion for the surgical treatment of congenital kyphosis, *Eur Spine J* 22:1368, 2013.

Demirkiran G, Dede O, Karadeniz E, et al.: Anterior and posterior vertebral column resection versus posterior-only technique: a comparison of clinical outcomes and complications in congenital kyphoscoliosis, *Clin Spine Surg* 30:285, 2017.

Hansen-Algenstaedt N, Gessler R, Goepfert M, Knight R: Percutaneous three column osteotomy for kyphotic deformity correction in congenital kyphosis, *Eur Spine J* 22:2139, 2013.

Helgeson MD, Shah SA, Newton PO, et al.: Evaluation of proximal junctional kyphosis in adolescent idiopathic scoliosis following pedicle screw, hook, or hybrid instrumentation, *Spine* 35:177, 2010.

McMaster MJ: Congenital kyphosis. In Bridwell KH, DeWald RL, editors: *The textbook of spinal surgery*, ed 3, Philadelphia, 2011, Wolters Kluwer/ Lippincott-Raven.

Reinker K, Simmons JW, Patil V, Stinson Z: Can VEPTR® control progression of early-onset kyphoscoliosis? A cohort study of VEPTR® patients with severe kyphoscoliosis, *Clin Orthop Relat Res* 469:1342, 2011.

Spiro AS, Rupprecht M, Stenger P, et al.: Surgical treatment of severe congenital thoracolumbar kyphosis through a single posterior approach, *Bone Joint J* 95:1527, 2013.

Tsirikos AI, McMaster MJ: Infantile developmental thoracolumbar kyphosis with segmental subluxation of the spine, *J Bone Joint Surg* 92B:40, 2010.

Zeng Y, Chen Z, Qi Q, et al.: The posterior surgical correction of congenital kyphosis and kyphoscoliosis: 23 cases with minimum 2 years follow-up, *Eur Spine J* 22:372, 2013.

PROGRESSIVE ANTERIOR VERTEBRAL FUSION

Bollini G, Guillaume JM, Launay F, et al.: Progressive anterior vertebral bars: a study of 16 cases, *Spine* 36:E423, 2011.

SPONDYLOLYSIS AND SPONDYLOLISTHESIS

Altaf F, Osei NA, Garrido E, et al.: Repair of spondylolysis using compression with a modular link and screws, *J Bone Joint Surg* 93B:73, 2011.

Beck NA, Miller R, Baldwin K, et al.: Do oblique views add value in the diagnosis of spondylolysis in adolescents? *J Bone Joint Surg* 95A:e65, 2013.

Bourassa-Moreau E, Mac-Thiong JM, Joncas J, et al.: Quality of life of patients with high-grade spondylolisthesis: minimum 2-year follow-up after surgical and nonsurgical treatments, *Spine J* 13:770, 2013.

Crawford 3rd CH, Larson AN, Gates M, et al.: Current evidence regarding the treatment of pediatric lumbar spondylolisthesis: a report from the Scoliosis Research Society Evidence Based Medicine Committee, *Spine Deform* 5:284, 2017.

El Rassi G, Takemitsu M, Glutting J, Shah SA: Effect of sports modification on clinical outcome in children and adolescent athletes with symptomatic lumbar spondylolysis, *Am J Phys Med Rehabil* 92:1070, 2013.

Fadell MF, Gralla J, Bercha I, et al.: CT outperforms radiographs at a comparable radiation dose in the assessment for spondylolysis, *Pediatr Radiol* 45:1026, 2015.

Fan J, Yu GR, Liu F, et al.: A biomechanical study on the direct repair of spondylolysis by different techniques of fixation, *Orthop Surg* 2:46, 2010.

Ghobrial GM, Crandall KM, Lau A, et al.: Minimally invasive direct pars repair with cannulated screws and recombinant human bone morphogenetic protein: case series and review of the literature, *Neurosurg Focus* 43:E6, 2017.

Ledonio CG, Burton DC, Crawford 3rd CH, et al.: Current evidence regarding diagnostic imaging methods for pediatric lumbar spondylolysis: a report from the Scoliosis Research Society Evidence-Based Medicine Committee, *Spine Deform* 5:97, 2017.

Leone A, Cianfoni A, Cerase A, et al.: Lumbar spondylolysis: a review, *Skeletal Radiol* 40:683, 2011.

Mac-Thiong JM, Duong L, Parent S, et al.: Reliability of the SDSG classification of lumbosacral spondylolisthesis, *Spine* 37:E95, 2012.

Mac-Thiong JM, Parent S, Joncas J, et al.: The importance of proximal femoral angle on sagittal balance and quality of life in children and adolescents with high-grade lumbosacral spondylolisthesis, *Eur Spine J* 27:2038, 2018.

Menga EN, Jain A, Kebaish KM, et al.: Anatomic parameters: direct intralaminar screw repair of spondylolysis, *Spine* 39:E153, 2014.

Menga EN, Kebaish KM, Jain A, et al.: Clinical results and functional outcomes after direct intralaminar screw repair of spondylolysis, *Spine* 39:104, 2014.

Nitta A, Sakai T, Goda Y, et al.: Prevalence of symptomatic lumbar spondylolysis in pediatric patients, *Orthopedics* 39:e434, 2016.

Rush JK, Astur N, Scott S, et al.: Use of magnetic resonance imaging in the evaluation of spondylolysis, *J Pediatr Orthop* 35:271, 2015.

Sakai T, Goda Y, Tezuka F, et al.: Characteristics of lumbar spondylolysis in elementary school age children, *Eur Spine J* 25:602, 2016.

Sakai T, Sairyo K, Mima S, Yasui N: Significance of magnetic resonance imaging signal change in the pedicle in the management of pediatric lumbar spondylolysis, *Spine* 35:E641, 2010.

Sakai T, Tezuka F, Yamashita K, et al.: Conservative treatment for bony healing in pediatric lumbar spondylolysis, *Spine (Phila Pa 1976)* 42:E716, 2017.

Selhorst M, Fischer A, MacDonald J: Prevalence of spondylolysis in symptomatic adolescent athletes: an assessment of sport risk in nonelite athletes, *Clin J Sport Med* 29:421, 2019.

Snyder LA, Shufflebarger H, O'Brien MF, et al.: Spondylolysis outcomes in adolescents after direct screw repair of the pars interarticularis, *J Neurosurg Spine* 21:329, 2014.

Sumita T, Sairyo K, Shibuya I, et al.: V-rod technique for direct repair surgery of pediatric lumbar spondylolysis combined with posterior apophyseal ring fracture, *Asian Spine J* 7:115, 2013.

Tanguay F, Labelle H, Wang Z, et al.: Clinical significance of lumbosacral kyphosis in adolescent spondylolisthesis, *Spine* 37:304, 2012.

Tofte JN, CarlLee TL, Holte AJ, et al.: Imaging pediatric spondylolysis: a systematic review, *Spine (Phila Pa 1976)* 42:777, 2017.

Tsirikos AI, Garrido EG: Spondylolysis and spondylolisthesis in children and adolescents, *J Bone Joint Surg* 92B:751, 2010.

Tsirikos AI, Sud A, McGurk SM: Radiographic and functional outcome of posterolateral lumbosacral fusion for low grade isthmic spondylolisthesis in children and adolescents, *Bone Joint J* 98:88, 2016.

KYPHOSCOLIOSIS IN MYELOMENINGOCELE

Altiok H, Finlayson C, Hassani S, Sturm P: Kyphectomy in children with myelomeningocele, *Clin Orthop Relat Res* 469:1272, 2011.

Ferland CE, Sardar ZM, Abuljabbar F, et al.: Bilateral vascularized rib grafts to promote spino-pelvic fixation in patients with sacral agenesis and spino-pelvic dissociation: a new surgical technique, *Spine J* 15:2583, 2015.

Flynn JM, Ramirez N, Emans JB, et al.: Is the vertebral expandable prosthetic titanium rib a surgical alternative in patients with spina bifida? *Clin Orthop Relat Res* 469:1291, 2011.

Ollesch B, Brazell C, Carry PM, et al.: Complications, results, and risk factors of spinal fusion in patients with myelomeningocele, *Spine Deform* 6:460, 2018.

Samagh SP, Cheng I, Elzik M, et al.: Kyphectomy in the treatment of patients with myelomeningocele, *Spine J* 11:E5, 2011.

Smith JT: Bilateral rib-based distraction to the pelvis for the management of congenital gibbus deformity in the growing child with myelodysplasia, *Spine Deform* 4:70, 2016.

Smith JT, Novais E: Treatment of the gibbus deformity associated with myelomeningocele in the young child with the use of the vertical expandable prosthetic titanium rib (VEPTR): a case report, *J Bone Joint Surg* 92A:2211, 2010.

UNUSUAL CAUSES OF SCOLIOSIS

MARFAN SYNDROME

Gjolaj JP, Sponseller PD, Shah SA, et al.: Spinal deformity correction in Marfan syndrome versus adolescent idiopathic scoliosis: learning from the differences, *Spine* 37:1558, 2012.

Haller G, Alvarado DM, Willing MC, et al.: Genetic risk for aortic aneurysm in adolescent idiopathic scoliosis, *J Bone Joint Surg Am* 97:1411, 2015.

Jiang D, Liu Z, Yan H, et al.: Correction of scoliosis with large thoracic curves in Marfan syndrome: does the high-density pedicle screwe construct contribute to better surgical outcomes, *Med Sci Monit* 25:9658, 2019.

Kurucan E, Bernstein DN, Ying M, et al.: Trends in spinal deformity surgery in Marfan syndrome, *Spine J* 19:1934, 2019.

Qiao J, Xu L, Liu Z, et al.: Surgical treatment of scoliosis in Marfan syndrome: outcomes and complications, *Eur Spine J* 25:3288, 2016.

Sponseller PD, Erkula G, Skolasky RL, et al.: Improving clinical recognition of Marfan syndrome, *J Bone Joint Surg* 92A:1868, 2010.

Zenner J, Hitzl W, Meier O, et al.: Surgical outcomes of scoliosis surgery in Marfan syndrome, *J Spinal Disord Tech* 27:48, 2014.

VERTEBRAL COLUMN TUMORS

Chunguang Z, Limin L, Rigao C, et al.: Surgical treatment of kyphosis in children in healed stages of spinal tuberculosis, *J Pediatr Orthop* 30:271, 2010.

Galgano MA, Goulart CR, Iwenofu H, et al.: Osteoblastomas of the spine: a comprehensive review, *Neurosurg Focus* 41:E4, 2016.

Hersh DS, Iyer RR, Garzon-Muvdi T, et al.: Instrumented fusion for spinal deformity after laminectomy or laminoplasty for resection of intramedullary spinal cord tumors in pediatric patients, *Neurosurg Focus* 43:E1 2, 2017.

Kim HJ, McLawhorn AS, Goldstein MJ, Boland PJ: Malignant osseous tumors of the pediatric spine, *J Am Acad Orthop Surg* 20:646, 2012.

Maheshwari AV, Cheng EY: Ewing sarcoma family of tumors, *J Am Acad Orthop Surg* 18:94, 2010.

Moon MS, Kim SS, Lee BJ, et al.: Surgical management of severe rigid tuberculous kyphosis of the lumbar spine, *Int Orthop* 35:75, 2011.

Rajasekaran S, Vijay K, Shetty AP: Single-stage closing-opening wedge osteotomy of spine to correct severe post-tubercular kyphotic deformities of the spine: a 3-year follow-up of 17 patients, *Eur Spine J* 19:583, 2010.

Ravindra VM, Eli IM, Schmidt MH, et al.: Primary osseous tumors of the pediatric spinal column: review of pathology and surgical decision making, *Neurosurg Focus* 41:E3, 2016.

Zhang HQ, Wang YX, Guo CF, et al.: One-stage posterior approach and combined interbody and posterior fusion for thoracolumbar spinal tuberculosis with kyphosis in children. , Available at orthosupersite.com.

OSTEOCHONDRODYSTROPHY

Absousmra O, Shah SA, Heydemann JA, et al: Sagittal spinopelvic parameters in children with achondroplasia, *Spine Defor* 7163, 2019.

Anissipour AK, Hammerberg KW, Caudill A, et al.: Behavior of scoliosis during growth in children with osteogenesis imperfecta, *J Bone Joint Surg* 96A:237, 2014.

O'Donnell C, Bloch N, Michael N, et al.: Management of scoliosis in children with osteogenesis imperfecta, *JBJS Rev* 5:e8, 2017.

Piantoni L, Noel MA, Francheri Wilson IA, et al.: Surgical treatment with pedicle screws of scoliosis associated with osteogenesis imperfecta in children, *Spine Deform* 5:360, 2017.

Wallace MJ, Kruse RW, Shah SA: The spine in patients with osteogenesis imperfecta, *J Am Acad Orthop Surg* 25:100, 2017.

Yilmaz G, Hwang S, Oto M, et al.: Surgical treatment of scoliosis in osteogenesis imperfecta with cement-augmented pedicle screw instrumentation, *J Spinal Disord Tech* 27:174, 2014.

SACRAL AGENESIS

Balioglu MB, Akman YE, Ucpunar H, et al.: Sacral agenesis: evaluation of accompanying pathologies in 38 cases, with analysis of long-term outcomes, *Childs Nerv Syst* 32:1693, 2016.

Ferland CE, Sardar ZM, Abduljabbar F, et al.: Bilateral vascularized rib grafts to promote spinopelvic fixation in patients with sacral agenesis and spinopelvic dissociation: a new surgical technique, *Spine J* 15:2583, 2015.

UNUSUAL CAUSES OF KYPHOSIS

MUCOPOLYSACCHARIDOSIS

Remondino RG, Tello CA, Noel M, et al.: Clinical manifestations and surgical management of spinal lesions in patients with mucopolysaccharidosis: a report of 52 cases, *Spine Deform* 7:298, 2019.

Roberts SB, Dryden R, Tsirikos AI: Thoracolumbar kyphosis in patients with mucopolysaccharidoses: clinical outcomes and predictive radiographic factors for progression of deformity, *Bone Joint J* 98-B:229, 2016.

Williams N, Challoumas D, Eastwood DM: Does orthopaedic surgery improve quality of life and function in patients with mucopolysaccharidoses? *J Child Orthop* 11:289, 2017.